The Nursing Profession

The Nursing Profession

A Time to Speak

Edited by

Norma L. Chaska, R.N., Ph.D., F.A.A.N.

Associate Professor
Chairperson, Nursing Administration
Coordinator, Nursing Research
School of Nursing
Medical College of Georgia

McGraw-Hill Book Company

New York   St. Louis   San Francisco   Auckland   Bogotá   Hamburg
Johannesburg   London   Madrid   Mexico   Montreal   New Delhi
Panama   Paris   São Paulo   Singapore   Sydney   Tokyo   Toronto

This book was set in Times Roman by Jay's Publishers Services, Inc.
The editors were David P. Carroll, John J. Fitzpatrick, and Stephen Wagley;
the production supervisor was Dennis J. Conroy.
The drawings were done by Jay's Publishers Services, Inc.
The cover was designed by Murray Fleminger.
R. R. Donnelley & Sons Company was printer and binder.

THE NURSING PROFESSION
A Time to Speak

2 3 4 5 6 7 8 9 0   DODO   8 9 8 7 6 5 4 3

ISBN 0-07-010696-7

Library of Congress Cataloging in Publication Data
Main entry under title:

The Nursing profession.   101494

Includes indexes.
1. Nursing. 2. Nursing—United States.
I. Chaska, Norma L. [DNLM: 1. Nursing. WY 16 N978]
RT82.N868   610.73   82-6620
ISBN 0-07-010696-7   AACR2

To
J. C.
A. S. F.
and my sisters and brothers,
Marjorie, Shirley, James, and Willard,
each of whom, in the depth of winter,
learned that within the self
there lay an invincible summer

Contents

1

PROFESSIONALIZATION

2
NURSING EDUCATION

3
NURSING RESEARCH

4
NURSING THEORY

5
NURSING PRACTICE

6

ADMINISTRATION: NURSING SERVICE AND EDUCATION

7

THE FUTURE OF NURSING

List of Contributors

MYRTLE K. AYDELOTTE, R.N.,
  Ph.D., F.A.A.N.
Former Executive Director
American Nurses' Association
Kansas City, Missouri

CONSTANCE M. BAKER, R.N., Ed.D.
Dean and Professor
College of Nursing
University of South Carolina
Columbia, South Carolina

DONALD A. BILLE, R.N., Ph.D.
Associate Professor
Department of Nursing
DePaul University
Chicago, Illinois

RITA BRAITO, R.N., Ph.D.
Associate Professor
Department of Sociology
University of Denver
Denver, Colorado

MYRTLE IRENE BROWN, R.N., Ph.D.,
  F.A.A.N.
Professor Emeritus
College of Nursing
University of South Carolina
Columbia, South Carolina

BONNIE BULLOUGH, R.N., Ph.D.,
  F.A.A.N.
Dean and Professor
School of Nursing
State University of New York at Buffalo
Buffalo, New York

RICHARD CASTON, Ph.D.
Assistant Professor
Department of Sociology
University of Denver
Denver, Colorado

NORMA L. CHASKA, R.N., Ph.D.,
  F.A.A.N.
Associate Professor
Chairperson, Nursing Administration
Coordinator, Nursing Research
School of Nursing
Medical College of Georgia
Augusta, Georgia

PEGGY L. CHINN, R.N., Ph.D.,
   F.A.A.N.
Editor
Advances in Nursing Science
and
Professor, School of Nursing
State University of New York at Buffalo
Buffalo, New York

LUTHER CHRISTMAN, R.N., Ph.D.,
   F.A.A.N.
Dean, College of Nursing
Vice-President of Nursing Affairs
Rush-Presbyterian—St. Lukes Medical
   Center
Chicago, Illinois

GLORIA M. CLAYTON, R.N., Ed.D.
Associate Professor
Chairperson, Adult Nursing
School of Nursing
Medical College of Georgia
Augusta, Georgia

VIRGINIA S. CLELAND, R.N., Ph.D.,
   F.A.A.N.
Professor
College of Nursing
Wayne State University
Detroit, Michigan

MARY E. CONWAY, R.N., Ph.D.,
   F.A.A.N.
Dean and Professor
School of Nursing
Medical College of Georgia
Augusta, Georgia

INGE B. CORLESS, R.N., Ph.D.
Program Director
St. Peter's Hospice
Albany, New York

FRANCES C. DALME, R.N., Ph.D.
Professor, Graduate Programs
College of Nursing
University of Arkansas for
   Medical Sciences
Little Rock, Arkansas

ANNE J. DAVIS, R.N., Ph.D.,
   F.A.A.N.
Professor
Department of Mental Health and
Community Nursing
School of Nursing
University of California
San Francisco, California

MILDRED A. DISBROW, R.N., Ph.D.,
   F.A.A.N.
Professor
Maternal and Child Nursing
School of Nursing
University of Washington
Seattle, Washington

SISTER ROSEMARY DONLEY, R.N.,
   Ph.D., F.A.A.N.
Dean and Associate Professor
School of Nursing
The Catholic University of America
Washington, D.C.

ANNETTE SCHRAM EZELL, R.N.,
   Ed.D.
Associate Dean of Academic Affairs
College of Nursing
University of Utah
Salt Lake City, Utah

CLAIRE M. FAGIN, R.N., Ph.D.,
   F.A.A.N.
Dean and Professor
School of Nursing
University of Pennsylvania
Philadelphia, Pennsylvania

JACQUELINE FAWCETT, R.N.,
   Ph.D., F.A.A.N.
Associate Professor
School of Nursing
University of Pennsylvania
Philadelphia, Pennsylvania

JUANITA W. FLEMING, R.N., Ph.D.,
   F.A.A.N.
Professor and

Assistant Dean for Graduate Education
and Director of Graduate Studies
College of Nursing
University of Kentucky
Lexington, Kentucky

MARYANN F. FRALIC, R.N., DrPh.
Assistant Professor
Department of Nursing Administration
University of Pittsburgh
Pittsburgh, Pennsylvania

DORIS FROEBE, R.N., Ph.D.,
  F.A.A.N.
Professor and Chairperson
Nursing Administration
School of Nursing
Indiana University
Indianapolis, Indiana

MARJORY GORDON, R.N., Ph.D.,
  F.A.A.N.
Professor
School of Nursing
Boston College
Chestnut Hill, Massachusetts

HELEN K. GRACE, R.N., Ph.D.,
  F.A.A.N.
Dean and Professor
College of Nursing
University of Illinois at the
  Medical Center
Chicago, Illinois

MARGARET HARDY, R.N., Ph.D.,
  F.A.A.N.
Associate Professor
School of Nursing
Boston University
Boston, Massachusetts

SUE T. HEGYVARY, R.N., Ph.D.,
  F.A.A.N.
Associate Dean/Assistant Vice-President
Rush-Presbyterian–St. Luke's
  Medical Center
Chicago, Illinois

SHAKÉ KETEFIAN, R.N., Ed.D.,
  F.A.A.N.
Associate Professor
Division of Nursing
New York University
New York, New York

JOHN F. KLEIN, R.N., Ph.D.
Associate Professor
Department of Sociology
John Carroll University
and
Staff Nurse
Department of Psychiatry
St. Luke's Hospital
Cleveland, Ohio

ELAINE L. LA MONICA, R.N., Ed.D.,
  F.A.A.N.
Associate Professor of Nursing
  Education
Director, Institute of Research and
  Service in Nursing Education
Teachers College
Columbia University
New York, New York

SOL LEVINE, Ph.D.
University Professor of Sociology and
  Community Medicine
Boston University
Boston, Massachusetts

PATRICIA MacELVEEN-HOEHN,
  R.N., Ph.D.
Research Fellow
Department of Parent and Child Nursing
School of Nursing
University of Washington
Seattle, Washington

DIANE O. MCGIVERN, R.N., Ph.D.,
  F.A.A.N.
Associate Dean
School of Nursing
University of Pennsylvania
Philadelphia, Pennsylvania

JANNETTA MacPHAIL, R.N., Ph.D.,
  F.A.A.N.
Dean and Professor
Frances Payne Bolton School of Nursing
Case Western Reserve University
Cleveland, Ohio

LOIS C. MALKEMES, R.N., Ph.D.
Patient Care Administrator
  and Professor
University Hospital
University of Arkansas Medical
  Science Campus
Little Rock, Arkansas

INGEBORG G. MAUKSCH, R.N.,
  Ph.D., Sc.D., F.A.A.N.
Consultant and Lecturer
Fort Myers, Florida
and
Distinguished Professor of Nursing
School of Nursing
Vanderbilt University
Nashville, Tennessee

GLORIA GILBERT MAYER, R.N.,
  Ed.D., F.A.A.N.
Senior Consultant
Health Management Systems Associates
Minneapolis, Minnesota

AFAF IBRAHIM MELEIS, R.N., Ph.D.,
  F.A.A.N.
Professor
Department of Mental Health and
  Community Nursing
School of Nursing
University of California at
  San Francisco
San Francisco, California

EDNA M. MENKE, R.N., Ph.D.
Associate Professor
School of Nursing
Graduate Department
Ohio State University
Columbus, Ohio

LUCILLE T. MERCADANTE, R.N.,
  Ed.D.
Assistant Administrator
International Hospital
Miami, Florida

REGINA L. MONNIG, R.N., Ph.D.
Associate Dean and Professor
Graduate Programs
School of Nursing
Medical College of Georgia
Augusta, Georgia

JUANITA F. MURPHY, R.N., Ph.D.,
  F.A.A.N.
Dean and Professor
College of Nursing
Arizona State University
Tempe, Arizona

B. JOAN NEWCOMB, R.N., M.S.
Doctoral Candidate
University of Chicago
Chicago, Illinois

MARGARET A. NEWMAN, R.N.,
  Ph.D., F.A.A.N.
Professor
Department of Nursing
Pennsylvania State University
University Park, Pennsylvania

KATHLEEN A. O'CONNELL, R.N.,
  Ph.D.
Assistant Professor
School of Nursing
University of Kansas
and
Associate Psychologist
Midwest Research Institute
Kansas City, Missouri

ANDREA O'CONNOR, R.N., Ed.D.
Assistant Professor
Department of Nursing Education
Teachers College
Columbia University
New York, New York

IRENE PALMER, R.N., Ph.D.,
  F.A.A.N.
Dean and Professor
Philip Y. Hahn School of Nursing
University of San Diego
San Diego, California

CAROL J. WILLTS PETERSON, R.N.,
  Ph.D., F.A.A.N.
Dean and Professor
College of Nursing
South Dakota State University
Brookings, South Dakota

SHARON J. REEDER, R.N., Ph.D.,
  F.A.A.N.
Professor
School of Nursing
Center for the Health Sciences
University of California at Los Angeles
Los Angeles, California

MARTHA E. ROGERS, Sc.D.,
  F.A.A.N., R.N.
Professor
Division of Nursing
New York University
New York, New York

SISTER CALLISTA ROY, R.N.,
  Ph.D., F.A.A.N.
Associate Professor and Chairperson
Department of Nursing
Mount St. Mary's College
Los Angeles, California

DOLORES SANTORA, R.N., Ph.D.
Associate Professor and Associate Dean
College of Nursing
Arizona State University
Tempe, Arizona

NANCY M. SARGIS, R.N., Ed.D.
Associate Professor
Loyola University
Chicago, Illinois

GRAYCE M. SILLS, R.N., Ph.D.,
  F.A.A.N.
Professor, Director

Advanced Psychiatric/Mental
  Health Nursing
School of Nursing
Ohio State University
Columbus, Ohio

RITA F. STEIN, R.N., Ph.D.
Former Professor and Director
  of Research
School of Nursing
Indiana University
Indianapolis, Indiana

BARBARA J. STEVENS, R.N., Ph.D.,
  F.A.A.N.
Director, Division of Health Services,
  Sciences and Education
Chairperson, Department of
  Nursing Education
Isabel Maitland Stewart Professor
Teachers College, Columbia University
New York, New York

MARY ANNE SWEENEY, R.N., Ph.D.
Associate Professor
School of Nursing
Boston College
Chestnut Hill, Massachusetts

DOROTHY M. TALBOT, R.N., Ph.D.,
  F.A.A.N.
Professor and Chairman
Department of Public Health Nursing
School of Public Health
University of North Carolina
Chapel Hill, North Carolina

DOROTHY JEAN WALKER, R.N.,
  Ph.D., J.D.
Attorney at Law
Professor, Graduate Program
Department of Nursing
George Mason University
Fairfax, Virginia

LORRAINE OLSZEWSKI WALKER,
  R.N., Ed.D., F.A.A.N.
Professor

School of Nursing
University of Texas at Austin
Austin, Texas

HARRIET H. WERLEY, R.N.,
    Ph.D., F.A.A.N.
Associate Dean (Research)
School of Nursing
University of Missouri
Columbia, Missouri

CAROLYN A. WILLIAMS, R.N., Ph.D.,
    F.A.A.N.
Associate Professor
School of Nursing
and
Department of Epidemiology

School of Public Health
University of North Carolina
Chapel Hill, North Carolina

JANET A. WILLIAMSON, R. N.,
    Ph.D.
Associate Professor
Department of Nursing
Pennsylvania State University
University Park, Pennsylvania

ROSALEE C. YEAWORTH, R.N.,
    Ph.D., F.A.A.N.
Dean and Professor
College of Nursing
University of Nebraska Medical Center
Omaha, Nebraska

Foreword

In producing this volume, Dr. Norma Chaska has made another useful contribution to the literature on the nursing profession. Even more ambitious and extensive than the book which she edited only a few years ago, this volume is a veritable handbook on practically any aspect of nursing which may be of interest to research investigators, educators, practitioners, administrators, and policy makers. And no wonder! Many of the major figures in the nursing field have contributed individual chapters to this volume.

The reader will not only find enlightening substantive reviews of the literature on specific topics; he or she will also encounter a range of competing action recommendations that are suggested by the data, recommendations that have to be pondered, weighed, and assessed. Because the book abounds with policy deliberations, the book could serve not only as a general reference book, but also a basic text for an advanced course on policy issues in nursing. The editor's introductory comments to each of the various chapters and questions for discussion are helpful and provocative and serve to maintain a thread of continuity throughout the book.

In future deliberations about health care and health personnel, we will certainly have to address the state of the nursing profession. By systematizing what is known in this broad field and in specifying the types of decisions we must make and the criteria we may use, this volume provides us with vital information and fruitful ideas for action.

Sol Levine, Ph.D.
University Professor of Sociology
and Community Medicine
Boston University

Preface

There is a season for everything, a time for every occupation under heaven:

A time for giving birth,
a time for dying;
a time for planting,
a time for uprooting what has been planted.
A time for killing,
a time for healing;
a time for knocking down,
a time for building.
A time for tears,
a time for laughter;
a time for mourning,
a time for dancing.
A time for throwing stones away,
a time for gathering them up;
a time for embracing,
a time to refrain from embracing.
A time for searching,
a time for losing;
a time for keeping,

a time for throwing away.
A time for tearing,
a time for sewing;
a time for keeping silent,
a time for speaking.
A time for loving,
a time for hating;
a time for war,
a time for peace.

Ecclesiastes, 3:1–8

This excerpt from chapter three of the book of Ecclesiastes presents a positive means for viewing the evolution of nursing as a profession. The first verse of this chapter provides the main theme for reflecting about the transition of nursing to the status of a full profession. Some verses are more applicable than others, specifically, "a time for speaking." Nursing has arrived at a stage where it may be most appropriate to speak.

In most respects, it has achieved the predominant attributes of a profession. Some are stronger and more evident than others; for example, the sanction by the community is substantial. There have been great advances in developing a systematic body of theory, but additional testing and refinement need to be completed. At the same time the profession is at risk in numerous ways through external forces impinging and challenging the strength of the profession. Particularly, it is at risk internally—for the professional culture that has been established is being weakened through the discontent and divisiveness among its members. The professional identity and unity of nurses and nursing are being threatened. This exposes a need for reflection.

Resolution and unity are essential for nursing to realize further gains in its endeavors as a profession. Ecclesiastes further states that: "What does a man gain for the efforts that he makes? I contemplate the task that God gives mankind to labor at. All that he does is apt for time; but though he has permitted man to consider time in its wholeness, man cannot comprehend the work of God from beginning to end" (Ecclesiastes 3:9–11). Verse thirteen advocates that when persons find happiness in their work, this is a gift from God.

Thus, the purpose of this book is to consider time in its wholeness, specifically in the wholeness of the profession. Though the profession may not comprehend the complete task that remains, it can reflect back and appreciate how much it has accomplished. The profession can assess its strengths, identify the areas where more attention is needed, prepare and plan for future direction. Periodic assessment of the profession is valuable, particularly in this society of ever-increasing change, stress, and action. In so doing, unity and further enjoyment in the labor of the profession may then result. To assist the process of reflection and assessment verses from Ecclesiastes have been chosen that appear relevant to each aspect of the profession and are presented prior to each part of the book.

This volume is a compilation of the knowledge of responsible professionals reflecting, questioning, searching for answers and positing solutions in the profession of nursing. As you can see in reading from the first through to the last page, a variety of personal and professional perspectives and issues are presented. There are obvious disagreements. However, it is of value to the profession to have each one's truth be heard, questioned, and tested in an open forum against the truth of others. As it was said in *The Nursing Profession: Views through the Mist* and repeated in this volume, "We need to appreciate diversity: a member of a single profession cannot find truth alone."

This book is a companion to *The Nursing Profession: Views through the Mist,* published by McGraw-Hill in 1978. The first text will remain available as long as there is a demand. This present volume is similar in format to the first; however, there are some major differences. It contains *original* chapters by contributors, with the exception of one chapter (15) which is an extension of the original paper that appeared in the first text. All of the contributors are doctorally prepared. Thirty-three of the contributors are nurse-sociologists. The other contributors have doctoral degrees representing the disciplines of nursing, psychology, education, philosophy, epidemiology, and law. The contributors are recognized leaders in the profession of nursing and/or other professions. Forty-one of the contributors are elected fellows in the American Academy of Nursing. This text has deleted the section Interdisciplinary Professional Relationships, which appeared in the first book. Discussion of those relationships is included throughout the majority of the individual chapters and all parts of the book. A section concerning nursing administration has been added. This was essential for all aspects of the profession to be represented. The editor has attempted to provide abstracts, rather than introductions, of each chapter in order to establish linkages throughout the book. In addition, far more questions for discussion are posed by the editor than in the last volume. This was done to ensure sufficient depth in reflecting on the chapters, and to make possible a comprehensive coverage of professional issues.

The book is divided into eight parts. The first seven parts contain chapters dealing with critical aspects of nursing as a profession: professionalization, nursing education, nursing research, nursing theory, nursing practice, administration: nursing service and education, and the future of nursing. To facilitate the process of reflection and dialogue, questions for discussion are raised by the editor at the end of each chapter. Part Eight summarizes in general the current state of the profession, presents some specific reflections, suggestions, and conclusions to stimulate additional questions and potential answers. A quotation from an essay by Albert Camus is applied in reflecting on the nursing profession. "In the depth of winter, I finally learned that within me there lay an invincible summer." (1968:169) The analogy of the tapestry is proposed for consideration of the nursing profession in this winter of discontent for the actualization of the profession as an invincible summer.

The questions that are posed throughout the volume may be helpful in a number of ways. Agencies or institutions employing nurses may use them in planning and establishing long-range goals. The questions may help identify and solve problems in organizations. They should provide a means for analyzing and formulation of nursing and health policy. It is hoped that they will greatly assist nursing educators at all levels in conducting discussion seminars for nursing students and, in addition, serve as the basis for specific course content. The questions should be of value to those interested in continuing education, whether they are instructors, practicing nurses, or nonpracticing nurses returning to practice. By reading the volume, reflecting on the questions, and positing possible answers, the reader should be able to gain a comprehensive perspective of the profession. The volume should help the reader to develop his or her own global view of the profession, to build a foundation for assessing possible future changes, and to enhance unity.

Two final comments are in order. First, the use of the feminine pronoun is used in the introduction to and Chapter 27 (Braito and Caston). This is not intended to be sexist, but it is made necessary by the nature of the research. The term "man" is used as a universal theoretical concept in discussions of nursing theory. Second, references concerning publications (not grants) of the Department of Health and Human Services (D.H.H.S.) that were published prior to 1979 are indicated as being publications of the Department of Health, Education and Welfare (D.H.E.W.).

ACKNOWLEDGMENTS

This volume owes its existence to a stimulating association of interest in and concern for nursing on the part of the contributors, who had the difficult task of reviewing broad areas of nursing within the confines of a few pages. Their patience and good will in responding to additional queries and stringent deadlines, and their understanding of necessary and unavoidable delays in the production process are appreciated.

It has been a formidable task to complete this volume, due to multiple changes and commitments related to changing location and assuming a new position. Nightingale's advice about the wisdom of small beginnings should have been heeded. In addition, it was a major challenge to locate appropriate secretarial assistance.

I am indebted to Elizabeth Heckathorn, R.N., M.S., chairperson of Intensive Care Nursing Services, Massachusetts General Hospital, who suggested the title and theme of this book and the summary chapter. Intellectual debt is due to Barbara Ponder, R.N., M.S., Assistant Professor School of Nursing, Medical College of Georgia and doctoral student at the University of Georgia, for insightful review and discussions concerning the chapters on nursing theory.

I am also indebted to Darton, Longman and Todd, Ltd., and Doubleday and Co., Inc., for permission to use excerpts from *The Jerusalem Bible,* from which the title and theme developed; and to Alfred A. Knopf Publishing Company for permission to use a quotation of Albert Camus, from which the title and theme of the summary chapter (Chap. 66) were developed.

I am much indebted to a vast pool of secretarial and administrative assistance personnel. All have other full-time positions in addition to the work they did for the editor in completing this volume. I am thankful for assistance of Mrs. Therese Bolf and Mrs. Charlotte Langley in the initial correspondence to contributors. Thanks are also due to the following: Mrs. Beth Jones for suggestions and some redesign of the text cover; Mrs. Georgia Foster for her faithful and skillful secretarial services in correspondence with the contributors, the maintenance of numerous changes in address, organizational aspects of developing the manuscript, and transcribing multiple pages of notes for the editor—at most irregular hours; Mrs. Claudia Geniton, who transcribed and returned to each contributor this editor's editing for review; Mrs. Marsha Holman for faithful and expert secretarial assistance at highly irregular hours required for the preparation of the manuscript; her consistency and effort in meeting incredible deadlines were most appreciated. With the tremendous time constraint, the manuscript process could not have been completed without the administrative assistance of Mrs. Daisy Arnold, R.N., M.S.N., Project Director for Nursing Service, University Hospital, Augusta, Georgia; she had a major responsibility for the primary review of the galleys and page proofs which was faithfully, thoroughly, and conscientiously completed. I am in particular debt to Mrs. Martha Fehrenbach, secretary for the Department of Nursing Administration, School of Nursing, Medical College of Georgia in Augusta; she greatly assisted in the management of the editor's time, and faithfully provided support, enabling the completion of commitments and responsibilities primary to the editor's faculty position while simultaneously finishing this volume.

Finally, I am greatly indebted to my family, friends, and colleagues in the School of Nursing, Medical College of Georgia in Augusta, for their sustained support, encouragement, and interest; without them this volume would not have been possible. My particular thanks are due to Mr. David Bass, Assistant Dean for Finance, School of Nursing, Medical College of Georgia, for arranging that the cost of materials utilized was reimbursed by the editor. This volume does not necessarily reflect the views of or opinions of the School of Nursing or of the Medical College of Georgia.

Mention is due in appreciation to the editor's support network, whose members have contributed significantly in the development of this manuscript. Particular thanks are due to Ms. Marilyn Moore and Dr. James Burks. In addition, acknowledgement of Mrs. Gervais Deutsch, Ms. Lillian Furtado, Dr. and Mrs. William Baldus, Mrs. Sharon Tennis, Mr. and Mrs. Thomas Kokesh, Mr. and Mrs. D. D. Thompson, Mr. and Mrs. John Jacobs, Dr. and Mrs. Neal Krupp, Dr. and Mrs. Laurence Gowan, Jr., Dr. and Mrs. R. G. Hahn, Dr. Leo F. Black, Reverend Daniel Corcoran, and Reverend Vern Trocinski is long overdue.

I wish to extend special appreciation to McGraw-Hill Book Company, and to David P. Carroll, Senior Editor, and Stephen Wagley, Area Editing Supervisor. Mr. Carroll's sustained support, encouragement, counsel, interest, and understanding throughout the unusual circumstances in completing this manuscript were important. Mr. Wagley's continued support, advice, interest, and editing of this author's writing were extremely helpful.

Norma L. Chaska

Introduction

I appreciate having been asked to introduce this book. Its potential readership is vast. Temporally, it addresses readers of today, and also of tomorrow. Boundarywise, it will exceed nursing considerably, because its content captures the interest of members of all health professions, has definitive appeal to consumers of health services, is rich in resources for the historian, and has much to say to health planners and to legislators on all levels! Thus, introducing this book can be likened to presenting a new princess to her realm—while her very birth assures her a place of note in many quarters, her potential impact is unfathomable, thus immeasurable!

Nursing has arrived at a rather critical period in its history. There are many reasons why this is so. To understand them is basic to coping with the problems to be faced, and which, if solved wisely, will provide for a productive transition into a new era of nursing care delivery.

What makes this a critical period for nursing? Principally, nursing's striving for change. The underlying dynamic for this is generated by the occupation's realization that nursing care of the sick and nursing's contribution to health maintenance, to the attainment of higher levels of health, and to the achievement of death with dignity are indeed essential, invaluable services to the society. As such, nursing insists, they must be planned, directed, and controlled by nurses. This has caused much opposition, particularly on the part of organized medicine, resulting in the creation of formidable barriers to autonomous, accountable nursing practice.

Furthermore, nursing, through its professional organization as well as through individual nurse activity, strives to attain its rightful place in the decision making arena of the health and illness care delivery system, be this in government or in the public or private sector. This new and undeterrable insistence has again met with opposition, even repression in many instances.

Nursing education has undergone major changes. It now appears that the relocation of nursing's educational site into the realm of higher education is about to be completed. Reorientation to this reality is painful to some, has elicited divisiveness, and certainly still requires a good deal of reeducation of many, within and outside the profession, before it ceases to be the still inflammatory issue. The significant commonality all these problems share is the issue of the profession's insistence on autonomy; the fact that other professional and occupational groups expect to share in decisions about nursing, yet are not willing to adopt the reverse, is no longer acceptable.

Let the record reflect, however, that not all circumstances surrounding nursing's transition to an autonomous accountable occupation are bleak. Through scholarship, nursing research, and attempts at theory building, much work has been done toward establishing nursing as a science. There is an ever growing cadre of nurse scholars and researchers whose work on ethical decision making, the occupation's heritage, and its values are shaping the discipline of nursing, thereby opening the way for the development of professional nursing practice.

We see incidents of approach between the two main establishments within our boundaries—education and care delivery; this will result in much improved communication between these two components, undoubtedly leading to higher standards of care, more realistic educational outcomes, and increasing unity of purpose.

As final example (not the last by any means) of nursing's determination to contribute autonomously to the health care of society, reference is made to the valiant activities of nurse-midwives and nurse practitioners who persist and gradually succeed in their efforts to provide needed and desired services, in the face of personal opposition, legal constraints, and economic sanctions.

Thus, this is a very timely book. It addresses the critical issues faced by nursing today. Boldly, its editor has secured original papers from a vast number of nursing's best thinkers: researchers, administrators, teachers, and clinicians. Foresightfully, the future constitutes a significant component of the book's orientation. Wisely, many issues are perceived through a variety of perspectives, opening new vistas of thought and vision. The choice of the subtitle for this volume encapsules the very essence of what nursing seems to have recognized as its task for today: A time to speak.

Ingeborg G. Mauksch, R.N., Ph.D., Sc.D., F.A.A.N.
Consultant and Lecturer
Fort Myers, Florida
and
Distinguished Professor of Nursing
School of Nursing
Vanderbilt University

Part One

Professionalization

There is a season for everything, a time for every occupation under heaven:
A time for giving birth, . . .
a time for tears, . . .
a time for laughter, . . .
a time for dancing

The time has come for nursing to actualize its complete status as a profession. Concerted effort has been made through individual and collective contributions of members in the profession to acquire the significant attributes of a profession. There are numerous struggles, tears and a long labor involved in the birth process of a profession. Throughout the process of evolving as a profession, there have been occasions when nursing appreciated humor more than other times. This has helped to soothe the frustrations in its serious effort to attain a goal. Finally, the legitimacy of nursing as a profession is being recognized. When nursing has fully achieved maturity as a profession, there will be a time for dancing.

The contributions to the first section of this volume reflect the essential evolution of nursing as a profession. Appropriately, the original history of nursing is reconsidered through the notes of Florence Nighingale. This is valuable in evaluating the current status of the profession and the degree nursing has maintained the original mission

1

of the profession. Direction for continued growth as a profession is targeted. Challenges in the pathway to maturity of the profession are stressed. The domain of nursing is more clearly defined. The territory of nursing is further clarified through the legal rights and responsibilities of nursing. In returning to the past and following through to the present, nursing can aptly guide the future of the profession. Evidence is provided in the following chapters for that guidance.

Chapter 1

From Whence We Came

Irene Sabelberg Palmer, R.N., Ph.D., F.A.A.N.
Dean and Professor
Philip Y. Hahn School of Nursing
University of San Diego
San Diego, California

It is significant that Irene Palmer's chapter is the first in this text. She clearly traces the current issues and concerns relevant to nursing to Florence Nightingale, who is acknowledged as the founder of modern nursing. In so doing, Palmer has chosen salient notes from the original writings of Nightingale to illustrate the beliefs, principles, and philosophy of Nightingale. The reader is able to recognize the extent to which these have been observed in the prevailing structure of nursing. Some of the many topics addressed are: the wisdom of small beginnings and an experimental approach to test new ventures; flexibility and nursing education; the definition, scope, and practice of nursing and medicine; professional associations; economic and general welfare programs for nursing; and the women's movement. Palmer cites examples of Nightingale's philosophy not being heeded and misinterpretations of Nightingale's tenets. She concludes that many of the founder's ideals have been realized as well as that others are yet to be drawn to fruition.

Nursing functions, responsibilities, authority, and place in the medical care system were forged in the crucible of the Crimean War and have been continuously reshaped ever since. Because of the far-reaching and long-lasting effects of her numerous efforts in social, hospital, medical, and military reform, Florence Nightingale is acknowledged as the founder of modern nursing and one of the greatest humanitarians produced in the nineteenth century. It would be quite safe to assert that few

The research for this paper was accomplished through support from a National Health Service Postdoctoral Fellowship #1F32 NU05352-01S1 awarded by the Division of Nursing, U. S. Public Health Service.

others have attained comparable greatness, and, while the nursing profession has produced many notable personalities, certainly no member has ever approached the luminosity of its founder.

As is well known, Nightingale and Sidney Herbert, Secretary at War in the British Cabinet, exchanged correspondence the weekend of October 14–15, 1854, about her going to the relief of the British wounded in the war with Russia. Fast friends who had enjoyed each other's confidence and respect ever since they had met in Rome the winter of 1847, they quickly realized their mutual objective of providing women nurses to help the beleaguered British Army care for its grossly neglected wounded and sick soldiers in the Crimean conflict.

The structure of nursing as an orderly work force was established as Herbert and Nightingale met at Harley Street the afternoon of Monday, October 16, and developed the Nightingale authority and the scope of the tasks, responsibilities, and positions of those who nursed. In the interim between October 16 and October 21, the first party of 38 women was organized and dispatched to the site of the war, arriving at Scutari November 4, 1854. Other groups followed at varying intervals.

Nightingale was officially appointed to the office of "Superintendent of the female nursing establishment in the English General Military Hospitals in Turkey" by unanimous action of the British Cabinet on Wednesday, October 18, and received her official appointment and instructions from Herbert the next day (Cook, 1913:155). The title "Superintendent of Nurses" was derived from Nightingale's office; that title—plus such variants as director, chief, administrator, and vice president—is still used to indicate a broad scope of authority and responsibility. Although the title "matron" was in vogue in civilian hospitals, Nightingale had selected the commanding title "superintendent" at Harley Street and continued its use to signify the definitive jurisdiction, responsibility, and position she was to occupy. She applied the title in subsequent years when she referred to military nursing, but in describing civilian nursing she reverted to the customary title, matron. As Nightingale was to write in *Subsidiary Notes:*

> There is much in a name; and in some respects, that of Superintendent would better denote her office, as regards nurses, would add to her authority, which is desirable, and would point her out as acting under the Superintendent General. (1858a:27)

A strong advocate of the principle of unity in command, Nightingale insisted that all women who would go as nurses would be under her authority. She seemed to have a prescience for the troubled seas upon which she was about to embark and believed that unless she went with appropriate authority, the operation was doomed. Other facts influenced Nightingale's determination about command. One was her own experiences as superintendent at Harley Street where she had to report both to a committee of ladies and to one of the medical doctors. Another influence was her religious studies and probings from 1848 to 1851; during these years she developed a "religion" for England's laborers in which she expressed her beliefs about the laws of nature and about a unifying system by which she perceived the universe was ordered (1860b). Her system of administration and authority related always to the identification of the one person who was in command.

Nightingale was a civilian agent of the British government, appointed with Cabinet approval by the War Office. Herbert spelled out Nightingale's scope of responsibilities in his instructions to her October 19. To ensure the success of the mission he also had instructions sent to Lord Raglan, the commander of the forces; to Mr. Wreford, the purveyor-in-chief; and to the principal medical officer with the forces in the east, Dr. John Hall, inspector general, stationed in the Crimea. Dr. Duncan Menzies, deputy inspector general, was principal medical officer at Scutari. Nightingale's instructions, which she assisted Herbert in drafting, specifically delineated the territory, geographical extent, authority, and command relationship of the superintendent. In clear, unequivocal terms, the communications stated:

> Miss Nightingale will undertake the entire management of the female nurses under the control of the Chief Medical Officer at Scutari. The nurses will be selected by her, or by persons whom she may appoint, and all will act under her supreme authority. (Pollock, 1910:385)

Herbert's letter of appointment instructed Nightingale to

...place yourself at once in communication with the Chief Army Medical officer of the Hospital at Scutari, under whose orders and direction you will carry on the duties of your appointment. (Herbert, 1854a)

These instructions eliminated any responsibility on her part for the sick or wounded in the army regimental hospitals, in the British Navy, or for female dependents of the British soldiers who, in limited numbers, were permitted to bring their wives to the war front. Nightingale's sphere of operation was specifically restricted to Turkey despite the fact that the British forces were waging battle on the soil of the Russian Crimean peninsula. Nor was any population other than the British soldier included in her charge.

Nightingale, described as a good Samaritan, had previously determined she would not countenance false barriers to providing succor to those in need. She had demonstrated her belief in ministering to people of varying social strata when she nursed villagers near her family's estates, particularly in the 1840s, in August 1854 when she nursed prostitutes and other victims of a cholera epidemic in London's Middlesex Hospital, and when she refused to work as superintendent at Harley Street if a test of religion was used as a criterion for admission (Cook, 1913:134). Nightingale's broad, compassionate humanitarian philosophy was already operational before she ever considered the Crimean experience. Therefore, it came as no surprise that Nightingale provided supplies for prisoners, established a hospital for the British soldiers' women and wives, and had British authority clarify her responsibility for their nursing operations on Russian soil (Cook, 1913:292; Blackwood, 1881). The traditional values of caring for humankind in need were operationalized once again in Nightingale's application of her authority and were thus reestablished as a basic philosophy for nursing.

Nursing was lodged firmly under medical authority under the terms of Nightingale's appointment and instructions. And, although the superintendent was charged with the selection and appointment of nurses, her official appointment stipulated,

Everything relating to the distribution of the nurses, the hours of their attendance, their allotment to particular duties, is placed in your hands, subject, of course, to the sanction and approval of the Chief Medical Officer.... (Herbert, 1854a)

The command responsibility to both medical care and hospital administration, which was a function of physicians and other personnel, such as the purveyor, was determined and firmly fixed by that historic instruction. Nurses in the Crimean experiment, while conveying official governmental approbation, were to be utilized and assigned to duties, tasks, work schedules, and responsibilities according to the preferences and opinions of the medical officer in charge of the hospital. In fact, the delegation of such authority reverted to the individual medical officers in charge of the respective wards. According to Nightingale,

The number of nurses admitted into each division of a hospital depended upon the medical officer of that division, who sometimes accepted them, sometimes refused them, sometimes accepted them after they had been refused, while the duties they were permitted to perform varied according to the will of each individual medical officer.... (1858b:152)

From these descriptions it will be seen that the physician was clearly in command and the nurse was a guest in the hospital, subject to acceptance or rejection by the physician. Tact and diplomacy were in great demand, and the superintendent required all the skills in interpersonal relations she had acquired through her social position, breeding, education, and foreign travel.

There were only three aspects of Nightingale's commission in which she held plenary power: the selection of nurses, their discharge or dismissal, and the prevention of religious proselytizing by her nurses. In all other matters, Nightingale was subordinate to the chief medical officer in the area or the principal medical officer in the hospital. The duties, functions, tasks, and assignments of the nurses required approval of the medical authorities.

The interpretation of the allocation of nursing duties and the distribution of nurses required constant attention. What was a large gray area then has continued to be clouded for the intervening century and a quarter, with a gradual redefinition of the scope of nursing functions and responsibilities occurring all the while.

The government's introduction of female nurses into army hospitals was interpreted by military and medical officers alike as an odious criticism of their own abilities to manage their respective spheres of responsibilities for the sick or wounded soldier. Nightingale's appointment and instructions came from lay officials in government, not military or medical officialdom, and that immediately created hostile barriers to the execution of her responsibilities. Obvious deficiencies in care were accurately and graphically reported by the war and diplomatic correspondents of the London *Times,* as well as by soldiers themselves and other witnesses. Although medical military authorities stoutly insisted "nothing was wanted," they were ultimately overridden by lay officials in London. Consequently, military bigotry and medical jealousy arose as physicians and other army personnel were commanded to accept women nurses under the authority of a woman who herself was outside military channels for appointment, promotion, and evaluation. This rankled deeply, and it is not to be wondered that Nightingale's reception was less than cordial.

As resentment among military officials and persons in key government positions mounted, Nightingale was subjected to a great deal of criticism and vilification from lay, military, medical, and political sources in the public press as well as in governmental and unofficial reports. Passive resistance and pettifogging were used in attempts to impede the Nightingale mission. But

as the success of the mission became known through soldiers and others who described the efficacy of her efforts, the Nightingale fame swelled and her popularity extended throughout the entire British social structure, from Queen Victoria to the common people.

Why did Nightingale place herself and her nurses under the absolute authority of the medical officers? Given the sympathetic and long-standing relationship between Herbert and Nightingale, it seems a logical assumption that she had an active role in designing the War Office instructions to her. While she did not hold medical men in awe, Nightingale clearly recognized their power, tried to avoid rousing their opposition, and was often conciliatory toward them publicly. Did she defer because she knew they perceived her mission as a reflection of their inadequacy to provide for the soldier? Was it because military management had objected to women nurses? Or, was the arrangement of authority an outcome of her Harley Street experience with a Committee of Physicians and a Committee of Ladies? Did she find it easier to work with physicians than with women? By her own admission, she found it easier to talk to physicians, for they did not have "that detestable nationality which makes it so difficult to talk to all Englishmen" (Cope, 1958:11). Moreover, certain members of the medical profession clearly recognized her as an authority. Did she perceive that the road to reform was accessible only through the prevailing organization, and if she traveled that road, she could later strike out independently?

What did Nightingale actually perceive about her mission to Scutari? She had much time to ponder her problems and her course of action as she observed the behavior of her charges during the 14 days of travel from London to Scutari. As early as 1840 Nightingale had seen the dangers of having untrained women, whether illiterate or well-bred, caring for the sick. A cadre of reputable, disciplined, knowledgeable women who could exercise sound nursing judgment and managerial expertise had yet to be produced. The prevailing status of women, the varying competence and morality of women who nursed, the management of the distribution of supplies from London rather than from the war zone, and the absence of definitive authority and responsibility all were to play a part in the organizational placement of nurses. The extraordinary number of sick and wounded and the number of hospitals to which the women were assigned were also significant factors.

It is possible that the resistance to nursing which is exhibited to this day had its inception in the Crimean conflict. The introduction of female nurses into hospitals, wherever occurring, has generally followed a pattern of rejection, resistance, and guarded acceptance. That response was observed in the United States as a few courageous souls, not to be deterred, first proved the efficacy of organized nursing in hospitals. Women successfully demonstrated to the laymen and physicians who operated hospitals the value of trained nurses. Those nurses proved to be the civilizing force that transformed hospitals from vicious sinks to hospitable havens. The introduction of nurses in new roles as well as innovative nursing practices still seem to be consistently challenged or rebuffed by a wide variety of skeptics, both internal and external to the profession, until an initial trial by fire is endured with varying measures of success (Mundinger, 1980).

Nightingale and her women, lay and religious, went as civilian nurses, all subject to military authority. The passage of several centuries had obliterated the memory of the male military nursing orders of the medieval era, orders such as the Hospitallers of St. John of Jerusalem (which ultimately became the Knights of Malta), the Hospitallers of St. Lazarus of Jerusalem, the Teutonic Knights, and the Hospitallers of the Holy Ghost (Frank, 1953). The prejudice against nurses in military hospitals had been raised earlier when the army rejected the notion of both men and women nurses because there were no suitable candidates (Roebuck Committee, 1855). The barrier against women nurses in the military was not

surmounted for almost 50 years. Despite the recognized advantages of assigning women nurses to military hospitals, nearly half a century was required before a female nurse corps was created in the U.S. Army, and almost a century was to pass before nurses were awarded rank, pay, and benefits equal to those of male officers and before male nurses were commissioned into the heretofore all-female nurse corps (Shields, 1981).

Other observations are merited here. In the British Army of 1854, pensioners were hastily enlisted as attendants for the sick and assigned haphazardly to nursing duties. Orderlies were also assigned with seeming lack of organization. These pensioners and orderlies were excluded from the Nightingale authority, thereby creating a cleavage in responsibility and authority over what were perceived to be nursing functions. Those assigned to orderly functions were under control of military medical authority and could be reassigned to other military duties as that authority deemed appropriate, while the nurses were under Nightingale's command. Although the nursing orderlies or pensioners so assigned were all men, it was stipulated in Nightingale's appointment that the nurses would be female.

The absence of men engaged in nursing duties in civilian or military institutions in Victorian England created a sexual onus that has been carried by nursing for more than a century. In the United States men desiring to function as nurses had such great difficulty finding educational opportunities in established schools that separate facilities for the training of men as nurses were established and maintained well into the second half of the twentieth century. Far into the twentieth century it was virtually impossible for trained male nurses to find employment except in such restricted situations as psychiatry and urology, and then they served almost exclusively on male wards. While nursing itself, as a predominantly female occupation, was slowly gaining a semblance of autonomy from male authority, male nurses likewise were slowly being accepted as colleagues by their female counterparts (Kalisch and Kalisch, 1978).

The transition was facilitated and hastened by the civil rights legislation of the 1950s and 1960s.

The entire scheme of sending Nightingale and her nurses to Crimea was proposed as an experiment to test the hypothesis that the introduction of female nurses in military hospitals would be of great benefit to the British soldier, would break through the prejudice against having female nurses in military hospitals, and would establish a worthwhile precedent. Nightingale realized all too well the desirability of keeping the number of nurses small enough to be manageable, but she was persuaded by Herbert to forego her preference for no more than 20 women and to accept 38 women, two short of his own desire for 40 nurses.

Throughout her writings, Nightingale expressed her belief in the wisdom of small beginnings to test new ventures, in the experimental approach, and in a minimum of rules. As she expressed her principles,

> Let nothing be done rashly. Let us not be fettered with many rules at first. Let us take time to see how things work; what is found to answer best; how the work proceeds. . . . it is essential to consider everything as tentative and experimental for some years to come. Do not be fettered by too many rules at first: try different things, and see which answers best. . . . But let there not be too many rules at first; see how things work, and take one step at a time. . . . A uniform system, as far as possible, and a little range to each, will answer best. But do not hurry the uniform system too much; take time: this is very important. . . . There is nothing so fatal to discipline as to require by regulation what is known and admitted cannot be performed. Such rules are made to be broken. (1858a:11, 44, 52, 55, 73)

The nursing profession did not heed some of these warnings. A proliferation of nursing schools swept the nation. Proscription and precisianism burgeoned in nursing schools, and nursing services were quickly encrusted with petty, meaningless, stifling regulations and prohibitions. Long after the need had passed to provide a safe, homelike environment for the would-be nurse in an attempt to shape and protect her moral character as well as to provide a facility for study, nurses' quarters remained mandatory residences, controlling and regulating the personal life of the nurse far beyond the needs of character formation or professional development.

However, the call for flexibility was heard by some, and that concept was paramount as nursing programs developed under a wide variety of auspices in the United States. One such system was that advocated by a Massachusetts physician, Alfred Worcester, who instituted a program of nurses' training in the homes of patients under the direction and supervision of medical doctors (Stewart and Austin, 1962). Another system prepared Red Cross nurses for disaster or war-time service, a system conducted by a physician assisted by a nurse. The benefits which accrued to hospitals conducting training schools and the pressures generated by state regulatory bodies and nursing educators seeking to enforce uniform educational standards resulted in the obliteration of such variants. These programs were deemed inappropriate educational models primarily because they violated two Nightingale principles: a person other than a trained nurse was in charge of training, and the program occurred outside a hospital organized for the purpose of training.

The principle of flexibility can also be seen in the development of such nontraditional programs as those in which the student is virtually self-directed, in the "university without walls," and in the "external degree" concept. Whether or not these programs have moved too far from the accepted educational format remains to be seen. The movement to lower passing scores for state board examinations, the development of licensing examinations by individual states, and permitting nursing students to write licensing examinations prior to their completion of an educational program are additional illustrations of questionable flexibility. Yet another aspect of this issue is awarding status as a professional nurse on the basis of experience or education in a subprofessional role. The value of experimentation seems to have been lost; Nightingale's admonition to wait for the efficacy of a new idea to be demonstrated before its widespread acceptance into practice seems no longer to be heeded.

Over the years, the struggle to upgrade educational programs continued. The effort was always to control the great variability of the product and to provide some measure of quality assurance for the public safety. As Isabel Hampton (Robb) expressed it:

> If the nurse had gone into . . . a hospital as a philanthropist it would be different, but she went there for the purpose of acquiring a certain kind of education. . . . the teaching methods of no two schools will be found to be alike, all varying according to the demands of the various institutions and their several authorities. Each school is a law unto itself. Nothing in the way of unity of ideas or of general principles to govern all exists, and no effort towards establishing and maintaining a general standard for all has ever been attempted. . . . (1893:6, 4)

Galvanized by Robb, the first nursing curriculum committee was appointed, and at the next annual convention of the Society of Superintendents a year later, Mary Agnes Snively (1895:24) presented the report, "A Uniform Curriculum for Training Schools." Superintendents and principals deliberated the desirability of creating a standard for recognizing those schools which provided a better system of education. Ultimately, through the leadership of Adelaide Nutting and under the auspices of the Committee of Education of the National League for Nursing Education, a *Standard Curriculum for Schools of Nursing* was published in 1917. This classic was revised in 1927 and 1937. What originated as a voluntary mechanism for upgrading nursing education was incorporated into mandatory standards for approval of schools by state boards of nursing.

Over several decades it became apparent that the *Standard Curriculum* was too rigid, permitting little flexibility in the arrangement and length of subject-matter courses required in the schools. Programs measured learning by counting: the number of times skills and tasks were performed; the number of hours of instruction students had in specific subject matter; the number of days, weeks, or months student nurses worked on various clinical services. As programs moved into other than hospital systems, the same degree of rigidity followed, reinforced by state boards charged with approving the operation of schools of nursing. The specified number of 1095 days spent in nursing school had to be shown on students' final records, with stipulated periods allowed for vacation and for illness, the latter generally being instituted after World War II. Periods of absence from clinical services had to be made up before the student could graduate or be eligible to write the licensing examination. Educators and nursing service providers came to realize the desirability of new approaches in the preparation of the post-World War II nurse, and more flexible methods in education resulted. Miss Nightingale's counsel for flexibility and experimentation was heard once again.

The desire and demonstrated need for quality as a means of protecting the public were illustrated in the long uphill struggle to develop and implement national educational standards through a voluntary process of accreditation. That goal was finally achieved in the 1950s with the establishment of the National Nursing Advisory Service and was subsequently lodged in the National League for Nursing. But another aspect of the inflexible nature of nursing education may be perceived in accreditation procedures—the rigid interpretation of qualitative criteria and the application of unwritten standards based on tradition—in the structure and implementation of educational models, and in the unyielding demands of state licensing agencies.

Nightingale frequently admonished her followers about the wisdom of few rules and of experimentation to determine what worked best. The concept of experimentation implicit in the Nightingale perspective would require a concerted thrust and herculean efforts by nursing's scholars and leaders before the idea of research-derived nursing knowledge would be accepted as a requisite for the profession, education appropriate to the development and acquisition of new knowledge would be available, and the dissemination of such knowledge would be widespread. For example, some of the women made remarkable observations about their experiences in Scutari. As Goodman (1862:132) expressed it, she quickly "learned that tact, training, and judgment are essentially necessary for those who fill the office of nurse." Another (Terrot, 1898) readily identified differences in the recovery rate of the wounded in one ward where the physician ordered a careful feeding system carried out by the nurses and in a ward where no such system existed. After the development of the Nightingale School at St. Thomas' Hospital, the passage of 100 years was required before American nursing embraced research in its national organizational structure, advocated use of research-derived knowledge as a basis of practice, and began to accept the system of university education for nursing.

Why was Nightingale selected as the first military nursing superintendent? What were Herbert's reasons for appointing Nightingale, since he had several persons from whom to choose? In describing the desirable personal qualities for which he was looking, Herbert observed:

> The difficulty of finding a woman equal to a task, after all, full of horrors, and requiring, besides knowledge and goodwill, great energy and great courage, will be great. The task of ruling them and introducing system among them, great; and not the least will be the difficulty of making the whole work smoothly with the medical and military authorities out there. This it is which makes it so important that the experiment should be carried out by one with a capacity for administration and experience. . . . (Herbert, 1854a)

Elaborating further, he identified the importance of familiarity with the nature of a hospital, of understanding the need for strict obedience to rule, especially in a military hospital, and of a capacity not to recoil from the work, or to be useless or in the way.

As Herbert expressed in his letter proposing the plan to Nightingale:

> Your own personal qualities, your knowledge and your power of administration, and among greater things your rank and position in Society give you advantages in such a work which no other person possesses . . . . (Herbert, 1854a)

From Herbert's caveats it appeared that he was not naive about the tempestuous seas on which he was launching the experiment. He noted the necessity, of cooperation as he seemingly foresaw the collision course on which Nightingale might be embarking. Perhaps he had a taste of the personalities and attitudes of both medical and military authorities from his service in the War Office. In any event he wanted a knowledgeable, proven administrator, one who was capable of organizing and managing a complex situation. And he wanted a person with good supervisory skills who would be able to direct and rule an admittedly difficult group of women of varying competence, as nurses were perceived to be.

From the outset it is obvious that Nightingale was Herbert's choice. He valued the extent of her knowledge and her administrative skills and powers, tested in the Harley Street establishment where she had been serving as Superintendent since August, 1853. It is important to realize that Herbert selected Nightingale because, in his opinion, she was the most experienced and learned figure in hospitals and nursing of her era, and he wanted to assure the success of the mission. All too often, missions in nursing have failed, generated undesirable effects, or achieved less than full success because persons lacking the requisite qualities of sound education and experience have been appointed to leadership positions.

The struggle against the rapid proliferation of training schools, the tremendous variability in learning-teaching opportunities, the lack of instructional personnel, and the appointment of superintendents or principals who had no training or preparation for their positions became the major concerns of the nursing leaders of the formative period. As Eliza Perkins, former superintendent of the Bellevue Training School in New York City, wrote on January 9, 1894, to Miss Darche, first secretary of the American Society of Superintendents of Training Schools for Nurses:

> I thank you for the invitation to attend the convention of Superintendents of Training Schools, especially as I have no claim to become a member of the society. . . . Though a Superintendent of the Bellevue Hospital for twelve years, I am not a graduate of any school. My assistant has always been a graduate, fully competent to give theoretical and practical instruction to the nurses, and upon me, with the advice and assistance of the managers, devolved the executive work of the school. Under this arrangement, the school increased and prospered, but it should not be considered a precedent, as the circumstances which rendered my appointment necessary at the time cannot probably occur again, and I entirely approve of the resolution that a superintendent should be a graduate of a training school of good reputation. . . . (American Society of Superintendents of Training Schools for Nurses, 1897:8)

Linda Richards, herself a product of a non-Nightingale training system, stated as president of the Society of Superintendents at the second annual convention, in referring to two superintendents,

> These women had done the best they could, but what woman with no training can be expected to properly manage a training school? Is it a wonder that the doctors pronounced it a failure and wished to return to the old order of things? (1895:20)

A century and a quarter after the Crimean experiment, nursing has yet to come to grips with the application of a national stipulation or acceptance of educational and experiential requirements for administrative positions, and the enforcement of minimal criteria for eligibility for professional practice.

The parameters of nursing's responsibilities were laid down in the Crimean crucible and can be categorized in two areas: those directly concerned with the soldier in hospital and those related to support and services requisite to his recovery. Although these areas blurred in Crimea they were still identifiable. For example, in the first category would be those areas of direct patient care which are still retained by nursing; in the second would be the ancillary activities of housekeeping, cooking, cleaning, and laundry, activities no longer retained. During her service as superintendent at Harley Street, Nightingale had brought order out of confusion by instituting comprehensive and economical systems of housekeeping that assured cleanliness and control of vermin, of procuring supplies, food, and drugs; and of assigning, training, and evaluating nursing and housekeeping personnel (Verney, 1970). While Nightingale's initial conviction of the great need for environmental control had been demonstrated earlier, her Crimean experiences forged her belief in the value of cleanliness into a rigid, inflexible dogma of sanitation. She observed the absence of a workable hospital laundry and the tremendous filth and vermin which characterized the hospital environment. A more stark observation was that the British soldiers hospitalized from battle wounds and diseases were hastened to their deaths because of starvation due to the lack of a diet that provided them with adequate consumable nutrients. Because there was no one else who seemed either able or willing to do so, Nightingale assumed responsibility for initiating a hospital laundry and for organizing the housecleaning duties of the hospital. Housekeeping activities such as making shirts, stump pillows, and slings filled duty hours as did stuffing ticking with straw for use as mattresses or pallets. Until Nightingale saw to these services, the British soldier in hospital lay on dirt or on concrete floors, in filth and vermin, and often as not died of starvation.

The preparation and serving of food was a recognized task of the English women at Scutari. Nightingale established diet kitchens and supplemented the army rations for the sick and wounded who more often than not were starving from the inability to feed themselves, from the inedible nature of the rations, or from the unavailability of food.

There also seem to have been some criteria for the assignment of personnel. The soldiers suffering slightly were attended by orderlies. The sisters and nurses cared for the extreme cases (Goodman, 1862:105). Simple nursing activities were carried out; the women moistened parched lips, adjusted blankets, and turned, bathed, dressed, and fed the patients. But the nurses' activities also involved the ministration of tasks related to biophysiological needs, tasks such as the application of heat, and cold poultices of linseed meal for frostbite, washing wounds, applying simple dressings and securing them with bandages, and dressing amputations. The psychosociological problems of patients also came under the nurses' jurisdiction; attendance at the bedside of the dying was an act the nurses performed often day and night in the corridors at Scutari. Also, patients suffering from depression and insanity benefited from the efforts and skills of the women who attempted to cheer the despondent and solace the mentally disturbed with soothing words. The delirious were also frequently ministered to by nurses who strove to keep these patients from tearing off dressings and otherwise damaging themselves. Another compassionate task was communicating with the soldier's people back home. Sisters, ladies, and nurses wrote letters home for soldiers unable to write, and letter writing to relatives of deceased soldiers occupied much of their labors. Esthetic consideration also influenced tasks, as the women spread handkerchiefs saturated with eau de cologne over loathsome wounds and foul-smelling dressings.

Management functions of the nurses included administration of medicines and control of dispensation of such dangerous substances as alcoholic beverages—porter, brandy, and wine—which were utilized as prescription items. The safeguarding of the patient's valuables was likewise entrusted to the nurses, since the soldiers believed these women were possessed of a greater sense of integrity than orderlies or fellow soldiers.

As Nightingale civilized Scutari, so did her followers affect civilian institutions both in England and the United States. But in following in Nightingale's footsteps, her adherents failed to recognize one essential difference. What she did in Scutari she did because it was an unprecedented war time emergency, not because she necessarily preferred that particular course or role. But the precedent was set and where there was no one else found to do menial tasks, nurses filled the void, providing a ready, willing, and able source of cheap labor.

Thus, nursing traditionally became charged with housekeeping functions, laundry activities, and dietary tasks. Nurses had great difficulty in identifying that their essential mission was ministering directly to patients. But the defining and redefining of nursing functions continued over time, and a century later nurses were able to make remarkable strides in determining that feeding patients was the sole remaining legitimate function from the corollary responsibilities Nightingale was forced to assume in Crimea. In her first definitive exposition of nursing she had written, "I conclude the Matron to have no cognizance of the laundry" (Nightingale; 1858b:99). Unfortunately it appears that except for the wisdom in *Notes on Nursing,* her followers took little cognizance of her other publications. When nursing insisted that the administration of medications and some treatments were uniquely its province, the founder's admonition seemed to be forgotten:

I use the word nursing for want of a better. It has been limited to signify little more than the administration of medicines and the application of poultices. It ought to signify the proper use of fresh air, light, warmth, cleanliness, quiet and the proper selection and administration of diet—all at the least expense of vital power to the patient. (Nightingale, 1860a:6)

The attendance of nurses on physician's rounds also was a Nightingale rule, implemented and enforced almost without exception. She insisted that the superintendent accompany the doctor on his visits, as she had done at Harley Street, to prevent mistakes, misunderstood directions, and forgotten or ignored instructions and orders. As a consequence, some nurses accompanied physicians on their ward rounds in Scutari and took their directions from them in the process. The rule of the written order, or at least the physician's order being heard by superintendent, can also be traced to Nightingale, who advocated that carrying out orders never heard by the nurse except from the patient was incompatible with good management and the nurse's duty to the hospital (Verney, 1970). The wisdom of the written order became manifest as discrepancies, misunderstandings, and misinterpretations of the intent of verbal instruction arose.

The professional roles we see today of psychological and physical comforting, of providing an environment conducive to recovery, of carrying out physicians' directives and assisting them in their work, and of managing a multitude of coordinating tasks came from the general framework for the activities of the nursing personnel in Scutari and created the bedrock of nursing practice.

As demands for nurses and nursing services grew, lesser trained persons of varying backgrounds and skills emerged and were utilized in direct services to the sick. Nursing assumed responsibility for more of the indirect aspects of care, the secretarial services, and the managerial functions of the agency. The assumption of such tasks moved the nurses further away from the recipient of care, while facilitating the business operation of the hospital, hospital services, and the work of physicians.

The reidentification and resumption of nursing's strategic role in health care became a major con-

cern in the mid-twentieth century as studies of nursing activities identified irrefutably that the bulk of the nurses' time was spent in activities which were rightfully those of other hospital departments. The quality of nursing and cost effectiveness of nursing models were assessed through experiment such as the nurse-operated Loeb Center in New York City, and impetus was given to the reaffirmation of nursing's primary purpose: the care of the sick and well.

Nightingale proposed that nursing was a significant way to improve the health of the British population. To achieve her idea of improved health, she developed a system of trained nursing in hospitals. Nightingale's primary objective was hospital reform. She explained:

> The main objective I conceive to be, to improve hospitals, by improving hospital-nursing; and to do this by improving or contributing towards the improvement, of the class of hospital nurses, whether nurses or head-nurses. This I propose doing, not by founding a Religious Order; but by training, systematizing, and morally improving as far as may be permitted, that section of the large class of women supporting themselves by labour, who take to hospital nursing for a livelihood, by inducing, in the long run, some such women to contemplate usefulness, and the service of God in the relief of man, as well as maintenance, and by incorporating with both these classes a certain proportion of gentlewomen who may think fit to adopt this occupation without pay, but under the same rules, and on the same strict footing of duty performed under definite superiors. These two latter elements, if efficient (if not, they would be mischievous rather than useless), I consider would elevate and leaven the mass . . . . (Nightingale, 1858a:1, 2)

Nightingale adapted her broad concept of reform when she identified that a way of preventing illness in the British soldier was to improve the health of the nation. To do this she formulated a precept that "since God did not mean mothers to be always accompanied by doctors" (1893:24), the health of the nation depended upon woman-kind, that women should be instructed in the art of health, and that the person to best accomplish this instruction was the nurse. Nightingale believed health teaching to be an inherent function of nursing.

Nursing's basic philosophy was defined by Nightingale (1860a:6), who asserted, "The same laws of health or of nursing, for they are in reality the same, obtain among the well as among the sick. . . . " Nightingale also identified the basic principles inherent in nursing, namely, creating those conditions in which the restoration and preservation of health and the prevention of disease and injury could be achieved. She established that it was nursing's obligation to help the patient to live. A second principle which Nightingale established was that "nursing is an art . . . requiring an organized practical and scientific training . . . (1882:1043).

The principles of health restoration, health maintenance, and disease prevention have long been introduced into the conceptual framework of the majority of professional nursing programs and form the bulwark of nursing's educational efforts. As technology developed through rapid and breathtaking scientific advances and as these advances were applied to medical and surgical therapeutics, the nurse's practice changed and more extensive preparation was required. But today's nursing programs still carry out the organized scientific training and the systematic clinical practice recommended by the profession's founder.

Nightingale's letters to her nurses are a rich source of data revealing her philosophy of nursing. The school she started at St. Thomas' Hospital had been in operation 12 years when she began to write letters of instruction, exhortation, and encouragement to the probationers there. Throughout the series—from 1872 to 1900, when the last was written—Nightingale clearly and frequently voiced her belief that nursing was a special vocational call to be followed in a religious spirit; that nurses must be learning all their lives; that nurses, willingly or not, exerted a moral influence;

and that nurses were expected continually to raise standards "to a common intelligence" (1872).

Nightingale identified a critical difference between nursing and other occupations when she wrote,

> The main, the tremendous difference is that nurses have to do with these living bodies and no less living minds; for the life is not vegetable life, nor mere animal life, but it is human life —with living, that is conscious forces, not electric or gravitation forces, but human forces. . . . (1893:34)

Shortly after initiating the school at St. Thomas', Nightingale also perceived that another system of protecting the health of the British population lay in the training of nurse-midwives. A school for midwives was created at King's College Hospital, in an attempt to provide greater safety to the parturient woman and to decrease the dreadful mortality rate resulting from childbirth. Though the school failed for many reasons unrelated to the training of nurses, Nightingale (1871) published a monumental statistical report on the subject of obstetrical mortality and emphasized the importance of nurse midwifery training "as a Career for Educated Women." Extending her concept of sick-nursing, she formulated the precept that "Health is not only to be well, but to be able to use well every power we have. . . . " She went on to explain that the purpose of nursing, whether care of the sick or of the well, was "to put us in the best possible condition for nature to restore or to preserve health—to prevent or to cure disease or injury" (Nightingale, 1893:26).

Florence Nightingale was always sympathetic to the idea of caring for the sick in their homes. It is likely that her own personal experiences as a young lady in her teens and twenties caring for villagers near her family's homes in Romsey or Lea played a decisive role, for it was during this time, in 1844, that she decided that nursing would be her life's work.

When Nightingale (1867a) first described the role of the district nurse in helping the sick or the family to help themselves maintain their independence, she established a critical principle, namely, that the nurse did not provide alms or relief. To do so would mean furthering dependence not independence. Nightingale elaborated more fully on the district nurse, pointing out that she required a fuller training and a better background than the hospital nurse because of the independent nature of her functions. Nightingale had herein described two primary functions of the nurse: district nursing, or the care of the well at home, and nursing the sick.

Nightingale (1882:1043) identified four areas of nursing which may be perceived as areas of specialization: hospital nursing; private nursing, namely, the care of one patient at home; district nursing, or nursing the sick poor at home; and midwifery nursing, or the nursing care of the healthy mother and of the infant after childbirth.

Specialization in nursing had its origins as Nightingale (1893:25) established the nurse-midwifery school, extended hospital nursing into district nursing, and identified the need of specialized emphasis in training for health teaching for mothers and their infants. In doing so, she formulated what would be identified today as a basis for both public health nursing and maternity child nursing: sanitation, the management of the health of infants, children, and adults—including women before and after childbirth—and health education. These goals would be accomplished through individualized instruction for mothers about home sanitation, "the essential principles of keeping the body in health, with reference to the skin, the circulation, and the digestion . . . " (1893:25), and first aid and emergency medical treatment.

In the vanguard of the high-level wellness movement, long before that concept was even defined, Nightingale perceived the nurse as the key in establishing a healthy, disease-free citizenry. The extension of nursing from acute hospital settings to the broadest concept of the community was expostulated by the founder of modern nursing.

Clearly and indisputably, Nightingale visualized the nurse as primary care agent, the nation's first bulwark in health maintenance, in the promotion of wellness, and in the prevention of disease. Nursing got sidetracked from this major, comprehensive objective, but through the pioneering efforts of Lillian Wald and others, the nurse's role in the broad area of public health was reasserted. Efforts of the profession since that time have been focused on the nurse in primary care, health teaching, health screening, and the management of individuals with nonacute health problems.

Theoretical instruction was incorporated into nursing curricula only after an uphill struggle from the very beginning, for even in the Nightingale school, theory was not a major focus. The same situation pertained in the American schools and was ultimately addressed only some 30 years after the first schools were established. The need to provide the nurse with a background of knowledge from which she could draw in developing creditable nursing judgments was a primary consideration of early nursing leaders.

As institutions of higher learning opened their doors to women toward the end of the nineteenth century and expanded their educational offerings, nursing leaders began to look toward them for the preparation of nurses. This expectation was furthered by the consequences of rapid industrialization, scientific breakthrough, and application of technological advances to medicine, surgery, pathology, and pharmacy, with resultant effects and alterations in nurses' practice. Efforts were directed to providing a system of postgraduate training for superintendents to better prepare them to manage training schools.

As modern medicine came to recognize the efficacy, efficiency, and desirability of attendance by trained nurses, they were given more responsibility and more serious duties, and a higher level of skill was expected of them. Those attributes generally ascribed to the professions—greater scientific understanding and inferential and analytical ability—were now required of nurses.

According to Robb, one of nursing's greatest leaders,

> ... medicine has taken the decision out of our hands, and has made trained nursing a profession, but how soon we shall attain to the full profession level depends upon ourselves entirely.... (1900:326)

Nightingale was not alone in perceiving the need for improved nursing. In 1841 Thomson, an English physician, addressed the question of the education of the nurse:

> It may appear a refinement to talk of the education of a nurse; but there is not a greater difference between noonday and midnight than between an educated and an ignorant nurse.... The old and ignorant nurse appeals to her experience: but what is the value of that experience? The educated nurse on the contrary acquires from experience the capacity of observing changes in the progress of the disease which calls her judgment into requisition.... the necessity of education and intelligence in the sick nurse cannot be doubted.... (132)

Nightingale was herself a very learned and intelligent woman; she valued education. Her basic educational philosophy can be summed up in the phrase *trained intelligence,* and her educational efforts and exhortations were directed toward the development of the nurse's intellect, a development which she perceived as a life-long process. Nightingale (1865) saw the preparation for and practice of nursing, as second in importance only to that of medicine, and, as she expressed it, she expected nursing to be trained up to its responsibilities.

Nightingale believed that nursing was an art, "a high calling," requiring constant effort and education. "To know whether we know our Nursing business or not is a great result of training" (1873). She also expected that nursing education would parallel the education trends of the general public, and she wrote to her nurses, reminding them that English law required every child between the ages of 5 and 13 to be in school and that

> It will be a poor tale, indeed, in their afterlife (as Matrons, Scholars, etc.) for nurses who cannot read, write, spell and cypher well and correctly ... now especially when the Nurse is often required to take the temperature of cases, and the like.... (1873)

Nightingale had given much thought to the development of her religious and philosophical treatise on the relationship between man, God, and universe. The concepts she put forth included her views of the nature of the universe, man's purpose in life, and God's laws and expectations for mankind. There is little evidence to suggest that these ideas were ever a part of any training she proposed for nursing. It seems evident that she neither recognized nor believed that her strong educational background was instrumental in her achievements, nor did those who followed her see its value, for more than a century would pass before the unifying theory Nightingale proposed as operational in the universe would be incorporated in the development of a science of nursing (Rogers, 1970).

Nightingale perceived two groups of nurses. Lady probationers, women from a higher class who were financially secure, would be trained for work as superintendents, matrons, home sisters, and head nurses. Paid probationers, women from the working and middle classes, were admitted to training to be prepared for general hospital nursing as ward nurses. Nightingale did not envision ultimate upward mobility when she said, "Many women are valuable as nurses, who are yet unfit for promotion to head nurses" (1858a:7). Those women being prepared as head nurses required a 2-year period of training. "Those probationers, who by education and otherwise are properly qualified, may become Matrons or Superintendents" (1867a, Appendix No. 2).

By 1882 Nightingale (1882:1039) had clearly defined that the first year's practical and technical training was to take place under those nurses who had been *"trained to train"* and that the second year of training as a ward nurse would include theoretical instruction. On the concept of "training to train," Nightingale (1882:1040) was very explicit: "To enable nurses to train nurses, a special training is required; and for this a longer period than a year, or even two years, in the hospital is necessary. To *train* to *train* needs a system . . . ." Nightingale proposed such a system; it consisted of an orderly course of reading; periods of study; oral and written examinations, including "essays on given subjects in nursing;" careful note taking on both classroom and clinical instruction and on the nurse's own clinical observations; opportunity to acquire "powers of expression to train others"; and clinical, managerial, and instructional experiences (1882:1040).

Nightingale's philosophy of nursing education was developed over a period of a quarter of a century.

> Training is to teach not only what is to be done, but how to do it. . . . *why* such and such a thing is done, and not such and such another; as also to teach symptoms. . . . and the 'reason why' of such symptoms. . . .
>
> Telling the nurse what to do is not enough and cannot be enough to perfect her. . . . The trained power of attending to one's own impressions made by one's senses . . . is the *sine qua non* of being a nurse at all. . . . Observation tells *how* the patient is; reflection tells *what* is to be done; training tells *how* it is to be done. Training and experience are, of course, necessary to teach us, too, *how* to observe, *what* to observe; *how* to think, *what* to think. Observation tells us the fact; reflection the meaning of the fact. Reflection needs training as much as observation. Otherwise the untrained nurse, like other people called quacks, easily falls into the confusion of "on account of,". . . . God's will is *not* that we should have our nurses, in whose hands we must leave issues of life or death, without training to fulfill the responsibilities of such momentous issues. (1882:1038)

Nightingale, in the years since the initiation of

the school at St. Thomas', had moved a long way from asserting the need for some lectures and keeping casebooks. It was her intent that the nurse should receive the fullest, richest preparation possible for the serious, weighty responsibilities she was to assume. The honing of the intellectual ability of the nurse, of her capacities for knowledgeable observation and intelligent reflection, would today be called critical thinking and analysis.

The financial independence of the Nightingale school made it possible to adhere to its educational ideals. Moreover, the school existed for the primary purpose of training the nurses, not for the pecuniary advantage of the hospital. Nightingale's original school was a separate and distinct entity. Therein lay the critical difference between the Nightingale system and the system developed in America. Furthermore, students under the Nightingale aegis were "trained to train," not trained to find work as private nurses as in the American system. With essential differences in control and in financial support, American nursing fell under the governance of hospital administrative bodies, and American nursing lost control of its educational standards, of the admission of recruits into the profession, and of its authority and scope of practice (Jacobi, 1976:vii). In addressing the annual convention of the Society of Superintendents, M. E. P. Davis, the president, said, "We are quite powerless to bring about sudden or radical changes without the co-operation of the managers of the training schools" (1896:4).

The chief problem about the system of nursing education Nightingale developed was its location in hospitals organized for that purpose. When the idea became popular, after the efficiency of the system was demonstrated, advocates neglected an essential principle of Nightingale education—namely, that hospitals be organized for the purpose of training—and they assumed that any hospital would suffice. Nightingale's exhortations as to experimentation, flexibility, matching societal trends in education, and training the nurse up to the responsibilities expected of her by medicine were largely ignored. Also ignored was her admonition that nursing was second in importance only to medicine (1865). Because of these lapses, education for nursing has been a long uphill struggle.

From the beginning, through the timorous acceptance of nursing education by universities, and through the pressure of nursing organizations concerned with the public safety as well as with the proper recognition of the nurse, the nursing profession gradually came to see the need for a uniform system of education. In 1960 the Committee on Current and Long-Term Goals of the American Nurses Association recommended to the House of Delegates that within the next 20 to 30 years the education for those entering the professional practice of nursing should be secured through programs providing intellectual, cultural, and technical components of a professional and liberal education. The Committee recommended that the baccalaureate degree become the basic educational foundation for professional nursing (ANA, 1976:184). Such a goal was seen as necessary in view of the explosive growth of knowledge, major theoretical discoveries, the technological revolution, and crucial and paramount changes in therapeusis.

Because of some of her statements about general educational trends, Nightingale has been described as an antieducationist. She cautioned against

> ...mak[ing] school and college education, all sorts of Sciences and Arts, even Nursing and Midwifery, a book and examination business, a profession in the low, not highest sense of the word. And the danger is that we shall be content to let the book and the theory and the words do for us. ... (1888)

But her major exhortations on the value of an informed intellect, "a trained intelligence," as she expressed it, of training the nurse up to her responsibilities, of specific education for specialty practice, of the dangers of the ignorant nurse, of continual learning throughout life seem more than

adequate evidence of the value she placed on education. Deploring any standards which would require

> ...a minimum of *practice,* which may substitute for *personal* progress in active proficiency, mere literary or word progress, instead of making it the material for growth in correct knowledge and practice. ... (1888)

Nightingale (1888) goes on to say, "The danger is lest she [the nurse] let the certificate be instead of her own never ceasing going-up-higher as a woman and a Nurse." By "practice," Nightingale (1888) meant not solely the ward performance, but "the development of each individual's thought & practice, character & dutifulness. ... "

> Let each one of us take the abundant & excellent food for the mind which is offered us, in our training, our classes, our lectures, our Examinations & reading– ...as bright & vigorous fellow-workers: working out the better way every day to the end of life. ... (1888)

Early on in her writings Nightingale decried the application of the word *profession* to nursing, asserting that nursing was not a profession but a calling. However, by 1865 she accepted that the study and practice of nursing as a profession was a universal need second only in importance to medicine itself; and by 1900 she was writing that "nursing has become a profession. Trained nursing is no longer an object but a fact. ... " Less well understood is her deep and abiding recognition of the need for a comprehensive grounding in clinical practice with the informed application of a keenly developed intelligence.

Nightingale established a basic principle of nursing education when she stated:

> Nursing proper can only be taught by the patient's bedside, and in the sick room or ward. Neither can it be taught by lectures or by books, though these are invaluable accessories, if used as such; otherwise, what is in the book stays in

the book. . . . Book learning is useful only to render the practical health of the health-work-shop intelligent, so that every stroke of work done there should be felt to be an illustration of what has been learned elsewhere. . . . (1893:24, 36)

Nightingale believed there were three essential motives requisite to everyone who would nurse: a natural or physical motive, or a love for nursing the sick; a professional or intellectual motive, which she interpreted as a consistent effort to do the work as well as it can be done; and a religious or spiritual motive, which she saw as necessary to meet the disheartening and devastating experiences which confront the nurse in her daily struggle with life, disease, and death. Since she believed the essential spirit or core of nursing had to exist in each one so engaged, Nightingale did not see the need for professional groups or associations.

Because of her deep-seated convictions about the religious nature of nursing, her belief that it was a vocational call, Nightingale rejected the idea that the advance of nursing was an economic problem to be addressed by the creation of unions, organizations, or societies. Those promoting the idea that good salaries would attract good nurses also desired to restrict women volunteers and prevent the untrained from earning a living by nursing. The public had no way of differentiating these groups. Because of the great variations in the skill and performance of the practitioner, public criticism arose which affected the "trained nurse." Hospitals and some members of British nursing wanted a differentiation made clear and proposed in 1886 that the nurse be qualified by an examination and the names of those qualified be placed on a register. Although Nightingale did not object to excluding the unfit or disreputable from nursing, she steadfastly and rigorously opposed any system of qualifying a nurse which did not take into account the nurse's personal character.

In her letter of May 16, 1888, to the probationer-nurses, Nightingale cited her opinions about organizations and certificates. She stated

that the "individual" makes the Association . . . [and] What the Association *is* depends upon each of its members. . . . [it] can never be a substitute for the individual nurse. . . . It is the individual that signifies. . . . (1888)

In this letter she expressed her firm belief that what the nurse did and how she lived was of the greatest importance, "not what she is certified for. . . . "

. . . you may have the most admirable circumstances and organizations and examinations and certificates, yet, if the individual allows herself to sink to a lower level, it is all but a "tinkling cymbal" for her. It is how the circumstances are worked that signifies. Circumstances are opportunities. (1888)

Nightingale expressed another concern about certifying the nurse, for she abhorred stagnation and constantly urged her nurses to grow. "No nurse can stand still. She must go forward or she will go backward every year. . . . It is a call to us, to each individual Nurse, to act up to her profession" (1888). She was of the opinion that no organization or system of registration could accomplish this.

As was described earlier, the identification of a nurse qualified to care for the sick had its origins in the instructions Nightingale and Herbert designed for the Crimean mission:

The persons so selected [by the Superintendent] will receive certificates from the Director-General and Principal Medical Officer of one of the General Hospitals, without which certificate no one will be permitted to enter the Hospital in order to attend the sick. (Herbert: 1854b)

Nursing's second attempt at certification occurred as a result of the methods of training at St. Thomas' Hospital. Upon the satisfactory completion of the year of training for hospital nursing, the probationers' names were entered on a register as certified nurses. However, a certificate was not given each, "to prevent them, in the event of misconduct, from using their certificates improperly" (1865:9).

As the growth of nursing schools spread and their graduates increased in number, the issue of differentiating the trained from the untrained worker in Britain became paramount. The method proposed to resolve the situation was the creation of an organization of trained nurses which would establish a national register of qualified nurses. Early in this movement, Nightingale, as quoted in the Privy Council, raised critical objections:

> You cannot select the good from the inferior nurses by any test or system of examination. But most of all, and first of all, must their moral qualifications be made to stand preeminent in estimation. All this can only be secured by the current supervision, tests, or examinations, which they receive in their training school or hospital, not by any examination from "a foreign body," like that proposed by the British Nurses Association. Indeed, those who came off best in such would probably be the ready and forward, not the best nurses. (1893:13)

Efforts to charter a national professional nursing organization continued, and in 1892, when the Privy Council sat again to debate the issues, formidable opposition was led, as it had been before, by the Council of the Nightingale Fund. Their petition was signed by Miss Nightingale herself, who voiced the belief that the register would be used by the public as an authoritative guide in the selection of nurses, that registration would be considered a sufficient and conclusive guarantee of competence, and that the association would exercise control over determining the qualifications of a trained nurse "and of regulating and controlling the Nursing and education of the whole body of nurses" (1893:26). The petition goes on to describe additional concerns of Miss Nightingale. The register, she said, would not provide

> ...the kind of information which is essentially required in the case of nurses for the sick, such as the possession of gentleness, tact, presence of mind, and other personal and moral characteristics without which no training can produce a good nurse. (1893:26)

Nightingale further asserted that the present base of about 25 years' experience was inadequate to make the decision and that insufficiently trained and inferior nurses would be included and considered on the same footing with "their rightly trained and thoroughly competent sisters." In short, the register would be untrustworthy; general standards would be lowered and incentives to advancement and improvement would be impaired. Raising additional objections, Nightingale took exception to limiting membership in the governing corporation exclusively to nurses. She deemed it necessary to include not only nurses, but training school bodies, governing bodies of hospitals, physicians, and other persons. Clearly Nightingale believed nursing was not able to direct and manage its own affairs, and she objected to allowing nurses alone to determine who was qualified to practice. She forgot that the very nature of the original struggle on which she embarked—namely, safeguarding the public safety—was again at stake. She forgot that a cadre of nurses, systematically trained, had been well received by the public and had become the nucleus for instigating the very nursing reforms she envisioned. In Great Britain, 30 years had to pass before national registration was finally achieved.

The determination to protect the public, and thereby the profession, by admitting to practice only those who had minimal standardized preparation called forth the first nurse licensing boards in the United States in 1903. Over a period of about 50 years, nursing standardized its system of national examinations and established minimum passing scores for eligibility for state registration and entry into practice. Recent clamor has been raised by foreign nurse-graduates and others, who want entry into registered nurse practice without benefit of a standard preparatory course, as well as by graduates from some state-approved programs. Agitation from such groups and recent legislative rulings have caused much consternation in nursing. Concern has arisen in several states as a result of state and national legislation stipulating that occupational, professional, and college entrance examinations must not be culturally biased or discriminatory. At this writing and with some regret, this author reports that the State of California Board of Registered Nursing is seriously considering removing itself from the State Board Test Pool Service, developing its own examinations, and lowering the minimum passing score—all in the guise of removing cultural bias and alleviating a nursing shortage. To proceed in this manner would pose the gravest threat to public safety and might be seen as discriminatory against those nurses who meet the national standards for practice in California and in the other 49 states. It would appear that nursing has come full circle and is about to enter a dark and dismal age.

The period since the end of World War II has been characterized by a rash of movements toward identifying persons from minimal to specialty qualifications in all fields of endeavor. Medicine has its diplomates, literature has its Pulitzer prizes, and nursing has its fellows in an academy. Nursing also has state registration, national certification in specialty areas, and state certification for public health nurses, school health nurses, etc. Then there is state approval for the operation of nursing schools and voluntary accreditation by regional and national bodies. Throughout these standard-setting and qualifying exercises run education systems with diplomas and associate, baccalaureate, master's, and doctoral degrees; and within the educational network, internal and external to graduate education, one sees programs preparing for specialty practice. Nor can one any longer ignore the proliferation of continuing education programs and the great variability in content, motive, and authorship

among them. Have we gone too far in such extensive searches to establish qualifications for practice? In the proliferation of all kinds of nursing programs? The lessons of the past have not been learned.

Nightingale never forgot the illustrations of depravity and immorality to which she had been exposed in her study and work in civilian hospitals as well as in Scutari. Nightingale knew that the success of her experiment to introduce trained nursing into hospitals depended upon upgrading the class of women who were nurses. She realized the great need to raise the morality of women who nursed as well as to protect the women subjected to demoralizing abuse while working in hospitals. Because of these conditions and because of the newness of her proposal to bring trained nurses into hospitals, Nightingale stipulated rigid rules regulating the nurse's personal life and work.

> None but women of unblemished character should be suffered to enter the work, and any departure from chastity should be visited with instant final dismission. All applications on behalf of late inmates of penitentiaries, reformatories, of all kinds and descriptions, should be refused. The first offence of drunkenness, should ensure irreversible dismissal. No nurse dismissed, from whatever cause, should be suffered to return. (Nightingale, 1858a:7)

In addition to providing a system of training, she determined that it was equally essential that nurses have a fit, secure, comfortable living environment. To achieve this, the "Nurses Home" was designed by Nightingale,

> . . . providing a real home, within reach of their work, for the nurses to live in—a home which gives what real family homes are supposed to give—materially a bedroom for each, dining and sitting rooms in common, all meals prepared and eaten in the home; morally, direction, support, sympathy in a common work;

further training and instruction in its proper rest and recreation . . . . (1876)

She believed that if nurses were to reform and recast the homes of the sick poor, the nurse herself had to have a proper place in which to live, and she recommended

> A garden for exercise and refreshment . . . rooms supplied with plain comfortable furniture. . . . A bed, arm-chair, and sofa; a chest of drawers, washstand table or shelf; bookcase or shelves; a little table, and a larger one, a couple of chairs, a footstool, and a cupboard with board shelves, the utmost that can be required. (Nightingale, 1858a:13)

Such facilities appear lavish when one compares the cell-like environment in the typical quarters which have been provided by hospitals since then. Nightingale likewise believed that "Every employer is bound to provide for the health of the workers" (1867a). Her concern for the nurse's comfort and safety seemed to have been forgotten in the proliferation of training schools more desirous of providing cheap hospital labor than a semblance of education, in the inadequacy of their living and educational facilities, and in the rate of invalidism resultant from laborious duties exacted in the guise of learning (Brown, 1940, 1948; Bridgman, 1953).

Nightingale believed in establishing high standards and modifying criteria as time and experience dictated. What was forgotten by her followers and those aspiring to leadership was reevaluation of existing conditions as a better class of women began to enter nursing and improvements were made in methods of instruction in training schools.

> Nurses trusted to do their duty in wards must be trusted to walk out alone if they choose, and I would not attempt to restrict it. . . . (Nightingale 1858a:116)

What may be less well recognized than Nightingale's stringent rules for nurses were her proposals for their economic security. The entire philosophy and rationale of the economic and general welfare program adopted by the American Nurses Association in 1946 had been outlined by Nightingale when she wrote,

> Besides,—a thing very little understood,—a good nurse has her professional pride in results of her Nursing quite as much as a good Medical Officer in the results of his treatment. There are defective buildings, defective administrations, defective appliances, which make all good Nursing impossible. A good Nurse does not like to waste herself, and, the better the Nurse, the stronger this feeling in her. Humanity may overrule this feeling in a great emergency like a cholera outbreak; but I don't believe that it is in human nature for a good Nurse to bear up, with an ever-recurring ever-useless expenditure of activity, against the circumstances which make her nursing activity useless, or all but useless. . . . It is a far greater pity to have a good Nurse wasting herself in this way than it would be to have a steam-engine running up and down the line all day without a train, wasting coals. Perhaps I need scarcely add that Nurses must be paid the market price for their labour, like any other workers; and that this is yearly rising. . . . (1867a:66)

To what extent did she perceive the altruistic motive as a determinant of the profession's growth? The altruistic philosophy undergirding all of nursing was expressed by Nightingale (1858a:2) when she described nursing as a service to mankind and thereby a means of serving God. Several years earlier she had defined that nursing under her auspices would not restrict its services to a test of religion. Since then the philanthropic motive has long been a hallmark of the profession, and its members have placed their own economic security, pecuniary rewards, and employment benefits secondary to their care for people.

Clearly, while Nightingale accepted the religious and vocational aspects of nursing as a calling and as a means of serving God by serving mankind, she was not advocating a selflessness and devotion implicit in accepting substandard working environments incompatible with safe, effective nursing practice. Nor was she advocating a rate of remuneration inconsistent with prevailing standards of living or inappropriate to the work, responsibility, and qualifications of the nurse. Granted, some of her recommendations seem rather pitiful today, as, for example, her suggestion in 1858 that an increase in salary might be given after 10 years' experience. However, her own ideas were revised from time to time and shortly thereafter she came to believe an annual merit increase more appropriate. Originally advocating a 2-week holiday annually, Nightingale revised this opinion also, for in 1882 she asserted that a "month's holiday was not too much." How many nurses working in 1981 are given a month's vacation annually? Nightingale's rationale for such terms was the responsible and burdensome nature of the work, a rationale which is surely relevant today and is reflective of her deep concern for the welfare of the nurse as a person. Another interesting concept developed when, in 1854, Nightingale and Herbert stipulated that the nurse's round-trip travel expenses to Scutari would be reimbursed upon satisfactory service. Only in exceptional circumstances are nurses reimbursed today for travel to places of employment or even to the interview appointment. To what extent does this benefit apply to other professionals, and hence to what extent is its absence discriminatory to nursing?

Nightingale might even be identified as an author of the idea of the day-care center, for she wrote of employing nurses who had dependent children:

> With regard to children we might look forward to a time when a school might be formed for the children, if any, of such of Her Majesty's Nurses as are widows. . . . I do not anticipate that it would be possible ever to have married women in the Service. . . . (1858a:24-5)

The establishment of a graduated pension plan for nurses was also a Nightingale recommendation. She observed,

> it is equally undesirable to turn faithfully worn-out servants adrift without any provision, or to retain them in duties for which they become unfit. It is a question whether there should not be a compulsory stoppage from wages, in order to entitle the nurse to pension under conditions. (1858a:14)

As hospitals began to employ nurses in great numbers, proper living and working conditions were disregarded and the justice of decent financial rewards and economic benefits largely ignored. Nurses began a struggle for improvements and started to organize. The creation of a national professional organization for nurses, the Nurses' Association Alumnae, came in 1897. Because of the deplorable employment conditions and abuses then prevalent, the association had as one of its objectives promoting the financial interests of the nursing profession. There were but a few isolated improvements, and ultimately a national program for the economic security of nurses was proposed in 1926 and adopted in 1946. Primary motivation for the establishment of a national economic security program for nurses was lodged in the conviction that a spirit of service was not incompatible with satisfactory working conditions. The profession was losing members. New recruits were not entering nursing because of the absence of economic incentives and of working conditions perceived to be equitable with those enjoyed by comparable workers in American society (ANA, 1976:169). Wandelt's (1980) study of the nursing shortage reidentified these problems and concerns.

In its formative years, from 1893 to 1900, the Society of Superintendents of Training Schools also expressed grave concerns related to the equality of financial remuneration of both women and men in nursing:

> The woman who nurses ought to be paid equally with the man who nurses. We all

know that men—even untrained ones—who nurse, command higher rates than women. . . . The old argument that women must be content to be underpaid, because they take men's work away from them, will not hold here, for it has always been undisputed that nursing is peculiarly a woman's work. Nor can it be maintained that a man must be paid more because he supports a family, for the young men in training schools have no families, but usually make nursing a stepping-stone to medicine, while, on the other hand, how many nurses do we not all know who help keep the home for a father or mother, or educate a young sister, or give a young brother his start in life? No. This inequality exists, but neither of these reasons explain why it exists, and not until nurses learn to take control of their affairs will it be different. (Dock, 1896:58)

The question of equal remuneration for men and women nurses was not a problem for Miss Nightingale, but it is one that has plagued American nursing to the present day. Federal legislation on equal rights was instrumental in trying to correct the situation, but the effects of discrimination can be seen in American nursing in the rapid advancement and promotion of men in favor of women. A 1981 court decision ruled that nurses did not receive remuneration equivalent to that obtained by men in occupations requiring similar skills and responsibilities but that to adjust the financial scale would disrupt the American economy!

As nursing moved forward in its efforts to obtain more equitable economic rewards, the profession struggled to relieve itself of nonnursing duties. As early as 1867, Nightingale was admonishing,

A good nursing staff will perform their duties more or less satisfactorily, under every disadvantage. But while doing so, their head will always try to improve their surroundings in such a way to liberate them from subsidiary work, and to enable them to devote their time more exclusively to the care of the sick. This

is, after all, the real purpose of their being there at all, not to act as lifts, water-carriers, beasts of burden, or steam engines—articles whose labour can be had at vastly less cost than that of educated human beings. . . . (1867a:68)

The altruism, humanitarianism, and philanthropy which have characterized nursing were not perceived by its founder as a justification for ignoring the personal needs of the nurses for respect, reward, recognition, and pride in proper utilization.

Concern about the legal status of women and their disenfranchisement was a current sociopolitical issue in Victorian England after the Crimean War. Martineau and Gaskill, two feminists, and male advocates, who included John Stuart Mill, campaigned for women's suffrage. Through an introduction by Edwin Chadwick, a notable contemporary sanitarian, Nightingale wrote to Mill asking his opinions about her recently privately published work on philosophy and religion (1860c). Apparently Mill had earlier read Nightingale's *Notes on Nursing,* for Chadwick had advised her that Mill took exception to her concluding remarks about women:

I would earnestly ask my sisters to keep clear of both the jargons now current everywhere (for they are equally jargons); of the jargon, namely, about the "rights" of women, which urges women to do all that men do, including the medical and other professions, merely because men do it, and without regard to whether this is the best that women can do; and of the jargon which urges women to do nothing that men do, merely because they are women, and should be "recalled to a sense of their duty as women," and because "this is women's work," and "that is men's," and "these are things which women should not do," which is all assertion and nothing more. Surely woman should bring the best she has, *whatever* that is, to the work of God's world, without attending to either of these cries.

For what are they, both of them, the one just as much as the other, but listening to the "what people will say," to opinion, to the "voices from without!" And as a wise man has said, no one has ever done anything great or useful by listening to the voices from without.

You do not want the effect of your good things to be, "How wonderful for a woman!" nor would you be deterred from good things, by hearing it said, "Yes, but she ought not to have done this, because it is not suitable for a woman." But you want to do the thing that is good, whether it is "suitable for a woman" or not.

It does not make a thing good, that is remarkable that a woman should have been able to do it. Neither does it make a thing bad, which would have been good had a man done it, that it has been done by a woman. (1860a:76)

Nightingale (1860c) responded and advised Mill that she "will alter the words in the next Edition," but it is apparent she never did, for subsequent editions still contain them. She further explained that her words did not mean that she believed women should be denied the liberty or freedom of working at certain occupations "merely because men do it." She (1860c) asserted that women in medicine "have made no improvement," to which Mill (1860) enjoined that, given the rare incidence of first-rate minds, it would hardly occur by chance that the first three women doctors would be exceptional. After an interval of 7 years, the subject of women's rights arose again in their correspondence, and Nightingale wrote

That women should have the suffrage, I think no one can be more deeply convinced than I. . . . (1867b)

She goes on to explain the characteristics of the disenfranchised women, especially married women who cannot own property, and emphatically questions that the entire set of inequitable "disabilities as to property and influence of women could be swept away by the legislature as it stands at present? And equal rights and equal responsibilities be given as they ought to be to both men and women?" (1867b).

Nightingale made no effort to conceal her belief that men had the obligation to give equal rights to women, especially since they expected them to pay taxes. She used the theme "taxation without representation" as the buttress for her argument that the evils pressing on women could be "*redressible* by legislation." Her rationale was that public agitation for corrective legislation would subject social reforms to political partisanship. The National Society for Women's Suffrage was founded in 1867 and Mill urged her to join. In her classic response Nightingale fell back upon her illness, the extreme press of her work, and the fact that she never gave her name to a cause for which she had no time to work. She denied ever wanting "personally political influence" and asserted that she worked better behind the scenes than out in front, although she believed that women's "political power" should be "direct and open." Mill's response was to the effect that this reticence was a general disposition among women. Mill drew her attention to his belief that political power is the only security against every form of oppression and that

it would be easier to attain political rights for women . . . than to obtain any other considerable reform in the position of women; and that there is . . . no danger of party spirit running high between men and women and no possibility of its making things worse than they are if it did. (Mill, 1867)

Mill further admonished Nightingale that she "joined in too few movements for the public good . . . " (1867). In 1871 she joined the Society but was never active in it.

Had Nightingale devoted some of her energy to forthrightly advocating women's reform and given it a fraction of the effort she gave military, medical, and nursing reform, the course of the women's movement may have been very different. It seems strange that she did not, because the very evils facing women which she began to address in nursing reform pressed upon all women. But Nightingale described herself as best working behind the stage, and she continued her reticence on this powerful issue.

In 1915 at its annual convention of the American Nurses Association, the House of Delegates altered its previous opposition and endorsed the women's suffrage amendment, which eventually became law in 1920 after a 45-year struggle. Shortly thereafter, the struggle for equal rights began in earnest. Unfortunately American nursing has not been in the vanguard of either of these women's movements and has not asserted itself in a leadership role.

Clearly, the prevailing structure of nursing in the United States can be traced to Nightingale's beliefs, precepts, and practices. The broadest, fullest scope of her vision was partially realized in her lifetime. Many of her comments are as practical today as a century ago. Many of the founder's ideals have come to fruition, but many have yet to be realized. For, to quote Miss Nightingale,

> Good nursing does not grow of itself; it is the result of study, teaching, training, practice, ending in sound tradition which can be transferred elsewhere. (1865:4)

and

> May we hope that, when we are all dead and gone, leaders will arise who have been personally experienced in the hard, practical work, the difficulties and the joys of organizing nursing reforms, and who will lead far beyond anything we have done.... (1893:37)

EDITOR'S QUESTIONS FOR DISCUSSION

What effects has Nightingale's placing herself and her nurses under the absolute authority of the medical officers had in the history and present relationship of nursing with medicine? How appropriate was Nightingale's apparent rationale for her subservience to medicine? How appropriate is it today for Nightingale's strategies for employment by nursing leaders? To what extent do Nightingale's writings suggest alternatives in modern nursing for the organization of authority, responsibility, and scope of functions?

Identify examples in nursing education and practice where Nightingale's principles of flexibility and experimental testing are not being followed. How can Nightingale's philosophy of nursing education and professional practice be reconciled with education and practice today? Currently, is the mission of nursing being defined differently than it was defined by Nightingale?

Since Nightingale originally appears to have viewed nursing as a "calling," not as a profession, to what extent should Nightingale's beliefs, tenets, and practices be followed in professional nursing? Identify the beliefs and practices of Nightingale which were essential in the development of nursing as a profession.

Identify any beliefs and practices espoused by Nightingale which have inhibited the development of the profession. Are there any beliefs and practices which should not be followed? If so, identify and justify the tenets which do not appear appropriate for this decade. To what extent has modern nursing deviated from the essential philosophy and spirit of Florence Nightingale? What lessons of the past has modern nursing not learned? If Nightingale were alive today, what might one project as suggestions she would offer for modern professional nursing? Would she advocate more directly than she did women's reform and equality? If so, what type of strategy or method might she suggest? What ideals of the founder have yet to be realized? What strategies might be suggested for achieving those ideals?

REFERENCES

American Nurses Association
1976 One Strong Voice: The Story of the American Nurses Association. Lyndia Flanagan (Comp.). Kansas City: ANA.
American Society of Superintendents of Training Schools for Nurses
1897 Annual Reports. Harrisburg: By the Society.
Blackwood, A.
1881 Narrative of Personal Experiences and Impressions during a Residence on the Bosphorus throughout the Crimean War. London: Hatchard.
Bridgman, M.
1953 Collegiate Education for Nursing. New York: Russell Sage Foundation.
Brown, E. L.
1940 Nursing as a Profession. 2nd ed. New York: Russell Sage Foundation.
1948 Nurses for the Future. New York: Russell Sage Foundation.
Cook, E. T.
1913 The Life of Florence Nightingale. Volume I. London: Macmillan.
Cope, Zachary
1958 Florence Nightingale and the Doctors. Philadelphia: Lippincott.
Davis, M. E. P.
1896 Address at Third Annual Convention of the American Society of Superintendents of Training Schools for Nurses. Harrisburg: By the Society.
Dock, L.
1895 "Directories for nurses" in First and Second Annual Conventions of the American Society of Superintendents of Training Schools for Nurses. Harrisburg: By the Society.
1896 "A National Association for Nurses and its Legal Organization." The Third Annual Convention of the American Society of Superintendants of Training Schools for Nurses. Harrisburg: By the Society.
Frank, Sister C. M.
1953 The Historical Development of Nursing. Philadelphia: Saunders.

Goodman, M.
1862 Experiences of an English Sister of Mercy. London: Smith Elder.
Hampton, I. A.
1893 "Educational standards for nurses," Pp. 1–12 in Isabel A. Hampton and others, Nursing of the Sick 1893. New York: McGraw-Hill reprint, 1949.
Herbert, S.
1854a Letter to F. Nightingale. Mss. 43393. British Library (reprinted in Cook).
1854b Instructions WO/43/97/155656/3. Public Record Office. London (reprinted in Cook).
Jacobi, E.
1976 Forward. In Lyndia Flanagan (Comp.), One Strong Voice: The Story of the American Nurses Association, Kansas City: ANA.
Kalisch, P. A. and B. J. Kalisch
1978 The Advance of American Nursing. Boston: Little Brown.
Mill, J. S.
1860 Letters to Florence Nightingale as printed
1867 in Hospitals, 1936.
Mundinger, M.
1980 Autonomy in Nursing. Maryland: Aspen.
National League of Nursing Education Standard Curriculum for Schools of Nursing.
1917 New York: The Society.
Nightingale, F.
1858a Subsidiary Notes as to the Introduction of Female Nursing into Military Hospitals in Peace and War. London: Harrison.
1858b Notes on Matters Affecting the Health, Efficiency, and Hospital Administration of the British Army Founded Chiefly on the Experience of the late War. London: Harrison.
1860a Notes on Nursing. London: Harrison.
1860b Suggestions for Thought to the Searchers after Truth among the Artizans of England. 3 Vols. London: Eyre and Spottiswoode.
1860c Letter to John Stuart Mill as printed in Hospitals, 1936.
1865 Suggestions on a System of Nursing for Hospitals in India.
1867a Suggestions on the Subject of Providing

Training and Organizing Nurses for the Sick Poor in Workhouse Infirmaries. Report of the Committee on Cubic Space of Metropolitan Workhouses with Papers submitted to the Committee.

1867b Letter to John Stuart Mill, as printed in Hospitals, 1936.

1871 Introductory Notes on Lying-in Institutions. Together with a Proposal for Organizing an Institution for Training Midwives and Midwifery Nurses. London: Longmans, Green.

1872 Address to the Probationer-Nurses in the "Nightingale Fund" School. London: Privately printed.

1873 Address to the Probationer-Nurses in the "Nightingale Fund" School. London: Spottiswoode.

1874 Address to the Probationer-Nurses in the "Nightingale Fund" School. London: Spottiswoode.

1876 "On Trained Nursing for the Sick Poor." Letter to the Times 14 April.

1882 Nurses, Training of, and Nursing the Sick in Quain's Dictionary of Medicine. London: Longman's, Green.

1888 Address to the Probationer-Nurses in the "Nightingale Fund" School. London: Privately printed.

1893 "Sick Nursing and Health Nursing." In Nursing of the Sick. New York: McGraw-Hill reprint, 1949.

1900 To My Dear Children, May 28, 1900. at the Nightingale School.

Pollock, C. E.
1910 "Original communications. Florence Nightingale." Journal of the Royal Army Medical Corps. XV:4, 385.

Privy Council
1893 The Battle of the Nurses. A Full Verbatim Report of the Actual Proceedings before the Privy Council. London: Scientific Press.

Richards, L.
1895 Address of Welcome at Second Annual Convention of the American Society of Superintendents of Training Schools for Nurses. Harrisburg: By the Society.

Robb, I. H.
1900 "A general review of nursing forces," Pp. 324–331 in Lyndia Flanagan (Comp.), One Strong Voice: The Story of the American Nurses Association. Kansas City: ANA.

Roebuck Committee
1855 Reports from the Select Committee on the Army before Sebastopol. Hansard.

Rogers, M. E.
1970 An Introduction to the Theoretical Basis of Nursing. Philadelphia: F. A. Davis.

Shields, E. A.
1981 Highlights in the History of the Army Nurse Corps. Washington, D. C.: U. S. Army Center of Military History.

Snively, Mary Agnes
1895 "A uniform curriculum for training schools," pp. 24–30. The Second Annual Convention of the American Society of Superintendents of Training Schools for Nurses. Harrisburg: By the Society.

Stewart, I. M. and A. L. Austin
1962 A History of Nursing. 5th ed. New York: Putnam's.

Terrot, S. A.
1898 Reminiscences of Scutari Hospitals in Winter 1854–55. Edinburgh: Stevenson.

Thomson, A. T.
1841 The Domestic Management of the Sick Room.

Verney, Sir H.
1970 Florence Nightingale at Harley Street. Her Reports to the Governors of her Nursing Home. 1853-4. London: Dent.

Wandelt, M.
1981 Conditions Associated with Registered Nurse Employment in Texas. The University of Texas at Austin, Center for Research, School of Nursing: The University of Texas at Austin.

Chapter 2

Prescription For Professionalization

Mary E. Conway, R.N., Ph.D., F.A.A.N.
Dean and Professor
School of Nursing
Medical College of Georgia
Augusta, Georgia

Mary E. Conway's chapter appropriately is in order after Palmer's notable tracing of Nightingale's philosophy, concepts, and practices in the development of nursing as a profession. At the present stage of professionalization, Conway targets the principal task for nursing as developing its knowledge base. The rationale offered is that possession of a distinct body of knowledge enables a discipline to control its practice field more than any other characteristic of a profession. Conway reviews some factors affecting the evolution of professions on a continuum from occupational to professional status. She cites reasons why the process of developing a knowledge base for nursing will be lengthy and indicates uncertainties to be encountered. Conway proposes a model to serve as a guide. The model requires a body of practitioners and theorists to singly and collaboratively share responsibilities for both generation and application of knowledge to practice.

Nursing is a profession which from a socioevolutionary perspective is still developing its professional identity. That is, it is continuing to define its parameters of practice and to delimit those parameters vis-à-vis other health professions. Thus, it seems appropriate—even necessary—to examine how nursing is proceeding in its pursuit of recognition as a fully qualified profession.

To some extent every profession can be viewed as more or less continuously in process of professionalization since the evaluations of practitioners and clients alike combine to bring about

This paper has benefited from a careful critique by Phyllis Kritek, Ph.D., University of Wisconsin-Milwaukee.

alterations in practices and/or public postures. Evaluation by clients focuses on the relevance and efficacy of the service provided, while practitioners tend to be concerned more with control of the profession itself. It is easy to see that both interests are inextricably linked; that is, serious dissatisfaction with a profession's performance on the part of those served is likely to result in legislation which gives more regulatory control of the profession to an outside agency such as a governmental unit. Historically speaking, the majority of professions have *evolved* from generic *work groups*. More about this concept will be said presently.

At several points in time over its historical

development every occupation is confronted with a *single* task which requires the concerted efforts of its scientists and practitioners if it is to make a measurable evolutionary advance. The task which confronts nursing—its most demanding task—is that of expediting the development of its knowledge base.

A number of assumptions about the present status of nursing as a science-based discipline may help to justify the case being made for concentration of effort on further development of a knowledge base. One of these is that nursing is a *work group* in sociological terms which can be classified as an occupation at one end of a continuum and a profession at the other (Pavalko, 1971:26). Another assumption is that nursing demonstrates a majority of the characteristics or criteria by which professions are commonly judged, but not all of these. A cameo of the ideal-typical profession includes at least the following characteristics: the acquisition of a body of knowledge in the discipline is an intellectual pursuit; there is a body of theory which guides the practice of members (Moore, 1970); members are unified in a community of shared values and goals (Goode, 1957); there is a code of ethics which guides the practice of individuals; members deal with matters of human urgency and significance (McGlothlin, 1964); and members exert control over the service arena in which they practice (Freidson, 1970). (Medicine and law frequently are cited as exemplary models of matured professions on the basis of possessing all these characteristics.) Of these characteristics, two for which nursing exhibits very little evidence to date are a recognizable body of theory and control of its practice arena. A third assumption is that leaders in the profession and a fairly representative number of its members recognize that the task, while already underway, needs to be given a high priority.

HISTORICAL PERSPECTIVE

A characteristic which has been noted to be common to all groups when comparing the evolution of occupations generally recognized as professions is that of a shift in emphasis over time from concerns of members for their individual job security to a concern with the service ideal. Yet acknowledging this feature may obscure a more subtle but important social reality. The fact is that many occupations which are universally acknowledged to be professions *simultaneously* exhibit some characteristics of *both* an occupation and a profession. That is, concern for bread-and-butter issues often coexists with concern for theory development, autonomy, a service ideal and/or with adherence to a code of ethics. Recent legislation in some states to permit advertising by members of the bar serves as a case in point. While members of the bar have a long-standing code of ethics, it is apparent that they feel a need to take steps to ensure their continuing income in the face of a substantial increase in the numbers of practicing lawyers. It may be that physicians will follow suit if an oversupply of physicians should occur as has been predicted.

Setting has proved to be an important determinant of both the nature and the pace of the evolutionary process which an occupation undergoes. Setting, more specifically the organizational position of the employee, has important consequences for the status of the individual worker. In general, although not always, those individuals who are self-employed tend to enjoy higher status than those who are employed in an organization. The historical evidence is that professionals have tended to be self-employed while blue-collar workers have been found more often in organizations (Braito and Prescott, 1978:52). More recently, increasing numbers of professionals, including physicians and lawyers, have come to be employed in organizations. In the aggregate these latter two professions have managed to retain much of the status and autonomy they achieved earlier. In this respect they differ from the more general pattern found among professionals employed within organizations, the difference stemming largely from the dominance both groups have exerted historically among all the professions. A recent finding raises some doubt about the generalization concerning the autonomy of physicians, particularly those employed within organizations. Engel (1970) has reported finding that physicians employed in a moderate-sized bureaucratic organization perceived themselves as having more autonomy than did physicians in solo practice. When the relative possession of autonomy among the professions is examined, nurses fit the more general pattern of professionals who possess limited autonomy. For the most part their practice has been under the supervision of physicians even when they are in solo practice, but more important, the majority of nurses have been and still are employed by organizations.

While in the aggregate nurses subscribe to a number of values and goal aspirations in common, nursing as a discipline fails to be a community in the sense Goode (1957) has described it. Rather than being a unified community of like-minded professionals, nurses comprise a *segmented* work group—that is, large numbers of nurses are concerned primarily with wages and conditions of employment while others are more concerned with advancing their professional status through certification for specialty practice, through involvement in research, and/or through greater involvement in the political process. If there is a single overt manifestation of community which links all these segments at the present moment in history, it may be the sense of militancy which is prevalent in public statements and contributions to the profession's journals.

That segment of the profession which exhibits the greatest concern with its conditions of employment comprises those nurses who provide the larger share of direct service to clients. In a real sense they are the most universally "visible" members of the profession. In contrast to this segment are those members of the profession who are involved in academic nursing—the teaching of nursing. These nurses form a *less* visible segment. They are fewer in number and they have little direct or sustained contact with recipients of care. Their contacts generally are limited to those which occur in the course of supervising students in the clinical laboratory. These profes-

sionals, as might be expected, are concerned primarily with realizing the ideal objectives set for students in their courses. The value differences which characterize these two segments are a continuing source of intraprofessional conflict.

EDUCATION AS PREPARATION FOR A DIFFERENT FUTURE

Inherent in the socialization plan of every profession is the recognition that the neophyte professional must be prepared for a practice field that is likely to be markedly different from the one he or she enters upon graduation from the preparatory institution. Roles which professional nurses will be called upon to fill in the future will demand nurses capable of highly independent (and interdependent) functioning in an increasingly wellness-oriented society. Thus, the response to this anticipated future on the part of many baccalaureate nursing programs has been to discard the so-called medical model of curriculum. In its place are curriculum models based on wellness since it is the latter arena of practice that nurses consider their domain.

Two important considerations are reflected in this deliberate curriculum revision. One is the recognition that concern for wellness has grown concomitantly with recognition of the finite limitations of medical technology. In addition the maximization of health is both economically and rationally defensible. Another consideration is the obvious reality that as some nurses move out of the medical model of practice, they will be associated less with physicians and more with other professionals, while their practice will be recognized as a separate and distinct type of health care practice. Thus, while educational programs develop curriculums to prepare graduates to practice in a field which differs from that which exists, at the same time graduates of these programs will *themselves be contributors* to the changes that will occur in the practice field.

While the wellness movement is likely to continue unabated for some time to come, there are uncertainties that will be encountered as nursing attempts to establish its domain. The costs of health care, increasing size of the older population cohort, and the proliferation of paraprofessional groups will have as yet unknown effects upon nursing.

One uncertainty is the extent to which nursing will be able to establish its primacy in wellness promotion. For example, although nursing increasingly is making public statements about its focus on preventive health measures and has established a number of so-called wellness centers, it cannot be assumed that physicians will accept a restriction of their practice to treating illness. In actual fact such a restriction is not possible since there is no objectively discernible demarcation in an individual's health status that can be called sick or healthy. The definition of one or the other of these statuses often rests on the determination made by the individual before seeking treatment.

Another uncertainty for nursing involves the aspirations of other health occupations. Health educators, for example, perceive themselves as having an important role in the field of health promotion, as do exercise physiologists and physical trainers. Supply and demand market forces will be an important determinant with respect to which profession—or professions—will become more preeminent in health promotion. In those geographic regions where the ratio of population to physicians is high, nurses will very likely become more dominant as health promotion practitioners; in regions where the reverse is the case, they are unlikely to do so. Given medicine's historical professional dominance in health care, actions on the part of organized medicine to limit nursing practice can be anticipated, at least in those instances where nurse practitioners may be perceived to be making incursions into the domain of medical practice.

A critical factor in determining the pace and ultimate success of nursing's claim to wellness-health as its sphere of practice is an economic one. In a number of instances university schools of nursing have established wellness centers or clinics in which services such as health screening,

hypertension monitoring, nutrition instruction, parenting classes, and life-style counseling are offered to clients without charge in order to permit nurses to establish their role in the provision of these services independently of physicians. However, no profession within a capitalist economy can afford to provide its services free, nor is it likely to be perceived as having anything of value to offer unless it demands payment for its services. The underlying strategy in such free-service centers is to move into a practice domain unobtrusively without raising the question of whether the provision of these services may be an intrusion into the territory of medical practitioners. It remains to be seen what form such centers will ultimately take and the numbers which will survive.

A CREDIBILITY GAP

As noted earlier, as a work group evolves from the occupation end of the continuum to the profession end, it tends to become increasingly concerned with its service ideal. Thus, the character or quality of the care provided by nurses, as this quality is perceived by clients, is linked to the rate at which professionalization occurs. Where the nature of service delivered and/or its quality are judged to be high, clients can be expected to give a positive evaluation and to support the claims of the profession to the prerogatives it demands. Client judgment and the professional's judgment of the type of care or service which *should* be provided in a given instance do not always coincide—nor should they necessarily.

This problem is not unique to nursing. Physicians, for example, often find themselves in the position of applying a remedy—or performing a test—for a symptom of which the patient is unaware rather than responding immediately to the patient's presenting problem. When any of these factors—quality, timing, or kind of service—fails to meet client expectations over an extended period of time, a *credibility gap* may follow. This credibility gap is best defined as the magnitude of the discrepancy that exists between the *ideal prescriptions* of the profession, as contained in its public statements and code of ethics, and the objective reality of its service at the point of application to the client.

The nursing profession internally is confronted with a contest between its practitioners and its scientists. For the so-called basic (laboratory) sciences this dilemma does not exist; the laboratory is the point of application for many discoveries and for the application of theoretical formulations. For the applied sciences, of which nursing is one, the dilemma is persistent and difficult to resolve. Practitioners tend not to value theory (or science) and in addition, the majority of nurses fail to perceive that research and its outcomes have any relevance for their practice (Ketefian, 1975).

The dilemma is further compounded in that one of the obvious approaches to bringing about a closer value consensus between practitioners and researchers—collaboration between both in the practice setting—is not widely encouraged. In addition, in the majority of settings where nurses practice, the dominant values are application of technology, adherence to routine, following established procedures, and "processing" clients in such a way as to speed their exit from the setting with a minimum cost. Knowledge as such is not valued. While there is increasing awareness that researchers and practitioners should collaborate to apply the benefits of newer knowledge in the service rendered to those that knowledge is intended to help, there are relatively limited dollars available for allocation to that goal.

If nursing's credibility as a profession lies ultimately in the value of its service to clients, what must be done seems clear; how it can be accomplished is somewhat less clear. What *must* be done is for practitioners and theorists to arrive at a consensus in regard to which of the problems based in the practice of nursing can be addressed through research and which, if researched, offer promise toward a reconceptualization of practice.

A concerted effort in this direction can be expected to generate knowledge exponentially. That is, as more problems are researched, hypotheses tested, and findings systematically applied and evaluated, other problems will be generated and thus generate additional research. Over time, as this self-perpetuating cycle becomes established, the theoretical formulations of nursing's theorists and the ideal prescriptive statements governing practice should begin to converge. Or, falling short of convergence, they should at least represent a closer link between the ideal and the reality than that which presently exists.

KNOWLEDGE BASE—THE CRITICAL ELEMENT

The task to which nursing as a professional body must devote its greatest efforts over the next several decades is the development of a knowledge base for its professional practice. For nursing as for every other learned discipline, its knowledge base is the *sine qua non* for its claim to professional status. This knowledge base will consist of a body of theoretical formulations derived from the generation and repeated testing of hypotheses and the application of findings from these tests to practice under carefully monitored and controlled conditions. At the present time the process of developing a knowledge base is well underway but the process undoubtedly will be lengthy and uneven.

There are a number of reasons to presume that the process will be a lengthy one. Nursing has been thwarted in its research efforts. This is due to a number of factors: for one, it competes with many other professions which have been able to command greater awareness of the need for monies to support research. It also competes with medicine for access to subjects (Conway, 1978). Furthermore those who control allocation of the scarce resources needed to support research have doubts about the competence of science in the social and behavioral disciplines (Schrag, 1968). Another important deterrent to an all-out effort in developing nursing science is the perception of a majority of nurses in practice that research is irrelevant to that practice. Each of these problems will have to be confronted individually as expanded research efforts continue.

To acknowledge that nursing is deficient in a body of theory is not to imply that there is a complete lack of evidence for theory. However such elements of theory as do exist are in a rudimentary stage and they have not been subjected to systematic testing. Nursing is forced to compensate for a deficit that exists because there is no heritage of earlier scientists in the discipline who, had they existed, would have laid the foundation blocks for the present generation of researchers to build on (Johnson, 1974). It is this hiatus that is largely responsible for the present lack of a clearly circumscribed body of knowledge identifiable as *nursing*. More importantly, as Johnson has noted, there is as yet no group of facts or empirical generalizations widely recognized and accepted as offering the rudiments of nursing science which can provide the foundation for further work. A part of the difficulty in attempting to establish empirical generalizations is that the parameters of nursing are not clearly defined (Johnson, 1974).

Theory building must continue concomitantly with other efforts to define the parameters of nursing. Both objectives—theory building and definition of parameters—may be viewed as essentially reciprocal events in a quasi-causal chain. That is, as theory contributes to an expanded knowledge base and as that knowledge is applied, tentative parameters should become more apparent. Some scholars have insisted that all efforts in theory building for nursing should be directed toward prescriptive theory (Dickoff and James, 1968). Yet, the history of theory development in science is replete with evidence that some of the most fruitful outcomes in terms of new knowledge have been those which are linked to earlier highly abstract, theoretical frameworks.

The lack of an earlier (historical) theoretical foundation in nursing is one antecedent that has accounted for the extended time lag between hypothesis testing and the statement of nursing's prescriptive theories. As a science which is essentially social in character, nursing reflects the dilemma in theory building which is faced by other social sciences: that is, there is no absolute agreement among researchers and theorists about which variables must be taken into account in specifying concepts and classification systems (Cleary, 1971).

Equally important to theory building-testing is the replication of earlier studies from which findings have been generated that offer promise for useful application in practice. Those research investigations which have been conducted under conditions of adequate control and methodological rigor offer the most likely possibilities for replication. Thus, while knowledge development in nursing should not be constrained by adherence to any single paradigm of research, there exists a justifiable concern among scholars that sufficient numbers of researchers attempt replication of the types of studies which ultimately *will result* in the prescriptive theories required for practice.

The point at which theoretical formulations, that is, generalizations, are systematically applied in practice is the critical end state for nursing. Explicated elsewhere (Conway, 1979) is a systems model which attempts to depict how knowledge develops in a science-based discipline. The model presumes a system in which the prerequisite or initial condition is the existence of a body of researchers and a body of practitioners. Inputs to the system include statements of theories, formulation of hypotheses, development of evidence, making of prescriptive statements, further testing of hypotheses, and systematic monitoring at the point of application. The model's output is the adoption of prescriptions into practice. A feedback loop from this point to the initial state of the model is also conceptualized. The end state, i.e., the point at which application is made of the generalizations developed through hypothesis testing, is the point at which nursing's practice is objectified for those who benefit (or fail to benefit) from it. This is the ultimate test for every science-based discipline. The discipline's practitioners must assure that its ideal prescriptive statements are *objectified* for clients by that practice. No discipline can hope to achieve or sustain credibility in the absence of this congruence between its ideal prescriptions and its practice.

FROM MODEL TO BLUEPRINT

The traditional separation of research from service in nearly all spheres of social endeavor is a rational one. The principle of rationality demands that institutions which are constituted for the purpose of providing services to people utilize all the resources available to them to provide such services. Rationality further presumes that service-providing organizations employ professionals, technicians, and administrators whose education and experience fit them specifically for the tasks assigned to them within the organization. The counter-proposition, still following the rationality principle, is that organizations, which are separate and distinct from service organizations and constituted for the sole purpose of conducting research can and will carry out that purpose more effectively than if they are a part of the service organization. Rationality is not universally applied to such an extreme as total separation in all cases. However, this can readily be noted by observing that there are many organizations which have a service function as the primary purpose and research as a secondary purpose. Hospitals and universities are foremost examples of such dual-purpose organizations.

Hospitals in recent years, unless a part of a highly endowed health science complex, have found it increasingly difficult to support research. This reality stems in large part from the stipulations of third-party payers, notably Medicaid and Medicare, who insist that only direct-service costs for patient care be included in reimbursement formulas. A long-standing "partnership" between government and academic health centers, which allowed more flexibility in allocating some research costs to the care "bill," has likewise deteriorated (Rogers, 1980) and needs reinforcement.

Similarly, universities, with a few notable exceptions, have experienced a decrease in support from federal sources for their research efforts over the past several years. Some of this decrease can be traced to inflation which has eroded "real" dollar purchasing power and some to actual loss in dollars appropriated by the Congress. Congressional actions have reflected disappointment on the part of the public that payoffs from government-supported research have not resulted in solutions to such pressing problems as depleted energy supplies, urban decay, and more accessible medical-health care. The present climate of disaffection with some of the national research effort related to human social problems presents an opportunity to nursing.

Nursing's research is directed to human problems; its results offer the promise of more beneficial interventions for these problems. A test of the model proposed above would be one strategy to speed research. That is, given both government and private foundation support, cohorts of nurse practitioners and researchers could be funded in several health science centers. A condition of qualifying for such funding would be the identification of a collaborative effort targeted to specific problems of client aggregates such as high-risk mothers, hypertensive adults, and teenagers at risk emotionally, to name but a few.

Collaboration between practitioners and researchers need not be, and should not be, restricted to health science centers. Collaborative research is needed in primary care delivery settings as well. Greater support of interdisciplinary research in primary care may well become a government priority as a matter of policy to implement the government's publicly stated intentions to bring about a higher level of personal health for an increased proportion of the population. Stringent guidelines and explicitly stated outcomes for those projects which are supported can be anticipated given federal policymakers' expressed intent to restrain the percent of the national budget which is allocated to health (Rogers, 1980).

Nursing is almost certain to find monetary

support for its intradisciplinary efforts in knowledge development—specifically for research—lessened and increasingly difficult to secure. More efforts at the national level to report both successes in research and the *application* of nursing's research should be undertaken. Public support is more likely to be encouraged as the public gains more awareness of nursing's contributions to improved health care. At the same time, the profession must inform its own members through increased reporting and sharing of new knowledge in its professional journals. This sharing must reach two professional groups: other researchers and practitioners. If it is to be shared with practitioners it will have to be communicated in terms understandable to them and therefore more relevant to them.

In this chapter the position has been taken that the principal task nursing as a discipline ought to undertake at this stage in its professionaliza-

tion is the development of its knowledge base. The rationale for this position is that the single characteristic which more than any other enables a discipline to control its practice field is the possession of a distinct body of knowledge which can be obtained only through intellectual endeavor. Some of the factors affecting the evolution of a profession—in this instance, nursing—on a continuum from occupational status to professional status have been reviewed. In addition, a model has been proposed which could serve as a guide to the development of knowledge for nursing. The model specifies as an initial condition a body of practitioners and a body of theorists who, singly and in *collaboration*, share responsibilities for both the generation and application of knowledge. The final condition is conceptualized as the application of knowledge to practice—the objective reality of nursing's purpose.

EDITOR'S QUESTIONS FOR DISCUSSION

To what extent would you agree with the assumptions indicated about the present status of nursing? Are there characteristics of the ideal-type profession—other than what was noted—lacking or of little evidence in nursing? What manifestations of community exist in nursing? What value differences may underlie intraprofessional conflict which may *not* be related to segmented work groups? What suggestions can be recommended to minimize value differences not related as well as those related to segmented work groups or practice settings?

What planning might occur to accomplish the long process of developing a knowledge base? What direction should be taken in the development of nursing theory? What purpose can abstract theories serve? Should prescriptive theory be the prime goal in theory development?

What strategies might be posed to effectively deal with the uncertainties in establishing nursing's domain? Indicate specific curriculum revision that will need to occur in preparing for the future. Suggest types of balance in content that might be offered. How can nursing practitioners assure that its ideal prescriptive statements are objectified for clients in practice?

Should the unification of research and service be encouraged? Would that be contrary to the principle of rationality? How can cohorts of nurse practitioners and researchers be developed? What avenues for financial support might be pursued? Illustrate how Conway's model might be utilized as a means in collaborative research.

REFERENCES

Braito, R. and P. Prescott
1978 "Rhetoric and behavior in conflict resolution: The professional employee." pp. 50–70 in N. Chaska (ed.), The Nursing Profession. New York: McGraw-Hill.

Cleary, F.
1971 "A theoretical model: Its potential adaptation for nursing." Image 4(1):14–20.

Conway, M.
1978 "Clinical research: Instrument for change." Journal of Nursing Administration 8(12):27–32.
1979 "Knowledge generation and transmission: A role for the nurse administrator." Nursing Administration Quarterly 3(4):29–41.

Dickoff, J. and P. James
1968 "A theory of theories: A position paper." Nursing Research 17(3):197–203.

Engel, Gloria
1970 "Professional autonomy and bureaucratic organization." Administrative Science Quarterly 30:12–18.

Freidson, Eliot
1970 Professional Dominance. New York: Atherton Press.

Goode, W.
1957 "Community within a community: The professions." American Sociological Review 22:194–200.

Johnson, D.
1974 "Development of theory: A requisite for nursing as a primary health profession." Nursing Research 23(5):372–377.

Ketefian, S.
1975 "Application of selected nursing research findings into nursing practice: A pilot study." Nursing Research 24(5):89–92.

McGlothlin, W. J.
1964 The Professional Schools. New York: Center for Applied Research in Education.

Moore, W.
1970 The Professions: Roles and Rules. New York: Russell Sage Foundation.

Pavalko, R. M.
1971 Sociology of Occupations and Professions. Itasca, Illinois: F. E. Peacock.

Rogers, D.
1980 "On preparing academic health centers for the very different 1980s." Journal of Medical Education 55:1–12.

Schrag, C.
1968 "Science and the helping professions." Nursing Research 17:486–496.

Chapter 3

Professional Territoriality in Nursing

Regina L. Monnig, R.N., Ph.D.
Associate Dean and Professor
Graduate Programs
School of Nursing
Medical College of Georgia
Augusta, Georgia

Defining the domain of nursing practice is vital for nursing as a profession. Regina L. Monnig explicates the concepts of territoriality and professional territoriality. She delineates how boundary demarcations can be further achieved through professional associations, legislation, and education. Monnig offers a means of defining the domain of practice through examining the extended scope of nursing practice. A survey of attitudes of a selected sample of nurse practitioners and physician preceptors and differences in perceptions of the functions of nurses and expectations of nurse practitioners is offered. The functions of teaching the patient and family, obtaining a health history, and identifying patient needs clearly are viewed within the domain of nursing. It is not clear regarding the decision as to who should meet certain patient needs. Specific functions such as prescribing medications and making a differential diagnosis are largely considered as belonging to the domain of medical practice. There is evidence in this survey that the two groups appear to be comfortable with overlap of functions between the two professions.

Historically, the concept of health care in America was synonymous with medical care. Legally, the Medical Practice Act gave physicians control of the domain of health care. Gradually other professions claimed portions of health care as their domain. Simultaneously, nurses began to expand their role to encompass functions traditionally performed only by physicians. The rise of physician's assistants stimulated the need for clarity of the nursing profession in its identity, accountability, and scope of practice.

In this chapter the concepts of *territoriality* and *professional territoriality* will be theoretically developed. Boundary demarcation as achieved by the nursing profession through its professional associations, legislation, and education will be explored. These three elements have been influential in changing the traditional boundaries between the nursing and medical profession. The scope of nursing practice will be viewed briefly through examination of attitudes of nurse practitioners and physician preceptors regarding functions of nurse practitioners, the contributions and handicaps expected through employment of nurses in an expanded role, and comparison of functions of nurse practitioners and physician's assistants.

As used in this paper, the phrase "expanded role of the nurse" refers to an extended scope of nursing practice which includes such responsibilities as obtaining a health history, assessing health-illness status, and entering a person into the health care system. Nurses functioning in an expanded role are frequently called *nurse practitioners* and have completed a special program of study. These nurses provide direct services, usually in conjunction with a physician, to individuals, families, and other groups in a variety of settings. The term *physician preceptors* refers to physicians who have served as mentors to nurses enrolled in a program of study to become nurse practitioners.

THE CONCEPT OF TERRITORIALITY

Behavioral scientists have borrowed ideas of *territoriality* from animal behavior and have adapted this concept to human behavior. One of the major authorities in this field has proposed that humans, like other animals, have an inherent need to acquire and defend space (Ardrey:1966). Ardrey also extends the idea of *territory* to a human space-time continuum which an individual or a cohesive group defends as an exclusive preserve.

The anthropologist Edward T. Hall (1966) describes territoriality as a basic evolutionary instinctual behavioral system characteristic of living organisms, including humans. Hall (1959:38) sees territoriality as a "primary message system which is a nonlinguistic form of the communicative process." According to Hall, territoriality meshes with cultural concepts in many different ways. Status, for example, is

indicated by the amount of space, type of space, or territory possessed. In humans, territoriality becomes highly elaborated, as well as very greatly differentiated from culture to culture.

Pilbeam (1973) replaces the concept of aggression and dominance among animals by a term he prefers for humans, *status-seeking.* His conceptualization of status-seeking includes prestige, which in turn accommodates the notion of values, rules, and norms.

Ardrey (1966:3–4) viewed motivation for territory as psychological, not physiological, claiming that it arises from twin needs for security and stimulation and that it is satisfied by the territorial heartland and the territorial periphery. He adds a third need called *identity* which territory satisfies; that is, identification with a unique fragment of something larger and more permanent than the individual per se, a place whether social or geographical, which belongs to that individual alone. Identity, stimulation, and security are seen by Ardrey as opposites to anonymity, boredom, and anxiety. A few years later, Altman (1970) and Joiner (1971) also recognized that territoriality provided the individual with security and identity.

Johnson (1979) perceived human territoriality as largely a passive affair based on mutual avoidance of personal spaces in accordance with social norms such as laws, rules, and customs. Human territoriality serves as an important organizer of behavior at several levels (Lyman and Scott, 1967) and promotes continuous association of person or persons with specific places, thus reducing stress of life and promoting adaptation (Edney, 1974).

In the process of describing territoriality as a psychological phenomenon, activities ranging from possession and guarding the area of space to security-ensuring behavioral adjustments are seen as territorial behavior. The ascribed functions of territoriality are mainly inferential and not scientifically proven in controlled experiments but do provide insights into human behavior. Therefore, it seems safe to agree with Carpenter (1964:411) that territoriality is of the nature of higher-order, complex, and dependent behavior systems which are organized upon numerous subsystems and behavioral determinants.

THE CONCEPT OF PROFESSIONAL TERRITORIALITY

Since ideas of territoriality are helpful in understanding human behavior, these ideas can be further extended to encompass the behavior of groups within a profession. Human needs for possession extend beyond the confines of physical territory to a defense of the individual's space, which includes "his institution, his role, his profession, and his area of operation" (Pluckham, 1972).

As a group, people organize to defend their professional or work territories from invasion by outsiders. According to Hediger (1961:36) "in order to occupy and defend a territory, or circumscribed region, it is necessary to render it recognizable by marking its borders." Professional territoriality, then, can be conceptualized as an area of work in which boundaries have been set through jurisdictional limitations and education under the control of an association. As professions have evolved, they have set up mechanisms for the establishment of boundaries and methods of protection of this territory from invasion by others outside the profession. Boundary demarcation has been achieved by a profession in three ways: professional associations, legislation, and education. The analogous territorial components of the profession taken together are self-regulation, licensure, and areas of authorized practice.

The establishment of boundaries is only one aspect of territoriality. Within these boundaries operate certain mechanisms which differentiate or characterize the territory. Carpenter (1958:242) listed 32 functions of territoriality, including the protection and evolution of the species. His list indicates the crucial nature of territoriality as a behavioral system. Personal and social functions associated with territoriality ,include reinforcement

of dominance, status, regulation of size of group, integration of groups, and provision of security. In competition for territoriality, individuals and groups are seen to pit their strengths and other behavioral capacities against others in a struggle which determines basic conditions of survival, especially recruitment and selection of members and access to rewards.

Likewise, the professions have certain characteristics which differentiate their territory. Professional characteristics, one or more of which are frequently discussed by a number of authors include the following: autonomy, altruism, colleague review, accountability, belief in public service, identity, body of knowledge, and belief in self-regulation (Cogan, 1953; Parsons, 1954; Goode, 1957; Wilensky, 1964).

Another characteristic *conflict*, also has appeared important in the study of professional territoriality. Professions experience a definite sense of conflict in the defense of boundaries from other occupations, in restraining the unqualified from areas of authorized practice, and in changing the territoriality through legislation. Autonomy, accountability, and identity have been identified as specific characteristics of professional territoriality. *Autonomy* is seen in self-regulation by professional associations and by the individual; *accountability* has roots in licensure through legislation; and *identity* is developed within areas of authorized practice as socialization occurs during the educational process.

BOUNDARY DEMARCATION IN NURSING

Boundary demarcation has been achieved in the nursing profession in three ways: professional associations, legislation, and education. Each will be discussed in more detail in this section. Over the years these boundaries have changed and will continue to change. The current expanded role functions of nurse practitioners is only one example of change in professional territoriality.

Stea (1969:41) formulated a hypothesis that "changing the defining characteristics of territory changes the behavior that occurs within it, and conversely, that changes in behavior lead to changes in territory." Changes in the nursing profession and behavior of nurses lend support to this hypothesis.

The Professional Association

In his study of evolution of professions, Carr-Saunders (1928:16) observed that as soon as a profession emerges, the practitioners are moved by recognition of common interests to form a professional association and mutually guarantee competence of qualified members as well as their honor. In his view, another motive leading to formation of a professional association is the desire to obtain proper recognition of its status in the larger society and a raise in the levels of renumeration.

The initial purpose of a professional association, as summarized by Schein (1972:19), is to protect and enhance the profession: through (1) defining its boundaries and setting entrance criteria; (2) providing autonomy or self-government by setting up and legalizing licensing procedures; and (3) conducting essentially public relation activities on behalf of the profession. Professional associations are distinguished by the degree to which they seek and establish minimum qualifications for entrance into professional practice and enforce appropriate rules and norms of conduct among members of the professional group.

Two major facts about professional associations are pointed out by Gilb (1966:109–110). First, the initial structuring of the association and the development and change of its structure are determined by the socioeconomic and political context into which the association fits, as well as by the dynamics within the association itself; and second, the structure of the association alters with the passage of time in ways that despite variations in detail appear to be similar for the different professional organizations, and these changes in turn alter relations with the public government.

In summary, the professional association has four main functions: (1) to set boundary lines, including lines of demarcation between qualified and unqualified persons; (2) to define the scope of practice and maintain high standards of professional practice; (3) to raise the status of the professional group; and (4) to promote recognition by society of its practitioners as the only ones fully competent to practice its particular skills.

Legislation

As a profession develops, it promotes legislation which legally establishes territoriality of the profession. Through licensure, an imprimatur of status is given. Licensing serves to label specialists and gives a person a right to function in a particular territory.

Territorial (or jurisdictional) limitations are inherent in licensing and self-regulation. An area of expertise, or area of *authorized practice,* is defined by statutes to correspond to competence without which professionals could not be licensed. The line between authorized and unauthorized practice is drawn by the professionals through their association. However, these boundaries may not be explicit and require further interpretation as problems arise.

According to Lieberman (1970), the jurisdictional boundary is twofold: it fixes and regulates the right of a particular person to engage in an act and it stakes off the area or kind of action involved. The first step is to prohibit all but the professional from practicing. For example, no one but a nurse may practice nursing. The next step is more difficult and involves a definitional crisis. The qualifications for becoming a nurse may be clear, but what is the practice of nursing?

Nurse practice acts set forth educational and examination requirements and provide for registration of the professional. The practice of the profession is described in broad general terms to provide the necessary freedom for interpretation of the law to cover new and innovative techniques and future conditions of practice.

Jurisdictional rights are crucial to the identity of the profession. Courts may be used to enforce boundary decisions but usually the professional association resolves internal disputes or collaborates with others in resolving disputes over territories. The most common problems in the health care system occur between medicine and nursing and are usually settled jointly through efforts of the medical association and nursing association.

Licensure is basically a means of protecting the public from incompetent practitioners and of protecting the competent from unfair competition. Lieberman (1970:38) states that defining unauthorized practice is a necessary concomitant of licensing. It is extended and refined by the power of self-regulation. The law tends to vest rather broad powers for self-regulation; yet the law of the respective state is the source of this power, and in a broad sense this is regulatory authority. The law established the Board of Nursing as the authority to regulate practice.

That the profession is not independent of the state is explicit in licensing requirements. The profession serves a public interest which the state may reasonably regulate. The public sees the profession subservient to the state because there is regulation, but the paradox is that the agency of regulation is self-regulation by the profession. Gilb (1966) in her study of complex relations between professions and government noted that in the licensing issue lies the key to community-professional relations. A truly powerful profession can usually gain control of the state regulatory apparatus and use it to its own advantage by using its expertise and influence to perpetuate a monopoly on the work. In addition, as Hughes (1958:78–87) notes, the profession must have the license to delve into the personal affairs of others or make impositions on them in ways unacceptable for the ordinary civilian; for these reasons, a profession must have the official backing of the state and community to do its work without danger to its members.

The delineation of professional boundaries is a decision of the profession and one that requires a continuing examination of the nature of that profession, the needs of society, and the functions of professionals in the delivery of services. For example, once the nursing profession has accepted a function as one falling into the sphere of nursing, then each nurse who carries out that function must obtain the systematic instructions needed to acquire the necessary knowledge and skill to support the practice of that function.

The real danger lies in the profession being swayed by urgency and assuming tasks on the basis of expediency, allowing them to fall into current practice. A pertinent example today is the tasks being assumed by nurses in the expanded role.

Statutes governing the practice of nursing define professional nursing in broad general terms which permits practice to advance into areas of expansion of skills which are supported by knowledge of underlying science. The difficult question is: Where are the legal safeguards for nurses who extend the periphery of their practice? Usually the limitations on procedures which a nurse may properly perform are governed by (1) the nature of the relationship between the medical and nursing profession in the community, (2) the scope of preparation offered in recognized nursing education programs, and (3) the training, experience and proficiency of individual nurses.

In a report on Nurse Practice Acts, Leitch and Mitchell (1977:19) noted two major changes: (1) the definition of nursing practice was being rewritten, and (2) provisions made in the rules and regulations permitted nurses to perform "additional acts." The essential question then became: Who will be recognized to perform "additional acts"? In many states education is not a prerequisite for performance of expanded role tasks. These states are looking to professional accreditation bodies to establish criteria for authorizing certain nurses to perform "additional acts," especially those acts which might require third-party payment.

Education

The profession, usually through its professional association, establishes and enforces standards of education through accreditation of schools, provides opportunities for students to gain field experiences, and admits entrants into the profession only on the basis of certain standards which can be met by graduation from approved schools. The approved schools then recruit, select, and educate students, certifying to the profession and the public through award of diplomas or degrees that these students have acquired the necessary knowledge and skills upon which professional competence can be developed through further experience and study. According to McGlothlin (1960:2–4) professional education has two aims: (1) providing professionally educated entrants to the profession in numbers adequate to society's needs and (2) maintaining or increasing the quality of entrants to the profession to satisfy society's needs. Briefly stated, professional education in nursing has the purpose of developing practitioners who are competent in the practice of nursing.

Knowledge on which the practice of the profession rests will continue to expand. The nursing profession, therefore, is concerned with encouraging research in sciences which underlie it and ensuring that its schools incorporate the newer knowledge in the instruction they provide. Professional education then constantly struggles with the necessity of incorporating new knowledge, consolidating other knowledge, and eliminating less useful experiences. Understanding of principles of practice and rules of manipulation of the discipline rather than mastery of skills of practice are emphasized, as well as education for flexibility and change. The functions that are specific to the nurse in the expanded role today will become a part of all nursing practice in the future.

The professional schools through research, investigation, and utilization of new knowledge serve as agents of change. Consequently professional schools cause changes in the territory shift by regulating the preparation of the practitioner as new tasks are added and others eliminated. These boundary shifts are being seen today as more nurses participate in the expanded role of the nurse and as basic education programs are broadened to include history taking, health assessment, and other skills that a decade ago were only taught to nurses preparing for an expanded role.

ATTITUDES OF NURSE PRACTITIONERS AND PHYSICIAN PRECEPTORS

The evaluation of nurses' expanded role has often been seen as a process of delegation by medicine, as a function of professional role identification, and as a means for career mobility. A more productive approach may be to address the apparent overlap between medicine and nursing through a theory of professional territoriality. Measuring attitudes regarding this overlap of territories provides insights into boundary demarcation between professions. Thus a questionnaire survey was mailed in 1979 to the two groups most involved with the expanded role of the nurse: selected samples of nurse practitioners and physician preceptors.

Nurse Practitioners

Fifty-seven nurses who had trained in an expanded role responded to the survey. Most of these nurses (74.4 percent) had practiced between 6 and 20 years. Only 2 percent had less than 2 years in nursing practice and 7 percent had more than 20 years in nursing practice. This distribution would indicate that nurse-practitioner programs appeal to nurses who have been actively engaged in nursing for several years but not to the older nurses. One-fifth of the nurses had a master's degree. Most likely these nurses had completed a nurse-practitioner program in their master's education. Diplomas were held by 50 percent and 2 percent were graduates of associate degree programs. Adult practitioners accounted for 68 percent and pediatric nurse practitioners for 28 percent. Of these nurses 50 percent practiced in cities of over 100,000 population and 30 percent were in rural areas (cities with fewer than 10,000 people). Contrary to expectations, one-third of nurses in the expanded role practiced in the hospital setting.

As anticipated, another one-third were located in offices or clinics. Nursing homes and public health agencies each accounted for one-tenth of the nurses functioning in an expanded role. The majority of nurses were very satisfied with their choice of nursing career. Only one nurse in the expanded role expressed dissatisfaction.

Physician Preceptors

Fifty-two physician preceptors responded to the survey. The highest proportion (30 percent) had practiced for more than 20 years. None had practiced for less than 2 years and only 5 percent for less than 5 years. The majority held an M.D. as highest degree (85 percent). Most of the preceptors were internists, family practitioners, and pediatricians. The physician preceptors were most frequently in large cities (77 percent), worked with six or more physicians (56 percent), and were very satisfied with their choice of medical career (64 percent).

Current Nursing Practice   Only a small percentage of nurses and physicians considered specific func-

tions such as prescribing medications and making a differential diagnosis as a part of current nursing practice (see Table 3-1). These functions were largely viewed as belonging to the domain of medical practice. As anticipated, the largest percentage of both groups believed that teaching the patient and family and obtaining a health history were nursing practice functions.

Nurses identified other areas of current nursing practice, such as counseling, health maintenance, prevention of chronic illness, well-child evaluation, and provision of emergency treatment, including suturing of minor lacerations. Physicians identified home calls, nursing home visits, well child physicals, blood drawing, intubation, and performing special studies as a part of current nursing practice.

Patient Needs   The identification of patient needs was clearly within the domain of nursing practice. The decision regarding how to meet these needs was less clear. The majority of physicians and nurses expected the nurse to identify patient needs. The percentage of those expecting nurses to independently decide how to best meet patient

Table 3-1   Attitudes of Nurse Practitioners and Physician Preceptors Regarding Functions Considered to Be Current Nursing Practice

Functions	Nurse practitioners (N = 57), %	Physician preceptors (N = 52), %
Teach patient and family	92.9	94.2
Obtain a health history	85.9	88.5
Supervise and manage care of normal pregnant women	68.4	59.6
Select therapy for specific problems	59.6	53.8
Perform physical examinations	75.4	44.2
Perform gyn exams and do Pap smears	56.1	26.9
Make a differential diagnosis	35.1	17.3
Prescribe medications	31.6	28.8
Other	15.8	19.2

Table 3-2 Expectations of Nurses to Meet Patient's Needs Held by Nurse Practitioners and Physician Preceptors

Patient's needs	Nurse practitioners (N = 57), %	Physician preceptors (N = 52), %
Proper positioning	96.5	86.5
Rest or sleep	94.7	76.9
Ambulation	92.9	69.2
Close observation of vital signs	89.5	84.6
Diet regulation	87.7	55.7
Bowel regulation	85.9	75.0
Range of motion exercises	84.2	80.7
Oxygen and facilitation of breathing	66.7	59.6
Fluid and electrolytes	29.8	25.0

needs was sharply lower (see Table 3-2). Only 29 percent of the nurses and 25 percent of the physicians believed that nurses could meet a patient's need for fluid and electrolytes. A significant difference in expectations of nurses meeting patient needs was found in the needs for rest or sleep, ambulation, and diet regulation.

Contribution of Nurse Practitioners In Table 3-3 the provision of a more comprehensive kind of health care and greater utilization of nursing skills were most frequently seen as the main contributions of nurse practitioners. The relief of physicians from routine tasks and provision of health care to more people were considered a contribution only by physicians. Written comments concerning contributions of nurse practitioners included: the utilization of judgment in observation and assessment in clinical areas; the freeing of nurses to think for themselves; and the provision of stimulating challenges.

Major Handicap of Nurse Practitioners Table 3-4 records that nurses believed the major handicap of employment as a nurse practitioner was the practice outside of the legal definition of nursing practice (10 percent). Over one-fourth of physicians believed the same. Another one-fifth of the physicians believed that greater legal liability was placed on the physician. Many nurses (68 percent) and physicians (42 percent) wrote in other comments. Nurses said that lack of acceptance by other nurses and physicians, reluctance of nurses to accept decision making, limited knowledge, and absence of protocol were also handicaps. Physicians identified lack of acceptance, fear of nurses to assume responsibility, inadequate education, difficulty with roles, reimbursement from third-party payments, and tradition as major handicaps.

Table 3-3 Main Contribution of Nurse Practitioners as Expressed by Nurse Practitioners and Physician Preceptors

Main contribution	Nurse practitioners (N = 57), %	Physician preceptors (N = 52), %
Provides more comprehensive kind of health care	50.9	21.2
Utilizes more completely his or her nursing skills	33.3	50.0
Relieves physicians from routine tasks	0.0	15.3
Provides health care to more people	7.0	7.7
Other	3.5	5.8
None	5.3	0.0

Table 3-4 Major Handicaps of Nurses Working as a Nurse Practitioner as Expressed by Nurse Practitioners and Physician Preceptors

Major handicap	Nurse practitioners ($N = 57$), %	Physician preceptors ($N = 52$), %
Practices outside legal definition of nursing	10.5	25.0
Places greater legal liability on physician	8.8	21.2
Requires too much supervision by a physician	3.5	11.5
Performs mainly medical functions	8.8	0.0
Other	68.4	42.3

Table 3-5 Willingness of Physician Preceptors to Delegate Functions to Nurse Practitioners or to Physicians' Assistants

Function	Delegate to nurse practitioners, %	Delegate to physician's assistants, %
Obtain health history	90.4	71.1
Provide emergency treatment	69.2	67.3
Sew up simple cuts	44.2	59.6
Select therapy for common illnesses	59.6	46.1
Perform physical examination	69.2	40.3
Order and interpret lab tests	50.0	40.4
Make adjustment on medications	48.0	26.9
Deliver a baby	28.8	26.9
Put a cast on a broken leg	26.9	25.0

Delegation of Functions The physician questionnaire contained a portion designed to compare the physician's preference and delegation of functions between the nurse practitioner and physicians' assistant (see Table 3-5). It is expected that the physician who preferred the nurse practitioner would have more positive attitudes toward the expanded role of the nurse. Physicians stated that they would delegate the suturing of simple cuts to the physician's assistant more frequently than to the nurse practitioner. Other functions would be delegated more willingly to the nurse practitioner. The majority of physicians were willing to delegate to both physician's assistants and nurse practitioners the following functions: obtaining a health history, providing emergency treatment, and performing physical examinations. The majority of physicians would not be willing to delegate the functions of applying a cast on a broken leg or delivering a baby to either physician extender.

Discussion

This survey of attitudes of nurse practitioners and physician preceptors demonstrates differences in perceptions of the functions of nurses and expectations of nurse practitioners. These differences did not provide evidence of a struggle between nurses and physicians for preservation of terri-

torial boundaries. Rather the two groups appeared comfortable with overlap of functions between the medical and nursing profession. Possible sources of future conflict between these professions can be avoided through continued exploration of professional territoriality. Professions can learn to function together in interdisciplinary teams and respect the territorial rights of others.

The work of the professional associations, legislation, and education must continue. Through the professional associations, the scope of practice can be delineated. Since boundaries are not explicit, the association can interpret practice, resolve disputes, and collaborate with other groups in reaching a settlement over territorial boundaries. Through legislation, an area of expertise can be defined by statutes to correspond to competence without which professionals cannot be licensed. Through education, functions of the professionals are learned. Since knowledge is expanding exponentially, professions are rapidly changing. This evolution of the professions adds further strain to territorial boundaries and conflicts within, as well as between, the professions.

EDITOR'S QUESTIONS FOR DISCUSSION

To what extent have professional associations of nursing defined the scope of nursing practice? Should it be the mandate solely of the American Nurses Association? How might attempts of associations within the profession of nursing be unified to define the scope of nursing practice? What boundary lines have been agreed upon within nursing and between nursing and medicine as being the domain of nursing and the domain of medicine? Wherein is the source or sources of conflict in legitimizing the demarcation between nursing and medical practice? To what extent can conflict regarding the issue of territoriality be positive from the point of view of the patient and the professions of nursing and medicine? What factors indicate continued strain regarding territorial boundaries? Why might there be comfort, as appears evident in Monnig's survey, in overlap of functions between nursing and medicine? How might exploring the overlap of functions be a means for nursing and medicine to resolve conflict between the two professions?

How can substantiation for jurisdictional rights in nursing practice via legislation be promoted? How have the role and functions of nursing been traditionally defined? What qualifications should persons possess who represent the state in regulation functions of the nursing profession? What qualifications should persons hold who are members of professional licensing and accreditation bodies?

What is the role of nursing education in defining the territory of professional nursing? To what extent is nursing education influential in delineating the scope of nursing practice? What factors in nursing education may promote and may inhibit the definition and characterization of nursing practice? What ethical responsibility do nursing education and nursing educators have for the scope of nursing practice?

REFERENCES

Altman, I.
1970 "Territorial behavior in humans: An analysis of the concept," Pp. 1-17 in L. Pastalan and D. Carson (eds.), Spatial Behavior of Older People. Ann Arbor: University of Michigan Press.

Ardrey, Robert
1966 The Territorial Imperative. New York: Atheneum.

Carpenter, C. R.
1958 "Territoriality: A review of concepts and problems," Pp. 224-245 in A. Roe and G. Simpson (eds.), Behavior and Evolution. New Haven: Yale University Press.
1964 Naturalistic Behavior of Nonhuman Primates. University Park, Pa.: Pennsylvania State University Press.

Carr-Saunders, A. M.
1928 Professions: Their Organization and Place in Society. Oxford: Clarendon Press.

Cogan, M. L.
1953 "Toward a definition of profession." Harvard Educational Review 23:33-50.

Edney, J.
1974 "Human territoriality." Psychological Bulletin 81:959-75.

Gilb, Corrinne L.
1966 Hidden Hierarchies: The Professions and Government. New York: Harper and Row.

Goode, W. J.
1957 "The librarian: From occupation to profession?" American Sociological Review 4:194-200.

Hall, Edward T.
1959 The Silent Language. Garden City: Doubleday.
1966 Hidden Dimensions. Garden City: Doubleday.

Hediger, H.
1961 "The evolution of territorial behavior," Pp. 66-78 in S. Washburn (ed.), Social Life of Early Man. New York: Viking Fund Publications in Anthropology.

Hughes, Everett C.
  1958 Men and Their Work. Glencoe, Ill.: The
         Free Press.
Johnson, Freddie L.
  1979 "Response to territorial intrusion by
         nursing home residents." Advances in
         Nursing Science 4:21–34.
Joiner, D.
  1971 "Social ritual and architectural space."
         Journal of Architect Research and Teach-
         ing 1:11–22.
Leitch, Cynthia and Ellen Mitchell
  1977 "A state by state report: The legal accom-
         modations of nurses practicing expanded
         roles." Nurse Practitioner 4:19–22.
Lieberman, Jethro K.
  1970 The Tyranny of the Experts. New York:
         Walker.
Lyman, S. and M. Scott
  1967 "Territoriality: A neglected sociological
         dimension." Social Problems 15:236–49.
McGlothlin, William J.
  1960 Patterns of Professional Education. New
         York: Putnam.
Parsons, T.
  1954 "The professions and social structure,"

in T. Parsons (ed.), Essays in Sociological
Theory. Glencoe, Ill.: Free Press.
Pilbeam, D.
  1973 "An idea we could live without: The
         naked ape." Pp. 110–121 in A. Montagau
         (ed.), Man and Aggression. New York:
         Oxford University Press.
Pluckham, Margaret L.
  1972 "Professional territoriality: A problem
         affecting the delivery of health care."
         Nursing Forum 11:302.
Schein, Edgar H.
  1972 Professional Education. The Carnegie
         Commission on Higher Education. New
         York: McGraw-Hill.
Stea, David
  1969 "Space, territory, and human move-
         ments." Pp. 37–42 in H. Proshansky, W.
         Ittelsen, and L. Rivlin (eds.), Environ-
         mental Psychology: People and Their
         Physical Settings. New York: Holt, Rine-
         hart and Winston.
Wilensky, H. L.
  1964 "The professionalization of everyone?"
         The American Journal of Sociology
         70:138–46.

Chapter 4

Legal Rights and Responsibilities of the Nurse

Dorothy Jean Walker, R.N., Ph.D., J.D.
Attorney at Law
Professor, Graduate Program
Department of Nursing
George Mason University
Fairfax, Virginia

After Monnig's prescription for explicating the domain of nursing, it is critical to be cognizant of the legal rights and responsibilities of the nurse. Dorothy Jean Walker clearly emphasizes critical legal aspects of nursing practice that are frequently misunderstood. She succinctly defines legal terms and concepts, and provides numerous examples of circumstances and court cases to illustrate legal implications in the practice of nursing. Walker discusses the legal rights of the nurse, the nature of the nursing license as a privilege and the need to protect the license from censure, and legal responsibilities of the nurse regarding the duty, standard, and degree of care. The bases of liability are thoroughly presented. She cites seven common types of circumstances for liability, indicating negligence as the most frequent grounds for liability. Trends in vicarious liability are particularly noteworthy. Walker's discussion of the doctrine of *respondeat superior,* corporate liability, and the independent contractor is essential to heed. Walker emphasizes that it is increasingly expected that the nurse will accept responsibility for accountability, including financial accountability, for her professional conduct. She offers four suggestions for nurses to best prepare to meet the rising demands of professional accountability.

It is needful for all nurses to understand their position in relation to the law—not that they may practice law, but rather that they may better practice nursing. Modern nurses often are called upon to make critical decisions in the performance of clinical or managerial functions which are wrought with legal implications for their clients, their employers, and/or themselves. It is important that they clearly understand their rights and responsibilities and, furthermore, that they recognize the situation in which legal counsel is needed so that they may seek such counsel in a timely fashion.

LEGAL RIGHTS OF THE NURSE

The Nurse's Rights as a Citizen

The nurse, on becoming a nurse, surrenders none of the rights of citizenship. Nurses are entitled to all rights granted citizens under federal and (applicable) state constitutions as well as those granted by federal and (applicable) state statutes. These include, among others, such rights as personal property rights and the right to privacy, equal protection, and due process. Whenever any right of a nurse has been violated, it becomes incumbent upon him or her (as it is upon any citizen) to allege the violation and assert his or her right to have the breach redressed.

In the case of *Swanson v. St. John's Lutheran Hospital* (Montana, 1979) a nurse-anesthetist brought action against the hospital upon the ground that she had been wrongfully dismissed from employment because she asserted her rights under the state conscience statute, which defined certain rights of medical persons confronted with sterilization procedures as part of their employment. The Montana statute (Montana, 1947) (1) mandates that no person can be compelled to participate in sterilization against his or her moral convictions or religious beliefs and (2) prohibits the firing of any person for refusing to participate in sterilization on such grounds.

Although a reading of the record indicates that Swanson may have been "an employee of questionable value" for a number of reasons, the single and only reason given in her letter of discharge was her refusal to participate in a tubal ligation which is protected conduct under the state statute. The Montana Court found that the plaintiff, having a statutory right to do so, had validly refused to participate in the sterilization procedure. Having done so, she was entitled to the further protection of the statute and her refusal should not have been a consideration in respect to staff privileges nor a basis for any discriminatory, disciplinary, or other recriminatory action against her. The Court held that Swanson would have been entitled to reinstatement to her position had the term of her employment contract continued to the time of the Court's decision. However, since the time of the contract had passed, the Court held that she was entitled "to monetary damages for injuries suffered" (Montana, 1979:711).

The Nature of the Nursing License

The nurse does not have a constitutional right to a nursing license. Licensure is a privilege. Each state, in response to its duty to protect the public health and safety of its citizens, has promulgated a nurse practice act which regulates licensure. Where licensure is mandated, no person, unless excluded by the act, may legally practice nursing as defined by said act within the respective jurisdiction absent a license to do so. Under the law of a few jurisdictions, one is only prohibited from practicing "as a registered nurse" without the nursing license. However, almost all states permit nursing actions without licensure by specific persons (such as parent, spouse, etc.) or under specific circumstances (such as in the case of an emergency).

Furthermore, the granting of a license privilege by one state does not create a right in another state. In *Scott v. State Ex Relatione Board of Nursing* (Nebraska, 1976) a nurse who held a license as a registered nurse issued by the State of New York and had previously worked as a nurse in New York, South Dakota, and, under a temporary license, in the city of Lincoln was denied a professional nursing license by the Nebraska Board of Nursing. The Board found evidence of "her unsafe nursing practices, her unsatisfactory work attendance, and her failure to utilize satisfactory judgment in administering nursing practices" (Nebraska, 1976:686). The evidence offered tended to show, among other things, that: (1) she had not rechecked the temperature of a 7-month-old child who reportedly had a temperature of 105°F prior to admission, nor did she notify the physician; (2) she had left the assigned area after coming on duty without notifying a supervisor; (3) she refused to follow through on procedures for admitting a patient; (4) she refused to attend in-service education programs; (5) she refused to follow employment policies, such as wearing designated uniform, appearing for duty at the designated time, giving prior notification if unable to report for duty, and refusing to accept and follow orders; (6) she conversed with patients in such an insensitive manner that the patient's anxiety level was increased; and (7) she was unwilling to accept supervision and guidance and did not cooperate with other nursing personnel. The Supreme Court of Nebraska held that the findings of the Board were not unreasonable or arbitrary and that it had acted within the scope of its statutory authority in denying licensure.

Not only is the nursing license a privilege, it is a privilege that is personal to the licensee. The actions of the nurse, and only those of the nurse, are legitimized by the license. The nursing license is not an umbrella which covers the nursing acts of others any more than a person's driver's license can be extended to cover the driving of an unlicensed friend. The clinical experiences of the student nurse are permitted under the license of the educational program, not that of the nurse instructor. Aides and orderlies work under the institution's license, not the nurse's. (However, the clinical nurse or the nurse instructor may be liable for his or her own negligent failure to assess and utilize staff according to its capabilities or to provide adequate instruction and supervision.)

Just as the nursing license does not permit the nurse to practice medicine, the medical license does not permit the physician to practice nursing. Each must conform to the appropriate act. It, therefore, follows that the nurse may not, at the direction of the physician, either omit or inaccurately record observations regarding the patient or patient care. The duty of the nurse to "accurately record" is understood in all jurisdictions and expressed in a number of nurse practice acts (see, for example, Maryland, 1967). Furthermore, while the employing institution may establish rules regarding the form of charting, it may not control the content of the record. A nurse who acquiesces in such effort (whether by institution or physician) may be left open to a felony charge of falsifying or conspiring to falsify legal documents.

It should never be overlooked that the privilege of the license extends to the nurse 24 hours a day, 365 days a year for a designated period of time (usually 1 or 2 years). The nurse is a licensed nurse during all that time and will be held to a nursing standard for her behavior even when her actions are undertaken voluntarily and done without compensation.

The Need to Protect the License from Censure

The nursing license makes it possible for nurses to practice their profession legally. Because of this it becomes the very key to their livelihood. They have a vested interest in seeing that their records remain clear of opprobrium inasmuch as reprimands, suspensions of license, or other forms of censure noted on their records will follow them thereafter. Effective protection of the nurse's license may necessitate the pursuit of remedies beyond the Board of Nursing.

In *Tuma v. Idaho Board of Nursing* (Idaho, 1979) the Supreme Court of Idaho reversed the license suspension of a nurse who allegedly had engaged in unprofessional conduct and interfered with the physician-patient relationship by advising a patient undergoing chemotherapy of alternative treatments for cancer, including laetrile. The Idaho Nurse Practice Act (Idaho, 1974) provided for the suspension of a nurse's license for "unprofessional conduct," and while it defined some conduct which would constitute unprofessional conduct, it left further definition to the Board. The Board failed to define the term on a basis broad enough to be applicable in the *Tuma* case. The Board argued that "professional conduct" need not be further defined since it is conduct which "is recognized to be unsafe or improper by the profession itself" (Idaho, 1979:716). The Court rejected the Board's contention, holding that due process requires that the Board may not exercise its discretion on a case-by-case basis and that the Idaho statute, unaided by Board rules and regulations, does not prohibit the conduct with which Tuma was charged.

LEGAL RESPONSIBILITIES OF THE NURSE

Duty of Care

In addition to defining and protecting the rights of the nurse, the law imposes certain specific responsibilities on the nurse with respect to both the duty of care and the standard of care to be given. It should be understood as a beginning proposition that there is no duty or obligation to tender care in the absence of a statutory provision requiring such care. An example of such statutory provision is the Vermont "good samaritan" law (Vermont, 1971) which imposes a positive duty on all persons—even those merely passing through the state—to provide reasonable assistance to any other person "exposed to grave physical harm." The statutory duty is neither limited to roadside accidents nor to health-care professionals. Furthermore, the statute (Vermont, 1971) provides for criminal penalties for failure to render assistance under conditions prescribed by the statute. In the absence of a statutory imposition of a duty of care, the legal duty grows out of the nurse-patient relationship, and such relationship is established by the act of providing nursing care whether the nurse's services are technically engaged or not. Once the duty of care arises, services cannot be negligently terminated to the detriment of the one who has relied on them.

Standard of Care

When nursing is undertaken, the law imposes upon the nurse legal responsibilities that are greater than the absolute duty on every person to act in a reasonable and prudent manner to avoid causing injury to another. The standard which applies is that of the *ordinary reasonable nurse under similar circumstances.* Courts have generally expressed this standard by stating that "in the performance of her professional duties, a nurse is required to exercise the degree of care and skill which a reasonably prudent nurse with similar training and experience practicing in the same community

would exercise under the same or similar circumstances" (Bernzweig, 1975:47).

Since nursing tends to follow the example of the medical profession regarding the acquisition of legal rights and responsibilities, nurses should be cognizant of recent court decisions regarding the standard of care of the medical profession with reference to customary practices within a geographic setting. The "strict locality" rule, i.e., the standard medical practices in the defendant's locality, has generally given way to the "same or similar locality" rule. Furthermore, the case of *Blair v. Eblen* (Kentucky, 1970) formulated an "accepted practice" rule which rejected locality rules in favor of the professional standard. These changes have occurred in response to, among other factors, the perceived need to avoid insulating pockets of substandard practice. It is not unreasonable to expect that the same principles will be applied to issues surrounding the standard of nursing practice.

The degree of care required of nurses is a relative one and their qualifications, experience, and education are always taken into consideration in determining whether they acted with reasonable care in a given situation. Nurse-specialists while, but only while, performing services in their specialty are held to a higher standard of care than general-duty nurses. The specialist must exercise the degree of care and skill customarily exercised by other nurses who practice that specialty. An important exception to the general rule regarding the standard of care to be used in measuring the nurse's conduct applies to student nurses. When nursing students perform nursing services which are customarily performed only by registered nurses, they will be held to the standard of care of the registered nurse (Bernzweig, 1975:51).

Bases of Liability

The nurse's liability may be predicated on any of a number of legal theories depending upon the circumstances surrounding the incident giving rise to the legal action (King, 1977:33–35). A breach of contract action might lie when the nurse agrees to care for the patient and later fails to perform or has promised specific therapeutic results that do not materialize. However, in most cases where nurse liability is charged it is grounded in the law of torts (King, 1977:9). Among potential theories of liability in tort are: false imprisonment, invasion of privacy, defamation, unauthorized disclosure of confidential information, battery, infliction of mental distress, and negligence. Of these negligence dominates the field, at least numerically (King, 1977:166–191).

False imprisonment occurs when there is an intentional and unprivileged nonconsensual confinement of an individual. A reasonable fear of force, rather than force itself, is all that is required. The tort of false imprisonment has been found in cases where patients (or newborns) have been detained in a hospital for failure to pay their bills. An actionable *invasion of privacy* occurs where one intentionally intrudes upon the solitude or seclusion of another or into his private concerns in a way that would be highly offensive to a reasonable person (e.g., permitting one who has no professional connection with the case to observe a procedure without the patient's express consent). Invasion of privacy also occurs when publicity is given to a matter concerning the patient's private life where the matter would be highly offensive to a reasonable person and is not of legitimate concern to the public (e.g., where information, photographs, x-rays, etc., are publicized without consent).

Liability for *defamation* may result from the communication to a third party of an untrue statement about another when the statement tends to lower the other's reputation and esteem in the eyes of the community (e.g., the imputation of a loathsome disease—usually venereal disease or leprosy—or one that might be incompatible with the performance of the plaintiff's occupation, such as epilepsy for a pilot). The nurse could be held liable for defamation even when holding a reasonable though erroneous belief in the truth of the statement.

Unlike defamation, liability for the *divulgence of confidential information* may be based on an entirely true statement. It differs from ordinary invasion of privacy (from which all citizens are accorded protection) inasmuch as less extensive publication and less offensive disclosure than might otherwise be required is actionable. The right of the patient to prevent disclosure is rooted in the patient–care provider relationship on the rationale that patients seeking health care should be free to reveal private matters without fear of unwarranted disclosure.

A *battery* may result from an intentional, unprivileged, and nonconsensual physical contact with plaintiff that would be offensive to a reasonable person in the plaintiff's position even when no harm results—indeed, even though some positive benefit may accrue to the patient. The disciplining of a minor patient or the restraining of a disoriented adult may give rise to a charge of battery. In *Leukhardt v. Commonwealth of Pennsylvania, State Board of Nurse Examiners* (Pennsylvania, 1979) the Board had found that the nurse defendant violated the professional nursing statute when she slapped the patient in an effort to induce him to release his grasp on her arm so that she, with the aid of other nursing personnel, might turn him in order to change his linen. The Court, finding that the nurse's action was reasonable in light of her need to have both arms free to care for the patient, reversed the Board's decision to formally reprimand the nurse. No battery had occurred.

Although an action for wrongful *infliction of mental distress* may be based on either intentional or negligent misconduct, the action will not lie for mere insults, indignities, threats, or annoyances. The intentional or reckless infliction of mental distress is sometimes referred to as the tort of "outrageous conduct." Perhaps the most graphic illustration of this tort in the health field is to be found in the case of *Johnson v. Woman's Hospital* (Tennessee, 1973).

Six weeks following the stillborn delivery of her premature infant, the mother, seeking clarification of a pathologist's report on her chart, sought information concerning the disposition of the child's body. She was taken to a hospital employee who allegedly presented her with a jar of formaldehyde containing the shriveled body of her infant. The Court characterized the tort as intentional because the employee had intentionally displayed the jar and held that a jury could find such conduct constituted an actionable infliction of mental distress.

Negligence is an unintentional tort. It is the failure to exercise the degree of care demanded by the circumstances. One may be held liable for such negligence whenever it causes harm or injury to the person or property of another. When the injury occurs in relation to a professional duty the tort may be referred to as *malpractice*. Negligence is not synonymous with carelessness. One may be careful and yet be legally negligent.

In *Massey v. Heine* (Kentucky, 1973) the hospital, nurse, and surgeon were sued in a negligence action. During the administration of an intramuscular antibiotic, the nurse struck the patient's sciatic nerve with the needle and caused damage to his right leg, including foot drop. The nurse and hospital settled the claim for $60,000. In the continuing suit against the surgeon, the jury found him not liable in negligence in entrusting the postoperative care of his patient to the hospital nursing staff.

In *Sandhofer v. Abbott-Northwestern Hospital* (Minnesota, 1979) the patient was admitted to the hospital with a comminuted fracture of the wrist. The fracture was surgically reduced and a circular plaster cast applied from above the elbow to the knuckles. During his hospital stay Sandhofer was treated by two staff physicians; the condition of his arm was observed periodically by nurses and aides and recorded in their notes on his chart. Several days after the operation, nurses observed and charted the fact that the patient's hand and fingers were swollen and dark blue. However, the attending physicians were not verbally notified regarding these significant changes. On the fifth day of hospitalization, the cast was split. At this point medical progress notes indicated ischemia. Two and one-half weeks later the patient discharged himself against medical advice. He was readmitted 10 days later and underwent surgery for displacement of the fracture and an open ulcer on the forearm. At this time, his condition was diagnosed as ischemic necrosis. Two months later Sandhoefer entered a second hospital where his arm was amputated below the elbow. In the ensuing legal action the failure of the nurses to notify the physicians of significant observable changes in the patient's condition was found to be culpable negligence. The Appellate Court refused to reverse the trial court's ruling in favor of the plaintiff even though the evidence might also have supported a finding that the doctors' negligence exceeded the negligence of the hospital nurses.

In order to escape liability the observing nurse must not only chart significant changes but must also be satisfied that the attending physician has read the notes or has been made aware of the changes by direct verbal communication. The nurse, at all times, must exercise reasonable care to safeguard and protect the patient from any known or reasonably foreseeable harm.

Trends in Vicarious Liability

Historically, the nurse has grown up with a sense of security fostered by the notion of being afforded some legal protection by the employing institution or physician. It is possible that the character of such protection has never been fully understood by the majority of nurses. In any event, as nurses move away from traditional roles and seek more independence in the practice of their profession, it becomes crucial that they each understand the principles on which legal responsibility is allocated among health care providers.

Vicarious liability is a broad legal concept

that refers to the imposition of liability upon one party because of the act or omission of another (King, 1977:225–249). It requires two fundamental preconditions: (1) The required relationship must exist between party A who is to be held vicariously liable and party B whose conduct triggered the liability. (2) B must have been acting within the scope contemplated by the relationship. This usually, though not always, involves a "master-servant" relationship wherein vicarious liability is based on the doctrine of *respondeat superior.* The doctrine holds an employer legally liable for the negligent acts of an employee which arise out of and in the course of the employment (Steffen, 1977:72–94). The *Massey* and *Sandhofer* cases (previously mentioned) are examples of circumstances wherein the "master" hospital may be liable for the acts of the "servant" nurse.

The doctrine of *respondeat superior* also may have legal implications for the procedural aspects of a case. In *Kambas v. St. Joseph's Mercy Hospital of Detroit* (Michigan, 1973), plaintiff was admitted to the defendant hospital for treatment following a heart attack. The doctor prescribed an anticoagulant drug and the injections were given by registered nurses employed by the hospital. Three days after admission, plaintiff began to experience swelling, discoloration, and disability of his arms. Thirty-three months later, he filed suit against the hospital alleging negligence in the administration of the drug.

The hospital claimed the action was barred by the 2-year malpractice statute of limitations. The Court found that no negligent acts were alleged against any physician or surgeon but only against nurses and other employees of the hospital and ruled that the action may not be deemed one for malpractice. The hospital's liability was predicated upon the doctrine of *respondeat superior.* The Michigan Court, having determined that nurses are not subject to the 2-year malpractice statute of limitations, concluded that the 3-year statute of limitations is applicable to injuries arising from the negligent act of a nurse and is equally applicable to the hospital

employer. In other words, unless nurses are specifically included in the statutory definition of malpractice, the common-law definition controls and neither they nor the employer-hospital will be given the added protection of the somewhat shorter malpractice statute of limitations. It is the employer-employee relationship and not the professional license that governs.

It should be clearly understood that the doctrine of *respondeat superior* has no legal effect on the personal liability of a wrongdoer. Nurses remain responsible for their own tortious conduct regardless of any agreement on the part of the employer (whether a physician or an institution in the person of a supervisor or administrator) to assume responsibility for the negligent acts of the nurse. The doctrine subjects the employer to liability for the nurse's negligence but does not relieve the nurse of personal liability for the conduct in question. Because the right has been infrequently exercised against nurses, many nurses fail to realize that the employer who is required (under the doctrine of *respondeat superior*) to pay damages because of the negligence of a nurse-employee has the legal right to recover the amount paid in a separate action against the nurse-employee.

A special application of the *respondeat superior* doctrine is the "borrowed servant" rule (Steffen, 1977:16–18; King, 1977:232–249). The borrowed servant rule provides that a temporary employer (who, in the health care setting, usually is a physician) is held liable for the negligent act of another when the act in question is done under his or her direction and control. The central question is: When is the master-servant relationship triggered by the borrowed servant rule in the absence of an actual employment relationship between physician and nurse? Earlier cases tended to impose liability on a physician who was present and had the right to exercise control; the recent trend has been to require that the physician have actually assumed or exercised control over the details of the work performed (King, 1977:242–249).

In *Burns v. Owens* (Missouri, 1970) a physician ordered intramuscular injections of Demerol every

4 to 6 hours if needed by a postoperative patient. The nurse allegedly administered the drug in the lower third of his left arm between the elbow and shoulder, i.e., in the wrong location. The patient's hand "went limp; went dead" (Missouri, 1970: 304), necessitating three subsequent hospitalizations and two operations in an effort to correct the situation. In affirming the directed verdict by the trial court in favor of the physicians, the Court held that the borrowed servant doctrine was inapplicable where the nurse was not acting under the direct and personal supervision and control of the physician.

In *May v. Broun* (Oregon, 1972) the patient was burned by an electric cauterizing machine during surgery. The evidence justified an inference that the machine was either incorrectly hooked up or improperly operated by the circulating nurse whose duty it was to set up the machine for the operation. At the request of the surgeon, the nurse checked the machine when it failed to work on the first two attempts. Although the purported negligence of the nurse occurred during surgery and in the presence of the doctors, the Court held that the surgeons were not vicariously liable for the acts of the nurse. The Court reasoned that the burden of defective equipment and negligent operators more properly rests with the hospital than with the surgeon. The hospital is charged with responsibility for the maintenance of the equipment and the selection and training of personnel to operate it. For this reason, the Court concluded that it was the hospital that would have the best opportunities for devising means to prevent like occurrences in the future.

Vicarious liability is quite different from *corporate responsibility*. Since a corporate entity can only act through individuals, at some point one or more individuals acting on behalf of the entity must have committed a wrongful act or omission. The conduct on which corporate liability is based is often more administrative than professional in nature. It frequently occurs in the form of failure of the governing board, administrative personnel, employees, and/or professional

staff to adopt or implement appropriate internal mechanisms to ensure the safe provision of services offered.

In the case of *Darling v. Charleston Community Hospital* (Illinois, 1965) the corporate liability of hospitals for failure to supervise and review the care administered by nonemployee staff members was recognized. The patient, an 18-year-old suffering from a football injury, was treated for a broken leg in the emergency room by the physician on call. A cast was applied. Thereafter, notwithstanding early obvious danger signals (great pain and swelling and discoloration of the toes) and the progressive worsening of the patient's circulation over the next 2 weeks, no doctor other than the attending physician was consulted until the leg became gangrenous and amputation was required.

The Illinois Supreme Court, in affirming a judgment for the patient, held that the jury's verdict against the hospital was supportable on either of two grounds: (1) The jury could have found that the hospital had negligently failed to have a sufficient number of trained nurses for bedside care of all patients at all times capable of recognizing and bringing to the attention of the hospital administration and the medical staff the progressively worsening gangrenous condition. (2) The jury could have concluded that the hospital surgical staff failed to review the treatment rendered to the patient by the attending physician and that the hospital had failed to require appropriate consultation or examination by the hospital surgical staff.

The thrust of the Court's holding was apparently based on the direct corporate liability of the hospital. The central premise seemed to be that a hospital through its administration, employees, and responsible staff collectively owes "certain responsibilities for the care of the patient" (Illinois, 1965:257) including the supervising of its medical staff members.

Another legal concept which relates generally to the topic of shared liability is that of the independent contractor. The term *independent con-*

tractor refers to a person who contracts "to do something for another" and is neither controlled by that other with respect to physical conduct in performance of the work nor subject to the other's right to control such conduct (Steffen, 1977:14–16). One nursing example of the independent contractor is the nurse in private practice. Such nurses are subject to the control of the persons with whom they have contracts only as to the result of the work but not as to the method by which the result is obtained. Since they do not fall under the *respondeat superior* doctrine, it is generally understood that if they were sued they alone would be responsible.

As the nurse moves away from the institutional setting and/or traditional contractual arrangements, there is an obvious increase in the judgmental aspect of the nursing practice. There also is a corresponding increase in the nurse's responsibilities and liability. The modern nurse may choose to negotiate an independent contractor agreement with a health care agency. Nurses and agencies entering into such arrangements would be well advised to review recent court decisions which have concluded that the *apparent authority* doctrine takes legal priority over contractual language about independent contractor status.

In *Arthur v. St. Peters Hospital* (New Jersey, 1979) the Superior Court of New Jersey, Law Division, held that, in cases where it can be shown that a hospital has created the impression that a particular physician is its agent, and where the patient has accepted treatment from the physician in the reasonable belief that the treatment is being rendered through a hospital employee, the hospital will be liable for the physician's negligence. The Court said: "Unless the patient is in some manner put on notice of the independent status of the professionals with whom he might be expected to come into contact, it would be natural for him to assume that these people are employees of the hospital" (New Jersey, 1979:447).

A CAVEAT TO NURSES

Nurses are becoming increasingly concerned about their own protection in relation to their professional activities. Many erroneously believe that they are protected under the employer's insurance policy. This is not necessarily the case and, in any event, an employer's insurance is likely to protect the nurse, if at all, only while she is on duty in the course of her employment. It would not protect nurses who, while off duty, respond to a request to assist a neighbor or friend or who volunteer their nursing services to community activity (such as a blood drive).

That all but a handful of nurses have escaped exposure to suits in the past is perhaps less the result of a perceived absence of liability on their part than a tacit recognition of their likely inability to pay—a condition known in legal parlance as being *judgment proof*. This situation is rapidly changing. Today it is expected that nurses will accept accountability (including financial accountability) for their professional conduct. They can best prepare to meet the rising demands of professional accountability by doing four things: (1) They can keep abreast of developments in their areas of nursing and nursing generally through recourse to the literature, formal and continuing education programs, and collegial dialogue. (2) They can maintain accurate, complete, and factual records of their professional observations and behaviors. (3) They can carry professional liability insurance for their own financial protection as well as for the protection of their clients. (4) They can seek legal counsel in a timely fashion whenever there is any indication that, within the realm of their professional lives, something has gone wrong or foreseeably might go wrong.

EDITOR'S QUESTIONS FOR DISCUSSION

How might potential conflicts between court and board of nursing rulings be prevented? What type of legal implications are there by virtue of inconsistent state nurse practice acts? What obligations does a professional nurse have regarding nurse practice acts? To what extent is "unprofessional conduct" defined by state boards of nursing? Discuss the pros and cons for broad definitions by State Boards of Nursing.

Differentiate the types of liability that a licensed professional nurse may have. Should nursing actions be permitted without licensure by specific persons? How can the professional nurse protect her license from censure?

How is the legal duty of care established? Once the duty of care arises, under what conditions may services be terminated without liability? Distinguish by examples in nursing practice the "strict locality" rule, "same or similar locality" rule, and the "accepted practice" rule. To what extent should any of these rules be a basis for the definition of nurse practice acts? What risks may be involved in following the "accepted practice" rule? Discuss justification for following an "accepted practice" rule. Are there safeguards that may be used in following an "accepted practice" rule? To what extent are "accepted practice" rules a basis for the definition of nurse practice acts? What is the process for developing statutes governing the practice of nursing?

What implications for nursing practice and nursing education are inherent in Walker's chapter? What legal responsibilities do nurse-educators and nursing students have regarding the standard and degree of care provided in a service setting? Discuss examples of bases for liability as presented by Walker and propose potential prevention strategies.

What risks are inherent for vicarious liability in independent nursing practice? To what extent can the risks be minimized or prevented?

How would the "borrowed servant" rule be applicable in the current situation of hospitals and service agencies utilizing supplemental (temporary) nurses from outside sources? To what extent may a supplemental nurse, a nursing department, or the outside source employer of the nurse be liable in circumstances of nursing practice? How can potential liability in utilizing supplemental nurses be minimized or prevented?

In the case of supplemental nurses, who might be considered the "independent contractor" — the nurse, the outside source employer of the nurse, or the service institution utilizing the nurse? What are the implications for the quality of care and nursing practice if any one of the above three parties could be considered the "independent contractor"? Discuss whether more than one contract may be involved and the legal implications of utilizing supplemental nurses.

REFERENCES

Bernzweig, Eli P.
 1975 The Nurse's Liability for Malpractice (2d ed.). New York: McGraw-Hill.
Idaho. Idaho Code, § 54-1422(2)(7), 1974.
Idaho. Tuma v. Board of Nursing, 593 P. 2d 711 (1979).
Illinois. Darling v. Charleston Community Memorial Hospital, 211 N.E. 2d 253 (1965).

Kentucky. Blair v. Eblen, 461 S.W. 2d 370(1970).
Kentucky. Massey v. Heine, 497 S.W. 2d 564 (1973).
King, Joseph H., Jr.
 1977 The Law of Medical Malpractice in a Nutshell. St. Paul, Minn.: West Publishing Company.
Maryland. Annotated Code of Maryland, Article 43, § 299(a)(3 and 5), 1967.
Michigan. Kambas v. St. Joseph's Mercy Hospital of Detroit, 205 N.W. 2d 431 (1973).

Minnesota. Sandhofer v. Abbott-Northwestern Hospital, 283 N.W. 2d 362 (1979).

Missouri. Burns v. Owens, 459 S.W. 2d 303 (1970).

Montana. Revised Codes of Montana, §69-5223, 1947.

Montana. Swanson v. St. John's Lutheran Hospital, 597 P. 2d 702 (1979).

Nebraska. Scott v. State Ex Relatione Board of Nursing, 244 N.W. 2d 683 (1976).

New Jersey. Arthur v. St. Peters Hospital, 405 A. 2d 443 (1979).

Oregon. May v. Broun, 492 P. 2d 776 (1972).

Pennsylvania. Leukhardt v. Commonwealth of Pennsylvania, State Board of Nurse Examiners, 403 A. 2d 645 (1979).

Steffen, Roscoe T.
1977 Agency-Partnership in a Nutshell. St. Paul, Minn.: West Publishing Company.

Tennessee. Johnson v. Woman's Hospital, 527 S.W. 2d 133 (1973).

Vermont. Vermont Statutes Amended, 12, §519 (Supp.), 1971.

Part Two

Nursing Education

A time for planting,
a time for uprooting what has been planted. . . .
a time for tearing,
a time for sewing

Nursing education is primarily concerned with the implementation of knowledge. In transmitting knowledge, previous learning frequently is disassembled and reorganized. This may be necessary in order to incorporate the most valuable additional knowledge that is available. Thus, critiquing and evaluation is a constant process in nursing education. At times knowledge, teaching strategies, the learning process, and modes of offering education are torn apart. The objective is to sew together all aspects of inculcating knowledge that will enable the nursing student to be the most competent, accountable, and effective professional in nursing practice, education, and research.

Nursing education has become increasingly complex. This is partly related to multiple issues which remain unresolved. The dilemma of three levels of education for entry into nursing continues to perplex the profession. Concern remains regarding the initial performance level of the new graduate. The proliferation of graduate programs in nursing without sufficient resources is an enigma. Some uncertainty in purpose of graduate programs exists as well as the role outcomes for their graduates. Numerous suggestions are offered to resolve these issues. The great decrease in federal funding for nursing education has hindered the profession.

Expectations are increasing for highly professional programs in nursing education. The quality of nursing education is carefully reviewed. Nursing curricula are being thoroughly examined and evaluated. Academic qualifications and standards for nursing faculty are greatly stressed. Faculty members are expected to fulfill multiple roles. The environment within which faculty members are appointed is explored. More nursing faculties are becoming role models for students as they combine education with nursing practice. Education for leadership in nursing is a source of concern. Throughout the ensuing chapters, the numerous changes, complexities, and challenges in nursing education are shown.

Chapter 5

Crisis in Academic Nursing

Janet A. Williamson, R.N., Ph.D.
Associate Professor
Department of Nursing
Pennsylvania State University
University Park, Pennsylvania

Given the many controversial issues in academic nursing, Janet A. Williamson offers a timely, challenging, and thought-provoking chapter. She addresses the historical evolution of the crisis in nursing, analyzes the current state of affairs, and proposes ideas she perceives would help to develop professional education in nursing and stature in academia. She discusses many issues such as: the dilemma of three levels of education for entry into nursing and the uncontrolled growth and direction of these programs as well as of graduate programs at the masters and doctoral level. Williamson emphasizes that there is no clear picture of what graduate education is, what its purpose is, or who is its product. She points out dangers in the violation of academic standards for faculty, the lack of financial control by deans, and the reliance on soft money. Williamson raises difficult questions throughout her chapter and argues strongly for the solutions she offers. One example: She urges redefining the current content for the baccalaureate degree and renaming it as a baccalaureate degree in nursing technology. She believes graduates of this program should need no other degrees for professional practice. Williamson clearly states her beliefs regarding graduate education at the masters and doctoral level and qualifications for faculty. Her explication of professional commitment as professional bonding is a new approach.

Crisis is a term connoting a crucial or decisive time or a turning point. Crises generally do not instantaneously appear; they are the result of a series of events or situations which finally reach a critical point. Decisions and events occurring at this critical point set the pattern for the success or failure of the crisis resolution.

In general, professional nursing in the early 1980s is facing a turning point. We are perceived as a weak, female occupation operating under the jurisdiction of the medical profession. We have not been able to demonstrate satisfactorily our unique role in health care, nor that we are a group powerful enough to be considered either singly or as a coalition. We are prone to develop our thinking for the future by idealizing a small step to be taken 20 years hence. We do not have a comprehensive plan for nursing for the future. And nowhere is the situation more acute and more reflective of the total picture than in academia. The academic crisis is a microcosm and forerunner of the crisis in nursing totally.

Academia is a world unto itself, having a language and culture not readily understood by those outside it. Even though the major part of nursing education is centered in academia, after 50 years or so it is still considered by many a neophyte. The present situation of nursing in academia is at a crucial stage and decisions are facing us, which, if sound, could pave the way for the true emergence of professional nursing.

The purpose of this chapter is to examine some of the important elements of the past that have contributed to this critical situation in academia, to analyze the current state of affairs, and to propose some ideas that would help to develop professional education in nursing and to increase its stature in academia.

HISTORICAL EVOLUTION OF CRISIS

The first baccalaureate nursing program in an institution of higher education was developed in the early 1900s. But the real thrust of generic nursing in these institutions occurred after World War II, and increased at the greatest rate in the 1960s and 1970s. At the same time, diploma programs gradually decreased and associate degree programs increased, resulting in the well-recognized dilemma of three levels of education offering entry into nursing.

From those years to the present the problem has been compounded by the large number of programs that did not meet the criteria for approval or accreditation, did not have upper-division nursing, and existed as an educational mill for the diploma graduate. Nursing was not able to control these programs, and, indeed, their graduates filled many of the faculty positions.

Graduate education, particularly at the master's level, did not gain momentum in nursing until the 1960s and rapidly expanded in the 1970s. The 1970s also saw an increased emphasis on doctoral education. However, graduate-level content in nursing was not developed to any great extent. Many programs focused on the nonnursing areas of administration or teaching; others, such as the

nurse-scientist programs, prepared nurses in other disciplines.

Throughout the checkered educational growth of nursing, no single pattern of preparation was developed and no clear-cut role was determined for the graduates of different programs. Uncontrolled growth and lack of direction produced confusion both for the public and for the profession.

Over these years, as nursing was growing in academia, it appears that academia was not sure just what to do with nursing. Nursing was placed in medical schools, in health science centers, and in traditional academic environments in colleges and universities. In many institutions nursing never became a central academic unit, but remained a cloistered unit outside the scholarly domain. Standards for nursing faculty were different from those for faculty of other disciplines.

Being a female profession has undoubtedly helped to determine the status of nursing in academia. The literature today abounds with the rhetoric decrying the results of discrimination against women and the second-class citizenship that has resulted. A large percentage of nurses, long socialized into roles controlled by the male-dominated medical profession or hospital administration, did not readily coalesce into a voice for women or for independent nursing. This criticism has been applied to diploma and associate degree graduates, but graduates of baccalaureate programs, as readily demonstrated by Kramer (1974), do not maintain professional ideals either.

The lack of control of nursing by nurses has also been apparent in many of the educational programs. Many deans have not controlled their nursing budgets, and have had no jurisdiction over capitation and other nursing monies. Yet their counterparts, mainly male, in the institutions have had control over their resources and probably would not have thought of accepting their positions without assurance of this control.

In addition to lack of resource control, another financial problem of nursing in academia has been the building of programs on a soft-money base. Nursing has had generous funding from outside sources, and nursing deans have utilized these funds for faculty positions and allotment expenditures without budgeting them against a hard-money base. The sole use of traineeships for graduate students is another example of reliance on soft money. The result has been that nursing has lagged far behind the rest of academia in the number of graduate assistantships (hard money) available to nursing majors, . . . Graduate assistantships are the lifeblood of a graduate program.

Federal funding has been generous for nursing but it has also been targeted to some very specific areas. For a long period, primarily in the 1960s, a majority of the funding went into awards for curriculum and program development, including construction of programs. Many institutions were able to receive funds to start up or enlarge nursing programs. But commitment to a program because there is outside money available to start that program is not necessarily a sound commitment.

The 1970s saw increased funding for graduate program development and traineeships. There was also a major effort to fund nurse-practitioner programs. Again, we saw nursing programs operate on the philosophy of "if the money is there, let's get it," even though the government required assurances of program continuation past the award period. The assurances, in many instances, have not been fulfilled.

But, in any crisis, the easiest part of analysis is to use hindsight to discuss the factors that probably contributed to the crisis. A harder task, because of the differing opinions on the current state of affairs, is to analyze the crisis state itself.

PRESENT CRISIS STATE

A crisis exists when a continuation along the present course would result in unacceptable consequences. What is there in present-day nursing in academia that can contribute to these unacceptable consequences?

Probably the most pressing turmoil today stems from the lack of clear-cut levels of nursing education. The familiar "1985 Proposal" (actually the "1965 Proposal") calling for two levels of nursing—professional and technical—has produced a plethora of rhetoric and emotionalism. The proposal has resulted in the formation of power coalitions on both sides of the argument which include, on the negative side, such nonnursing groups as the American Hospital Association.

But this is not the crux of the issue. This proposal is once again a small step which will produce problems in the future. We are struggling to differentiate between "professional" and "technical" when the majority cannot even determine what "professional" means. What is professional education in nursing? What is professional practice apart from medicine? What level of education is *necessary* for the profession of nursing? To decide, at this stage in nursing's evolution, upon baccalaureate education as our professional entry level is certain to invite the return of this same turmoil 10 or 20 years from now.

And what of graduate education? Graduate education is another part of the sometimes perplexing, sometimes erratic, always confusing system of nursing education. Most of the emphasis and attention in the system today is directed toward initial educational preparation, but we need to be equally as concerned with graduate education which is drifting toward the same confused state as the entry level.

We have a large number of accredited master's programs in nursing, with such varying degree titles as master of science, master of nursing, and master of arts. (As an aside, it should be understood that a degree title in most instances is determined by the university offering that degree.) These degrees in nursing are offered by both colleges and universities. The subject areas of the degrees range from medical model titles such as medical or psychiatric nursing to the developmental titles such as geriatric, pediatric, etc., and we have also degrees in nursing administration and nursing education. The titles we give the graduates of these programs range from "clinical specialist," "clinician," and "practitioner" to "administrator," "educator," and yes, even "researcher," at the master's level.

We have programs that provide "something" both in a clinical area and in a so-called functional area of administration or education. And we have programs which utilize unqualified faculty, i.e., master's prepared, to teach at the master's level.

Several forces are operating positively and negatively on master's programs today. First, we have an obvious need for individuals with advanced knowledge to perform beyond the baccalaureate level. Second, we have an accreditation process that, in the definition of functional area, equates practice, administration, education, and research. Third, we have several national organizations making statements, profound ones, on the content and outcome of graduate education—and these statements are not all harmonious. Fourth, we have nursing faculties in colleges moving onto the bandwagon of graduate education even though these institutions do not have university or research status. Fifth, we have the confusion as to what constitutes entry-level education for nursing. Sixth, and most important, we have not clearly delineated nursing and nursing practice apart from medicine.

If we look at nursing education on the master's level today, there is no clear picture of its purpose or its product. This problem in graduate education is closely aligned with another—the lack of adherence to academic standards.

Academia existed many years before it embraced nursing. Academic standards and culture were established and, in the main, adhered to by its elements. As a new discipline developed in academia, it added to the culture and conformed to standards; it did not violate them.

Many programs in nursing do violate university standards and make it extremely difficult for the nursing programs which try to maintain the standards. The basic credential for a faculty position in academia is a doctoral degree, and certainly this degree is required for tenure, for the professorial rank, and for teaching at the graduate level. Yet across the country, individuals with masters' degrees and individuals with doctorates, but with no background in research or scholarly activity,

are teaching in graduate programs and are being awarded tenure and professorial rank. One hears the argument that we do not have enough nurses with doctorates, and therefore we have to utilize individuals with lesser preparation. The argument does not stand, for unqualified faculty can not expect to be accepted fully by academia, and programs thus staffed should never be started (or continued).

The lack of adherence to basic credential and tenure standards allows for justifiable criticism of nursing by other disciplines. It also places nursing outside the mainstream and relegates it to a position of little power. Nurses with masters' degrees and minimal or no research activity sitting on university committees with scholars from other disciplines are not among equals, and they are not qualified to be there.

We plead for respect, nay, we demand the respect given to any academic discipline. But we must earn this respect, and we must utilize qualified faculty and administrators as a beginning step to our rightful place in academia. We must speak the language and accept the customs; otherwise we should move out.

Another current problem producing a crisis state is the reduction in external funding for nursing. As stated earlier, many nursing programs have been built and continued on government support. As this support is reduced and specifically targeted, many nursing educators feel that the university should replace the funds. Yet we know the difficult economic straits of higher education, and we recognize that these funds are not easily forthcoming.

Nursing was built on soft money and will now have to deal with the consequences. Graduate students may be without the "no strings" funding; special programs built as appendages to the regular programs may have to close; faculty soft-money positions will collapse; and indeed some total programs may have to close. All of these may not be negative consequences.

For example, one of the results of traineeships has been a lack of the need for students to function as research or teaching assistants and to thereby benefit from the mentor concept. Faculty have also lacked these assistants. With different, and more stringent, funding from university sources and from research grants, graduate students and faculty may develop closer and more scholarly mentor relationships.

Nursing may no longer be a financially "privileged" group. Nursing faculty will have to enter the larger, more competitive arena for research monies where credentials and track records are important. A problem is arising as universities look at the comparable data on outside funding brought in by the various disciplines and find that nursing's data no longer include large amounts of capitation, traineeships, and program development monies. Our weakness is being exposed.

There are other elements in the crisis: male domination of the institutions; enrollment stability and perhaps decline; "whispers" one hears of a power play by others for the control of nursing; divisions over accreditation and credentialing; replacement and loss of strong nursing administrators in many institutions; and the continuing lack of a strong central educational policy for nursing. All these elements, along with the ones discussed before, have played a role, major or minor, in contributing to the present state of academic nursing.

But we can bemoan the past and the present just so long. We must seek solutions, credible and far-reaching, to diminish the unacceptable consequences of the present state.

CRISIS RESOLUTION

Decisions made for one component of nursing have ramifications for all components. Decisions regarding nursing education will impact profoundly on nursing practice. Yet education is the place to start to plan for the future of nursing.

The graduates of today's programs—baccalaureate, associate degree, and diploma—perform a much-needed service to society. This service is a technical service based on a composite of medical and nursing technology. The content of the three programs is primarily concerned with supporting this composite technology and allowing the graduates to perform at the technical level.

We should (1) allow the continued phase-out of diploma programs; (2) redefine the content of the associate degree to a narrow sphere of technology and/or workplace, such as intensive care; (3) rename the current baccalaureate degree a "baccalaureate degree in nursing technology" and maintain current licensure for this degree. This would be a terminal degree for technical but not professional practice. It should not be necessary to have a baccalaureate degree in nursing technology as an entrance requirement to a professional nursing program. Persons with a baccalaureate degree from other disciplines should be permitted to enter the professional program for nursing.

This approach allows for the development of the professional degree in nursing such as the professional doctorate (for e.g., Nursing Doctorate, or N.D.) at the postbaccalaureate level. The basic content for professional practice should be conceptualized from the laws of health in the expanding field of nursing theory and should also include the content of the technology from the current baccalaureate programs. From my perspective, we have developed technical baccalaureate programs and technical practice. We have not developed professional programs nor professional practice. This postbaccalaureate degree (N.D.) should be the basic preparation for professional practice and the graduates of this program should need no other degree for professional practice, specifically not a graduate degree. Additionally, we must clearly articulate the parameters of nursing practice apart from medical practice and teach this only at the professional postbaccalaureate level.

The purpose of a master's-level program in nursing education should be to provide knowledge in a specialized area (subdiscipline) of nursing in order to enhance practice. Nursing, as a professional discipline, educates for the discipline at the entry level, and it educates in the subdisciplines at the graduate level. Nursing practice per se is not the focus at the master's level, nor at the doctoral. The focus here is advanced knowledge in nursing and any new skills inherent in that knowledge. The degree should reflect the subdiscipline, and the higher the educational level, the more narrow the knowledge area.

There is only one level of nursing practice—the professional level. The structure of this practice should obviously be taught through professional education. There have been very few attempts to articulate the structure of nursing practice, yet this is an absolute necessity. Once the structure is taught and implemented, it is not retaught at a higher educational level. There is really no such creature as an advanced practitioner, there is only a specialized practitioner. The master's degree should not be conceived as a second professional degree, a continuation of the first professional degree. That first degree is a terminal degree, and one should need no further formal education to practice professionally. The master's degree should be an academic degree which adds knowledge in a very specific area, but which does not change the role of the practitioner.

Individuals with career goals in other fields, such as administration and education, should enter programs in those fields, i.e., health care administration or higher education, and not seek to realize those goals through nursing. This approach allows for a more in-depth course of study in the preferred area and allows much more career mobility. We should not be wasting our scarce resources teaching in areas that are not nursing.

Preparation for a career in research requires the minimum of a doctoral (Ph.D.) degree, the focus of which is research. This is an academic doctorate. Practice is not the focus of these doctoral programs, which should offer only the development of research expertise in a narrowly defined subdiscipline of nursing. We should offer only the Ph.D. with title in a subdiscipline.

Since graduate education relies upon the scholarly and research activities of an institution and on collaboration between disciplines, this education should occur only in research institutions with faculty prepared at the doctoral level, faculty who are continually engaged in research and scholarly activity. It is time for nursing to exert some collective power and wisdom and set rigorous standards for the development of graduate programs.

These standards and other decisions made in such professional organizations as the American Association of Colleges of Nursing, the Council of Baccalaureate and Higher Degree Programs, and the American Nurses Association—organizations that deal with graduate education—should be made only by individuals with doctoral degrees. Unless one has experienced the totality of the educational process, one cannot make informed decisions on the advanced process.

In conjunction with the clear articulation of professional and graduate education in nursing, academic rigor for both students and faculty has to be maintained. Standards for students, such as intellectual curiosity, academic achievement, seriousness of purpose, and career commitment, need to be enhanced. Standards for faculty, such as proper credentials, a strong commitment to and a proven track record in research and scholarly activity, and practical expertise, need to be enforced. Those who are not qualified should be denied tenure, denied professorial rank, and denied a faculty position in a professional program. This is one aspect of professional commitment.

Another aspect of professional commitment is the support for one's fellow professionals. A professional is a member of a collective whole, a totality which is responsible for meeting the goals of the profession. Each member has a responsibility for and to the other members, a commitment to one another that might be termed professional bonding. Strength emerges when the professional bonds of the unit, or its subunits, remain unbroken. Disagreements and problems may arise in a subunit, but a true bond will hold the members within the group. Nurses need to act professionally, not just speak professionally.

Professional actions speak louder than professional words. A crisis resolution requires action on the part of the profession to diminish the severity and intensity of the crisis state. Individual opinions will differ as to exactly what is wrong and exactly what should be done. But we must break out of our current self-imposed restrictions and try to solve the whole problem, else we will move from crisis to crisis. We in nursing must broaden our horizons; we must seek a rightful place in society—a place of value for ourselves. As the physicist David Bohm says, "Thinking within a fixed circle of ideas tends to restrict the questions to a limited field. And, if one's questions stay in a limited field, so also do the answers" (Watson, 1979:12).

EDITOR'S QUESTIONS FOR DISCUSSION

How accurate is Williamson's evaluation of the crisis in academic nursing? What other factors might have contributed to the crisis? To what extent do you agree with Williamson's analysis of the present crisis state? What evidence is there for the analysis that is presented? What is professional education in nursing? What level of education is necessary for the profession of nursing?

Discuss the pros and cons of the six forces indicated as impacting on master's education. What approach might be suggested for dealing with those forces?

To what extent do you agree with Williamson's answers to the argument that since we do not have enough nurses with doctorates, individuals with lesser preparation need to be utilized in graduate programs? Are there other criteria that should be considered for meeting the needs for graduate education in underserved geographical areas?

Discuss Williamson's belief that the lack of adherence to basic credential and tenure standards is a significant factor in nurses not being accepted as an equal with scholars from other disciplines. If it is not present, how can respect for the discipline of nursing be earned? Is the issue of faculty academic standards unique to nursing?

Debate the solutions Williamson proposes to resolve the crisis. Should licensure be the same for nurses who have graduated from associate degree programs as for those with a baccalaureate degree in nursing technology? What program content, degree, and length is proposed for entry level into professional practice? Should nurses who have graduated from diploma programs be considered as having the requisites for baccalaureate degree in nursing technology and/or prerequisites to enter the professional program for nursing? Should prerequisites be required for entry into the nursing professional program for persons who have a baccalaureate degree in other disciplines?

Should a master's degree be needed for professional practice? Do you maintain the same belief regarding the focus of doctoral programs? What should be the defined advanced knowledge for masters and doctoral programs? What would be the purpose of focusing on advanced knowledge? What implications might such programs have for nursing practice?

Discuss the issue of the appropriateness of graduate education in administration and teaching in schools of nursing. Under what conditions can one justify nurses seeking graduate education in administration and teaching completing programs other than in schools of nursing? Debate the issues implied in Williamson's chapter regarding graduate education.

Discuss Williamson's concept of professional bonding. To what extent is this the critical issue in the profession? How might professional bonding be promoted?

REFERENCES

Kramer, Marlene
  1974   Reality Shock. St. Louis: Mosby.

Watson, Lyall
  1979   Lifetide. New York: Simon and Schuster.

Chapter 6

Anarchy and Revolution Within Educational Organizations of Nursing

Annette Schram Ezell, R.N., Ed.D.
Associate Dean of Academic Affairs
College of Nursing
University of Utah
Salt Lake City, Utah

In Annette Ezell's chapter a different aspect of crisis in academia is analyzed: anarchy and Machiavellian behavior in colleges of nursing. She examines the three decision-situation properties of organized anarchies: ambiguous goals, unclear technology, and fluid participation. The "garbage can" theory is explained whereby decision making is dependent on a setting possessing the properties of an organized anarchy. Ezell describes colleges of nursing as being reflective of both organized anarchies and "garbage can" decision making. Emphasis in this chapter is on factors influencing organizational choice. Ezell delineates four combinations of faculty participation in organizational decision making. Ezell further analyzes the use of power within schools of nursing and demonstrates the relationship of power to manipulative behavior. A model demonstrating individual manipulation orientations is presented. Finally, Ezell illustrates a schema of organized anarchy in which the clustering effect of Machiavellian participant behaviors, the organizational setting, and social interactions is shown. She urges faculty to understand the events resulting in anarchy. Ezell suggests tactical strategies for controlling anarchy and predicts colleges of nursing will remain in spite of the ambiguity that is present.

Varying states of anarchy exist within all educational systems, including colleges of nursing. This chapter will explore the concept of anarchy and revolutionary (Machiavellian) behavior within organizations, specifically within colleges of nursing. Analyses of the personal characteristics and strengths of current and future leaders, as well as of the situational elements in colleges of nursing which contribute to environmental constraints will be presented, and strategies for purposeful decision making and distribution of power will be discussed. Since colleges of nursing often operate within turbulent environments, the individuals and groups who make up these educational systems frequently find themselves in conflict with appointed leaders and rarely understand the nature of the organizational conditions. In this light, the author will describe the characteristics of anarchy in schools of nursing and the effect of manipulative (Machiavellian) administrative behaviors on directing policy, formalizing organizational goals, and facilitating the decision making of educational organizational structures.

The author suggests that these patterns of organizational behavior are not unique to nursing and that deans and faculty should be aware of the underlying organizational behaviors and the patterns of interaction that are known to influence anarchic, or revolutionary, behavior in educational institutions and, hence, in colleges of nursing in the 80s. In describing what she sees as the present situation in administration in some educational organizations of nursing, the author will not judgmentally evaluate the moral nature of the situation, but will recommend alternative patterns of administrative behavior, i.e., personal and situational decision-making strategies, which might be implemented.

SOME ORGANIZATIONAL ASSUMPTIONS

Predictable Organizations

Most people appear to believe that the organizations of which they are a part are predictable, stable, and constant, that they have a low level of risk taking, and that they engage in rational decision making. Organizations are seen as having firm boundaries which create an artificial separation in the environment. Within an organization, order rules through procedural and operational routines, and hierarchies and departments search for balance in power and authority. There is an orderly and highly selective admission of participants. There is judicious allocation of rewards and resources. There are rational decisions about organizational goals and about utilization of time toward meeting these goals. This is the thinking, and the hidden wish, of the majority of people involved in an organization. Let us, they say, maintain an organizational system of stability and safeness—both within and without—and, by all means, use only rational decision making.

"Garbage Can" Model[1]

The model of organization proposed by Cohen et al. (1972), called the "garbage can," postulates that the predictability of the system cannot be assumed. This type of organization is organized anarchy. A classic and current example of such an organization is seen in a study by Sproul et al. (1978) of the creation of the National Institute of Education in 1972. This agency was to support research and development in education throughout the United States. Cohen et al. have elicited three key properties of the decision situation in organized anarchies (1972:1). These properties are (1) ambiguous goals, (2) unclear technology, and (3) fluid participation.

Ambiguous goals in anarchic organizations remain measurable; however, there are problematic preferences regarding agreement. Generally, the goals are known through a loose collection of ideas rather than in a coherent structure. The organization is viewed as discovering preferences through action rather than acting on the basis of preferences.

An *unclear technology* is one in which there is low probability of identifying or describing courses of action that have an intended impact upon a previously specified problem (Sproul et al., 1978). Most operations are seen as trial-and-error and as pragmatic inventions of necessity.

Fluid participation refers to the participation of people inside and outside the organization who have limited time and energy. The degree of involvement of these people varies from time to time, and the boundaries of the organization become very uncertain. The audience and the decision makers change capriciously, and often no single participant dominates the choosing acts.

Therefore, Cohen et al. describe the organiza-

---

[1] Intellectual debt is owed to Michael Cohen, James March, John Olsen, and their colleagues, who have contributed to this insightful theory of organizational choice.

tion setting as a "garbage can" collection in which choices are fundamentally ambiguous. An organization is a set of procedures for argumentation and interpretation as well as for solving problems and making decisions. A choice situation is a meeting place for issues and feelings looking for decision situations in which they may be aired, solutions looking for issues to which there can be an answer, and participants looking for problems or pleasure. (1976:25)

In this alternative and novel view of organizations, a stream of *problems, solutions, participants,* and *choice opportunities* are funneled through the organizational and social structure. *Problems* are found in organizational ideology; group relations; and distribution of status, jobs, and money. *Solutions* are considered to be answers looking for questions. *Participants* enter and exit the organization relatively easily and participation is largely time-dependent. Lastly, *choice opportunity* is the organizational behavior which results in decisions, e.g., contracts signed; people hired, promoted, or dismissed; and money allocated. These four elements of the "garbage can" model are greatly influenced by their interrelated linkage, allocation of people-energy, and time patterns.

Organized Anarchies

These major characteristics—ambiguous goals, unclear technology, and fluid participation—may be viewed in any organization. In particular, governmental organizations, educational institutions (especially universities), and social-policy institutions operate under these conditions. Such organizations are also referred to as organized anarchies; that is, they are loosely coupled units (Weick, 1976). Because of these unique characteristics, organizational decisions cannot be fully explained by rational intentions.

The essence of the organized anarchy is ex-plained by behavioral theories of organizations and a closed system of organizational choice (March and Olsen, 1976b:13; Turner, 1977). Participants generally sense some discrepancy between what they think ought to be and what actually is, and this discrepancy produces behavior that is aggregated into organizational choices or actions. External criteria are used to judge the discrepancy and its inherent effectiveness. This closed system of organizational choice contains four cyclic elements:

1 Preferences of participants affect their behavior.
2 Individuals participate in choices.
3 Organizational choices affect the environment.
4 Environmental acts in turn affect preferences of the participants.

Most organization theory is purposeful. It is assumed that behavior and participation follow belief and attitude. In the "garbage can" model, "participation" merely refers to a broad base of activities without considering individual motivation. These attentive activities include seeking information, discussing, attending meetings, voting, and competing for office. Such activities are limited and incomplete when the organization cycle is disrupted. The disruption is frequently referred to as "loose coupling" (Weick, 1976). This notion relates to the idea of Cohen et al. (1972) that there is considerable variation in individual choice among organizational participants, that changes can be reflected over time, and that there is variation in the quality of attention given to a problem. Hence, the time and energy an individual must devote to decisions becomes a scarce resource and one from which the highest utilitarian return is expected (Becker, 1965). We find that individuals, in this case the faculty, attend to those decisions that translate into specific obligations, personal interests, and following the rules. March and Olsen conclude that attitudes and beliefs may or may not represent behavioral implications and that there may exist some interplay between behavior and self-interest (1976c: 38-53).

Organizational choices are also seen as being derived, although somewhat loosely, from individual actions. It may be seen that organizational choices may not be related to organizational action, e.g., in specific dean or assistant dean appointments and in policy selections. Hence, organizational choices are more often related to allocation of status, to maintenance of or change in friendships, to loyalties, and to multiple selections of group or self-interest. Therefore, organizational choice may be viewed as highly time-dependent, variable, and subject to actions not anticipated nor necessarily desirable.

The environment must also be understood as a major shaper of the interaction between events, actors, and structures. This interplay may result in minimal or maximal relationship between environmental response and organizational decision.

Lastly, individuals and organizations operate under myths, fictions, and legends. Their ideologies are transmitted and reported by the organizational participants (Kamen, 1977). This occurs because the organizational actors and events are often ambiguous, and participants must rely on the interpretations of others. The myths are infused into all levels of organizational policy and decision making.

Concerning these limitations and flaws, March and Olsen suggest some areas of confusion that need to be recognized in analyzing organizations. They set out certain assumptions as operational:

What appeared to happen did happen.
What happened was intended to happen.
What happened had to happen. (1976b:20)

These assumptions underlie this chapter. Interest has arisen in individual and group pursuit of objectives and the reflected organizational choices as a result of March and Olsen's assumptions. Cohen et al. conclude that:

in situations in which the load is heavy and the structure is relatively unsegmented, intention is lost in context-dependent flow of problems, solutions, people, and choice opportunities. Indeed, outcomes are frequently sufficiently dependent on elements of exogenously determined timing as to make the differences between what happens and what does not happen deceptively significant. (1976:37)

Structure of the Anarchic Organization

Organizational choice via the "garbage can" model, as previously mentioned, is essentially a meeting place for problems, solutions, participants, and choice opportunities. This theory underlies the structure and development of organized anarchies. In summary, decision making in organized anarchies is dependent upon ambiguous goals, unclear technologies, and part-time participants.

Olsen has cited the interrelationship of three models of decision-making behavior in explaining the organized-anarchy proposition (1976a:82–139). These are the rational or entrepreneurial model; the conflict-resolution model; and the artifactual, or nondecision model. Each of these models can be briefly described.

Rational or Entrepreneurial Model This model exemplifies the willed product and utilitarian function. Intellectual aspects are emphasized to link organizational (seen as a single unit) means to ends. This assumes that participants know their preferences and how to get what they want through use of power and knowledge.

Conflict-Resolution Model This model describes decision-making behavior of individuals and subgroups with competing interests. Here no single alternative organizational event will suffice for all the participants. This model permits the emergence of coalitions bargaining for resources. The resultant decision making becomes problematic.

Artifactual or Nondecision Model This model is considered the opposite of the other two models.

Here decision outcomes are an unintended product of processes having dynamics of their own. In other words, events happen which force participants to describe the decisions *post factum*; they do not make goal-oriented decisions through a structural process.

According to Olsen (1976a:82–139), these models are intertwined. Six other criteria are necessary to explain how the models interact to form organized anarchies. The six criteria are part-time participants, ambiguity, decision time, organizational slack, style of decision making, and external, or contingency, factors.

1 *Part-time participants.* Rarely does an organizational decision demand the attention of all the participants, except in constitutional and policy decisions. Often the participants are overloaded with the work of the organization (e.g., teaching and research) and simply cannot devote large amounts of time to decision-making efforts. Therefore, variations in participation patterns are critical. It is relatively easy to document the number of participants (i.e., faculty) activated, the types of participants involved, the nature of participant activity (e.g., reacting or generating solutions), and the extent of turnover or attrition.

2 *Ambiguity.* Organizations have a process or a set of procedures into which participants are gathered to make choices. There is also an abundant supply of choices as well as methods for making decisions. The process includes looking for problems to fit solutions and looking for issues and feelings which can be attached to decision situations. This "garbage can" mixture of issues, activities, and feelings generates the production of extraneous factors which contribute to the ambiguity in choice (decision) opportunity.

3 *Decision time.* Decision-time is a critical factor affecting both process and outcome. Generally, the longer a choice remains unresolved, the greater the range of issues that are defined as relevant. Also, the longer the time, the more the number of participants increases and, hence, the greater the complexity. The more complex the situation, the more the participants will postpone decision making and early commitment, becoming less agreeable and less attracted to the leadership role and the generation of solutions. It is also known that issues and other choices often become loosely coupled with the original choice opportunity, thus compounding the problem.

4 *Organizational slack.* Slack is a term defined by Cyert and March (1963) to show the discrepancy between organizational resources and activated demands. The more slack, the easier to find satisfactory solutions, the fewer participants involved, and the less delay. However, sometimes the organization will not know the extent of the slack, and so it becomes a trial-and-error situation. When slack is reduced, more participants are activated, and often there are not ways to meet the demands. Issues are couched in a political style.

5 *Decision-making style.* Again, decision-making styles coincide with the organizational models. The entrepreneurial style assumes that objectives and goals are shared; there is a rational search for the one alternative. In the political style, there is disagreement in organizational goals. In the conflict-resolution style, solutions which do not require the operational cohesion of a community of goals are sought. In the nondecision style, choices are the extraneous products of "other" activities which were not planned.

March and Simon (1958) have predicted that political processes can disrupt by placing strain on the status and power systems. Therefore, it is appropriate to approach all decisions as if they were analytical problems. The analytical process assumes goal (value) agreement, which enlarges potential resources and results in organizational integration.

Features noted in bargaining in the political process are competition of values, distribution of resources, and resolution by decisive action (polarizing). Fiction and rumors increase, since participants tend to spend time and talk with those who agree rather than those who disagree. Information is generated and processed in subgroups (anarchy), and meanings which have limited comparison with reality are read into situations.

Nondecision style is always vulnerable. Dissatisfaction becomes predominant. There is an attempt to change the leadership, or participants begin to leave the organization.

6 *External, or contingency, factors.* These contingency factors result in competition for participant resources—time, energy, and attention. If one assumes that most organizational participants are operating near capacity, an increase in any area will produce heightened response. Either the length of time must be extended (longer deadlines), the number of persons involved must be increased, or the total amount of attention by participants must be reduced. Therefore, many organizations, organizations like colleges of nursing, become crisis- and deadline-oriented; the participants are heavily burdened with external factors and tend to make decisions only when they have to.

Each of the above criteria has been carefully described in Olsen's report of a study of the appointment of a new dean to a school at a major public university (1976a:82-139). The study analyzes the anarchy inherent in the system. The college setting is described as one with a great deal of freedom for students and individual faculty members (subgroups). The decision-making process is described as one in which the dean would consult with the faculty and then announce the decision. Few important joint decisions were made in the organization. The school was externally viewed as an innovative college—but it was not universally supported in the university. There was internal tension between the dean and some of the faculty. The college was nondepartmentalized, as are many colleges of nursing, and therefore was not organized along traditional disciplinary lines. The choice of a new dean became a critical organizational choice. In this, the similarities are remarkably congruent with the administrative state of the art in nursing, especially in higher educational systems in the United States.

COLLEGES OF NURSING AS ANARCHIC ORGANIZATIONS

A recent work (March and Olsen, 1976a) on university decision making has categorized the university and university units (such as colleges of nursing) as being organized anarchies. University decision making has largely been classified as the "garbage can" variety. It is the belief of this author that colleges of nursing are models of both organized anarchy and "garbage can" decision making. The "garbage can" theory asserts that organized anarchy is typified by unclear goals, poorly understood technology, and variable participation. In this model, the decision process is likely to produce an outcome which is a by-product of decision processing rather than rational problem solving. The organization is not required to reach or solve problems by a specified time. The organization (e.g., the college of nursing) merely works on decisions until they are made. Neither the beginning nor the end of the process can be well-defined. Decisions already made may be unmade. It is often unclear, except in retrospect, when things started. Often there is little saliency or importance to decisions; this state is referred to as the "importance of the unimportant." The participants are few, and many have other things on their minds to draw their energy and attention. In general, the actors are part-time and changing, a condition evident in nursing faculties. It seems as though the persons filling the administrative positions as deans and department chairs change more quickly than the issues are resolved. In one instance, the assistant dean of baccalaureate programs in a college of nursing at a major university changed 7 times in 5 years.

March and Romelaer state that there are three conditions underlying organizational choice in organizations like American universities. They state that there is a relatively small number of active participants; that there is interaction of position in the decision structure, i.e., there is a trade-off of authority for time and commitment; and that there is orderly drift (1976:268-269). In this author's opinion, the events and decisions, or choices, made in colleges of nursing have been consistent with what is discerned throughout higher education in the United States.

It has also been shown that participants are not equal in their impact on the organizational choice process. Influence on organizational choice has been seen to be dependent on two factors—presence and position (March and Romelaer: 1976:272-273). Regarding the issue of *presence*, it has been cited that few people are involved, that they often wander in and out, and that those who are willing to spend time in decision making become very influential. Throughout the decision process, individuals on the faculty are obligated to respond to memoranda and to acknowledge specific choices. If faculty participants are willing to be involved, the college will be prone to give considerable latitude in determining which "garbage" will be used and which will be left in the can. Long delays are characteristic of infrequent presence.

The impact of *position* is also remarkable. It has been repeatedly observed that the chairperson or dean can exercise discretion in blocking initiatives. Actions often require positive approval from an administrative official, a requirement which serves as a delay or denial tactic. Leverage is exercised by persons in authority positions to pursue senior appointments, to make judgments on tenure, to spend extra resources, and to set agendas.

One can often see an interrelationship of position and presence. The major office holders—chairpersons, deans, provosts—spend more time on organizational choices. However, their attention is often divided among a large variety of concerns. In colleges of nursing, which are largely non-departmentalized, there is a major trade-off between position and presence, a trade-off which is extremely political. When the chairperson or dean is limited in the amount of attention and energy that can be devoted to any one question, the issues of priorities and values become paramount.

COLLEGE GOVERNANCE

Formal hierarchy plays little part in the colleges of the United States today. Clark (1977: 64-78) states that the university is a composite of multiple subcultures, intense professionalism, federation structures, and bureaucratic coordination. Since universities have grown so much in the last 30 years, the diversity of subunit growth has led to ambiguous and multipurpose goals, e.g., those which inspire centers for specific study, colleges of liberal arts, scientific research units, and professional schools such as colleges of nursing. The ambiguity, discontinuity, and overlap of goals has led Clark (1977) to categorize colleges as loosely joined federations.

Multiple subcultures in the universities have sprung up around the individual disciplines—so there may be as many value systems as there are departments. The work of the academic person has become intensely specialized. Clark reaffirms that the academic professional is on the ascendant ladder of research and scholarship; there is "a new rise in commitment to create knowledge" (1977: 68). This also creates the need for the professional to have a high degree of autonomy, to be innovative, and to be critical of established ways. As a result of these major changes in academe, there has been a lessened need for a community of scholars; instead the professor tends to be seen as one who is in the position of entrepreneur. Kerr (1963) agrees with Clark to the extent that he suggests that the power of the individual faculty member—power based on the rewards of consultation, competition in the job market, and resources from the federal government and private foundations—is going *up*, while the power of the collective faculty is going *down*.

All of these factors contribute to the increasingly widespread view of the college as a bureaucratic organization. Specialists, or administrators, are appointed throughout the organization to handle all kinds of work. For example, the registrar handles grades; the business officer, purchasing; the officer of academic affairs, faculty hiring, promotion, and tenure, and rules and procedures. Clark concludes that faculty structure is gravitating toward federal structure and that authority is moving to individual or group clusters in possibly anarchic fashion. Thus one may sometimes speak of the university as "a lawless place where power lies around loose" (Clark, 1977:77).

These characterizations are also true of colleges of nursing. Some are now departmentalized (clusters of experts) and some are not. The trend in colleges of nursing has been to create budget officers of academic affairs and student affairs. Colleges with doctoral programs seem to be adamantly imbued with the idea of generating new nursing knowledge. Thus, many colleges of nursing can be regarded as having all the characteristics of anarchy—ambiguous goals, unclear technology, and fluid participation.

Schools of nursing often have *ambiguous goals*, and there is wide disparity according to the particular participant asked. The goals of baccalaureate programs differ from those of associate degree programs. The goals of the college of nursing become problematic preferences, and often the organization is not quite sure what is actually being done. Different members see different goals or give different priorities to the same goals. There are both internal (faculty) and external (professional nurses) forces which continually disrupt the organization and create ambiguity in goals.

Unclear technology is typical of all educational nursing organizations. Faculty is usually hard put to know what student nurses have learned and certainly are unclear about how the learning took place. Faculty often bases teaching styles and techniques on trial-and-error methods rather than on scientific cause-and-effect methods. Some prefer simulated situations. Others are adamant about one-to-one faculty-student contact, hence low faculty-student ratios. In reality the faculty-student ratios are high, i.e., 1-10 and 1-15; however, the learning process does continue, learning does take place, and faculty measures the learning (as much for their own peace of mind as well as to ensure patient safety) in terms of student scores on state board examinations.

Another anarchic characteristic of nursing education organizations is the *fluid participation* of faculty members. In an ideal organization there is concern for equal and continuous participation of all members. Colleges of nursing write by-laws and charters that describe which faculty may

participate and in what activities and how. The various members also give limited attention to the decisive activities of the organization. Baccalaureate programs are plagued by high faculty turnover rates, rates probably related to family responsibilities. Baccalaureate faculty women who are married tend to move with their husbands more often than married faculty women who teach in graduate programs. In any event, it is evident that great variations exist in the manner in which faculty participates in organizational decision making and in how much time and energy they devote to the process.

Olsen analyzes university governance on the basis that nonparticipation may be viewed as exclusion of choice (1976b:277). In other words, faculty participation and leadership activities may be seen as responsibilities that some teachers seek under some circumstances and avoid under others. Olsen delineated four categories of faculty and classified them as seen in Fig. 6-1 (1976b:279). He views leader (dean, assistant dean) behavior on a continuum from resisting to soliciting nonleader (faculty) participation. Conversely, nonleader (faculty) behavior is viewed as an effort to obtain or to avoid participation.

Each of these categories can be described in a nursing context in order to better understand faculty participation in decision-making activities. The combinations of behaviors are dependent upon two premises: (1) the organization provides for individual satisfaction and (2) the individual faculty member is able to affect the allocation of rewards (e.g., salary increases, sabbatical leaves, and research money). The more important the organizational choices, the stronger the demand for participation. If decision making is not considered important and is not tied to rewards, faculty will avoid or greatly reduce the time and energy invested in participation.

Usually colleges of nursing are highly process-oriented, and values and beliefs are thought to be similar among the faculty. Often, choice is made by consensus, and it is considered a duty to participate. Another form of choice behavior is

FACULTY   DEANS, ASSISTANT DEANS

Nonleader (faculty) demand for participation	Leader (deans, assistant deans) resistance to participation by nonleaders	
	High	Low
High	I Power struggle	II Circulation of elites
Low	III Stable organization	IV Burdensome organization

Figure 6-1 Four combinations for level of demand and resistance to participation in decision-making.

I   High demand, high resistance   Where: I = Power struggle
II   High demand, low resistance   Where: II = Circulation of elites
III Low demand, high resistance   Where: III = Stable organization
IV   Low demand, low resistance   Where: IV = Burdensome organization

Source: Adapted from J. Olsen, "University governance: Non-Participation as exclusion or choice," Pp. 277-313 in J. March and J. Olsen, Ambiguity and Choice in Organizations, Sweden: University of Bergen, 1976.

seen in collective decision making. Though arrangement is often cumbersome and time-consuming, the faculty often prefers the long discussions, the development of reports and minutes, the lobbying for votes, and the act of voting when it means it can truly allocate specific rewards within the college. There are times when a faculty member may choose not to participate because there are better external rewards (tenure, federal grants, consultation, prestige, professional competence). A great portion of professional schools, including nursing schools, have this type of faculty member—the prima donna who takes a less and less active role in the formal decision making of the organization. Such faculty members are often not bound by organizational decisions, and they conform less to demands for participation.

Combination I—high demand and high resistance—aptly describes the classical power struggles

seen in colleges of nursing. Power struggles occur when both leaders and nonleaders value organizational choices, when neither group has any alternative to formal participation, and when there is little chance of moving from a nonleader to a leader position or vice versa. This promotes a strained situation in the organization. The formal distribution of power, authority, and status becomes very visible. Leaders may emphasize their power to control resources and affirm their legitimacy in making organizational choices. Nonleaders may try to force leaders to leave, and leaders may try to force nonleaders to leave. Tension is high and criticism is prevalent. Clashes usually peak when the organization—the college of nursing—begins to experience a damaged reputation, reduced financial support, or reduced ability to provide certain types of educational programs. The power struggle generally goes on until one group or the other is forced away (Chaska, 1979). Combination I behavior is frequently seen today in colleges of nursing throughout the country.

In Combination II—high demand, low resistance—leaders and nonleaders value organizational choices differently. It is usually nonleaders who consider choice opportunities more important. In this *elitist* model, the leaders generally have more alternatives for formal participation than do nonleaders. There is assumed to be a steady stream of leaders, but the new leaders are required to have some of the characteristics of the old leadership. Where this is not true, the beginnings of a power struggle (Combination I) may become evident. Often structural reorganization will take place in order to change the legitimacy of power and yet not change the day-to-day operations. The power structure changes will come in slow, continuous, incremental stages. Colleges of nursing have experienced many Combination II types of faculty participation.

In Combination III—low demand, high resistance—organizational choices are valued by leaders but not by nonleaders. Here the nonleaders may have alternatives to participation. This is especially true in nursing where so many nonleaders have access to external funding or have high prestige expertise relative to their specialized area of knowledge. In this more or less *stable* organizational setting, leaders plan to stay leaders, while some nonleaders may anticipate becoming leaders through promotion and other organizational increments. Thus, nonleaders spend time in other areas of the organization, e.g., research and writing, in order to increase their qualifications for leadership positions. This situation results in decreasing demands by the leader for participation. Because relative numbers must be maintained between leaders and nonleaders, reorganization efforts are small and organizational climate is generally good. But if lack of progress toward professional competence is seen, dissatisfactions rise quickly. When nonleaders sense that organizational choices

are more important to the leaders, there is an actual decline in the ability of nonleaders to gain leadership positions. Here, too, a power struggle (Combination I) may erupt.

Leadership is considered a *burden* in Combination IV—low demand, low resistance. Organizational choices are not very important and there are other alternatives to formal participation. In this instance, leaders do not have a potential for growth but nonleaders do. Therefore, leadership is seen as a burden by both. The traditional elite groups are not in power, and leaders are not necessarily representative of their faculty. Often there are leader positions which are filled by rotation arrangements. In colleges of nursing that are not departmentalized, responsibility for a program of study or for a cluster of faculty can become burdensome, and the quasi-administrative position often carries little reward.

In each of the four combinations of faculty participation, it is possible to identify examples from colleges of nursing. The power struggles that are being experienced in nursing are also occurring in other colleges on campuses. Colleges of nursing have hardly been studied from the perspective of androgyny. However, Sanger and Alker (1972) do report on research which indicates that young radicals (e.g., some in the women's liberation movement) tend to make decision choices closely aligned with society at large and that their personalities become fused with their politics. This seems to be a good omen for nursing, since nursing is currently involved in recognizing and analyzing female oppression and is supporting a major cultural and economic revolution in the United States. Behind much of the conflict in institutions of nursing appears to be a quest for collective social action, for increased economic rewards, for opportunities to gain leadership status, and for professional autonomy. Therefore, the anarchy and revolution observed in nursing's higher education organizations is predictable according to the three major anarchic criteria of Cohen et al. (1976:24-37). However, this author believes that the female-oppression issues have not been addressed in studies of colleges of nursing. These concluding sections will focus on the use of power and manipulation in colleges of nursing. Though no specific attention will be given here to the oppression issues, it is recognized that they do exist.

ORGANIZATIONAL POWER

Normative ideology emphasizes that value resides in consistency with external authority and standards. Most theories of administration conclude that leaders in an organization have a basic ideology similar to that of the organization. However, in anarchic organizations, multiple ideologies are prevalant and their presence leads to conflict. Such conflict of ideologies may be seen in colleges of nursing, even though these schools are generally considered somewhat humanistic.

Studies of ideology by Alker and Popper (1973:665) and Loye (1977) have included both humanistic and normative ideologies, as well as Machiavellianism. The conclusion of these studies is that both the principled moralist and the Machiavellian have striking commonalities, in that their choices in decision making are uniquely personal. These choices may be morally creative or selfishly opportunistic, and both may be free of conventional morality. These approaches afford diffusion of responsibility and are authentic. Both the normative and humanistic ideologies are prepackaged, or fused in personality (Sanger and Alker, 1972) and represent ready-made solutions to decision choices. It has been asserted that humanism, as well as normativism, provides escape from the burden of making a free and personal choice through acceptance of authority and power. Throughout most colleges of nursing there is a rather high consensus on the distribution of power and authority—or so it is believed.

These authorities seemingly conclude that the Machiavellian person is not unauthentic in making choices. Isaiah Berlin also documents support of this thesis (1971:20–32). He argues that Machiavelli was a principled moralist since he was totally committed to the use of power in leadership in order to unify Italy (ca. 1500 A.D.) and to improve the welfare of citizens.

The use of power within schools of nursing has not been well analyzed, nor has the relationship of power to manipulative behavior been documented. Nagel (1975) resorts to solving the definition of power by first denoting that the study of likes, desires, wants, values, intentions, and purposes involves the concept of *preference*. Preference, in rational choice theory, would be inferred from behavior (choice) and would not be identified with outcome, specifically, because preference is the disposition to make choice and is not considered an act of choice itself. Therefore, an empirical definition of influence would be a power relation—actual or potential—so that actual or potential causal relationships would exist between the preferences of an actor, i.e., the faculty member, regarding an outcome and the outcome itself. Outcomes are then considered variables indicating the state of another social entity, e.g., manipulation via lobbying (the attempt to change the preferences of those which lobbyists perceive to have power and influence).

Actual and potential power as manipulative behavior is schematically shown in Fig. 6-2 when the behavior of A (the dean) is the proximate cause of B's (the assistant dean's) response, and when A's preference directly results in B's response and is regarded as the actual influence on B's behavior. However, in anticipated reaction or potential power, B's anticipation is substituted for A's behavior.

The intent of this organizational analysis of power is to look at the differences in power assigned or perceived by the participants, i.e., faculty and administration. This area of study—the theory and measurability of power within organizations—remains a controversial issue. However, faculty members, as participants in colleges of nursing, do believe that they hold power (to a lesser degree) as do others (to a greater degree), who may or may not be in hierarchical positions. Faculty members also share some preferences for organizational

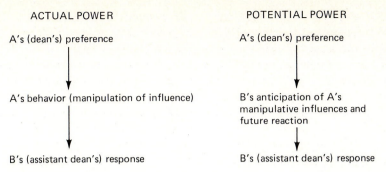

Figure 6-2 Schemation of actual and potential power and manipulative behavior.

choices, and they understand the means-ends connections.

Again the literature cites many conflicting theories in decision process versus outcome in establishing models of decision making. Riker (1964:341-349) has identified one major difference among the power theorists for defining the postulated object of power. To differentiate stability and nonstability relative to the object of power, Riker utilized the ego-direct (inner- and other-directed) characterizations. Inner-directed refers to characterizations in which an individual has early incorporated principles which reflect learning from parents and authorities similar to parents. As faculty, these individuals are guilt-directed, but they tend to remain stable even when the reinforcement of social approval is not available. Other-directed refers to characterizations in which the individual responds to a wider circle of persons rather than primarily to parents. As faculty, this grouping is more cosmopolitan, lacks the inner capacity to go it alone, and responds poorly to diffuse anxiety. Both inner- and other-directed individuals are known to use manipulative behaviors in order to cope with their environment.

In translating these concepts to power relationships, Riker has identified ego-oriented power as that in which the object is to increase utility for ego (1964:341-349). It is essentially indifferent to others as long as ego wins. Power is measured as a chance to occupy a uniquely valuable position

in the process by which one makes final choices in outcomes.

For other-oriented power, the object is to decrease another's utility. In other words, power is measured as the ability to force others to do what one wishes. However, the theoretical difference is not so much related to manipulating people and outcomes as it is to determining whether or not power always exists. Riker contends that power *always* exists and that ego-oriented structures preserve power and are stable systems for the study of power (1964:341-349).

Ebert and Mitchell (1975) have clearly stated that an individual's power can be conceptualized as a function of the types of organizational choices mediated. They have also demonstrated that a wide variety of effective outcomes, rather than traditional rewards and punishments, comprise power bases. High-powered individuals are frequently liked, communicated with, listened to, and modeled. The general bases of informal power arise primarily from unique personal characteristics of the individual or from his or her location or position within the organization. The decision-maker, who needs compliance of others in decision making or who needs to influence the decisions of others, has a wide variety of outcomes as options. Decision choices can be more effectively determined when environmental factors and social group influences are not opposed to the decision-maker's goals.

Enderud also concluded that faculty members

with formal status talk a lot, belong to committees, and feel that they are close to the action (1976: 395). These persons are generally perceived as powerful. Interestingly enough, those members who are relatively dissatisfied with organizational decision outcomes tend to be the most active and are subsequently viewed as the most powerful.

For years controversy has existed over studies of power because measurement techniques emphasized outcomes which contained manipulative elements. Was the element being manipulated the outcome or the individual? Rational-choice theory clearly denotes that bargaining, negotiating, and choice making are based on the assumption that participants will use all strategic possibilities open to them in the best and most productive way. This includes manipulation—both overt and covert. Therefore, beliefs about power and influence may best be understood by observing the process of organizational decision—how the choice is made—rather than by observing the outcome. Essentially, this is the position held in the study of anarchic organizations.

MANIPULATION IN DECISION CHOICE (MACHIAVELLIANISM)

The theory of organized anarchies suggests that choice opportunity is one in which there is permeability of solutions, problems, and participants who move in and out and that the energy of the participants is directed toward choosing. The major effect of increased participation by certain teachers within colleges of nursing will certainly be to increase their competence, power, and experience in dealing with problems. This competence serves as a mechanism for including some teachers more frequently in organizational choice—and limiting access by others. Such participation actions are one form of manipulation commonly experienced by faculties of all kinds, including those in schools of nursing.

When power is used in this context, it is defined as a purposeful, directional force in decision making. And Machiavellianism is defined as one form

of manipulation and referred to as an individual's manipulative orientation via Machiavellianism (Ezell, 1977). Much work in the biological and social sciences has involved means-ends as a method of causal experience—hence, direct or indirect manipulation. However, manipulation, in the sense of Machiavellianism, in most circles of society is characterized by overtones of illegal power and immorality, evoking puppetlike actions from others.

Christie and Geis (1970) speculated that in the early 70s individual orientations to manipulating others and Machiavellianism (Machs) were visibly increasing in society. Numerous research studies have shown that manipulative behavior is becoming more prevalent (Ezell, 1977; Gold et al., 1976; Whetton, 1971; Gutterman, 1970; Schwendiman, 1971; Gleason et al., 1978). Others have also indicated that Machiavellianism might be an antecedent to effective social control and to individual power within various bureaucratic organizations, including colleges of nursing.

Can manipulative intentions be measured? Christie believed this to be possible (Christie, 1970; Christie and Geis, 1970). Christie developed a scale derived, in part, from excerpts of Machiavelli's *The Prince*. The scale, Mach V, consists of 20 triads of items which derive scores of Machiavellian attitudes and social desirability. Christie and others have demonstrated that people who score high on the scale *do* actually behave in a more manipulative (Machiavellian) fashion than those who score low. Scoring for Machiavellianism is dichotomized into high Machs and low Machs.

To demonstrate individual manipulation orientations, Geis has conducted many studies (1970: 130-160). One study elucidated the bargaining characteristics of individuals. High Machs had an acute opportunistic sense of timing in social situations. Their behavior did not appear to be based upon being sensitive to the needs or wishes of other persons. It appeared more likely to be based upon a construct of acting in a way that works at a given point in time. Certain characteristics in specific situations may facilitate or mask

Table 6-1   High-Mach and Low-Mach Orientations

High machs: The "cool" syndrome	Low machs: The "soft touch"
Resistance to social influence	Susceptibility to social influence
Orientation to cognitions	Orientation to persons
Initiating and controlling structure	Accepting and following structure

Source: Adapted from R. Christie and F. Geis, *Studies in Machiavellianism* (New York: Academic Press, 1970), p. 285.

dispositional differences between high and low Machs. These characteristics surfaced in face-to-face interaction and in latitude for improvisation. The personal characteristics are clustered and account for the differences in outcomes for high and low Machs. (See Table 6-1.)

These characteristics and similar behaviors have also been observed in innovative educators interested in creating organizational change. Some deans and administrative leaders in colleges may be known as "cool," while others are "soft." Both high- and low-Mach administrators may succeed, but the means-ends will differ depending upon the individual administrator's repertoire of knowledge and skill, the situational context and boundaries of the organization, and the interaction of participants, i.e., faculty. Administrators in nursing who use a rational (entrepreneurial) model of decision making know what their preferences are and how to achieve those preferences by utilizing personal power and knowledge of ambiguity within the school.

Another important feature of successful manipulation and high Machs is their ability to put on whatever "face" is necessary during an encounter (Miles, 1975). The low Machs will become distant and alienate themselves from interaction because of emotional commitment and personal identity concerns. Low Machs will generally withdraw when demands on their identity are unsettling; they have less ability to manipulate because of their insensitivity to situational subtleties. High Machs, by comparison, demonstrate that all public behavior—deference, flattery, ingratiation, dependence, freedom allowed to others—is consistent with their definition of teamwork.

This analysis of high Machs coincides with other data which indicate that high Machs are not easily caught at manipulation. They are not necessarily more competitive, but they have a wide repertoire of interpersonal strategies available for quick recourse and can organize and exploit whatever organizational resources are available. At least, they do this better than low Machs. The advantage that high Machs have in manipulating others is that they appear to be more accurate in their interpretation of vulnerable characteristics in other participants. Low Machs tend to permit themselves to be overrun and outmaneuvered by high Machs. Low Machs persistently cling to idealistic interpretations of how people should behave.

Figure 6-3 demonstrates the clustering effect of Machiavellian participant behaviors, the organizational setting, and the social interactions which result from such combinations. The Machiavellian or manipulative orientations of leaders and non-leaders, especially in high-Mach behavior, can significantly impact upon already organizing anarchies. Organized anarchies must be administered by new and innovative theories, theories which will be able to handle ambiguous goals, unclear technology, and fluid participation of faculty. All of these factors combined will help to point out the limitations of participant behavior in rational choice in organizations and will begin to call into question the interplay of behavior and self-interest. It is through understanding appropriate means-ends that organizational life in colleges of nursing can be understood.

Christensen concludes that faculty in organized anarchies (1) are primarily concerned with the decision process rather than with the decision

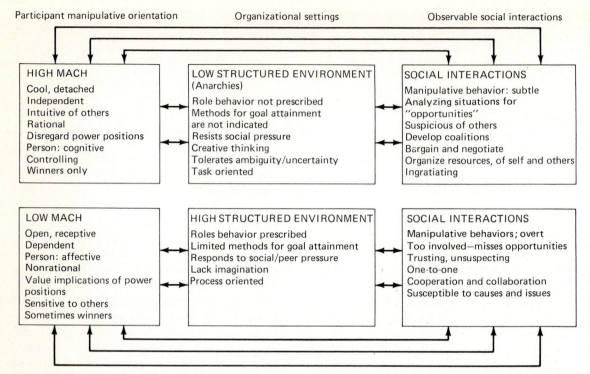

Figure 6-3 Schemata of organized anarchy.

outcome; (2) are concerned that the collective decisions which are implemented involve active collaboration of bureaucrats (deans and administrative types); (3) are fearful that the particular combination of participant (faculty) energy and attention for a particular decision will most likely not be sustained; and (4) are quick to provide other problems and solutions (new crisis) to absorb the attention of the organization (1976: 378). Any of these four factors can contribute to disparities between the decision and its implementation. However, the flow of participants (faculty and administrators) often becomes so fluid that distrust and loss of integration result, enhancing anarchic behavior.

MANIPULATIVE ADMINISTRATIVE BEHAVIOR AND CONSTRUCTIVE TACTICS

Cohen and March declare that a pervasive egalitarian ideology contributes to making status (dean or department chair) a scarce organizational resource in places like universities (1976:204). The dean and other administrative officials have more power than others, but the power is often placed in a rigid controversial managerial world. Still, focusing on beliefs about power is important and necessary in order to understand participant reports on power distribution, actual and perceived. Therefore, some administrators, including those in colleges of nursing, have resorted to common manipulative management strategies. Dyer (1976: 129-134) acknowledges that leadership strategies developed over the years may be interpreted as "ways of getting people to do what you want them to do!" Dyer (1976:129-134) suggests the following manipulative typology:

The Illusionary Democratic Participant: The leader presents the problem, cites the parameters, and suggests some solutions to the problem. The committee is supposed to derive the decision choice—when more than likely it is already nearly implemented.

The Benevolent Autocrat: The leader becomes the "wise one," or at least the "most wise." Decisions are made and announced.

The Pseudo Family: The leader is concerned about group identity versus integration. Feelings of intimacy, whether relevant or not, are fostered to assist group work. Essentially the leader is able to "sell" ideas to the group.

The Managerial Facade: The leader feels out the situation and the decision climate. The leader organizes a group of allies, presents the problem and solution, and gets a group consensus.

The Phony Proposer: Using a tactic in which the "motions" of participative management are performed, the leader often forces decisions by asking for a vote on one of two favorable alternatives.

The Public Praiser: The leader gives abundant praise to coworkers, even though he or she has often made the decision, asked for suggestions, and then implemented what was first intended.

The Impotent Committee: The leader assigns decision work to committees for choice action. All of the choices are then routed through an "executive committee." The committee is given too short a time frame or is simply designated as only a recommending body.

Dyer concludes that there is a *guise* of participation. Hence, colleges of nursing and other institutions become more anarchic as participants move in and out of decision-making opportunities and are limited by the amount of time and energy they are able to devote. Dyer also states that "as opposed to the autocratic leader who apparently has certain needs to dominate, the Machiavellian is an unabashed manipulator of superb expertise" (1976:134).

What can faculty and administrators of colleges of nursing do to cope with the anarchic organization? There are several things. First, faculty—all participants—must understand the events that produce anarchy (ambiguous goals, unclear technology, and fluid participation). These conditions are present in all colleges and universities. The organizations of nursing are environments which

support multiple goal attachments, a permissive atmosphere for creative thinking, and participant behavior loosely prescribed.

Second, the faculty must accept the fact that some people enjoy being in anarchic organizations. Most participants in organized anarchies are members because they perform best in ambiguous settings. Our colleges are full of high and low Machs.

Faculty members can analyze organizational choice in their own particular colleges, looking for the formal power and noticing decision opportunities. Typically, university decision making will be describable in terms of the "garbage can" decision process. Often neither the beginning nor the end of the process will be well-defined. Decisions that have been made will be changed, and exactly when decisions are settled will be quite hazy. Such analysis will lead to understanding and hopefully will prevent resentment and anger.

For administrators of colleges, Weiner advocates some tactical strategies:

1 Distract the opposition. Since participants (faculty) have limited attention and energy, assign opponents to work on issues that have competing elements. If no such issues are under debate, create one. This tactic absorbs the energy of enemies in a creative and productive fashion.

2 Be selective in your ambition. Participants in organized anarchies should limit the number of decision choices under consideration at any point in time. There are limits to the time and energy of opponents and allies alike.

3 Impose deadlines judiciously. Care must be taken so that all sides of an issue can be heard. Committees and task forces should contain both opponents and allies. Since participation depends on energy and time, extend or relax deadlines that have been created. If you are not able to create deadlines, seek the cooperation of others; use external sources, e.g., vice presidents, the university senate, etc.

4 Use friends in the organization (environment) as a resource. Advisory committees of insiders and outsiders can be helpful in expanding the ranks of allies for decision making. In an orga-

nized anarchy that is overloaded with problems, the significance of formal position for the outcome of decisions is depressed (1976:248-249).

Another novel tactic called "protest absorption," has been proposed by Leeds (1964:115-135). Protest absorption has been prescribed in those organizational situations where there are a number of participants who are considered recalcitrant, nonconformist, or anarchic. Such groups may be able to contribute to the goals of the organization, so a structural approach is used to legitimatize a subunit. The process could take a year or several years to accomplish. Organizational structural changes are made to legitimatize the authority and power of some of the anarchic participants. Generally these anarchic individuals or groups are led by a charismatic leader with strong loyalties to the anarchist leader.

Most of Leed's work on protest absorption has been done on military and religious groups. However, the appropriateness for nursing is striking, since the profession of nursing has evolved from both the military and the church. These nonconformists (anarchists) do not hide their disagreement with the prevailing norms. All activities are open; they are simply nonconforming and in opposition to the majority. Leeds advocates protest absorption over condemnation, avoidance, or expulsion from the organization.

During protest absorption processes, which are lengthy, internal battles involving several levels of hierarchy will erupt. Anarchists typically oppose those persons who are their immediate supervisors. Administrators will find that closing communications with the charismatic leader and the hierarchy, restricting members' movements, and reducing resources will create an even more enthusiastic and cohesive group. As is generally known, when barriers are raised via regular channels, the anarchist leader will develop his own route to the top, either directly or through an intermediary or perhaps by personal attractiveness and Machiavellianism tactics (Singer, 1964: 128-150).

Administratively, protest absorption can be evaluated as successful when the top hierarchy recognizes the anarchists and directs communications back to the appropriate administrative position. The anarchy group must then agree to certain organization stabilizers—rules of behavior—both within the new subunit and within the organization as a whole. The anarchist activities are hence limited to the specific organizational unit and will continue to support the organizational goals. Therefore, from the perspective of top administration, the anarchist group has been encapsulated.

Finally, administrators may control anarchists by using joint decision making as a form of socialization. Through these efforts, careful attention can be given to different decision choice opportunities and appropriate behaviors associated with them—e.g., negotiation, co-optation, cooperation, compromise, collaboration, and bargaining. Discussion process should be separated from decision outcome, since process is the way organizations, including colleges of nursing, interpret and reinterpret their goals. Procedures can be established to identify and clarify the varied ideologies and beliefs about the technology of nursing education. Then, a plan can be developed to communicate their preferences as participants in nursing organizations. During this time, manipulative participant behaviors, whether high Mach or low Mach, can be openly identified, acknowledged, and used as organizational assets rather than liabilities. These efforts of organizational learning may decrease ambiguity and organizational uncertainty.

SUMMARY

Nursing schools as educational organizations have historically been understudied. Additionally, few nursing leaders (Chaska, 1979; Leininger, 1974; Torres, 1981) have been courageous enough to look at nursing from within—to analyze what nursing organizations are, what they do, and what they wish to be.

This chapter has been written to support a "new view," one which specifically analyzes nursing educational organizations of today as anarchic organizations.

Nursing leaders and nonleaders alike need to be encouraged to study the bureaucracy of higher education and to review critically organizational choice theory as one strategy of decision making. Even Cohen et al. are careful to cite limitations of organizational choice, and yet they request that critical thinkers look at the

systematic interrrelatedness of organizational phenomena which are familiar, even common, but which have previously been regarded as isolated and pathological. Measured against a conventional normative model of rational choice, the garbage can process does seem pathological, but such standards are not appropriate. (1972:16)

Christensen also reminds us that "we should make note of the one thing that might easily become lost. During the ritual and struggle for meaning, the school [college of nursing] went on. There was a program, and it changed from time to time. Students went to school and met teachers (faculty). The world neither collapsed nor stayed constant" (1976:384). Colleges of nursing will endure in spite of the ambiguity and uncertainty that is present in the organization.

By acknowledging our participation in an anarchic organization, teachers, who are predominently females, will become more familiar with their participation in revolutionizing organizations like colleges and universities. Faculty members as participants can be prepared for evolutionary action, be aware of a revolutionary consciousness, be cognizant of Machiavellian manipulative skills of leaders and nonleaders, and be ready to use these forces to improve nursing educational organizations during the 80s.

EDITOR'S QUESTIONS FOR DISCUSSION

How applicable is Ezell's description of organized anarchies to colleges of nursing? What factors are essential for organized anarchy? What assumptions are frequently made in analyzing organizations? Is there evidence for validating these assumptions? What interrelationships exist between the three decision-making behavior models described and organized anarchies? How do the six criteria described by Ezell interact with the three models of decision-making behavior? Justify the extent to which you perceive colleges of nursing reflect "garbage can" decision making. Are there other factors not indicated by Ezell which may contribute to "garbage can" decision making and anarchy in colleges of nursing? To what extent do you agree with Ezell's classification of faculty and participation in decision making? Identify examples in colleges of nursing of each combination of faculty participation in decision making.

What patterns of faculty and administrative behavior may be unique to colleges of nursing? What patterns may be common to other educational institutions? To what extent can the concepts of anarchy and Machiavellian behavior be applied to service settings? Are there factors inherent in one type of setting versus another that more likely promote anarchy and manipulative behavior?

How applicable is Ezell's organizational analysis of power to colleges of nursing? What effect can ego (inner directed) persons in administrative positions have on faculty in power relationships? In Ezell's description of power could both inner- and other-directed individuals use power primarily to serve ego needs rather than for altruistic reasons? Are there inconsistencies in the description of the characteristics of high and low Machs? Can Ezell's description of ego (inner and other directed) persons be compared with characteristics of high- and low-Mach individuals? What variables are not accounted for in the measurement of manipulative intentions?

Can characteristics be identified in potential administrators that may indicate a disposition to develop specific manipulative orientations? To what extent do you perceive specific situations facilitating the development of a particular manipulative orientation versus basic personal characteristics? Can manipulation be considered a positive effective behavior? Under what conditions is manipulation a negative behavior? What ethical issues are involved with utilizing manipulation? Do you agree with Ezell that faculty members enjoy being in anarchic organizations? What alternatives can you suggest for controlling anarchy in academia?

REFERENCES

Alker, H. and P. Popper
1973 "Personality and ideology in university students." Journal of Personality 41 (4):653–671.

Becker, G.
1965 "A theory of the allocation of time." The Economic Journal 75:493–519.

Berlin, I.
1971 "The question of Machiavelli." The New York Review of Books 27(7):20–32.

Chaska, N.
1979 "The 'cooling out' process in a complex organization." Journal of Nursing Administration 9(1): 22–28.

Christensen, S.
1976 "Decision making and socialization." Pp. 351–385 in J. March and J. Olsen (eds.), Ambiguity and Choice in Organizations. Bergen, Norway: University Press.

Christie, R.
1970 "The Machiavellians among us." Psychology Today, November: 82–85.

Christie, R. and F. Geis
1970 Studies in Machiavellianism. New York: Academic Press.

Clark, B.
1977 "Faculty organization and authority." Pp. 64–78 in G. Riley and U. Baldridge (eds.), Governing Academic Organizations. Berkeley: McCutchan.

Cohen, M. and J. March
1976 "Decision, residents, and status." Pp. 174–205 in J. March and J. Olsen (eds.), Ambiguity and Choice in Organizations. Bergen, Norway: University Press.

Cohen, M., J. March, and J. Olsen
1972 "A garbage can model of organizational choice." Administrative Science Quarterly 17(1):1–18.
1976 "People, problems, solutions and the ambiguity of relevance." Pp. 24–37 in J. March and J. Olsen (eds.), Ambiguity and Choice in Organizations. Bergen, Norway: University Press.

Cyert, R. M. and J. March
1963 A Behavioral Theory of the Firm. Englewood Cliffs, N.J.: Prentice-Hall.

Dyer, W.
1976 Insight to Impact: Strategies For Interpersonal and Organizational change. Provo, Utah: Brigham Young University Press.

Ebert, R. and T. Mitchell
1975 Organizational Decision Process. New York: Crane, Russak.

Enderud, H.
1976 "The perception of power." Pp. 386–396 in J. March and J. Olsen (eds.), Ambiguity and Choice in Organizations. Bergen, Norway: University Press.

Ezell, A.
1977 "Power, via Machiavellianism in educational decision-making: A study of selected educators, state officials and lobbyists in the 1975 Nevada legislative session." Unpublished doctoral dissertation. Provo, Utah: Brigham Young University. (University Microfilms order no. 77-17, 624; Dissertation Abstracts International 38/Z-A, 566.)

Geis, F.
1970 "Bargaining tactics in the con game."
Pp. 130–160 in R. Christie and F. Geis
(eds.), Studies in Machiavellianism. New
York: Academic Press.
Gleason, J., F. J. Seaman, and E. P. Hollander
1978 "Emergent leadership processes as a function of task structure and Machiavellianism." Social Behavior and Personality
6(1):33–36.
Gold, A. R., R. Christie, and L. N. Freedman
1976 Fists and Flowers. New York: Academic
Press.
Gutterman, S.
1970 The Machiavellians: A Social Psychological Study of Moral Character and Organizational Milieu. Lincoln: University of
Nebraska Press.
Kamen, D.
1977 "Legitimating myths and educational
organization: The relationship between
organizational ideology and formal structure." American Sociological Review
42:208–219.
Kerr, C.
1963 The Uses of the University. Cambridge,
Mass.: Harvard University Press.
Leeds, R.
1964 "The absorption of protest: A working
paper." Pp. 115–135 in W. W. Cooper,
H. J. Leavitt, and M. W. Shelley II (eds.),
New Perspective in Organizational Research. New York: Wiley.
Leininger, M.
1974 "The leadership crisis in nursing: A
critical problem and challenge." The
Journal of Nursing Administration 4(2):
28–34.
Loye, D.
1977 The Leadership Passion: A Psychology
of Ideology. San Francisco: Jossey-Bass.
Machiavelli, N.
1947 The Prince. T. Bergin (trans.) Northbrook,
Ill.: AHM.
March, J. and J. Olsen
1976a Ambiguity and Choice in Organizations.
Bergen, Norway: University Press.
1976b "Organizational choice under ambiguity."
Pp. 10–23 in J. March and J. Olsen (eds.),
Ambiguity and Choice in Organizations.
Bergen, Norway: University Press.
1976c "Attention and the ambiguity of self-
interest." Pp. 38–53 in J. March and J.
Olsen (eds.), Ambiguity and Choice in
Organizations. Bergen, Norway: University
Press.
March, J. and P. J. Romelaër
1976 "Positions and presence in the draft of
decisions." Pp. 251–276 in J. March
and J. Olsen (eds.), Ambiguity and Choice
in Organizations. Bergen, Norway: University Press.
March, J. and H. Simon
1958 Organizations. New York: Wiley.
Miles, R.
1975 Theories of Management: Implications
for Organizational Behavior and Development. St. Louis: McGraw-Hill.
Nagel, J.
1975 The Descriptive Analysis of Power. New
Haven: Yale University Press.
Olsen, J.
1976a "Choice in an organized anarchy." Pp.
82–139 in J. March and J. Olsen (eds.),
Ambiguity and Choice in Organizations.
Bergen, Norway: University Press.
1976b "University governance: Non-participation
as exclusion or choice." Pp. 277–313 in
J. March and J. Olsen (eds.), Ambiguity
and Choice in Organizations. Bergen,
Norway: University Press.
Riker, W.
1964 "Some ambiguities in the notion of
power." American Political Science Review 58:341–349.
Sanger, S. and Henry Alker
1972 "Dimensions of internal-external locus of
control and the women's liberation movement." Journal of Social Issues 28(4):
115–129.
Schwendiman, G.
1971 "Machiavellianism as a predictor of success in bargaining under high/low incentive conditions." Unpublished doctoral
dissertation. Provo, Utah: Brigham Young
University. (University Microfilms order
no. 71-12,110; Dissertation Abstracts
International 31/11-B, 6881.)

Singer, J.
 1964 "The use of manipulative strategies: Machiavellianism and attractiveness." Sociometry 27(2):128–150.
Sproul, L., S. Weiner, and D. Wolf
 1978 Organizing an Anarchy: Belief, Bureaucracy and Politics in the National Institute of Education. Chicago: University of Chicago Press.
Torres, Gertrude
 1981 "The nursing education administrator: Accountable, vulnerable, and oppressed" Advances in Nursing Science 3(3):1–15.
Turner, Colin
 1977 "Organizing educational institutions as anarchies." Educational Administration 5(2):6–12.

Weick, K.
 1976 "Educational organizations as loosely coupled systems." Administrative Science Quarterly 21:1–19.
Weiner, S. S.
 1976 "Participation, deadlines, and choice." Pp. 225–250 in J. March and J. Olsen (eds.), Ambiguity and Choice in Organizations. Bergen, Norway: University Press.
Whetton, D.
 1971 "The effect of human relations training on the Machiavellian personality." Unpublished master's thesis, Brigham Young University.

Chapter 7

Overview of Issues in Nursing Education

Carol J. Willts Peterson, R.N., Ph.D., F.A.A.N.
Dean and Professor
College of Nursing
South Dakota State University
Brookings, South Dakota

Carol J. Peterson presents a significant challenge to nursing education. She poses extensive, insightful questions and issues which direly need to be resolved. Her chapter can be viewed as a prime introduction to the following chapters in this section which focus more in depth on some of the numerous queries Peterson presents. Peterson reviews trends — such as consumer awareness of health care, increasing costs and an aging population, and emphasis on wellness — and identifies health care needs. She examines the implications of health care trends and issues for nursing education. Curriculum design for quality and relevance is emphasized. She states that nursing programs seem obsessed with curriculum revision, rigid implementations of behavioral objectives, and strict ideas about ratios, assignments, and hours. Peterson indicates that this presents problems of relevance in learning and contributes to the education of products with a fractionalized view of nursing practice.

Peterson highlights serious implications for the profession and nursing education related to decreased enrollments, the critical shortage of nurses, decreased funding, the entry into practice question, new pressures impinging on faculty, and competition for academically qualified faculty. She cites the threats to control in practice and in academia as a salient issue of the profession. Peterson challenges the reader to contrast the disparities in nursing education and nursing practice in a unique manner. Finally, in spite of the documented problems, Peterson acknowledges that few professions have shown such dramatic rapid building in their evolution as nursing.

INTRODUCTION

This chapter is intended to be a broad survey of issues in nursing education. No one issue is covered in depth; rather a framework of issues and questions is provided. The reader may find some of the issues treated in greater detail in other individual chapters. Hopefully other issues introduced will stimulate readers to do their own in-depth study. Issues will be presented under these major headings:

Impact of future health care on nursing education

Curriculum design for quality and relevance

Students of the 1980s and 1990s
Delivery of instruction and programs
Politics, power, dynamics
Faculty of the future
Preparation for leadership

IMPACT OF FUTURE HEALTH CARE
ON NURSING EDUCATION

An active observer of nursing and the health care scene the past few years would likely concur with these trends or issues in health care.

1 There is an increasing dissatisfaction with the current health care system, its high cost, unequal access, and its emphasis on disease and cure.

2 Consumer awareness and activism are marked by a growing scrutiny of the system and the practitioners within the system. In particular, the medical profession no longer enjoys the unquestioned, uncontrolled, and lauded dominance over the health care of increasingly knowledgeable persons.

3 The costs of health care must be controlled. The pressures to contain costs will continue, particularly in view of the need to increase access without having cost become a disrupting, potentially bankrupting national concern.

4 There is increasing awareness of the need for and activism to establish a preventive health theme in our society and to promote health. This is evidenced by movements within some professions, priorities in federal legislation, consumer movements, and the establishment of health education promotion centers. The recent themes *wellness* and *patient self-activation* particularly imply this trend in its popular sense.

5 Some form of national health care insurance is inevitable. The philosophical developments of recent years within our society, particularly embodied in the concepts that health care is a basic right and that there must be reasonable access for all persons, make this a humanitarian and political necessity.

Given these trends, what are some of the continuing health care needs in our society? Again the active observer and reader of the past decade would probably agree with these points as some of the major ones.

1 There continues to be, in spite of legislative priorities in recent programs, professional movements, and widespread publicity on the matter, maldistribution of health care professionals and the services they deliver. Access to health care, particularly primary care, is still a serious problem for some persons in our society.

2 Certain illnesses related to high-risk factors and the level of our societal and industrial development will continue. Problems associated with cardiovascular stress, injuries, overweight, pollution, and substances in the internal and external environment whose effects on the body are not immediately known are among these. New or altered forms of infectious diseases may be on the increase. Some observers would say our lax attitude about old contagious diseases may result in renewed problems.

3 Our aging population is already a serious health care concern in some communities. It will become increasingly so as the national percentage of persons over 65 continues to rise in the next few decades.

4 The potential psychopathology and physiopathology related to changing family and community patterns are still not clearly known to us. At times we seem totally oblivious to them as we anticipate current and future health problems.

What are the implications of these trends and issues for nursing education? Examination of curriculum materials from a sample of nursing programs at various levels would likely reveal acknowledgment of these trends and issues and more. But do our curricula really incorporate these so that graduates are being impacted?

The pressures on nursing programs place them in a quandary. The nursing profession and various elements within the health care scene philosophize about health promotion, yet disease and cure dominate agencies and delivery mechanisms. Baccalaureate degree nursing programs in particular are attempting to place more emphasis on prevention, primary care, and health promotion. While some policy makers and employers laud this, others criticize sharply the product of such programs because they are less oriented toward secondary and tertiary care in traditional hospital scenes.

Part of the solution rests with clearer definition of care settings and a coordinated educational system. This has been well explained in the work of the Southern Regional Educational Board (SREB, 1976) and by the Department of Health, Education, and Welfare (U.S. DHEW, 1976). In particular the definitions of primary, secondary, and tertiary care provided by these sources are helpful. Primary care refers to the point of entry into the health care system and emphasizes health promotion and prevention of disease. In contrast, secondary and tertiary care focus on persons in the system with either fairly clearly specified, common problems (secondary care) or the more complex or complicated needs requiring special (tertiary) care. The work of the SREB then meshes a nursing education system with these definitions, suggesting the type of care that would be emphasized within different levels of nursing education.

The problem continues to be one of implementation of such concepts. Struggling within the dilemma of the entry into practice issue, the various types of programs seem fearful of implementing a focused system such as that suggested in the SREB reports. A candid critique of nursing programs suggests that graduate programs do not consistently capture in depth the primary care or tertiary care foci that seem appropriate. Many baccalaureate degree programs give lip service to primary care, yet are disappointingly burdened with traditional disease content. Further, as associate degree and diploma programs confront the entry-into-practice issue, one often sees them inappropriately include community primary care experiences to emulate the so-called professional curricula.

In addition to this matter of focus on health rather than illness, a number of questions about nursing education as it relates to trends and issues in health care delivery come to mind.

1 Nursing is logically and historically suited to respond to the increasing demands for access, primary care, and economical service. Will it do so with a unified response or will the internal struggles in the profession disable it to the point of missing this challenge of the 1980s?

2 The nurse-practitioner movement seems to hold much potential for nursing to make the necessary response to the trends and issues outlined above. Yet nursing's expanding role is being actively fought by the medical profession. Will nursing education, through its preparation of advanced practitioners of primary care, succeed in impacting health care as this potential implies?

3 Although nursing education is meeting some of the special needs of the elderly, are the new graduates really interested in the care of this segment of our population? Employment patterns of new graduates and nursing home staffing needs would suggest that very limited progress is being made in this area. What are the barriers to motivating nurses to meet the challenges of the elderly population?

CURRICULUM DESIGN FOR QUALITY AND RELEVANCE

Nursing curriculum development during the past several decades has been marked by several distinct trends.

1 Movement away from blocked curricula to ones with integration of content around broad themes or threads.

2 General progression away from the medical, systems model to a conceptual, nursing-care-process model.

3 Development of curricula based on conceptual models. More recent developments are beginning to include emphasis on better developed theories as the basis for curriculum, including the emphasis on testing frameworks used by faculty and students.

4 Increased emphasis, particularly in baccalaureate and graduate curricula, on the research process and use of research findings in planning care.

5 Inclusion of themes such as standards of

care, care planning, and quality assurance within undergraduate professional curricula.

6 Derivation of curricula from a detailed framework of goals and objectives.

7 Implementation of the academic model of the laboratory in the clinical component of the curriculum.

8 Increased use of the techniques and strategies of individualized and independent instruction.

Curriculum design: What impact does it have on the graduate's practice? The design of integrated curricula around carefully explicated conceptual frameworks has produced some ideal models from a curriculum point of view. Few professions can claim similar expertise in the application of curriculum theory itself to program development and design. This writer would classify nursing as the leader in that respect.

But the questions and concerns continue. Some critics of nursing education complain that the graduates of these programs are not competent. The criticism is that students' exposure to an integrated program with a process orientation does not prepare them for the real world of work. Because of the traditional framework of licensing examinations, concern about state board performance also enters into such arguments about curriculum design. Questions related to this issue and others cited above are:

1 What problems do specialty-oriented faculty have teaching in an integrated curriculum?

2 Have some integrated curricula that call heavily upon conceptual models from other disciplines lost a nursing focus?

3 Do the most sophisticated curriculum designs based on conceptual models adequately blend content on health and illness? Do they assure adequate competence of the graduate to reduce the level of reality shock experienced upon graduation?

4 Have nursing curricula that heavily use behavioral objectives fractionalized the content-science of nursing to the point that students fail to synthesize the essence of nursing knowledge and practice?

5 Is today's model of clinical laboratory viable? Or does it, too, fractionalize the experiential learning to the point that a true picture of nursing practice in its totality is not gained by the student? One can speculate that this then contributes to reality shock for the new graduate.

STUDENTS OF THE 1980s AND 1990s

Nursing, too, will experience the national decline in numbers of college-age students. Projections of general enrollments in higher education across the country for the next several decades are down dramatically. These forecasts are relatively accurate, influenced only by shifts of population in the country and by increases of nontraditional, older students into the higher education arena.

Recent statistics published by the National League for Nursing seem to already illustrate this trend. Overall enrollments in schools of nursing preparing persons for R.N. licensure declined 1.9 percent from October 1978 to October 1979 (NLN, 1980). What important questions and/or factors relate to this issue?

1 College-bound females have many more professions open to them now. This factor is and will continue to affect the attractiveness of nursing to talented female students.

2 The dilemmas within the profession such as low salaries, entry into practice, collective bargaining, power conflicts with medicine and hospital management, control of practice in the expanded role, and the high incidence of burnout among nurses are becoming more widely publicized and known to the general public. What impact will this have on enrollments in nursing education?

3 In the face of a continuing critical shortage of nurses, the declines in enrollments pose serious threats to the profession. At a time of vulnerability, issues such as these seem to appear again:

   a Pressure to sustain or reopen weak diploma programs in nursing, thus delaying nursing's steady movement into the higher education mainstream

   b Arguments against the requirement for a two-level system

    c Increased agitation by health care agencies and hospital administration for institutional licensure

    d Training and certification of new types of auxiliary personnel to meet critical shortages for professional practitioners

    e Increased political pressures to reduce the control of the profession from within and increased controls on nursing from legislation and management

What other than a decrease in students can we expect in the next several decades?

• Faculty and programs will need to continue to place emphasis on the recruitment and retention of minority persons. Although some progress has been made in this area the past decade, the profession is still dominated primarily by white middle-class females. Ethnic persons of color, males, and older students still make up a small minority in the total picture of enrollments and graduation.

• More adult nontraditional students will appear on the scene. Some of these will be first career seekers; others will be persons already established in one field seeking a new or complementary career through nursing. How do curricula and methods need to be adapted to meet his group's needs?

• Assuming that economic conditions and power and influence of positions can be improved in the profession, nursing has the potential of attracting a greater share of the highly talented, motivated students.

• Students will be increasingly demanding of relevance and adequacy of role modeling in their programs. Increased sophistication about the cost of education, the job market, and the potential for reality shock will make students increasingly concerned about clinical competence and relevance. Faculty members can expect to feel this pressure from students to a greater extent than now.

A strong student force for which nursing education must prepare more realistically is the educational mobilist. While there continues to be much overt argumentation about the entry-into-practice issue, there is growing covert movement for resolution of this matter. Nurses at all levels are increasingly sensitive to the pressures for more preparation. Licensed practical nurses will be seeking the associate degree level in greater numbers and nondegree R.N.s will be a growing force to contend with in the baccalaureate arena. These students are increasingly vocal and capable of exerting pressure on the educational system for relevant, reasonable, accessible upward mobility programs. If nursing education programs do not respond to this force, particularly in a time of decreased generic enrollments and critical nursing shortages, they will miss the greatest opportunity of the century to further along the resolution of the entry-into-practice question.

DELIVERY OF INSTRUCTION AND PROGRAMS

One must speculate why it is that nurse educators adopt new trends and themes in curriculum and instruction and become such zealous perpetuators of these. At times this occurs to the extent that the trend or innovation loses all flexibility and becomes a structure or barrier that fosters a continuing rigid system of education. Is it related to nurse educators' own educational backgrounds? How is it perpetuated within the profession and through educational and service agencies?

In view of the above observation, a critical review of nursing education in the past decade leads one to express these concerns.

1 Nursing programs seem obsessed with curriculum revision. Curricula are constantly being revised, funding for large curriculum revision projects is sought, curriculum revision coordinators are named, and deans and directors seek extra internal funds to release faculty to work on curriculum matters. This writer knows of no other health profession characterized by this ongoing, zealous curriculum development. From a curriculum theory and development point of view nurse-educators have developed model programs. However, what impact does this continual emphasis on curriculum revision have on students, budgets, relevance, faculty satisfaction, and retention?

2 Nursing education has adopted the behavioral objective movement in a rather widespread fashion. Some programs are characterized by literally hundreds of very specific behavioral objectives. Faculty members write objectives until the finiteness of the statements borderlines on the ridiculous. Tests are blueprinted religiously according to objectives and items coded according to objectives and cognitive level. This writer believes that this rigid implementation of an educational trend has contributed to the education of products with a fractionalized view of nursing practice.

3 As with behavioral objectives, nursing education has readily become involved in the individualized, modular, self-paced instruction movement. Large funded projects during the late 1960s and 1970s focused on converting curricula to modularized, self-paced approaches. Competency-based instruction and mastery learning were concepts intertwined with these developments. In some instances these approaches have since been abandoned because the methodology became so structured and cumbersome that the espoused potential benefits of the technologies were lost.

4 Strict interpretation of the academic clinical laboratory model has been a by-product of nursing education's movement out of the apprenticeship model and into the academic model. This methodology too has become so structured that it presents problems of relevance. Rigid ideas about ratios, assignments, hours, and student-teacher relationships have at times caused educators to overlook some of the most relevant learning in the clinical setting. Some reconsideration of use of role models, carefully controlled preceptorships, and better integration into the real clinical scene seem urgent at this time to bridge the gap between nursing education and nursing service.

What potential is there for rebirth of certain methodologies in nursing education? Questions relevant here are as follows:

1 How can nursing education use a well-rounded blend of practice laboratory, simulation, closely controlled clinical laboratory, and preceptorships that capitalize on the positive aspects of apprenticeship education?

2 How can multimedia, video and telecommunications be used to reach extended clinical sites and persons needing continuing education and for faculty development? Could generic programs share more human and material resources this way?

3 How can computer technology be more accessible for teaching process and decision making?

4 Can independent study experiences and materials be freed from the heavy structure imposed by some curricula so that they truly contribute to flexible education for growing numbers of nontraditional students?

5 What is the potential for greater use of the cooperative education model in nursing?

POLITICS, POWER, DYNAMICS

Because of the breadth of this section, a review of pertinent questions has been selected as the framework for highlighting the key issues. Questions are raised under these headings: funding for nursing education; resources—new frontiers and limitations; entry into practice; the issue of control in practice and academe; and the great disparities.

1 Funding for Nursing Education

• What is the future of federal funding for nursing education?

• Will future funding sources recognize the priority need for bachelor's degree and master's degree prepared persons?

• What threats are there to nursing programs, particularly at the bachelor's and master's levels, because of their high cost?

• Will nursing research be adequately funded as an integral part of academic nursing?

• How can graduate nursing education be funded to sustain the development of teachers and researchers for the profession?

• Can modern nursing education survive without federal funding?

2 Resources: New Frontiers and Limitations

• How can clinical facilities be used more effectively to reduce the disparity between learning and the real world of practice?

• Will faculty be able to develop creative but sound ways of bridging the gap between nursing service and nursing education?

• As attempts are made to bridge the self-produced gap between nursing education and nursing service, will accrediting agencies allow innovative solutions?

• Can the positive aspects of apprenticeship education and preceptorships be capitalized on to solve the reality shock problem without undermining the quality of nursing education?

• What broadened use of clinical experiences will strengthen even more the community, prevention, primary care skills of the bachelor's or master's prepared persons?

• In times of inflation, shrinking enrollments, and limited funding, will various programs and levels of nursing education be able to work together to maximize resources?

• What threats are there to nursing education related to clinical agencies demanding compensation for the use of their clinical experiences?

3 Entry into Practice

• Opposition and conflict continue to be associated with the overt entry-into-practice question. Yet there are many signs of a covert resolution of the matter as evidenced by prospective students and nurses themselves. How can this be nurtured and maximized? Is the nursing profession making the mistake of "talking to itself" rather than to the prospective student and consumer on this matter?

• What problems are associated with the issue that there are supporters of the master's (M.N.) degree or doctor of nursing (N.D.) degree as the entry points into professional practice rather than the bachelor's degree?

• Will the profession be able to implement both a two-level system and a reasonable mobility system between levels without creating complete disunity within its ranks?

• What responsibility do the two major organizations have for providing more creative leadership to resolve the entry-into-practice question? To what extent will vision overcome vested interests and fear of organizational demise so that the major nursing organizations will work together in the solution rather than in conflict?

• Will the entire profession be "brought along" in resolving this issue? Or should the leadership recognize certain segments of the profession that will not change and that should be ignored rather than be addressed with undue energy and effort? Is it heresy to suggest that perhaps an almost "new profession" has to be created to accomplish the development goals?

4 The Issue of Control: In Practice and Academe

• The hard-earned position of colleges and schools of nursing in academic settings appears to be under attack. Several schools have experienced serious threats to their legitimate autonomy the past several years. Will this continue? Is academic medicine regaining the upper hand where nursing has developed relative autonomy? Will university and college administrators capitulate to these renewed pressures? In what way is this another manifestation of the problems of achieving affirmative action goals for women in higher education in general?

• To what extent is the burnout among nurses associated with increasing industrial-type management perspectives in hospital administration?

• Can one assume that history will prevail? That is, will nurses, like all suppressed, ego-diminished groups, respond with a significant and somewhat violent revolt? Or will societal forces, self-images, and the power of management increase the dominating forces affecting professional nurses?

• Will society's genuine need and demand for more nurses in expanded roles supersede medicine's increased efforts to counter nursing's growing visibility and power in this arena?

• To what extent are hospital administration's and medicine's organized efforts operating to undermine nursing's professional development? How extensively will they fight the entry-into-practice movement?

• What are the long-range implications of re-affirmation of diploma programs by some elements in the hospital industry?

• To what extent will the nursing shortage be misused by medicine and hospital administration to counter nursing's professional evolution, particularly the press for greater preparation for entry into practice?

5 The Great Disparities

As one considers the power and control questions in the previous four subsections, one is reminded about the great disparities in nursing education and in nursing practice. A key question related to the professional evolution of nursing is: Can these be resolved or reconciled some way? Think for a moment about these disparities.

• Contrast the associate degree program in a small rural junior college with the baccalaureate degree program in a large, complex metropolitan university. Consider the differences in faculty, learning experiences, institutional press, and intellectual stimulation.

• Contrast the graduate of a single-focus, somewhat traditional diploma program with that of a baccalaureate graduate in a large university.

• Contrast the relatively experienced bachelor's prepared faculty member in a practical nursing program with his or her doctorally prepared, research-oriented counterpart in a school of nursing in one of the Big Ten universities.

• Contrast the 1950 diploma graduate working in a small 50-bed rural hospital with a recently graduated master's-prepared clinician in a large medical center.

• Contrast the esteem, assertiveness, and independence of the above diploma nurse with a baccalaureate graduate working in a joint practice project in a 500-bed acute care setting.

• Contrast the ideas about nursing education of the 10 best-known nurse educators in the country with the ideas of the average small-town consumer or physician.

The disparities are vivid and one could continue to list many others equally pointed. Confrontation

with them has two sides. One one hand, such disparities emphasize the revolution occurring in this profession. On the other hand they are frightening. All these persons view themselves as involved in or knowledgeable about the nursing profession. The fiber of their thoughts and being is so different that one questions if we are dealing with one or two professions. Can these disparities be reconciled through evolutionary development or do they require a different approach?

FACULTY OF THE FUTURE

In addition to the matter of increased academic preparation, new pressures are impinging upon faculty. As the problems of reality shock and lack of competence to function within the demands of the real world continue to become more intense for new graduates, faculty will feel more pressure from outside agencies and will be compelled to face the disparities between nursing education and demands of nursing service. Related to this is the need to be involved in their own practice and to emerge as better role models and to retain credibility. Continued shortages of qualified faculty, budget austerity leading to greater teaching loads, and decrease in federal support for nursing education are factors countering progress in this area.

In spite of faculty shortages now and in the near future, nursing must also plan for an era of less faculty growth and turnover. The dramatic decreases in higher education enrollment, coupled with greater popularity of other fields for talented women, may affect the internal vitality of some faculties. Lack of resources for creative activities that contribute to personal and professional development, meshed with more stable faculties, will pose a challenge to schools of nursing to keep their faculty vital and current.

Although one must cite the potential problems noted above, the here and now problem continues to be one of achieving adequate leadership and stability in nursing faculties. Deans, directors, and department heads of all sizes and types of nursing programs continue to be plagued with problems such as these:

- Intense competition for doctorally prepared persons for leadership and senior faculty positions
- In some regions, significant competition for master's prepared faculty
- Faculty who have the academic credentials but are obsolete clinically or do not have teaching skills
- High turnover rates in faculties related to job market, career-family conflicts, and problems with professional commitment
- Increasing competition for master's and doctorally prepared persons from service agencies

In spite of the documented problems in faculty availability, continuity, and qualifications, one must praise the nursing faculty of this country who have been engaged in a historic bootstrap-type operation to pull nursing education out of the apprenticeship past into the academic arena of the present. Few professions can show such a rapid dramatic building effort in their evolution toward maturity.

PREPARATION FOR LEADERSHIP

This review of issues in nursing education would not be complete without some mention of the leadership crisis in nursing. Leadership is used here to refer to the characteristics that all professional practitioners must have. It refers to the ability to utilize one's own talents and to encourage and promote the abilities of others so that the needs and goals of the profession are realized. It is not to be confused with the terms *management* and *administration*. Education and socialization for leadership are among our most crucial needs. How do we socialize baccalaureate program students so that they will stand up to the dominance of hospital management and medicine? How can we instill in every student that a lifetime commitment to professional involvement, not just an intermittent involvement in nursing, is crucial if he or she is going to contribute to the viability of this profession? What more can we do to assure that master's prepared clinicians and practitioners can make the changes in health care delivery we believe so important? Other professions have more successfully socialized their products to maintain a level of commitment and involvement that fosters a strong professional community. Nursing's very viability is dependent upon similar accomplishments. The designers of nursing curricula and the faculty of the future are faced with a great challenge indeed.

EDITOR'S QUESTIONS FOR DISCUSSION

What other implications of the health care trends and issues cited by Peterson exist for nursing education? What problems exist in the implementation of current concepts in health care into curriculum? How can one assist faculty in the acceptance and adoption of nursing conceptual frameworks? To what extent can a medical, systems model be reconciled with conceptual, nursing care models in curriculum development? How can the design of integrated curricula around specific nursing conceptual frameworks produce some ideal models for practice?

Should curricula be developed on the basis of a single theory, model, or conceptual framework, or integration of the three? What alternatives are there for nursing education in dealing with decreasing nursing student enrollments and lack of financial support for students?

What can nursing education do concerning the threats posed by Peterson associated with the critical shortage of nurses? What obligation or responsibility does nursing education have in resolving the nursing shortage? How can nursing educators assure relevance and adequacy of role modeling in their programs?

How has the behavioral objective movement in nursing education contributed to the education of students with a fractionalized view of nursing practice? What is the basis for the seeming obsession with curriculum revision? Indicate examples of too much structure in curricula and suggest alternative methodologies. How can nursing education reconcile the issue of clinical agencies requesting compensation for the use of their clinical facilties and experiences?

How can colleges/schools of nursing prevent or deal with the threat to their autonomy? What societal, professional forces and power of management might increase the dominating forces affecting professional nurses? Keeping in mind Williamson's statements in Chap. 5, what strategies and methods can be utilized by faculty to meet and maintain academic standards? How can the issue of hiring or maintaining faculty who possess clinical expertise but not a doctoral degree be effectively faced? How can faculty realistically meet the increasing simultaneous expectations to teach, practice, publish, and conduct research?

REFERENCES

National League for Nursing
   1980   Assuring a Goal-Directed Future for Nursing. Publication No. 52–1814. New York: National League for Nursing.
Southern Regional Educational Board
   1976   S.R.E.B.'s Nursing Curriculum Project: Summary and Recommendations. Atlanta, Georgia: Southern Regional Educational Board.
U.S. Department of Health, Education, and Welfare (HRA)
   1976   Trends Affecting U.S. Health Care System. Publication No. 76-14503. Washington, D.C.: U.S. Government Printing Office

Chapter 8

Conceptual Frameworks of Undergraduate and Graduate Nursing Programs[1]

Dolores Santora, R.N., Ph.D.
Associate Professor and Associate Dean
College of Nursing
Arizona State University
Tempe, Arizona

After Peterson's entreaty for curriculum design of high quality and relevance, this chapter by Dolores Santora is enlightening. According to Santora, no view of a profession can be complete without an examination of its present educational premises. Thus, Santora presents an unique descriptive study of the existing conceptual frameworks used in the curricula of 61 schools of nursing in 36 states that have both a baccalaureate and master's degree program.

First, Santora reviews the background and some issues concerning conceptual frameworks. She discusses the criterion established by NLN in 1972, the belief by educators that conceptual frameworks are essential curricular components to provide rationales for the selection of content in a discipline, the confusion and difficulty for faculty in identifying frames of reference, reviews three conceptual frameworks proposed for nursing education and three studies of the use of conceptual frameworks. Santora clearly defines and differentiates the appropriate use of the terms: "concept," "theoretical," "propositions," "conceptual model," and "framework." Santora's findings indicate six categories by which conceptual frameworks can be classified.

One-third ($N=41$) of the programs had either none or ambiguous conceptual frameworks, while two-thirds utilized adaptation, multiple, systems, or developmental as conceptual frameworks. Adaptation was the most frequent conceptual framework on which programs were based. Although no statistically significant trends were discernible, Santora presents captivating conclusions and implications that may be alarming for professional nursing education programs and the profession.

---

[1] Santora, D., Condensed from Conceptual Frameworks Used in Baccalaureate and Master's Degree Nursing Curricula. League Exchange Publication, no. 126 New York: National League for Nursing, 1980.

The future of any profession or discipline is inextricably woven into its present educational programs since viable educational programs are, of necessity, future-oriented. Thus, no view of a profession is complete without an examination of its present educational premises—an examination which can logically be expected to yield a fascinating glimpse into the future of that profession.

A current curricular problem plaguing educators in baccalaureate and master's degree nursing programs is the selective utilization of content from the various professional and "bio-psycho-socio-cultural" disciplines which contribute to the complex knowledge base of nursing. The problem is compounded, moreover, by the knowledge expansions which have characterized those fields as well as the nursing field itself throughout the third quarter of the twentieth century.

Thus, nursing curricula have tended to become increasingly additive and complex. In 1972, therefore, the National League for Nursing (NLN), as the accrediting agency for all nursing education programs in the United States, added a new criterion measure for evaluating nursing curricula leading to baccalaureate or master's degrees. In essence, the new criterion requires that nursing schools identify the conceptual frameworks of their curricula and that the conceptual frameworks be consistent with the stated philosophy, purposes, and objectives of the program(s) (National League for Nursing, 1972). The main objective of the new requirement for delineation of conceptual frameworks is the belief that conceptual frameworks do, indeed, provide "a systematic ordering of selected facts, concepts, and propositions that direct curriculum work and provide a basis against which to evaluate the curriculum" (Chater, 1975: 431). Conceptual frameworks, therefore, are viewed by educators as essential curricular components which help provide the rationales for the selection of content through the identification of the key concepts in a discipline or profession (King and Brownell, 1966).

As a consequence of the new NLN requirement, nursing educators have been involved in laborious searches to identify and specify their programs' unique conceptual frames of reference. The searches have been difficult and time-consuming for faculty for two main reasons: first, as Kelly (1975:15) has pointed out, "considerable confusion exists over what is meant by 'a conceptual framework'"; second, faced with the magnitude of the knowledge explosion,

faculty feel caught in the nightmarish impasse of how to add more to the curriculum within the constraints imposed by budget, institutional guidelines, student-faculty ratios, and the like. (Chater, 1975:428)

Furthermore, considerable ambiguity surrounds the issue of the types of conceptual frameworks used by professional nursing education programs to organize the knowledge and practice of nursing.

This study, therefore, was designed to identify and classify the existing conceptual frameworks used in the curricula of baccalaureate and master's degree nursing programs in the United States. The study also sought to identify the conceptual elements of the conceptual frameworks and to describe the relationship between baseline demographic variables and the conceptual frameworks of the nursing programs in the study. The following questions were posed:

1 What are the conceptual frameworks used by baccalaureate and master's degree nursing curricula?
2 Which concepts are incorporated into the conceptual frameworks?
3 Are the conceptual frameworks of the baccalaureate and master's degree programs related?
4 Do the conceptual frameworks of the baccalaureate and master's degree nursing programs vary according to enrollment size, faculty size, existence of a university hospital, or year of application for NLN accreditation?

REVIEW OF RELATED LITERATURE

A review of the literature concerning curriculum development reveals that crucial terms are often defined loosely and inconsistently, dictating the need for a more disciplined language based upon "careful and consistent use of technical terminology" (Beauchamp, 1968:58).

An example of such a pivotal curricular term is *concept*, a frequently misused and inappropriately defined term inextricably related to conceptual frameworks. In this study concepts are defined as abstract generalizations based on perceptions about general classes of objects or events which have common attributes (Kaplan, 1964; Hoult, 1969). Weinberg (1970) supported the above definition by pointing out that universality is a feature only of concepts, not ideas, and thus the two terms are not necessarily synonymous as is often found in the literature. Furthermore, Weinberg explained that concepts "have universality only insofar as they are capable of representing indifferently the things of which they are a similitude" (1970:30). Similarly, Kaplan, in a cogent discourse on concepts, pointed out that concepts are impersonal and timeless and serve to "mark out the paths by which we may move most freely in logical space" (1964:52).

Kaplan (1964) also identified several functions of concepts which have relevance for an understanding of conceptual frameworks; for example, he explained that concepts: (1) serve as norms; (2) identify natural classes; (3) contribute to the disclosure of relationships that exist; (4) identify those categories which are more revealing about a subject than any other categorical sets; and (5) bring order to the vast diversity of empirical phenomena, thereby permitting generalizations and comparisons. The latter function is basic to theory development and has led Nye and Berardo to conclude that concepts are "the most important of all sociological research tools" (1966:4).

From a curriculum development perspective, selected, interrelated multidimensional concepts combine to form cohesive, supporting linkages known as *conceptual frameworks*. These unique linkages of concepts into conceptual frameworks possess symbolic values since they represent a form of invisible togetherness which is not obvious

without proper interpretation. Proper interpretation, of course, demands an understanding of the form or structure of conceptual frameworks as well as the functions of those frameworks, for there is a reciprocal relationship between structure and functions (Grava, 1969).

Much of the confusion which exists among higher education faculties in nursing concerning conceptual frameworks may be traced to inconsistent usage of the term and to subsequent misunderstandings concerning the structure and functions of conceptual frameworks. A review of the nursing literature reveals a trend toward more careful usage of the term *conceptual framework*.

Nevertheless, among the gamut of terms misused by authors as being synonymous with conceptual frameworks, the most frequent misuse is that of "theoretical" for "conceptual" and "model" for "framework." "Theoretical" refers to theory, which is a symbolic construction composed of a set of concepts and a set of "systematically interrelated propositions" (Zetterberg, 1965:28). Propositions, in turn, are statements that a relationship exists between two or more objects or events. Zetterberg further explained that

> the saving quality of a theory is to coordinate many methodologically imperfect findings into a rather trustworthy whole in the form of a small number of information-packed sentences or equations. Moreover, some of the bits and pieces coordinated into this trustworthy whole can be . . . far from trivial propositions. (1965: vii–viii)

Thus, theoretical frameworks represent a higher level of abstraction than conceptual frameworks and contain empirically interpretable concepts through the postulation of relationships, descriptions, explanations, or predictions. In addition, these empirically interpretable concepts are "narrowly bounded, specific, and explicitly interrelated" (Fawcett, 1978:19). In contrast, the type of concepts which are generally incorporated into conceptual frameworks are highly abstract and multidimensional.

Distinctions are also evident between "models" and "frameworks" in curriculum usage. Models have value connotations and are used by researchers as being analogous to some aspects of phenomena in order to develop ideas for systematizing relationships in the phenomena observed. However, Phillips observed:

> One of the dangers of dealing with models is that they may be taken literally and come to be treated not as an hypothesis but as the reality itself. Reification of models leads to several different types of errors. If the model is accepted as the reality rather than as a tentative statement about reality, the investigator may be led to close the door on further research. Or he may incorporate in the model factors that are irrelevant to the phenomena under investigation or exclude factors that are important. . . . An important principle in developing models is the clear differentiation between the model and the reality being modeled. (1966:59)

Frameworks, meanwhile, are purely structural devices "for supporting, defining, and enclosing selected parts for a larger cohesive whole" (Chater, 1975:428). Insofar as frameworks provide the matrix by which selected parts are unified, they are, indeed, reality-oriented, thereby providing a further distinction between them and models.

The literature reveals a general consensus regarding the functions of conceptual frameworks despite the fact that, in the approximately 30 years since Tyler (1949) first proposed the need for some type of conceptual frameworks for curriculum development, curriculum theorists have only intermittently pursued exploration of the subject of conceptual frameworks. Taba summarized the general functions of conceptual frameworks for curriculum designs by stating that conceptual frameworks are

> . . . a way of organizing thinking about all matters that are important to curriculum development: what the curriculum consist of, what its important elements are, how these are chosen

and organized, what the sources of curriculum decisions are, and how the information and criteria from these sources are translated into curriculum decisions. (1962:420)

King offered the following list of some functions of conceptual frameworks specifically for nursing:

1 Provides basic structure for the curriculum

2 Provides a system for classifying the knowledge, skills, and values of the field of nursing

3 Provides a way of ordering facts into a system that organizes subject matter into levels of functions in systems

4 Shows relationships in the content essential for nursing (1978:29)

King further specified some functions of conceptual frameworks for curriculum development in nursing:

1 Identifies the goal(s) of nursing

2 Shows behavioral objectives and content organization in harmony with the school's philosophy and objectives

3 Gives a set of guidelines for developing instructional materials

4 Provides schema for evaluation of the graduates and of the curriculum (1978:29)

The need for identification of key supporting concepts in a discipline or professional field such as nursing has steadily gained recognition in curriculum development, primarily because of the accelerating growth of knowledge—the irreducible element of a curriculum (King and Brownell, 1966). For the purposes of this study, the conceptual frameworks *adaptation, developmental,* and *the family as an open system* will be briefly reviewed as they pertain to professional nursing education.

Adaptation as a conceptual framework for nursing professes that nursing is concerned chiefly with man as a total being somewhere along the health-illness continuum and therefore that the function of nursing is to support and promote patient adaptation. Thus, this framework views the nurse's role in promoting adaptation as involving both assessment and intervention. Assessment includes evaluating a man's position on the health-illness continuum, the forces impinging on man and the effectiveness of his coping strategies. Intervention, meanwhile, includes selection of nursing strategies designed to promote adaptation in the patient, a process whereby the patient's energy is conserved, making energy available for the healing process (Roy, 1970).

Developmental, as a conceptual framework for nursing education, views man as moving through the life cycle from conception to death while he is undergoing real developmental changes. Thus, the nursing process in this framework must give full consideration to the developmental status of individuals and groups. According to this framework,

> . . . development generally is discussed in terms of biological, sociological, psychological and cognitive aspects which encourage or impinge upon development. Nursing process and theory can be viewed from its relationship to any of these aspects during any life period. (Branstetter, 1969:21)

The conceptual framework of *the family as a system* provides a view of the family as a whole entity interacting with the unified whole of the environment, thereby encouraging the nurse to work with the family as a whole. According to Fawcett

> . . . it fosters a more comprehensive view of family life, and consequently, a more comprehensive plan of intervention. . . . The family and the nurse, as part of the family's environment, are open to mutual, simultaneous interaction. (1975:116)

This brief review of three conceptual frameworks proposed for nursing education indicates

the diversity of concepts which are incorporated into the respective frameworks and their potential significance for the development of program objectives, selection of content, and overall curriculum design in higher education.

The first study of the use of conceptual frameworks in baccalaureate nursing curricula was done by Torres and Yura (1974) to identify concepts commonly held by nursing faculty and the terms in which the concepts were expressed. The sample included 50 baccalaureate nursing programs accredited by the NLN during 1972 to 1973. The conceptual frameworks delineated in the self-evaluation reports of the programs in the study were examined for components, themes, topics, and threads. These were then grouped and classified according to similarities, commonalities, and subgroupings. Results indicated that most of the curricula in the study reflected the use of more than one concept, for the average was three or four concepts. The major concepts were found, in most of the programs in the study, to be man, society, health, and nursing. However, the development, emphasis, and priority given the concepts differed, as did the identification, clarification, and development of subconcepts.

In a recent study, Tiedt (1978) designed a conceptual framework curriculum model which she distributed to a sample of 68 curriculum coordinators or chairpersons of baccalaureate nursing programs who were asked to respond, by means of a questionnaire, to each of the elements in the model. Tiedt's results yielded the following list of conceptual framework elements with which respondents agreed strongly or very strongly:

1 Nature of nursing and the delivery of nursing care

2 Nature of the teaching/learning process

3 Nature of man, death, and health care delivery

4 Role of giver and recipient of care

5 Goals of nursing action

6 Focus of intervention

7 Responsiveness to society's current and changing needs

A third, related research study was conducted by Hill and Hansen (1960) of the Minnesota Family Study Center to identify conceptual frameworks used by marriage and family researchers. Hill and Hansen did a content analysis of hundreds of studies and abstracted out of the concepts utilized those which referred primarily to structure, to process, to solidarity, to development over time, and to spatial arrangements. The authors found that

> ... the most significant elements in differentiating one framework from another are the underlying assumptions which each makes about the nature of man, the family, and society. (Hill and Hansen, 1960:308)

METHODOLOGY

The subjects for this descriptive study were the 61 schools of nursing with both a baccalaureate and a master's degree program which had applied for continuing accreditation to the NLN between fall 1972 and spring 1978. The schools were located in 36 states. These schools represented 122 programs (61 baccalaureate and 61 master's degree programs).

Data were collected for this study by using the statements by the schools concerning their conceptual frameworks in their self-study reports submitted to the NLN. Demographic data were obtained from the fact sheets in the self-studies and from the *Education Directory—1977–78* (Podolsky and Smith, 1978).

Data analysis consisted of a content analysis of the data. The content analysis was at the manifest level of analysis and involved the development of two category sets based on the researcher's interaction with the data and review of the literature. Furthermore, the category sets were designed to answer the research questions. The category sets were unidimensional, since they were derived from a single frame of reference of the subject or content aspect of professional nursing education. The first category set was designed to classify the conceptual

frameworks into six broad categories, and the second category set classified the major concepts within the conceptual frameworks into nine categories. The indicators of each of the categories, in both sets, were specified. The researcher then coded the written statements of the schools into the two category sets. A second coding of the written statements followed and was done by a judge who was knowledgeable, experienced, and skilled in the area of higher education nursing curriculum design. The judge was trained, prior to coding, in order to familiarize her with the category sets, their indicators, and the unit boundaries. All the programs ($N = 122$) in the study were coded by the judge. The percentages of intercoder agreement, in both category sets, were calculated as reliability indices and were corrected for the number of categories, as well as for the frequency with which categories were used (Scott, 1955). The reliability indices were .97 for the first category set and .985 and .986 for the two parts (baccalaureate and master's degree concepts) of the second category set. Disagreements between the coders were settled by a second judge, who served as a referee and who was also a higher education nursing curriculum expert, trained by the researcher regarding the category-set indicators and coding procedures. The second judge's decisions were incorporated into the final tabulations.

RESULTS

The findings of this study revealed six categories by which the conceptual frameworks could be classified: none, ambiguous, multiple, adaptation, systems, and developmental. As shown in Table 8-1, one-third ($N = 41$) of the programs had either none or ambiguous conceptual frameworks, while the remaining two-thirds had adaptation, multiple, systems, or developmental as conceptual frameworks. The largest category of the conceptual frameworks was adaptation ($N = 35$), and the smallest category was developmental ($N = 2$). However, analysis of the six combinations of frameworks, within the multiple category, revealed

Table 8-1   Frequencies and Types of Conceptual Frameworks in Baccalaureate and Master's Degree Nursing Curricula

| Conceptual framework | Nursing curricula | | Total | |
	Bacca-lau-reate	Master's degree	N	%
None	2	14	16	13
Ambiguous	17	8	25	20
Multiple	13	15	28	23
Adaptation	20	15	35	29
Systems	8	8	16	13
Developmental	1	1	2	2
Total	61	61	122	100

Table 8-2   Frequencies of Subcategories within the Multiple Conceptual Framework Category of the Nursing Curricula

| Multiple conceptual framework subcategories | Nursing curricula | | Total |
	Bacca-lau-reate	Mas-ter's degree	
Adaptation plus developmental	1	—	1
Adaptation plus health	4	6	10
Adaptation plus systems	5	2	7
Adaptation plus developmental plus health	2	5	7
Adaptation plus developmental plus systems	—	1	1
Adaptation plus developmental plus health plus systems	1	1	2
Total	13	15	28

that developmental appeared 11 times in combination with other frameworks (see Table 8-2). Similarly, health, as a conceptual framework, appeared in 19 multiple combinations, but had not appeared as a singular framework. A total of 28 programs was listed in the multiple category—a category which revealed that adaptation was in all 28 combinations.

Further analysis revealed that, in 32 (52 percent) of the schools of nursing, the baccalaureate and master's degree programs had the same frameworks. It was also found that a significant relationship existed between the types of conceptual frameworks and their use in baccalaureate or master's degree curricula. In addition, a high degree of association was found to exist between the frameworks and the curricula.

Nine concepts: man, nursing, nursing process, health, illness, family, community, social systems, and environment were in the second category set (see Table 8-3). Four of the concepts: man, nursing, nursing process, and health occurred more frequently than any of the other concepts in the baccalaureate program as well as the master's degree programs, but a fifth concept, environment, also appeared as frequently as the other four in the master's degree programs. Man was the most

Table 8-3   Frequency Distribution of Concepts Among Baccalaureate and Master's Degree Programs with Conceptual Frameworks

| Concept | Programs with conceptual frameworks | | | |
| | Baccalaureate N = 59 | | Master's degree N = 47 | |
	N	%	N	%
Man	58	98	46	98
Nursing	49	83	42	89
Nursing process	53	90	40	85
Health	51	86	39	83
Illness	40	68	31	66
Family	37	63	27	57
Community	35	59	29	62
Social systems	34	58	32	68
Environment	42	71	39	83

Note: The frequencies are not mutually exclusive; therefore, the % columns do not total 100%.

frequently (98 percent) appearing concept in all the conceptual frameworks.

No statistically significant relationship was found to exist between the demographic variables of enrollment size, faculty size, or existence of a university hospital and the types of conceptual frameworks in the baccalaureate or master's degree programs. Finally, no statistically significant relationship was evident between the year of application for continuing NLN accreditation and the conceptual frameworks.

CONCLUSIONS

The following conclusions were reached as a result of the study:

1 Considerable confusion exists among the leadership in nursing schools in its attempts to define a conceptual framework.

2 Among the programs which did specify frameworks, adaptation, either as a singular framework or in combination with other frameworks, was the most frequent conceptual framework on which the programs were based.

3 The diversity of the existing frameworks in nursing programs is an indication of strength and creativity within the profession.

4 A strong relationship within individual schools of nursing exists between the consistency of conceptual framework classification in both the baccalaureate and master's degree programs.

5 Baccalaureate nursing programs tend to have large numbers of ambiguous frameworks and low numbers of programs with frameworks in the none category, while master's degree programs reverse those findings, with large numbers in the none category and low frequencies in the ambiguous category.

6 Nurse educators involved with master's degree programs have more difficulty, both in specifying concepts and identifying their organizing frameworks, than do nurse educators involved with baccalaureate programs.

7 Professional nursing education programs are focusing more on the phenomenon of man himself as an overriding entity, requiring emphasis

above and beyond the concepts of social systems, community, and family.

8 The concept of environment, with its broad, health-oriented ramifications, is replacing the more traditional, structural concepts of social systems, community, and family.

9 No statistically significant trends are discernible concerning the frequencies of the various frameworks in nursing programs at the baccalaureate or master's degree level during the 1972 to 1978 period.

10 Conceptual frameworks are not related, in any way, to the demographic variables of enrollment size, faculty size, or presence of a university hospital.

IMPLICATIONS

The findings of this study have implications for professional nursing education programs in institutions of higher education and thereby for professional nursing practice. Foremost among the implications of this study for professional nursing education programs is its contribution to the scarce amount of research findings available concerning conceptual frameworks in nursing education. Thus, the findings will prove useful to those curriculum planners involved in curriculum revisions or to those curriculum planners among the 219 baccalaureate programs without master's degree programs who may be considering expanding their offerings to include master's degree programs. For both the former and the latter, the findings of this study will contribute to a better understanding of the conceptual elements within conceptual frameworks and how other schools have chosen to delineate them.

To those schools which are having problems specifying a framework, it will be comforting to realize that they are not alone. However, the study indicates that baccalaureate nursing faculties may tend to identify concepts in isolation from some organizing schema, whereas master's degree program faculties may tend to simply not identify a framework in their frustration from coping with a myriad of clinical or functional program specialties. For this latter group, a unifying multiple schema may be best. For the baccalaureate group, to function with a multiplicity of concepts lacking a cohesive linkage is confusing to both students and faculties. The study findings indicate that it might be productive for baccalaureate nursing faculties to identify those major concepts which support their philosophy of nursing and thus direct them toward the conceptualization of a specific framework.

EDITOR'S QUESTIONS FOR DISCUSSION

What significance may there be for nursing as a profession with NLN adding the criterion for conceptual frameworks? Whose responsibility is it to define criteria for a profession and its professional education programs? To what extent should representatives who are not members of the discipline be responsible and accountable for establishing criteria for a specific profession?

Discuss examples of how conceptual frameworks provide the rationale for the selection of content in professional education programs? What traditionally has been the rationale for content in nursing education programs? What forces promoted a change in rationale? What evidence is there of the impact of utilizing conceptual frameworks in professional nursing programs on nursing practice, nursing students, nursing faculty, and the profession? How would you define and apply a specific conceptual framework in nursing practice? How would you discuss with a colleague in nursing practice the utilization of a conceptual framework in practice? How can colleagues in nursing practice contribute to the development of conceptual frameworks for practice and education? From what base or source should conceptual frameworks be derived in order to be effective? What strategies might be considered for implementation of a conceptual framework in nursing practice and in education programs? To what extent may the findings of Santora's study be different in 1982? What alternative explanations might be offered for her findings? Would you recommend replication of Santora's methodology? What alternative methodologies might be considered? What implications might be suggested regarding 52 percent of the schools utilizing the same conceptual framework?

What questions can be posed for professional nursing education and the profession regarding Santora's conclusions? Why might nurse educators involved with master's degree programs have more difficulty in identifying their frameworks than those faculty in baccalaureate programs? What further implications are there of this study?

REFERENCES

Beauchamp, G. A.
  1968 Curriculum Theory (2d ed.) Wilmette Illinois: Kagg Press.

Branstetter, E.
  1969 "Theory is not enough," Pp. 18-22 in C. M. Norris (ed.), Proceedings—First Nursing Theory Conference. Lawrence: University of Kansas Medical Center, Department of Nursing Education.

Chater, S.
  1975 "A conceptual framework for curriculum development." Nursing Outlook 23(7): 428-433.

Fawcett, J.
  1975 "The family as a living open system: An emerging conceptual framework for nursing." International Nursing Review 22(4):113-116.

  1978 "The 'what' of theory development." In National League for Nursing, Theory

Development: What, Why, How? New York: National League for Nursing, pp. 17–33.

Grava, A.
1969 A Structural Inquiry into the Symbolic Representation of Ideas. The Hague: Mouton & Co., Printers.

Hill, R. and D. Hansen.
1960 "The identification of conceptual frameworks utilized in family study." Marriage and Family Living 22:299–311.

Hoult, T. F.
1969 Dictionary for Modern Sociology. Totowa, New Jersey: Littlefield, Adams & Co.

Kaplan, A.
1964 The Conduct of Inquiry. San Francisco: Chandler Publishing Company.

Kelly, J.
1975 "The conceptual framework in nursing education," in National League for Nursing, Faculty-Curriculum Development: Part VI, Curriculum Revision in Baccalaureate Nursing Education. New York: National League for Nursing, pp. 15–21.

King, A. R. and J. A. Brownell
1966 The Curriculum and the Disciplines of Knowledge. New York: Wiley

King, I.
1978 "How does the conceptual framework provide structure for the curriculum?" In National League for Nursing, Curriculum Process for Developing or Revising Baccalaureate Nursing Programs. New York: National League for Nursing, pp. 23–34.

National League for Nursing
1972 Criteria for the Appraisal of Baccalaureate and Higher Degree Programs in Nursing. New York: National League for Nursing.

Nye, F. I. and F. M. Berardo.
1966 Emerging Conceptual Frameworks in Family Analysis. London: Macmillan.

Podolsky, A. and C. R. Smith
1978 Education Directory—1977–78. U.S. Department of Health, Education, and Welfare, National Center for Educational Statistics. Washington, D.C.: U.S. Government Printing Office.

Phillips, B. S.
1966 Social Research—Strategy and Tactics. New York: Macmillan.

Roy, S. C.
1970 "Adaptation: A conceptual framework for nursing." Nursing Outlook 18:42–45.

Scott, W. A.
1955 "Reliability of content analysis: The case of nominal scale coding." Public Opinion Quarterly 19:321–325.

Taba, H.
1962 Curriculum Development. New York: Harcourt Brace Jovanovich, Inc.

Tiedt, E.
1978 A Model to Achieve Organized Integration of the Conceptual Model for Nursing Practice Within the Total Curriculum Development Process. Unpublished doctoral dissertation, Ohio State University.

Torres, G. and H. Yura
1974 Today's Conceptual Frameworks: Its Relationship to the Curriculum Development Process. New York: National League for Nursing.

Tyler, R. W.
1949 Basic Principles of Curriculum and Instruction. Chicago: University of Chicago Press.

Weinberg, J. R.
1970 Ideas and Concepts. Milwaukee: Marquette University Press.

Zetterberg, H. L.
1965 On Theory and Verification in Sociology (3d ed.). Totowa, N.J.: Bedminster Press.

Chapter 9

Upper-Division or Completion Programs for R.N.s

Nancy M. Sargis, R.N., Ed.D.
Associate Professor
Loyola University
Chicago, Illinois

The educational model of a B.S.N. upper division or "completion program" for registered nurse students has become as controversial as the whole issue of entry level into the profession. Nancy Sargis adeptly addresses critical points regarding completion programs. Insightful arguments pro and con from the perspective of nurse educators and R.N.s seeking a B.S.N. degree are specified. The dilemma of R.N.s and nurse educators is clearly made apparent. Sargis cites factors stimulating the growth of completion programs, describes the various types of curriculum patterns, and illustrates the lack of standardization in fundamental variables of programs. She discusses the impact of N.L.N. accreditation and the implications for R.N.s who enter a non-N.L.N. accredited program. Sargis notes the lower graduation rates of R.N.s from generic programs and increasing number of R.N. graduations from programs for R.N.s only. Finally, Sargis raises vital questions and offers concrete means to resolving the issue.

The educational preparation of nurses in this country continues to present the nursing profession with a serious conflict that must be resolved. There is no question that the continued fight on the issue of the entry level into the profession is distracting nurses from their major responsibility which is, after all, service to the public.

The question before the profession is, When will the baccalaureate degree in nursing (B.S.N.) be required for licensure to practice nursing? If one considers the fact that currently 78.3 percent of registered nurses do not have a B.S.N. then the seriousness of the question is apparent (ANA, 1979). The literature is beginning to identify the sense of disenfranchisement experienced by those registered nurses who do not have a degree. In addition, perceived threats to economic security in terms of job marketability have given impetus to a back-to-school movement among these nurses. The irony in the return of licensed health workers to school to obtain preparation they are told they do not have must give us pause!

One educational model that has appeared on the scene in response to the R.N.'s expressed needs is the so-called B.S.N. completion program, or the upper-division baccalaureate nursing program for registered nurses only. These completion programs seem to herald a new phase in our nursing education, much as the associate degree programs represented a new pattern in our educational system in the sixties. Reported enrollments of registered nurses in baccalaureate programs for R.N.s show dramatic growth over the past decade and suggest that this educational model may not be transient. Therefore, it behooves us to consider the history that led to the creation of these programs, the nature of these programs, and the implications of these programs for the profession.

HISTORY OF THE "1985 PROPOSAL"

The "1985 Proposal" of the New York State Nurses Association was an attempt in 1974 to legislatively revise the Nurse Practice Act of that state so that, by 1985, a baccalaureate degree in nursing would be required for licensure as a registered nurse. The initial 1985 Proposal also called for an associate degree in nursing for licensure as a practical nurse (NYSNA, 1975). In 1978, the language in the legislative bill was changed to read that the B.S.N. would be requried to practice professional nursing under the title "nurse," and that the associate degree in nursing would be required to practice associate nursing under the title "associate nurse" (NYSNA, 1978).

The 1985 Proposal calling for two distinct careers in nursing based on academic training was not a seminal concept adopted by the voting membership of the New York State Nurses Association at the 1974 Convention in Lake Placid, New York. Indeed, a careful review of the literature documents that, since the Josephine Goldmark Report of 1923, a significant study has been conducted every decade on the state of "the fledgling profession." A dominant theme of these reports, buttressed by recommendations, is that nursing should put its educational house in order and that the preparation of its practitioners should take place in colleges and universities.

A significant turning point in nursing education occurred with the American Nurses Association's position statement in 1965, which brought closure to the controversial "Goal Three," which had been introduced to the House of Delegates at the 1960 convention in Miami Beach. The purpose of Goal Three was:

> To insure that within the next 20–30 years the education basic to nursing on a professional level, for those who then enter the field, shall be secured in a program that provides the intellectual, technical and cultural components of both professional and liberal education. Toward this end, the ANA shall promote the baccalaureate program so that in due course it becomes the basic educational foundation for professional nursing. (ANA, 1960:55)

The position paper issued by the American Nurses Association in 1965 stated that "minimum preparation for beginning technical nursing practice be baccalaureate education for nursing," and that "minimum preparation for beginning technical nursing practice be associate degree education in nursing" (ANA, 1965). As reiterated through our history, the leadership in nursing was calling for standardization of educational requirements. From 1965 until the present, the literature is replete with outcries from special interest groups articulating grievous antagonism toward the baccalaureate degree as entry level into the profession of nursing. In light of this ever-present opposition, it is of interest to note, the American Nurses Association's House of Delegates at convention in 1978 reaffirmed its commitment and support of the B.S.N. for entry into the practice of nursing. While the 1980 House of Delegates supported the B.S.N. entry issue, it postponed its decision on titling until 1982, at which time the ANA Commission on Nursing Education will have completed its work on competencies of the two categories.

WHAT ARE THE ARGUMENTS?

The Protagonists

The proponents of a baccalaureate degree in nursing for licensure established their argument on the premise that the public need *will* best be served by this program. The thesis is that, through standardization and elevation of educational requirements, one can improve standards of nursing practice. The continuation of multiple types of basic nursing education programs which qualify their graduates to sit for the *same* licensing examination will only perpetuate existing public confusion. The protagonists' lament is "a nurse is *not* a nurse is *not* a nurse."

Increasingly complex demands of the health care system, coupled with the explosion of knowledge at an exponential rate, necessitate more than a technical preparation essentially concrete in nature and dealing with the "here and now." The true professional nurse must be the one who is comfortable in the world of abstraction, problem-solving, and futuristic thinking. The foundation of the liberal arts and sciences in the BSN program not only educates the individual in conceptualization, that is, in "thinking nursing," it serves as a very real means of personal enrichment. The protagonists also argue that nursing will not receive professional respectability until its practitioners, "though somewhat different in the amount of practice" are minimally credentialled at the baccalaureate level, as is the case with physicians, lawyers, dentists, clergy, engineers, and teachers. Lastly, they argue that, without professional credibility, nursing will not acquire the power to determine its destiny.

The Antagonists

The antagonists of the call for a baccalaureate degree in nursing for licensure establish their argument on the premise that the public need *will not* be served this way. The thesis is that there is no proven connection between academic preparation and quality care. The existence of multiple educational pathways to registered nurse licensure provides educational options that allow for career mobility and advancement. Further, the antagonists argue, there is no evidence to the claim that multiple kinds of basic nursing programs have resulted in public confusion. They would argue

that the public is concerned only with outcome of care and not with the basic program from which the registered nurse comes. Thus, "a nurse *is* a nurse *is* a nurse."

The antagonists would view the proponents as "ethereal educators," who have lost sight of the day-to-day, highly technical performance demands made of the nurse, demands which can only be met through mastery of specific concrete information and related hospital experiences. They view the baccalaureate-prepared nurse as one who is steeped in theory to the point of being rendered incompetent in the practice domain. They frequently cite the dearth of performance testing and research that would give credence to the protagonist's assertion that baccalaureate education impacts positively upon nursing care. Lastly, the antagonists argue that the economic cost of baccalaureate education for all is prohibitive, and if it were the only type of basic nursing preparation, one would not be able to produce the needed supply of nurses. In addition, eliminating our current three-tiered system of preparing nurses would discriminate against disadvantaged ethnic and socioeconomic groups, many of who could not afford baccalaureate education. The protagonist's rejoinder is that the three-tiered system is economically wasteful and that it exploits disadvantaged ethnic and socioeconomic groups by suggesting that the poor are neither intellectually capable nor worthy of seeking baccalaureate education.

AGAINST THIS BACKDROP

With some 85 percent of the nation's registered nurses lacking a baccalaureate degree in 1965, it is not surprising that colleges seeking new audiences moved quickly to accommodate these R.N.s.

Specifically, the shrinking pool of students in small private liberal arts colleges prompted these institutions to go into the "nursing education business" for survival. Thus, the registered nurse population was an attractive source of degree candidates for small colleges, as well as for larger universities who sought to offset declining populations in the traditional colleges of arts and sciences.

Unfortunately, many of these baccalaureate programs for registered nurses were housed in colleges and universities that were having their *initial* encounter with nursing education. Ignorance of what should be involved in bona fide baccalaureate nursing education and institutional economic constraints led schools to aggressive recruitment of registered nurses into academic programs that did not have nursing as a major field. The ethos was to offer the nurse a program of studies that was inexpensive and that could be completed in a short time span. The baccalaureate degree was obtained in such fields as biology, psychology, anthropology, health education, and applied science. The rationale for the nonnursing major was that the R.N. already had basic preparation in nursing, and what was now educationally needed were courses in the liberal arts and sciences that would embellish the nurse's background. In support of this rationale, large blocks of blanket college credits (without validation) were given for prior nursing work in a hospital school, for life experiences, and for having a registered nurse license. The notion in nursing practice that "a nurse is a nurse is a nurse" was now being translated into nursing education as "a degree is a degree is a degree."

This questionable educational practice led the Board of Directors of the National League for Nursing to issue its statement on the matter in October, 1971.

> The National League for Nursing notes with concern the growth in the number of collegiate programs that have no major in nursing but are designed to appeal specifically to potential and enrolled nursing students and registered nurses. Publicity about these programs leads students to believe that they offer preparation for advanced positions in nursing or provide the base needed for further education in nursing when this is not the case. (NLN, 1971: 760)

Then again, in 1977 Epstein and Friesner (1977:470-472) alerted registered nurses to the dangers of a nonnursing degree. In speaking for the National League for Nursing, they stated that the purpose of the upper-division nursing major is to provide nursing theory and related clinical experiences essential for beginning practice as a professional nurse. The nonnursing degree, they said, does not give the student the nursing expertise needed to be an independent practitioner and to assume a leadership role. Further, the prospects of acceptance into an accredited master's program in nursing for those holding a nonnursing bachelor's degree were remote. They concluded the NLN's position by stating,

> In summary, the benefits of a nonnursing degree to the employer, the nurse, and the consumer appear limited and the risks and implications considerable. (Epstein and Friesner, 1977:472)

Those registered nurses who chose to pursue a nonnursing degree had their story to tell. Many stated strong skepticism about the notion of baccalaureate nursing courses expanding already acquired nursing knowledge and skills. Many registered nurses perceived their basic preparation as being eminently better than the generic B.S.N. preparation, and they truly believed that concentration of study in a nonnursing field would make them better nurses. Many nurses expressed feelings of "professional burnout" and disillusionment and viewed a new field of study as a source of excitement that would perhaps renew their interest in nursing. Many nurses, embittered, deliberately chose to attain a nonnursing degree because they had given up on the profession and had no aspirations for career advancement, further professional development, or graduate education in nursing.

Many of those registered nurses who truly sought a B.S.N. degree experienced incredible frustion at attempting to overcome obstacles, a frustration which finally resulted in their decision to seek a degree outside of nursing. Perceived factors impeding attainment of their initial goals were: (1) no opportunities for part-time study, (2) no opportunities to challenge nursing courses, (3) no mechanisms for advanced placement, (4) insensitivity to the R.N. as an adult learner with needs different from those of the generic student, (5) long waiting lists for admission, (6) a period of full-time residency, and (7) direct and indirect educational costs exceeding the R.N.'s economic capability (Allen, 1977:468–469).

In commenting on the plight of those frustrated registered nurses who implied that the leadership in organized nursing was making it hard to get the bachelor's degree, Lewis (1977:369) chided the profession for having done so little to translate the rhetoric of the ANA position statement of 1965 into action. Lewis also expressed compassionate understanding of the situation when she stated:

> Who could have said in 1965 to those thousands of diploma nurses then making up the backbone of hospital nursing services, "You are not appropriately prepared for professional nursing practice?" Yet, implicity, and in one way or another, this is what we have been saying ever since. (1977:369)

More importantly, Lewis and others have observed that the saddest part of this paradoxical situation is that the B.S.N. to wit, attainment of the credential, has become an end in itself rather than a means to educational opportunity for professional and personal enrichment.

BSN PROGRAMS FOR R.N.s ONLY— SEPARATE BUT EQUAL?

Data released by the National League for Nursing's Research Division for the academic year 1978–1979 tells us that there is a steady growth pattern of registered nurses working toward B.S.N. degrees, both in generic nursing programs and in programs for R.N.s only.[1]

In 1970, the reported R.N. enrollments in generic programs were 6144, while the reported enrollments in BSN programs for R.N.s only were 1548. Reported R.N. enrollments in generic programs showed increases to 16,676 in 1978 and to 17,347 in 1979. Enrollment of registered nurses in B.S.N. programs for R.N.s only soared to 8887 in 1978 and to 10,686 in 1979 (NLN, 1980b:46). One variable that may explain this marked increase in enrollment in R.N.-only B.S.N. programs is the growth of such programs in this country. As of January 1, 1980, the data released by the NLN in their publication *State-Approved Schools of Nursing–R.N.* (1980a) show 330 generic baccalaureate programs and 99 baccalaureate programs designed exclusively for R.N. students. Today B.N.S. programs for R.N.s constitutes less than one-fourth (23 percent) of baccalaureate nursing education.

One of the factors stimulating growth of these programs was the trend toward investigating nontraditional approaches to nursing education. Nurse-educators were beginning to think about and talk about different categories of learners achieving different career goals through different modes of learning. In 1970 the National League for Nursing created an Open Curriculum Project in Nursing Education, which culminated in the first Conference on Open Curriculum in 1973. The proceedings of that conference were published in 1974.

The open curriculum system used in the NLN study was defined as

> . . . one which incorporates an educational approach designed to accommodate the learning needs and career goals of students by providing flexible opportunities for entry into and exit from the educational program, and by capital-

---

[1] The phrase "B.S.N. programs for R.N.s only," or "completion programs" refers to those programs which admit only students who are registered nurses.

izing on their previous relevant education and experience. (NLN, 1974:145)

Further, the NLN study identified four distinct open curriculum patterns.

1 A previously licensed student is admitted into a program especially designed to build on his or her prior level of nursing education. The student is already either a licensed practical nurse or a registered nurse from a diploma or associate degree program.

2 The student with some past education and experience in nursing or health-related programs is admitted with advanced standing into the regular basic nursing program. Such advanced standing may be achieved through transfer or credit examinations or other means.

3 The student is admitted to a specially designed program which prepares for multiple exit credentialing. This type of system may be referred to as a career ladder.

4 The student is awarded a degree or certificate on the basis of successful demonstration of acquired knowledge, rather than attendance and completion of a particular program. This may be referred to as the external degree in nursing (NLN, 1974:145).

While the numbers of R.N. students were increasing in generic programs, there was a strong call for curricula designed specifically for the R.N. student. In a survey conducted by Slaninka (1979: 1095), it was found that 71.3 percent of the respondents of NLN-accredited baccalaureate programs in the United States still do not have such programs. But, as baccalaureate programs for R.N.s flourished during the seventies so did the curricula, so to speak. It would appear that no two programs were the same. Indeed, there was a variety in educational purposes and goals, in approaches, and in teaching strategies. We had a range of curricula simulating the traditional generic models that presented basic content and a variety of nontraditional curricula that presented advanced professional theory and practice. What was quickly learned by the pioneers who

chose to teach R.N. students was how noticeably disparate the R.N. students were from the basic students. Muzio and Ohashi (1979:528–532) describe the R.N. student as one with unique characteristics and needs. They state that the practice of fitting R.N.s into the generic model of baccalaureate education is not desirable because of their differences in knowledge and experience, thinking patterns, and prior socialization. They argue that meeting the needs of this special group of baccalaureate candidates demands making significant changes in the structure and processes of current baccalauareate education.

It was not until these R.N.-only programs sought National League for Nursing accreditation that attention was signaled to the fundamental dissimilarities between the generic model and the myriad patterns of B.S.N. programs for R.N.s. The variables that seemed to be lacking in standardization were admissions criteria, challenge examinations, advanced standing, full- and part-time study, clinical experiences, and the time required for completion of the program. As was stated earlier, no two programs were the same.

More importantly, a crucial departure from what the accrediting body (NLN) saw as the role of baccalaureate education was to present some serious problems for the architects of these developing programs. The NLN philosophy of baccalaureate education is that the curriculum is to prepare a generalist who can render competent care to individuals and groups in a variety of practice settings (NLN, 1979:1). A case was being built to depart from the traditional NLN program goals and to allow for greater specialization at the baccalaureate level. The rationale was that one would honor past basic nursing knowledge and experience and capitalize on the R.N.'s motivation to pursue a practice area of interest, thereby developing nursing expertise in a particular role.

The notion of specialization on the baccalaureate level was not new. During the decades of the forties and fifties, many fine schools of nursing offered strong baccalaureate programs to R.N.s in the functional areas, e.g., bachelor of science in nursing education (B.S.N.Ed.), bachelor of science in nursing service (B.S.N.Sc.), and in the practice areas, e.g., bachelor of science in public health nursing (B.S.PH.N.). But the point remains that, if the profession is seeking to elevate standards by mandating college education for entry level, then, as is the case with academic disciplines, specialization in nursing should take place on the master's level.

As of January 1, 1980, 23 of the 99 baccalaureate programs for registered nurses, or 23.2 percent were accredited by the National League for Nursing, whereas the League had accredited 285 of the 330 generic baccalaureate programs or 86.3 percent (NLN, 1980a). No data are available at the present time to explain the marked discrepancy between the accreditation status of these two types of B.S.N. programs. However, consideration of the following factors does allow us to speculate about the matter.

First, as has been noted, these upper-division programs for R.N.s are new. Some of the 99 programs may not have graduated their first class and thus are not eligible to seek the accreditation. Some programs determined at the outset that they would not actively seek the accreditation because they lack the academic, professional, and economic resources to do so. Some programs that sought initial accreditation and were denied chose not to reapply, and some programs that sought initial accreditation and were deferred may not have been able or chose not to address the recommendations for final accreditation determination by the NLN Board of Review.

Second, a lack of clarity of purpose of baccalaureate nursing education for the individual with prior nursing preparation resulted in program designs that could not be defended as quality education. Individualizing the curriculum for registered nurses as adult learners who brought diversity of background and circumstances to the program may have weakened academic vigor. Faculty efforts to be creative and innovative when planning new learning may have resulted in an absence of order and logical progression in the curriculum. Further, presentation a[...] of knowledge and competency fo[...] may have been sacrificed in atte[...] unnecessary repetition of prior expe[...]

Third, perceived difficulty by some nurse-educators in utilizing the NLN "Criteria for the Appraisal of Baccalaureate and Higher Degree Programs in Nursing" when designing the program may have had negative bearing on the accreditation outcome. If the NLN criteria were not viewed as relevant and useful for the planning of an educational program for R.N.s, then their importance was undervalued and not properly understood. A real dilemma confronts those nurse-educators who are proponents of the open curriculum and of nontraditional approaches to nursing education. They see themselves in a predicament when asked to adhere to the standards set forth in the NLN criteria, which, they state, restrains them from meeting expressed needs of R.N.s whose motivation and orientation toward higher education differ significantly from the younger beginning generic students.

Whatever the reasons for the low percentage of NLN-accredited B.S.N. programs for R.N.s, one point is strongly evident. At the present time in nursing education in this country, the National League for Nursing accreditation is synonymous with quality education. Furthermore, the absence of said accreditation places the reputation of the college or univeristy, administration, and nursing faculty in a tenous and awkward position.

To appreciate the full impact and ramifications of the NLN accreditation is to understand why a voluntary procedure is, in point of fact, a mandatory accreditation for the nursing profession. Specifically, the R.N. who enters a non-NLN-accredited program may not have access to scholarship monies or student loans earmarked for accredited programs. Furthermore, the R.N. who enters a non-NLN-accredited program jeopardizes his or her chances to enter an NLN-accredited master's degree program, since 60 percent of these graduate programs require an NLN-accredited B.S.N. degree for admission (NLN, 1976). The graduate of a non-NLN-accredited program will also be ineligible for enlistment as a nurse in the Armed Forces of the United States, although the nurse could enlist as a civilian. Finally, many employers of nurses—hospitals, public health agencies, community health care facilities, and federal governmental agencies—reserve the right to recognize or reject the graduate of a non-NLN-accredited BSN program.

SOME CONCLUDING THOUGHTS

While the enrollment of registered nurses in both generic and R.N.-only programs has been relatively high, recent data show low graduation rates of R.N.s from generic programs. In 1972 approximately 17 percent of the total graduates from NLN-accredited baccalaureate programs were R.N.s (Dineen, 1972). This figure alerted us to the trend of goal-oriented R.N.s wishing to earn the B.S.N.

In the academic years 1974-1975 and 1975-1976, the growth rate of R.N. graduations from generic programs exceeded 25 percent. However, it is interesting to note that while graduations continue to increase the growth rate is waning. There was only a 14 percent increase in 1976-1977, a 13 percent increase in 1977-1978, and a 5 percent increase in 1978-1979. On the other hand, R.N. graduations from programs for R.N.s only increased steadily from 15.8 percent of the total R.N. graduations for the year 1974-1975 to 38.2 percent in 1977-1978, then dropped slightly to 36.7 percent in 1978-1979 (NLN, 1980c:86).

Whereas graduations of basic students are predictable, graduations of R.N.s in baccalaureate programs are not. It is difficult to monitor graduation data for a large population of R.N. students who attend school on a part-time basis. In addition, withdrawal and reentry into the program because of personal circumstances prolongs graduation target dates.

Wilson and Levy (1978) studied factors relevant to nursing school attrition in one western baccalaureate nursing program that was designed for R.N. students only. Their data indicated that the R.N.s' personal characteristics—self-image, values, knowledge, and capabilities—were crucial in adjustment to the pressures of changing roles and academic or clinical requirements. Given the obvious participation of R.N.s in undergraduate nursing education, it is both reasonable and necessary to expect that more attention will be given to the areas of attrition and retention strategies in B.S.N. programs.

There is no disagreement as to the provision of educational opportunity for those registered nurses desirous of pursuing a B.S.N. degree. There is disagreement, however, on the route which should be taken by these motivated nurses who, for various reasons, have chosen to return to school.

Some educators believe if the R.N. sincerely seeks an education, then the path to take is to enroll in an NLN-accredited generic baccalaureate program (Reed, 1979). Other educators defend the B.S.N. Program for R.N.s only as a legitimate and viable model of higher education for these adult learners in nursing. But the current multiplicity of patterns of programs for R.N.s, a multiplicity emanating from differing philosophies and goals, has caused some uneasiness. Some programs have been designed to be a capstone experience in which the upper-division nursing major is built upon the lower division-nursing major obtained through either an associate degree program or a diploma program. The design is not acceptable to those who subscribe to the notion that the only appropriate foundation for graduate education in nursing is the upper-division major in a generic baccalaureate nursing program (Sorenson, 1976). Some programs have been designed to allow the R.N. to specialize, e.g., as an independent nurse practitioner, or to develop further some chosen area of specialization that the student is currently practicing. This latter design runs counter to the notion that the purpose of baccalaureate education in nursing is to prepare a generalist who can function in hospitals, homes, and communities.

A fundamental question to be addressed is: Should content (theory) and learning experiences in B.S.N. programs for R.N.s only be similar to that provided in generic baccalaureate nursing programs in order to guarantee comparability of educational offerings? There seems to be misguided thinking among some nurse-educators that what we teach is synonymous with how we teach. Emphasis might better be placed on varying teaching strategies and approaches, rather than subject matter, when teaching registered nurse students.

Be that as it may, the educational model of a B.S.N. completion program for registered nurses has become as controversial as the whole issue of entry level into the profession. That is, the profession seeks to standardize nursing education and to upgrade standards of practice by mandating the BSN degree as the minimum credential to practice as a professional nurse. However, it is being asserted that B.S.N. programs designed for registered nurses may prove counterproductive to the attainment of standardization. Specifically, will two prototypes of B.S.N. degree programs present us with a special set of problems for resolution in the future? It is the author's intuitive sense that they will.

To accommodate a special audience of learners, we may have prematurely introduced yet another nursing educational blueprint. Is it not in order to consider now the systematic study of the place and ambit of these B.S.N. programs for R.N.s only within our educational system? For nurse-educators to do less during these critical times in our history is to shirk a major responsibility, the responsibility to provide the best possible nursing education for all.

EDITOR'S QUESTIONS FOR DISCUSSION

To what extent would you agree and/or disagree with the arguments proposed by the proponents and antagonists of a baccalaureate degree in nursing for licensure? How can one demonstrate a linkage between a conceptual base in academic preparation and the public need being served? How would you define quality care to serve the public need? What evidence is there that the public is concerned only with outcomes of care?

From the perspective of a profession, what response might be made to the charges of discrimination regarding nursing's current "three-tiered" system of preparing nurses? Wherein is the responsibility of the nursing profession to provide educational opportunity for those registered nurses desirous of pursuing a B.S.N. degree? What is the evidence that the R.N. with a nonnursing degree differs in nursing practice from those with a generic baccalaureate degree? What options might be considered for resolving the upper division ("completion program") dilemma for R.N.s and nurse educators?

What are the implications and relationships between Williamson's, Peterson's, Santora's, and Sargis's discussions in their chapters regarding program designs for quality nursing education?

What suggestions might be offered for nurse-educators who find themselves in conflict between adhering to the standards set forth in the NLN Criteria and meeting expressed needs of R.N.s who differ from generic students? Discuss differences in learning needs and teaching strategies required for R.N.s seeking a B.S.N. degree and generic baccalaureate students. How might B.S.N. programs designed for registered nurses prove counterproductive to the attainment of standardization in education? For what variables and to what extent is standardization desirable in nursing education programs? What future potential problems might be presented to be resolved by the nursing profession with two prototypes of B.S.N. degree programs? What preventive measures might be suggested to offset potential problems?

After reflecting on Santora's and Sargis's chapters and questions posed, discuss further the significance of NLN accreditation. What are the implications of Sargis's comment that though it is a voluntary procedure in essence it is a mandatory accreditation for the nursing profession?

REFERENCES

Allen, Marcia Divoll
1977 "Yes, I have my degree, but . . ." American Journal of Nursing 77:468–469.

American Nurses Association
1960 "Report of the Committee on Current and Long-term Goals of the ANA." Proceedings 1960 House of Delegates and Sections. 42nd Convention, American Nurses Association, Miami Beach, Florida, May 2–6, 1960. New York: By the Association.
1965 Educational Preparation for Nurse Practitioners and Assistants to Nurses: A Position Paper. Publication No. G–83. Kansas City, Missouri: By the Association.
1979 "National Sample of Registered Nurses 1977." American Nurse 11:1.

Dineen, Mary A.
1972 "The open curriculum: Implications for further education." Nursing Outlook 20: 770–774.

Epstein, Rhoda B. and Arlyne Friesner
1977 "Caution! This baccalaureate may be hazardous to your health." American Journal of Nursing 77:470–472.

Lewis, E. P.
1977 "The baccalaureate degree." Nursing Outlook 25:369.

Muzio, Lois G. and Julianne, P. Ohashi
1979 "The R.N. student—unique characteristics, unique needs." Nursing Outlook 27: 528–532.

National League for Nursing
1971 "A statement of concern about degree programs for nursing students that have no major in nursing." Nursing Outlook 12:760.
1974 Proceedings—Open Curriculum Conference 1. A Project of the NLN Study of the Open Curriculum in Nursing Education.
Publication No. 19–1534, Division of Research. New York: By the League.
1976 Masters Education in Nursing: Route to Opportunities in Contemporary Nursing—1976–1977. Publication No. 15–1312. New York: By the League.
1979 Characteristics of Baccalaureate Education in Nursing. Publication No. 15–1758. New York: By the League.
1980a State-Approved Schools of Nursing—R.N. Division of Research, June.
1980b Nursing and Health Care. Official Publication of the National League for Nursing 1:46
1980c Nursing and Health Care. Official Publication of the National League for Nursing 1:86.

New York State Nurses Association
1975 Proposal Regarding Implementation of Resolution of Entry into Professional Practice Through Revision of Article 139, Nursing, Title VIII, Education Law. The Association. Albany, New York: By the Association.
1978 Proposal Regarding Implementation of Resolution on Entry into Professional Practice Through Revision of Article 139, Nursing, Title VIII, Education Law. New York: The Association Guilderland.

Reed, Fay Carol
1979 "Education or exploitation." American Journal of Nursing 79:1259–1261.

Slaninka, Susan C.
1979 "Baccalaureate programs for R.N.s." American Journal of Nursing 79:1095.

Sorenson, Gladys
1976 "Sounding board . . . in support of the generic baccalaureate degree program." Nursing Outlook 24:384–385.

Wilson, Holly Skodol and Judith Levy
1978 "Why R.N. students drop out." Nursing Outlook 26:437–441.

Chapter 10

Identification of Professional Competencies

Gloria M. Clayton, R.N., Ed.D.
Associate Professor
Chairperson, Adult Nursing
School of Nursing
Medical College of Georgia
Augusta, Georgia

Competency-based curriculum is considered one of the means for accountability in education. Emphasis in competency-based education is on the achievement of clearly specified objectives. Accountability is possible when the consumer, the educational system, and the learner are aware of clearly delineated behaviors that are necessary for professional practice.

Gloria Clayton examines the trends of competency-based education and the necessity for congruence on competency expectations between nursing educators and nursing practitioners. Clayton presents her survey to determine a defensible list of competencies. She utilizes a random sample of 1000 registered nurses and all faculties in nursing programs in Georgia. A list of 68 competencies under 11 categories is employed in the study. It is a model similar to that developed by Florida educators and practitioners. The investigator's findings indicate that with the exception of two rejected competencies all others received an approval rate of at least 80 percent from both practitioners and faculties. Clayton's study is an effort to move forward the development of a nationally accepted list of entry-level competencies for registered nurses.

Accountability is one of the most frequently used terms in education today. Colleges are expected to be accountable to accrediting bodies and to students, the consumers of their services. In nursing and other professional disciplines, the heavy hand of accountability also extends to clients as future recipients of the services of graduates.

In response to demands for accountability, a trend toward competency-based curriculum began

about 8 years ago (McDonald, 1974). Competency-based education is predicated on the enumeration of definitive behaviors which characterize competence in a given field. The emphasis in competency-based education is on the achievement of clearly specified objectives. In a competency-based program, specific observable behaviors are identified so that the person whose competency is being judged will know exactly what standards of performance are expected. Accountability becomes more than an educational term when the consumer, the educational system, and the learner are cognizant of clearly delineated behaviors which are generally accepted as necessary for professional practice.

Lessinger (1975) clarifies the rationale for marrying accountability to competency-based curriculum in his definition of accountability. He defines it as a "... process designed to insure that an individual can determine for himself if the educational goals have been met." Competencies, once articulated, can be presented to any concerned party as criteria for measuring educational progress. Competencies can become the basis for evaluation.

It is apparent that the first task in competency-based education is to determine what is relevant both to the learner and to society. Despite the obvious importance of a nationally accepted list of professional competencies for registered nurses, at the present time no such list exists. Nursing educators in a variety of groups and settings, from the national level to individual faculty units, have attempted to delineate those critical competencies demanded in the practice of nursing. The problem is compounded by the multiple educational alternatives leading to licensure as a registered nurse.

Currently there exist three types of educational programs for nurses. The most traditional form of nursing education is the three-year diploma program which is operated primarily by hospitals. In the early 1900s nursing education was initiated in institutions of higher learning. These programs are 4 years in length, and graduates are awarded a baccalaureate degree. In the early 1950s community college programs were begun for the purpose of educating nurses. These programs are 2 years in length, and graduates are awarded an associate degree. The National League for Nursing, the accrediting agency for nursing education programs, currently publishes three different sets of accreditation criteria based on the three types of educational programs.

At the present time there is obvious ambiguity as to the relative qualifications of the three types of graduates. Graduates of any of the three types of programs are eligible to take state board examinations for registered nurses. Successful completion of such an exam entitles a nurse to practice. Each type of educational program purports to prepare nurses who have skills and characteristics specific to that type of program, but there has been little differentiation in the roles graduates of the various programs fill when they enter actual practice (Hassenplug, 1965). At the present time, employers in health care facilities generally make no differentiation in job classification and responsibilities for graduates of the three types of programs. This is evidenced in job descriptions, nursing assignments, and performance evaluation (Johnson, 1966). Consumers also do not recognize the various educational levels. They are concerned only with the nursing care they receive.

Nursing is currently in the process of delineating levels of practice which will be based on the differing educational programs and their differing emphasis on different specific competency criteria. The Southern Regional Education Board (S.R.E.B.) recently completed a study which is an example of this effort. The Board's goals were to "define the characteristics of practice for the different levels of workers envisioned," and to "determine the competencies needed by each level of provider" (S.R.E.B., 1976). While the value of this endeavor is obvious, the project was not designed to settle the basic issues involved in accountability. For all nurses to be held accountable, it is necessary to delineate those major competencies which are required of registered nurses as they enter the labor force.

In 1975, Hale tested the abilities of two groups of nurses. One group was composed of associate degree graduates, and the other group consisted of graduates of baccalaureate programs. She studied the nurses' abilities to identify nursing problems, state care objectives, and specify nursing actions, and she compared the performance of the two groups. She found no significant differences and determined that the existing description of nursing functions is ambiguous.

In 1967 Brandt et al. compared the performance of practicing nurses with behavioral objectives delineated by nursing studies. While this study yielded no definite conclusions, it did confirm that some confusion exists. This confusion is also indicated in a study done by Coe in 1967. While studying the importance of selected educational objectives to groups of staff nurses, Coe found that nurses disagree among themselves as to which nursing functions are significant.

In the early 1970s the department heads of community colleges in Florida formed an informal group to delineate competencies for associate degree graduates. This document, a theoretical model for associate degree practice, has been shared at meetings and other informal occasions with nurses who represent both education and practice. The competency list has been continually revised and now enjoys the acceptance of Florida nurses. As an attempt to delineate professional competencies, this document is one of the most promising efforts to date. Its value is enhanced by the fact that it has been developed by educators and practitioners working together. A version of the Florida list was used in the data collection for this present study.

While the Florida list has been accepted by Florida nurses, neither it nor any other list has been widely disseminated for sanction by nurses throughout the United States. But a second large group is currently working to establish national standards of professional competencies in nursing. This group consists of the faculties in all nursing programs. While such a group represents a large number of people working to establish competencies, these people are working in small, rather isolated clusters.

Individual faculties must delineate the terminal objectives for their specific programs. Montag (1969) speaks of this task as a teaching function: "Perhaps the most difficult aspect of the teacher's job is to select the content and learning experiences which are appropriate and necessary for he must accept the fact that he cannot teach everything."

A third group expressing interest in delineating competencies is found among practicing nurses and future nurses. According to Burnside and Lenburg (1970:161), "A growing number of students now want a voice in decisions which affect them; they want an education which prepares them to live in a contemporary society, but one which is not dehumanizing in the process."

To gain general agreement as to competencies necessary to practice in contemporary society, it is necessary to have input in the formative stages from nursing educators and nursing practitioners. Research indicates that these two groups do not always concur on behaviors needed for nursing practice (Brendt, 1967). It is erroneous to assume automatic agreement among nurse-educators and nurse practitioners. A study which questioned students, faculty, staff nurses, and nursing supervisors found lack of congruence among the groups concerning eight nursing behaviors. Coe (1967:145) found that "there is confusion in the minds of nurses as to which are the most important functions of a staff nurse."

After a partial review of the professional literature related to the issue of professional competencies in the practice of nursing, three conclusions seem apparent. First, consumers expect all professional disciplines to be accountable for the services they render, and they expect the educational systems preparing the practitioners to be accountable for their products. Secondly, although many nurses, both in groups and as individuals, are currently concerned with delineating competencies, very little material has been compiled to show progress toward that goal. And finally, if delineated competencies are to be used as a means of accountability, it is essential that consensus exist between nursing educators and nursing practitioners.

Recognizing that the development of a list of nationally accepted professional competencies is an ultimate goal in nursing, the present investigator instigated a study using a limited population of nurses to identify such competencies. These findings were then used to compile a defensible list of those professional competencies which should be required of registered nurses. The following questions formed the base of the study:

• What are the professional competencies identified by registered nurses in Georgia?
• What are the professional competencies identified by faculties in nursing programs in Georgia?
• To what extent does congruency exist between competencies identified in the previous two questions?

In order to develop a defensible compilation, it appeared reasonable to survey both registered nurses currently practicing the competencies and faculty in programs preparing future nurses for practice. Conceptually at least, these two sources should yield the information required.

The investigator developed a competency list, using a Florida list as a model, and ascertained acceptance or rejection of each competency from the two groups. The research was conducted according to the following plan:

1 Two groups, registered nurses in Georgia and faculties in nursing programs in Georgia, were given a questionnaire designed by the present investigator to determine acceptance or rejection of the specific competencies enumerated. Subjects were to indicate acceptance, i.e., the competency is imperative as an entry-level skill, or rejection, i.e., the competency is unnecessary at the point of entry into the profession.

2 Responses of the two groups were tabulated to determine congruence.

3 A defensible list of competencies based on the responses of the two groups was formulated, with those competencies which were unacceptable to 70 percent of the respondents in either group being deleted from the defensible list.

Two sample-selection processes were necessary. The first process involved the selection of practicing nurses for participation in the study. The second process was the determination of nursing faculty members for inclusion in the study. There are presently 32,000 registered nurses in Georgia.

An arbitrary decision was made to survey 1000 of them. Subjects for the group of registered nurses were randomly selected from the files of the State Board of Nursing for Georgia.

For the second group the investigator decided to survey the faculty as a body in all the nursing programs in Georgia. A listing of all the current programs (31 in 1978) was obtained from the State Board of Examiners for Nurses in Georgia. A copy of the same questionnaire sent to the registered nurses was sent to the dean, department head, or director of each of the 31 schools. An attached letter explained the nature of the investigation and requested that the questionnaire be completed according to faculty consensus. The dean, department head, or director was asked to chair a meeting of the faculty or of a representative group of the faculty if all members could not be present, and complete the questionnaire according to group decisions.

A three-part questionnaire was constructed for distribution to individual participants and faculty participants. Part I was designed to provide descriptive and demographic data. The respondents were asked to check the appropriate categories under seven headings: sex, age, highest degree held, basic educational preparation, employment status, field of employment, and type of position. According to Bevis (1978:67), nurses may vary drastically on these demographic points, according to geographical area. In view of this, the demographic section was seen as vital in order to ensure that the present investigation would serve to develop nationally accepted competencies. A summary of this demographic information is presented in Table 10-1.

Seven hundred and twenty nurses of the 1000 polled returned valid questionnaries. The data collected in the demographic section revealed that 680 of the registered nurses responding are female and 40 are male. Nursing is still a predominantly female profession; in the present investigation, approximately 95 percent of the participants in the registered nurse group are female and approximately 5 percent are male.

Table 10-1 Summary of Demographic Information Concerning Registered Nurse Participants

Sex		Employment	
Male	40	Employment status	
Female	680	Not employed	101
Age		Employed full-time	
20–25	119	in nursing	481
26–30	192	not in nursing	14
31–40	178	Employed part-time	
41–50	77	in nursing	117
51–60	119	not in nursing	7
Over 60	35	Employment field	
Education		Clinic	8
Basic education		Self-employed	9
Diploma	395	School nurse	13
A.D.	166	Occupational health	16
B.S.N.	159	Nursing home	19
Highest degree held		Nursing education	31
Diploma	317	Office nurse	50
A.D.	150	Private duty	51
Baccalaureate		Community health	64
B.S.N.	195	Hospital	459
Other field	2	Position held	
Master's		Health planner (nonnurse position)	1
Nursing	89	Nurse-anesthetist	4
Other field	14	Independent practice	6
Doctorate	0	Clinical specialist	14
		Consultant	14
		Faculty in nursing program	21
		Administrator or assistant	39
		In-service education faculty	42
		Head nurse or assistant	77
		Supervisor or assistant	105
		Staff or general duty	397

The second category in the demographic section revealed age patterns. Six age ranges were offered to the participants. Of the 720 participants, 489, or approximately 67 percent, classified themselves in the lower three age categories. Two hundred thirty-one, or approximately 33 percent, indicated that their ages were in the upper three categories.

In the third category of this section, highest degree held, the largest number of participants indicated that the diploma is their highest degree. Of the 720 respondents, 318 hold diplomas from nursing programs. The number holding associate degrees and baccalaureate degrees are almost equal—150 and 147 respectively. Only 89 partici-

pants cited a master's degree in nursing and 16 listed degrees in other fields.

The largest percentage of respondents had received their basic educational preparation in diploma programs. Three hundred ninety-five, or approximately 55 percent of the registered nurse group are diploma graduates. Comparing degrees held with how degrees were obtained revealed that 77 participants originally completed diploma programs and subsequently earned higher degrees. The remainder of the respondents were divided fairly evenly between graduates of associate degree programs (166) and of baccalaureate programs (159).

The fifth category concerned current employment status. A large majority of the participants (481) were found to be employed full time in nursing. Only 21 of the employed participants are employed outside the nursing profession. The final two categories, field of employment and position of employment, indicated some diversity among participants. As would be expected, the largest percentage of respondents are employed at the staff level (397).

Part II of the questionnaire was the actual list of competency statements. This section was formulated using the model developed by the Florida nurses, a model utilized for several reasons. First, it is considered one of the most promising attempts to date to delineate professional competencies. Second, it has been submitted to the National League for Nursing for consideration as a possible national model by the Florida members of the Council of Associate Degree Programs. It was felt that using the same competencies in the present investigation in a geographical area other than Florida would certainly advance the available information in the area of professional competencies. Third, the competencies in the model are specific and are stated in behavioral terms. According to Dobbert (1976:3) these are necessary criteria in the actual writing of competency statements. Fourth, although the model was developed as a competency list for graduates of associate degree programs, it should also be useful as a professional entry-level model. Since the associate degree program is the shortest route to licensure as a registered nurse, it can be assumed that the graduates of the two more extensive educational programs should certainly be able to meet the minimal or entry-level criteria established for graduates of the associate degree program. Finally, the Florida document was developed jointly by nursing educators and nursing practitioners. As indicated by Coe (1967), agreement between the two groups cannot be assumed without actual investigation.

The actual competency statements in Part II are divided into 11 categories, categories which include safety, hygienic care, activity and rest, nutrition, elimination, respiration, medication and

specific therapeutics, assessment, communication, organization, and self-development. Under each category is a varying number of competency statements relating to that category. A total number of 68 competency statements appeared in Part II as it was distributed to the participants. Table 10-2 shows the form in which the questionnaire was presented to the subjects.

Table 10-3 lists all 68 of the competencies as presented under the 11 categories. Frequency of acceptance was tabulated for each statement. The number of positive responses and the corresponding percentage of acceptance were tabulated for each of the statements. Those tabulations can be seen in Table 10-3.

The data reveal several points or possible indicators which warrant discussion. Initially, it is important to recall the individuals from whom the data were collected. Responses were gathered from 720 of the 32,000 registered nurses in Georgia. It cannot be assumed, therefore, that these responses reflect the entire registered nurse population. A large majority of the respondents are female (680). The majority are from younger age categories— 26–30 or 31–40. Over half of the respondents (395) received their basic education in a diploma program. Only 89 of the respondents hold a master's degree in nursing, and none has earned a doctorate. Approximately two-thirds (481) of the respondents are employed in nursing on a full-time basis. A large majority (459) are employed in a hospital setting, and a majority (397) of them work in a staff position. With that population in mind, several pieces of data warrant futher consideration.

First, rate of agreement on most of the competencies is very high. Seven of the 68 competencies listed received 100 percent endorsement from both groups. Fifty-three of the 68 statements, or close to 78 percent, were approved by 90 percent or more of all respondents. In fact, with the exception of the two rejected competencies discussed below (and marked in Table 10–3), all competency statements received an approval rate of at least 80 percent from both groups.

In accordance with the original study plan, any

Table 10-2 Form Used for Part II of Questionnaire Submitted to Georgia Nurses*

Directions. Listed below are competencies or skills which may be necessary for the practice of nursing. Please check Yes for each skill which you determine *IS* a necessary entry skill and No for each skill you determine *IS NOT* a necessary entry skill.

Yes	No	Competencies
		Safety
——	——	1.1 Maintains a safe environment
——	——	1.2 Exercises appropriate physical control (e.g., restraints)
——	——	1.3 Carries out medical asepsis (e.g., transmission control, skin prep)
——	——	1.4 Carries out surgical asepsis (e.g., wound care, gowning and gloving)
——	——	1.5 Uses proper body mechanics (self-patient)
——	——	1.6 Recognizes changes in patient's condition and intervenes as necessary
——	——	1.7 Prepares and cares for patients undergoing diagnostic tests
——	——	1.8 Cares for the surgical patient (pre- and postop)
——	——	1.9 Checks blood products for proper identification
——	——	1.10 Recognizes and reports transfusion reactions
——	——	1.11 Functions in appropriate role in fire/disaster procedure

*Table 10-3 (pp. 128–132) gives complete list of 68 competencies under their 11 categories.

competency rejected by 70 percent of either group was to be eliminated from the list. The only two statements which failed to make the defensible list were:

1 Assesses nutritional status
2 Utilizes O_2 analyzer to correctly determine O_2 concentration in Isolette or neonatal environment.

These two statements were the only two on which the groups disagreed. Both statements were approved by the nurse faculty group but rejected by the registered nurse group. The rationale for disapproval by the registered nurse group was not determined by this study. Perhaps because nutritional assessment is done in most acute care settings by a nutritionist, the registered nurse group has disowned that skill. Since the second rejected competency would primarily occur in a specialized area, the majority of staff nurses would perhaps not be familiar with the task. Both skills are apparently included in curricula since the nurse faculty group endorsed them.

This study was conducted to determine a defensible list of entry-level competencies for registered nurses. The list includes all competencies from the Florida list with the two aforementioned exceptions. The participants represent only a small sample of nurses in one geographic area. Additional studies surveying larger numbers of nurses from a variety of locations are needed. A single list of competencies with general agreement from registered nurses would serve the profession and the general public well. Professional autonomy could be more easily developed with such an agreement. Through education, consumers could become more insightful about expectations regarding registered nurses.

Table 10-3   Response to List of Competencies by Groups

	Competency	Response			
		Registered nurse group		Nurse faculty group	
		Positive responses	% of total	Positive responses	% of total
Safety					
1.1	Maintains a safe environment	720	100	20	100
1.2	Exercises appropriate physical control (e.g., restraints)	671	93.2	19	95
1.3	Carries out medical asepsis (e.g., wound care, gowning, and skin prep)	713	99	20	100
1.4	Carries out surgical asepsis (e.g., wound care, gowning and gloving)	720	100	20	100
1.5	Uses proper body mechanics (self-patient)	713	99	20	100
1.6	Recognizes changes in patient's condition and intervenes as necessary	713	99	20	100
1.7	Prepares and cares for patients undergoing diagnostic tests	684	95	19	95
1.8	Cares for the surgical patient (pre- and postop)	705	98	20	100
1.9	Checks blood products for proper identification	650	90.3	20	100
1.10	Recognizes and reports transfusion reactions	699	97	20	100
1.11	Functions in appropriate role in fire/disaster procedure	692	96	18	90
Hygienic care					
2.1	Administers and/or supervises oral care	699	97	20	100
2.2	Administers and/or supervises skin care	720	100	20	100
2.3	Administers and/or supervises care of hair, hands, and feet	699	97	20	100
Activity and rest					
3.1	Makes beds (e.g., occupied, unoccupied, surgical)	635	88	20	100
3.2	Maintains body alignment (e.g., includes positioning and use of devices to maintain alignment)	713	99	20	100
3.3	Directs and assists with ambulation	685	95	20	100
3.4	Directs and assists with transfer activities	705	98	20	100
3.5	Maintains immobilization (e.g., casts, traction, splints, special beds, and frames)	692	96	20	100
3.6	Maintains supports (e.g., slings, bandages, binders)	699	97	20	100

Table 10-3 Continued

Competency	Registered nurse group		Nurse faculty group	
	Positive responses	% of total	Positive responses	% of total
Activity and rest continued				
3.7 Teaches and supervises use of assistive devices (e.g., cane, crutches, walkers, braces)	628	87	19	95
3.8 Administers, teaches, and supervises activities of daily living, including range of motion	692	96	20	100
Nutrition				
4.1 Assesses nutritional status	195	27	17	85
4.2 Assists with feeding	657	91	20	100
4.3 Performs gastric gavage	643	89.3	17	85
4.4 Assists in maintenance of hyperalimentation	657	91	17	85
4.5 Incorporates diet therapy in care	656	91	20	100
Elimination				
5.1 Inserts, irrigates, and removes tubes (e.g., rectal, urinary, levine)	706	98	19	95
5.2 Performs continuous and intermittent bladder irrigations	636	88	19	95
5.3 Collects specimens (e.g., urine, sputum, stool)	690	95.8	20	100
5.4 Gives enemas	664	92.2	20	100
5.5 Identifies and removes fecal impaction	626	86.9	19	95
5.6 Participates in bowel and bladder retraining	670	93	17	85
5.7 Performs ostomy care	678	94.1	19	95
5.8 Anticipates elimination problems and intervenes appropriately	699	97	20	100
Respiration				
6.1 Positions patient for optimum ventilation	705	98	20	100
6.2 Maintains patent airway	713	99	20	100
6.3 Suctions (e.g., oral, nasal, or via tracheostomy or endotracheal tubes)	699	97	19	95
6.4 Administers resuscitation: a) introduces oropharyngeal airway b) uses Heimlich maneuver and CPR techniques	692	96	18	90
6.5 Cares for tracheostomy (e.g., cuffed and uncuffed)	671	93.1	18	90
6.6 Cares for chest tubes	664	92.2	18	90
6.7 Positions for postural drainage	671	93.1	18	90

Table 10-3 Continued

	Response			
	Registered nurse group		Nurse faculty group	
Competency	Positive responses	% of total	Positive responses	% of total
Respiration continued				
6.8 Supervises coughing and deep breathing exercises	698	96.9	20	100
Medications and specific therapeutics				
7.1 Applies heat and cold treatments	692	96	20	100
a) heat lamp				
b) ice cap				
c) ice collar				
d) hot water bottle				
e) sterile compresses				
f) cradle				
g) electric hot water pack				
h) moist heat and cold				
7.2 Prepares and administers medications safely for patients of all ages, as prescribed by the physician so as to maintain asepsis, prevent tissue damage and complications which could arise from the way in which the meds were prepared and administered	706	98	19	95
a) oral medications				
b) topical medications				
c) parenteral medications (including piggyback I.V. and secondary I.V.s)				
d) inhalant medications				
e) suppositories				
f) nose, eye, and ear drops				
g) instillations				
7.3 Adds medications to I.V.s according to established policy	706	98	20	100
7.4 Administered O_2 using prescribed method (e.g., mask, catheter, cannula)	713	99	20	100
*7.5 Utilizes O_2 analyzer to correctly determine O_2 concentration in Isolette or neonatal environment	216	30	16	80
7.6 Administers therapeutic baths (e.g., Sitz, alcohol)	664	92.2	20	100
7.7 Assists with common diagnostic and therapeutic procedures (e.g., thoracentesis, lumbar puncture, or paracentesis)	713	99	19	95
7.8 Performs venapuncture for I.V. infusion on a training arm	671	93.1	20	100

Table 10-3 Continued

		Response			
		Registered nurse group		Nurse faculty group	
	Competency	Positive responses	% of total	Positive responses	% of total
Assessment					
8.1	Measures, monitors, and records: a) temperature b) pulse c) respiration d) blood pressure e) weight f) body measurement	706	98	20	100
8.2	Observes, monitors, and records: a) skin color and temperature b) level of consciousness (e.g., orientation, pupil reaction) c) secretions and excretions d) intake and output e) results of specified tests	713	99	20	100
8.3	Recognizes and intervenes in life- threatening situations	713	99	19	95
8.4	Identifies and intervenes in deviations from normal behavior	706	98	20	100
Communication					
9.1	Initiates and maintains indivi- dualized nursing care plan	712	98.8	20	100
9.2	Communicates observations both orally and in writing	720	100	20	100
9.3	Identifies and interprets verbal and nonverbal communication	713	99	20	100
9.4	Utilizes therapeutic communication skills (e.g., interviewing, health teaching, clarification of information)	706	98	20	100
9.5	Interacts constructively with other members of the health team as the client advocate	713	99	19	95
9.6	Participates in the referral process to health/social agencies	671	93.1	18	90
Organization					
10.1	Plans and gives total nursing care to 4-6 patients	643	89.3	19	95
10.2	Participates as a member of the nursing team; has beginning skills in leading a nursing team of 2 or 3 health personnel in the total nursing care of 8-10 patients	692	96	20	100
10.3	Participates in team conferences;	692	96	20	100

Table 10-3   Continued

	Response			
	Registered nurse group		Nurse faculty group	
Competency	Positive responses	% of total	Positive responses	% of total
Organization continued				
has beginning skills in leading team conferences				
10.4 Finds and consistently uses appropriate resources	706	98	18	90
Self-development				
11.1 Demonstrates commitment to self-growth	720	100	20	100
a) Accepts responsibility for his/her own behavior				
b) Takes responsibilities for continued learning				
c) Recognizes and initiates constructive action for his/her own limitations				
11.2 Practices within the framework of the profession's legal ethical, and organizational responsibilities	720	100	20	100
11.3 Suggests constructive changes in the health care delivery system through appropriate channels such as:	692	96	17	85
a) nursing service				
b) legislation				
c) professional organizations				

*Competency rejected by 70% of registered nurse group and deleted from defensible list.

EDITOR'S QUESTIONS FOR DISCUSSION

How can the arguments and rationale for competency-based education presented by Clayton be reconciled with outcomes of the behavioral objective movement cited by Peterson in Chap. 7? What other pros and cons might be cited of competency-based curriculum? What alternatives exist for compromise and/or resolution of potential conflict in the development of curriculum?

To what extent do you agree with the competencies identified in this study as essential for entry into practice? Are there any additional competencies you perceive essential? What are the implications of this study for nursing education and nursing practice? What other explanation might be posed for the two rejected competencies deleted by the registered nurse group? What is the relationship between this study and findings in Monnig's survey as presented in Chap. 3?

What are the strengths and limitations of this study? How typical might the respondents in this study be of registered nurse practitioners and faculties in other states? What suggestions might be offered regarding additional research questions and methodology in studying competency-based curriculum and the identification of professional competencies?

REFERENCES

Bevis, Em Olivia
  1978 Curriculum Building in Nursing: A Process. Saint Louis: Mosby Company.
Brandt, Edna M., Bettimae Hastie, and Delores Schumann
  1967 "Comparison of on-the-job performance of graduates with school of nursing objectives." Nursing Research XVI, No. 1: 50–61.
Burnside, Helen and Carrie B. Lenburg
  1970 "Nursing in the decade ahead." Pp. 161 in Edith P. Lewis (ed.), Changing Patterns of Nursing Practice. New York: The American Journal of Nursing Company.
Coe, Charlotte
  1967 "The relative importance of selected educational objectives in nursing." Nursing Research XVI, No. 2: 141–145.
Dobbert, Daniel J.
  1976 "Short answers to frequent questions about competency-based curriculum." Unpublished. ERIC document #Ed 124–039.
Hale, Evelynn Stephens
  1975 "Identification of the range of functions performed by graduates of associate degree programs and graduates of baccalaureate degree programs." Ed.D. dissertation, University of Alabama.
Hassenplug, L. W.
  1965 "Preparation of the nurse practitioner." Journal of Nursing Education XXIX, No. 4.
Johnson, Dorothy E.
  1966 "Competency in practice: Technical and professional." Nursing Outlook XIV: 30–33.
Lessinger, Leon
  1975 "Accountability and the new realities." By Robert R. Ramsey. Southern Regional Education Board 26th Meeting of the Council on Collegiate Education for Nurses. Atlanta, Georgia.
McDonald, Frederick J.
  1974 "The national commission on performance based education." Phi Delta Kappan 55, No. 5: 296–298.
Montag, Mildred
  1969 "The associate degree nursing program: Its philosophy and objectives." Workshop for Teachers in Associate Degree Nursing Programs. DeKalb, Illinois.
Southern Regional Education Board.
  1976 Nursing Curriculum Project: Summary and Recommendations. Atlanta, Georgia: By the Board.

Chapter 11

Nursing Students and the Development of Professional Identity

by Frances C. Dalme, R.N., Ph.D.
Professor, Graduate Programs
College of Nursing
University of Arkansas for Medical Sciences
Little Rock, Arkansas

Faculty members as significant referents of behavior are critical to students' socialization process and adoption of professional values. Frances Dalme's exploratory study tests whether there is a correlation between nursing students' perception of the influence of peers, faculty, and staff nurses and the professional identity nursing students develop. Identity development and reference group theory is the framework for this research. The investigator uses a 73 item Likert-type scale. The empirical indicator of professional identity is 10 items which measures students' attitudes toward the nursing profession. Students' perceptions of peers, faculty, and staff nurses' influence are each measured by 21 items. The sample consists of 250 students in their first and second year from four baccalaureate nursing programs. The findings reveal that the perception scales correlated statistically significantly with the professional identity scale. Partial correlations indicate that peers are the only group influence that appears to remain constant for the grouped data. Dalme further separately examines the first- and second-year nursing students. Her findings indicate that first-year students are influenced by peers. Peers continue to significantly influence the second-year students' development of professional identity. However, evidence is provided that faculty and staff nurses also began to significantly influence the second-year students. In addition, Dalme analyzes the two groups of students regarding their different response to 21 questionnaire items. This research reflects the importance of student culture in the mediation of values transmitted by faculty and staff nurses.

This research was supported in part by a Special Nurse Research Fellowship awarded by the Division of Nursing, U.S. Public Health Service and a research award from Sigma Theta Tau.

A special thanks to Veronica McNeirney, M.S.N., who was helpful in many ways in the preparation of this manuscript.

The primary focus of this study was the development of a professional nursing identity, or that part of a student's social identity which is specific to self-identification with the nursing profession. An attempt was made to identify a relationship between the professional identity nursing students develop, as measured by their attitudes toward the nursing profession, and the perceptions held by these same students, of specific groups of people as influences in the clinical educational environment. The three groups who, in this study, were considered to exercise some influence on students' developing identities were peers, faculty, and staff nurses.

THE PROBLEM

Professional nursing education takes place in a complex setting of social interrelationships among many persons and groups. Some of the persons and groups with whom nursing students interact are patients, peers, physicians, staff nurses, auxiliary personnel, faculty, and visitors. These relationships may exist in any number of learning environments—classrooms, hospitals, community health facilities, and neighborhood health agencies—all of which are considered to offer clinical experiences. This study was limited to nursing students' perceptions of peers, faculty, and staff nurses as environmental influences, without regard to the locus of the interaction, as long as that locus was a clinical learning environment.

This exploratory study was specifically designed to test the hypothesis that there is a correlation between nursing students' perceptions of environmental influences and the professional identity these nursing students develop.

FRAMEWORK

The framework for this study was derived from two theories—the theory of identity development and reference group theory—both of which were used as the basis for an analysis of the human developmental process in relation to the educational goals of professional nursing schools. Identity, according to Erikson (1950:263), is the self-identification that one develops from the "soil of social organization." He has hypothesized a continuous thread of life which shapes one's identity, beginning at birth and ending with death. Identity of the individual emerges from all human interactions, shifting to accommodate the multiplicity of human roles that one assumes during a lifetime.

Erikson (1950) has further postulated an interrelated chronological pattern of eight stages of man out of which evolve the component parts of personal identity. The individual identifies with roles appropriate for his or her age level, and thus personal identity is extended through the socialization process.

Erikson discusses the crises which occur when new roles or tasks are encountered at each stage of development. Adolescent crises arise at that time in life when the individual must

> struggle to make sense out of what has gone before in relation to what he now perceives the world to be, in an effort to find a persistent sameness in himself and a persistent sharing of some kind of essential character with others. (Erikson, 1960:47)

Although each stage of development is a potential crisis period, the adolescent is most prone to identity crises. The later years of adolescence, the age of most nursing students, are characterized by a period which Erikson (1968:128) labels a "moratorium." During this time the individual must synthesize sexual, ethnic, social, and professional role definitions. It seems logical to this investigator that the sexual, ethnic, and social roles are not completely new components of self-identity of the adolescent; it is only the professional role identity that is the new ingredient.

Professional nursing education may be viewed as a potential crisis period for the young nursing student. It is during this period that the student attempts to define norms, attitudes, and standards of the profession he or she has chosen. New expectations must be integrated, and, through observation and participation in the role behaviors of nursing, the total self-identity must be modified to encompass a professional identity. In short, some sense must be made of what the current situation is perceived to be. The positive or negative character of the developing identity is determined more by environmental influences than by the inherent personality structure.

Erikson (1960:48) does not treat attitudes as positive or negative per se, but refers to negative identity in terms of antisocial behavior. Conversely, a positive identity is manifested by acceptable social behaviors. In this study, a negative professional identity was operationally defined in terms of the negative attitudes a student expressed toward the nursing profession, while the more positive the attitudes a student held toward the nursing profession, the more positive the professional identity of that student was assumed to be. Problems of identity formation are minimized in the developmental process if the individual is "able to identify with new roles of competency and invention and to accept an implicit ideological outlook" (Erikson, 1968:130).

The essence of reference group theory is that an individual who wishes to become a part of a particular group adopts the values and attitudes of that group. That is, members of the group serve as models or referents of behavior for the aspirant (Merton, 1957:289-290). As the nursing student moves into the learning environment, he or she interacts with other nurses and experiences the role of a nurse through practicing nursing behaviors; that is, the student identifies with the group to which he or she hopes to belong.

OTHER STUDIES

In the clinical learning environment, faculty and staff nurses provide students with models of the nursing roles; they are the reference groups, the models of standards, as well as of behaviors, for professional nursing. Merton and associates (1957:

287) have suggested that faculty becomes important in guiding the student toward identification with the profession. These same authors and others have pointed out that faculty is the most significant role model for molding certain professional values of students (Merton et al., 1957:287; Davis and Olesen, 1964:13; TenBrink, 1968:149; Pease, 1967:65). However, Quarantelli et al. (1964:43) have noted that this is not the case in dental school. There are no studies in schools of nursing that would clarify these two positions, even though the assumption is made that teachers who practice nursing could serve as role models for nursing students (Christman, 1979:9; Mauksch, 1980:23).

Staff nurses have been described as having an influence on professional development. However, student references to staff nurses as role models center around perceived conflicts in nursing roles. The argument is that staff nurses, with a different orientation, provide the student with alternatives to the orientation presented by the faculty (Smith, 1965:202; Copp, 1968:213-214; Christman, 1979:8). For at least 20 years it has been a belief that the faculty is more oriented to the ideal type of care, or the type of care that *should* be carried out, while the staff is more oriented to the way care *can be* and *is* carried out (Corwin, 1961:614). Kramer (1974:196) provides evidence that the student holds an image of the nurse's role that is more ideal than real. Nonetheless, after much experience in the role and through exposure to many role models and many other influences within the clinical educational setting, the student achieves a reorganization of his or her perception of the nurse's role.

Upon entering an educational program, the learner is exposed to stimuli from several groups of people. The peer group provides feedback in terms of the appropriateness of behavior in the learning environment. Peers provide support during difficult times in the process of learning; peers provide solutions to problems in the process of learning; and indeed, peers provide reinforcement for behaviors experienced in the learning process (Hughes et al., 1967:522-527). Olesen and Whitaker (1968) have also suggested that the peer group is a significant force in shaping the professional. In their study of medical students, Merton et al. (1957:180–181) reported that less-advanced students looked to upperclass students for cues in "professional behavior."

Waltz (1978:96) reported that student bias toward nursing faculty is influenced by the faculty member's reputation among fellow students. Furthermore, students' preferences for practice are influenced by their perceptions of the reputations of faculty members. From this study it seems possible that peers are more influential than faculty in the practice preference of their classmates.

METHODOLOGY

To test the hypothesis that there is a correlation between nursing students' perceptions of selected environmental influences and the professional identity nursing students develop, a Likert-type scale questionnaire was developed by the investigator (Dalme, 1971; 1979). The empirical indicator of professional identity was student response to 10 items which measured positive or negative attitudes toward nursing as a profession. Likert-type scales of 21 items each were developed to measure students' perceptions of the influence of peers, faculty, and staff nurses upon nursing students in the clinical educational environment.

The 73-item instrument was drawn from a list of 173 items originally submitted to rigorous validity and reliability studies. These studies, which included factor analysis, communality coefficients, homogeneity ratios (HR), Cronbach's alpha computations, and test-retest reliabilities, were all applied before the scales were used to collect data. Eighty-nine students, juniors and seniors at two southern universities, participated in the reliability studies. After the first tests were administered, only those items which yielded the highest communality readings were retained. Analysis of the retest result revealed that three of the four item-clusters—faculty, staff nurses, and professional identity—exceeded the minimum homogeneity

ratios (HR) and reliability criteria established for the study. The item-cluster designated as peers met the minimum criterion of reliability but not the criterion established for HR. Test-retest reliabilities were above .83 for all scales except the peers scale, which was .58.

An additional 17 items of the research instrument were designed to elicit biodemographic characteristics, how the respondents ranked nursing as compared with other professions, their general beliefs about their educational experiences, and their role model preferences.

SETTING AND SAMPLE

This study was conducted in four baccalaureate nursing programs located in one midwestern state. Because these schools were located within a 50-mile geographical radius, the data could be gathered within a 1-week time span.

Schools A and B were both state universities, the latter a medical center campus with a large nursing student enrollment and a graduate nursing program. Schools C and D were small private schools, Catholic and Protestant respectively.

Two hundred and fifty subjects, approximately 66 percent of the total nursing student population (377), participated in this study. One hundred and eighteen were students in the first year of clinical nursing and 132 were in the second year. A summary of the total number of nursing students enrolled, the number participating in the study, and the number of participants in each year of clinical work is reflected in Table 11–1.

The 250 nursing students who participated in this study were remarkably homogeneous in background and biographical characteristics. Eighty-five percent of the subjects were between 20 and 23 years of age; 97.2 percent were unmarried; 57.3 percent had been reared in rural or small metropolitan areas; and 75 percent were from the middle to upper socioeconomic levels. There were no significant differences in first-year and second-year clinical students with regard to their background and biographical characteristics.

Table 11-1   Number of Nursing Students Enrolled in Schools A, B, C, D, Number and Percent Participating in Study, and Number Participating from First and Second Year of Clinical Nursing

Schools	Students in clinical nursing			Number of participants by year of clinical nursing	
	Number enrolled	Number participating	% participating	First year	Second year
A	114	102	89.1	50	52
B	158	80	51.9	40	40
C	48	28	58.3	15	13
D	57	40	70.1	13	27
Totals	377	250	66.3	118	132

ANALYSIS

The intercorrelations among scales obtained from the responses of the 250 subjects are presented in Table 11-2.

Grouped Data

The grouped data as reported in Table 11-2 reveal statistically significant correlation between each perception scale and the professional identity scale. The two perception scales, peers and faculty, yield correlations with the professional identity scale that are significant ($P < .001$), and the staff nurses scale, too, is statistically significantly correlated ($P < .01$) with the professional identity scale. These findings affirm the hypothesis of the

Table 11-2   Intercorrelations among the Perception Scales of Peers, Faculty, Staff Nurses and Professional Identity
(Grouped Data $N = 250$)

Perception scale	Peers	Faculty	Staff nurses	Professional identity
Peers	.658	.388	.252	.392*
Faculty		.862	.289	.276†
Staff nurses			.836	.185‡
Professional identity				.880

*6.53 $P < .001$
†4.60 $P < .001$
‡3.08 $P < .01$

study. There is a correlation between students' perceptions of learning environmental influences and the professional identity students develop. The magnitude of the correlation coefficient between the perception scales with the professional identity scale is progressively decremental from peers to staff nurses.

Since all three perception scales are statistically significantly correlated with the identity scale, the methodological question of interaction of one scale with another arose. To determine the effect of one scale on the correlation of another scale with the scale of professional identity, partial correlations were calculated. The results of these calculations reveal that only the highest interscale correlation (peers with professional identity, .392) remains statistically significant ($P < .001$) with the effects of the other scale variables removed. Peer influence is the only group influence that appears to remain constant for the grouped data.

The data were then examined from the standpoint of group variability. It was suspected that in the two different clinical years there may have been different environmental influences operating.

Comparison of First-Year and Second-Year Clinical Students

In examining the data from the two groups separately it was found that first-year clinical nursing students ($N = 118$) attained a significant ($P < .01$)

Table 11-3 Correlation Coefficients for Perception Scales with the Professional Identity Scale and the Partial Correlations*

Perception scale	Correlation with PI scale	Scale partialled	Partial correlation coefficient
Clinical year I (*N* = 118)			
Peers	.280	Faculty	.276[†]
Peers	.280	Staff	.267[†]
Clinical year II (*N* = 132)			
Peers	.473	Faculty	.376[‡]
Peers	.473	Staff	.433[‡]
Faculty	.478	Peers	.381[‡]
Faculty	.478	Staff	.451[‡]
Staff nurses	.303	Peers	.235[§]
Staff nurses	.303	Faculty	.248[§]

*Partial correlations were calculated for those scales that were statistically significantly correlated with the professional identity scale. In the first-year class the faculty-professional identity correlation was .070 and the staff nurses–professional identity correlation was .085. Since the effect of these two scales was so small, it was assumed that the effects on the other scale relationships would be negligible. Conversely, a much higher correlation was obtained for all scales with the professional identity scale for second-year students than for the first-year students; therefore, each scale was submitted to partial correlations.

[†] .239 *P* < .01
[‡] .265 *P* < .001
[§] .214 *P* < .01

correlational value (.280) of the peer perception scale with the professional identity scale, as indicated in Table 11-3. The correlations between the other two perception scales, faculty and staff nurses, with the scale of professional identity yielded values that were no greater than could be expected by chance. This evidence suggests that peers do influence first-year nursing students' professional identity development.

To ascertain if this trend of peer influence observed in the first year continues and if or how it is affected by other environmental groups, the data from the second-year clinical nursing students were examined. The scores of second-year clinical nursing students (*N* = 132) show significant (*P* < .01) correlations between all the perception scales (peers, faculty, and staff nurses) and the professional identity scale. Furthermore, the relationship of the peer influence with professional identity that is observed in the analysis of the first-year students actually seems greater in the second

year, as demonstrated by a higher correlation coefficient (.473). In the second-year group, all correlations of environmental influence perception scale scores with those of professional identity are statistically significant (*P* < .01–.001).

The peer influence continues into the second year, and the second-year faculty and staff nurses begin to significantly influence the students' development of professional identity. Spuriousness that might have been attributed to the confounding of one scale with another was ruled out by partial correlations. The partial correlation coefficient gives a truer value of the actual relationship of one variable with another (Glass and Stanley, 1970: 182–186).

In Table 11-3 it can be seen that the partial correlation coefficient (.276) obtained for the peer-professional identity scales for first-year students is smaller than the original correlation (.280), while holding constant (partialling out) the contribution made to this relationship by the faculty scale. The partial coefficient obtained was .276, which means that the faculty scale contributed only .004 to the peer-professional identity scale correlation for first-year clinical nursing students. The partial relationships between the perception scales and professional identity are smaller than the original correlations for both first- and second-year students, but they remain statistically significant at the .01 level. These results are reported in the partial correlation coefficient column in Table 11-3.

A study of scale means, as reported in Table 11-4, for first-year and second-year clinical students shows the latter had higher scale means than the former on every scale except the professional identity scale. The scale mean for the professional identity scale is lower for second-year students than for first-year students. The lower mean, though not statistically significant, indicates a more negative attitude on the part of the respondents.

The differences in the means, although not statistically different using the *t*-test, suggest that the two groups may have differed in their responses to specific items. All 73 items were submitted to the chi-square test and first-year and second-year clinical groups responded differently to 21 items. These results are reported in Table 11-5.

As seen from the responses to the 21 items, the groups differed, according to year in school, in their perceptions of peers, faculty, and staff nurses

Table 11-4   Scale Means and Standard Deviation for First- and Second-Year Clinical Nursing Students
(*N* = 250)

Perception scale	First-year		Second-year	
	Mean	S.D.	Mean	S.D.
Peers	51.9	6.9	52.7	7.6
Faculty	51.8	11.0	56.2	9.8
Staff nurses	42.9	10.6	44.8	9.2
Professional identity	32.3	5.7	31.7	6.4

as influences, and in their attitudes toward their education for the profession. Similarly they differed in their selection of a role model. A final item of the research instrument was designed to have the students indicate the title of the person who possessed those characteristics and attributes that they would most like to have.

Faculty members were more frequently chosen as role models by both student groups (39.1 percent). However, if head nurses, supervisors, and staff nurses are considered together, then first-year students more frequently (39.8 percent) selected a role model other than a faculty member (32.2). Moreover, first-year students more often (28 percent) than second-year clinical students (18.5 percent) indicated that they had "no preference" as to a role model.

DISCUSSION

The findings of this study indicate that the longer the nursing student is in the clinical arena, the more different groups of people significantly influence his or her attitudes toward the profession. This finding supports both the hypothesis of this study and Erikson's (1950) theoretical proposition that there is a relationship between environmental influences and the identity one develops.

It also seems apparent that the student culture mediates how the values of faculty and staff nurses are transmitted (Merton et al., 1957:296; Hughes et al., 1967:522-527; Waltz, 1978:96). If peers are the mediating group, then it seems logical that the first influential group relationship that is developed in nursing school may be with peers; and relationships with other groups significant in the development of professional identity follow.

Table 11-5 indicates some salient findings. First-year students agreed that there was "group spirit in caring for patients" and that there was "interest in studying and learning" more frequently than did their second-year classmates. In the second year there appeared to be a shift from group spirit to a more competitive peer relationship, a perception revealed by the fact that a larger percentage

Table 11-5 Percentage Agreement or Disagreement of First- and Second-Year Students on Items Reflecting Statistically Different Responses

Item no.	Content of item*	Clinical year	Disagree (%)	Agree (%)	χ^2	d.f.[†]
1	Classmates would do what they could to prevent staff from hurting patient	1 2	65.1 39.1	34.9 60.9	17.93	2
6	Classmates have group spirit when caring for patients	1 2	41.5 53.5	58.1 46.6	8.73	3
7	Students pay little attention to how well they do relative to others	1 2	64.9 84.6	34.1 15.4	17.19	4
9	Class has been successful in changing course content	1 2	44.9 29.4	55.1 70.6	24.58	3
10	Classmates suggest their own learning experiences	1 2	17.1 6.1	82.9 93.9	15.18	2
12	Classmates are interested in studying and learning	1 2	26.4 20.7	73.6 79.3	10.84	4
22	Instructor would label crying "unprofessional"	1 2	47.7 68.4	52.3 31.6	12.06	2
23	Teachers are too watchful	1 2	60.6 83.1	29.4 16.9	10.97	3
24	Faculty would think public protest of social problems unprofessional	1 2	41.2 60.0	58.8 40.0	8.97	3
25	Teachers do not allow students opportunity to plan course content	1 2	52.9 72.1	47.1 27.9	12.74	3
32	Teachers encourage students to express views about social problems	1 2	21.9 14.6	68.1 85.4	12.15	3
34	Faculty encourages students to undertake independent projects	1 2	52.1 39.2	47.9 60.8	15.24	3
36	Well-reasoned student's report is accepted if different from view of teacher	1 2	48.7 43.2	51.3 56.8	11.97	4
38	Faculty helped crystallize a desire to become a nurse	1 2	40.3 23.2	59.7 76.8	9.34	3
40	Teachers encourage interest in social problems	1 2	46.2 29.2	53.8 70.8	10.45	3

continued

Table 11-5 Continued

Item no.	Content of item*	Clinical year	Disagree (%)	Agree (%)	χ^2	d.f. †
42	Faculty is well qualified to help students achieve goals in nursing	1 2	31.1 24.0	68.9 76.0	27.31	4
46	Students can depend on staff nurses for help	1 2	46.1 31.7	53.9 68.3	17.24	4
47	Staff nurses are eager to find out new ideas of patient care	1 2	63.8 45.4	36.2 54.6	9.31	3
50	Staff nurses are willing to teach new procedure	1 2	53.7 49.7	46.3 50.3	6.51	2
59	Being closely watched by staff nurses causes tension	1 2	71.8 86.6	27.7 13.4	10.27	4
71	Being in nursing school is an unpleasant experience	1 2	86.5 69.2	13.6 30.8	16.47	4

*Item is not repeated verbatim here, but the idea is conveyed.
†Probabilities are read as follows:

d.f.	P value	P <	P value	P <	P value	P <
2	13.85	.001	9.201	.01	5.991	.05
3	16.27	.001	11.345	.01	7.815	.05
4	18.465	.001	13.277	.01	9.488	.05

By using the BMDO2S computer program the decision was made as to the best way to collapse the tables. Expected frequencies in some cells were sometimes too small to be acceptable for the calculation of chi-square, hence these small cells were collapsed into other cells. The entire table, given on the original printout, was put into a 2 X 2 table (by the investigator) for this report. However, the original degrees of freedom (d.f.) are reported also; the response categories were dichotomized into "agree (A)" or "disagree (D)" rather than the original five response categories as were given on the questionnaire, or the 2 X 3, 2 X 4, or 2 X 5 categories that were given in the collapsed tables on the computer printout.

Percent of agree and disagree were rounded to the nearest tenth and may result in not equaling exactly 100 percent.

of the second-year students (85 percent) disagreed with the statement that "students pay little attention to how well they do relative to others."

Students also seem to assume more control over the methods of the socialization process as they progress, in that the older students consider themselves "successful in changing course content." The confidence of the nursing students in the faculty's capacity to guide, to motivate, and to accept them into the profession is evident in the responses given by second-year clinical students to specific items. In contrast to first-year nursing students, second-year students reported that teachers "give opportunity to plan course content," "encourage them to take independent projects," "help crystallize desire to become a nurse," and "are qualified to help students achieve goals."

First-year students did not appear to trust or to have the confidence in faculty or in staff nurses that their second-year classmates expressed. First-year nursing students did not believe they could count on staff nurses "for help" or "to teach new procedures." More frequently than the second-year clinical students they reported that staff nurses made them "tense" and staff nurses were not "eager to find out new ideas about patient care." This lack of trust and confidence is evident in their perception of faculty influence. Even so, there is a fairly even distribution, regardless of clinical year, in student selection of faculty (39.1 percent) or nursing personnel (37.9 percent) as role models.

Less than one-third (28.6 percent) of the nursing students from four baccalaureate nursing programs in one midwestern state agreed that they would be prepared to practice nursing when they finished the nursing program. It is noteworthy that a larger percentage of second-year clinical students (30.8 percent) than of first-year students (13.6 percent) agreed that "being in nursing school [was] an unpleasant experience." These findings may simply indicate that neither first-year nor second-year students could be regarded as having been fully socialized into the profession. The conclusion was that both groups were in the continuing process of socialization.

CONCLUSION

The genesis of professional identity formation seems apparent. The nursing student first achieves a kind of sociability with peers, then becomes involved in a competitive apprenticeship with and among the peer group. The evidence from this study suggests that faculty and staff nurses become significant to the development of professional identity some time during the student's second clinical year.

Faculty relationships help the nursing student to internalize norms of the profession and to begin to have a sense of belonging to the group. As the student progresses in the nursing program he or she adopts the values of the professional group, and the faculty members become more and more significant referents of behavior.

Staff nurses, too, become significant referents

of behavior late in the educational sequence. This evidence supports the argument for model clinical settings for student learning.

IMPLICATIONS

Since the student's perception of faculty and staff nurses seems to be related to professional identity development, there is a need to have the student associate with faculty and staff nurses who demonstrate excellence in the practice setting and who can serve as appropriate role models. In addition, since peers are the first group to exert some influence upon the development of professional identity, faculty needs to have input into the peer group very early in the clinical learning experience.

One way to accomplish this would be to have small peer group discussions directed by faculty toward the goal of professional identity development. In these discussions other questions raised by this study could be addressed. For instance, are there groups in the learning environment besides faculty, staff nurses, and peers, who influence attitudes toward the profession? Practical nurses and aides are significant to the new graduate during the process of "reality testing" (Kramer, 1974:97). Although these two groups and others in the learning environment have no direct responsibility for professional formation, they may influence the student's perception of the nursing role. What attitudes are transmitted by these other groups and adopted by the nursing student?

Discussions with students about their clinical experiences could explore their perceptions of the roles of other groups and how these roles are complimentary to the role of the professional nurse. If such discussions are to be productive, it seems imperative that faculty practices in the learning environment. Only teachers who deal with the conflicts of the real practice setting and who are an integral part of the learning milieu can assist students in identifying, evaluating, and adopting attitudes that are "professional."

EDITOR'S QUESTIONS FOR DISCUSSION

How can faculty members further develop themselves as role models for nursing students? What variables in an education setting affect role modeling by students? How might faculty positively influence the impact of peers on students' evolution of a professional identity?

What are the implications for the profession if students' peers are more influential than faculty in the development of professional identity? If references to staff nurses as role models for students center around creating conflict in nursing roles, what effects in nursing practice might be reflected after graduation? What might account for the negative change in professional identity between the first- and second-year nursing students? If the majority of students in this study continue to perceive that they would not be prepared to practice nursing by the time they complete their nursing program, what might be the implications for nursing practice and nursing education programs?

To what extent might the findings of this study be typical of other nursing students? How appropriate was the process for the development of the research instrument? Does the reliability of the peers' scale need to be kept in mind in interpretation of the findings? What was the purpose of calculating partial correlations? What additional research questions does this study suggest?

REFERENCES

Christman, Luther
  1979 "The practitioner teacher." Nurse Education 4:8–11.
Copp, Mary Carol
  1968 The Student as a Marginal Person. Unpublished doctoral dissertation. Boulder: University of Colorado.
Corwin, Ronald G.
  1961 "The professional employee: A study of conflict in nursing roles." American Journal of Sociology 66:604–615.
Dalme, Frances Carolynn
  1971 A Study of the Relationship of Nursing Students' Perception of Selected Environmental Influences and the Students' Development of Professional Identity. Unpublished doctoral dissertation. Boulder: University of Colorado.
  1979 "Learning environment questionnaire." in Mary J. Ward and Mark E. Fetler (eds.), Research Instruments for Use in Nursing Education Research. Boulder, Colorado: WICHE.
Davis, Fred and Virginia Olesen
  1964 "Baccalaureate students' images of nursing: A study of change, consensus and consonance in the first year." Nursing Research 8:8–15.
Erikson, Erik
  1950 Childhood and Society. New York: Norton.
  1960 "Youth and the life cycle." Children 7:43–50.
  1968 Youth and Crises. New York: Norton.
Glass, Gene V. and Julian Stanley
  1970 Statistical Methods in Education and Psychology. Englewood Cliffs, New Jersey: Prentice-Hall.
Hughes, Everett C., Howard Becker, and Blanche Geer
  1967 "Student culture and academic effort." pp. 522–527. in Nevitt Sandord (ed.), The The American College. New York: Wiley.
Kramer, Marlene
  1974 Reality Shock: Why Nurses Leave Nursing. St. Louis: Mosby.
Mauksch, Ingeborg
  1980 "Faculty practice: A professional imperative." Nurse Educator 5:21–24.
Merton, Robert K.
  1957 Social Theory and Social Structure. New York: The Free Press.

Merton, Robert K., George D. Reader, and Patricia L. Kendall
1957 The Student Physician. Cambridge, Massachusetts: Harvard Press.

Olesen, Virginia L. and Elvie Whittaker
1968 The Silent Dialogue. San Francisco: Jossey-Bass

Pease, John
1967 "Faculty influence and professional participation of doctoral students." Sociological Inquiry 9:63–70.

Quarantelli, Enrico, Margaret Helfrich, and Daniel Yutsey
1964 "Faculty and student perceptions in a professional school." Sociology and Social Research 49:32–45.

Smith, Kathryn M.
1965 "Discrepancies in the role-specific values of head nurse and nursing educators." Nursing Research 14:196–202.

TenBrink, Carol Lee
1968 "The process of socialization into a new role: The professional nurse." Nursing Forum 1:146–160.

Waltz, Carolyn Feher
1978 "Faculty influence on nursing students preference for practice." Nursing Research 27:89–96.

Chapter 12

Doctoral Education in Nursing: Dilemmas and Directions

Helen K. Grace, R.N., Ph.D., F.A.A.N.
Dean and Professor
College of Nursing
University of Illinois
at the Medical Center
Chicago, Illinois

Having focused upon the basic education of the nursing student in previous chapters it is crucial to also present an in-depth discussion of doctoral education in nursing in order to have an overall view and approach to nursing education. Helen K. Grace clearly reviews the history of doctoral programs in nursing, defines the issues, and offers substantial direction. She describes four early program models. Grace addresses numerous issues that have never been resolved, such as the type of doctoral programs nurses should complete. She cites the conflict of programs caught between preparing researcher-scholars and maintaining ties to the clinical practice of nursing. Grace discusses the separate paths of education and practice as well as unrealistic expectations. Having emphasized doctoral preparation for nurse researchers, Grace believes it is time for nursing to prepare clinician-teachers and clinician-practitioners. In viewing the education and practice domains, she advocates a need for two patterns of doctoral preparation for nurses and proposes a curriculum model for a two-track approach to doctoral education.

The decade of the seventies may well be described by future nurse historians as one in which doctoral education *in* nursing came to the fore. In 1960 only 4 doctoral programs in nursing existed; by 1980 this number had grown to a total of 21. Given this proliferation of doctoral programs, it is timely to review the process of doctoral program development in nursing, identify the dilemmas confronting doctoral education in nursing, and propose new directions.

As all higher education faces a constricting economic climate, the focus on quantity is waning in the eighties, with an emphasis on preservation of quality. This poses serious difficulties for nursing education where the need for doctorally prepared nurses continues, despite the constraints which are being placed upon the entire system of higher education. Given this economic climate, nursing education must find a way of meeting the needs for production of doctorally prepared nurses adequate to the needs of the field, while simultaneously being able to speak to the qualitative issues of doctoral nursing programs. In order to do this, it is crucial that nursing be clear about the goals and direction of the profession. Patterns of doctoral education in nursing must be appropriate to the practice dimensions of the discipline as well as to the goals of generation and transmission of in-depth nursing knowledge. With these ends in mind, a careful review of the rationale surrounding doctoral education in nursing is warranted.

NATURE OF DOCTORAL EDUCATION

Prior to the sixties, doctoral education in nursing and for nurses emanated predominantly from settings directed toward the preparation of educators. Then in the early sixties development of professional nurse doctoral programs, e.g., the D.N.Sc. at Boston University and at the University of California, San Francisco, began. Next, federal funding for the nurse-scientist programs opened up avenues for nurses to pursue doctoral study in other scientific disciplines and served to stimulate the flow of nurses into doctoral study. By the mid-sixties the first of a series of conferences speaking to direction for doctoral education in nursing was held at Case Western Reserve University. Issues identified in the mid-sixties still surround doctoral education in nursing today. Jean Berthold, the moderator of that conference, posed these issues in her introduction:

> At the present time nursing is confronted with four general but overlapping issues related to doctoral preparation. First, . . . what are the goals of doctoral preparation for nurses?
>
> Second, who are the "some nurses" who need to be prepared at the doctoral level in order to fulfill their role responsibilities adequately? . . .
>
> Next, what type of doctoral programs should nurses undertake? . . .
>
> Lastly, when should a nurse be encouraged to go into a doctoral program? (1966:48)

As a participant in this 1965 conference Peplau distinguished the nature of two doctoral pathways:

> In psychiatric nursing, the Ph.D. would mean that the nurse has depth knowledge in human behavior, drawn from selected behavioral sciences and from psychiatric nursing researches, and that she has an intense interest in further clinical research in a piece of such knowledge. . . . The D.N.Sc. would mean that the nurse has pursued depth clinical training for expert psychiatric nursing practice. While the exposure to research methods would be required—for this sharpens clinical investigation—the main concern would not be with evolution of new basic knowledge but rather with the practical knowledge or new knowledge developed by others. The emphasis would be on procedures for the application of knowledge. This is not to say that both nurses would not be competent to practice, or that the nurse with the D.N.Sc. would not, perhaps incidentally, originate some new ideas concerning psychiatric pathology. The difference is one of emphasis in the educational program. The Ph.D. emphasizes theory and the production of original new knowledge; the D.N.Sc. emphasizes applications of established theory, some of it "hot off the press," but derived by others. Accordingly, the D.N.Sc. would require the student to complete a thesis having to do with the testing of a theoretically based practice. The Ph.D. would require the nurse to complete an original study leading to a new knowledge. (1966:57-67)

Peplau clearly identifies the need for at least two distinctively different patterns of doctoral education for nurses to address the practice domain of the profession.

Schlotfeldt, in the same conference and speaking to the same point proposed yet a different model (1966). In arguing that preparation of nurses at the doctoral level must appropriately be within basic science disciplines, Schlotfeldt is a proponent of the model of medicine.

> In medicine, knowledge is being constantly

advanced by investigators who are at once physicians and scientists prepared in the basic disciplines. They are engaged in scientific work which advances medical knowledge. In addition, the specialist-clinician collaborates with the physician-scientists and with scientists who are not physicians, and the knowledge derived from that collaboration is extensive. Nursing could profit from similar collaboration. (1966:74)

While the model proposed by Schlotfeldt differs from that of Peplau, both are directed toward the same end, bridging the generation and transmission of knowledge with the practice domain. These issues were identified early in the development of doctoral programs in nursing but the content of doctoral programs currently in existence shows that approaches toward addressing those issues have not been appreciably clarified.

In tracing the history of doctoral program development in the United States it is interesting to note the diversity within the first doctoral programs for nursing. Early programs such as that at Teachers College, Columbia University were based upon an Ed.D. model and were tailored as were other education degrees. The Ph.D. at New York University developed out of a College of Education framework into a Ph.D. in Nursing Science. A third program model, that of the D.N.Sc., was developed at Boston University. This program was initiated in 1960 and was based upon the development of "nursing theory" as the focal point of a practice discipline. This program produced 10 graduates before being restructured into a more traditional mold (Mellow, 1966:71). Yet another approach was that of the University of Pittsburgh, with its Ph.D. program in Maternal and Child Nursing, which focused upon clinical research in nursing. While these original progam models were distinctively different, as time has gone on the distinctions between these programs have become muted. Program models across the country, be they D.N.Sc. or Ph.D. models, are remarkably the same, with most having fallen into a trap that Matarazzo so eloquently cautioned

against in his paper presented at a conference on "Future Directions for Doctoral Education," sponsored by the Nursing Division of HEW in 1971. In speaking to the problems faced by nursing in moving aggressively toward the establishment of doctoral programs in nursing, Matarazzo spoke to nurses' romanticized view of science.

In articles, debates, and conferences, nurses engaged in agonizing soul-searching and stock-taking about practice derived from principle and scientific theory in its relation to practice. These articles read like sophomore level textbooks ... Nurses talk and talk and talk about science instead of doing it ... Science ... has little relationship to practice. Why is nursing so set on establishing a relationship between science and practice, when no other field has been able to carry it off? Why do members of nursing faculties not stop talking about scientific method and research strategies and instead go take a good look at a scientifically active colleague in any other discipline? ... What they would learn is that what the scientist does is the very antithesis of the nonsense they write in their articles about the relationship between nursing and science. U.S. Dept. of HEW, Division of Nursing. (1971:5–11)

Doctoral programs in nursing are caught up in the cross currents of on the one hand preparing research and scholars and on the other hand maintaining ties to the clinical practice of nursing. In attempting to achieve all things within our doctoral programs, the emphasis increasingly is placed upon rote learning of research methods and nursing theoretical frameworks rather than upon the process of conceptualization of significant research questions and the excitement of the investigative process. This serves to seriously hamper the viability of our research enterprise.

Secondly, since currently no well-developed clinical doctoral program models exist, we are not addressing the needs of the practice domain for nurses prepared at the level of the doctorate as nurse clinician-investigators. Although a number of authors speak to the need for a true professional doctorate, there is little evidence that such a program model has, as yet, been developed.

Professional doctorates are of two types: (1) those based upon a generalized baccalaureate degree plus additional years of professional education leading to a first professional degree such as the M.D. or J.D.; and (2) programs based upon a generic first professional degree program such as a B.S.N. with clinical specialization and research at the doctoral level. In nursing these two degrees would be the D.N. and the D.N.Sc. degrees. While both types of professional degrees are currently being offered, the distinctions between program models are not clear. Cleland in support of professional doctorates writes:

> I personally favor the development of the professional doctorate. It will be essential for the recognition of nursing's role in patient care management in the health service setting. We must be clear, however, about our expectations and goals. The professional doctorate is designed to prepare a utilizer of research rather than an investigator, and its primary focus should be upon expert clinical practice. (1976:632)

Downs, speaking to similar issues, makes a plea for clarification of programmatic goals and directions:

> If we believe that doctoral education for nurses is worth the huge investment in time, energy, and money that we believe it is, we need to move as rapidly as possible to clarify the nature and goals of that course of study. Otherwise, degree recipients may discover they have been offered hollow promises of a professional future that will not exist by the time they reach it. Experience has taught us that this kind of educational dilemma can happen. It is absolutely essential that future movements into doctoral education be guided by the explicit assumptions underlying them and by some kind of consensus regarding their meaning within the context of professional function. No prospective student can be expected to make an intelligent career decision without such information. (1978:60)

The need for clarification of programmatic goals and directions is clearly identified, and remains the challenge of the 1980s. With 21 doctoral nursing programs in place, we have a sufficient critical mass of programs from which programmatic distinctions can be drawn. Before delineating a possible model for program differentiation at the doctoral level, a hard look at the particular dilemmas nursing as a profession must confront in charting its course is perhaps warranted.

DILEMMAS CONFRONTING NURSING

Nursing, in the course of its development as a profession, has constantly been in a position of being controlled by a variety of outside forces. Nursing education, in attempting to gain autonomy by moving out of the context of hospital settings and into the educational mainstream, has been caught up in another struggle, that of gaining respectability in the halls of academe. Nursing practice, on the other hand, has struggled along a separate path, with education and service frequently at odds with one another. Issues related to doctoral education in nursing are integrally tied to these larger contextual issues. A first priority for doctoral programs in nursing was that of producing a sufficient number of doctorally prepared nurses to fill faculty positions in academe so that nursing education would meet the same standards of qualification as that of other university disciplines. In our endeavors to get a sufficient number of doctorally prepared faculty members we have frequently lost sight of the nature of both of the clinical teaching and practice of nursing.

Our models for doctoral education have predominantly been drawn from the disciplines in which most nursing educators have received their doctoral preparation, i.e., education and the biological and social sciences. While we recognize the need for a cadre of capable and active nurse researchers to develop the body of nursing knowledge upon which education and practice rest, it is of equal importance that nurse-educators and clinicians be prepared to incorporate this knowledge base into educational programs and service delivery. Our emphasis in doctoral education to date has been upon preparing a cadre of nurse-researchers; this emphasis should in no way be diminished, but the time is ripe for the development of doctoral level programs geared to prepare clinician-teachers and clinician-practitioners. Our questions now need to turn from production of sufficient numbers to considering what types of education and experiential backgrounds are needed to meet the diversified demands of the nursing profession in its education and practice domains.

At a conference convened by the Nursing Division of HEW in June of 1974, it was proposed that all nurse faculty teaching at the baccalaureate level, all directors of nursing service in health science teaching centers, and coordinators of research within these settings ultimately be doctorally prepared (U.S. Dept. of Health, Education, and Welfare, Division of Nursing, 1974). In addition the need for doctorally prepared nurses functioning in service delivery roles was clearly identified. It was suggested that in nursing, as in other fields, 1 to 2 percent of the entire population of nurses be doctorally prepared. Given this large and diversified a number, it is reasonable to assume that within nursing we need more than one program pathway to meet the needs of the profession. To reach clarification as to the needs of the profession it is perhaps best to look carefully at the dilemmas faced by the groups of nurses identified as needing doctoral preparation.

First, consider the nursing faculty group. The types of roles and functions performed by nursing faculty are highly diversified. Teachers in a small baccalaureate program housed in a liberal arts setting have a very different role in the teaching process than do those who teach within a complex, large educational program housed within a health science teaching context. There are currently some 250 baccalaureate programs in nursing; faculty within these programs totals about 10,000. To prepare this large number in a traditional research-oriented mold would, first of all, be impossible given our current capabilities and would not be appropriate preparation for all faculty given the roles and functions it is to perform.

Within this group, we need both a cadre of well-prepared research scholars and teachers and a cadre of well-prepared clinicians-teachers if the quality of nursing education is to be maintained. Currently, baccalaureate nursing education is being conducted by faculty prepared primarily at the master's level, with clinical specialization and expertise. These members need great depth of preparation in their clinical specialization area. In addition, they need to be participants in the research process but because of the constraints of undergraduate teaching they are unable to function as principal investigators. Their involvement in clinical practice should be a central component of their teaching role.

Other faculty members with depth of preparation in research need to be actively involved as principal investigators in the research process in collaboration with clinician-teachers and clinician-practitioners, while also engaged in teaching in their area of specialization at all levels of the educational program. Moreover, nursing educational administrators of academic programs certainly also need preparation in nursing doctoral programs that will provide them with a sound grounding in research. Similarly, administrators of nursing services in complex health science settings need a sound base in research as well as the substantive content related to their specialization. A rigorous preparation in research is especially necessary for nurses employed as coordinators of nursing research in clinical settings. Nurse-clinicians prepared at the doctoral level, on the other hand, more appropriately should be prepared in strong professional doctoral programs with intensive clinical specialization as the focus. In looking at both the educational and practice domains, the need for two patterns of doctoral preparation for nurses seems evident.

What then, makes it difficult for us to move into some clear, distinctive patterns of doctoral education? It is of interest to note that in the 1960s the program at Boston University was clearly a clinical doctoral program. Its demise as such was attributed to there not being sufficient content in the clinical specialty area to warrant a doctoral program. Mellow rebutted this assumption and instead offered the explanation that the clinical practice field that provided the site for preparation of doctorally prepared nurses in "nurse therapy" collapsed; hence the program could not be continued (1966:71). In any event, it is apparent that the timing for the development of this program was not right.

In developing the doctoral program at the University of Illinois, I have previously argued that there is a need first for the development of sound research doctoral programs in nursing focused upon the generation of new knowledge. Once these programs are firmly established, there is a need for the development of clinical doctoral programs focused upon testing out of knowledge in the clinical practice area. The time is now for this next step of doctoral program development. What precludes us from making this next step? The problem of the self-esteem of nurses has been identified by Matarazzo as a problem that plagues us to this day.

There are many facets to this phenomenon. One is the "Avis" phenomenon of "We try harder," perceiving ourselves to be second best. This is evidenced by our holding to the belief that all nurses can and should do everything equally well. Assuming that nurses can be researchers, expert clinicians, and teachers simultaneously imposes a burden found in very few other academic disciplines. In fact, there is some rather good evidence coming out of the psychology profession that those with a bent to research, as contrasted to the expert clinicians, are different groups of students with distinctively different psychological attributes and modes of thinking. Doctoral programs in psychology clearly differentiate a clinical and research track that are comparable but different. An example that I am particularly fond of is drawn from the arts.

In most music departments of universities there are two types of faculty—the scholar-theoreticians

and the performing artists. Certainly there are instances in which faculty combine these areas, but most frequently the most brilliant theoretician or music historian is not the most competent performer. In nursing we need both our scholar-theoreticians and our performing artists, the clinicians. And most certainly there needs to be carefully constructed communication between groups lest they begin to track off in different directions, thus producing a cacophony.

In addition to expecting too much of one another, our nursing educational programs, as they are currently constructed, place too great an expectation upon the student. Since the initial discussions regarding doctoral education it has been advocated that graduate programs be constructed on a continuum; to date we have few program models that are so constructed. Content of master's programs has been progressively expanded, and in many instances a master's program takes years to complete. Even at that, the student's program is overly loaded, with little room for electives or courses outside of nursing. In some instances, a master's program prepares clinical specialists at the master's level and has a heavy research requirement, in many instances a master's thesis. Tremendous amounts of time and energy on the part of both students and faculty are expended, in many instances nonproductively, in meeting these herculean demands.

As nursing educators struggle with heavy teaching loads and attempt to prepare qualified nurses at the baccalaureate and graduate level, they frequently become isolated from the nursing practice setting. In many instances, as teachers become increasingly divorced from clinical practice, they develop self-doubts about their abilities to perform in the clinical arena. The clinical practice setting is deprived of the expertise that faculty could provide to the setting. The presence of nurse-clinicians prepared in clinical doctoral programs within the practice setting would allow for sharing the responsibility of teaching students with these prepared clinicians in exchange for faculty involvement in some aspects of nursing practice. By developing such a system of exchanges between the education and practice settings, both teaching and service would benefit. Given this as a rationale and the need, what then might be the program models that would prepare nurse research scholars and clinician-teachers?

FUTURE DIRECTIONS FOR DOCTORAL EDUCATION IN NURSING

With 21 doctoral programs in place, some of them 20 or more years of age, it is now appropriate to take stock of the accomplishments of these programs as well as to propose new directions. For those programs whose goal is that of producing research scholars and teachers it is important to appraise the success in accomplishment of this goal. If our Ph.D. programs are not producing active and vigorous nurse-researchers, it is important to raise the question of why, and take the necessary corrective action. It is my fear that in many instances doctoral work has become yet another series of course taking and mastery of content rather than the independent and creative enterprise it needs to be if the end product is that of an investigator seeking to expand the bounds of nursing knowledge. Our catalogs are cluttered with courses and our faculty is occupied in developing curricular models and syllabi rather than being engaged in research, which is the crux of the educational process within a Ph.D. program. And for those programs that offer a professional nursing doctorate (D.N.Sc.), are they designed to produce a different type of product, a most highly qualified professional in nursing?

The Association of Graduate Schools and the Council of Graduate Schools have clearly articulated differences between the Ph.D. and a professional degree:

The demonstration of the ability to carry out meaningful research and to discover new knowledge is now recognized by the award of the degree of Doctor of Philosophy (Ph.D.), . . . The professional doctorate is granted only to those who have satisfactorily completed advanced studies that are comparable in rigor to existing doctoral experiences of high quality such as the professional programs leading to the Doctor of Medicine or the research-oriented programs leading to the degree of Doctor of Philosophy . . . The professional doctoral program . . . prepares the student for professional practice and related activities. (1971:1-4)

While the Ph.D. and the professional doctorate are directed toward different ends, it is important to note that they should be equal in rigor.

How might such programs be constructed? There are some important principles to keep in mind. First, doctorally prepared nurses, be they researcher-scholars or clinician-teachers, need a broad base of understanding of nursing. Ironically, much of what is currently being taught at the doctoral level as nursing theory would more appropriately form the base for all graduate education. Our current models are designed so that students become highly specialized at the master's level, with minimal attention to issues related to nursing on a broader, more conceptual level. Table 12-1 depicts a proposed curricular model for a two-track approach to doctoral education in nursing.

Within this proposed model nurses enrolled in graduate study in nursing would share a common base. The first year, in essence, would constitute the core or foundation upon which the student subsequently builds expertise either in the practice of nursing or in research. Within this model most of the first year of graduate study would be generalized, rather than specialized, but with some content in a specialty area such as psychiatric-mental health or medical-surgical nursing. A philosophy of science course is extremely helpful in developing the conceptual abilities of students so necessary both for researchers and practitioners. Research methods and statistics are essential for both the clinician-teachers and the researchers. In the second year students in both the professional and Ph.D. programs share in learning the

Table 12-1

	Professional doctorate track	Research doctorate track
Year I	Generalized content in nursing and in a specialty field of nursing Nursing theory Philosophy of science Research methods Statistics	
Year II	Content in specialized area of study Support courses from related science fields Practicum experience in the specialty area	Content in specialized area Support courses Research seminars Independent study
M.S.N.	(Clinical paper)	M.S. (Research project)
Year III	Clinical seminar in specialty area Practicum experience Clinical research project formulation	Research seminars Independent research
Year IV	Internship Completed doctoral Clinical paper D.N.Sc.	Completed doctoral dissertation Ph.D.

content of their specialty fields and the supporting sciences from which their particular specialty area builds. Branching between groups occurs with clinical practicum experiences for those within the professional track and research seminars and involvement in research projects on the part of the Ph.D. students. Nurses who do not wish to proceed to the completion of the doctorate could terminate at this point with either an M.S.N. degree or an M.S., depending upon the track in which they are engaged. In the third and fourth years of the program doctoral students within each of the tracks would become increasingly specialized, with those in the professional program becoming proficient in the clinical speciality areas and those in the research tract developing their research projects and maintaining active involvement in research seminars with faculty mentors.

In the fourth year of the program, those within the professional tract would be engaged in an internship experience and be expected to develop a clinical research study designed to demonstrate their application of knowledge within the practice domain. Those in the Ph.D. program would be expected to complete a piece of original

research designed to develop and test new knowledge. While this model is specifically addressed to clinical specialization, it is assumed that doctoral students, be they in the professional or Ph.D. program, would avail themselves of courses related to functional areas of nursing, teaching, and administration.

While this model has been drawn with the assumption that two program tracks might be offered within one university, there is no reason why they need to stand side by side within one university. However, if we looked carefully at our current master's education programs and redesigned them to be part and parcel of an overall approach to doctoral education, we could accomplish much more with our current resources of both faculty and students. Programs providing depth of experience in clinical practice would do much to enrich and build closer ties with nurses in practice settings, and as nurses with in-depth clinical practice preparation enter teaching and practice roles, the current chasm between nursing practice and nursing education could appropriately be bridged.

In summary, the need for program models designed to prepare both nurse-researchers and expert practitioners of nursing has been recognized since the initiation of doctoral programs in nursing. Our current doctoral programs constitute a critical mass sufficient for us to begin to construct distinctively different program models directed toward explicit goals. Within the discipline of nursing we need a cadre of research scholars devoted to building the knowledge base upon which teaching and practice rest. A parallel group of expert practitioners of nursing are needed for the clinical teaching of nursing as well as its practice. These nurses may be expected to validate nursing knowledge in the practice setting. At this stage it is important to carefully evaluate our current doctoral offerings, look critically at the way in which graduate education is structured with our overemphasis on master's education, and develop new program models that would address the diversity of goals of the nursing profession.

EDITOR'S QUESTIONS FOR DISCUSSION

What differences exist today between Ph.D. programs in nursing and D.N.Sc. programs? How would you respond to a statement that there is not sufficient content in a clinical specialty to warrant a doctoral program? How can content be clearly defined to address the needs of the practice domain and prepare nurses at the doctoral level as nurse/clinicians? Should the clinical specialist be prepared at the doctoral level instead of at the master's level? What content would you propose for doctoral preparation of faculty and nurse administrators in education and service? How would you respond to Dr. Matarazzo's question: "Why is nursing set on establishing a relationship between science and practice?"

What distinctions should be made between the two types of professional doctorates? Should the D.N. degree be the basis for entry into practice? Should "advanced" preparation for practice be expected beyond a D.N. degree? What relationship exists between Grace's discussion and what Williamson advocates in Chap. 5?

If nursing education and practice are on separate paths as Grace suggests, how can they really be united? What forces might have influenced faculty to lose sight of clinical teaching and practice? What type of education and experiential backgrounds are needed in nursing as a profession in order to meet the demands of the public? What different pathways might be considered for doctoral programs to meet the needs of the profession?

What is the role and status of external degree doctoral programs for nursing? Are enrollments in those programs increasing due to other avenues not being available for some nurses? What are the implications for the profession of nurses completing external degree doctoral programs?

REFERENCES

Association of Graduate Schools and Council of Graduate Schools in the United States
  1971 The Doctor's Degree in Professional Fields. Washington, D.C.: Council of Graduate Schools in the United States
Berthold, Jean
  1966 "A dialogue on approaches to doctoral preparation." Nursing Forum 5:2, 48.

Cleland, Virginia
  1976 "Developing a doctoral program." Nursing Outlook 24:10, 631–35.
Downs, Florence
  1978 "Doctoral education in nursing: Future directions." Nursing Outlook 26:1 56–69.
Mellow, June
  1966 "Nursing therapy as a treatment and clinical investigative approach to emotional issues." Nursing Forum 5:3, 64–73.

Peplau, Hildegarde
  1966 "Nursing's two routes to doctoral degrees." Nursing Forum 5:2, 57–67.
Schlotfeldt, Rozella
  1966 "Doctoral study in basic disciplines: A choice for nurses." Nursing Forum 5:2, 68–74.
U.S. Department of Health, Education and Welfare, Division of Nursing

  1971 "Future Directions of Doctoral Education for Nurses."
U.S. Department of Health, Education and Welfare, Division of Nursing, Health Resources Administration
  1974 Invitational Conference on Doctoral Manpower Requirements in Nursing, June 19–21.

Chapter 13

Continuing Education for Nursing's Leaders

Andrea B. O'Connor, R.N., Ed.D.
Assistant Professor
Department of Nursing Education
Teachers College, Columbia University
New York, New York

It is appropriate to end this section on nursing education with this chapter by Andrea O'Connor in which a strong plea is made for preparation and continuing education for nursing leaders. Andrea O'Connor reflects Barbara Stevens' view that nurse leaders are in mediated role positions. O'Connor advocates graduate education at the master's and doctoral level to prepare nurses for mediated roles. Three elements of graduate preparation considered essential by O'Connor are explored. These are: advanced study of the discipline and practice of nursing; study of the discipline supporting the mediated role; and synthesis of the nursing and supporting discipline in the development and enactment of the mediated nursing role. She asserts that the nature of advanced study of nursing in the curriculum is determined by the role selected and knowledge necessary for its successful enactment. O'Connor delineates five specific skills leaders must possess to influence nursing. She outlines the components of continuing education to be general nursing and specialty content appropriate to the leader's setting, as well as content related to the selected mediated role. Continuing education is to be pursued to ensure sufficient up-to-date knowledge, skill, and competence to successfully enact the leadership role. O'Connor urges that for the nursing leadership group continuing education be reconceptualized based on role demands. She advises that continuing education for nurse-leaders be based on their identified needs and cannot be restricted to a clinical focus. Finally O'Connor approves nontraditional formats for nurse leaders that may not necessarily comply with accreditation requirements.

Nurses in positions of leadership in health care facilities, institutions of higher education, government, professional societies, and health-related industries such as publishing facilitate the direct care provided by other nurses. Although nurse-leaders influence health care delivery and the advance of the nursing profession, little attention has been directed to identifying the best ways to prepare these leaders for the roles they will assume or to providing for their continued learning once they are practicing in these roles. While education of the nurse-leaders on the undergraduate and graduate level provides a substantive base in nursing, these programs may not adequately prepare such nurses for the practice of the complex roles they eventually assume, roles that require the synthesis of the discipline of nursing with other supporting disciplines. Regardless of the nature of initial role preparation, in this era of rapid technological advance, continuous change, and growth of knowledge at an exponential rate, high-level role function demands continued learning. If the nursing profession is to advance in its ability to provide high quality health care, the capacity of the profession's leaders to guide and direct that advance must be ensured. This is a role for continuing professional education.

LEADERS IN NURSING: WHO ARE THEY?

Nurse-leaders are those who influence the nursing profession through such activities as educating practitioners, facilitating direct care, establishing health care policy, advancing knowledge, and promoting communications in the field. They hold positions as nursing service executives; educational program administrators; nursing educators in basic, graduate, staff development, and continuing education programs; editors of professional journals and texts; executives of professional organizations, government executives and representatives; researchers; and consultants. Nurse-leaders in these positions are able to improve health care delivery and alter patterns of professional nursing practice, because the decisions they make and actions they take affect large groups of nurses and entire health care systems.

Traditionally, leadership positions in nursing have been labeled "functional," occupied by nurses who function as educators, administrators, and so forth. In this view, the nurse is seen as filling a somewhat alien role, and much of the available preparation for such functional roles has done little to overcome this alienation. The nurse is left with the task of synthesizing the functional discipline with the primary nursing discipline while retaining a self-image of "nurse." Perhaps it

is this failure to synthesize that has led many nurses to denigrate the positions they fill, failing to recognize their inherent potential for power and influence.

Stevens (1979:775) views leadership positions as "mediated roles" and claims that these roles "have more power to bring about good one-to-one care than has the hands-on role itself." The nurse-leader's decisions have the capacity to affect the care of thousands; the nurse practicing in a direct care role has a more limited sphere of influence. Such a view does not devalue the direct care role, but underlines the power of the mediated role, a power that has not been fully activated nor adequately exploited. Preparation for the mediated role proceeds from a common core of nursing incorporating its theories, practice, modes of inquiry, and professional enactment. Such preparation provides ample exposure to and study of the theories, practice, modes of inquiry, and professional enactment of those disciplines fundamental to mediated-role performance and promotes synthesis of the discipline of nursing with the adapted disciplines to yield the knowledge and skills characteristic of the mediated-nursing role and necessary to its successful enactment.

Houle identifies positional leaders as "facilitators," persons who maintain career identification but do not practice their profession directly. "They teach, do research, study, organize, administer, regulate, coordinate, and engage in other activities that advance the profession" (1980:160). In these positions, facilitators reinforce the major professional activites of direct practitioners; they may or may not influence that practice. In Houle's view, a profession's influentials—those who pursue new knowledge in unique and unconventional ways and those who lead in the application of new knowledge to practice—are as likely to be drawn from the ranks of its practitioners as from the leadership elite (Houle, 1976). In nursing, however, influentials are most likely to be drawn from the positional leadership group. The 71 nurse influentials identified in Vance's (1977) study held positions as academic educators and administrators, researchers, nursing service administrators, professional organization officers and executives, editors, and government officials. Only 18 of these influentials were identified as such because of their clinical practice roles, and only one was identified solely as a clinician.

EDUCATION OF NURSING'S LEADERS

Education for leadership positions in nursing begins with basic professional education. Upon graduating from the basic educational program, the nurse usually engages in professional practice for some time, beginning in direct care roles and, perhaps, eventually undertaking lower-level mediated roles. For the nurse who aspires to a leadership position, the demands of the employment situation or a desire for a shift to a mediated role prompts a return to the educational setting for advanced professional education and mediated-role preparation on the graduate level. While aspects of the selected role can be understood on the basis of experience and much on-the-job training does occur, preparation for a mediated role demands graduate level education in nursing and in the disciplines supporting the mediated-nursing role to achieve the synthesis necessary for successful role enactment. Once prepared at the master's or doctoral level, the nurse-leader must pursue continuing professional education through a lifetime of practice.

Professional nursing education is rooted in the liberal arts, not only because such an education is broadening and humanizing, but because much of professional practice derives from this base. Matejski (1979:80) notes that nurses "are in a unique position to utilize the vast stores of knowledge provided by the humanities." Benoliel (1977:108-109) claims that "the art of nursing practice rests in a judicious and thoughtful application of insights and inferences drawn from many fields of human endeavor, including the arts, the humanities and the physical, biological, and behavioral sciences." Zbilut (1977:67) argues that such nonscientific aspects of nursing as "care" and "concern"

might best be studied using the theories, methods, and understandings of the humanities.

In addition to the humanities, professional nursing education is rooted in the natural and behavioral sciences, for these disciplines contribute to and support the professional discipline of nursing in its development of theories and technologies and in its practice. Knowledge of the dominant theories, modes of inquiry, and understandings of those disciplines supporting nursing is necessary to the effective use of this knowledge in the practice of nursing. Donaldson and Crowley (1978:118) note that "in delivering health care, practitioners must in fact draw from many disciplines. ... Rarely, if ever, does the skilled clinician rely only on knowledge from one discipline or even rely solely on scientific knowledge."

Education in the primary discipline of nursing proceeds from initial acquisition of the content upon which it is built and involves mastery of the major conceptualizations of the discipline, its primary theories, and its modes of inquiry; the skills used in the practice of nursing; the societal context within which nursing practice occurs and its purposes; and the mores and values surrounding professional practice.

Thus, basic professional education introduces the student to the basic disciplines supporting nursing, their content, theories, and modes of inquiry; focuses on the understandings, theories, practices, modes of inquiry, and behavioral expectations that are nursing; and promotes synthesis of these elements to enable the nurse to appropriately select and apply knowledge needed to successfully enact the professional practice role.

Graduate preparation of nurse-leaders contains three elements: advanced study of the discipline and practice of nursing; study of the discipline supporting the mediated role; and synthesis of the nursing and supporting discipline in the development and enactment of the mediated-nursing role. Such preparation ideally occurs on the doctoral level, but may occur at the master's level.

Grace (1978:22-23) identifies three patterns of doctoral education for nurses: functional education, with emphasis on knowledge and methods related to the selected functional role; science education, with emphasis on advanced preparation in one of the social or biological sciences supporting nursing; and nursing education, with emphasis on substantive knowledge of the discipline and the development and application of its theory through research. Master's education generally parallels these patterns, although substantive content in the discipline of nursing and its clinical practice forms a major component of the curriculum (NLN, 1979).

The advanced study of nursing is an essential thread in any graduate nursing curriculum. While this is clearly true for programs preparing nurses for clinical specialty roles, it is equally true for programs preparing nurses for mediated roles. Indeed, if the nursing component is missing from the master's curriculum, it is difficult to imagine meaningful study of the mediated role or successful synthesis of the supporting discipline with nursing. The nursing component in such programs, however, need not be specialized or even clinical. Advanced generalist preparation in nursing theory, in the analysis of professional issues and trends, in the application of knowledge and skills in the care of persons at various stages of the life cycle and phases of the health-illness continuum, and in alternative modes of health care delivery may be the most meaningful content to support the mediated-role preparation of the nursing service executive, professional organization executive, government representative, or consultant. Thus, the nature of advanced study of nursing in the graduate curriculum preparing nurse-leaders for mediated roles is determined by the role selected and the knowledge necessary for its successful enactment.

Study of the mediated role requires the adoption and adaptation of a second discipline in addition to nursing. For example, for the nursing educator the adapted discipline is education, while for the nurse-executive it is management science. In preparing for a mediated role, the nurse must master the content, theories, practices, modes of inquiry, and accepted professional behaviors of the second discipline before synthesis of the new discipline with nursing can occur. Such mastery also entails the study or reexamination of those basic disciplines upon which the adapted discipline is built and the ways in which their content is used. For example, psychology supports the disciplines of nursing, education, and management science, but each applies psychological content and theories in unique ways. Therefore, the nurse must investigate seemingly familiar content from the perspective of the second, adapted discipline.

Too often, study in the mediated discipline is appended to the advanced study of nursing. Any synthesis between the two disciplines occurs within the individual nurse or not at all. Such a curricular approach assumes that content is the only difference between the teaching of nursing and of geography, or that industrial models can be transferred intact to hospital settings. True mediated-role preparation must provide opportunities for the exploration of how the content, theories, and practices of the mediated discipline are applied in a nursing context and how the mediated role is enacted for nursing. Furthermore, because nurses in mediated roles are also those most likely to lead the profession, their preparation must enable them to perform the full range of activities expected of such leaders.

LEADER ROLE ENACTMENT

Clearly, responsibilities related to the nurse-leader's selected role dictate, to a great degree, the nature of role enactment. For example, the nursing education role carries traditional expectations of classroom and clinical instruction, student advisement, service to the educational and professional communities, and scholarship. The nurse who would succeed in a given role must fulfill expectations accruing to that role. Furthermore, the nurse-leader must also maintain authenticity and credibility as a member of the nursing profession; students, coworkers, and subordinates all must acknowledge the nurse-leader as a nurse as well as a leader.

Position-specific responsibilities, however, do not necessarily exhaust the nurse-leader's role responsibilities. In order to influence nursing and health care delivery, leaders must be skilled in communication, innovation, inquiry, consultation, and advocacy.

Effective oral and written communication is essential if the nurse-leader is to influence health care delivery and the nursing profession. The nurse-leader must be able to communicate not only with nursing colleagues within and outside the employment setting, but also with members of other discipline groups and with the public.

Innovation is another key leadership skill. The nurse-leader who would influence the profession must propose new directions for its growth. Innovation involves the conception, recommendation, implementation, and evaluation of creative solutions to existing situations and imaginative strategies for dealing with potential situations. Innovation also involves the transformation of new knowledge from other disciplines for use in nursing.

Inquiry and consultation are necessary elements in the nurse-leader's repertoire of skills. Inquiry involves the posing of research questions and their systematic investigation as well as the application of research findings in the health care setting. Inquiry aids the process of innovation by enabling the nurse-leader to methodically formulate and test new conceptions of practice and expand the boundaries of the nursing discipline.

Consultation takes the products of innovation and inquiry to those who will implement them. In the consultative process the nurse-leader shares knowledge and skills and promotes the acceptance of the new, thus influencing the growth of the profession and its modes of practice.

As an influential, the nurse-leader must be prepared to address broad concerns related to the nursing profession and health care generally. Advocacy entails skills in identifying central issues and analyzing their impact, as well as in formulating and expressing stances in relation to these issues. Advocacy requires more than the voicing of an opinion; it demands thoughtful deliberation of issues from multiple perspectives and the capacity to forecast the consequences of proposed resolutions.

CONTINUING PROFESSIONAL EDUCATION FOR NURSE-LEADERS

Houle (1976:45–57) has identified the purposes of continuing professional education as follows: to keep up with new knowledge required to perform responsibly in the chosen career; to master new conceptions of the career itself; to keep up with changes in the relevant basic disciplines upon which the profession's theory is built; to prepare for changes in a personal career line; to maintain freshness of outlook on the work performed; to continue to grow as a well-rounded person; to retain the power to learn; and to effectively discharge the social role imposed by one's professional membership.

For nurses practicing in direct care roles, this interpretation of the scope of continuing education requires a major educational effort. Indeed, formal continuing education has been largely directed toward nurses who are currently practicing in clinical roles or who are returning to such positions following a period of absence from practice. This is appropriate, since the great majority of nurses practice in direct care roles, and it is the profession's responsibility to ensure that health care needs are met by currently competent practitioners. Yet, if the profession's leaders are to influence the quality of health care provided by direct care practitioners, the leaders' currency and competence must also be ensured. This, too, is a role for continuing professional education. Unfortunately, nurse-leaders find that they advocate continuing professional education through a lifetime of practice to prevent professional obsolescence, but have little guidance and few resources for the pursuit of their own continuing education.

Houle's conceptualization of continuing education is a staggering one for the nurse in a mediated role, who must remain up to date in at least two fields, nursing and the mediated-role field; keep abreast of advances in the disciplines supporting these fields; achieve synthesis between the fields to permit optimum functioning in the mediated-nursing role; and gain and maintain those skills characteristic of the nurse-leader. Consider the nature of continuing professional education for one type of leader in nursing—the director of staff development.

As a nurse, the director of staff development must keep up to date in the knowledge and skills necessary to competent performance of the direct care role. Without this basic understanding, the director is ill-equipped to select relevant content for staff development education programs. Further, lack of currency in the nursing discipline and its practice decreases the director's credibility and authenticity as a nurse, hampering efforts at staff development. In pursuing continuing education in nursing content, the director must consider knowledge and skills related to general nursing as well as the specialty content appropriate to the director's practice setting. For example, continuing education to maintain practice competence in general nursing might involve mastery of the nursing process, including skill in nursing diagnosis; analysis and application of various nursing theories in the delivery of client care; skill in techniques of interpersonal communications; and other such topics. Continuing education to ensure maintenance of specialized nursing knowledge and skills would vary depending on the setting. In an orthopedic hospital, the staff development director would have to keep abreast of new knowledge and skills related to the nursing care of the orthopedic patient; the director in an acute care general hospital would have different needs for specialized continuing nursing education.

In addition to maintaining currency in both general and specialized practice, the staff development director must constantly consider what directions nursing will take in the near and distant future, Houle's (1976:48) "new conceptions of the career," if educational programs are to be

geared as much toward advancing practice as maintaining it. For example, the director must determine the extent to which nurses' skills in health assessment will be used by the agency and must plan educational programs to ready nurses for expanded roles. In this regard, the director must recognize emerging issues that have the potential to affect nursing practice, forecast their effects, and plan programs to prepare nurses to respond to future practice demands.

A major neglected area of continuing education for professionals involves keeping up with changes in supporting disciplines that may affect professional practice. In relation to the nursing discipline, for example, the staff development director must know what is going on in the biophysical and social sciences as well as in medicine, pharmacology, and other contributing disciplines, as advances in these areas may impact nursing in the future. In the recent past, research in the physiology of pain has altered the treatment of persons with chronic pain, including their nursing care. Theories advanced by behavioral psychologists resulted in the application of behavioral modification techniques in a variety of nursing care situations. It is only by keeping abreast of changes in relevant supporting fields that the nurse-leader can recognize which advances have applicability for nursing practice and devise means of communicating these to other practitioners and promoting their transformation to and adoption in nursing care settings.

In addition to the continuing education demands imposed by membership in the nursing profession, the nurse-leader must also pursue continuing education related to the selected mediated role. The staff development director has blended two roles, educator and administrator, with nursing.

As an educator, the staff development director has adopted the major discipline, education, with a focus on the specialty discipline, adult education. The priority knowledge and skills needed by adult educators were elicited by Rossman and Bunning (1978:146-148) using the Delphi technique in a survey of adult education professors. Their results indicated needs related to role performance, such as knowledge of learning theories in nursing practice, evaluation methods, and program design and skills in diagnosing educational needs, using educational resources, and counseling adults; needs related to future trends, such as awareness of the changing nature of the adult and societal trends affecting adult education; as well as awareness of trends in supporting disciplines such as psychology of the adult and philosophy of education. While much of this specialized content is learned during a graduate program preparing the nurse for a leadership role as a staff development educator, the same forces that are responsible for the explosion of knowledge in nursing and promoting the need for continued learning in that field are also affecting the discipline of education, necessitating continued learning for the educator role.

As an administrator, the staff development director has further need for basic and continuing education related to the management role, such as in budgeting skills and marketing expertise, in educational administration, such as in computer technology, and in organizational psychology.

Further, since the mediated role is more than a mere appending of a second or third discipline to the primary discipline, nursing, continuing education for the nurse-leader requires advanced content related to the knowledge and skills essential to the competent performance of the mediated-nursing role. Thus, the director of staff development must synthesize knowledge and skills in educational evaluation. For example, an understanding of the unique problems of clinical performance evaluation is essential in order to devise appropriate means for determining outcomes of clinical instruction. Also, general approaches to marketing must be revised and adapted in the development of materials promoting educational programs for nurses.

Added to this is the need to develop and maintain skills in communications, innovation, inquiry, consultation, and advocacy, skills which are built upon specific disciplines and which require transformation for use in the context of nursing leadership. Even the nurse-leader who is a skilled

and effective communicator must learn to expand these skills in the light of technological advances, perhaps for use in writing a television script or consulting via satellite. The nurse-researcher will continually review the literature of supporting science disciplines to identify new techniques for the study of nursing problems.

Evidence of the far-reaching and varied continuing education needs of nursing leaders can be found in the few reported surveys of leaders' needs. Abruzzese (1975) identified planning for change, legal aspects of nursing, psychology of motivation, leadership methods, group dynamics, and counseling and evaluation as learning needs of directors of hospital nursing in-service education. Binger (1979) cited professional writing, legislative strategies, communications strategies, leadership principles, and business law as learning needs of nursing education program administrators. Chase (1975) found conduct and utilization of research, survival strategies during times of change, and involvement of consumers in decision making to be among the learning needs of hospital nursing service administrators. Vance's (1977) nurse influentials indicated that they had received insufficient formal education in the following areas to perform effectively in their roles: administration-management theory, political science and processes, economic theory, research training, writing skills, and health systems planning.

WHY BOTHER?

Houle (1970; 1976; 1980) views professionals as ranged along a normal probability curve in terms of their readiness to innovate and adopt new practices, to learn and to apply what is learned to practice situations. Innovators, at the extreme right of the curve, tend to be in the vanguard of the profession, pursuing new knowledge in unique and, at times, unconventional ways. Pacesetters, to the left of innovators but still above the mean, are quick to see the implications of new knowledge, usually brought to their attention by innovators, and to apply it. Majority adopters, ranged across the middle of the curve, follow the lead of the pacesetters with various degrees of delay. The laggards, at the extreme left of the curve, fail to improve practice. Two concerns of organized continuing professional education are how to accelerate learning by majority adopters and how to reach laggards.

In his early work on continuing professional education, Houle (1970:13) identified positional leaders in a profession, leaders he labeled the "reinforcers," as a fifth group distinct from practicing professionals. Later, Houle (1976) revised his picture of the reinforcers, indicating that they are drawn from the larger practitioner group and, therefore, include among their ranks laggards, majority adopters, pacesetters, and innovators. Still later, Houle (1980:160) renamed the reinforcers, calling them "facilitators," but his notion of their varying responsiveness to and influence on change and growth of the profession remained the same.

If positional leaders are the influentials for the nursing profession, as Vance's (1977) study indicates, one must consider the effects on the profession's growth and development if a significant number of its influentials fail to remain sufficiently up to date in either the nursing discipline or in the knowledge and skills needed to successfully enact the positional leadership role. Within this group too lies a challenge to continuing educators to reach laggards and motivate majority adopters. The challenge is best met by offering programs vital to the nurse's performance as leader.

Central to any characterization of professionalism is the existence of a systematized body of knowledge, the practical application of which constitutes the professional's practice. The professional applies knowledge in the solution of social problems, solutions oriented toward community interest rather than self-interest. The esoteric nature of the professional's knowledge is such that only members of the profession can adequately evaluate problems in their domain and the appropriateness of solutions posed. Therefore, society grants to the profession a measure of control over

its practice in exchange for formal assurances and continued evidence of ethical behavior. Because knowledge is integral to the professional's practice and to fulfillment of a commitment to society, maintaining and improving professional knowledge and competence is a part of fulfillment of that commitment. The alternative is professional obsolescence.

Changing social values and the consumer movement have led to public distrust of professions. The public has questioned the legitimacy of licensure laws that bestow lifetime practice privileges on the basis of a single test of knowledge upon entry into the profession's ranks and the validity of internal controls imposed by professional organizations. Despite a surfeit of credentialing mechanisms, the public has remained unconvinced of the continuing competence of professionals. One proposed means of ensuring that professionals maintain practice competencies is the requirement of continuing education for relicensure.

An initial flurry of activity promoting mandatory continuing education for a variety of professional groups, including nursing, has subsided. Both professionals and consumers now question the cost-benefit ratio of such education, the relation of continuing education to health care outcomes, and the relevance of particular continuing education activities to the professional's role functions. Clinically focused continuing education may not always be the most appropriate type of education for the nurse in a leadership position. However, state boards may refuse to acknowledge alternative educational experiences as acceptable for relicensure purposes.

For the nursing leadership group, continuing education must be reconceptualized based on role demands. Continuing professional education can offer the nurse-leader endless opportunities for professional growth and enrichment. Programs may be developed to build upon a base in theory, provide practical know-how for immediate application in the employment situation, and promote the leader's ability to innovate. To accomplish these ends, continuing education for nurse-leaders must be based on their identified needs. A needs analysis is derived from models of leader-role enactment against which the individual can assess proficiencies and deficiencies. The development of leader models is a first challenge for the profession if meaningful continuing education for the leadership group is to be devised.

Continuing education for nurse-leaders cannot be restricted to a clinical focus or a review of content the nurse already knows. This means that nurse-leaders, and those who counsel them in their pursuit of continued learning, must be aware of educational resources not labeled "nursing" that may expand knowledge and skills related to the mediated-role discipline and its supporting fields. Identification of appropriate continuing

education resources is crucial to developing an individualized continuing education curriculum for the nurse-leader.

Finally, continuing education programs for nurse-leaders may not conform to traditional formats and, therefore, may not necessarily comply with stringent accreditation or approval requirements. Continuing nursing education for leaders may involve sharing of problems, exploration of possible solutions, brainstorming, and innovative programs designed by the learners themselves. The educator working with nurse-leaders must be able to tolerate such ambiguity in program offerings, catalyze the discovery process, and support the nurse-leaders' innovations in continuing education designed to meet their own needs.

EDITOR'S QUESTIONS FOR DISCUSSION

What has been the effect within nursing education and the profession in using the term "functional" for persons being prepared for or in the role of educator or administrator? If every nurse is provided an advanced general-knowledge base in nursing as proposed in Grace's model (Chap. 12) for the first-year graduate student, to what extent should master's and doctoral programs in nursing provide content that is specifically clinical for those who are preparing for a mediator role, content from the discipline supporting the mediated role, and content synthesizing the primary nursing discipline with a "functional" supporting discipline? What is the difference between "mediators" and "facilitators" in the nursing roles of practice, education, and research?

What content can be defined as the advanced study of nursing? To what extent do you agree with O'Connor's suggestion for determining the nature of advanced study of nursing in graduate programs preparing nurse leaders for mediated roles? What avenues may be employed for a synthesis of the content of nursing and the mediated discipline in programs? At what level and/or to what extent should the nurse leader maintain current clinical knowledge and competence through continuing education?

What differences are there in the identified patterns of doctoral education O'Connor attributes to Grace (1978) with the patterns proposed by those in her Chap. 12? To what degree is there congruence between O'Connor's beliefs regarding basic professional education, support of mediated role preparation at the graduate level, and what Williamson advocates in Chap. 5 and Grace offers in Chap. 12? Does O'Connor's discussion of professional nursing education imply support for the N.D. degree as the basis for advanced preparation in mediated roles?

REFERENCES

Abruzzese, Roberta S.
1975 "Continuing education needs of directors of hospital nursing inservice education in New York State." Doctoral dissertation. Columbia University.

Benoliel, Jeanne Q.
1977 "The interaction between theory and research." Nursing Outlook 25:108–113.

Binger, Jane L.
1979 "Perceived learning needs and resources of undergraduate and diploma program directors." Journal of Nursing Education 18:3–7.

Chase, Beatrice A.
1975 "Self-assessment of learning needs of hospital nursing service administrators." Doctoral dissertation. Columbia University.

Donaldson, Sue K. and Dorothy M. Crowley
1978 "The discipline of nursing." Nursing Outlook 26:113–120.

Grace, Helen K.
1978 "The development of doctoral education in nursing: In historical perspective." Journal of Nursing Education 17:17–27.

Houle, Cyril O.
1970 "To learn the future." Medical Clinics of North America 54:5–18.

1976 "The nature of continuing professional education." In Robert M. Smith (ed.), Adult Learning: Issues and Innovations. DeKalb, Illinois: ERIC Clearinghouse in Career Education.
1980 Continuing Learning in the Professions. San Francisco: Jossey-Bass.

Matejski, Myrtle P.
1979 "Humanities: The nurse and historical research." Image 11:80–85.

National League for Nursing.
1979 Characteristics of Graduate Education in Nursing Leading to the Master's Degree. New York: NLN.

Rossman, Mark H. and Richard L. Bunning.
1978 "Knowledge and skills for the adult educator: A Delphi study." Adult Education 28:139–155.

Stevens, Barbara J.
1979 "Improving nurses' managerial skills." Nursing Outlook 27:774–777.

Vance, Constance N.
1977 "A group profile of contemporary influentials in American nursing." Doctoral dissertation. Columbia University.

Zbilut, Joseph P.
1977 "Nursing research and the humanities." Nursing Research 26:67.

Part Three

Nursing Research

A time for searching, . . .
a time for throwing stones away,
a time for gathering them up

The systematic method of inquiry utilized by nurse researchers is indeed a searching process. Most often there are obstacles to be overcome in conducting research that demand ingenuity and persistance. Nurse researchers are prepared to throw away preconceived ideas regarding the simplicity of addressing a research question; choosing appropriate research designs; and collection, analysis, and interpretation of data. Many questions for research are thrown away due to the complexities in attempting to reliably and validly address a problem. The time for independent research is past. Nurse researchers are gathering new methods in approaching and conducting research. Qualitative and quantitative methods are being utilized, as well as experimental, quasiexperimental, and nonexperimental (descriptive and exploratory) designs. Collaborative and interdisciplinary research is being advocated.

Research to identify the knowledge base of nursing is emphasized, although the need for relevance of research for nursing practice has significantly increased. The awareness of the value of nursing research as grown, partly due to closer relationships between nurse researchers and clinicians of nursing. Nurse clinicians are becoming more directly involved in the research process. Mentorships in nursing research are developing. Master's-prepared nurses are more frequently collaborating with nurses who have doctoral degrees. Ethical issues concerning the conduction of nursing research have multiplied. A serious factor that is influencing the quality and quantity of nursing research is the decreased federal funding for research. In spite of the problems that exist considerable advances that have been made in nursing research are noticeable. The chapters that follow represent a broad spectrum of issues concerning the investigative process in nursing research and questions addressed through utilizing the research process.

Chapter 14

Contemporary Nursing Research: Its Relevance for Nursing Practice

Jacqueline Fawcett, R.N., Ph.D., F.A.A.N.
Associate Professor
School of Nursing
University of Pennsylvania
Philadelphia, Pennsylvania

The primary purpose of nursing research is to generate and validate the knowledge needed for practice. Inherent in the data of nursing research is the basis of theory development for explicating a body of knowledge for nursing and practice. Research derived from nursing practice enables the genesis of theory building in a hierarchical and cumulative manner. Helen K. Grace made the point in Chap. 12 that if the prepared nurse researcher from Ph.D. doctoral programs is not conducting research, the question should be asked, "Why not?" An additional question is raised by this editor: If the prepared Ph.D. nurse-researcher is conducting research, what is the theoretical base for the research being conducted? Both questions are partly answered through a quest which Jacqueline Fawcett pursues in this chapter. She investigates whether contemporary research is indeed generating and validating the knowledge needed for practice. Fawcett answers three critical questions concerning nursing phenomena, the types of knowledge about these phenomena, and the validity, reliability, and relevance of nursing knowledge needed before it can be utilized by practitioners. The relevant phenomena of the discipline of nursing are represented by the abstract concepts person, environment, health, and nursing and linked in a general way through specification of nursing's metaparadigm. The major focus of Fawcett's chapter is on the consideration of four types of nursing knowledge: scientific (empirical), ethical, esthetic (the art of nursing), and personal knowledge of the therapeutic use of self.

She reviews three schemas of the knowledge needed for practice and notes the research related to each. The Dickoff and James hierarchy is thoroughly examined as the most frequently cited schema of nursing knowledge. Fawcett concludes that prescriptive theory can be considered as a combination of scientific and ethical knowledge, and not as a distinct form of knowledge. She notes that the greatest flaw in nursing research is the failure of investigators to clearly explicate where and/or how their study fits into the building and testing of a given theory. In answering the third critical question posed, Fawcett offers three sets of criteria proposed by Haller, Reynolds, and Horsley (1979) which identify the conditions necessary for transferring knowledge from scientific research to practice situations. The focus in the first set of criteria is on evaluation and integration of related studies; for the second set attention is on the clinical relevance of studies; the third set concerns the potential for evaluation of a new intervention in the clinical setting. She expresses concern that few, if any, of 10 proposed practice innovation protocols are based on explicit, consistent theory. The protocols represent the 10 areas of nursing research identified as being directly relevant for nursing practice that meet all the sets of criteria developed by Haller and her associates. Fawcett concludes with a challenge for nursing to develop series of related studies that build and test the knowledge needed for practice.

The advancement of the discipline of nursing, and hence nursing practice, rests on development of distinctive knowledge about relevant phenomena. However, to be useful for nursing practice, such knowledge must be tested and validated in the real world of nursing. And only research can do this. Indeed, research is the only route to the generation, refinement, and enlargement of nursing knowledge.

The purpose of this chapter is to consider whether contemporary nursing research is generating and validating the knowledge needed for nursing practice. This requires answers to three questions. First, what are relevant nursing phenomena and does contemporary nursing research focus on them? Second, what types of knowledge about these phenomena are needed, what kinds of research can provide this knowledge, and is this research currently being conducted? But not all valid nursing knowledge can or should be applied to nursing practice. Thus, the final question asks: What additional information is required before knowledge can be utilized and is nursing research now providing this information?

THE PHENOMENA OF NURSING

The first question requires us to identify nursing's metaparadigm, that is, the individuals, groups, situations, and events of interest to us and our distinctive view of these phenomena. Currently, there is a growing consensus that the relevant phenomena of nursing's metaparadigm can be represented by the abstract concepts *person, environment, health, nursing* (Bush, 1979; Fawcett, 1978a; Yura and Torres, 1975). The connections

among these four concepts are explicated in the following statement by Donaldson and Crowley (1978:119): "Nursing studies the wholeness or health of humans, recognizing that humans are in continuous interaction with their environments."

The concepts and linking statement clearly summarize the parameters of nursing and provide a general focus for nursing research. What is needed next are the more specific conceptual, theoretical, instrumental, and methodological rules required for empirical investigations of nursing's phenomena. Such rules will help us to identify research questions, formulate hypotheses, and select research strategies that are appropriate for investigation of person-environment interactions related to health. Different versions of these rules are suggested in the conceptual models of nursing put forth in recent years by several scholars (Nursing Theories Conference Group, 1980; Riehl and Roy, 1974, 1980).

While there should be little doubt that contemporary nursing research focuses on one or more of the four concepts representing phenomena of interest to nursing, a distinctively nursing perspective is not always obvious. In fact, only a few studies have been derived explicitly from a conceptual model of nursing. One example is Kearney and Fleischer's (1979) work on development of an instrument to assess clients' abilities for self-care, a component of Orem's (1980) model. Other examples, guided by Rogers's (1970) conceptual system, are Fawcett's (1977) investigation of couples' shared body image changes during and after pregnancy, and Fitzpatrick's (1980) studies of temporal experience. Still other examples are Fawcett's (1981) and Kehoe's (1981) exploratory studies of the needs of cesarean birth parents, which used components of Roy's (1976) model for content analysis categories.

The importance of using conceptual models of nursing as guides for nursing research needs to be emphasized. These models provide distinctive perspectives of the person, the environment, health, and nursing goals and process. Thus, their use can increase researchers' confidence that what they are doing is nursing research—not research in another discipline, such as medicine, psychology, or sociology. This is not to say that the findings of nursing research cannot or will not add to the general body of knowledge about human beings, but that the contribution will be within the identified parameters of the discipline of nursing, and therefore should have more direct relevance for nursing practice.

In summary, the relevant phenomena of the discipline of nursing have been identified and linked in a general way through specification of nursing's metaparadigm. The emerging conceptual models of nursing are presenting diverse views of these phenomena and contain the precursors of the specific rules needed for empirical study of the phenomena. Contemporary nursing research does reflect a focus on concepts representing the phenomena of interest to nursing but often lacks the distinctive perspective of nursing that can be provided by using a conceptual model as an organizing framework for a study.

TYPES OF NURSING KNOWLEDGE

The second question raised at the beginning of this chapter requires consideration of types of nursing knowledge and how that knowledge is generated.

The most frequently cited schema of nursing knowledge is the Dickoff and James (1968) hierarchy. These philosophers have proposed that practice professions such as nursing require four levels of knowledge, each presupposing the next lower level.

The lowest level, *factor-isolating theory*, involves description and classification of phenomena. This

type of knowledge is developed by descriptive research. Such studies attempt to identify and describe the specific characteristics of particular people, groups, situations, or events when nothing or very little is known about them (Payton, 1979: 44). Nursing research designed to develop factor-isolating theory focuses on descriptions and classifications of the person, environment, health, and nursing.

One descriptive design used for development of factor-isolating theory is the *grounded theory approach*, which is especially useful when formation of specific concepts and their categories is needed. This strategy was first described by Glaser and Strauss (1967). An overview of the method and discussion of a nursing study using it was recently presented by Stern (1980).

Other descriptive designs focus on description of concept categories. One of the most clear-cut examples of an attempt to categorize a concept is the current work on nursing diagnosis (Chinn, 1979). Other recent work, while not focused explicitly on the generation of factor-isolating theory, does provide the needed data for theorizing at this level. Examples of nursing studies whose findings provide such data include the following titles:

Comparison of primiparas' perceptions of vaginal and cesarean births (Marut and Mercer, 1979)
Changes in mental states in older adults with four days of hospitalization (Roslaniec and Fitzpatrick, 1979)
Personality factors of contemporary baccalaureate nursing students: A descriptive study (Mansell and Porter, 1979)
Situational stress and temporal changes in self-report and vocal measurements (Brockway, 1979)

The second level in the Dickoff and James (1968) schema is *factor-relating* or *situation-depicting* theory. This type of knowledge describes relations among various phenomena and is developed by descriptive and correlational studies. Such research is appropriate when the essential characteristics of study variables have already been adequately explained and relationships need to be established (Payton, 1979:44). Nursing research designed to develop factor-relating theory involves attempts to discover relations among various aspects of the person, the environment, health, and nursing.

Many current nursing studies seek to establish the relations among variables, although the generation of factor-relating theory is not always an explicit goal. Examples of investigations providing the needed data for this level of theory are:

Health care workers' role conceptions and orientation to family-centered child care (Porter, 1979)

Relationship of psychological factors in pregnancy to progress in labor (Lederman, Lederman, Work, and McCann, 1979)

Life events, emotional support, and health of older people (Fuller and Larson, 1980)

Type A (coronary-prone) behavior and transient blood pressure change (Sparacino, Hansell, and Smyth, 1979)

Dickoff and James's (1968) third type of theory is termed *situation-relating*. Knowledge at this level focuses on explanation and prediction. Whereas factor-relating theory seeks to discover the relations among phenomena, situation-relating theory proposes or predicts specific kinds of relationships among particular variables (Diers, 1979: 46–47). Thus, factor-relating theory generates hypotheses while situation-relating theory building tests them. Correlational and experimental studies can develop this type of theory. These research designs are appropriate when relations among concepts have been found and causal statements are of interest (Payton, 1979:45). Nursing research designed to generate situation-relating theory emphasizes such things as identification of antecedent conditions in the person and/or the environment that lead to consequences in health status, the effects of nursing care on the person's health, and so on. Examples of nursing studies of this type are:

Effects of orientation information on spouses'

anxieties and attitudes toward hospitalization and surgery (Silva, 1979)

Effect of structured preparation for transfer on patient anxiety on leaving coronary care unit (Toth, 1980)

Duration experience for bed-confined subjects: A replication and refinement (Smith, 1979)

Altering patients' responses to surgery: An extension and replication (Johnson, Fuller, Endress, and Rice, 1978)

The fourth level of the Dickoff and James (1968) knowledge hierarchy is *situation-producing* or *prescriptive* theory. This kind of theory specifies the actions needed to realize goals identified within the theory. It also includes theories at the lower levels. While scientific knowledge in any discipline includes the three previous levels, Dickoff and James maintained that nursing and other disciplines having a practice component must have prescriptive theories that clearly identify goals to be achieved and the activities required to achieve such goals. These theories include statements of who or what performs the activity, who receives it, the context in which the activity is performed, how it is performed, why it is performed, and the desired end result of the activity.

Diers (1979:53) noted that this level of theory can be generated by what she called *prescription-testing* research designs. However, she further noted that the methodological aspects of this kind of research remain to be developed. This well-known proponent of prescriptive theory has presented the most comprehensive description of this level of knowledge available in the literature (Diers, 1979: 47–54, 199–200). What is clear from her discourse is that examples of research designed to generate prescriptive theory do not exist and that applied research is not the same as prescription-testing research.

While the aim of applied research certainly is to achieve a particular goal (Kerlinger, 1979:283), this is done through application of knowledge generated by non-goal-oriented, or basic, research. In fact, applied research does not generate new knowledge. Rather, it is directed toward determination of the extent of applicability of knowledge in practical situations and of the pragmatics of implementation of knowledge. In other words, applied research seeks to determine if the boundaries of knowledge generated in controlled laboratory settings extend to the real world of practice and how such knowledge can be used by practitioners (Donaldson and Crowley, 1978). Prescription-testing research, in contrast, would be directed toward development of new knowledge at a higher level than other forms. While this type of knowledge would incorporate lower levels of theory, its most predominant characteristic "is the explicit inclusion of professionally defined goals for the prescribed activities" (Diers, 1979:47).

The validity and utility of the knowledge hierarchy proposed by Dickoff and James, and especially the need for distinct prescriptive theory, have been questioned by Beckstrand (1978a, 1978b, 1980). She argued that prescriptive theory is not required for a comprehensive body of nursing knowledge. Beckstrand based her position on the proposition that practice must take into account the conditions that exist in a given situation, the conditions that need to be changed, the outcomes that are scientifically and practically possible to achieve in the situation, the value of changes and outcomes in terms of desired ends, and the choice of one from among all possible outcomes in terms of the greatest good that might be achieved in the situation.

She then maintained that:

> The conditions identified as being relevant in practice depend on the scientific and ethical knowledge of the practitioner. The values used to determine needs for change and desired outcomes in particular situations are determined by the knowledge of ethics. The knowledge of the changes that will realize these outcomes is scientific, and the value ascribed to outcomes of the changes depends again on the ethical theory of value and scientific relationships. Finally, the question of the greatest good is related to the knowledge of moral right, non-moral value, and scientific possibility under conditions of uncertainty (Beckstrand, 1978b: 178–179).

Thus, scientific knowledge, which includes descriptive, explanatory, and predictive theory, and ethical knowledge, which focuses on explication of values, are completely sufficient for practice. Therefore, special knowledge, or prescriptive theory, is not needed by the practitioner. Beckstrand's position is strengthened by Diers's (1979: 200) statement that prescriptive theory includes descriptive, explanatory, and predictive theory, i.e., scientific knowledge, and that it is "normative theory; that is, it contains within the theory conceptions of desirable states to be manufactured, or norms or goals." Diers also commented that these goals are defined by the practice discipline and reflect professional values. It should be obvious that such values are articulated in the ethical knowledge of the discipline. Thus, prescriptive theory can be thought of as a combination of scientific and ethical knowledge, and not as a special or distinct form of knowledge.

The research strategies needed to develop scientific knowledge were discussed earlier, and examples of current nursing studies were cited. It should be noted, however, that few nursing investigations have presented clear explications of the theories being formulated or tested. As pointed out previously, many nursing research reports contain the data needed for theory development. What remains, then, is for those nurses interested in an explicit body of knowledge for nursing to formalize the findings of these studies into specific theories. Such efforts will be facilitated by application of theoretical "substruction" (Hinshaw, 1979b) and various inductive, deductive, and retroductive techniques of theory construction (Burr, 1973).

Ethical knowledge is developed through philosophic inquiry. While scientific research emphasizes empirical investigations designed to formulate or test hypotheses, philosophic inquiry uses critical discussion to organize phenomena into coherent systems (Smith, 1980). Thus, the ethical dimensions of professional nursing practice, the values held by members of the discipline of nursing, are established through philosophic inquiry. Nurses are only beginning to establish formal systems of ethical knowledge. In fact, a review of all research published between January 1979 and June 1980 in *Nursing Research, Research in Nursing and Health*, and the *Western Journal of Nursing Research*[1] revealed no articles that could be classified as philosophic inquiry.

However, a doctoral dissertation recently completed by Judith Smith (1979) at New York University serves as an exemplar. Smith reviewed writings about health since ancient times. This search of the literature led to her formulation of four ideas of health that reflect the values and interests of different disciplines. One such idea is the *clinical model*, which considers a person to be well if symptoms of disease or disability are absent. This model clearly reflects the values of medicine. Another idea is the *role-performance model*, which defines health as the ability to perform social roles, thus encompassing the interests of sociology. Another idea is the *adaptive model*, emphasizing ability to adapt to the changing environment and reflecting the values and interests of many disciplines. The fourth idea, called the *eudaimonistic model*, views utmost health as self-actualization and exuberant well-being. This model most clearly explicates the values of psychology as well as other disciplines. Smith's inquiry raised many questions regarding the implications of these ideas of health for nursing education, research, and practice, as well as for development of ethical knowledge related to the person and the environment.

In concluding her work, Smith (1979:160) noted that while the clinical and role-performance models are clearly exemplified in traditional and current medical and nursing practice, the implications of the adaptive and eudaimonistic models

[1] The issues of the journals included in this review are: *Nursing Research*, Vol. 28, Nos. 1–6; Vol. 29, Nos. 1–3; *Research in Nursing and Health*, Vol. 2, Nos. 1–4; Vol. 3, Nos. 1–2; *Western Journal of Nursing Research*, Vol. 1, Nos. 1–4; Vol. 2, No. 1.

"carry a certain urgency because they are, in fact, anticipations of changes in practice which would result from a widespread adoption of these two models as directives of health care." It seems obvious that nursing needs to further develop this and other components of their ethical knowledge. What is needed are theories that explicate moral obligation, including standards for deciding what one ought to do in a given situation; moral value, including standards for evaluation of the goodness or badness of people and their attributes; and nonmoral value, including value judgments based on custom or utility (Beckstrand, 1978a:134–136).

The two schemas of nursing knowledge discussed thus far have characterized nursing as a rational science, a conscious application of scientific knowledge in practical situations deemed appropriate by the personal and collective ethics of members of the discipline. Such a viewpoint denies the intuitive aspects of nursing as well as the skillful use of the tools and techniques of nursing technology. These aspects of nursing, as well as the scientific and ethical components, are encompassed by Carper's (1978) typology of nursing knowledge. Carper (1978:22) maintained that nursing "depends on the scientific knowledge of human behavior in health and in illness, the esthetic perception of significant human experiences, a personal understanding of the unique individuality of the self and the capacity to make choices within concrete situations involving particular moral judgments." Thus, nursing practice requires four kinds of knowledge—scientific, or empirical, knowledge; ethical knowledge; esthetic knowledge, or the art of nursing; and personal knowledge of the therapeutic use of self.

The characteristics of scientific and ethical knowledge have been discussed already, as have the methods of inquiry used to generate these types of nursing knowledge. Moreover, examples of research designed to develop this knowledge in the current nursing literature have been noted. Carper (1978:16–17) stated that esthetic knowledge extends well beyond manual and technical nursing skills to perception of particulars rather than universals. It involves the perception of what is significant in a client's behavior, the recognition of what need is actually being expressed by that behavior; clearly, empathy is an important aspect of this type of knowledge. While it is certainly possible to measure empathy, development of knowledge regarding the art of nursing through empirical research seems difficult, if not impossible. In fact, the empirical methods of scientific research are not appropriate for formulation of a way of knowing that focuses on the "specific and unique rather than exemplary" (Carper, 1978:16) aspects of a situation. However, insights arising from particular situations may serve as the basis for development of empirical knowledge. Indeed, many discoveries in science reflect the creativity inherent in esthetic knowledge.

Personal knowledge of the therapeutic use of self is "concerned with the knowing, encountering, and actualizing of the concrete, individual self" (Carper, 1978:18). Since this type of knowledge emphasizes "wholeness and integrity in the personal encounter" (Carper, 1978:20) between nurse and client, it is most characteristic of what nurses mean when they say that nursing deals with the whole person or that the focus of nursing is holism. Clearly, personal knowledge is concerned with the quality of the interpersonal process. While it is probable that much of this type of knowledge cannot be subjected to the methods of empirical science, certain aspects of the interpersonal relationship between nurse and client have been studied. One of the most outstanding examples of nursing research designed to develop this type of information is Diers and Schmidt's (1977) work on analysis of nurse-patient interactions. Other current work includes the following:

Postpartum perceptions of touch received during labor (Penny, 1979)

The use of verbal and tactile comfort to alleviate distress in young hospitalized children (Triplett and Arneson, 1979)

These last titles reflect the overlap in Carper's categories of knowledge, which are not conceived of as mutually exclusive. Thus, the research cited above may be thought of as development of empirical knowledge about the therapeutic use of self. The ideas for the research reflect perception of the client's need for certain interactions with the nurse at certain times or for esthetic knowledge. And the knowledge that such interactions should be engaged in by nurses comes from ethics.

Carper's schema provides a comprehensive overview of the knowledge needed for nursing practice. In effect, her work extends Beckstrand's position that the prescriptive level of theory advocated by Dickoff and James is not needed by practitioners. Rather, what is needed is a synthesis of empirical, ethical, esthetic, and personal knowledge. Such a mix could take the form of application of the findings of science in situations generally deemed appropriate by nursing's articulated values and particularly as necessary by esthetic perception of the significance of the client's behavior, through knowledge of the most therapeutic use of self.

In summary, three schemas of the knowledge needed for nursing practice have been reviewed and the research related to each has been noted. While many current nursing studies provide data that can be used to develop nursing knowledge, few researchers have presented their findings in a formal, theoretical manner. Thus, development of a body of distinctive nursing knowledge progresses slowly. Given nursing's historical lack of interest in formal theory, it is unlikely that the pace will increase until theory development is valued more highly and rewarded more generously by more than a handful of nurses.

UTILIZATION OF NURSING KNOWLEDGE

The last question posed at the beginning of the chapter requires an examination of the information about the validity, reliability, and relevance of nursing knowledge needed before such knowledge can be used by practitioners. Perhaps the best answer to this question is provided by the criteria for development of research-based protocols for nursing practice innovations set forth by Haller, Reynolds, and Horsely (1979).

Three sets of criteria proposed by these investigators identify the conditions required for transferring knowledge developed by scientific research to practice situations (Haller, Reynolds, and Horsley, 1979:47-51). The first set of criteria focuses on evaluation and integration of related studies, and the first consideration is replication. Repeated study of the same research question in different settings using different samples or populations and conducted by different investigators helps to establish the generalizability of findings. While replication is commonplace in most disciplines, nursing research rarely is of this kind. The paucity of replication of nursing studies is clearly documented in the literature. In fact, of the 145 articles published between January 1979 and June 1980 in *Nursing Research, Research in Nursing and Health*, and the *Western Journal of Nursing Research*, only 5 could be identified as replications. The titles of these studies are:

Topical application of insulin in decubitus ulcers (Gerber and Van Ort, 1979)

Duration experience for bed-confined subjects: A replication and refinement (Smith, 1979)

A follow-up study of the reliability and validity of the Motor Activity Rating Scale (Fitzpatrick and Donovan, 1979)

A survey of health needs of older adults in northwest Johnson County, Iowa (Franck, 1979)

Nurse practitioners', public health nurses' and physicians' performance on clinical simulation tests: COPD (McLaughlin, Cesa, Johnson, Lemons, Anderson, Larson, Gibson, and Delucchi, 1979)

The second consideration is evaluation of the scientific merit of a study. The standard elements of the research critique are used, with emphasis on the demonstrated corroboration of findings in clinical situations with actual clients of nursing (cf. Jacox and Prescott, 1978; Norbeck, 1979). Although assessment of the theoretical structure of a study is part of any comprehensive critique, Haller

et al. (1979) failed to make this crucial aspect of scientific merit explicit. Given the hierarchical arrangement of theory (Dickoff and James, 1968; Payton, 1979), it is important that each study contain an explanation of where it fits into the building and testing of a given theory. This is the single most common flaw in nursing research (Batey, 1977:325). Perhaps the recent attention to the relation between theory and research and the need for developing theory in a cumulative manner (Chinn and Jacobs, 1978; Fawcett, 1978b, 1980), coupled with discussion of techniques for analysis of the theoretical structure of studies and for assessment of the logical consistency of the theoretical, design, and analysis structures of investigations (Hinshaw, 1979a, 1979b), will serve to strengthen this aspect of nursing research.

The third consideration in the evaluation of studies is the assessment of the risk-benefit for the client. Certainly any practice that might have risks associated with it requires a stronger, more established research base than does an intervention carrying no identified risk. Thus, the extent of replication and the integration of related studies having different findings must be taken into account.

In other words, how much replication is enough for a given research problem? And, how are conflicting findings explained? Are these due to differences in the scientific merit of the studies or is the explanation less obvious? While the answers to these questions finally depend on subjective judgment, objectivity may be introduced through application of *metaanalysis*. This refers to the comprehensive statistical analysis of the results from related studies. The technique requires calculation and comparison of the effect sizes (i.e., the standardized measures of the magnitude of differences between group means or of associations between variables) of study findings. Thus, by considering the meaningfulness as well as the statistical significance of findings, conflicting results can be synthesized (Glass, 1977; Pillemer and Light, 1980).

The second set of criteria proposed by Haller, Reynolds, and Horsley (1979) focuses on the clinical relevance of studies. The first consideration examines the clinical merit of research, that is, "the degree to which the research base addresses a problem of significance to the practice setting or the degree to which the suggested innovation will be potentially useful" (Haller, Reynolds, and Horsley, 1979:49). There should be little doubt that most, if not all nursing research derives from and ultimately relates to nursing practice. However, not all research findings are immediately ready for application in the clinical arena. As noted repeatedly throughout this chapter, theory building is hierarchical and cumulative. This is a slow and tedious process requiring determination and commitment. "It means sticking to some particular area of inquiry long enough to produce related findings or contrasting explanations of phenomena and then to formulate links among them" (Downs, 1975:7). It also means resisting the urge to make premature leaps to practice implications. As Ketefian (1980:430) observed, "nursing has not recognized that a scholarly inquiry or research generally is not immediately ready to be applied, and that most frequently it needs to be recast into new molds, reconceptualized, and developmental activities carried out, replicated, and so on, before it can be safely used in patient care."

While some study findings clearly are not ready for clinical application, others may appear to be ready for immediate utilization. Unfortunately, many of these lack a clear theoretical base and therefore contribute little, if anything, to nursing knowledge. Clinical merit of a study therefore must be balanced with scientific merit, especially that related to theory. This is because a collection of empirical "facts" is unsystematic and usually not applicable outside the specific situation and setting in which they were first observed. Indeed, the most impractical knowledge is that which is atheoretical. Thus, although the approximation of a research question to a clinical goal must be considered, this must be done within the context of the theoretical contributions of the study. Regrettably, this is not always the case. In fact, "the extent to which . . . practice innovations have

actually been subjected to the scientific rigor of [basic research] is often more questionable than the ordinary professional consumer realizes" (Downs, 1979:85).

The second consideration is the nurse's ability to control both independent and dependent variables. This is especially problematic, since nurses frequently are not the only ones who determine their practice. Thus, the practitioner may not be able to implement certain interventions or may not be able to measure the effect of nursing practice, as when measurement techniques are medical procedures such as cystoscopy. These constraints may be overcome, however, by clearly defining nursing practice. This is greatly facilitated by designing and implementing nursing activities within the context of a conceptual model of nursing. Just as research guided by a nursing model helps the investigator to focus on the phenomena of interest to nursing, so practice guided by such a conceptualization helps the practitioner to provide *nursing* care.

The next consideration in this set of criteria evaluates the feasibility of implementing research in a given clinical nursing setting. Here, resources such as time, personnel, expertise, and equipment must be assessed, as well as the politics of change. As Stetler and Marram (1976:563) pointed out, the time and effort needed to overcome the real and usual obstacles to change may be worthwhile only if the change will produce meaningfully different outcomes in clients' health. Clearly, nurses must learn to assess the health care delivery systems in which they work and to become more political.

The final consideration related to clinical relevance is the actual dollar cost of implementing a given innovation. This involves assessment of the financial resources of the agency and the willingness of those who control these resources to spend the money. Haller et al. (1979:50) point out that the "costs of materials, laboratory expenses, personnel development, and staff time [must be balanced] against such benefits as reduced incidence of complications and patient or staff satisfaction." Thus, nurses must also learn to consider the economic issues related to nursing practice.

The third set of criteria for utilization of nursing knowledge concerns the potential for evaluation of a new intervention in the clinical setting. The crucial consideration is the possibility for evaluation of the results of implementing a given practice. Although there are differences in the context of a systematic research project and the real world of clinical practice, clinical evaluation of an innovation can be thought of as a form of replication in the clinical setting. It is, in fact, applied research. As noted earlier in this chapter, this kind of research is directed toward establishing the boundaries of knowledge in clinical practice settings and identifying how practitioners can use the knowledge to solve practice problems.

Haller et al. (1979:47) noted that the project staff of CURN (Conduct and Utilization of Research in Nursing) have been able to identify 10 areas of nursing research they think meet all criteria mentioned above sufficiently to warrant development and testing of nursing practice innovation protocols. These are:

1 Structured preoperative teaching
2 A lactose-free diet
3 Sensation information: distress reduction
4 Sensory information: recovery rate
5 Nonsterile intermittent urinary catheterization
6 Prevention of catheter-associated urinary tract infections
7 Intravenous cannula change regimen
8 Prevention of decubiti by means of small shifts of body weight
9 Mutual goal setting: goal attainment
10 Deliberative nursing: pain reduction

CONCLUSIONS

The above protocols are the areas of nursing research that have been identified as directly relevant for nursing practice. While this is certainly encouraging, it is also a cause for concern. This concern lies in the fact that few, if any, of these protocols are based on explicit and logically consistent theory. Although the theoretical explanations probably exist, they have not been articulated. Until that is done, nursing will not have a distinctive body of knowledge.

Although the foregoing may sound discouraging, it is important to note that nursing is an emerging discipline that is only now beginning to recognize the need for studies that build on one another from the descriptive theory building stage to that of clinical evaluation. Furthermore, only now is nursing starting to produce the numbers of doctorally prepared nurses who have the knowledge, skill, and commitment needed to initiate and continue programs of nursing research. The challenge for the future of nursing research should be clear: Develop series of related studies that build and test the knowledge needed for practice.

EDITOR'S QUESTIONS FOR DISCUSSION

With research purported to be essential for developing and testing theory for nursing's knowledge base and practice, why have there been so few studies explicitly derived from a nursing conceptual or theoretical base? Are there clear differences between prescription testing and applied research? Is it important to distinguish between knowledge generated by non-goal-oriented research and knowledge obtained by identifying the specific actions needed to realize goals in order to apply knowledge for practice? In determining the extent knowledge is applicable in practice (applied research) may an outcome be generation of new knowledge? Why are there no examples of research designed to generate prescriptive theory? Is it possible for applied research to be a final step in the development of knowledge after prescriptive-theory testing? Do you agree with Beckstrand's position that prescriptive theory is not necessary for a comprehensive body of *nursing* knowledge in that it focuses on the conditions that exist in a given situation? What is *nursing* knowledge? Does prescriptive theory concern itself with external variables in the *application* of nursing knowledge and not *development* of nursing knowledge in itself? If you agree, then to what extent can prescriptive theory testing be considered the same and/or part of applied research?

What factors may influence the conditions required for transferring knowledge developed by scientific research to practice situations? Why is it a common failure of nurse-researchers not to indicate where their study fits into the building and testing of a given theory? What implications does this have for the further development of nursing as a profession? How can utilizing a nursing conceptual or theoretical base to design and implement nursing activities clearly define nursing practice? What relationship is there between using a nursing conceptual or theoretical base to the nurse-researcher's ability to control both independent and dependent variables for clinically relevant studies?

Why were the 10 protocols indicated as relevant for testing of nursing practice not clearly based on explicit and logically consistent theory? Is there a base and/or rationale for the 10 defined areas of research and protocols to be legitimately accepted as contributing to the knowledge of nursing? Is the acceptance of protocols which are not based on theory an indicator of an actualized chasm between research and protocols that are identified as relevant for nursing practice and those which are specifically designed to develop the knowledge base of nursing? Does this imply there can be research relevant for nursing practice that need not be derived from a nursing theoretical base? If so, what are the implications for the practice of nursing and the profession?

REFERENCES

Batey, Marjorie V.
1977 "Conceptualization: Knowledge and logic guiding empirical research." Nursing Research 26:324–329.

Beckstrand, Jan
1978a "The notion of a practice theory and the relationship of scientific and ethical knowledge to practice." Research in Nursing and Health 1:131–136.
1978b "The need for a practice theory as indicated by the knowledge used in the conduct of practice." Research in Nursing and Health 1:175–179.
1980 "A critique of several conceptions of practice theory in nursing." Research in Nursing and Health 3:69–79.

Brockway, Barbara F.
1979 "Situational stress and temporal changes in self-report and vocal measurements." Nursing Research 28:20–24.

Burr, Wesley R.
1973 Theory Construction and the Sociology of the Family. New York: Wiley.

Bush, Helen A.
1979 "Models for nursing." Advances in Nursing Science 1(2):13–21.

Carper, Barbara A.
1978 "Fundamental patterns of knowing in nursing." Advances in Nursing Science 1(1):13–23.

Chinn, Peggy L. (ed.)
1979 "Nursing diagnosis." Advances in Nursing Science 2:1:1–100.

Chinn, Peggy L. and Maeona K. Jacobs
1978 "A model for theory development in nursing." Advances in Nursing Science 1(1):1–11.

Dickoff, James and Patricia James
1968 "A theory of theories: A position paper." Nursing Research 17:197–203.

Diers, Donna
1979   Research in Nursing Practice. Philadel-
       phia: Lippincott.
Diers, Donna and Ruth L. Schmidt
1977   "Interaction analysis in nursing research,"
       Pp. 77–132 in P. J. Verhonick (ed.),
       Nursing Research II. Boston: Little,
       Brown.
Donaldson, Sue K. and Dorothy M. Crowley
1978   "The discipline of nursing." Nursing
       Outlook 26:113–120.
Downs, Florence S.
1975   "Nature of relationship between theory
       and practice." Pp. 1–9 in S. Ketefian (ed.),
       Translation of Theory into Nursing Prac-
       tice and Education. New York: New York
       University Division of Nursing.
1979   "Clinical and theoretical research," pp.
       67–87 in F. S. Downs and J. W. Fleming
       (eds.), Issues in Nursing Research. New
       York: Appleton-Century-Crofts.
Fawcett, Jacqueline
1977   "The relationship between identification
       and patterns of change in spouses' body
       images during and after pregnancy."
       International Journal of Nursing Studies
       14:199–213.
1978a "The 'what' of theory development." in
       Theory Development: What, Why, How?
       New York: National League for Nursing,
       pp. 17–33.
1978b "The relationship between theory and re-
       search: A double helix." Advances in
       Nursing Science 1(1):49–62.
1980   "A declaration of nursing independence:
       The relation of theory and research to
       nursing practice." Journal of Nursing
       Administration 10(6):36–39.
1981   "Assessing and understanding the cesarean
       father." Pp. 143–156 in C. F. Kehoe (ed.),
       The Cesarean Experience: Theoretical and
       Clinical Perspectives for Nurses. New
       York: Appleton-Century-Crofts.
Fitzpatrick, Joyce J.
1980   "Patients' perceptions of time: Current
       research." International Nursing Review
       27:148–153, 160.
Fitzpatrick, Joyce J. and Michael J. Donovan
1979   "A follow-up study of the reliability and

validity of the Motor Activity Rating
       Scale." Nursing Research 28:179–181.
Franck, Phyllis
1979   "A survey of health needs of older adults
       in northwest Johnson County, Iowa."
       Nursing Research 28:360–364.
Fuller, Sarah S. and Sandra B. Larson
1980   "Life events, emotional support, and
       health of older people." Research in
       Nursing and Health 3:81–89.
Gerber, Rose Marie and Suzanne R. Van Ort
1979   "Topical application of insulin in decubi-
       tus ulcers." Nursing Research 28:16–19.
Glaser, Barney G. and Anselm L. Strauss
1967   The Discovery of Grounded Theory:
       Strategies for Qualitative Research. Chi-
       cago: Aldine.
Glass, Gene V.
1977   "Integrating findings: The meta-analysis
       of research." Pp. 351–379 in Review of
       Research in Education. Volume 5. Wash-
       ington, D.C.: The American Educational
       Research Association.
Haller, Karen B., Margaret A. Reynolds, and
       Joanne Horsley
1979   "Developing research-based innovation
       protocols: Process, criteria, and issues."
       Research in Nursing and Health 2:45–51.
Hinshaw, Ada S.
1979a "Planning for logical consistency among
       three research structures." Western Jour-
       nal of Nursing Research 1:250–253.
Hinshaw, Ada S.
1979b "Theoretical substruction: An assessment
       process." Western Journal of Nursing
       Research 1:319–324.
Jacox, Ada and Patricia Prescott
1978   "Determining a study's relevance for
       clinical practice." American Journal of
       Nursing 78:1882–1889.
Johnson, Jean E., Sarah S. Fuller, M. Patricia
       Endress, and Virginia S. Rice
1978   "Altering patients' responses to surgery:
       An extension and replication." Research
       in Nursing and Health 1:111–121.
Kearney, Barbara Y. and Barbara J. Fleischer
1979   "Development of an instrument to mea-
       sure exercise of self-care agency." Re-
       search in Nursing and Health, 2:25–34.

Kehoe, Carole F.
  1981 "Identifying the nursing needs of the post-partum cesarean mother." Pp. 85–141 in C. F. Kehoe (ed.), The Cesarean Experience: Theoretical and Clinical Perspectives for Nurses. New York: Appleton-Century-Crofts.
Kerlinger, Fred N.
  1979 Behavioral Research. A Conceptual Approach. New York: Holt, Rinehart and Winston
Ketefian, Shake
  1980 "Using research in practice: Selected issues in the translation of research to nursing practice." Western Journal of Nursing Research 2:429–431.
Lederman, Regina P., Edward Lederman, Bruce A. Work, Jr., and Daisy S. McCann
  1979 "Relationship of psychological factors in pregnancy to progress in labor." Nursing Research 28:94–97.
Mansell, D. Moira and Karen K. Porter
  1979 "Personality factors of contemporary baccalaureate nursing students: A descriptive study." Western Journal of Nursing Research 1:85–98.
Marut, JoAnne S. and Ramona T. Mercer
  1979 "Comparison of primiparas' perceptions of vaginal and cesarean births." Nursing Research 28:260–266.
McLaughlin, Frank E., Thomas Cesa, Harold Johnson, Mary Lemons, Sara Anderson, Patricia Larson, Josephine Gibson, and Kevin Delucchi
  1979 "Nurse practitioners', public health nurses' and physicians' performance on clinical simulation tests: COPD." Western Journal of Nursing Research 1:273–295.
Norbeck, Jane S.
  1979 "The research critique: A theoretical approach to skill development and consolidation." Western Journal of Nursing Research 1:296–306.
Nursing Theories Conference Group
  1980 Nursing Theories. The Base for Professional Nursing Practice. Englewood Cliffs, N.J.: Prentice-Hall.
Orem, Dorothea E.
  1980 Nursing: Concepts of Practice. 2d ed. New York: McGraw-Hill.

Payton, Otto D.
  1979 Research: The Validation of Clinical Practice. Philadelphia: F. A. Davis.
Penny, Karen S
  1979 "Postpartum perceptions of touch received during labor." Research in Nursing and Health 2:9–16.
Pillemer, David B. and Richard J. Light
  1980 "Synthesizing outcomes: How to use research evidence from many studies." Harvard Educational Review 50:176–195.
Porter, Luz S.
  1979 "Health care workers' role conceptions and orientation to family-centered child care." Nursing Research 28:330–337.
Riehl, Joan P. and Sr. Callista Roy
  1974 Conceptual Models for Nursing Practice. New York: Appleton-Century-Crofts.
Riehl, Joan P. and Sr. Callista Roy
  1980 Conceptual Models for Nursing Practice. 2d ed. New York: Appleton-Century-Crofts.
Rogers, Martha E.
  1970 An Introduction to the Theoretical Basis of Nursing. Philadelphia: F. A. Davis
Roslaniec, Anita and Joyce J. Fitzpatrick
  1979 "Changes in mental status in older adults with four days of hospitalization." Research in Nursing and Health 2:117–187.
Roy, Sr. Callista
  1976 Introduction to Nursing: An Adaptation Model. Englewood Cliffs, N.J.: Prentice-Hall.
Silva, Mary C.
  1979 "Effects of orientation information on spouses' anxieties and attitudes toward hospitalization and surgery." Research in Nursing and Health 2:127–136.
Smith, Judith Ann
  1979 The Idea of Health. Unpublished Doctoral Dissertation, New York University.
  1980 "The idea of health: A philosophical inquiry." Advances in Nursing Science, 3(3):43–50.
Smith, Mary Jane
  1979 "Duration experience for bed-confined subjects: A replication and refinement." Nursing Research 28:139–144.

Sparacino, Jack, Stephen Hansell, and Kathleen Smyth
1979 "Type A (coronary-prone) behavior and transient blood pressure change." Nursing Research 28:198-204.

Stern, Phyllis N.
1980 "Grounded theory methodology: Its uses and processes." Image 12:20-23.

Stetler, Cheryl B. and Gwen Marram
1976 "Evaluating research findings for applicability in practice." Nursing Outlook 24:559-563.

Toth, Jean C.
1980 "Effect of structured preparation for transfer on patient anxiety on leaving coronary care unit." Nursing Research 29:28-34.

Triplett, June L. and Sara W. Arneson
1979 "The use of verbal and tactile comfort to alleviate distress in young hospitalized children." Research in Nursing and Health 2:17-23.

Yura, Helen and Gertrude Torres
1975 "Today's conceptual frameworks within baccalaureate nursing programs." Pp. 17-25 in Faculty-Curriculum Development Part III. Conceptual Framework—Its Meaning and Function. New York: National League for Nursing.

Chapter 15

Nursing Practice: A Decade of Research

Kathleen A. O'Connell, R.N., Ph.D.
Assistant Professor, School of Nursing
University of Kansas
Kansas City, Kansas
and
Associate Psychologist
Midwest Research Institute
Kansas City, Missouri

There is an unique opportunity to evaluate the change in nature and direction of nursing practice research during the past decade through the results of a content analysis by Kathleen A. O'Connell. This chapter represents a replication and extension of the original efforts by O'Connell and Duffey to analyze research in nursing practice that has been published in the journal *Nursing Research*. She includes an appendix of all the studies reviewed from 1970 to 1979. In addition, O'Connell compares the studies published from 1970 to 1974 with those published in 1975 to 1979 to identify changes. She also briefly compares the first two volumes of the journal *Research in Nursing and Health* with *Nursing Research* for the proportion of studies published in nursing practice. To be classified as a study of "nursing practice" and included in the review, the research had to deal with the *interaction* of nurses, acting as nurses, and clients—well or ill. O'Connell differentiates between studies of "nursing practice," "laboratory," and "clinical" studies. During the 10-year period, 145 (28 percent) of the studies published in *Nursing Research* were classified as studies of nursing practice. This research was conducted by 303 investigators, the majority of whom had master's degrees.

Some of the changes noted when the second half of the decade was compared with the first are as follows: an increase in the number of investigators, nonnurse investigators, and the proportion of investigators with Ph.D.s; an increase in collaborative research among nurses and with nonnurses. Studies funded by federal research grants increased from 14 percent to 38 percent. A change in emphasis was apparent. More studies were related to chronic illness, the elderly, obstetrics, outpatients, psycho-

This chapter is an extension of the chapter by Kathleen O'Connell and Margery Duffey, "Research in Nursing Practice: Its Present Scope," in N. Chaska (ed.), *The Nursing Profession: Views Through the Mist* (New York: McGraw-Hill, 1978), pp. 161–174.

logical needs, and needs assessment. The content of the research was more nonaggregated. Far more experimental designs were utilized, and the number of descriptive studies was greatly reduced. Provocative explanations are offered for the changes. O'Connell notes that, although there was not an increase in the number of studies for the second half of the decade, there appeared to be a greater concern with reliability and validity of the instruments. She concludes that the findings suggest a definite improvement in the quality of the research conducted.

This chapter presents an analysis of the research in nursing practice which has been published by *Nursing Research* during the 10-year period from 1970 to 1979. The research is described according to (1) the characteristics of the investigators, (2) the funding sources of the studies, (3) the content of the studies, and (4) the research methods employed. The results of this analysis enable us to identify the nature and direction of research in nursing practice. The content areas that researchers emphasized, as well as those that they neglected, are described. The analysis also gives some indication of the relative sophistication of the research methods. In addition, the studies published in the first half of the decade are compared with those published in the second half to identify possible changes in the characteristics of the research.

In an article in a 1975 issue of *Nursing Research*, Dickoff et al. contended that nursing research has left nursing practice virtually untouched. As if to prove the point, *Nursing Research* editors followed the article with a study by Ketefian (1975), in which only one of 87 nurses knew the correct placement time for taking oral temperatures. Experiments by Nichols and others (1966; 1967; 1972) that determined the correct placement time had been reported in *Nursing Research* and in the *American Journal of Nursing*.

The lack of impact of nursing research was attributed to different causes in the two articles. Ketefian held that there was a lack of communication between researchers and practitioners. Dickoff et al., on the other hand, maintained that nursing researchers were so preoccupied with "pseudo-technical research methodology" that they lost sight of the real problems in nursing. The research findings, they said, are either obvious generalities or inapplicable minute points. However, in a more recent discussion of the development of nursing research, Gortner (1980) has said that this preoccupation with methodology has done much to increase the rigor of research. In addition, she pointed out that practice-related research demonstrated considerable growth in the 1970s.

This chapter enumerates and describes a sample of studies that concern the practice of nursing. The sample was selected from studies of nursing practice published in *Nursing Research* from 1970 through 1979. (An appendix to this chapter lists the 145 studies which made up the sample.) *Nursing Research* is not the only publisher of studies of nursing research; however, because it is a refereed journal, it was felt that the sample would be representative of the best studies available. In addition, the studies in *Nursing Research* are presented in enough detail to allow adequate classification. And, because of its close relationship with recognized leaders in nursing research, the journal's editorial policies, with respect to publication of studies in nursing practice, are likely to reflect the values and priorities of leaders and policy-makers in nursing.

A study of "nursing practice" has been defined as a study which in any way deals with the interaction of nurses, acting as nurses, and clients, be they well or ill. This definition was designed to include studies of nurses in extended roles and studies that deal with the use of nursing assessment tools. The definition excludes studies of nurses in isolation from patients and studies of patients in isolation from nurses.

The variables of the studies were examined to determine if any of them related to the interaction of nurses and patients. If no such variables were found, the study was excluded from the sample. For instance, a study by Muhlenkamp et al. (1975) dealt with the perception of life-change events by the elderly. Because the study was focused on clients, rather than on nursing personnel, students, or educators, it met one criterion of the definition. However, because the variables considered did not include interaction between the clients and nurses, the study was excluded from the sample. Similarly, studies that correlated preoperative patient anxiety with variables such as number of days in the hospital, number of complications, and number of analgesics were not included in the sample, unless a specific nursing action, such as preoperative teaching by a nurse, was among the variables considered. Studies that concerned patients' attitudes toward specific nurses or patients' satisfaction with care were included in the sample, since these variables presuppose interaction with nurses. If a study encompassed many variables and at least one of them concerned the interaction between nurses and patients, the study was included in the sample.

It should be noted that a study of "nursing practice" is not necessarily a "clinical study." Some of the studies in the present sample were carried out in laboratories. The laboratory studies included research on the reliability of monitoring techniques and on methods of applying elastic bandages, of administering oxygen, and of increasing tolerance for pain. Such studies have direct relevance for nursing practice because they concern behaviors that are generally recognized as nursing care. However, they may be considered laboratory rather than clinical studies. On the other hand, some of the studies that might be of a clinical nature, e.g., the study of the perception of life-change events by the elderly, were not considered studies of nursing practice.

The sample of studies was classified along a number of dimensions. The investigators were categorized according to whether or not they were nurses and according to their educational attainment. A revision of the classification system devised by Simmons and Henderson (1964) for classifying nursing studies was used as a basis for categorizing the content of the studies. Each study's content was classified according to four different perspectives: general diagnostic category of the subjects, the procedure or technique investigated, the specific needs of patients on whom the research focused, and the state or condition of the subjects. The studies were also categorized according to the research methods that were employed. These methods included the types of subject samples, the design of the studies, the types of variables manipulated, and the instruments employed.

During the period from 1970 through 1979, *Nursing Research* published about 520 studies. For purposes of this analysis, 145, or 28 percent, were deemed studies of nursing practice. Table 15-1 shows the number of studies of nursing practice published each year. The sharp decline in the number of studies in 1977 can be attributed to an editorial policy of publishing a variety of review articles to commemorate the silver anniversary of *Nursing Research*. Because of limitation of space, the journal published fewer research reports of all

Table 15-1 Number of Studies of Nursing Practice by Year

Year	Number of studies
1970	14
1971	16
1972	15
1973	12
1974	14
1975	17
1976	14
1977	7
1978	14
1979	22
1970–1974	71
1975–1979	74
Total	145

types in 1977. However, in 1979 the journal published 22 articles on nursing practice. Therefore, the number of studies of nursing practice published in the first 5 years of the decade (71) was virtually the same as the number published in the second 5 years (74).

CHARACTERISTICS OF INVESTIGATORS

The 145 studies were carried out by 303 investigators. While the number of studies increased by only three from the first half to the second half of the decade, the number of investigators increased from 131 to 172. This greater number of investigators indicates more studies in which collaboration was necessary. Several of these studies were associated with the Western Interstate Commission on Higher Education, which has supported collaborative research among nurses in the western part of the United States.

The collaborative nature of the research is also reflected in the increase in the number of nonnurse investigators (see Table 15-2). The second half of the decade also demonstrated an increase in the number and proportion of investigators with Ph.D.s and a slight decrease in the proportion of investigators with other types of doctoral preparation (e.g., Ed.D., M.D., D.P.H., D.N.Sc.). The proportion of investigators with masters' degrees remained stable across the two halves of the decade

and represented the educational preparation of the majority of the investigators.

FUNDING SOURCES

Table 15-3 displays the funding sources of the studies in the sample. Over half of the studies indicated no source of funding. While many of these studies probably represent research carried out to fulfill educational requirements, many other studies reflect the commitment of practicing nurses and educators to carrying out research without funding sources. Nevertheless, a comparison of the studies in the first half of the decade to those in the second half demonstrates dramatic changes in funding sources. Studies funded by federal research grants increased from 14 percent to 38 percent. Most of these grants were from the Division of Nursing. In addition, funding from "other" sources doubled. "Other" sources included intramural sources and state and private agencies. Meanwhile, studies funded by federal training grants decreased from 14 percent to 1 percent. These trends reflect the federal policy shift which occurred during the 1970s (Gortner, 1980) in the Division of Nursing. The federal emphasis changed from personnel development (training grants) to research resource development (program grants) and finally to support of individual research studies.

Table 15-2   Professional and Educational Background of Investigators

	Years					
	1970–1974 (N = 131)		1975–1979 (N = 172)		1970–1979 (N = 303)	
	N	%	N	%	N	%
Profession						
Registered nurses	113	86	139	81	252	83
Nonnurse	18	14	33	19	51	17
Educational preparation						
Bachelor's degree or less	16	12	16	9	32	11
Master's degree	78	60	103	60	181	60
Ph.D.	20	15	37	22	57	19
Other doctorates	17	13	16	9	33	11

Table 15-3   Number of Studies by Type of Funding Source*

Funding source	1970-74 (N = 71)		1975-79 (N = 74)		1970-79 (N = 145)	
	N	%	N	%	N	%
Federal training grant	10	14	1	1	11	8
Federal research grant	10	14	28	38	38	26
Nursing	4	6	2	3	6	4
Other	5	7	11	15	16	11
None noted	45	63	35	47	80	56

*Six studies had more than one funding source.

CONTENT

Diagnostic Category of the Subjects

The 145 studies in the sample were classified according to the (medical) diagnostic category of the subjects. Studies in which all subjects were less than 17 years of age were classified in the "pediatrics" category, regardless of the diagnosis of the subject. However, studies related to the effect of labor, delivery, or prenatal activities on the infant and studies of teenagers who were pregnant were categorized as "obstetrics." Studies in which the subjects were healthy or in which subjects did not fit in any of the diagnostic categories were classified as "other." The "diverse" category included studies in which the subjects were in more than one category.

As Table 15-4 shows, the "diverse" category accounted for nearly one-fourth of the studies, a greater proportion than any of the other categories. There were no studies of patients with communicable diseases and only two reports on patients with orthopedic diagnoses. There was a shift in the types of diagnostic categories studied in the last half of the decade compared with the first. Surgical patients were the most frequently studied group during 1970 to 1974, while patients with chronic diseases and disabilities were most frequently studied in the latter half of the decade. In addition, there was a threefold increase in the

Table 15-4   Diagnostic Categories of the Subjects

Category	1970-74 (N = 71)		1975-79 (N = 74)		1970-79 (N = 145)	
	N	%	N	%	N	%
Obstetrics	3	4	9	12	12	8
Pediatrics	8	11	10	14	18	12
Acute medicine	1	1	5	7	6	4
Surgery	13	18	7	9	20	14
Orthopedics	2	3	1	1	3	2
Communicable diseases	0	0	0	0	0	0
Chronic disease/disability	5	7	14	19	19	13
Mental health	8	11	6	8	14	10
Other	9	13	9	12	18	12
Diverse	22	31	13	18	35	24

number of studies in the obstetrics category in the second half of the decade compared with the first half.

The use of diverse patient groups is indicative of the investigators' concern with problems that are common to a wide variety of patients. The change of emphasis to chronic illness may reflect the investigators' response to the need for research on this growing group of patients and to the realization that nursing measures may have greater impact on this group than on any other.

Procedures and Techniques

The 145 studies were classified according to the procedures and techniques which were investigated. "Monitoring techniques" refer to procedures for measuring physical indices such as vital signs. "Psychiatric treatments" refer to specific treatments of psychiatric patients. Studies dealing with emotional support and communication with physically ill patients are classified in the "other" category. "Assessment techniques" refer to the process of determining an individual patient's needs for nursing care. The category "organization of staff" refers to studies of the effect on patients of special nursing care programs or staffing procedures.

As Table 15-5 shows, 14 percent of the studies did not deal with any procedure or technique. Most of these studies were concerned with patients'

attitudes towards their nursing care in general. The relatively low number of studies dealing with psychiatric treatments reflects the relatively few studies done on this group. As the decade progressed, there was an increase in studies of physical treatments. In addition, the number of studies of techniques that were in the "other" category doubled. These studies include procedures designed to increase communication and relaxation and may reflect an increasing interest in the use of nontraditional techniques for meeting patients' needs.

Specific Needs of Patients

The 145 studies were classified according to the specific needs of the patients studied. The categories concerned both physical and nonphysical needs. The category "protection" refers to the need for prevention of infection or other complications. The "communication" category includes studies of verbal and nonverbal communication that do not expressly relate to the relief of anxiety or tension. Studies relating to the relief of these conditions are categorized under "emotional support." Nineteen of the studies concern more than one type of need. The "other" category was used to classify studies that were concerned with many (more than four) needs or with the assessment of needs. "Other" also includes studies on

Table 15-5 Procedures and Techniques Studied*

	Years					
	1970–74 (N = 71)		1975–79 (N = 74)		1970–79 (N = 145)	
Techniques	N	%	N	%	N	%
Monitoring techniques	11	16	6	8	17	12
Physical treatments	11	16	16	22	27	19
Psychiatric treatments	4	6	6	8	10	7
Teaching techniques	12	17	10	14	22	15
Assessment techniques	9	13	10	14	19	13
Organization of staff	3	4	8	11	11	8
Other	9	13	19	26	28	19
None	15	21	5	7	20	14

*Some studies dealt with more than one procedure.

Table 15-6 Number of Studies Focusing on Specific Needs*

| | Years | | | | | |
| | 1970–74 (N = 71) | | 1975–79 (N = 74) | | 1970–79 (N = 145) | |
Needs	N	%	N	%	N	%
Physical						
Food and nutrition	3	4	3	4	6	4
Rest and sleep	3	4	3	4	6	4
Cleanliness	2	3	1	1	3	2
Body mechanics	1	1	2	3	3	2
Elimination	3	4	3	4	6	4
Respiration	5	7	2	3	7	5
Relief of pain	5	7	4	5	9	6
Protection	8	11	12	16	20	14
Medication	0	0	4	5	4	3
Nonphysical						
Emotional support	11	16	16	22	27	19
Communication	7	10	10	14	17	12
Recreation	0	0	1	1	1	1
Occupation	0	0	0	0	0	0
Religious	0	0	0	0	0	0
Other	4	6	21	29	25	17
No specific needs studied	26	37	8	11	34	23

*Nineteen studies dealt with more than one need.

the need for touch, for sex, for feeling of control over one's life, and for information.

As Table 15-6 indicates, approximately one-fourth of the studies were classified as "no specific need studied." Most of these studies concerned monitoring techniques, measurement of attitudes, and teaching that was not directed at specific needs. Approximately one-fifth of the studies concerned emotional support, the need studied most frequently in this sample. The "other" category, which included studies of needs in general, contained 17 percent of the studies. Relatively little attention was given to physical needs. The practicing nurse spends a great deal of time meeting patients' needs for medication, cleanliness, nutrition, rest and sleep, and pain relief. Yet each of these needs was studied in fewer than 6 percent of the investigations reviewed. Comparing the first half of the decade to the second, there was little change in the number of physical needs studied by investigators. However, there was an increase in the number of studies of emotional support. In addition, the decrease in the "none" category was accompanied by an increase in the "other" category as the decade progressed. This is indicative of the increasing emphasis on the assessment of needs in general.

State or Condition of the Subjects

The studies were also classified according to the state or condition of the subjects. Thirty-two of the studies were concerned with more than one state. Many of these concerned the anxiety of patients about to undergo surgery. The "other" category refers usually to very specific states, such as pregnancy, labor, cardiac myopathy, or cancer, or to more general states, such as being in a nursing home. The "reactions to nursing" category refers to studies of patients' attitudes toward nursing care or toward specific nurses. As Table 15-7

Table 15-7   Number of Studies That Focused on Specific Patient States*

Patient state	Years					
	1970–74 (N = 71)		1975–79 (N = 74)		1970–79 (N = 145)	
	N	%	N	%	N	%
Anoxia	0	0	1	1	1	1
Anxiety or fear	11	16	6	8	17	12
Bedfastness	2	3	6	8	8	6
Dying	0	0	1	1	1	1
Fever	6	8	0	0	6	4
Healthy	7	10	10	14	17	12
Hyperactivity or hypoactivity	1	1	0	0	1	1
Incontinence or constipation	1	1	1	1	2	1
Infection/inflammation	6	8	2	3	8	6
Insomnia/sleep deprivation	4	6	2	3	6	4
Malnutrition	0	0	1	1	1	1
Nausea	0	0	0	0	0	0
Pain or distress	10	14	7	9	17	12
Preop, postop states	14	20	10	14	24	17
Reactions to nursing	10	14	7	9	17	12
Psychological maladaptation	9	13	6	8	15	10
Unconsciousness or disorientation	4	6	4	5	8	6
Other	3	4	18	24	20	14
None	9	13	6	8	15	10

*Thirty-two studies dealt with more than one state.

indicates, the most frequently studied state related to surgery. Reactions to nursing care, pain or distress, and anxiety and fear were also studied relatively frequently. There were, on the other hand, few studies of clients who were anoxic, dying, hyper- or hypoactive, constipated or incontinent, malnourished, or nauseated. Compared with the first half of the decade, the last half showed a decrease in the studies of patients who were anxious and an increase in the study of a variety of specific states represented in the "other" category.

RESEARCH METHODS

Characteristics of Subjects

The studies of nursing practice were classified according to the subject's status (inpatient, out-

patient, etc.) and age. Tables 15–8 and 15–9 display the results of the classification. Sixteen of the studies dealt with subjects in more than one category. Over two-thirds of the studies used inpatients as subjects, while less than one-fifth used outpatients. Approximately 10 percent of the sample used both health professionals and patients as subjects. The studies of outpatients more than double during the last half of the decade compared with the first half. Nearly half of the studies used adults exclusively. However, as Table 15–9 indicates, the studies appear to span the age groups rather well. This situation is impressive, especially when compared with the large number of studies in the behavioral sciences, for instance, which use college-age subjects. Studies of the elderly increased sixfold in the last half of the decade compared with the first half.

Table 15-8   Number of Studies by Status of Subjects*

Status	1970–74 (N = 71)		1975–79 (N = 74)		1970–79 (N = 145)	
	N	%	N	%	N	%
Inpatients	55	78	44	59	99	68
Outpatients	8	11	20	27	28	19
Healthy	9	13	11	15	20	14
Nurses and other health professionals	8	11	6	8	14	10

*Sixteen studies dealt with subjects in more than one status.

Table 15-9   Number of Studies by Ages of Subjects*

Age group	1970–74 (N = 71)		1975–79 (N = 74)		1970–79 (N = 145)	
	N	%	N	%	N	%
Neonate	3	4	3	4	6	4
Children	5	7	8	11	13	9
Adults (of varying ages)	40	56	27	37	67	46
Elderly (all subjects over 55)	2	3	13	18	15	10
Not specified or spans categories	21	30	23	31	44	30

*Percents do not equal 100 because of rounding error.

Sample Size

Table 15-10 summarizes the sample sizes employed in the 145 studies. A wide variety of sample sizes were employed. Over half of the studies used 50 subjects or fewer. There was a slight tendency for the sample sizes to increase as the decade progressed. More than one-fourth of the studies in the second half of the decade had over 100 subjects each.

Research Design

Table 15-11 shows the frequency of the studies with different research designs. Experimental studies were those that manipulated one or more variables. Correlational studies showed relationships between variables but did not manipulate

Table 15-10   Number of Studies of Various Sample Sizes*

Number of subjects	1970–74 (N = 71)		1975–79 (N = 74)		1970–79 (N = 145)	
	N	%	N	%	N	%
10 or fewer	9	13	7	9	16	11
11 to 30	17	24	22	30	39	27
31 to 50	16	22	13	18	29	20
51 to 70	6	8	6	8	12	8
71 to 100	6	8	6	8	12	8
Over 100	15	21	19	26	34	23
Not reported	2	3	1	1	3	2

*Percents do not equal 100 because of rounding error.

Table 15-11   Number of Studies by Research Design*

Research design	Years					
	1970–74 (N = 71)		1975–79 (N = 74)		1970–79 (N = 145)	
	N	%	N	%	N	%
Experimental	33	46	46	62	79	54
Correlational	16	22	13	18	29	20
Descriptive	12	17	5	7	17	12
Reliability	10	14	10	14	20	14

*Percents do not equal 100 because of rounding error.

them. Descriptive studies presented frequency counts and percentages without showing relationships between variables studied. Reliability testing had to do with studies that were solely concerned with testing the reliability of measurement instruments. If a study was both experimental and correlational, it was categorized as experimental.

Over half of the studies used experimental designs. This probably reflects the practice orientation of the studies reviewed. Experimental studies increased from 46 percent in the first half of the decade to 62 percent in the second half, while descriptive studies were reduced from 17 percent to 7 percent in the same period. Although the number of studies of reliability of instruments

remained constant between the two 5-year periods. studies in the first half of the decade concerned reliability of monitoring techniques, while studies in the second half of the decade were more likely to concern reliability of paper-and-pencil instruments.

Variables Manipulated

As reported above, 79 of the studies were experimental. Table 15-12 illustrates the classification of the studies according to the nature of their independent variables. The "other" category concerned manipulation of nonphysical aspects of care such as techniques for reducing anxiety or for giving emotional support. This category accounted for the greatest proportion of studies. Physical care techniques and teaching techniques were also frequently manipulated variables. Compared with the first half of the decade, the last half showed an increase in the proportion of studies that manipulated physical care techniques and a decrease in studies that did not manipulate variables.

Instruments

The instruments used to measure the phenomena studied are critically important to the validity of the findings. As Table 15-13 shows, the 145 studies

Table 15-12   Number of Studies by Types of Variables Manipulated*

Independent variable	Years					
	1970–74 (N = 71)		1975–79 (N = 74)		1970–79 (N = 145)	
	N	%	N	%	N	%
Physical care technique	8	11	14	19	22	15
Psychiatric treatment	3	4	7	9	10	7
Assessment technique	3	4	2	3	5	3
Monitoring	0	0	2	3	2	1
Teaching	11	16	9	12	20	14
Other	10	14	14	19	24	17
None	38	54	28	38	66	46

*Four studies had more than one type of independent variable.

Table 15-13   Number of Studies Using Various Types of Instruments*

Instruments	Years					
	1970–74 (N = 71)		1975–79 (N = 74)		1970–79 (N = 145)	
	N	%	N	%	N	%
Physical measures	27	38	24	32	51	35
Interviews	14	20	17	23	31	21
Self-report of attitudes, feelings, behaviors	19	27	30	40	50	34
Knowledge measures	3	4	11	15	14	10
Observer rating scale	25	35	31	42	57	39
None	6	8	3	4	9	6

*Fifty-eight studies used more than one type.

were classified according to the types of instruments used in the studies. Fifty-eight of the studies used more than one type of instrument. Approximately one-third of the studies used some type of physical measure. The measures were approximately equally divided between those that nurses usually perform, e.g., central venous pressure readings, and those not usually performed by nurses, e.g., galvanic skin response. Approximately one-fifth of the studies used the interview as a data-collection technique. The interviews were largely devised by the experimenters and were not typically subject to reliability testing procedures. The remaining instruments are paper-and-pencil measures. These include self-reports of attitudes, feelings, or behaviors, knowledge tests given to patients or clients to assess knowledge of particular areas, and observer rating scales. Approximately one-third of the sample of studies used measures of attitudes, opinions, or behaviors, and nearly 40 percent used observer rating scales. Only 10 percent of the studies used knowledge measure. Compared with the first half of the decade, the second half of the decade showed an increase in the use of paper-and-pencil measures and a decrease in the use of physical measures. A separate analysis indicated an increase in the use of previously developed scales during the last half of the decade compared with the first half. This trend toward the use of previously developed instruments reflects a growing

concern among nurse-researchers about the validity and the reliability of measures.

SUMMARY AND CONCLUSIONS

This chapter presented the results of a content analysis of 145 studies in nursing practice published over a 10-year period in *Nursing Research*. Most of the studies were carried out by nurses with masters' degrees. The group of studies represented research on a wide variety of diagnoses, needs, and conditions. A little over half of the studies used experimental designs. The studies focused mainly on inpatients and on psychological rather than physical aspects of care.

A comparison of the studies published during the first half of the decade with those published in the second half disclosed some interesting trends. Although Gortner (1980) described the 1970s as a time of expansion in practice research, this expansion was *not* reflected in an increase in the number of studies of nursing practice published in the second half of the decade. This finding may represent an editorial policy, an artifact related to the silver anniversary of the publication, or a problem of publication lag.

A similar analysis of the first two volumes of *Research in Nursing and Health* revealed that of the 33 studies published, 12, or 36 percent, were studies of nursing practice. This proportion is slightly greater than the proportion of studies of nursing practice published by *Nursing Research*. However, *Research in Nursing and Health* published only 12 studies of nursing practice in the first 2 years of publication (1978, 1979), while *Nursing Research* published 36 such studies in the same period. There was a definite increase in the number of studies (22) published in *Nursing Research* in 1979. However, it is yet to be determined if this increase will continue into the 80s.

Although the quantity of the studies did not appear to change over the decade, there appeared to be a definite change in the quality of the studies. The studies in the latter half of the decade appeared to be more sophisticated. There was increased evidence of collaboration among nurses and collaboration with nonnurses. There appeared to be greater concern with reliability and validity of the instruments, and experimental designs were used in a greater proportion of the studies.

It should be noted that an increase in the use of the experimental design may not necessarily produce better research. Downs (1980), editor of *Nursing Research*, reported an abundance of experimental studies that produce "astoundingly low" correlations among variables. Downs attributes this trend to the neglect of descriptive research on which experimental studies should be based.

In addition to the increased sophistication of the research methods over the decade, the content of the research also changed. There was a greater emphasis on chronic illness, on the elderly, on outpatients, on psychological needs, and on needs assessment in the second half of the decade compared with the first half. This change of research emphasis may be attributable in part to the recognition by nurses of the failure of the traditional medical model to deal adequately with nonacute, nonhospitalized clients experiencing long-term health problems.

The changing emphases and the increased sophistication of the studies in the second half of the decade may also be related to the increase in the number of funded studies. Because the research

plans of most funded studies are reviewed by experts before they are carried out and because funding provides resources for gathering more comprehensive data on a greater number of subjects, increases in the number of funded studies should increase the quality of the research produced. In addition, funding sources may have priorities related to specific areas, such as chronic illness or the elderly, and may influence researchers to design studies in these areas. Thus, the funding source may have direct effect on the content area of the studies. It should be reiterated, however, that 56 percent of the studies reviewed here reported no funding sources, and that at least some of the change in emphasis in the latter part of the decade cannot be attributed to funding sources.

Another change in the content of the studies in the latter half of the decade was made apparent because of the type of classification system used. As mentioned above, the system was based on one devised by Simmons and Henderson (1964). It was thought to be more useful than an empirically devised classification system because it could point out the areas of nursing practice which were neglected as well as those which were emphasized. However, when the content of the studies of the first half of the decade were compared with the content of the second half, an increase was seen in each of the classification groups of the "other" category.

This finding may be partially due to an outdated classification scheme. However, efforts to generate new categories in which to classify the studies were unsuccessful because the content areas covered varied widely, sometimes within the same study. The Simmons and Henderson classification scheme assumed that nursing research would concern itself with areas of broad interest rather than with specific concerns. Gortner (1980:205) has noted, however, that an onlooker might characterize most nursing investigations as "discrete, non-aggregated studies of empirical phenomena" for which an underlying explanatory theory is either unknown or undefined. The results presented here indicate that the content of the studies of nursing practice became more nonaggregated as the decade progressed. This finding may reflect a temporary situation signifying growth. However, if a research area is to be useful to the practice of nursing it must be studied systematically in order to increase its construct validity and its replicability. In their development of research-based protocols, Haller et al. (1979) used replication and construct validation as major criteria for utilization of research in nursing practice. The present analysis indicates that, although a few content areas are intensively studied, an increasing amount of research effort is being focused on disparate content areas. It remains to be seen whether this represents brief and unproductive excursions which dissipate research energy or whether some of these disparate areas represent creative and nontraditional approaches to the practice of nursing which will be studied and explored by ever-increasing numbers of investigators and which will engender significant advances in the science and in the practice of nursing.

EDITOR'S QUESTIONS FOR DISCUSSION

What other explanations might be offered for the lack of increase in the number of studies published the last 5 years of the decade? What might account for the increased evidence of collaboration among nurses and with nonnurses? What are the advantages and disadvantages for research and the profession in such collaboration?

What are the implications of the increase in investigations by those who have a Ph.D. and decrease by those with other types of doctoral preparation? What is the significance of the apparent increased quality of studies, given that the majority of the investigators possess masters' degrees? How might you account for the increase in previously developed scales? What is the significance of the increase in experimental studies and decrease in descriptive research? What differences in educational and experiential backgrounds might be related to the type of research design chosen by the investigator?

What is the significance for nursing practice and the profession of funding sources establishing priorities related to specific areas of research? What might be expected regarding the future funding of research?

Discuss the validity and reliability of the type of classification system utilized in this study. What suggestions can you offer regarding a classification system for research?

What is the significance for the future development of nursing research of the increasing amount of research focused on disparate content areas? What areas and content would you suggest for study in nursing research? To what extent do you agree with O'Connell's definition of nursing practice research? What other explanations might be offered for the change in the content of research?

REFERENCES

Dickoff, J., P. James, and J. Semradek
　1975　"8-4 Research Part 1: A stance for nursing research—tenacity or inquiry." Nursing Research 24:84–88.
Downs, F.
　1980　"The relationship of findings of clinical research and development of criteria: A researcher's perspective." Nursing Research 29:94–97.
Gortner, S.
　1980　"Nursing research: Out of the past and into the future." Nursing Research 29: 204–207.
Haller, K. B., M. A. Reynolds, and J. A. Horsley

1979   "Developing research-based innovation protocols: Process, criteria, and issues." Research in Nursing and Health 2:45-51.

Ketefian, S.
1975   "Application of selected nursing research findings into nursing practice: A pilot study." Nursing Research 24:89-92.

Muhlenkamp, A. F., L. D. Gress, and M. A. Flood
1975   "Perception of life change events by the elderly." Nursing Research 24:109-113.

Nichols, G. A. and D. H. Kucha
1972   "Taking adult temperatures: Oral measurements." American Journal of Nursing 72:1090-1093.

Nichols, G. A., M. M. Ruskin, B. A. K. Glor, and W. H. Kelly
1966   "Oral, axillary, and rectal temperature determinations and relationships." Nursing Research 15:307-310.

Nichols, G. A. and P. J. Verhonick
1967   "Time and temperature." American Journal of Nursing 67:2304-2306.

Simmons, L. W. and V. Henderson
1964   Nursing Research. New York: Appleton-Century-Crofts.

RESEARCH STUDIES OF NURSING PRACTICE IN NURSING RESEARCH BY YEAR

Nursing Research, Volume 19, 1970

Bluemle, Madeline L.:
"Tracheal bacterial counts of patients following suctioning," 116-121.

Cohen, Roberta:
"The effect of specific emotional support on anxiety levels prior to electroconvulsive therapy," 163-165.

Forster, Brenda, Diane C. Adler, and Mardell Davis: "Duration of effects of drinking iced water on oral temperature," 169-170.

Glor, B. A. K. and Zane Estes:
"Moist soaks: A survey of clinical practices," 463-465.

Glor, B. A. K., E. F. Sullivan, and Zane E. Estes:
"Reproducibility of blood pressure measurements: A replication," 170-172.

Graffam, Shirley R.:
"Nurse response to the patient in distress—development of an instrument," 331-336.

Guberski, Thomasine and Mary Ellen Campbell:
"The effects on leg volume of two methods of wrapping elastic bandages," 260-265.

Hamdi, Mary Evans and Carol M. Hutelmeyer:
"A study of the effectiveness of an assessment tool in the identification of nursing care problems," 354-359.

Larson, Elaine:
"Bacterial colonization of tracheal tubes of patients in a surgical intensive care unit," 122-128.

Lowe, Marie L.:
"Effectiveness of teaching as measured by compliance with medical recommendations," 59-63.

Putt, Arlene M.:
"One experiment in nursing adults with peptic ulcers," 484-494.

Triplett, June L.:
"Characteristics and perceptions of low-income women and use of preventive health services," 140-146.

Waligora, Sr. Barbara Marie:
"The effect of nasal and oral breathing upon nasopharyngeal oxygen concentration," 75-78.

Whitner, Willamay and Margaret Thompson:
"The influence of bathing on the newborn infant's body," 30-36.

Nursing Research, Volume 20, 1971

Aiken, Linda H. and Theodore F. Henrichs:
"Systematic relaxation as a nursing intervention technique with open heart surgery patients," 212-217.

Ankenbrandt, Marguerite D. and Linda K. Tanner:
"Role-delineated and informal nurse-teaching and food selection behavior of geriatric patients," 61-64.

Balthazar, Earl E., George E. English, and Ronald M. Sindberg: "Behavior changes in mentally retarded children following the initiation of an experimental nursing program," 69-74.

Bliss, Ann, Lila Decker, and Wayne O. Southwick:
"The emergency room nurse orders X-rays of distal limbs in orthopedic trauma," 440-443.

Chastko, Helen E., Ira D. Glick, Edward Gould, and William A. Hargreaves: "Patients' post-hospital evaluations of psychiatric nursing treatment," 333-338.

Cleland, Virginia, Frank Cox, Helen Berggren, and M. R. MacInnis: "Prevention of bacteriuria in female patients with indwelling catheters," 309–318.

Cross, Joanne E. and Carol R. Parsons: "Nurse-teaching and goal-directed nurse-teaching to motivate change in food selection behavior of hospitalized patients." 454–458.

Foley, Mary F.: "Variations in blood pressure in the lateral recumbent position," 64–69.

Lagina, Suzanne M.: "A computer program to diagnose anxiety levels," 484–492.

Lindeman, Carol and Betty VanAernam: "Nursing intervention with the presurgical patient—the effects of structured and unstructured preoperative teaching," 319–332.

McCaffery, Margo: "Children's responses to rectal temperatures: An exploratory study," 32–45.

McFadden, Eileen H. and Elizabeth C. Giblin: "Sleep deprivation in patients having open-heart surgery," 249–254.

Mikulic, Mary Ann: "Reinforcement of independent and dependent patient behaviors by nursing personnel: An exploratory study," 162–165.

Nield, Margaret Ann: "The effect of health teaching on the anxiety level of patients with chronic obstructive lung disease," 537–542.

Palmer, Edwina M. and Elizabeth W. Griffith: "Effect of activity during bedmaking on heart rate and blood pressure," 17–24.

Van Meter, Margie and Patricia W. Mitchell: "Reproducibility of blood pressures recorded on patients' records by nursing personnel," 348–352.

Nursing Research, Volume 21, 1972

Brink, Pamela J.: "Behavioral characteristics of heroin addicts on a short-term detoxification program," 38–45.

Diers, Donna, Ruth Schmidt, M. A. B. McBride, and Bette Davis: "The effect of nursing interaction on patients in pain," 419–428.

Elms, Roslyn: "Recovery room behavior and postoperative convalescence," 390–397.

Harper, Mary, Betty Marcom, and Victor Wall: "Abortion—do attitudes of nursing personnel affect the patients perceptions of care?" 327–331.

LaFargue, Jane P.: "Role of prejudice in rejection of health care," 53–58.

Lindeman, Carol: "Nursing intervention with the presurgical patient," 196–209.

Marshall, Jon C. and Sally S. Feeney: "Structured versus intuitive intake interview," 269–272.

Nichols, Glennadee A.: "Time analyses of afebrile and febrile temperature reading," 463–464.

——, Rosemarie Mahoney, and Delores Kucha: "Rectal thermometer placement times for febrile adults," 76–77.

——, Ruth Kulvi, Nancy Christ, and Hazel Life: "Measuring oral and rectal temperatures of febrile children," 261–264.

Ross, S. A.: "Infusion phlebitis," 313–318.

Walker, Betty Boyd: "The postsurgery heart patient: Amount of uninterrupted time for sleep and rest during the first, second, and third postoperative days in a teaching hospital," 164–169.

White, Marguerite: "Importance of selected nursing activities," 4–14.

Williams, Anne: "A study of factors contributing to skin breakdown," 238–243.

Woods, Nancy F.: "Patterns of sleep in postcardiotomy patients," 347–352.

Nursing Research, Volume 22, 1973

Anderson, Catherine J.: "Use of videotape feedback as a psychotherapeutic nursing approach with long-term psychiatric patients: A pilot study," 507–515.

Chamorro, Ilta L., Mary L. Davis, Dora Green, and
Marlene Kramer: "Development of an instru-
ment to measure premature infant behavior
and caretaker activities: Time sampling meth-
odology," 300–309.
Cornell, Sudie A., Laura Campion, Susan Bacero,
Judith Frazier, Mary Kjellstrom, and Susan
Purdy: "Comparison of three bowel manage-
ment programs," 321–328.
Gosnell, Davina J.:
"An assessment tool to identify pressure
sores," 55–59.
Hedberg, Allan G. and Audrey Schlong:
"Eliminating fainting by school children during
mass inoculation," 352–353.
Lindeman, Carol and Steven L. Stetzer:
"Effect of preoperative visits by operating
room nurses," 4-16.
Mansfield, Elaine:
"Empathy: Concept and identified psychiatric
nursing behavior," 525–530.
McPhetridge, L. Mae:
"Relationship of patients' responses to nursing
history questions and selected factors: A pre-
liminary study," 310–320.
Midgley, Jan W. and Sr. Ruth Ann Osterhage:
"Effect of nursing instruction and length of
hospitalization on postoperative complications
in cholecystectomy patients," 69–72.
Mulcahy, Rae Ann and Nancy K. Janz:
"Effectiveness of raising pain perception
threshold in males and females using psycho-
prophylactic childbirth technique during in-
duced pain," 423–427.
Pienschke, Sr. Darlene:
"Guardedness or openness on the cancer unit,"
484–490.
Schmitt, Florence E. and Powhatan Wooldridge:
"Psychological preparation of surgical patients," 108–116.

Nursing Research, Volume 23, 1974

Budd, Suzanne P. and Willa Brown:
"Effect of a reorientation technique on post-
cardiotomy delirium," 341–348.
Burgess, Ann W. and Lynda L. Holmstrom:
"Crisis and counseling requests of rape victims,"
(3):196–202.

Castle, Mary, and Suydam Osterhout:
"Urinary tract catheterization and associated
infection," 170–174.
Cornell, Sudie A.:
"Development of an instrument for measuring
the quality of nursing care," 108–117.
Drake, Joyce Johnson:
"Locating the external reference point for cen-
tral venous pressure determination," 475–482.
Eoff, Mary Jo Fike, Robert S. Meier, and Carol L.
Miller: "Temperature measurement in infants,"
457–460.
Foster, Sue B.:
"An adrenal measure for evaluating nursing
effectiveness," 118–124.
Jensen, Judith L. and W. Leona McGrew:
"Leadership techniques in group therapy with
chronic schizophrenic patients," 416–420.
Johnson, Jean E. and Virginia Hill Rice:
"Sensory and distress components of pain,"
203–209.
McCorkle, Ruth:
"Effects of touch on seriously ill patients,"
125–132.
Murray, Jacquelyn E.:
"Patient participation in determining psychia-
tric treatment," 325–333.
Nunnally, Diane M. and Martha B. Aguiar:
"Patients' evaluation of their prenatal and
delivery care," 469–474.
Pender, Nola J.:
"Patient identification of health information
received during hospitalization," 262–267.
Rodgers, Beckett, Julian Ferhold, and Carol
Cooper: "A screening tool to detect psycho-
social adjustment of children with cystic
fibrosis," 420–426.

Nursing Research, Volume 24, 1975

Aspinall, Mary Jo:
"Development of a patient-completed admis-
sion questionnaire and its comparison with the
nursing interview," 377–381.
Beard, Margaret T. and Patsy Y. Scott:
"The efficacy of group therapy by nurses for
hospitalized patients," 120–124.
Brown, Marie Scott and Joan T. Hurlock:
"Preparation of the breast for breast feeding,"
448–451.

DeWalt, Evelyn M.:
"Effect of timed hygienic measures on oral mucosa in a group of elderly subjects," 104–108.

Durand, Barbara:
"Failure to thrive in a child with Down's syndrome," 272–286.

Dyer, Elaine D., Mary A. Monson and Maxine J. Cope: "Increasing the quality of patient care through performance counseling and written goal setting," 138–144.

Felton, Geraldene:
"Increasing the quality of nursing care by introducing the concept of primary nursing: A model project," 27–32.

Hampe, Sandra O.:
"Needs of the grieving spouse in a hospital setting," 113–120.

Hefferin, Elizabeth A. and Ruth E. Hunter:
"Nursing assessment and nursing care plan statements," 360–366.

Johnson, Jean E., Karin T. Kirchhoff, and M. Patricia Endress: "Altering children's distress behavior during orthopedic cast removal," 404–410.

Keener, Mary Lou:
"The public health nurse in mental health follow-up care," 198–201.

Kramer, Marlene, Ilta Chamorro, Dora Green, and Frances Knudtson: "Extra tactile stimulation of the premature infant," 324–334.

Leonard, Calista V.:
"Patient attitudes toward nursing interventions," 335–339.

Moore, Diane S. and Karen Cook-Hubbard:
"Comparison of methods for evaluating patient response to nursing care," 202–204.

Risser, Nancy L:
"Development of an instrument to measure patient satisfaction with nurses and nursing care in primary care settings," 45–52.

Volicer, Beverly J. and Mary Wynne Bohannon:
"A hospital stress rating scale," 352–359.

Wolfer, John A. and Madelon Visintainer:
"Pediatric surgical patients' and parents' stress responses and adjustment," 244–255.

Nursing Research, Volume 25, 1976

Amborn, S. A.:
"Clinical signs associated with the amount of tracheobronchial secretions," 121–126.

Baltes, M. M. and M. B. Zerbe:
"Reestablishing self-feeding in a nursing home resident," 24–26.

Brockway, B. F., O. B. Plummer, and B. M. Lowe:
"Effect of nursing reassurance on patient vocal stress levels," 440–446.

Champion, V. L.:
"Clean technique for intermittent self-catheterization," 13–18.

Downs, F. S. and J. J. Fitzpatrick:
"Preliminary investigation of the reliability and validity of a tool for assessment of body position and motor activity," 404–408.

Freihofer, P. and G. Felton:
"Nursing behaviors in bereavement: An exploratory study," 332–337.

Geertsen, H. R., M. Fors, and C. H. Castle:
"The subjective aspects of coronary care," 211–215.

Van Ort, S. R. and R. M. Gerber:
"Topical application of insulin in the treatment of decubitus ulcers: A pilot study," 9–12.

Haussmann, R. K. and S. T. Hegyvary:
"Field testing the nursing quality monitoring methodology: Phase II," 324–331.

Jeanes, K. R. and J. R. Grant:
"Children's retention of dental hygiene instruction," 452–454.

Komaroff, A. L., K. Sawayer, M. Flatley, and C. M. Browne: "Nurse practitioner management of common respiratory and genitourinary infections, using protocols," 84–89.

Mills, M. E., S. A. Thomas, J. J. Lynch and A. H. Katcher: "Effect of pulse palpation on cardiac arrhythmia in coronary care patients," 378–382.

Moore, D. S. and C. S. Bauer:
"Effect of Prepodyne® as a perineal cleansing agent for clean catch specimens," 259–261.

Rottkamp, B. C.:
"A behavior modification approach to nursing therapeutics in body positioning of spinal cord-injured patients," 181–186.

Nursing Research, Volume 26, 1977

Brown, M. M., J. K. Boosinger, M. Henderson, S. S. Rife, J. K. Rustia, O. Taylor, and W. W. Young: "Drug-drug interactions among residents in homes for the elderly," 47–52.

Dittmar, S. S. and T. Dulski:
"Early evening administration of sleep medication to the hospitalized aged: Consideration in rehabilitation," 299–303.

Fortin, F. and S. Kerouac:
"Validation of questionnaires on physical function," 128–135.

Keck, V. E. and L. S. Walther:
"Nurse encounters with dying and nondying patients," 465–469.

Meyer, R. M. S. and P. T. Morris:
"Alcoholic cardiomyopathy: A nursing approach," 422–427.

Stetler, C. B.:
"Relationship of perceived empathy to nurses' communication," 432–438.

Vincent, P. and J. R. Price:
"Evaluation of a VNA mental health project," 361–367.

Meleis, A. I. and L. A. Swendsen:
"Role supplementation: An empirical test of a nursing intervention," 11–18.

Mitchell, P. H. and N. K. Mauss:
"Relationship of patient-nurse activity to intracranial pressure variations: A pilot study," 4–10.

Owens, J. F., C. S. McCann, and C. M. Hutelmyer:
"Cardiac rehabilitation: Patient education program," 148–150.

Salter, A.:
"Birth without violence: A medical controversy," 84–88.

Tamez, W. G., M. J. Moore, and P. L. Brown:
"Relaxation training as a nursing intervention versus pro re nata medication," 160–165.

Williamson, Y. M.:
"Methodologic dilemmas in tapping the concept of patient needs," 172–177.

Nursing Research, Volume 27, 1978

Daubenmire, M. J., S. S. Searles, and C. A. Ashton:
"A methodologic framework to study nurse-patient communication," 303–310.

Dracup, K. A. and C. S. Breu:
"Using nursing research findings to meet the needs of grieving spouses," 212–216.

Flaherty, G. G. and J. J. Fitzpatrick:
"Relaxation technique to increase comfort level of postoperative patients: A preliminary study," 352–355.

Goodman, H. C. and E. C. Perring:
"Evening telephone call management by nurse practitioners," 233–237.

Huber, C. J., S. R. Stangler, and D. K. Routh:
"The BOEL test as a screening device for otitis media in infants," 178–180.

Levine, J. I., S. T. Orr, D. W. Sheatsley, J. A. Lohr, and B. M. Brodie: "The nurse-practioner: Role, physician utilization, patient acceptance," 245–254.

Lum, J. L., M. Chase, S. M. Cole, A. Johnson, J. A. Johnson, and M. R. Link: "Nursing care of oncology patients receiving chemotherapy," 340–346.

Majesky, S. J., M. H. Brester, and K. T. Nishio:
"Development of a research tool: Patient indicators of nursing care," 365–371.

Nursing Research, Volume 28, 1979

Applegate, J., A. D. Haverkamp, M. Orleans, and C. Taylor: "Electronic fetal monitoring: Implications for obstetrical nursing," 369–371.

Atkinson, L. D.:
"Prenatal nipple conditioning for breast-feeding," 267–271.

Brower, H. T. and L. A. Tanner:
"A study of older adults attending a program on human sexuality: A pilot study," 36–39.

Carey, R. G. and E. J. Posavac:
"Holistic care in a cancer care center," 213–216.

Doerr, B. C. and J. W. Jones:
"Effect of family preparation on the state anxiety level of the CCU patient," 315–316.

Fitzpatrick, J. J. and M. J. Donovan:
"A follow-up study of the reliability and validity of the motor activity rating scale," 179–181.

Friedeman, J. S.:
"Development of a sexual knowledge inventory for elderly persons," 372–374.

Gerber, R. M. and S. R. Van Ort:
"Topical application of insulin in decubitus ulcers," 16–19.

Hammon, E. A. and P. K. Begley:
"Screening for glaucoma: A comparison of opthalmoscopy and tonometry," 371–372.

Hester, N. K.:
"The preoperational child's reaction to immunization," 250–255.
Hogstel, M. O.:
"Use of reality orientation with aging confused patients," 161–165.
Ipema, D. K.:
"Rape: The process of recovery," 272–275.
Kinney, A. B. and M. Blount:
"Effect of cranberry juice on urinary pH," 287–290.
Krueger, J. C., J. Hassell, D. B. Goggins, T. Ishimatsu, M. R. Pablico, and E. J. Tuttle: "Relationship between nurse counseling and sexual adjustment after hysterectomy," 145–150.
Kruszewski, A. Z., S. H. Lang, and J. E. Johnson: "Effect of positioning on discomfort from intramuscular injections in the dorsogluteal site," 103–105.
Lamb, K.:
"Effect of positioning of postoperative fractured-hip patients as related to comfort," 291–294.

Linde, B. J. and N. M. Janz:
"Effect of a teaching program on knowledge and compliance of cardiac patients," 282–286.
Minckley, B. B., D. Burrows, K. Ehrat, L. Harper, S. A. Jenkin, W. F. Minckley, B. Page, D. J. Schramm, and C. Wood: "Myocardial infarct stress-of-transfer inventory: Development of a research tool," 5–10.
Stricklin, M. L. V.:
"Mental health patient assessment record: Interobserver reliability," 11–15.
Sullivan, J. A. and F. Armignacco:
"Effectiveness of a comprehensive health program for the well-elderly," 70–75.
Timm, M. M.:
"Prenatal education evaluation," 338–342.
Williams, M. A., J. R. Holloway, M. C. Winn, M. O. Wolanin, M. L. Lawler, C. R. Westwick, and M. H. Chin:
"Nursing activities and acute confusional states," 25–35.

Chapter 16

The Research Mentor: A Missing Element in Nursing?

Harriet H. Werley, R.N., Ph.D., F.A.A.N.
Associate Dean (Research)
School of Nursing
University of Missouri
Columbia, Missouri
     and
B. Joan Newcomb, R.N., M.S.
Doctoral Candidate
University of Chicago
Chicago, Illinois

Mentorship for the process of conducting research is a relevant means to advance the profession. Harriet H. Werley and B. Joan Newcomb offer a timely chapter on mentor relationships in nursing as an avenue to accelerate the development of both nursing research and nurse researchers. They differentiate between the concepts of mentor, master-apprentice, and role-model relationships. The major difference is in the commitment of the mentor in working with and for the protégé. Master-apprentice relationships afford the student an opportunity for a "hands-on" learning of nursing skills and techniques with the teacher. A role model can be someone merely to emulate and admire. Werley and Newcomb indicate that the seeds of mentorship can be nurtured in the fertile undergraduate student years as well as explain the possible evolution from the master-apprentice into a mentor-protégé relationship. Numerous interpersonal and organizational factors are cited that deter the operationalization of mentor-protégé relationships. The need and tendency for newly doctorally prepared nurses to propel into administrative positions, without first establishing themselves as researchers-scholars is one of the factors discussed. Werley and Newcomb indicate this fact has had a deleterious effect on the support for nursing research. They report preliminary A.N.A. data, that predict the components of high research productivity, and alarming findings. It is significant to the deterrents of mentor-protégé relationships that more than 60 percent of the newly graduated nurse doctorates had no contact with other researchers in their first positions after completion of the doctoral program.

The meaningfulness of the preliminary findings offered by Werley and Newcomb is provocative and challenging. In addition they present their data from 20 of the 21 doctoral programs which indicate opportunities do exist for faculty-student collaboration in research, but there are few collaborative publications. Strong advocates for the development of research, Werley and Newcomb offer an insightful analysis of the problems and suggest positive means for resolution.

Literature dealing with socialization in the scientific, academic, and business worlds (Levinson et al., 1978; Sheehy, 1976; White, 1970; Zuckerman and Cole, 1975) suggests that in addition to the intellectual and technical proficiency acquired during the training period, students are also initiated into an informal network of colleagues and advisers (the so-called "old boy" network) who "shortcut corporate formalities and help each other up the success ladder" (Henry, 1980:11). However, a corollary to the old boy network is not as readily apparent for women who occupy positions in academic and corporate structures. Why this is so is the subject of both speculation (Kelly, 1978; Krueger, 1980; Levinson et al., 1978; Sheehy, 1976) and an increasing amount of investigation (Barhyte, 1977; Kundsin, 1974; National Research Council, 1979; Vance, 1979), because this type of system is viewed as highly influential in ensuring successful competition for increasingly responsible and prestigious positions.

We are interested in the *mentor* concept and its potential for accelerating the development of both nursing research and nurse-researchers. Therefore we have undertaken an analysis of current information on the occurrence of mentor relationships in nursing, particularly among nurses engaged in research. In this paper we will: (1) explore the means by which the seeds for mentorship are sown in the course of education for research in nursing and certain other fields; (2) speculate on why nursing has been slow in making operational mentor relationships in the research area; (3) discuss potential benefits for the profession and society if conscious efforts were made to structure mentor-protégé mechanisms and (4) share data that describe the extent to which the mentor concept may be operative in the 21 nursing doctoral programs throughout the country.

THE SEEDS OF MENTORSHIP

Socialization

Since we view mentorship as a type of role phenomenon, it seems appropriate to begin discussion of it with a review of some tenets of socialization, a concept under which mentorship can be subsumed. Inkles stated that "socialization refers to the process whereby individuals acquire the personal system properties—the knowledge, skills, attitudes, values, needs and motivations, cognitive, affective and conative patterns—which shape their adaptation to the physical and sociocultural setting in which they live" (1969:615-616). According to Zigler and Child, "socialization is a broad term for the whole process by which an individual develops, through transactions with other people, his specific pattern of socially relevant behavior and experience" (1973:36). Thus, socialization involves transmitting the norms and values appropriate to actualizing a role (Conway and Glass, 1978:425).

The process of this transmission is influenced by the organizational setting in which it occurs and the individuals who perform in the roles dictated by organizational structure. Therefore, the socialization of nursing students is influenced by the type of educational programs in which they are enrolled, the underlying philosophies of the associated health care institutions in which they practice, and the personal values and philosophies of their faculty members. Neophyte nurses are socialized to their professional role (health care practitioner) by clinical instructors and staff members of the hospitals and agencies in which they obtain field experience. Students enrolled in university or college-based programs are exposed to the norms and values of academia as well. At the graduate level, the emphasis on development of clinical specialists, master teachers, administrators, and researchers requires further role differentiation and the concomitant adoption of attitudes, values, and behaviors associated with those roles.

This characteristic of differentiation of roles was described by White, who emphasized the informal and implicit nature of socialization that begins during professional life. Once launched on a career, a neophyte must learn "the roles, the informal values and attitudes, and the expectations which are an important part of real professional life" (1970:413). More importantly, in the process the individual gains a firmer image of self as competent and adequate through appraisals of one's work by others. However, "[m]any people are unaware of this period of role learning in scholarly, scientific, or academic professions, and fail to realize how important such a stage is, and how lengthy it has become because of the increased complexity of professional life. . . . There are elaborate social systems in all parts of academic and business life, and purely technical training is rarely enough. The aspiring young scientist must be knowledgeable about many aspects of institutions, journals, professional meetings, methods of obtaining source materials, and funding grant applications. Knowing how to command these technical and institutional facilities requires numerous skills, many unanticipated by the young student. But once gained, such skills often seem very simple in retrospect and even thoughtful professionals forget that they were once not second nature. This is the kind of learning we speak of as 'caught,' not 'taught,' and it is a valued by-product of acceptance and challenging association with other professionals" (White, 1970:414).

Thus, socialization as described by White suggests a system whereby "juniors" learn the ropes by observing and working with "seniors" within a given institutional setting. Inherent in the junior-senior dichotomy is the concept of mentorship, the situation in which a promising student or junior colleague is coached or groomed for advancement to a higher-level position by an established member of the system. As described by Vance, the mentor system is a type of "patron-protégé system, whereby those more experienced and further along in their careers serve as role models, teachers, promoters, supporters, and door openers for the newer, less experienced people in the profession" (1979:40).

The Mentor Relationship

Perhaps the broadest and most comprehensive definition and description of the mentor relationship was offered by Levinson et al. (1978) who highlighted its significance in adult development. In addition to encompassing functions of teacher, adviser, or sponsor, the mentor must also "foster the young adult's development by believing in [the person], sharing the youthful Dream and giving it his [or her] blessing, helping to define the newly emerging self in its newly discovered world, and creating a space in which [the protégé] can work on a reasonably satisfactory life structure that contains the Dream. . . . The mentor represents a mixture of parent and peer . . . must be both and not purely either one" (Levinson et al., 1978:99). The mentor is usually older than the protégé by half a generation and in the usual course of events the relationship becomes more mutual. The mentor "represents skill, knowledge, virtue, accomplishment—the superior qualities a young [person] hopes someday to acquire" (Levinson et al., 1978:333). When the relationship terminates, the mentee may take the acquired qualities of the mentor more fully into self and the person's personality is enriched. The internalization of significant figures is a major source of development in adulthood.

One aspect of Levinson et al.'s description deserves attention. It is the *character* of the relationship rather than formal role prescriptions that distinguish the mentor from the role model, preceptor, or master as in a master-apprentice relationship. Kelly (1978) addressed this distinction in proposing mentor relationships as a means of purposefully preparing promising nurses for influential positions. And, in responding to Kelly's exhortation, Pilette underscored the subtle difference that characterizes the mentor relationship when she stated that the mentor "is a transitional figure that helps one grow in personal and professional power" (1978:473). The mentor, unlike the preceptor, master, or role model, takes a personal interest in the growth of the protégé and makes a personal investment in the individual's growth.

Thus, mentors provide students more than academic counseling and advice. In academe, the mentor is one who provides the student the opportunity to participate in his or her research or to work on a related project, to join in research planning and discussion of methodology and results, and to assist in writing and presenting research reports and articles (Chicadonz, 1980). According to Fawcett, mentors "guide their protégés through school and then through the scientific community by recommending them for choice positions in the professional world and by sponsoring their membership in honorary societies and on important committees. Students repeatedly turn to their mentor for advice about taking a new position, about current and projected work, and about the political climate of the scientific community" (1980:51).

In graduate education, where the student-faculty ratio is more favorable and where there is more faculty involvement in the individual work of the student, mentor relationships can develop more easily. Indeed, there is evidence (Mullins and Mullins, 1973) that the senior figures stand to gain also from working with energetic and imaginative students under their tutelage. Lack of such stimulation by bright students or mentees is believed to play a major role in the failure of some budding theories to reach full maturity and of timely ideas to be explored to their logical conclusions.

Effective use of students as collaborators in research was described recently in a *New York Times* report of a genetic breakthrough. In explaining the productivity of the scientist credited with the discovery, a colleague was quoted thus: "He is very clever in devising strategies for mapping the chromosomes of man. But those strategies wouldn't do him much good if he did not have a large clutch of graduate students who want to work with him and provide essential manpower so that he can get something done (Severo, 1980:8). A former graduate student analyzed this scientist's popularity with his students by stating, "I think he had a real genius for getting the best out of people who worked with him. . . . He would be critical of the work but in a very helpful and constructive way. No one ever felt antagonized by his suggestions" (Severo, 1980:8).

Levinson et al.'s analysis (1978) derived from their study of adult development in men; they emphasized the scarcity of female mentors. Sheehy (1976) echoed this observation when reporting that most of the women interviewed in her study of adult development did not know what she was talking about when she asked about their mentors. Yet some studies of women considered to be successful (Hennig and Jardim, 1977; Kundsin, 1974; Vance, 1979) indicated that, at least for this elite group (i.e., women viewed as successful), which is relatively small when compared with a man's world, mentorlike relationships did occur and were viewed as significant. This appears to be the case with the 70 female "nurse-influentials" studied by Vance (1979) in her doctoral research. These women "attested to the importance of mentorship and the support of others throughout their professional careers. Eighty-three percent reported having mentors, while 93 percent reported consciously being mentors to others. . . . They reported that their mentors helped them through: (1) career promotion, door opening, and creating opportunities; (2) professional career role modeling; (3) intellectual and scholarly stimulation; and (4) inspiration" (Vance, 1979:40-41).

The latter attribute of the mentor is reflected in Schorr's editorial in which she quoted from Aydelotte's obituary for Katharine Densford Dreves: "She is remembered as a mentor who saw in us potential of which we ourselves were often unaware" (Schorr, 1978:1873). The discussion of mentorship that accompanied this quotation inspired a response from an anonymous nurse who described poignantly the qualities of an instructor who had guided and inspired her throughout her undergraduate studies. These testimonials serve to suggest that perhaps Levinson et al. (1978) were referring to male-dominated professions in which there were relatively few women in leadership positions to serve as sponsors of protégés within the ranks.

In situations where there are few or no potential female mentors, it often develops that parents, spouses, and male supervisors or bosses provide the guidance and inspiration that ensure success in a woman's career. This was documented by Kundsin (1974) in summarizing biographical data on a small group of women invited to participate in a conference on women and success sponsored by the New York Academy of Science, and by Hennig and Jardim (1977) in their study of managerial women. Some career women also claim to have found or identified mentors who are in other settings but with whom they maintain contact, seeking counsel or advice and on occasion returning to work in the research mentor's well-established research laboratory.

Mentor versus Master or Role Model

Perhaps the closest thing to the mentor-protégé relationship is that of the master-apprentice, in which student and teacher engage in a learning experience that affords the student the opportunity for "hands-on" involvement. The master-apprentice term conjures up the vision of the students actively engaged in learning skills and techniques. For those in the health professions, this usually means mastering treatment procedures or acquiring technical competence in using equipment. Indeed, traditional nursing education relied heavily on this mode of interaction in which clinical instructors, head nurses, supervisors, and physicians oversaw student nurses' activities in the clinical area.

Similarly, in educational programs in other fields there are reports (Cowles and Csanyi, 1963; Maeroff, 1976; Worthen and Roaden, 1975) of efforts to enhance research learning by involving

students in departmental research being conducted by faculty. This type of involvement is viewed by many as critically important in developing researchers. As stated by Sibley, "No amount of formal instruction in methods and no amount of discussion of others' research can take the place of the first hand experience of undertaking to translate an unstructured situation into a problem or problems amenable to scientific investigation, and then proceeding to seek solutions" (1963:37). And according to Taylor, Garner, and Hung, "Research is learned by doing and taught by contagion" (1959:179). Indeed, testimony (Bailey, 1971) and occasionally data (Rickard and Siegel, 1976; Worthen and Roaden, 1975; Zuckerman, 1977) have been offered in praise of apprenticeship as a means of introducing novice scientists to the social system of science; it is viewed as a prerequisite for productive research and creativity.

Master-apprentice relationships occasionally evolve into those of mentor-protégé depending on certain intangibles inherent in the situation. According to Williams, "Achieving a mentor relationship with an older person is like falling in love—you can't force it to happen, and it only works if the chemistry is right. You can, however, make yourself receptive to such a relationship by displaying a teachable attitude and an eagerness to learn" (1977:179).

In addition, Kelly stated, "The apprentice has to show that she is someone worth investing in, someone who will show a measure of return by success in the field. On the other hand, a role model can be merely that—someone to emulate and admire, even with minimal contact. Some apprenticeships are carried out with almost total impersonality" (1978:339). The role model might be any admired teacher, practitioner, scientist, or other illustrious individual who inspires students to follow his or her example.

Thus, if a master-apprentice or student-teacher relationship is to evolve to that of mentor-mentee, there must be mutual exchange of ideas and aspirations relative to the protégé's career plans, or what is characterized by Levinson et al. (1978) as "the dream." What this implies is that the protégé will, in the main, imitate or draw from the role performance of the mentor. Further, there is an element of collegiality inherent in mentorship which must be fostered through opportunities to work together on projects in which both share ideas and work toward a common goal. There is in addition a personal investment and commitment to the success or achievement of the mentee on the part of the mentor.

In summary, then, as Table 16-1 indicates, the difference between mentor and master lies in the commitment of the mentor to providing

Table 16-1 Behavioral Characteristics of Two Styles of Professional Guidance

Master-apprentice	Mentor-protégé
Ensure competence and standard of practice; learn by doing; rehearsal and practice (e.g., treatment, video tape); peer review process	Participate in realization of the career goals—the Dream; mentor makes personal investment and commitment to mentee
"Research caught, not taught" (Taylor, Garner, and Hung, 1959)	Socialization to the informal organization, e.g., grant writing, professional meetings, locating resources (White, 1970)
Research learned by doing, rather than just by course work (Sibley, 1963)	Patron-protégé system; door opening, coaching, creating opportunities on a one-to-one basis (Vance, 1979)
Students become productive researchers by assisting with faculty research in all its phases (Worthen and Roaden, 1975)	Sponsor development through interpersonal support (Levinson, et al., 1978)
Preparation for conflict resolution is accomplished better through apprenticeship than course work (Bailey, 1971)	Experiential learning and collaboration with senior scientists with gradual transition to independence enhances productivity (Chicadonz, 1980)
Research productivity increases when students work with faculty researchers (Cowles and Csanyi, 1963)	Guidance versus criticism of young nurses by older nurses (Schorr, 1978; Kelly, 1978)
Danger of exploitation of students by teachers through appropriation of their work (Hagstrom, 1965)	Faculty work with students to increase their publications before graduation (Richard and Siegel, 1976)
Apprentice enjoys benefits of master's experience (Williams, 1977)	Emotional support of parents and spouses enhances chances for success (Kundsin, 1974)
	Intimate nature of mentorship makes opposite sex mentor-protégé relationships problematic (Sheehy, 1976)
	Helping juniors learn rules of the game has payoffs for both junior and senior individuals (Conway & Glass, 1978; Mullins and Mullins, 1973)
	Provide guidance, recommend for positions, sponsor in honor societies and on committees, and provide advice (Fawcett, 1980)
	Teach you how to deal with or solve problems; guide one along; counsel and teach younger person; take under wing (of older person); give valuable insights into . . .; help smooth career climb; mentor receives satisfaction of watching student grow; act as a sounding board for decision making; help pave the way (Williams, 1977)
	Give mentee sharpened sense of what matters in research; enhance protégé-visibility to scientists who distribute opportunities and rewards; learn by collaborating with sponsor; learn from sponsor's productivity; get students started publishing (Reskin, 1979)

guidance to the junior by working *with* and *for* the mentee, affording a variety of experiences, exposing the junior to developments in the field, making possible contacts with leaders in the field, pulling strings, and putting in a good word. The mentor-protégé relationship grows out of an earlier structured interaction between student and teacher, boss and employee, senior and junior faculty, investigator and research assistant or associate, and senior and junior collaborators or coauthors.

In nursing, the seeds of mentorship as they pertain to research are sown in classrooms, clinical sites, collaboration on research or writing, and other endeavors in which the opportunity exists for testing compatibility, mutual admiration, and desire to work together. Mentorship can begin in undergraduate educational experiences where talents and special interests are identified, be they in clinical areas such as pediatric or gerontological nursing, in the challenges of organization and administration of a unit or clinic, or in working to plan, conduct, and report research. The nursing student research assistantship, especially in the undergraduate years, can be a fertile time during which to stimulate interest in research (Werley, Murphy, and Newcomb, 1981) and to help students become excited about research.

DETERRENTS TO MENTOR-PROTEGE RELATIONSHIPS IN NURSING RESEARCH

Nursing has been slow in operationalizing research mentor-protégé relationships basically because nursing has been late in developing its research and its researchers. Although nursing struggled long and hard to get nursing education established within institutions of higher education, once this goal was attained there was no immediate effort to develop research dimensions within nursing and nursing education. Faculty energies were devoted to developing and revising curriculum and to supervising the clinical practice of students in the field. Despite the fact that nursing's heritage derived largely from Florence Nightingale, who was known

for her investigations (Grier and Grier, 1978; Seymer, 1954), emphasis on development of research is a relatively recent phenomenon in nursing. The beginnings of this movement have been documented elsewhere (Abdellah, 1970a, 1970b, 1970c; Gortner and Nahm, 1977; Vreeland, 1964; Werley, 1976). Since most nursing faculties earlier did not have research-prepared professors, it is understandable that the focus on research, research-based instruction, and research learning experiences for students did not receive prime attention. There also was insufficient interest in and emphasis on developing the science of nursing, and there was a lack of emphasis on the need to publish. In retrospect, these were serious oversights.

However, being interested increasingly in meeting the educational requirements for university faculty appointments, nursing recognized the need for doctoral preparation of its faculty. Unfortunately, the degree of choice for the majority of nurses seeking their doctorates was the Ed.D. rather than the Ph.D., or research degree. Thus, many of the doctorally prepared nurses were not capable of conducting research or providing students with research learning experiences, for that had not been part of their own educational program. And not having been socialized themselves to value, participate in, and develop research in nursing, these faculty members could not demonstrate to their students how the researcher role could be developed in nursing. Therefore, the nurse with a desire to carry out clinical or theoretical investigations related to nursing practice or health care was not likely to find a research mentor among nurse faculty.

Another reason for which nurses interested in developing research and nursing knowledge might not find mentors among nurse faculty was the fact that those newly graduated with doctorates were desperately needed to help make nursing education programs academically respectable. Thus, new doctorally prepared faculty members were drawn into administration and/or carried overwhelming teaching loads, leaving no time for developing research questions and projects, becoming accomplished researchers themselves, and guiding students in research. More recently, this situation should have been relieved somewhat, for, as Aydelotte (1980) has pointed out, since 1972 approximately 100 nurses have earned doctoral degrees each year. In introducing the recently updated *Directory of Nurses with Doctoral Degrees,* Pender (1980:1) stated that there is now a population of 2348 known doctorally prepared nurses in the United States, 1956 of whom are listed in the directory. However, if the approximately 2400 doctorally prepared nurses were interspersed among the 12,180 faculty members of the baccalaureate and higher-degree nursing programs across the country (National League for Nursing, 1978:56), their research talents would still be spread quite thin and their impact would be minimal.

Data from this latest survey of nurses with doctoral degrees will become available through an American Nurses' Association publication of the final report of the project. Preliminary examination and discussion of these data with the project director (Skoner, 1981) show clearly that certain factors are facilitative or predictive of high research productivity. These are: contact with researchers (nurse or nonnurse) in the first position after the doctorate; differential types of environments in which employed (schools of nursing or other health professional schools and academic departments); amount of teaching; average percentage of time for work-related activities (administration, clinical practice, other, including meetings, teaching); and time allocated for research. High research productivity was more likely for those whose research contacts were nonnurses; the largest numbers of highly productive nurse researchers were found in other health professional schools and academic departments as opposed to being in schools of nursing, where about two-thirds of the nurse doctorates are employed; time allocated for research in the first position after the doctorate was less in the 1970s than before the 1960s; and, sadly, more than 60 percent of the newly graduated nurse doctorates had *no* contact with other researchers in their first positions after doctoral

program completion. These facts speak strongly to the deterrents of establishing proper research mentor-protégé relationships in nursing and warrant nursing's greatest attention.

The fact that research traditionally was not considered part of nurse faculty functioning meant that for years nursing's leadership was not fighting for research support locally and nationally, and often was not even receptive to granting one or two faculty members time for carrying out research as part of their workload. Therefore, those faculty members who may have had relatively good research training soon lost their skills through nonuse; many gave up the idea of conducting research, as they became mired down with teaching, curriculum revision, committee meetings, and administrative duties.

Because the profession had such desperate needs for doctorally prepared nurses in educational administration, many so prepared went that route, without first establishing themselves as researcher-scholars. Thus, the fact that many deans themselves were not experienced first as researcher-scholars and not widely published prior to going into administration further retarded the research movement; they had not been socialized to value scientific investigation as a legitimate role of the nurse. Further, they did not understand what was involved, and they did not seek aggressively the type of support systems needed for researchers.

The fact that newly graduated nurse doctorates did not for the most part find situations in which they could develop themselves as researchers or align themselves with compatible scholars further led to their ineffectuality as scientists in the larger scientific community. Even when some nurses managed through heroic efforts to obtain small grants to carry out research or follow a lead from their dissertation research, it often was not viewed as pilot work which would then lead to a larger-scale proposal for external funding to lay the groundwork for a program of research. Some of this was due to lack of support by administration and naiveté on the part of newly graduated nurse doctorates with no support systems, including no other nurses who had "made it" as productive teacher-researchers. Thus, nursing still suffers from the fact that nurses are not generally competing in the larger scientific community for research funds for proposals that include provision for graduate students and appropriate support staff, such as computer programmers, certain types of technical personnel, and consultants. Not having the benefit of research monies which prepared researchers should obtain for themselves, developing nurse-researchers do not have that "clutch" of graduate students who could help to move research programs along. Even more tragic is the fact that few nurse researchers maintain and extend their own research skills and capabilities needed to attract a cadre of bright, research-interested students and to provide them with increasingly sophisticated research leadership, while they themselves are becoming better, more recognized investigators.

Nursing has been slow to promote the idea of postdoctoral research appointments for nurse-researchers, although these are now available through the Division of Nursing of the U.S. Department of Health and Human Services (USDHHS). The delay in promoting the postdoctoral research movement among nurses in understandable, for indeed there are a few nurse-researchers well enough developed themselves as investigators to serve as mentors for postdoctoral research experiences. There is no reason, however, why some nurses cannot seek postdoctoral experiences with researchers of other disciplines from whom they can learn how to: (1) become productive researchers themselves, (2) develop research programs, (3) obtain external funding, and (4) build teams of students and coinvestigators who will contribute to developing productive research situations that will attract additional promising students and research-committed faculty.

If nursing is truly interested in doing the best it can to improve nursing and the health care delivery system, it must look critically at what should be done to develop its successive generations of nurse-researchers who may make more of an impact through research productivity and who may thus be qualified as research mentors to bright students. A number of years ago steps leading to research productivity were discussed by Werley and Shea (1973), Werley (1975), Fuller (1976), and Stevenson (1979); they are as applicable today as when the papers were written.

POTENTIAL PROFESSIONAL AND SOCIETAL BENEFITS FROM ESTABLISHED RESEARCH MENTOR-PROTEGE RELATIONSHIPS IN NURSING

It is in the interest of both the profession of nursing and society for nurses to work toward developing mentor-protégé relationships among its prepared researchers and promising students. Through these relationships students will experience some of the excitement of science and join their faculty in conducting research, raising further research questions, and generally participating in advancing the frontier of nursing and health care knowledge. Thus, there would be greater research productivity—both original and replication to verify findings in different settings and under different conditions.

As more sound and rigorous research is planned and conducted, nursing will become recognized for its contributions to health science and health care, and nurses will be sought increasingly to collaborate with members of other disciplines and professions in tackling some of the complex unresolved health problems. With resolution of problems based on soundly conceived and conducted research, health care, and related policies will gain more credibility because of being research-based. Eventually, as more nurses compete favorably in obtaining research grant monies, there will be greater respect for nursing research within the scientific community, and funding agencies will welcome their proposals. Overseeing groups, such as the National Research Council (1978) of the National Academy of Sciences, will become aware of nursing's research contributions, and they will no longer need to be concerned about the proliferation of nursing doctoral programs without sufficient numbers of actively involved nurse-researchers capable of serving as sponsors and research mentors for doctoral students.

Nursing schools and nursing service settings will increasingly become recognized as institutions with funded nursing research programs of high caliber, thus adding a mark of distinction to these institutions and credibility to the nurse-researchers themselves. And, as nurse-researchers in these settings increase the number of large-scale funded research projects, more provision will be made for student research assistants to have needed research learning experiences; the mentor-protégé network will grow.

As nursing assembles increasing numbers of research-prepared faculties, some possibly with common research interests, and as nurse-researchers become more capable of competing for research grant funds, there is a likelihood that certain schools of nursing will become known for specific research programs, as opposed to simply conducting isolated studies. Small isolated studies generally do little toward moving the boundaries of knowledge or toward building research programs. As long ago as the 1950s, Margaret Arnstein (1962) of the U.S. Public Health Service Division of Nursing urged nurses to look toward developing series of studies that would hang together or be linked in some way, instead of conducting isolated studies that appear like single cookies on a baking tin. In recent years, personnel of the USDHHS Division of Nursing (1979a, 1979b) have again attempted to help nurses move further in the direction of research program planning, this time through the influence of available nursing research program grants and later nursing research emphasis grants for those schools with doctoral programs in nursing. The research emphasis grants were made available on a one-time basis only.

MAKING OPERATIONAL THE MENTORSHIP CONCEPT IN NURSE DOCTORAL PROGRAMS

It is our belief that mentorship is a desirable and potentially beneficial construct which could enhance the development of nursing research. We also recognize that the development of mentor-protégé relationships hinges on intangible, interpersonal factors as well as on organizational variables. Even so, it seems likely that certain environmental characteristics might relate to and perhaps facilitate the growth and development of a milieu in which research would flourish. The investigators involved in research would conceivably influence students and colleagues to share in this endeavor and thus elaborate a network of colleagues, apprentices, protégés, and assistants.

In an effort to learn how many underlying structural and interactional features to foster research mentor relationships are already in place in nursing's 21 current doctoral programs, we sent a short questionnaire to the directors in mid-1980. Knowing that the term *mentor* was not fully understood by women in Kundsin's (1974) research, we did not ask questions per se about mentors; rather, we aimed to elicit explicit actions or behaviors from which mentor-protégé relationships might be inferred. Twenty responded with completed questionnaires. Of those, 18 (90 percent) provide opportunities for students to assist faculty with their research. Students can receive academic credit for this involvement in 12 instances (60 percent), they can earn wages in 16 (80 percent), or they may be rewarded with coauthorship in 6 (30 percent) of the schools. In 13 (65 percent) of the programs, their assistance can be volunteered as a means of gaining research experience. Junior faculty members have the opportunity to assist senior members with research in 14 (70 percent) of the institutions.

While 17 (85 percent) of the programs report having an identifiable unit within the school as a focal point for research (e.g., office, department, or center), only 13 (65 percent) claim to have developed a specific research program of related studies in one or more content areas. However, this can be expected to change since the USDHHS Division of Nursing encouraged such development through its recent program of research emphasis grants.

Number of faculty associated with the doctoral

programs in nursing ranges from 7 to 35, averaging 17.5 for the 17 schools responding to the question. The number at the upper end of the range seems high, but possibly the question was not specific enough. Sixteen (80 percent) of the schools report having faculty engaged in research supported by extramural funds, 18 (19 percent) have faculty working on studies receiving intramural support, and 13 (65 percent) cite faculty engaged in research for which no external support is being provided. The maximum number of studies reported to be underway in any one school is 19, and in all but one school at least some research activity on the part of the faculty is reported, even though it may be self-supported research.

Although respondents indicate engagement of faculty and students in research, relatively few can point to collaborative faculty-student publications based on their joint research. While one school cites 24 such publications, only 4 other programs note any at all based on either faculty, student, or cooperative research. Yet, as shown in Table 16–2, when asked to rate the importance of various attributes and learning conditions believed to influence development of productive researchers, "opportunity to work with a productive researcher" is rated as very important and ties in importance with the "ability to express ideas clearly." Table 16–2 shows the order of importance ascribed to eight attributes suggested on the questionnaire

Table 16-2 Mean Ratings of Variables Considered Important in Developing a Productive Researcher

Variable	Score
Opportunity to work with a productive researcher	17
Ability to express ideas clearly	17
Personality characteristics	16
Ability to collaborate with others	13
Good thesis experience	10
Clinical nursing expertise	9
High grades in research courses	6
Academic major in basic science	2

Note: Scores are based on the sum of responses to the two highest categories on a 5-point scale.

distributed to directors of nurse doctoral education programs.

Thus, it would appear that interactional and structural factors are in place within nursing doctoral programs to promote faculty-student collaboration in research. The opportunities exist. What we cannot measure from this brief survey, however, are the actual dynamics within these educational programs and the extent to which students are being inspired and coached to assume responsible positions within the research community. This will no doubt become more evident as nurses become more involved in postdoctoral fellowship experiences. Currently available within only three nursing programs, such fellowships provide the opportunity to practice the use of research techniques, develop a productive work style, expand one's publication record, develop a colleague network in one's research area, and generally consolidate previous learning acquired during the research period. However, if such learning opportunities are to expand to meet nursing's need for well-trained researchers, there must be established, experienced researchers to serve as faculty and as research mentors for the aspiring students willing to make sacrifices to extend their education, in the hope of ensuring more productive research careers.

With the steady growth of scholarship and scientific investigation within nursing, opportunities for collaboration between junior and senior researchers will multiply. With that growth will come opportunities for role modeling, preceptorships, apprenticeships, and mentor relationships —the whole gamut of interpersonal-intellectual dynamics that characterize science and its practitioners. A certain number of these relationships will make a critical difference in the course of the individual development of one or both members and perhaps of the profession and the world of health care. We can only hope that nurses at every stage of development will be open to the prospect of benefiting from the development of research mentor-protégé relationships, for their own sakes and for all of nursing.

EDITOR'S QUESTIONS FOR DISCUSSION

What are the issues of concern in research collaborative efforts between faculty members, faculty with a student's individual work, and students with a faculty member's research? What are the ethical responsibilities of each person in collaborative research? At what time in the research process should negotiations be clearly made regarding the role, responsibility, and authority each person has, and the authorship of publications? What guidelines would you suggest for defining role relationships, responsibility, and authority in collaborative research?

How might you account for the lack of collaborative faculty-student publications from schools that indicated joint research was being conducted? Should faculty be indicated as a coauthor in publications based on student's individual research? If so, what guidelines might be suggested?

Given the student-faculty ratios, how can faculty capitalize on the fertile years of undergraduate students to nurture mentor-protégé relationships? How can faculty members be encouraged to develop mentor-protégé relationships with other faculty members?

What is the significance of the preliminary findings from the A.N.A. survey? Are there other explanations that might be offered for the findings?

Given the great role demands for doctorally prepared faculty, what preventive measures can be suggested to avoid the fate outlined by Werley and Newcomb for newly doctorally prepared faculty?

To what extent do you agree that the factors presented by Werley and Newcomb are deterrents to nursing research and the profession? Are there other factors that might be considered? What alternatives can be suggested for effectively dealing with the factors? To what extent is it the responsibility of deans and/or faculty members to find avenues to conduct research? What type of support systems needed for research might deans and/or faculty seek? Should every faculty member be expected to conduct research? How might deans and faculty together realistically resolve the dilemma of faculty work loads and the inclusion of time to conduct research as part of the workload? What is the significance and implication for the profession and society of doctoral programs being developed without sufficient numbers of actively involved nurse researchers?

REFERENCES

Abdellah, Fay G.
1970a "Overview of nursing research, 1955–1968, Part I." Nursing Research 19:6-17.
1970b "Overview of nursing research, 1955–1968, Part II." Nursing Research 19: 151-162.
1970c "Overview of nursing research, 1955–1968, Part III." Nursing Research 19: 239-252.
Arnstein, Margaret G.
1962 "Research in public health nursing." Pp. 444–472 in Harriet H. Werley (ed.), Report on Nursing Research Conference, 24 February–7 March 1979. Washington, D.C.: Walter Reed Army Institute of Research.
Aydelotte, Myrtle K.
1980 "Preface." P. v in Directory of Nurses with Doctoral Degrees. Kansas City, Mo.: American Nurses Association.
Bailey, Stephen K.
1971 "Preparing administrators for conflict resolution." Educational Record 52: 233-239.
Barhyte, Diana Young
1977 Ph.D. deployment in biochemistry: Role of the dissertation mentor." Paper pre-

sented at the American Sociological Association Meeting, Chicago, September.

Chicadonz, Grace
1980 "Leadership in action: The mentor system and research." Reflections 6:8-9.

Conway, Mary E. and Laurie K. Glass
1978 "Socialization for survival in the academic world." Nursing Outlook 26:424-429.

Cowles, John T. and Jenny L. Csanyi
1963 Research Training of Medical Students: A Survey of Faculty and Students at 13 Schools within USPHS Experimental Training Grants. Pittsburgh: University of Pittsburgh.

Division of Nursing
1979a Nursing Research Emphasis Grants for Doctoral Programs in Nursing (NRE/DPN). Unpublished Guidelines. Hyattsville, Md.: U.S. Department of Health and Human Resources, November.
1979b "Nursing research program grants." National Institutes of Health Guide for Grants and Contracts 8 (September 26):47.

Fawcett, Jacqueline
1980 "On development of a scientific community in nursing." Image 12:51-52.

Fuller, Ellen
1976 "Research Q and A: How does the doctorally prepared nurse develop into a productive researcher?" Nursing Research 25:110-111.

Gortner, Susan R. and Helen Nahm
1977 "An overview of nursing research in the United States." Nursing Research 26:10-33.

Grier, James Brown and Margaret R. Grier
1978 "Contributions of the passionate statistician." Research in Nursing and Health 1:103-109.

Hagstrom, Warren O.
1965 The Scientific Community. New York: Basic Books.

Hennig, Margaret and Anne Jardim
1977 The Managerial Woman. New York: Doubleday.

Henry, Gina
1980 "The 'good old girl' strategy: Networking your way to contacts." United Mainliner 24:11-12,14.

Inkles, Alex
1969 "Social structure and socialization." Pp. 615-632 in David Goslin (ed.), Handbook of Socialization Theory and Research. Chicago: Rand McNally.

Kelly, Lucie Young
1978 "Power guide—the mentor relationship." Nursing Outlook 26:339.

Krueger, Janelle C.
1980 "Women in management: An assessment. Nursing Outlook 28:374-378.

Kundsin, Ruth B.
1974 "To autonomous women: An introduction." Pp. 9-12 in Ruth B. Kundsin (ed.), Women and Success. New York: William Morrow.

Levinson, Daniel J., Charlotte N. Darrow, Edward B. Klein, Maria H. Levinson, and Braxton McKee
1978 The Seasons of a Man's Life. New York: Ballantine.

Maeroff, Gene Irving
1976 "Use of undergraduates in research is hailed by M.I.T.", New York Times, January 11, 1976, section 4, p. 44.

Mullins, Nicholas C. and Carolyn J. Mullins
1973 Theories and Theory Groups in Contemporary American Sociology. New York: Harper and Row.

National Research Council
1978 Personnel Needs and Training for Biomedical and Behavioral Research. Washington, D.C.: National Academy of Sciences.

National Research Council, Commission on Human Resources
1979 Climbing the Academic Ladder: Doctoral Women Scientists in Academe. Washington, D.C.: National Academy of Sciences.

National League for Nursing
1978 NLN Nursing Data Book (Publication Number 19-1751). New York: Author.

Pender, Nola J.
1980 "Introduction." P. 1 in Directory of Nurses with Doctoral Degrees. Kansas City, Mo.: American Nurses' Association.

Pilette, Patricia Chehy
1978 "The mentor relationship." Nursing Outlook 26:473.

Reskin, Barbara F.
  1979 "Academic sponsorship and scientists' careers." Sociology of Education 52: 129-146.
Rickard, Henry C. and Paul S. Siegel
  1976 "Research—apprenticeship training for clinical psychologists: A follow-up study." Professional Psychology 7:359-363.
Schorr, Thelma M.
  1978 "The lost art of mentorship." American Journal of Nursing 78:1873.
Severo, Richard
  1980 "Geographer of small world of genes: Dr. Francis Hugh Ruddle." New York Times, September 3, 1980, page 8.
Seymer, Lucy Ridgely (Buckler)
  1954 Selected Writings of Florence Nightingale. New York: Macmillan.
Sheehy, Gail
  1976 Passages: Predictable Crises of Adult Life. New York: Bantam.
Sibley, Elbridge
  1963 The Education of Sociologists in the United States. New York: Russell Sage Foundation.
Skoner, Martha M.
  1981 Personal communication, January 6.
Stevenson, Joanne S.
  1979 "Support for an emerging social institution." Pp. 39-66 in Florence S. Downs, and Juanita W. Fleming (eds.), Issues in Nursing Research. New York: Appleton-Century-Crofts.
Taylor, Donald, Wendell R. Garner, and Howard F. Hung
  1959 "Education for research in psychology." The American Psychologist 14:167-179.
Vance, Connie N.
  1979 "Women leaders: Modern day heroines or societal deviants?" Image 11:37-41.
Vreeland, Ellwynne M.
  1964 "Nursing research programs in the Public Health Service." Nursing Research 13: 148-158.
Werley, Harriet H.
  1975 "Research Q and A [on research-prepared nurses conducting research]." Nursing Research 24:453-454.
  1976 "Nursing research in perspective." Pp. 17-42 in Round Table Discussion, Nursing in Illinois: A Bicentennial Glimpse. Chicago: University of Illinois College of Nursing.
Werley, Harriet H., Patricia A. Murphy, and B. Joan Newcomb
  1981 "Student research assistant: Tomorrow's nurse researcher." Pp. 180-192 in Sidney D. Krampitz and Natalie Pavlovich (eds.), Readings in Nursing Research. New York: Mosby.
Werley, Harriet H. and Fredricka P. Shea
  1973 "The first center for nursing research: Its development, accomplishments, and problems. Nursing Research 22:217-231.
White, Martha
  1970 "Psychological and social barriers to women in science." Science 170:413-416.
Williams, Marcille G.
  1977 The New Executive Woman: A Guide to Business Success. Radnor, Pa: Chilton Books.
Worthen, Blaine R. and Arliss L. Roaden
  1975 The Research Assistantship: Recommendations for Colleges and Universities. Bloomington, Ind.: Phi Delta Kappa.
Zigler, Edward F. and Irvin L. Child
  1973 Socialization and Personality Development. Reading, Mass.: Addison-Wesley.
Zuckerman, Harriet
  1977 Scientific Elite: Nobel Laureate in the United States. New York: Free Press.
Zuckerman, Harriet and Johnathan R. Cole
  1975 "Women in American Science." Minerva 13:32-102.

Chapter 17

The Clinical Nurse-Researcher: Role-Taking and Role-Making

Gloria Gilbert Mayer, R.N., Ed.D., F.A.A.N.
Senior Consultant
Health Management Systems Associates
Minneapolis, Minnesota

Like Werley and Newcomb, Gloria Mayer is a strong advocate of collaborative research. She views collaboration as an ideal means for "role-taking" and "role-making." Mayer specifically focuses on the development of nursing research roles in the clinical setting. She cites the lack of research models, identifies the phases of role-making and provides valuable suggestions for the genesis of the role-making process. Some of the facilitative examples indicated are: critiquing studies and validating findings on the nursing unit, collaboration with departments of staff development in research programs, and application of appropriate research findings for continuing education credit. Mayer shows the importance of the nurse-researcher's position in the hierarchy of nursing administration. She suggests strategies to obtain administrative and physician support for nursing research as well as for effectively confronting conditions that promote role ambiguity. Mayer emphasizes the significance of a job description for the clinical nurse-researcher. A formal example is illustrated, and guidelines endorsed by the American Society for Nursing Service Administration for the formation of a nursing research program within a clinical facility are indicated.

Although research in clinical nursing has been advocated since the time of Florence Nightingale, only recently has it achieved legitimacy. Maturation of clinical nursing research could be facilitated by the employment of nurse-researchers by clinical facilities, for example hospitals, but this has been a slow process. In fact, to date, there are fewer than 40 nurses who have identified themselves to an American Nurses Association's special interest group as nurse-researchers employed by clinical facilities (Steckel,

1979). Although a few institutions have invested in the establishment of this role, currently this could not be considered a major national trend.

The recency of the position of the clinical nurse-researcher and the paucity of persons in these positions necessitates pioneering risk-taking efforts in order to create roles and relationships that facilitate accomplishment of goals. There are few tested role models to emulate. This position is not only new to the profession of nursing, but it is also new to the institutions, new to nurses, and new to other researchers. Therefore, the nurse employed as a researcher in a clinical setting may find role development a frustrating task.

The examination of role theory may provide a perspective with which to approach the establishment of the role of the clinical nurse-researcher. In this paper, the sociological concepts of *role-taking* and *role-making* will be elaborated upon, with special emphasis given to methods of succeeding in this newly established role.

Kramer (1974:52) states that "a role is a set of expectations about how a person in a given position in a particular social system should act." Two categories of roles are those ascribed and those achieved. *Ascribed roles* are those over which we have no control, such as age and sex. *Achieved roles* are those that can be personally controlled, and the clinical nurse-researcher has achieved this role through professional and educational level, competition, and personal effort. However, the success of this achieved role will be determined by many operational factors, including the effectiveness of the nurse in utilizing the concepts of role-taking and role-making to develop this expanded role of nursing.

Role-taking has been defined by Turner (1956: 316) as "a process of looking at or anticipating another's behavior by viewing it in the context of a role imputed to that other." Role-taking is a process in which one person puts him- or herself in the other's place for the purpose of being able to obtain the other person's perspective to function in a specific position, i.e., nurse-researcher. This allows one to anticipate the other's behavior and then act accordingly (Contu, 1951:181). In performing this task, the role incumbent can develop understanding and empathy and can better predict how behavior will affect others.

Taking the role of others can be extremely useful in the development of a new role and occurs through the process of social interaction. Through interaction individuals learn both their own responses to others and the responses of those others with whom they interact (Brim,

1966:10). In learning self-other roles, the individual obtains needed information by direct instruction, by observing interactions as a participant, or by observing interactions as a bystander (Heiss, 1976:6–7).

Clinical nurse-researchers, in attempting to develop their roles as researchers, may find social interaction with researchers in other disciplines and nurse-researchers in academic institutions a useful activity. Factors such as the extent of social experience with a particular role either as an actor or observer and ability to remember and utilize these experiences affect an individual's role-taking ability (Hurley, 1978:44). Therefore spending deliberate time with established researchers can assist in the process of creating and modifying people's concepts of their own, unique role. This activity cannot be overemphasized as a means of role development.

The process of role-taking may prove helpful in situations of others' acceptance of the role of the clinical nurse-researcher. Gramse (1971: 31) points out that the nursing profession itself is one of the greatest obstacles nurse-researchers frequently face. The nurse-researcher frequently is a department unto him- or herself and must successfully interface with both managerial and staff nurses in the establishment and implementation of the nurse-researcher role. The clinical nurse-researcher may be isolated and often feels like a marginal person with a foot in two camps, neither fully accepted nor fully rejected by either one.

Staff nurses have a long history and their role is clear—patient care. This is sometimes the primary mission of the institution and must be respected by nurses in peripheral roles. Nurse-researchers must be empathetic to this, especially in times of staff shortage, but must not lose sight of the importance of their contributions to the health care of these very same patients. A true understanding of the staff nurse's role, with subsequent appropriate behavior and effective communication, can prove extremely beneficial in the joint effort of providing quality patient care—the goal of all nursing personnel. Role-taking activity can assist in this very essential process.

The term role-making refers to the interpretation of one's own role and emphasizes the positive process of role development (Hardy, 1978: 96–97). Conway (1978) describes the five distinct phases that occur in the sequential process of role-making as: (1) initiator behavior; (2) other-response; (3) interpretation by actor and other; (4) altered response pattern; and (5) role validation. The majority of this chapter further addresses these phases and related issues of role ambiguity and role conflict.

When the five phases of role-making are used to examine the role of the clinical nurse-researcher, the initiator behavior may be: (1) the research process itself, a function not usually associated with nursing; or (2) the process of obtaining a position as a clinical nurse-researcher, a position that may raise questions in times of budgetary restraints. An example of the other-response may be staff nurses and physicians questioning the legitimacy of this practice by nursing. The staff nurse and physicians may accept a detailed explanation of the clinical nurse's research position and its potential for improving patient care. From these interactions, the clinical nurse-researcher may be accepted as a research-nurse-scientist, and as this altered role begins to demonstrate its contributions to the patient, validation will occur.

Although the process of role-making has been clearly defined by Conway (1978), the modification of a role can be difficult. One problem identified by Davis (1968:167) is difficulty in establishing identity as a clinical nurse-researcher. A related problem is the lack of nurse research role models.

A role model can enhance the socialization process by providing assistance on how a role is to be performed. Lum (1978:142) states that "the availability of a role model facilitates the acquisition of an adequate level of performance." As previously stated, role models for the clinical

nurse-researcher are few and far between. Although research in nursing has been performed for many years, many times these researchers were not nurses or were nurses who obtained higher degrees in areas outside of nursing and have identified with their new discipline. The research nurse who is employed by a clinical institution and is engaged in research directly related to the practice of nursing and patient care may be at a loss to find other professional colleagues and role models. Davis (1968:168) notes the benefits she experienced from the association with social scientists in the development of a research identity.

In phases 2 and 3 of the role-making process, other responses and interpretations are identified as being crucial in the eventual establishment and validation of the role. The "others" that may have to be dealt with are other nurses at all levels, administrators, and physicians. Each of these "others" will be discussed with practical suggestions which may assist in the role-making process.

To obtain support and understanding from other nurses, involvement in the research program within the institution is essential. Obviously, not everyone could or should become a research nurse, but every professional nurse can become knowledgeable about the research process as well as a consumer of the research product. This is an area where staff involvement can be maximized.

A method of developing further knowledge of research is to collaborate with the in-service department in the presentation of research material. During in-service programs concerning clinical topics, research findings can be presented to validate the procedure and treatment being discussed. Appropriate research articles can be made available on the clinical unit to encourage utilization of research findings. This is especially helpful in any specialty area where new treatments and procedures are constantly being introduced, for example, neonatal intensive-care units. Informal discussions with the research nurse concerning the study serve to clarify the protocol, answer questions relating to methodology and the utilization of research findings, and demonstrate the practical aspect of nursing research. This activity is an effective means of obtaining staff nurse involvement and eventual support.

Another method of obtaining staff nurse involvement in research is the introduction of the nurse to the method of critiquing studies and applying appropriate findings. At one institution, an independent study module dealing with this topic was developed that was awarded two continuing-education contact hours. The purpose of this exercise was for the nurse to become adept at the interpretation and utilization of germane research. The participant selected a relevant research study and, following specific guidelines, critiqued the study and described how the findings could be utilized clinically or why they could not be used. The guidelines suggested by Krueger (1978:7) on the utilization of nursing research are included in the exercise and used in the determination of the appropriateness of the study findings for the particular clinical setting.

Another technique utilized in gaining support for nursing research by the staff is the establishment of a nursing research committee. The stated purpose of our research committee is "to promote nursing research and make recommendations for the application of nursing research findings into clinical practice" (Minneapolis VA Policy 118-32: 19-80). In addition to the stated purpose, the committee has served as a vital element in the public relations realm of nursing research. Membership on this committee is open to all interested persons, and participation in some research program is highly encouraged. Since all staff may serve as members, the mystique of nursing research has been eliminated and an appreciation of the contributions of nursing research has been established.

The nursing research committee sponsors a yearly nursing research conference. The specific focus of this conference is determined by the members, and all members become involved in the planning and implementation of this conference. Again, this is a technique utilized to gain support and establish visibility of our nursing research program.

A nursing research newsletter is also a device to gain visibility and is published biannually by the nursing research committee. In the newsletter, individuals are recognized for specific contributions. This has been met with positive response throughout the hospital. The conference and the newsletter are made available to all disciplines in the health care facility, thereby creating a communication channel focusing on nursing research.

Physicians usually view nursing research with great suspicion. This may be different in each institution, depending upon the philosophy of the institution and its general commitment to research in general. In a research institution, the nurse-researcher may be viewed as a competitor in the arena of patient access. Physicians have always found difficulty in understanding the different levels of nursing, and the doctorally prepared nurse-researcher adds to this confusion. Membership on the human subjects study committee or the hospital research committee may be useful in establishing credibility. Appropriate questioning of submitted research proposals can demonstrate that nursing can offer valuable input to the research process.

Collaboration on studies with other disciplines increases rapport and understanding of each discipline, including nursing. Collaboration means equal cooperation in terms of goal setting and in action (Mundinger, 1980:23). It is not merely cooperating in data collection. True collaboration implies an equal respect for all parties involved with the project, with the potential of equal rewards and frustrations. Mundinger (1980:23-24) states, "Collaboration may be the strongest means of providing nursing's unique yet subtle service: collaboration with physicians, clients, and most of all, with our fellow nurses."

Cooperating on various research projects should

not be discouraged, but it should be recognized that there is a difference between cooperation and collaboration. Assisting in the research process can be a valuable experience for the novice researcher. In addition, this endeavor can be a forerunner to the establishment of true collaborative efforts between disciplines.

It is crucial that nursing administration support the role of the clinical nurse-researcher. Chance and Hinshaw (1980:32) state that "if a research program is to succeed, the nursing director must value research and fact-gathering for administrative and clinical decision making." This support must extend to all parties including the hospital administrator, physicians, and other nurses.

In some situations, a nursing director sees the role of the researcher as a person to solve many reoccurring clinical and administrative problems. In other instances, the director may see the role of the nurse-researcher as the head of a quality assurance program. Still other nursing administrators may expect the nurse-researcher to bring in large amounts of grant monies. These expectations of the role must be made extremely clear from the onset if role conflict is to be avoided. Role conflict occurs in a situation in which two or more sets of expectations operate, and the usual result is some degree of tension and anxiety (Lindgren, 1969:175). Therefore it becomes crucial to define one's role and obtain endorsement from the chief administrator of the service.

Another important factor to consider is the placement of the position of the clinical nurse-researcher on the organizational chart. In considering this aspect of role development, it is helpful to think of positions in the categories of *line* and *staff*. Persons in line positions are part of and contribute to a basic hierarchical function in the nursing service department, for example, primary nurse, head nurse, or supervisor. The organizational chart directly reflects the hierarchical authority. A staff position is one in which the person provides advice, consultation, and/or service to aid persons in the hierarchical line or-

ganization to perform their duties. Usually, the organizational chart *indirectly* reflects staff positions via "dotted" lines, linked to someone with direct hierarchical authority and responsibility. The clinical nurse-researcher usually occupies a staff position and therefore has little power or authority. The functions of staff personnel in the organization usually include activities such as providing information, rendering analysis, giving assistance, and providing coordination. Implicit in these activities may be some form of indirect power, especially if the nurse-researcher is a member of an executive board. However, a staff position does not carry any direct authority.

The placement of the clinical nurse-researcher within the organization in a staff position is both positive and negative. Because researchers do not evaluate nurses, they are not viewed as a threat. Many times they are utilized as "sounding boards" and problem solvers by others in the organization, and this may prove helpful in identifying areas of potential research. The negatives of a staff position are similar to those of any person who may have responsibility but no power or authority to carry out functions. However, the determination of placement within the organization is something to be negotiated prior to job acceptance.

One example of a formal job description of a clinical nurse-researcher is included in Table 17-1.

Recently, the American Society for Nursing Service Administrators of the American Hospital Association issued a statement entitled, "The Role of the Nursing Service Administrator in Nursing Research" (1980). This document presents the following guidelines in the formation of a nursing research program:

1 Establishment of an advisory committee
2 Establishment of a hospital nursing research committee (comprising staff nurses and a coordinator-facilitator)
3 Implementation of the research process
4 Integration of findings into clinical practice
5 Evaluation

Table 17-1   Clinical Nurse-Researcher: Job Description

I. Role

The clinical nurse-researcher has overall program accountability for all aspects of research within nursing service. He or she is a professional nurse who has achieved a doctoral degree. This person assumes the responsibility for the organization and administration of the component of nursing research defined by the philosophy, objectives, and concepts of patient care management. The nurse-researcher should have a sound basis of clinical nursing experience, a high degree of knowledge and skill in nursing research, expertise with interpersonal relationships, experience in teaching, and evidence of interest related to health care, nursing practice, and education.

II. Functions and responsibilities

A Clinical practice

1 Establishes clinical nursing research priorities

2 Assists nursing staff in the identification of potentially researchable clinical practice-patient care problems

3 Identifies and develops systematic ways in which the observed clinical practice-patient care problems may be studied or resolved

4 Assists nursing staff in the appropriate analysis, reporting, and dissemination of their research findings

5 Assists nursing staff to seek out and plan for the use of research findings for validating or improving clinical practice

B Administration

1 Develops short- and long-range goals related to nursing research and contributes to overall nursing service objectives

2 Participates in establishing hospital and nursing policies

3 Establishes and maintains avenues of communication between nursing research, nursing service, nursing education, and other hospital staff

4 Designs, maintains, and evaluates an effective record system for documentation of nursing staff research activities

5 Assists in obtaining time for nursing staff to conduct research

6 Supervises and evaluates performance of nursing service research staff

7 Seeks funds for nursing research studies

8 Participates as an active member on various intra- and extrahospital committees and task forces

C Research

1 Identifies current and potentially researchable problems and questions relevant to nursing practice, administration, and education

2 Develops and implements study protocols focused on identified research priorities

3 Participates in nursing research studies

4 Develops research and program evaluation proposals appropriate for nursing service

5 Acts as research-evaluation consultant to the nursing service and the community in the development of research activities, projects, and funding

6 Assists nursing staff in the development of techniques and instruments for program evaluation

7 Assists nursing staff in the development and conduct of scientific studies to provide a basis for making and validating nursing decisions

8 Assesses the feasibility of nursing staff proposals

9 Collaborates with members of other health disciplines in the development, conduction and evaluation of research activities and care programs

10 Coordinates the research efforts of community individuals (students, faculty, etc.) as these relate to nursing service through:

a Providing information concerning research policies and procedures

b Assisting in the preparation of research protocols for hospital committees

c Making appropriate arrangements for the conduct of hospital-approved projects

d Monitoring the progress of these projects

e Assisting in the preparation and presentation of final study reports

Table 17-1 Continued

D Education
  1 Acts as research consultant to nursing service in the planning, development, and evaluation of projects and programs
  2 Provides an orientation for new staff, nursing faculty, and students to the role and functions of the nurse-researcher and the program in general
  3 Designs, teaches, and evaluates selected intra- and extrahospital workshops and seminars
  4 Establishes and maintains relationships with local universities and colleges through adjunct faculty appointments
  5 Assists in the development and evaluation of nursing educational programs

Source: Adapted from the Minneapolis Veterans Administration Medical Center, "Roles, Responsibilities, and Functions of the Associate Chief Nursing Service for Research," 1979.

This statement lends support to the establishment of a nursing research program within a clinical facility. If an outside accrediting agency recognizes the need for nursing research and its application to patient care, the nursing administrator can certainly justify and support the implementation of the program.

Kahn et al. (1964:22–23) have suggested three organizational conditions that significantly contribute to role ambiguity: (1) organizational complexity, (2) rapid organizational change, and (3) managerial philosophies about communication. The nurse employed as a researcher in a health care facility will probably face all three conditions. By the very nature of a hospital that would employ a nurse-researcher, complexity and size would have to be major factors. The complexity of a health care center lends itself to organizational change, which includes personnel movement. This becomes significant when the director of nursing leaves the institution and a new top nurse executive arrives. If the nurse-researcher's role has been clarified with the first director, a new director may

have different expectations. The preestablished role may be invalidated by new nurse-executives. This becomes a particularly significant in institutions where mobility of top management is a requirement.

Restriction of communication at all levels, intentional or not, is another contributor to role ambiguity. This coupled with personnel changes and organizational complexity certainly contributes to dissatisfaction with the role of the clinical nurse-researcher. Therefore, the need for a well-defined job description and expectations cannot be overemphasized. In addition, the formation of a long-range plan related to nursing research and specific objectives can help to bridge the gap for new management.

Role conflict can also occur when one is required to fill simultaneously two or more roles that present inconsistent, contradictory, or even mutually exclusive expectations (Getzels and Guba, 1954). This situation may be faced by the nurse-researchers as they conduct clinical field studies and find themselves at the patient's bedside for other purposes than patient care. On busy days, the urge to assist in patient care may be overwhelming but may be contradictory to the research protocol. Staff nurses may pressure the researcher to assist with patient care and may not be able to understand the research limitations in doing this. Resolution of this type of situation is crucial for effective role development.

Once the nurse-researcher has defined, developed, and implemented his or her role within the clinical setting, altered responses will eventually pursue. The staff will eventually recognize that the researcher cannot assist in patient care if the protocol requires nonparticipant observation and eventually will not seek this type of behavior. As the nurse-researcher persists in this realigned role over time, the staff, physicians, and administration will accept the role and eventually it will be validated.

This chapter has briefly summarized the concepts of role-taking and role-making and has presented several strategies that may be useful in establishing the role of the clinical nurse-researcher. This process may take several years, and the implementation of a well-functioning research program within a clinical setting may take even longer.

However, the rewards are significant, and as more nurse-researchers begin to develop their role within clinical facilities, the eventual effects on patient care will make the process well worth the effort.

EDITOR'S QUESTIONS FOR DISCUSSION

How can nurse-researchers in clinical settings develop support systems for research? What suggestions might be offered in seeking collaborative research relationships with multidisciplinary health professionals in clinical settings? What other approaches can be proposed for obtaining acceptance of the clinical nurse-researcher? What might be suggested for ensuring that recommendations made for the application of nursing research findings are actually tested, evaluated, and implemented into clinical practice? What strategies can be used to effectively demonstrate the application of appropriate research findings and its effects on the quality of care provided? How might cooperation and interest of the nursing staff in the process and implementation of nursing research be elicited? What means can be utilized in an institution to disseminate the results of applied research findings in patient care?

What are the purposes and appropriate functions for research committees in clinical settings and in academe? What suggestions do you have for operationalizing the functions of those research committees? What is the significance and role of the clinical nurse-researcher as a member on the human subjects study committee or hospital research committee?

With what types of protocols, under what circumstances, and by whom should clinical nursing research proposals be directly supervised? What suggestions might be offered for clinical nurse-researchers and nursing students in obtaining formal approval of appropriate nursing research protocols without representation and/or direct supervision of their studies by a member of the medical profession?

What considerations need to be kept in mind in order to increase nursing administration support for clinical nursing research? How can the influence of clinical nurse researchers in "staff" rather than "line" positions be increased to advance research? Keeping in mind Fawcett's discussion and editor's questions in Chap. 14 concerning the lack of a theoretical base in many nursing practice protocols, how can the clinical nurse-researcher be the facilitator to bridge the chasm? To what extent is the clinical nurse-researcher in an unique position to develop protocols to advance the knowledge base of nursing as well as the practice of nursing?

REFERENCES

American Society for Nursing Service Administrators
  1980 "The Role of the Nursing Service Administrator in Nursing Research." Chicago: American Hospital Association.
Brim, O. G., Jr.
  1966 "Socialization through the life cycle." Pp. 1–48 in O. G. Brim, Jr. and S. Wheeler (eds), Socialization After Childhood: Two Essays, New York: Wiley.
Chance, H., C. and A. S. Hinshaw
  1980 "Strategies for initiating a research program." Journal of Nursing Administration 10:32–39.
Contu, W.
  1951 "Role-playing vs. role-taking: An appeal for clarification." American Sociological Review XVI:1951:180–187.

Conway, M. E.
1978   "Theoretical Approaches to the Study of Roles." Pp. 24–27 in M. Hardy and M. Conway (eds.), Role Theory, Perspectives for Health Professionals, New York: Appleton-Century-Crofts.

Davis, M. Z.
1968   "Some problems in identity in becoming a nurse researcher." Nursing Research 17:166–168.

Getzels, J. W. and E. G. Guba
1954   "Role, role conflict and effectiveness: An empirical study." American Sociological Review 19:164–175

Gramse, C. A.
1971   "Progress and research in nursing." The Journal of Continuing Education in Nursing 9:30–34.

Hardy, M. E.
1978   "Role stress and role strain." Pp. 73–109 in M. E. Hardy and M. E. Conway (eds.) Role Theory, Perspectives for Health Professionals, New York: Appleton-Century-Crofts.

Heiss, J.
1976   "An introduction to the elements of role theory." Pp. 3–30 in J. Heiss (ed.): Family Roles and Interaction: An Anthology, 2d ed. Chicago: Rand McNally.

Hurley, D. A.
1978   "Socialization for roles." Pp. 29–71 in M. E. Hardy and M. E. Conway (eds.) Role Theory, Perspectives for Health Professionals, New York: Appleton-Century-Crofts.

Kahn, R. L., D. M. Wolfe, R. P. Quinn, J. D. Snock, and R. A. Rosenthal
1964   Organizational Stress: Studies in Role Conflict and Ambiguity. New York: Wiley.

Kramer, M.
1974   Reality Shock. St. Louis: C. V. Mosby.

Krueger, J. C.
1978   "Utilization of Nursing Research: The Planning Process." Journal of Nursing Administration 7:6–9.

Lindgren, H. C.
1969   An Introduction to Social Psychology. New York: Wiley.

Lum, J. L. J.
1978   "Reference groups and professional socialization." Pp. 137–156 in M. E. Hardy and M. E. Conway (eds). Role Theory, Perspectives for Health Professionals. New York: Appleton-Century-Crofts.

Minneapolis Veterans Administration Medical Center
1980   Nursing Service Policy, Number 118–32.

Mundinger, M. O.
1980   Autonomy in Nursing. Germantown, Md.: Aspen.

Steckel, S.
1979   "Nurse Researchers Employed in Clinical Settings." Sub-interest group of the Council of Nurse Researchers, American Nurses' Association.

Turner, R. H.
1956   "Role-taking, role standpoint and reference group behavior." American Journal of Sociology 61:316–329.

Chapter 18

Conducting Interdisciplinary Research: Gratifications and Frustrations

Mildred A. Disbrow, R.N., Ph.D., F.A.A.N.
Professor, Maternal and Child Nursing
School of Nursing
University of Washington
Seattle, Washington

Since little research has been conducted on interdisciplinary projects, Mildred A. Disbrow's treatise is uniquely valuable. It appropriately follows the contributions by Werley and Newcomb (Chap. 16) and Mayer (Chap. 17). Disbrow provides further insight into the discourse upon collaborative research and replies to numerous questions raised for discussion by those chapters. She justifies the need for interdisciplinary research by making clear six criteria related to complex study problems due to interaction of persons in multiple environments. Disbrow describes the process, method, stages, and salient issues in evolving interdisciplinary studies. The portrayal is based predominantly on her personal experience with a team that worked together for 7 years to develop measures to predict child abuse. She cites the capability to study research questions that could not otherwise be studies as a major gratification of interdisciplinary research. Other satisfactions are: increased access to research sites, subjects, and the broadening of one's research perspective. The predominant frustrations are related to the number of personnel, recruitment of qualified team members, and communication. Disbrow candidly describes the sources of difficulty in organizing and executing interdisciplinary research. Problems related to the status concordance of the group, conflicts between a member's research and clinical role, data production, analysis, and publication of findings are explicated. Success factors for conducting interdisciplinary studies are indicated.

The field of interdisciplinary research is not a new arena for nurses; nurses have been involved in this type of research for a long time. The difference today is that more nurses are the principal investigators or the coinvestigators responsible for conducting such studies. Nurses are now experiencing directly the rewards and problems associated with interdisciplinary research. In the past most nurses had lesser roles, less impact on the research process, and probably less gratification and frustration.

What is interdisciplinary research? Most authorities consider research interdisciplinary when two or more persons from different disciplines pool and integrate their knowledge and resources to investigate a problem that could not be addressed as effectively by an individual working alone (Mar, Newell, and Saxberg, 1976; Luszki, 1957; Benoliel, 1973). This implies that all investigators share equally in all decision making. Since such a highly ideal situation is rarely found, Mar et al. (1976) chose to delineate what they saw as four prevailing modes of mixed discipline research: (a) the multidisciplinary group, where roles are so defined that each investigator conducts his or her own research, (b) the cross- or bidisciplinary group, where two persons from separate but related disciplines collaborate on a study, (c) the interdisciplinary staff and student group, where one individual brings together persons from separate disciplines and directs them, and (d) the multidisciplinary individual who, through formal or informal study, has acquired preparation in several disciplines and applies this knowledge to a research problem. For this chapter a research group representing a combination of these modes will be addressed.

The interdisciplinary nature of a research group will be evident not only in the investigators but also in others, such as research associates, whose varied backgrounds provide both strengths and weaknesses for the project as they collect data and become involved in group decision making.

An interdisciplinary approach to research is justified when no single discipline can adequately handle the problem, when the problem falls theoretically between disciplines, when conceptual integration of formerly distinct conceptual frameworks is needed, when the problem is large and complex, when relevant disciplines appear ready to collaborate, when multiple research methods are needed, and when broad interdisciplinary application is desirable (Blackwell, 1955; Milgram, 1969; Sherif and Sherif, 1969). Questions concerned with how persons interact with their environments frequently fit these criteria, since human beings have multiple

environments—social, psychological, physical, cultural, and psychological.

Two problem areas, areas too broad to be handled by one discipline alone and areas in which persons have difficulty interacting with their environments, are problems of the elderly and child abuse. In each of these areas, both research and treatment have been interdisciplinary in nature.[1]

When working with old people, it is difficult to separate the physiological factors from the social, cultural, physical, and psychological factors involved in the aging process. There is much interaction between all the aspects, and interdisciplinary research teams composed of physicians, psychologists, sociologists, and sometimes nurses have conducted much of the research on older people. Research can focus on the societal or the individual level (McTavish, 1971). The societal approach has been used to study the level of regard in which the elderly are held by society and the social consequences of this view. How others regard old people is influenced by personal experience with the elderly, by cultural values, and by what the elderly themselves bring to the situation. Satisfied, happy, well-adjusted older people differ in many respects from the less satisfied, unhappy elderly who cannot adapt (Adams, 1969; Peterson, 1971). Money or the lack of it, type of housing, and the adequacy or inadequacy of social support systems interact in the lives of the elderly with the physiological factors of disease (Woodruff and Birren, 1975).

In child abuse, many of the same problems exist, and the same type of broad-based research is needed. Parke and Collmer (1975) have suggested three models for studying child abuse, models based on child-abuse etiology. These are the psychiatric, the sociological, and the social situa-

[1] The interdisciplinary research group described in this study has produced "Measures to Predict Child Abuse: A Validation Study." That research was supported by a Maternal and Child Health (Social Security Act, Title V) Grant, MC-R-530351.

tional models. The psychiatric approach has been used to study parents, their personality characteristics, and how they were reared as children (Kempe, 1973; Steele and Pollock, 1968). The sociological model focuses on cultural norms, social class, housing and living conditions, family size, social isolation, and social stress (Elmer, 1977; Gelles, 1973; Gil, 1970). Findings from these approaches have not been very helpful in either preventing or treating child abuse. Research using the third model, the social situational, looks at the effects on the child, at parent-child interaction, and at everyday family interaction (Burgess and Conger, 1978; Patterson, 1974), and this last model appears to be a more productive approach. Belsky (1980), in speaking of the three alternative models of child-abuse etiology, proposed integration of the models since child abuse is multiply determined. Belsky recommended four levels of analysis. He proposed studying the abuse situation in terms of (a) ontogenic development, or what parents bring with them to the situation; (b) the microsystem, or the immediate context—the family setting; (c) the exosystem, or the social structures, including support systems, which impinge on the child and adult(s); and (d) the macrosystem, or the cultural values and belief systems that foster abuse and neglect through influence on the other three levels. In most of these approaches the research teams are composed of physicians, social workers, social scientists, and sometimes nurses.

Our research in developing measures to predict child abuse utilizes all four of Belsky's levels of analysis, plus measurement of parents' physiological response to child-related behaviors.[2] Disciplines

and professions represented on the team include nursing, clinical psychology, sociology, social work, and physiology (Caulfield et al., 1977; Disbrow et al., 1977).

Research questions in many other problem areas can and should be studied using an interdisciplinary approach. Problems of the elderly and child abuse are simply examples of large, complex problem areas where it is necessary to take into consideration interaction with several environments and interaction between environments.

The capability of studying certain research questions that can not otherwise be studied is only one of the gratifications of conducting interdisciplinary research. Collaborating with persons in other professions or disciplines can also facilitate access to desired research sites or subjects (Benoliel, 1973). Stimulating interaction with others interested in the same problem can increase the breadth of perspective and give a wider range to, and ensure a more effective application of, the research findings. Such rewards, however, seldom accrue without payment of a certain price; frustrations do frequently occur when persons from several disciplines collaborate.

Interdisciplinary research, because of its very nature, tends to grow complex and lead to larger studies requiring more personnel. Recruitment of qualified personnel may be difficult, and retaining such personnel until the end of a long project may be very difficult. This is particularly true when funding agencies require yearly review and when notification of continued funding is late. Review committees for funding agencies question gaps in a proposed personnel list, but equal opportunity employers do not permit personnel recruitment until monies are guaranteed.

A type of Peter principle (Peter and Hull, 1969) may be in operation in interdisciplinary

---

[2] Our child abuse research has been conducted in two stages, a developmental stage completed in 1977 and a current validation stage conducted from 1977 to 1981. In the current stage, 551 families, stratified on social class, were screened through the battery of measures developed in the first stage of the research. The 100 high-risk and 100 low-risk families selected from the screening were tested at 6 to 12 month intervals until the children were 2½ years of age. Testing included

interviews, questionnaires, videotaped behavior observation and physiological response to child-related behaviors.

projects. Investigators may elect to work with one another because of their respect for each other's individual research ability. How one conducts independent research, however, is not necessarily a good predictor of how that person will work with team members. Communication may also be a problem. Members of a research team must be able to evaluate and criticize their peers, but it takes a long time for members of a newly created team to become comfortable with one another. When persons from three or more disciplines are involved, it may take as long as a year for them to become acquainted with one another's way of thinking and use of terminology. The longer the group works together, the better will be its chances of high performance (Mar et al., 1976; Birnbaum et al., 1979).

Creative people whose conceptual schemes are logical and whose decision making is rational are not always apolitical. Power and economy struggles frequently exist in team research. Dubin (1969) pointed out that science progresses through competition, not consensus. Benoliel (1973) suggested that the slow development of research in nursing may be tied to a lack of competitive spirit among nurses who tend to comply rather than challenge. Lack of agreement, stimulating at one point in time, may become devastating to the project if prolonged, particularly when important issues are involved.

ISSUES AT VARIOUS STAGES OF THE RESEARCH

Some issues remain the same throughout the project; other issues, and their handling, differ according to the stage of the research.

Conceptualization and Design Stage

Interdisciplinary research teams may evolve out of discussion of common interests or may be intentionally recruited according to what each collaborator can contribute to a preselected research question. Regardless of how the team originates, the goal is the assembling of a group of qualified, highly motivated individuals who, working together, can solve a research problem that no one of them could effectively address alone. Issues that would pose barriers to the efficacy of the group are important throughout the life of the research project but are of more serious nature in the conceptual or proposal stage. Mar et al. (1976) differentiated between the nurtured group, formed for a particular research project, and the pooled group whose members have had prior experience in working together. Improper formation of a nurtured group may cause it to disintegrate.

The importance of status concordance for effecting group unity has been pointed out by Gillespie and Birnbaum (1980:44) who defined this concept as "matched-equal ranks between members' university-position/discipline-prestige and their team position." In concordant teams, senior members of higher-prestige disciplines headed teams of junior members and lower-prestige disciplines. If the external status of a team member was not in accord with his or her status on the team, discordance existed. Gillespie and Birnbaum found concordance to be more salient in early team interaction for defining tasks, allocating resources, and guiding communication. After funding or firm establishment of the team, the expertise of individual members relevant to particular problems becomes more important. Funding agencies take team concordance into consideration and may question a principal investigator's ability to motivate and direct team operations if that person holds a lower faculty position or belongs to a less prestigious discipline than other team members.

Nursing has experienced this particular problem. Well-prepared but inexperienced nurse-scientists may select research questions which can best be studied by an interdisciplinary team. They then recruit persons from other disciplines with the necessary expertise to supplement their own. Since the nurse-scientist has selected the problem, done the recruiting of other investigators, and designed the major portion of the study, the nurse becomes the principal investigator. At this point the faculty affiliation of the principal investigator also becomes very important, since it is the investigator's school or discipline to which extramural funds are awarded and to which biomedical research support grants are also awarded, when there has been sufficient federal funding to permit such awards. Many proposals are rejected because funding agencies frequently underestimate the abilities of the nurse-scientists to direct team operations.

Pooled teams obviously need less lead time to get organized and have higher credibility with funding agencies. When schools have research support grants, seed money can be allocated to groups of faculty to form research teams for pilot studies. Some universities provide seed funds as part of each school's budget, an obviously desirable practice.

The kind of leadership the team has is crucial. If the leader is a prima donna who tends to dominate, the research becomes the leader's project and others lose interest. There must be a clear division of labor with each member's role spelled out. This includes the role of the leader. Team members differ according to scholarly productivity, motivation, and ability to work as members of the team. Some persons need autonomy; others become overly dependent on the group. An effective leader will help the group map out each individual's responsibility for the research based on his or her expertise (Luszki, 1957; Benoliel, 1973; Gillespie and Birnbaum, 1980).

Since interdisciplinary research usually requires a large staff, there are really two leaders to be considered for most projects—the principal investigator, who is responsible for administering the whole project, and a project coordinator, who organizes data collection, keeps the subject records, and generally provides the lubricant to keep the day-to-day operations running smoothly. The leadership style and personality of the coordinator are just as important to the project as are those of the principal investigator.

Communication among team members may be difficult at first. Disciplines differ according to values, expectations, perspectives, and semantics. Channels of communication must be provided and kept open. Regularly scheduled staff meetings, seminars, and conferences must be arranged. Bennis (1956) referred to a contemporaneity between cultural products which interdisciplinary research infers. He warned that this might take time and, in some cases, might never occur. Blackwell (1955) recommended the use of position papers and the preparation of a glossary of selected terms, explicitly defined, to bridge the communication gap between members of different disciplines.

Definitions of research itself differ from discipline to discipline. In some, research that is not experimental is not considered research. There may not be consensus on sampling. For certain disciplines, an in-depth study of a convenience sample may be acceptable. For others, it is important to be able to generalize the findings beyond the sample. In experimentation, some will accept the use of a small sample tested over time with each person serving as his or her own control; others will insist on a control group with before-and-after testing. Descriptive and exploratory studies are considered to be research in some disciplines while in others, hypotheses must be tested. Such differences should be taken into consideration when assembling the research team, and decisions made on the issues.

Ultimately, agreement on major issues is necessary, but forcing premature agreement may be detrimental to the project. Fantasy is necessary at the conceptual stage of the research, but in a group interruptions by colleagues may intrude on fantasy and change the conceptualizer's direction (Luszki, 1957). Planned time for individual reading and thinking is important, but channels of communication must also be provided for sharing. Dubin (1969:67) warned that collaboration might force team members to "sing out of the same prayer book" and might thereby extinguish creativity. The end result could be the use of ideas and tools from the dominant discipline or a compromise under which the lowest common denominator of the analytic tools of several disciplines would be selected. When various portions of the research utilize data from differing levels, comparisons of those data frequently use analytic measures with low power.

In the preproposal stage of our child-abuse study, the three investigators for the developmental stage met regularly to discuss one another's ideas about the conceptual framework, the testing of hypotheses, the handling of a mixed design where part of the research would be experimental and part descriptive, and the methodological issues which such a design would provoke. Consultants, local and national, were utilized. Now, after 7 years of working together, the two investigators who remained with the validation stage of the research no longer feel the need to meet on a regularly scheduled basis, meeting now only when it is felt necessary.

There are still regular meetings of the two research teams that work together on a daily basis for data collecting and processing. One team works with collecting and processing self-report, behavioral observation and chart review data, the other team works with physiological data. One or both investigators meet with these groups. These meetings are used for sharing and working out solutions to problems, for keeping the investigators up to date on project progress, and for sharing information about other child-abuse studies. Suggestions from these two teams are utilized when the investigators meet for policy decisions. The whole research team of 12 meets periodically for social functions. Requests for presentations of the research at local, state, and regional meetings are shared with members of the team who decide which one(s) will make the presentation. When visitors come to the project, any team members who are available meet with them. The library on child abuse is housed in the offices of research associates, and material is readily available to all.

Data Production Stage

Some persons refer to this stage as data production rather than data collection, since data, unlike fruit or vegetables, are not readily available for collecting.[3] Researchers must institute procedures for producing the data. Successful use of such procedures is greatly influenced by the persons using them, and training is essential.

In the child-abuse study, it was assumed that some training would be necessary for interviewing, administering questionnaires, videotaping, and applying electrodes. What was not expected was that so much training would be necessary. Nurses, social workers, and counselors were recruited as research associates. Such persons from the helping professions have been taught to help, and when patients or clients ask questions, practitioners and therapists tend to give them complete answers in terms they can easily understand. Therefore, when subjects in our study asked questions about child abuse, parenting, or what we were looking for in videotaped parent-child interactions, our research associates showed a tendency to respond, offering help to parent-subjects who appeared to be having difficulty. Subjects had been told at the time of recruitment that they could ask any questions they wished, but it has been assumed that questions about the outcomes of specific procedures could be fielded during the testing period simply by promising a copy of the findings at the end of the study.

Conflicts between the research role and the clinical role are frequent when practitioners from the helping professions are recruited as research associates. Such personnel have not had much training in research, particularly with respect to the effects produced by the researcher and those due to subject awareness. In some research fields the answer is to recruit persons who do not have much knowledge about the

[3]Credit for the idea of data production should be given to Herbert Costner, Associate Dean, College of Arts and Sciences, University of Washington, who devised the idea while teaching methods courses in sociology.

subject being studied. However, these persons are hired strictly as staff and not as research faculty, since research faculty must be well read in the subject area in order to be able to make presentations at professional and community meetings and to share in publishing the findings.

In nursing research, involving practitioners as research assistants is seen as an important way of encouraging interest in research. Therefore, our solution was to use practitioners, but to provide longer training at repeated intervals. All interviews were taped, and, in the beginning, the project coordinator, who had had extensive interviewing experience, listened to the tapes and discussed them with the interviewers involved. Research associates listened to and recoded tapes of their colleagues' interviews. Effective research techniques were also discussed at weekly team meetings, with emphasis being placed on the possible effects that subject awareness would have on the findings.

Another source of difficulty in the data production stage was the local publicity given to the project. When the research being done has interest to the public, as in the case of child abuse, parenting, or problems of the elderly, or when team members from different disciplines are known in the community, there are frequent requests for interviews by reporters from newspapers, magazines, radio, and television. Local groups, such as professional societies, business groups, parent-teacher associations, high schools and colleges, request speakers on the topic. We were very careful about this in the data collection stages of our research, but there was one source we did not control well enough. At the start of the validation study a local social scientist had asked permission to do secondary analysis of some of our videotapes from the original study to test his nonverbal communication scale. He was given permission for this as well as permission to publish his findings in a small communications journal. Unfortunately, this person felt he could also share his research findings with a local newspaper reporter, who then wrote a

half-page article which appeared in a Sunday edition. In the article the reporter named the project and the principal investigator and described in some detail what we were looking for in parent-child interaction as well as what the social scientist was looking for. We could not determine the effect of this publicity on our subjects, since none of them mentioned having read the article and we hesitated to call it to their attention. At the debriefing 2½ years later, parent-subjects could not remember the incident.

Data Analysis Stage

Problems can also occur during the data analysis stage. The first issue in this stage of the research usually involves the choice of statistics. Ideally, decisions about statistics would be made in the preproposal period. But since very few research projects proceed in an ideal manner, alternative decisions as to what to do with the data are usually considered at the time of analysis. Problems may include use of parametric versus nonparametric statistics. In some disciplines, there is rigid adherence to the use of only those more powerful parametric statistics whose assumptions can be met; for others, regardless of the assumptions, the use of the less powerful nonparametric statistics is frowned upon.

For some disciplines, casual inferences are drawn only when the research is experimental. Others, like Blalock (1964), permit conclusions on causality using regression analysis. Regression analysis is usually considered appropriate only when data are continuous and meet the assumptions necessary for parametric correlation coefficients. Even this last statement is now being questioned, with consideration being given to the use of path analysis for ordinal data (Blalock, 1976; Leik, 1976).

A third problem may involve the use of inferential statistics. For some investigators, little attention is given to the assumption of randomness necessary for determining the statistical significance of findings; for others, there is strict compliance to that assumption (Morrison and

Henkel, 1970). An even more troublesome problem in interdisciplinary research occurs when different segments of the research produce different kinds of data.

In the child-abuse study, the measuring of subjects' physiological responses to child-related behaviors involved two types of experimentation, one where baseline data were collected and subjects served as their own controls, and the other where the version of the stimulus tape used was randomly selected for each subject. Data were of interval level and the choice of using parametric and inferential statistics was easily made. The self-report measures, behavioral observation and chart reviews, produced data which ranged from dichotomous to 7-point Likert scales for which nonparametric and descriptive statistics were indicated. Since we were testing the predictive validity of a battery of measures, comparison of data from all the variables was necessary. In our first study, Kendall's tau was used for intercorrelations of all variables and for generating beta weights for the path analysis. As we near the end of the second study, there is a tendency to become less pure and use more powerful statistics for comparisons.

The second issue in the data analysis stage concerns generalizations of the findings. Again, flexibility may be discipline related. For many reasons, among them attention to human subject protection, it is becoming very difficult to recruit a random sample for prospective research. Comparing sample characteristics with the same characteristics in the population from which they were selected is frequently the best one can do. All team members may not agree with this, and some may insist that generalizations of findings be restricted to the sample. Since interdisciplinary research usually involves practical societal problems and is costly, applying such restriction to the findings may not be pragmatic.

The Sharing of Reporting Stage

Sharing of findings can be done through papers presented at meetings, through publications, or through press releases—formal and informal. The budget for extramural funding usually includes travel for presentation of papers at national meetings. Most funding agencies allocate travel sparingly, and sometimes the number of trips requested for presentation at named meetings is restricted. Procedures must be set up to decide who can utilize the travel funds. For large teams, all members may not have funded travel. In the preproposal stage, it might be good strategy to check with funding agencies to which the proposal will be submitted to learn their policies.

Another problem with giving papers based on research findings is the tendency to publish proceedings of national and international meetings. When proceedings are published, the one who presented the paper is usually the senior author. To have the research findings published as proceedings of a meeting may prevent publication in refereed journals, most of which do not accept material which has been published or submitted elsewhere. This affects all team members.

Decisions about publications, the type of articles, papers, and monographs to be prepared, where to submit manuscripts, order of authors' names on publications, how to give recognition to junior as well as senior staff, whether single author articles will be permitted, and how findings can be divided for publication should all be made early in the collaboration, even at the time of recruitment of team members (Bennis, 1956; Benoliel, 1973; Blackwell, 1955). For some projects, all of the investigators are included as authors with the order of names rotated; for other projects, only those investigators particularly involved with the portion of the research reported are included. Staff members who are not investigators may be asked to write a particular portion of the research, or they themselves may request permission to analyze parts of the data in ways not conceptualized in the proposal. In these cases, negotiations for single authorship may be appropriate. Whatever the publication rules, they should be formal and should be shared among all research staff.

SUMMARY

Conducting interdisciplinary research can be gratifying. As a group it is possible to study research problems which an individual researcher could not address alone. Access to sites and subjects may be facilitated. Collaborating with others can be stimulating, can provide a broader perspective, and can give a wider and more effective range to the application of the findings. Such an endeavor can also be frustrating, with discipline-related problems occurring at each stage of the research. These can be problems of conceptualization, design, data production and analysis, and sharing of the findings once the research is completed.

There has been very little research done on interdisciplinary projects. Much of what has been written has been based on personal experience, not on well designed studies of the research process. One exception to this is the recently completed project at the University of Washington which studied interdisciplinary research teams both within and outside of the university (Newell et al., 1980). Six success factors were delineated in this study:

1 Recognition by the scientific community. Highest ratings were given when investigators were full professors with national reputations.

2 Funding agency involvement. Highest ratings were given in the case of prior contracts with the agency or when the team had been contacted by the agency for the current research or for other research funded by the agency.

3 Group interaction. Teams of long duration rated the highest, followed by current teams having completed previous research and with regularly scheduled formal meetings.

4 Degree of interdisciplinary participation. Ten or more principal investigators (P.I.s) drew highest rating, followed by three to six P.I.s.

5 Size of proposed research. A budget of at least $300,000 rated highest, followed by a budget of at least $250,000.

6 Concept development. Concepts proven via prior research rated highest, then concepts emerging from preliminary research, and, finally, concepts developed in the proposal.

Most of these factors reflect successful team interaction which results from working together over a period of time. It would appear to be highly desirable to facilitate formation of research teams. Some universities have seed funds for this purpose, and biomedical research support grants have been used in some cases. The Nursing Research Emphasis grants from the Division of Nursing, recently awarded to some schools of nursing, have similar purposes, i.e., to provide a climate for collaborative research among faculty members and between faculty and doctoral students.

Another source of funds useful for training nurses for collaborative research is the National Research Service Awards. The Division of Nursing has made three of these institutional awards —one at Teachers College, Columbia University, under the direction of Elizabeth Hagen, one at University of California, San Francisco, under the direction of Anselm Strauss, and one at the University of Washington under the direction of Kathryn Barnard and Mildred Disbrow. These awards provide funds for postdoctoral research fellowships for nurses. The postdoctoral training includes experience in working with existing research teams as well as in developing individual research projects.

The author would like to add to the success factors delineated by Newell et al. (1980), her own list of prerequisites for persons conducting interdisciplinary research. This list would include a dedication to studying the research question, a flexibility with respect to accepting the views of others, a thickness of the epidermis, and a sense of humor. These are all essential requisites, particularly the last. There has been heavy emphasis on the frustrations of conducting interdisciplinary research, but when the cost-benefit ratio of the research is calculated, it usually comes out positive.

EDITOR'S QUESTIONS FOR DISCUSSION

What questions previously raised for discussion by Chaps. 16 and 17 are spoken to by Disbrow? What relationship is there between Werley's and Newcomb's (Chap. 16) concept of a mentor-protégé relationship and concordant teams?

In organizing a study team what queries regarding potential team members should be explored? What criteria might be suggested for selecting who should be the principal investigator and who should be the project coordinator? What predictive factors might be identified as indicators for effective working relationships of a group? What strategies can be proposed to effectively deal with potential personality difficulties among the group?

What are the advantages and disadvantages of recruiting persons to produce the data who do not have as much knowledge about the subject being studied? What considerations are essential in the resolution of conflicts between a team member's research and clinical roles? When should the clinical role supersede the research role in conducting research?

In conducting large studies, what preventive measures can be utilized to protect the privacy and rights of human subjects and the research team? What kinds of situations might arise that could result in an infraction of those rights? What should be done when there is a known violation of those rights during the research process?

What are the essential considerations for choosing parametric and nonparametric statistics in data analysis? To what extent should an investigator indicate the limitations of a statistical test employed in interpretation of data? What legitimate alternatives are there to increase the generalizability of findings? Regarding the publication rules that have been established early in organizing the study team, what situations can arise where renegotiation of the rules is in order? What process should be followed in renegotiating?

REFERENCES

Adams, David
 1969 "Analysis of a life satisfaction index." Journal of Gerontology 24:470–474.
Belsky, Jay
 1980 "Child maltreatment: An ecological integration." American Psychologist 35:320–335.
Bennis, Warren G.
 1956 "Some barriers to teamwork in social research." Social Problems 3:223–335.
Benoliel, Jeanne Q.
 1973 "Collaboration and competition in nursing research." Pp. 1–11 in M. Batey (ed.), Communicating Nursing Research: Collaboration and Competition. Boulder, Colorado: Western Interstate Commission for Higher Education.

Birnbaum, Philip H., William T. Newell, and Borje O. Saxberg
 1979 "Managing academic interdisciplinary research projects." Decision Sciences 10:645–665.
Blackwell, Gordon W.
 1955 "Multidisciplinary team research." Social Forces 33:367–374.
Blalock, Hubert M.
 1964 Causal Inferences in Non-Experimental Research. Chapel Hill: University of North Carolina Press.
 1976 "Can we find a genuine ordinal slope analogue?" Chap. 7 in D. R. Heise (ed.), Sociological Methodology. San Francisco: Jossey-Bass.
Burgess, Robert L. and Rand D. Conger
 1978 "Family interaction in abusive, neglectful

and normal families." Child Development 49:1163–1173.

Caulfield, Colleen, Mildred Disbrow, and Michelle Smith
1977 "Determining indicators of potential for child abuse and neglect: Analytical problems in methodological research." Pp. 141–162 in M. Batey (ed.), Communicating Nursing Research—Optimizing Environments for Health: Nursing's Unique Perspective. Volume 10. Boulder, Colorado.

Disbrow, Mildred A., Hans Doerr, and Colleen Caulfield
1977 "Measuring the components of parents' potential for child abuse and neglect." Child Abuse and Neglect: The International Journal 1:279–296.

Dubin, Robert
1969 "Contiguous problem analysis: An approach to systematic theories about social organization." Pp. 65–76 in M. Sherif and C. Sherif (eds.), Interdisciplinary Relationships in the Social Sciences. Chicago: Aldine.

Elmer, Elizabeth
1977 Fragile Families, Troubled Children. Pittsburgh: University of Pittsburgh Press.

Gelles, Richard J.
1973 "Child abuse as psychopathology: A sociological critique and reformation." American Journal of Orthopsychiatry 43:611–621.

Gil, David
1970 Violence Against Children: Physical Child Abuse in the United States. Cambridge, Massachusetts: Harvard University Press.

Gillespie, David F. and Philip H. Birnbaum
1980 "Status concordance, coordination and success in interdisciplinary research teams." Human Relations 33:41–56.

Kempe, Henry C.
1973 "A practical approach to the protection of the abused child and rehabilitation of the abusing parent." Pediatrics 51:804–812.

Leik, R. K.
1976 "Monotonic regression analysis for ordinal variables." Pp. 271–275 in D. R. Heise (ed.), Sociological Methodology. San Francisco: Jossey-Bass.

Luszki, Margaret B.
1957 "Team research in social science: Major consequences of a growing trend." Human Organization 16:21–24.

Mar, Brian W., William T. Newell, and Borje O. Saxberg
1976 Interdisciplinary Research Issues in a University Setting. Working paper number 7. Research Management Improvement. Seattle: University of Washington.

McTavish, Donald G.
1971 "Perceptions of old people: A review of research methodologies and findings." The Gerontologist 11:90–101.

Milgram, Stanley
1969 "Interdisciplinary thinking and the small world problem." Pp. 103–120 in M. Sherif and C. Sherif (eds.), Interdisciplinary Relationships in the Social Sciences. Chicago: Aldine.

Morrison, Denton E. and Ramon E. Henkel
1970 The Significance Test Controversy. Chicago: Aldine.

Newell, William T., Borje O. Saxberg, Brian W. Mar, and Sheila A. Adams
1980 Guidelines for Applied Interdisciplinary Research in the University: How to Manage the University's Role in Solving Society's Problems. Project report number 11. Research Management Improvement. Seattle: University of Washington.

Parke, Ross D. and Candace Whitmer Collmer
1975 "Child abuse: An interdisciplinary analysis." Pp. 509–590 in E. M. Hetherington (ed.), Review of Child Development Research. Volume 5. Chicago: University of Chicago Press.

Patterson, G. R.
1974 "A basis for identifying stimuli which control behaviors in natural settings." Child Development 45:900–911.

Peter, Lawrence F. and Raymond Hull
1969 The Peter Principle. New York: Morrow.

Peterson, Warren A.
1971 "Research priorities on perceptions and

orientations toward aging and toward older people." The Gerontologist 11:60–63.

Sherif, Muzafer and Carolyn W. Sherif
  1969 "Interdisciplinary coordination as a validity check: Retrospect and prospects." Pp. 3-20 in M. Sherif and C. Sherif (eds.), Interdisciplinary Relationships in the Social Sciences. Chicago: Aldine.

Steele, Brandt F. and Carl B. Pollock
  1968 "A psychiatric study of parents who abuse infants and small children," Pp. 89-133 in R. Helfer and C. H. Kempe (eds.) The Battered Child. Chicago: University of Chicago Press.

Woodruff, Diana S. and James E. Birren (eds.)
  1975 Aging: Scientific Perspectives and Social Issues. New York: D. Van Nostrand.

Chapter 19

Judging Ethical Issues in Nursing: Research Strategy and Selected Correlates

Shaké Ketefian, R.N., Ed.D., F.A.A.N.
Associate Professor
Division of Nursing
New York University
New York, New York

Research directed to critical aspects of clinical practice is the substance of this chapter and the four that follow by Chaska, Mercadante, Stein, Sweeney, and Gordon. In a time when professional nurses are increasingly overwhelmed with dilemmas in moral decision making, Shaké Ketefian's research is extremely relevant. Her essay focuses on approaches to values education—specifically the development of moral reasoning as a tool to measure moral behavior. Emphasis is on reasoning about moral choice, not content of the choice. Due to the fact that ethical resolutions to matters lies within a professional's individual conscience and morality, Ketefian views it as critical to explicate the process of moral reasoning and determine whether the process is related to actual decisions a professional would make in conflict situatior s. The three conceptual levels: preconventional, conventional, and postconventional (principled reasoning) are clearly defined. Each level includes two stages, logical and moral. The logical stage sets limits to the moral stage an individual can attain. There are three characteristics of the stages which pertain to consistency, a tendency to move forward, and incorporation of lower-stage thinking into a higher level. Ketefian reviews pertinent literature. One study shows that four academic groups of students in the same nursing program were not significantly different in their moral reasoning levels.

Ketefian discusses the methodological difficulties in constructing a tool to measure moral behavior in nursing. She describes her strategy to devise an instrument in which the Code for Nurses is utilized as a standard against which moral choices made by nurses can be assessed and measured. The instrument, called "Judgments about Nursing Decisions" (JAND), is a self-administered, 48-item objective test with seven stories of ethical dilemmas that frequently occur. Two variables are measured: knowl-

This is an expansion of the original article "Moral reasoning and moral behavior among selected groups of practicing nurses," Nursing Research 30(3):171–176.

edge and valuation of ideal moral behavior and perception of realistic moral behavior in nursing dilemmas. The vital validation process for the tool included the utilization of eight nationally recognized authorities in nursing ethics who are closely associated with the Code of Nurses.

Ketefian shows the findings of her correlational study with 79 practicing nurses in which the JAND tool was utilized. The data indicate a significant discrepancy between educational groups for ideal values but not for likely action scores. The data support the theory that the process of moral reasoning is related to moral behavior.

The data indicate that type of education in nursing, critical thinking, and moral reasoning are predictor variables. In explaining the findings, Ketefian cites many other variables that are likely to influence nurses' decisions and behavior. Factors such as organizational policy, the degree of professional autonomy, and the relationship of nurses with other health care providers are discussed. With education being a crucial variable in the finding, Ketefian focuses on the implications for nursing education and the manner in which ethical issues are taught in nursing curricula. She concludes that moral reasoning can be enhanced by specific learning experiences in curriculum and approach at the institutional level.

INTRODUCTION

Societal and technological changes, along with changes occurring in nursing, have forced the profession to confront controversial issues. Abortion, right to die, rights of clients to claims of self-determination about what will be done to their persons—these problems have pressed themselves on the consciousness of society at large and professionals alike. Such issues as these have overlapping legal and ethical implications as they demand resolution in specific conflicts. Courts have been leading the way in recent years, and headlines have abounded about decisions rendered that are viewed as authoritative and binding. The locus of the *ethical* resolutions to such matters, however, tends to reside within individual professionals, their realms of competence, authority, and power, and above all, their individual conscience and morality. External pressures from the society at large, combined with internal pressures within the disciplines themselves, have caused rethinking of the adequacy of traditional values and codes of conduct that most service professionals have had.

The teaching of ethics and values in American higher education has had an uncertain fate in the past century and has depended on factors at play in the society at large, as well as those having to do with the development of the state of knowledge in the fields of natural and social sciences (Sloan, 1979). A renewed interest in the roles of ethics and values in a complex and technological society is manifest. While much is written about the teaching of ethics, suspicion prevails that this may be tantamount to *indoctrination* of specific values. Perhaps as a result, despite the concern for the area the teaching of ethics does not appear to be a fundamental component of university curricula.

An important component in the teaching of ethics relates to the development of a personal and professional sense of responsibility; this involves creating such awareness as is needed to distinguish issues that are moral from those that are not, as well as strategies involved in developing analytic and problem-solving skills to enable a professional to approach a moral dilemma rationally and cognitively rather than intuitively.

These two areas—that having to do with what values are taught or comprise the content of ethical decisions, and that having to do with the teaching of strategies which enable a person to reason, analyze, and offer appropriate justifications for actions taken—have frequently been dichotomized in the literature, implicitly or explicitly. The fact remains, however, that they are interwoven in their implementation and tend to influence one another, even though they can be, and often are, conceptually dealt with as separate domains of inquiry.

In an effort to enhance understanding of the way analytic and reasoning strategies influence the nature of values held and the type of ethical decisions professionals make in ethical dilemmas, this chapter draws on relevant literature, presents a recently developed research strategy to measure moral behavior, describes its use in a correlational study, with implications for the profession, and suggests next steps.

REVIEW OF LITERATURE

Moral Development

At present, a major approach to values education is that of moral development. Its primary goal is to stimulate the development of moral reasoning. Placed within the tradition of cognitive-developmental psychology, it provides a portrait of perceiving human beings where "the human psyche develops through sequential stages, each of which is characterized by higher capacity for logical, abstract thought than the stage preceding it" (Samples, 1978:221).

Building on the ideas of Dewey and the research of Piaget, Kohlberg refined and validated a hierarchical scheme of moral development. His research encompassed longitudinal and cross-cultural studies over a 20-year period. Moral development focuses on the person's *reasoning* about moral choice, rather than the content of the choice. Such reasoning is said to reveal the *structure* of the person's moral judgment. Kohlberg (1978:50-51) conceptualized three levels of moral development, with two stages within each level, for a total of six stages.

At the preconventional level of moral reasoning, externally established rules determine right or wrong action, interpreted in a pragmatic way. In moving toward the conventional level a person is mindful of the expectations of family and group; loyalty and conformity to the existing social order are considered important. At the highest, or postconventional, level of moral reasoning, the individual autonomously examines and defines moral values and principles apart from the group norms or that of the culture. This level is also referred to as *principled reasoning.* Kohlberg (1978:39) posits that moral reasoning is centered on 10 universal values or concerns: punishment, property, roles and concerns of affection, roles and concerns of authority, law, life, liberty, distribution of justice, truth, and sex. A conflict between two or more of these values necessitates a moral choice and its subsequent justification by the individual, requiring systematic utilization of the person's problem-solving and other cognitive capabilities.

Stages in moral development theory have three characteristics: (1) they are "structured wholes," organized systems of thought in which people are *consistent* in their levels of moral judgment; (2) they have "invariant sequence," where people tend to move forward; and (3) they are "hierarchical integrations," where higher-stage thinking incorporates all levels of lower-stage thinking (Rest, 1974a:242). At higher levels of moral development, there is an increasing adequacy for solving complex moral problems whereby the scope of the person's conceptualization of moral issues is more universal and less situation-bound (Rest, 1974b).

Cognitive development is related to moral development in that the former facilitates the latter (Keasey, 1975). Specifically, the concept of "structural parallelism" suggests that as cognitive transformation takes place developmentally, thinking on moral issues changes as well (Piaget, 1965). Kohlberg (1973) maintains that while cognitive development is a *necessary, prerequisite* condition, placing a ceiling on moral development, it is *not a sufficient condition*. More recently, Kohlberg tried to depict the complex nature of the relationship between cognitive thought and moral reasoning as follows:

> Since moral reasoning clearly is reasoning, advanced moral reasoning depends upon advanced logical reasoning; a person's logical stage puts a certain ceiling on the moral stage he can attain. A person whose logical stage is only concrete operational is limited to the preconventional moral stages (Stages 1 and 2). A person whose logical stage is only partially formal operational is limited to the conventional moral stages (Stages 3 and 4). While logical development is necessary for moral development and sets limits to it, most individuals are higher in logical stage than they are in moral stage. As an example, over 50 percent of late adolescents and adults are capable of full formal reasoning, but only 10 percent of these adults (all formal operational) display principled (Stages 5 and 6) moral reasoning (1978:38).

In the last few years a number of nurse investigators have studied moral reasoning among nurses. Murphy (1976) found that 95 percent of her sample of 120 nurses were at the conventional level of moral reasoning. When Munhall (1979) studied moral reasoning levels of 15 nurse faculty and of groups of freshman, sophomore, junior, and senior nursing students, she found no significant differences among the four student groups, although there were significant differences between students and faculty. Students tended to be at the conventional level, while faculty was at the principled level. Findings from these two studies are not directly comparable because of differences in types of samples utilized, and most importantly, because of differences in the tools used to measure moral development.

Ketefian utilizing a sample of practicing nurses, found a significant and positive correlation between critical thinking and moral reasoning ($r = .5326$, $p = .001$), which confirmed Keasey's, Piaget's, and Kohlberg's contentions (1981a).

Factors other than cognitive and intellectual development are thought to affect moral development. Social and educational climates are said to be crucial; environments that provide opportunities for participation, shared decision making, and assumption of responsibility for consequences of action tend to stimulate moral judgment development (Kohlberg, 1971:183). Also, if the educational process intentionally creates cognitive conflict and disequilibrium by showing inadequacies of a person's mode of thinking, the individual is stimulated to seek higher and more adequate levels of moral reasoning (Rest et al., 1969).

Individuals can respond to and assimilate verbalizations of concepts that are one stage above their own (Rest et al., 1969). That is, the teacher who is to create the cognitive disequilibrium needed to assist the upward movement of students' moral development must be at a higher level of moral reasoning. While the majority, though not all, of the nurse instructors in Munhall's (1979) study were at the principled level, their direct impact is difficult to assess from that study. The faculty sample was small and while they *may* have been instrumental in helping upward stage movement in the students, the design and one-time measurement might have failed to detect such change. To depict change and to assess how enduring such change might be, longitudinal studies are needed. The distressing point remains that the four academic groups of students in the *same* nursing program were not significantly different in their moral reasoning levels. This finding is especially important in view of the fact that education has been demonstrated to account for the greatest part of the variance in moral development through numerous studies (Kohlberg, 1973; Rest, 1975:79; Rest, 1976).

The centerpiece of Kohlberg's work on moral reasoning and of the works of authors mentioned so far relates to the *reasoning process* about moral choice, as opposed to the *content* of the choice. Thus, it is possible for two persons to be at the same moral developmental stage and yet indicate completely different answers to a moral dilemma.

For example, in a typical story in which a man is faced with the possibility of stealing a drug to save his wife's life, one respondent might say, "Yes, he should steal," while another might say, "No, he should not steal." Depending on the nature of the justifications they offer and the reasons they give, both persons may be at the same stage or they may be at different stages.

Moral Reasoning and Moral Behavior

An implicit assumption prevails in the literature that persons at higher moral reasoning stages are more likely to act "morally" than those who are at lower stages. Such an assumption appears to be inherent in the definition of postconventional, principled reasoning rather than based on a body of empirical evidence. Thus, the suggestion has been advanced that a nurse who is at the principled level of moral reasoning "questions authority, and abides by social norms insofar as they serve human values, which is the essence of moral obligations" (Munhall, 1979:30). Similarly, Murphy (1976) contends that movement to principled thinking enables a nurse to act as a morally responsible agent and as advocate for patient rights. These statements, and others similar to them, suggest at once that an inference is being made from the thought process to the content of the moral choice or to the nature of the moral act itself. They also point up the perennial philosophical and unresolved question: Is ethics grounded in process, content, or a combination of the two, or does it reside elsewhere?

It is not the intent of the present essay to resolve this philosophical dilemma. Rather, given the nature of our complex health care delivery system and the importance of the nurse's role in that system, it is proposed that the public has a right to expect that nurses practice "morally," according to some established standards, and further, that they do so with thought and reflection—in essence, that they act "morally" for the "right" reasons (as opposed to actions based on intuition, self-interest, pragmatic considerations, etc.)

Fenton (1978) addressed the relationship between moral reasoning and moral action in a suggestive study. An experimenter requested subjects to fill out and return a form, for which a stamped, addressed envelope was provided; the experimenter told the subjects that failure to return the form on time would result in her failing a course. Only 30 percent of subjects at stages 2 and 3 returned the form on time, while 70 percent of stage 4 subjects and 100 percent of stage 5 subjects did so. The study, though revealing, is hardly conclusive.

Kohlberg (1971) and Wilson (1978) have contended that the teaching of values is ineffective and constitutionally and philosophically unjustifiable. Perhaps partly as a result of such thinking, many authors who write on the aims and purposes of education have emphasized the need for developing problem-solving strategies and decision-making capabilities and for enabling the individual to learn principles and to perform "synthesizing operations" (Rest, 1974a:242).

Similar ideas about the aim of professional education are expressed by nurse-educators in dealing with theoretical and research-based knowledge (Rogers, 1970:138) to develop intellectual skills and operations so that the practitioner can assess a broad range of cues (Schlotfeldt, 1965); engage in complex problem-solving (Johnson, 1968); and practice autonomously in decision making, action, and assumption of individual responsibility for consequences of one's acts (Kohnke, 1978). These very qualities valued for professional nurses are those that, according to Murphy (1976), would enable a person to engage in postconventional moral reasoning and to act as a morally responsible agent.

Based on such support found in the literature, it has been contended that if in fact professional nursing programs emphasize the development of qualities mentioned, nurses from these programs will have higher levels of moral reasoning; therefore, a descriptive study was designed and was replicated recently with a different sample of practicing nurses, hypothesizing that there will be a relationship between educational preparation, critical thinking, and moral judgment (Ketefian, 1981a). In both studies, which used completely different samples, there was a significant relationship between education and moral judgment (at the .01 level), and between critical thinking and moral judgment (at the .001 level). It was further found that education and critical thinking *together* accounted for 32.8 percent of the variance in moral reasoning.

Yet, the question remains as to how, and whether, moral reasoning, which addresses the *process* of reasoning, is related to the actual decisions a professional would make in ethical conflict situations.

Despite views advanced by certain authors about the inadvisability or unconstitutionality of teaching values, society expects that professionals practice with certain ethical standards—values, if you will. To this end, more established professions have evolved a code of ethics according to which its members are expected to practice. That these codes endorse certain values which a given professional group contends to uphold is clear. Some of the questions that have continued to be debated, however, relate to: What are the most effective methods or strategies to inculcate and teach these codes and values in the professional curriculum? How can a profession most effectively monitor violations of its code by its members?

The nursing profession first endorsed a code for professional conduct in 1950. Since then the code has been periodically revised and updated to meet the demands of evolving practice. As the code has evolved, one of the major shifts has been away from a prescriptive approach, addressed to the personal conduct of the nurse, toward endorsement of universal ethical values that are intended to be applicable to a wide range of situations. The present Code for Nurses (American Nurses' Association, 1976) is intended to serve as a general guide to nurses for resolving ethical conflicts that arise in practice.

Such review and beginning research evidence led to the postulation that three selected variables—namely, the nature of nurses' educational preparation, critical thinking, and the level of moral judgment—would help predict nurses' moral behavior or ethical decision making in simulated moral dilemmas in nursing.

Measuring Moral Behavior

The major problem, therefore, was to devise a tool to measure moral behavior in nursing. Given the normative nature of this construct and the inherent difficulties in making operational normative aspects of behavior, it was not surprising that no measuring device was available. In constructing a tool, the decision was made at the outset to utilize the Code for Nurses as the standard against which moral choices made by nurses would be assessed and measured. Given that the Code is the official statement of the professional association intended to "provide a framework for the nurses to make ethical decisions and discharge responsibilities to the public, to other members of the health team, and to the profession" (American Nurses' Association, 1976:1), the document seemed a logical choice to serve the purpose expressed above.

Seven stories were constructed, depicting a nurse in an ethical dilemma. While the stories are hypothetical, they were drawn from a pool of over 100 stories practicing nurses provided from their own experiences. A group of nurse clinicians assessed the dilemmas in the stories to ascertain that they represent realistic occurrences in nursing practice situations. No effort was made to include all possible kinds of dilemmas that nurses might encounter. Effort was made to avoid certain ethical issues such as those dealing with termination of life support systems or with genetic engineering, since such situations do not occur on a daily basis. The seven stories confront issues, such as: threats to patient safety as a result of understaffing; incompetent and/or unethical conduct of nurse colleagues or other professionals; demands from clients for the "truth" about their condition where the nurse knows the patient has been lied to; and client self-determination in the face of other demands on the nurse.

After the stories were constructed and their representativeness ascertained, 12 practicing nurses subsequently discussed the dilemmas and generated a series of nursing actions for each story. Following this step, eight nurses, who are nationally recognized authorities in nursing ethics and who are closely associated with the Code for Nurses, rated *each* nursing action, for *each* story, on a scale of 1 to 5, the degree to which the nursing action embodied ethical nursing behavior advocated in the Code. As a result of this validation process each nursing action was assigned a weight for later scoring.

Validity The instrument has content and face validity in two respects; first, it includes a reasonably representative sampling of the domain of ethical nursing conflicts; second, all the items in the tool were assessed and evaluated by experts in terms of the extent to which each embodies the tenets of the Code, which served as the standard for moral behavior.

Reliability The instrument was administered to 63 nurses in a pilot and an internal consistency test was done using coefficient a; this yielded an a of .70. Item analysis led to further refinement and elimination of a few weak items.

The instrument is called *Judgments about Nursing Decisions* (JAND) and is a self-administered, 48-item, objective test with seven stories of ethical dilemmas. Following each story is a list of nursing actions, ranging five to eight in number. Respondents are asked to check "yes" or "no" for each nursing action twice: first, in column A, where they are asked whether they thought the nurse experiencing the dilemma in the story *should* or *should not* engage in that action; second, in column B, which ask whether or not they thought the nurse experiencing the dilemma is *likely* to engage in the nursing action. JAND therefore measures two variables instead of one. One variable is called *knowledge and valuation of ideal moral behavior in nursing dilemmas*

and is the respondent's score on column A; the second is called *perception of realistic moral behavior in nursing dilemmas* and is the respondent's score on column B.

The instrument was utilized in a correlational study with 79 practicing nurses as respondents; 43 nurses had a baccalaureate degree, 36 either a diploma or associate degree. The predictor variables were type of education in nursing, critical thinking, and moral reasoning; the criterion variables were the two columns in Judgments about Nursing Decisions: knowledge and valuation of ideal moral behavior in nursing dilemmas (column A scores), and perception of realistic moral behavior in nursing dilemmas (column B scores).

The details of this research are presented elsewhere (Ketefian, 1981a, 1981b). After a brief presentation of the findings, their ramifications for research and for the profession at large will be discussed.

Table 19-1 presents a correlation matrix for the study variables; Table 19-2 compares the mean differences for columns A and B for the entire sample, as well as differences between and within the two educational groups.

The theory that the *process* of moral reasoning is related to moral behavior—using the Code for Nurses as the standard for the latter—is supported by these data. This relationship was stronger with the "knowledge and valuation" component of moral behavior than for "perception of realistic moral behavior." Data also supported existing research evidence that moral reasoning *is reasoning* (Kohlberg, 1978:38), as seen by the high magnitude of correlation between critical thinking and moral reasoning (.53). It can be seen from Table 19-1 that educational preparation and moral reasoning account for varying amounts of variance in the study variables.

Table 19-2 highlights two important facts. The first is that there were significant differences between educational groups for column A scores but *not* for column B scores. Second, for the

Table 19-1   Correlation Matrix Presenting the Pearson Product Moment Correlation Coefficients for Five Variables (N = 79)

| | Study variables | | | | |
| | | | | Moral behavior | |
Study Variables	Educational preparation*	Moral reasoning	Critical thinking	Column A	Column B
Educational preparation	1.00				
Moral reasoning	-.33‡	1.00			
Critical thinking	-.21†	.53‡	1.00		
Moral behavior					
Column A	-.36‡	.28‡	.19†	1.00	
Column B	-.19†	.19†	-.003	.18†	1.00

*Minus sign is a function of dummy variables created for educational preparation.
† $p = .05$.
‡ $p = .01$.

entire sample and for the two educational groups, there were significant differences between column A and B scores, indicating that nurses generally had a different response pattern for column B than they did for column A.

IMPLICATIONS

Discrepancy between Knowledge and Valuation and Perception of Realistic Moral Behavior

It is important to note that while Table 19-1 shows a modest positive correlation between column A and B, this is deceptive. A t-test (Table 19-2) showed significant differences between the

means of *all* respondents. Why did such discrepancy exist between nursing actions that nurses indicated they knew and valued, as opposed to what they thought was likely to be implemented? The possible explanations may be both theoretical and methodological in nature.

Inherent in the nursing actions in the JAND is a combination of values, beliefs, knowledge, and attitudes endorsed personally and professionally. No effort was made to parcel out these dynamic elements in the construction of the items. In column A, respondents were asked to check what they thought nurse X in the story should do. Here, there is a good likelihood that their responses reflect their own beliefs, values, and

Table 19-2   Comparison of Mean Differences for Moral Behavior for Entire Sample, and *Between* and *Within* Educational Groups, by *t*-Test

Group	N	t value	Degrees of freedom	p Value
Entire sample (for col. A vs. B)	79	12.45	78	< .01
Professional nurses (for col. A vs. B)	43	9.49	42	< .01
Nursing technicians (for col. A vs. B)	36	7.98	35	< .01
Professional vs. technician (for col. A)		-3.39	77	< .01
(for col. B)		-1.73	77	> .01

knowledge of what they knew to be professionally appropriate behavior. On the other hand, in column B nurses were asked what they thought nurse X in the story was likely to do. This may have placed the nurses in the position of predicting someone else's behavior, or giving their *assessment* of what they thought would actually happen, as opposed to what they themselves would do in the dilemmas. If this is the case, the validity of any inferences from such an assessment to what the respondent might actually do is open to question, and this aspect would require further methodological investigation. McGuire et al. (1976) provide a strong case for the validity of simulations and inferences drawn from them; it is not clear, however, whether an inference could more validly be made if the question asked for column B were "If you were nurse X, what would you do?" as opposed to the question that was asked, "What do you think nurse X is realistically likely to do?"

Also, despite the documented validity of simulations and their relative convenience as measurement devices, the question of the correspondence between a person's responses to hypothetical situations versus the individual's behavior in real-life situations must be posed. Given the complex and normative nature of moral behavior, many variables are likely to come into play that might influence nurses' decisions and behavior. Factors such as organizational policy, the degree of professional autonomy and authority nurses may possess, and the relationship of nurses vis-à-vis other health care providers may vary in settings. The simulated situations in JAND mostly address the ethical dimensions of nurse-client relationships and the imperatives that arise in the case of unethical or incompetent behavior of another professional (nurse or other), but they do not address the three factors mentioned above. The instrument does, however, provide the respondent the opportunity to consider these factors under column B, which calls for "likely" action.

Beyond these inherent methodological difficulties, an examination of sample items presented in Tables 19-3 and 19-4 may suggest additional explanations. A close scrutiny of the items in Table 19-3 where there is no, or minimal, discrepancy between columns A and B reveals these to be actions that involve one-to-one dealings with a patient; further, these are actions that do not entail risk taking or entering into negotiations

Table 19-3   Sample Items Indicating General Agreement Between Column A and Column B*

	Column A (Should do)		Column B (Likely to do)	
	Yes, %	No, %	Yes, %	No, %
1 Allow Mrs. J to talk out about how she feels about consenting (to an autopsy) and explore her reasons. Whatever decision Mrs. J finally makes, the nurse supports.	97.5	2.5	94.9	5.1
2 Ascertain if the mother understands the implications of her offer to donate a kidney (to her son).	97.5	2.5	94.9	5.1
3 Postpone *all* nonessential tasks so that everyone can focus on patients' safe care.	98.7	1.3	89.9	10.1
4 Help Mr. T problem-solve, i.e., explore with him the implications of having surgery and of not having surgery.	96.2	3.8	88.6	11.4
5 Support Mr. T in whatever decision he makes.	94.9	3.8	88.6	10.1

*N = 79.

Table 19-4   Sample Items Indicating General Disagreement Between Column A and
Column B *

	Column A (Should do)		Column B (Likely to do)	
	Yes, %	No, %	Yes, %	No, %
1 Write a signed letter to the medical board stating her concerns (about an alcoholic physician).	86.1	12.7	25.3	72.2
2 She need do nothing; it is not nurse M's responsibility to "clean up" medical practice.	5.1	93.7	48.1	49.4
3 Speak to Dr. Z privately, and express concern about his health and patient safety.	83.5	15.2	36.7	62.0
4 Tell the supervisor that safe care cannot be assured and that she (nurse P) will not accept responsibility. Also tell her this will be documented on Katie's chart.	70.9	27.8	46.8	51.9
5 Ask to have a conference with Mr. T, family, herself, the head nurse, and the physician to discuss the matter.	84.8	15.2	17.7	79.7

*N = 79.

with others. They are supportive, expressive of understanding of the patient's predicament. The item "postpone *all* nonessential tasks so that everyone can focus on patients' safe care" also suggests that the nurse has control over the situation. A similar scrutiny of Table 19-4, where there is high or moderate degree of discrepancy between columns A and B, reveals nursing actions that require varying degrees of risk taking, negotiating, and possible confrontation with others, some of whom may be perceived as authority figures. From these data in Table 19-4 it may be possible to speculate that nurses perceive large organizations as presenting constraints to their practice, substantially diminishing their professional control over their own practice. Such perception of these constraints may stem from hierarchical structuring of authority, from work pressures, or from existing rules and regulations. This discrepancy between ideal values and likely action may also reflect uncertainty among nurses as to the amount of support that might be forthcoming from peers or nursing administration if they did engage in

risk-taking behavior or challenged authority figures.

In any case, it is interesting to note such patterns as indicated from the examples above among the agreement and disagreement items—especially in view of the methodological point raised earlier, that is, were these nurses implicitly responding to column B in terms of what they themselves would do, or were they predicting someone else's behavior? If the former is the case, the presence of organizational constraints or lack of control nurses may have over their practice needs to be considered seriously. If the latter is the case, then perhaps nurses tend to regard other nurses negatively, or in any case as being less principled than themselves. All these elements need to be better understood and viewed as impinging on the behavior of nurses in ethical dilemmas.

There may also be an indication for the practice arena to clearly distinguish areas of responsibility and functions for nursing personnel that are commensurate with the educational preparation, knowledge, and skills of the individual nurse, so that each may utilize her or his strengths and preparation background to the client's fullest advantage and in a manner which provides greater satisfaction for the nurse.

Another area for investigation that merits attention relates to personality characteristics of nurses as a group and how these may be affecting their practice, their behavior in ethical conflict, and indeed, the professionalization and professional image of nursing. Variables such as degree of assertiveness, ego development, willingness to take risk, and the degree to which nurses feel they can direct and control what happens to them (internal locus of control) as opposed to feeling that fate or others determine what happens to them (external locus of control) all merit consideration in this context.

Implications for Nursing Education

Another important finding with clear implications for the educational process in nursing is that type of educational preparation was an important variable in relation to both moral reasoning and moral behavior. Professionally prepared nurses were shown to have higher levels of moral reasoning and more adequate levels of moral behavior. Interestingly, while critical thinking was highly correlated with moral reasoning and accounted for 28.3 percent of variance in moral reasoning, it was only weakly related to moral behavior (column A only). It is possible that critical thinking—used as an index of cognitive development—is an important mediating or intervening variable, and its impact on moral behavior may be reflected via moral reasoning. Both Piaget (1965) and Kohlberg (1976) propose that moral reasoning levels reflect an interaction between cognitive development and social-educational experiences. While variations in moral reasoning tend to occur within samples at similar educational and age levels, Kohlberg (1973) reported that moral reasoning tends to stabilize at the time the person leaves the educational environment, and that subjects who did not

attend college did not develop principled moral reasoning. This indicates that education is a crucial variable. However, it cannot be regarded as automatically enhancing moral reasoning, but rather, to do so it must have certain qualities and provide certain experiences. Learning experiences and opportunities that are new and different can stimulate and help restructure the thought process (Rest, 1974b). Group participation and discussion reflecting on social and moral issues and conflicts have been known to stimulate moral reasoning. Participation in democratic decision making, assumption of responsibility, and accountability for one's own behavior also provide opportunities for enhancing moral reasoning.

Given the random way in which ethical issues are taught in nursing curricula at present (Aroskar, 1977), there may be indications for more focused attention aimed at stimulating moral development; systematic strategies need to be explored, such as dilemma discussion, ways of creating cognitive disequilibrium so the student can see the inadequacy of his thought process. Also, nurse-educators may need to consider the governance structures of their institutions and the degree to which students are involved in the day-to-day educational process as active, participating agents, as well as the degree to which they contribute to the formation of educational and institutional policies that affect them. Patterns of thought and behavior begin forming while at school. If students experience the educational environment as authoritarian and are engaged only in a passive way, it is hard to see how such individuals will be able to deal with difficult practice situations in a creative, assertive, and responsible manner upon beginning their employment. It is important to note then that enhancing moral reasoning involves both inclusion of specific learning experiences in the curriculum and a total approach at the institutional level. The findings from the present study seem to suggest that when moral reasoning is enhanced, a person is more likely to behave adequately in ethical conflicts.

Future Steps in Research

The tool utilized to measure moral behavior is new; further refinements are indicated, with special attention to strengthening its reliability and building a continuing case for its construct validity. These efforts are currently under way. It may also be worthwhile to study what influence the instructions to the participants may have on their responses. For instance, if the subjects were asked, "If you were nurse X what should you do?" and, "If you were nurse X, what would you actually do?"—would these questions elicit more truthful and valid responses than were obtained from the present set of instructions?

Alternative approaches to measuring moral behavior may be considered. Given the present state of meager empirical data in this area, alternative and exploratory approaches may point to fruitful insights and directions.

EDITOR'S QUESTIONS FOR DISCUSSION

What societal and professional factors have contributed to the increased need for the teaching of ethics? Does the establishment of ethical values precede, follow, or interact with principled moral reasoning in moral development? Does principled moral reasoning preclude conflicts evolving between two or more values? How does focusing on a professional's reasoning about moral choice reveal the structure of a person's moral judgment? To what extent can consistent modes of thought be a predictor of moral judgment? How is it possible for two persons being at the same moral developmental stage to indicate completely different answers to a moral dilemma? Can the assumptions that persons at higher moral-reasoning stages are more likely to act "morally" than those who are at lower stages be validated? How can the public's expectations that nurses act "morally" for the "right" reasons be assured?

Can a student's logical stage in reasoning be changed retrogressively and/or progressively? What factors inhibit advanced logical reasoning? What might account for most individuals being higher in the logical than the moral stage of reasoning? What impact can faculty have on students if their level of moral reasoning is higher than or lower than the students? What qualities of nursing education programs enhance or inhibit nurses to develop higher levels of moral reasoning? What variables might account for the finding in one study that four groups of students in the same nursing program were not different in their moral reasoning levels? What strategies might be used to increase the internalization of ethical values by students? When might ethical issues most effectively be taught in a university curriculum? What other implications does Ketefian's study have for nursing education?

What are the implications for nursing practice and the profession in supporting risk-taking behavior? How, to what extent, and by whom should risk-taking behavior be encouraged? What other explanations might be offered for Ketefian's findings?

To what extent are there limitations in utilizing the JAND tool? How can the reliability and construct validity of the tool be strengthened? How would you respond to her final query concerning increasing the possible validity of the "ideal" and "actual" questions? How can the validity of inferences drawn from simulations be increased? What alternative approaches to measuring moral behavior might be considered?

REFERENCES

American Nurses' Association
1976 Code for Nurses with Interpretive Statements. Kansas City, Mo.: American Nurses' Association.

Aroskar, M.
1977 "Ethics in the nursing curriculum." Nursing Outlook 25:260–264.

Fenton, E.
1978 "Moral education: The research findings." Pp. 52–59 in P. Scharf (ed.), Readings in Moral Education. Minneapolis: Winston Press.

Johnson, D. E.
1968 "Professional practice and specialization in nursing." Image 2:2–7.

Keasey, C. B.
1975 "Implications of cognitive development for moral reasoning." Pp. 39–56 in D. DePalma and J. Foley (eds.), Moral Development: Current Theory and Research. New York: Wiley.

Ketefian, S.
1981a "Critical thinking, educational preparation and development of moral judgment in selected groups of practicing nurses." Nursing Research 30(3):98–103.
1981b "Moral reasoning and moral behavior among selected groups of practicing nurses." Nursing Research 30(3):171–176.

Kohlberg, L.
1971 "From is to ought: How to commit the naturalistic fallacy and get away with it in the study of moral development." Pp. 151–235 in T. Mischel (ed.), Cognitive Development and Epistemology. New York: Academic Press.
1973 "Continuities in childhood and adult word development revisited," Pp. 179–204 in P. B. Boltes and K. W. Schaie (eds.), Life-Span Developmental Psychology, Personality and Socialization. New York: Academic Press, 1973.
1976 "Moral stages and moralization: The cognitive developmental approach," in T. Lickona (ed.), Moral Development and behavior. New York: Holt, Rinehart and Winston.

1978 "The cognitive-developmental approach to moral education." Pp. 36–51 in P. Scharf (ed.), Readings in Moral Education. Minneapolis: Winston Press.

Kohnke, M. F.
1978 The Case for Consultation in Nursing: Designs for Professional Practice. New York: Wiley.

McGuire, C. R., L. M. Solomon, and P. G. Bashook
1976 Construction and Use of Written Simulations. New York: The Psychological Corporation.

Munhall, P.
1979 Moral Reasoning Levels of Nursing Students and Faculty in a Baccalaureate Nursing Program. Unpublished doctoral dissertation, Teachers College, Columbia University.

Murphy, C. P.
1976 Levels of Moral Reasoning in a Selected Group of Nursing Practitioners. Unpublished doctoral dissertation, Teachers College, Columbia University.

Piaget, J.
1965 The Moral Judgment of the Child. New York: The Free Press. (Originally published, 1932.)

Rest, J.
1974a "Developmental psychology as a guide to value education: A review of Kohlbergian programs." Review of Educational Research 44:241–258.
1974b "The cognitive developmental approach to morality: The state of the art." Counseling and Values 18(2):64–78.
1975 "Recent research on an objective test of moral judgment: How the important issues of a moral dilemma are defined." Pp. 75–93 in D. DePalma and J. Foley (eds.), Moral Development: Current Theory and Research. New York: Wiley.
1976 Moral Judgments Related to Sample Characteristics. Minneapolis: University of Minnesota.

Rest, J., E. Turiel, and L. Kohlberg
1969 "Levels of moral development as a determinant of preference and comprehension of moral judgments made by others." Journal of Personality 37:225–252.

Rogers, M. E.
    1970 The Theoretical Basis of Nursing. Phila-
          delphia: F. A. Davis Publishing Co.
Samples, R.
    1978 "Psychology, thought and morality:
          Some limitations of Piaget and Kohlberg."
          in P. Scharf (ed.), Readings in Moral Edu-
          cation. Minneapolis: Winston Press.
Schlotfeldt, R. M.
    1965 "A mandate for nurses and physicians."
          American Journal of Nursing 65:102–105.

Sloan, D.
    1979 "The teaching of ethics in the American
          undergraduate curriculum, 1876–1976."
          Hastings Center Report 9(6):21–41.
Wilson, R. W.
    1978 "A new direction for the study of moral
          behavior." Journal of Moral Education
          7:122–130.

Chapter 20

Program for Mild Chronic Obstructive Pulmonary Disease and Compliance

Norma L. Chaska, R.N., Ph.D., F.A.A.N.
Associate Professor
Chairperson, Nursing Administration
Coordinator, Nursing Research
School of Nursing
Medical College of Georgia
Augusta, Georgia

Although the current emphasis in providing health care is on collaboration with the patient, eliciting the motivation of clients to continue with the agreed upon recommendations continues to be an issue. Norma L. Chaska offers a new approach to the problem.

She selected all of the attitudes found to be statistically significant in studies related to compliance. The majority of the attitudes predominantly are associated with the Health Belief Model. Following this initial step, she combined the attitudes to formulate a scale, which was tested and labeled "Compliance Aptitude Response Profile" (CARS). The scale is used in a study to measure and determine whether one can predict the likelihood of decreasing or ceasing smoking, and to evaluate the effectiveness of a patient education program to encourage decreasing or ceasing smoking. A questionnaire was developed for the study that, in addition to the Likert-scale items measuring attitudes (CARS), also included items to obtain demographic data, the smoking history of the patient, and queries pertaining to the patient education program. The study was completed over a three-year period. It was experimental in design. The sample consisted of patients who currently were cigarette smokers, diagnosed and tested as having mild chronic obstructive pulmonary disease (COPD). Originally there were 322 patients each in the control and experimental group.

All patients who were initially seen at a medical center in a specific time frame, who met the above criteria, agreed to participate, completed the pretest questionnaire, and were entered into the study. After 1 year, both experimental and control groups were mailed a posttest questionnaire. The final sample included 199 patients in the control and 187 in the experimental group. The experimental group viewed an educational videotape, were seen by a nurse who addressed their questions, and encouraged them to decrease or cease smoking.

The findings indicate there were no statistically significant differences between the control and experimental group in education, income, and occupation. There were slightly more males and more heavy smokers in the experimental than control group. The experimental group decreased their smoking habits significantly more than the control group after one year. There were no significant decreases for women in either group. Males tended to decrease their smoking habits if their spouses did not smoke but tended to stop smoking when their spouses smoke.

"Susceptibility" was the key attitudinal factor indicated as a predictor for compliance. The experimental group had a statistically significant higher score for that factor, and there was a tendency for those who smoked less or who stopped to have a high score for "susceptibility." It was difficult to clearly define an association between the patient education program and changes in smoking although the predominant reasons cited for quitting smoking were areas of information emphasized in the audiovisual tape. It should be noted that data were not accessible as to whether the reasons for not quitting or quitting differ between the experimental and control group, nor attainable for further analysis of the findings. Chaska emphasizes that there were no significant differences between the groups regarding females who were heavy smokers either in smoking habits or in attitudes. She concludes that they may be a high-risk population who are more difficult to influence change in smoking habits.

Health education is more and more frequently utilized as a means to increase compliance among patients (Davis, 1968b; Stimson, 1974; AGPA, 1976). However, health education programs need to be assessed in order to determine the variables which are the most influential in increasing compliance. Patient education and evaluation of intervention strategies are integral to inducing a positive behavioral response. Intervention strategies to increase compliance include patient education about the illness, the treatment, and the risk factors, such as smoking, that predispose to illness. Sequential intervention is often more effective than dependence on only one strategy, particularly if the goal is to alter a long-term pattern of behavior. For example, in this study audiovisual instruction about a prospective illness is followed by a discussion with a nurse in which patients' questions are answered. Close follow-up or monitoring by the physician of the effect of the intervention is essential. In evaluating the intervention for compliance, one can look for a change in, or reinforcement of, the attitudes that are related to a positive outcome.

Compliance is a major perplexing behavioral issue concerned with the delivery of medical care.

Reviewers (Blackwell 1973; Davis, 1968b; Stimson, 1974) agree that at least one-third of the patient population in most studies fail to follow physician's recommendations, and in some studies noncompliance is reported to be in excess of 60 percent (Becker et al., 1972b; Bergman and Werner, 1963; Gordis et al., 1969; Vincent, 1971). Thus far writings about empirical findings generally appear to be more substantial than the findings themselves. The findings to date have not been consistent, either in direction or in strength, and there have been few attempts to coordinate results or to account for apparent disparities. Factors contributing to this situation are varying methodologies, differing medical care systems, the lack of refined standardized measures of compliance, and the rhetoric of interpretation. In order to determine what inducements are needed for compliance, research should be done to determine why patients do and do not comply.

One approach to the problem of compliance is the development of a scale to predict compliance, a scale based on the measurement of all the significant attitudes indicated from previous research. The process of developing such a scale was a major part of this study. The scale has been labeled *The Compliance Aptitude Response Profile*. The perfection of such an instrument could be a valuable asset to the professional who is responsible for the administration of any treatment program in which the patient has an active role. The test could be utilized for four purposes: to aid the professional in deciding whether the patient is attitudinally amenable to entering a treatment program; to determine the extent to which a patient might comply with the treatment program; to determine what attitudes need to be reinforced or changed to ensure compliance with a treatment program; and to determine the intervention necessary by patient-education programs to increase the likelihood of compliance.

PURPOSES OF THE STUDY

The purposes of this study were to determine whether one can predict compliance behavior on the basis of attitudinal measurement via the development of the Compliance Aptitude Response Profile scale; to measure, via a questionnaire through a self-report method, compliance in decreasing or ceasing smoking; and to evaluate the effectiveness of a patient-education program to encourage compliance in not smoking. The study was initiated in January 1976 and was completed in September 1979.

HYPOTHESES

Three hypotheses were formulated:

1 Compliance to recommendations will be greater by subjects who have participated in an education program than by subjects who have not participated.
2 Compliance to an intervention program for lung disease is greater with subjects having a high positive attitude and knowledge-of-lung-disease score than with subjects having a low negative attitude and knowledge score.
3 Attitudes related to health and health care can be used to predict compliance behavior.

METHODOLOGY

The Instrument

The following variables for attitudinal measurement were suggested for questionnaire development from a review of the literature and previously reported significant research findings.

- Health beliefs and knowledge of a particular disease (Becker and Malman, 1975; Rosenstock, 1966; Kirscht et al., 1976)
- Motivating factors such as concern about health matters (Becker et al., 1972a; Kasl and Cobb, 1966)
- Willingness and intention to comply (Davis, 1968a; Kegales, 1963; Knutson, 1965; Senior and Smith, 1973; AGPA, 1976)
- Susceptibility or vulnerability to heart disease (Davis, 1967; Haefner and Kirscht, 1970; Davis and Eichhorn, 1963)
- Belief in the diagnosis (Becker et al., 1972a)
- Perceived severity of lung disease (Heinzelmann, 1963)
- Perception of the doctor-patient relationship and communication (Davis, 1968b; Korsch et al., 1968)
- Advice of influential persons such as relatives and friends (Davis, 1968b).

In addition to the above variables from which Likert-scale items measuring the knowledge of lung disease and attitudes related to compliance behavior were developed, the questionnaire consisted of items to obtain demographic data and the smoking history of the patient.

Pilot Study

A pilot study was accomplished for assessment of reliability and validity of the instrument. The sample consisted of 34 patients who were cigarette smokers and diagnosed as having mild chronic obstructive pulmonary disease (COPD). The reliability was determined to be .86 using the coefficient alpha formula. Factor analysis was completed. Five factors were indicated as being measured in the instrument. The cumulative eigenvalue for the five factors was .492. In order of importance, the five factors were the quality of the physician interaction, the patient's belief concerning his or her susceptibility, the seriousness of COPD, the prevention of COPD, and the importance of following the advice of a professional. Patients had no difficulty in understanding the questions.

SAMPLE

The criteria applied to the study sample were:

1 Patients were currently cigarette smokers.
2 Patients had been diagnosed and tested as having mild chronic obstructive pulmonary disease according to MMF L/S (maximal midexpiratory flow rate) values criteria established by the medical center where the study was conducted.
3 MMF L/S values designating mild chronic obstructive pulmonary disease were defined by age and sex.

All patients who met the above criteria and were seen at the medical center from January 1976 through September 1978 entered into the study. A timing factor was involved that prevented the control and experimental group samples from being simultaneously obtained. The patient-education program that was being developed was not complete for utilization until January 1977. Thus all patients seen at the medical center from January 1976 through January 1977 who met the above criteria constituted the control group. The total number of patients in this control group was 322. After January 1977 patients who had pulmonary function test results designating mild chronic obstructive pulmonary disease according to the defined criteria and who were cigarette smokers were entered into the study as the experimental group until there were an equal number of patients to compare with the control group. This process of collecting the experimental sample was completed in September 1978, and data collection for the study was completed in September 1979.

PROTOCOL AND FINAL SAMPLE

Both the control and experimental group subjects were asked to complete the pretest questionnaire while they were at the medical center. This form was completed before patients were told that they had an abnormal pulmonary function test. After 1 year, both the experimental and the control groups were mailed posttest questionnaires. One follow-up questionnaire was mailed to those who did not respond after a month.

Of the original 322 patients included in each group, 123 patients from the control group and 135 patients from the experimental group were eliminated from the study because they did not return their posttest mailed questionnaires. The response rate on the posttest mailed questionnaire was 62 percent for the control group and 58 percent for the experimental group. These figures are higher than the average response rate (48 percent) reported for mailed questionnaires (Vincent, 1971; Heberlein, 1978:457). Thus the final sample consisted of 199 patients in the control group and 187 in the experimental group.

PATIENT-EDUCATION PROGRAM

The experimental group, after completing the pretest questionnaire, viewed an educational videotape pertaining to chronic obstructive pulmonary disease. The tape, developed by a physician who specialized in thoracic diseases, presented specific information regarding the cause, treatment, and prevention of COPD. The information was presented empathetically and conveyed an understanding of the difficulty in quitting smoking. The presentation made no effort to instill fear of the consequences of smoking or of COPD.

After reviewing the videotape, the patients were seen by a nurse who addressed questions to them concerning the videotape. She elicited the patients' reasons for smoking and encouraged them to decrease or cease smoking. Common reactions of the patients were anticipated by the nurse and responded to in such a way that, insofar as it was possible, each patient was given a similar response. For example, a common reason indicated for smoking was that it reduced tension. And the appropriate response to that was the suggestion that the patient take some slow, deep breaths when the urge to smoke was strong.

FINDINGS AND DISCUSSION

Data were analyzed to determine the comparability of the two groups, the changes in smoking habits after 1 year, and whether or not it made a difference if spouses smoked. Analysis of the data also included isolating and examining the data of "heavy" smokers, of those who smoked less, and of those who ceased completely. Attitude scores were examined to determine whether there were relationships between attitudes and compliance. Finally, the effectiveness of the patient-education program was examined. It should be noted that discrepancies in figures on the tables are due to the fact that some persons did not always respond to all of the questions.

DEMOGRAPHIC FINDINGS

There were no statistically significant differences between the control and experimental groups in education, income, and occupation. Data are as follows:

Education Forty-nine percent of the subjects in both groups had more than a high school education. In the control group 18 percent had less than a high school education and 33 percent had a high school diploma. In the experimental group 17 percent of the subjects had less than a high school education and 34 percent had completed a high school education.

Income Fifty-eight percent of the control subjects earned less than $20,000 per year while 42 percent earned $20,000 or more per year. In the experimental group 50 percent of the subjects earned less than $20,000 per year and 50 percent earned $20,000 or more.

Occupation There was considerable variation in occupations between the two groups, especially in the number of subjects categorized as "professional," and the number catagorized as "housewives." Of the subjects in the control group 26 percent were classified as professional, 5 percent as clerical, 20 percent as workers-craftsmen or laborers, 4 percent as farm-related workers, 17 percent as retired, and 28 percent as "other." Twenty-two percent out of the 28 percent listed in the "other" category were housewives.

Of subjects in the experimental group 41 percent were professional, 22 percent clerical, 11 percent workers-craftsmen or laborers, 2 percent farm-related workers, 16 percent retired, and 8 percent were categorized as "other." There were no housewives indicated in this latter group.

COMPARABILITY OF GROUPS

Data were analyzed to determine the comparability of the experimental and control group. Table 20-1 indicates there were slightly more males in the experimental group. This was not significant when the chi-square test was utilized. Table 20-2 indicates that the experimental group had statistically significantly more subjects who were heavy smokers. A heavy smoker was defined as a person who smoked one or more packs per day. In interpreting the results of the study it is important to recall how the two groups differed.

CHANGES IN SMOKING HABITS

Comparisons were made between the two groups regarding changes in smoking habits after 1 year. Table 20-3 indicates graphically packs-per-day smoked on the pretest in comparison with the posttest for members of the experimental group. The figures within the accented boxes indicate the

Table 20-1 Sample Groups Compared According to Sex
$(X_1^2 = 3.362, p = < .07)$

| | Sex | | | |
| | Male | | Female | |
Group	N	%	N	%
Experimental 187 (48.45%)	125	66.84	62	33.16
Control 199 (51.55%)	115	57.79	84	42.21
Combined 386 (100%)	240	62.18	146	37.82

Table 20-2 Comparison of Sample Groups According to Smoker's Habits
$(X_1^2 = 4.213 \quad p = < .0401$

| | Amount Smoked | | | |
| | Less than 1 pack | | 1 or more packs | |
Group	N	%	N	%
Experimental 190 (48.84%)	40	21.05	150	78.95
Control 199 (51.16%)	60	30.15	139	69.85
Combined 389 (100%)	100	25.71	289	74.29

Table 20-3 Comparison of Pretest and Posttest Smoking Habits of Experimental Group

| Pretest | | Posttest | | | | | |
| | | Number of persons by number of cigarettes per day | | | | | |
Number of cigarettes smoked per day	Number of persons	None	1 cig	1 cig–1/2 pack	1/2 pack–1 pack	1–2 packs	2+ packs
1 cig	4	1	2	0	1	0	0
1 cig–1/2 pack	12	4	1	2	5	0	0
1/2–1 pack	24	5	0	3	13	3	0
1–2 packs	104	17	3	2	29	48	5
2+ packs	46	11	0	0	1	12	22

Accented boxes = no changes
Everything above to the right = smoked more on posttest than pretest
Everything below to the left = smoked less on posttest than pretest

number of patients who had no change in their previous smoking habits. The figures to the right of the accented boxes indicate the number of patients who increased, and those to the left the number who decreased their smoking. It appears that the experimental group smoked considerably less on the posttest than on the pretest.

Table 20-4 indicates a similar comparison for the control group. Table 20-5 compares the changes statistically between the experimental and control groups in smoking habits. The experimental group had decreased its smoking significantly more than the control group after 1 year. Note that 46.84 percent of the experimental group smoked less in comparison with 37.69 percent of the control group.

The question is . . . Who decreased their smoking more? Males in the experimental group decreased their smoking significantly more than those in the control group, as indicated in Table 20-6. There was no significant decrease for women in either group.

CHANGES RELATED TO SMOKING OR NONSMOKING OF SPOUSE

It was decided to examine the difference a nonsmoking spouse made, since behavior of significant others may influence the smoker's behavior. Table 20-7 indicates that, when spouses were nonsmokers, the experimental group decreased its smoking more than the control group did. Note

Table 20-4   Comparison of Pretest and Posttest Smoking Habits of Control Group

Pretest		Posttest						
		Number of persons by number of cigarettes per day						
Number of cigarettes smoked per day	Number of persons	None	1 cig	1 cig–1/2 pack	1/2 pack–1 pack	1–2 packs	2+ packs
1 cig	3	2	1	0	0	0	0
1 cig–1/2 pack	9	3	1	3	0	2	0
1/2–1 pack	48	9	0	7	27	4	1
1–2 packs	104	14	1	5	20	60	4
2+ packs	35	3	0	0	0	10	22

Accented boxes = no change
Everything above to the right = smoked more on posttest than pretest
Everything below to the left = smoked less on posttest than pretest

Table 20-5   Changes in the Amount Smoked after 1 Year
$(X_1^2 = 3.34, p = < .05)$

	Amount smoked after 1 year					
	Less		Same		More	
Group	N	%	N	%	N	%
Experimental 190 (48.84%)	89	46.84	87	45.79	14	7.37
Control 199 (51.16%)	75	37.69	113	56.78	11	5.53
Combined 389 (100%)	164	42.16	200	51.41	25	6.43

Table 20-6　Changes in the Amount Smoked by Males
($-X_1^2 = 7.13, p < .01$)

	Amount smoked after 1 year					
	Less		Same		More	
Group	N	%	N	%	N	%
Experimental	66	52.80	48	38.40	11	8.80
125 (52.08%)						
Control	41	35.65	66	57.39	8	6.96
115 (47.92%)						
Combined	107	44.58	114	47.50	19	7.72
240 (100%)						

Table 20-7　Changes in the Amount Smoked by Group Members Whose Spouses Were Nonsmokers
($-X_1^2 = 4.47, p = < .05$)

	Amount smoked after 1 year					
	Less		Same		More	
Group	N	%	N	%	N	%
Experimental	45	52.33	38	44.19	3	3.49
86 (52.44%)						
Control	28	35.90	46	58.97	4	5.13
78 (47.56%)						
Combined	73	44.51	84	51.22	7	4.27
164 (100%)						

that the percentages indicate more improvement for the experimental group than the control group in all three of the categories. Data relating to the male heavy smoker who smoked less were analyzed in more depth to determine whether or not it made a difference whether or not the spouse smoked. Table 20-8 indicates that a statistically significant number of heavy smokers whose spouses did not smoke decreased their smoking. As indicated in Table 20-9, the findings also show a decrease for heavy smokers whose spouses did smoke, but the decrease was far less.

Data relating to the male heavy smokers who *stopped* smoking were then analyzed. The subject had to have ceased smoking for 1 month or more to be considered as "stopped." It was further examined whether or not there was a difference between those males whose spouses smoked and did not smoke. As shown in Table 20–10

there was a statistically significant difference for males who stopped smoking whose spouses smoked. However, there were no significant differences found for males who stopped smoking whose

Table 20-8　Comparison of Changes in the Amount Smoked by Heavy Smokers Whose Spouses Were Nonsmokers
($-X_1^2 = 6.035, p = < .01$)

	Amount smoked after 1 year			
	Same or more		Less	
Group	N	%	N	%
Experimental	16	38.10	26	61.90
42 (56%)				
Control	22	66.67	11	33.33
33 (44%)				
Combined	38	50.67	37	49.33
75 (100%)				

Table 20-9   Comparison of Changes in Amount Smoked by Heavy Smokers Whose Spouses Were Smokers
($-X_1^2 = 3.022, p = < .05$)

Group	Amount smoked after 1 year			
	Same or more		Less	
	N	%	N	%
Experimental 44 (53.66%)	23	52.27	21	47.73
Control 38 (46.34%)	27	71.05	11	28.95
Combined 82 (100%)	50	60.98	32	39.02

spouses did not smoke. In the latter category only one of eight stopped in the experimental group and one of 13 stopped in the control group. Thus, only two male heavy smokers whose spouses did not smoke stopped, compared with 15 whose spouses did smoke who stopped.

In conclusion, males who were heavy smokers tended to *decrease* their smoking if their spouses did *not* smoke. However, more males tended to *stop* smoking when their spouses were smokers. Other extraneous variables may account for the findings. For females who were heavy smokers there were no significant relationships between changes in smoking habits and whether or not their spouses smoked. Tables 20–11 and 20–12 summarize the findings of the above relationships.

Table 20-10   Comparison of Males Who Stopped Who Had Been Heavy Smokers and Whose Spouses Smoked
($-X_1^2 = 2.858, p = < .05$)

Group	Did not stop		Stopped	
	N	%	N	%
Experimental 44 (53.66%)	33	75.00	11	25.00
Control 38 (46.34%)	34	89.47	4	10.53
Combined 82 (100%)	67	81.71	15	18.29

Table 20-11   Relation of Spouses' Smoking to Heavy Smokers' Abilities to Decrease Smoking

	Males	
Spouses	Did not decrease	Did decrease
Smoked	N.S.	< .05
Did not smoke	N.S.	< .01
	Females	
Spouses	Did not decrease	Did decrease
Smoked	N.S.	N.S.
Did not smoke	N.S.	N.S.

Table 20-12   Relation of Spouses' Smoking to Heavy Smokers' Abilities to Stop Smoking

	Males	
Spouses	Did not stop	Did stop
Did smoke	N.S.	< .05
Did not smoke	N.S.	N.S.
	Females	
Spouses	Did not stop	Did stop
Did smoke	N.S.	N.S.
Did not smoke	N.S.	N.S.

COMPARISON OF COMPLIANCE ATTITUDES

Further analysis was completed to compare the pretest attitudes of the experimental and the control groups in relation to compliance in ceasing to smoke. Table 20–13 indicates there was a significant difference between the two groups in one attitude factor—susceptibility. The degrees of freedom ranged from 390 to 392. Those in the experimental group believed there was a greater likelihood that they could develop a lung disease than did those in the control group.

The attitude scores were also analyzed for those patients who decreased their smoking and those who stopped. Table 20–14 indicates that there was no significant difference in the attitude factor "susceptibility," between those who smoked less and those who did not decrease their smoking. The degrees of freedom ranged from 383 to 385. This finding could have occurred by chance. The same attitude factor has a tendency to be signifi-

Table 20-13   Pretest Attitude Factor Scores by Groups

		Data							
		Experimental			Control		Correlation analyses		
Factors	N	Mean	STD dev	N	Mean	STD dev	t-test	df	P value
Interaction	191	3.87	.66	201	3.84	.67	0.4	390	N.S.
Susceptibility	192	3.49	.54	202	3.08	.65	6.7	392	< .001
Seriousness	191	4.21	.42	201	4.14	.43	1.5	390	N.S.
Prevention	191	3.44	.61	202	3.34	.51	1.7	391	N.S.
Advice	191	4.23	.45	202	4.19	.44	0.9	391	N.S.

Table 20-14   Attitude Factor Scores for Those Who Smoked Less

		Data							
		Did not smoke less			Smoked less		Correlation analyses		
Factors	N	Mean	STD dev	N	Mean	STD dev	t-test	df	P value
Interaction	224	3.85	.65	161	3.83	.67	0.4	383	N.S.
Susceptibility	225	3.24	.63	162	3.36	.64	1.8	385	< .08
Seriousness	224	4.19	.45	161	4.14	.38	1.1	383	N.S.
Prevention	224	3.43	.54	162	3.34	.59	1.4	384	N.S.
Advice	224	4.18	.44	162	4.23	.45	1.2	384	N.S.

cant when the scores of those patients who stopped are compared with the scores of those who did not stop smoking. This is shown in Table 20-15. The degrees of freedom ranged from 383 to 385. It appears that "susceptibility" may be a more important attitude factor than the other four.

FINDINGS AND DISCUSSION OF THE PATIENT-EDUCATION PROGRAM

Finally, an attempt was made to examine the effect of the patient-education program. Data were ana-

lyzed from the total sample of 386 patients as to reasons for not quitting smoking, reasons for quitting, and the number of months quitters had not smoked.

From Table 20-16 it appears that the predominant reasons for not quitting are related to motivation and need for tension relief. Table 20-17 shows that the predominant reasons for quitting are related more to health than to specific attitudes. As noted in Table 20-17, not all of the respondents who ceased smoking provided a reason. Table 20-18 shows the length of time the

Table 20-15   Attitude Factor Scores for Those Who Stopped Smoking

		Data							
		Did not stop			Stopped		Correlation analyses		
Factors	N	Mean	STD dev	N	Mean	STD dev	t-test	df	P value
Interaction	317	3.85	.63	68	3.81	.77	0.4	383	N.S.
Susceptibility	318	3.26	.65	69	3.42	.53	1.9	385	< .06
Seriousness	316	4.18	.44	69	4.14	.34	0.6	384	N.S.
Prevention	319	3.40	.55	67	3.36	.63	0.6	384	N.S.
Advice	317	4.19	.44	69	4.26	.43	1.1	384	N.S.

Table 20-16   Reasons for Not Quitting Smoking (As Given by 152 of the 306 Patients Who Did Not Stop Smoking)

Reason	N	%
No will power	28	18
Needed for tension relief	25	16
Cannot break habit	14	9
Still trying to quit	13	9
No reason indicated	13	9
Did not know why	9	6
Too hard to quit	9	6
Enjoy smoking	8	5
Do not want to quit	8	5
Quit but restarted	8	5
Other health problems	5	3
Smoked too long to quit	4	3
Gain weight without smoking	3	2
Smoking causes no harm	2	1
Quit smoking off and on	1	1
Procrastination	1	1
M.D. who told me to quit smokes	1	1
Total	152	100

Table 20-17   Reasons for Quitting Smoking (As Given by 37 of the 70 Patients Who Stopped Smoking)

Reason	N	%
Physical changes	12	32
Maintain health and not get worse	5	14
Better health	4	11
Fear of getting worse	4	11
Physician influence	3	8
Patient decided to quit	3	8
Audiovisual program	3	8
Belief in susceptibility	2	5
Family influences	1	3
Total	37	100

patients had stopped smoking. Not every respondent of the 70 who actually stopped indicated a length of time. There were no statistically significant differences between the control and the experimental groups, though the median time was slightly greater for the experimental group.

It is difficult to clearly define an association between the patient-education program and

Table 20-18   Length of Time Patients Had Stopped Smoking*

Group members who stopped	Time in months		
	Minimum	Maximum	Median
Experimental 36	1	14	10.3
Control 30	1	12	8

*Not all respondents indicated time

changes in smoking. As shown in Table 20–16, the predominant reasons provided for not quitting were, in general, issues which the nurse addressed in sessions with the experimental group patients after they had seen the audiovisual tape. As shown in Table 20–17, only three subjects specifically cited the audiovisual program (with follow-up counseling by the nurse) as the reason for ceasing smoking. However, the predominant reasons for quitting, i.e., physical changes and health maintenance, were related to information provided in the audiovisual tape. Data are not accessible to indicate whether the reasons for not quitting or quitting differ between the experimental and control groups. Nor are data available for further analysis of the findings of the study.

HYPOTHESES TESTING

The t-test was used to test the three hypotheses. The first hypothesis was accepted; compliance was greater for the experimental than the control group. Males in the experimental group decreased their smoking habits significantly more than females. The second hypothesis was partially accepted; the experimental group did have a statistically significantly higher score for the susceptibility factor. There was also a tendency for those who smoked less or ceased smoking to have a high score for susceptibility. The third hypothesis was partially accepted; in this study susceptibility was the key attitudinal factor indicated as a predictor for compliance behavior. There may be other attitudes not included in this study that are also significant predictors of compliance.

CONCLUSIONS AND INDICATIONS

In general, males in the experimental group who were heavy smokers improved, either by decreasing or ceasing their smoking, more than did those in the control group. The experimental group also showed a significant attitude difference regarding susceptibility. It appears that only males who are heavy smokers are more likely to smoke less or to stop if exposed to a patient-education program. Because there were more males and more heavy smokers in the experimental group, caution is urged in interpreting the data.

Finally, it should be noted that for females who were heavy smokers there were no significant differences between the groups, either in smoking habits or in attitudes. Females who are heavy smokers may form a high-risk population that proves to be difficult to influence through a patient-education program.

Thirty-two percent of those who stopped (12 of the 70) indicated "physical changes" as the predominant reason for ceasing to smoke, and physical changes were emphasized in the videotape viewed by the experimental group. However, there is insufficient evidence to judge the effectiveness of the patient-education program.

If one were to develop further educational programs aimed at decreasing smoking, it appears that such programs should include motivation issues, aids to reduce tension, and factors related to the health-belief model, particularly susceptibility. It also appears that sequential periodic reinforcement methods should be utilized in a patient-education program for compliance.

EDITOR'S QUESTIONS FOR DISCUSSION

What are the implications and issues concerning the use of the term "compliance" in regard to the provision of health care? What more appropriate term can be suggested? What nursing conceptual or theoretical base could have been utilized for this study?

What methods can be utilized to increase the validity of self-report research instruments? How valid and reliable is the "Compliance Aptitude Response Profile"? What is the significance of cumulative eigenvalues in factor analysis? In obtaining the sample for this study, what are the implications concerning validity due to the timing factor that could not be controlled?

What are the explicit limitations of this research? Contrast an "ideal" versus "realistic" methods in obtaining subjects and data for this study. What are the advantages and disadvantages of conducting research in clinical settings where pragmatism is essential? What constraints may exist that need to be negotiated and accepted by virtue of the ideal or desirable settings in which studies can be conducted?

What considerations need to be evaluated in attempts to increase response rates for mailed questionnaires? How valuable and pragmatic would it be to explore the reasons patients did not return mailed questionnaires? What effects of history and maturation does one need to consider in longitudinal studies?

What other attitudes not included in this study may more currently be significant predictors of compliance? To what extent should such variables measuring the appropriateness of "timing" for a behavioral change be included in similar studies? What would you suggest to further reinforce the impact of patient education programs?

What are the implications for interpretation of these data due to the fact that the experimental and control groups differed? What other variables might account for the fact that male heavy smokers tended to decrease their smoking habits if their spouses did not smoke, but more males tended to stop if their spouses smoke? What explanations can be offered regarding the finding of no difference between the groups in smoking habits or in attitudes of females? How could an association between the patient education program and changes in smoking more clearly be defined? If the data from this study were accessible, what further analysis would you suggest? What alternative explanations can be offered for the findings of this study?

REFERENCES

American Group Practice Association
1976 "Patient education update." The Association Newsletter, December 10.

Becker, M. H., R. H. Drachman, and J. P. Kirscht
1972a "Motivations as predictors of health behavior." Health Services Reports 87:852.
1972b "Predicting mother's compliance with pediatric medical regimens." Journal of Pediatrics 81:843.

Becker, M. H. and L. A. Malman
1975 "Sociobehavioral determinants of compliance with health and medical care recommendations." Medical Care 13: 10-24.

Bergman, A. B. and R. J. Werner
1963 "Failure of children to receive penicillin by mouth." New England Journal of Medicine 268:1334.

Blackwell, B.
1973 "Drug therapy: Patient compliance." New England Journal of Medicine 289: 249.

Davis, M. S.
1967 "Predicting non-compliant behavior." Journal of Health and Social Behavior. 8:265-271.
1968a "Physiologic, psychological and demographic factors in patient compliance with doctors' orders." Medical Care 6: 115.
1968b "Variations in patients' compliance with doctors' advice: An empirical analysis of patterns of communication." American Journal of Public Health 58:274.

Davis, M. S. and R. L. Eichhorn
1963 "Compliance with medical regimens: A panel study." Journal of Health and Human Behavior 4:240.

Gordis, L., M. Markowitz, and A. M. Lilienfeld
1969 "The inaccuracy of using interviews to estimate patient reliability in taking medications at home." Medical Care 7:49.

Haefner, D. and J. P. Kirscht
1970 "Motivational and behavioral effects of modifying health beliefs." Public Health Reports 85:478.

Heberlein, Thomas A. and Robert Baumgartner
1978 "Factors affecting response rates to mailed questionnaires: A quantitative analysis of the published literature." American Sociological Review 43:457.

Heinzelmann, P.
1963 "Factors in prophylaxis behavior in treating rheumatic fever: An exploratory study." Journal of Health and Human Behavior 4:240.

Kasl, S. A. and S. Cobb
1966 "Health behavior, illness behavior, and sick role behavior: I—Health and illness behavior." Archives of Environmental Health 12:246.

Kegales, S. S.
1963 "Some motives for seeking preventive dental care." Journal of the American Dental Association 67:90.

Kirscht, J. P., M. H. Becker, and J. P. Eveland
1976 "Psychological and social factors as predictions of medical behavior." Medical Care 14:422.

Knutson, A. I.
1965 The Individual, Society, and Health Behavior. New York: Russell Sage Foundation.

Korsch, B. M., E. K. Gozzi, and V. Francis
1968 "Gaps in doctor-patient communication: I. Doctor-patient interaction and patient satisfaction." Pediatrics 42:855.

Rosenstock, I. M.
1966 "Why people use health services." Milbank Memorial Fund Quarterly 44:94.

Senior, B. and B. A. Smith
1973 "The motivation of the patient as a neglected factor in therapy." Journal of Medical Education 48:589-591.

Stimson, G. V.
1974 "Obeying doctor's orders: A view from the other side." Social Science and Medicine 8:97.

Vincent, P.
1971 "Factors influencing patient noncompliance: A theoretical approach." Nursing Research 20:509.

Chapter 21

The Relationship of Selected Characteristics of Nurses and Their Attitudes toward Elderly Patients

Lucille T. Mercadante, R.N., Ed.D.
Assistant Administrator
International Hospital
Miami, Florida

Improving retention of nurses in settings, particularly where the majority of patients is elderly, is a growing professional concern. Lucille Mercadante approaches the issue by determining whether relationships exist between individual and clinical group characteristics of registered professional nurses and their attitudes toward elderly persons. The literature indicates a dearth of studies correlating length of employment with nurses' attitudes toward a particular group of patients. Mercadante's survey includes a convenience sample of 180 nurses employed in a 700-bed Southeastern Medical Center Hospital. Kogan's "Old People Scale," designed to measure attitudes toward elderly persons with respect to norms and individual differences, is utilized in the study. In addition, she includes the independent variables: length of employment at the hospital, age, type of nursing education, and length of experience working with elderly patients.

In data analysis, tetrachoric correlation coefficients are calculated for comparisons between mean Kogan's Scale scores of clinical groups and the independent variables. The major findings indicate that as a total group there was no relationship between the independent variables and respondents' performance on Kogan's "OP Scale." However, there was a tendency for nurses in this survey, who held more positive attitudes toward elderly patients, to be older, have less education preparation, more experience working with the elderly, and increased longevity working at the medical center.

Mercandante concludes with specific implications of the study for recruitment, selection, and assignment of nurses and for preservice and in-service nursing education programs. She recommends program content and creative experiences to assist in the development of positive attitudes toward elderly patients and positive aspects of gerontological nursing. Mercadante concludes that administering Kogan's OP Scale questionnaire to all nurses seeking employment at this specific medical center would be an effective screening process.

INTRODUCTION

Most critical problems confronting nursing service administrators revolve around recruitment and retention of registered professional nurses. The 700-bed Southeastern Medical Center utilized in this study, like other hospitals, experiences a high turnover of nurses, which occurs particularly during the first year of employment. Because many hospitals experience similar problems, improving current procedures used for recruitment and selection of nurses and improving retention through reduced turnover rank high in priority for nursing service administration. Achieving this goal requires knowledge and understanding of the covert as well as the overt factors contributing to turnover.

Because of its location, 73 percent of this Southeastern Medical Center's patients range from 65 to over 90 years of age. In any setting delivering patient care, a major concern exists regarding the extent to which negative attitudes of nurses are conveyed to patients and positive attitudes not expressed appropriately. Studies indicate that attitudes of health care givers relate directly to the quality of care provided. If the challenge of providing quality care to rapidly increasing numbers of elderly patients admitted to health care institutions is to be met, procedures utilized in selecting nurses for employment must be analyzed critically.

REVIEW OF LITERATURE

Nurses have never been as mobile as they are today. Factors contributing to this mobility include new and/or expanded roles for nurses, increased job opportunities created by additional health services, and increases in nursing education programs, particularly at the graduate level and in continuing education, requiring more nurse faculty (*American Journal of Nursing*, 1979). Although hospitals still employ the largest number of professional nurses, recruitment and retention have intensified as major critical issues for nursing service administrators. Reduction of turnover ranks high in priority because of its costly and disruptive effects in hospitals, where safe, adequate, and appropriate care to patients depends upon sufficient and well-qualified nurses. Additionally, the expanding role of federal, state, and local governments in controlling costs of health services magnifies these concerns.

During the last decade, nurses have been the subject of many studies focused on employee-employer-related aspects of job dissatisfactions leading to turnover. Additionally, a number of studies reported in the literature relate to attitudes held by health professionals, primarily nurses toward elderly as well as psychiatric, alcoholic, and drug-addicted patients (Campbell, 1971; Futrell and Jones, 1977; White, 1977). The literature fails to reveal studies, however, correlating length of employment with nurses' attitudes toward a particular group of patients. A study conducted by Brief (1976) suggests that the underlying causal factor contributing to high turnover rate exhibited by nurses stems from nurses' dissatisfaction with the work itself. While some of the dissatisfiers identified in other employee-employer relationship studies related to shift preference and salary, Campbell (1971) finds that stereotyped attitudes concerning elderly persons exist among nursing care personnel, and neither salary increase nor shift preference increases willingness to work with elderly patients. In a survey conducted by Godfrey (1978a), it is reported that 24 percent of nurse respondents identify as most repugnant, physical tasks such as caring for incontinent patients, trimming toenails, giving mouth and eye care, bathing, and trying generally to keep the elderly, senile patient clean. Other studies reported by Heller and Walsh (1976) indicate that nurses prefer to avoid working with the aged because of their complaining, demanding, incontinence, and inability to care for or feed themselves. Heller and Walsh note further that while nurses are committed to providing the best possible nursing care to patients, professional ethics conflict with emerging social patterns of rejection, isolation, intolerance, and neglect of elderly persons. Neglect shown the elderly ill by professionals reflects a general unwillingness to face problems that remain unsolvable or continue for long periods (Butler and Lewis, 1973).

In nursing, perhaps more than any other health profession, the problem of attitudes and resultant behaviors rank significantly high. Many stereotypes of old age prove negative. Therefore, failure to see the elderly patient as an individual occurs frequently (Lore, 1979). These negative attitudes toward older persons evince themselves in health professionals' tendencies to segregate elderly persons and impatience with their way of doing things (White, 1977). Perhaps this tendency to segregate elderly patients manifests itself in the more acceptable behavior of changing place of employment, commonly referred to as turnover.

Preference in working with elderly persons is an indicator of nurses' attitudes. DeLora and Moses (1969) find that students in baccalaureate nursing programs place geriatrics as their last choice of work. Constant turnover, therefore, may imply that nurses either lack adequate basic nursing educational preparation in caring for elderly patients or lack the attitudinal characteristics essential for the job. Although nursing service comprises the largest single component in provision of care to elderly persons, most nursing education programs either omit or interject haphazardly aspects of geriatrics and gerontology in the nursing curricula (Elmore, 1964; Moses and Lake, 1968; Brower, 1977). After establishing a minisemester clinical elective in

gerontological nursing at the University of Maryland, Brock (1977) found no specific requests for an elective in the area of gerontological nursing. She concludes that this lack of interest reflects "limited and inadequate exposure of students to the elderly patients during their educational experience" (Brock, 1977:28).

In a study of nursing students' attitudes toward the elderly patient, Gunter (1971) finds that students express more negative attitudes toward elderly patients at the end of the course in geriatrics than at the beginning. To change these attitudes and motivate nursing students to see and accept the challenge in geriatric care, Brock (1977) emphasizes the need to plan creative experiences focusing on the positive aspects of geriatrics. Brower (1977:41) notes that "perhaps the most pressing need to stimulate young nursing students into service for the elderly is a nucleus of enthusiastic, informed teachers." Results of a study conducted by Wilhite and Johnson (1976) support Brower's statement. These researchers find that a positive correlation exists between attitudes of faculty members and the mean student group attitude change. They conclude that change in nursing students' stereotypic attitude toward elderly persons relates functionally to attitudes of the nursing faculty.

Equally significant findings result from studies of registered professional nurses' attitudes and their relationship to care for elderly persons. Utilizing Kogan's Old People Scale (1961), Hatton (1977) found that nurses with more favorable attitudes exhibited a high percentage of positive interactions with elderly patients. Also using Kogan's scale, Futrell and Jones's study (1977:45) demonstrated that older, better-educated, and more experienced nurses evince more positive attitudes toward elderly patients than younger, less experienced, and less educated nurses.

In contrast to Futrell and Jones's findings, Taylor and Harned (1978) found that nurses under 40 years of age, nurses with fewer than 10 years' experience working with elderly persons, and nurses who work in hospitals demonstrated more positive attitudes toward elderly people as measured by their scores on Kogan's Old People Scale. Since a lower mean score reflects a more positive attitude, these nurses achieved scores below the group mean.

The field of geriatric and gerontological nursing is relatively new. A review of the literature on attitudes nursing students and nurses hold toward the aged demonstrates a need for further study to determine whether relationships exist between specific characteristics of nurses and their attitudes toward elderly persons. Lore (1979) points out that nurses caring for elderly patients may feel threatened by what they see as an omen of their future, and their own level of maturity may affect their ability to care for these patients. Solomon and Vickers (1979) report that attitudes are conveyed to patients, and positive attitudes not expressed appropriately remain of major concern to nursing service administrators (White, 1977).

PURPOSE OF STUDY

Determining whether relationships exist between characteristics of registered professional nurses employed at the Medical Center's Nursing Department and their attitudes toward elderly persons constituted a major purpose of the study. Data was collected from two instruments: Kogan's Old People Scale and a biographical data sheet designed for the study. Biographical data included respondents' length of employment at the Medical Center, age, type of nursing education, and length of experience working with elderly patients. Four research questions were addressed: Does length of employment at the medical center correlate with nurses' attitudes toward elderly persons? Are attitudes toward elderly persons influenced by educational preparation of nurses? Does a relationship exist between age of nurses and their attitudes toward elderly persons? Does length of experience working with elderly patients correlate with nurses' attitudes toward elderly patients?

PROCEDURE AND METHODOLOGY

Utilizing regularly scheduled staff meetings, nurses employed in the nursing department received the opportunity to participate voluntarily in the study; 180 nurses participated. Thus the sample was a convenient rather than a randomized one. A trained data gatherer explained the study's purpose and instructions for filling out biographical data sheets and responding to the survey instrument. To promote valid responses, emphasis regarding purpose of the study focused on use of data to plan continuing education programs in the care of elderly patients for nurses employed in the medical center's nursing department. Consent forms were obtained from all participants.

In 1961, Kogan developed an instrument with a Likert-type scale designed to measure attitudes toward elderly persons with respect to norms and individual differences. Commonly referred to as Kogan's *Old People (OP) Scale,* the instrument contains items in the form of positive-negative pairs. The instrument was tested adequately for reliability and validity. The reliability coefficients and interscale correlations ranged from .66 to .85 (Kogan, 1961:48). The content of the items focuses on feelings of discomfort in the presence of elderly persons, residential aspects of old peoples' lives, and their personal attributes, e.g., degree of independence, intelligence, wit, etc. Primarily indicating group attitude, individual scores are interpreted in relation to the distribution of scores made by other respondents in a test group. Respondents were asked to score each item by placing a check mark in the column which best expressed their opinion. Additional instructions were not to leave any item blank and to mark only one response per item.

Respondents were grouped according to the clinical area where they work: critical care, medical-surgical, pediatric-obstetrics, and "other or unidentified." The latter category included such areas as operating and postanesthesia recovery rooms, emergency department, outpatient clinics, and nursing education. Each respondent's score on Kogan's scale appeared next to her or his individual characteristics regarding years of employment at the medical center, years of experience working with elderly patients, age, and type of nursing education.

Since one of the independent variables, educational preparation, does not qualify as an interval scale, a numerical code was established for diploma, associate, baccalaureate, master's, and doctoral educated respondents. Analysis of the distribution of the respondents' educational levels of preparation revealed that one held a master's degree and none held a doctoral degree. Based on further analysis, all degreed respondents were placed into one category identified by code number 2. Code number 1 represents graduates of hospital-based diploma programs. No specific statistical analysis was performed. The data were tabulated by determining frequency of responses for each numerical code and converting totals to percentages.

The results of Kogan's scale were scored by utilizing his methodology, which requires adding individual item scores for the OP+ and OP– scales and converting the sums to mean scores. Following Kogan's methodology, positive mean scores were subtracted from 8.0 to make both scales comparable. Using this method, higher scores reflect more unfavorable attitudes and lower scores more favorable attitudes toward elderly persons (Kogan, 1961:45–45). To characterize the performance of the group, each individual total score was added and the sum divided by the number of respondents to establish the group mean.

Mean scores of all respondents and clinical area groupings were computed for Kogan's scale, length of employment at the medical center, length of experience working with elderly patients, age, and type of nursing education. The tetrachoric correlation coefficient statistical method was used to calculate correlations between respondents' specific characteristics and group mean scores on Kogan's OP scale.

RESULTS AND DISCUSSION

Results of this study cannot be generalized. This study was a survey in one medical center that has a high population of elderly patients. Limitations exist in the study, owing partly to the design of the study and factors beyond control for the study. Since involvement in the survey was voluntary, a specific limitation is that only nurses with favorable attitudes toward elderly persons may have volunteered to respond to the questionnaire. Another limitation beyond control relates to respondents' favorable or unfavorable experiences with elderly persons.

As shown in Table 21-1, mean length of employment at the medical center for the entire group of respondents was 4.99 years. Critical care nurses remained well below the mean, averaging 3 years. This finding correlates with national surveys reporting a high turnover rate among nurses working in intensive care–critical care areas (Brief, 1976; Godfrey, 1978a and b). Comparing time employed with the group's mean on Kogan's scale, critical care nurses with 6.21 scored well below the overall group mean of 6.35.

The nature and purpose of critical care–intensive care units may explain why results of critical care nurses' scores reflect more favorable attitudes toward elderly persons. Patients admitted to these areas are in an acute, critical stage of illness requiring immediate and intensive care. When they pass this stage of illness (3–5 days), they are transferred to a medical-surgical unit. Average length of hospitalization for elderly patients in this medical center's medical-surgical units is 9.5 days. The comparatively "rapid" patient turnover in critical care units limits the length of time critical care nurses spend with elderly patients. This factor coupled with the nurse's favorable scores on Kogan's scale support other findings which reflect a relationship between

Table 21-1   Individual Characteristics of Respondents and Group Means of Kogan Scale Scores

Independent variable (characteristics)	Critical care (N = 31)		Medical-surgical (N = 83)		Pediatrics-obstetrics (N = 31)		Other or unidentified (N = 35)		All respondents (N = 180)	
Time employed at medical center	3.00		5.76		4.60		6.63		4.99	
Experience working with elderly patients	5.34		6.37		4.06		10.3		6.51	
Age	28.5		33.8		31.8		35.1		32.3	
Education and preparation	N	%	N	%	N	%	N	%	N	%
Code 1 (diploma)	15	48	47	57	14	45	20	57	96	54
Code 2 (ADN, BSN, MSN)	16	52	33	40	16	52	13	37	78	43
No answer			3	3	1	3	2	6	6	3
Dependent variable (Kogan's scale scores)	6.21		6.33		6.58		6.31		6.35	

less experience with elderly persons and more positive attitude scores (Taylor and Harned, 1978).

Pediatric-obstetric nurses scored second lowest for length of employment at this medical center, with a mean of 4.60 years. Unlike the critical care nurses, however, their group mean on Kogan's scale (6.58) proved well above the overall mean of 6.35. Possible reasons for these results may be that nurses select specific clinical areas because of their interest in, and desire to work with, certain types of patients. Nurses selecting pediatrics do so because of their desire to work with children or their desire to avoid working with elderly patients. Nurses selecting obstetrics (maternity nursing) do so because they enjoy seeing new life come into the world. They may avoid working with elderly patients because they perceive the specter of death in their countenance. Preference (or avoidance) in working with elderly persons presents an indicator of nurses' attitudes toward these persons (Delora and Moses, 1969).

Respondents grouped under "other or unidentified" areas represent nurses working in emergency, outpatient, or nursing education departments, surgical suite (operating room), and postanesthesia recovery rooms. As shown in Table 21–1, mean length of employment for these nurses was 6.63 years. This score ranks highest of all individual

clinical groups and well above the overall mean of 4.99 years. The finding is consistent with some studies showing that nurses working in these areas usually have more longevity than nurses working in other areas of a hospital (Godfrey, 1978b). The group's mean on Kogan's scale (6.31) ranked slightly below the overall mean of 6.35 and second lowest in comparison with the critical care nurses' group mean of 6.21 and the medical-surgical group mean of 6.33. Mean length of employment for the medical-surgical nurses' group was 5.76 years.

The pediatric-obstetric nurses' group received the lowest score for length of experience working with elderly patients, with a mean of 4.06. This is not surprising in view of previous observations regarding why nurses choose to work in specific clinical specialties. These nurses apparently selected working in pediatric or obstetric units. Therefore, they would not have as much experience working with elderly patients as their counterparts in medical-surgical, critical care, and "other or unidentified" areas where elderly patients predominate. The group's performance on Kogan's scale placed it well above the overall mean of 6.35, with a score of 6.58. This score ranked highest among all clinical groups. As noted previously, preference (or avoidance) in working with elderly persons presents an indicator of nurses' attitudes toward these persons (Delora and Moses, 1969).

The third characteristic subjected to determination of means was respondents' age. Following previous format, mean age was determined for individual clinical groups and the total group (all respondents) (Table 21-1). Mean age for all respondents was 32.3 years. Critical care nurses proved the youngest group with a mean age of 28.5 years. On Kogan's scale, this group scored well below the mean, with 6.21, reflecting more favorable attitudes toward elderly persons. Pediatric-obstetric nurses, the second youngest group, demonstrated a mean age of 31.8 years. Their score on Kogan's scale ranked above the mean with 6.58, reflecting more unfavorable attitudes toward elderly persons. They were the only group that scored above the mean on Kogan's scale. Two groups scored above the mean age, medical-surgical and "other or unidentified." Medical-surgical nurses demonstrated a mean age of 33.8 years and their mean score on Kogan's scale was 6.33. "Other or unidentified" nurses represent the oldest group, with a mean age of 35.1 years. They scored 6.31 on Kogan's scale.

Respondents' type of nursing education represents the fourth independent variable (Table 21-1). Ninety-six, or 54 percent of all respondents, graduated from hospital-based diploma programs. This finding proves consistent with educational preparation of nurses employed in most hospitals; diploma programs reflect the traditional method of nursing education. Medical-surgical and "other or unidentified" respondents from hospital-based diploma programs represented 67 or 70 percent of all respondents who participated in the survey. The medical-surgical and "other or unidentified" groups evinced similar performances on Kogan's scale, scoring slightly below the mean of 6.35 with respective scores of 6.33 and 6.31. Additionally, both groups scored above the means on length of employment at the medical center and age.

Contrasting the critical care and pediatric-obstetric groups, of the 31 respondents in each group, 52 percent were code 2, or graduates of associate, baccalaureate, or master's degree nursing programs. Except for scores on Kogan's scale, the critical care and pediatric-obstetric groups demonstrated similar findings on all independent variables. They scored below the means on length of employment at the medical center, length of experience working with elderly patients, and age.

The dichotomy described in the literature proved evident throughout the study. There was no relationship to length of employment at the medical center, length of experience working with elderly patients, age, type of nursing education, and respondents' performance on Kogan's scale as a total group. In comparison, analysis of performance of clinical groups revealed higher correlations between Kogan's scale scores and respondents' specific characteristics. Table 21-2 displays results of the calculated tetrachoric correlation coefficient ($r\hat{t}$) for all groups.

Table 21-2 Results of Calculated Tetrachoric Correlation Coefficient for All Groups

Independent variables	Critical care nurses N = 31	Pediatric/ obstetric nurses N = 31	Medical/ surgical nurses N = 83	Other or unidentified nurses N = 35	All respondents N = 180
Time employed at MSMC	−.35	+.31	−.04	−.25	−.04
Experience working with elderly	−.35	−.09	+.08	+.01	−.05
Age	−.13	+.36	−.09	−.12	−.06
Education preparation	−.25	+.71	−.20	+.02	+.01
Dependent variable (Kogan scale scores)	6.21	6.58	6.33	6.31	6.35

Higher correlations between dependent and independent variables achieved by critical care and pediatric-obstetric nurses' groups are apparent. Results reveal that although the critical care nurses' group scored lower on Kogan's scale, the critical care and pediatric-obstetric nurses' groups as a whole demonstrated higher correlations between Kogan's scale scores and length of employment at the medical center, length of experience working with elderly patients, age, and educational preparation than their counterparts in the medical-surgical and "other or unidentified" nurses' groups. Noting that the respondents may not represent the medical center's critical care and pediatric-obstetric nurses accurately because of voluntary participation in the study, these findings suggest that younger nurses with more educational preparation and less experience working with elderly patients possess more unfavorable attitudes toward elderly persons. The findings suggest also that unfavorable attitudes toward elderly persons may contribute to the pediatric-obstetric nurses' short length of employment at the medical center.

Contrasting the data for the pediatric-obstetric nurses' group with those of the critical care, medical-surgical, and "other or unidentified" nurses' groups, the findings show that the latter three groups scored lower on Kogan's scale (reflecting more favorable attitudes toward elderly persons). However, the medical-surgical and "other or unidentified" groups scored higher than the critical care and pediatric-obstetric groups in years employed at the medical center and experience working with elderly patients, were older, and had less educational experience. The findings reveal that nurses working in the medical center's medical-surgical units, emergency and outpatient department, and operating and postanesthesia recovery rooms possess more favorable attitudes toward elderly persons. With the exception of the critical care nurses who held the highest positive attitudes on Kogan's scale, the nurses who participated in this survey and held more positive attitudes toward elderly patients tended to be older, evinced less education preparation, had more experience working with elderly patients, and more longevity working at the medical center.

IMPLICATIONS AND RECOMMENDATIONS

It has been estimated that by the turn of the century over 30 million people will be 75 years of age and older. Approximately 20 percent will be institutionalized and will require professional nursing care. Because this medical center services a high percentage of elderly patients, it may be that the findings of this study have implications for a larger community of providers of health care services to elderly patients. The implications concern recruitment, selection and assignment of nurses, preservice and inservice nursing education programs, and need for further studies.

Favorable attitudes toward elderly persons reflect a desirable characteristic for employment. Administering Kogan's OP Scale questionnaire to all nurses seeking employment at this medical center would be an effective screening process to identify nurses with more unfavorable attitudes toward elderly persons. Although pressures to fill positions often take precedence over effective screening procedures, identification of those nurses who lack positive attitudes toward elderly persons enhances the nursing service administrator's ability to focus in-service education programs for them. To assist these nurses in developing and maintaining supportive and realistic attitudes toward elderly patients, extensive orientation and attitudinal development programs should be implemented. Program content should include the process of normal aging as a positive experience and discussions regarding nurses' self-image in this process, as well as the dynamics of aging and the care of elderly patients.

While in-service education may effect change in attitudes toward elderly patients, the appropriate place to start is at the preservice education level. The literature review showed that nursing students are not exposed sufficiently to creative experiences focusing on positive aspects of geriatric nursing. Basic nursing education programs should emphasize geriatrics. To accomplish this, however, we need more graduate programs preparing enthusiastic and informed gerontological nurse-educators.

This study and others generate questions requiring further study. Follow-up studies of this medical center's nurses should be conducted to determine whether their attitudes toward elderly persons influence the quality of care their patients receive. Both preliminary and follow-up attitudinal surveys should be conducted to determine the effects of workshops specifically focused on attitudinal change and increased knowledge in geriatric-gerontological nursing. Additional studies should determine whether similarities exist in life experiences of nurses with favorable versus unfavorable attitudes toward elderly patients. Acceptance of elderly persons and our attitudes toward them may be reflective of how we will accept ourselves as elderly persons.

EDITOR'S QUESTIONS FOR DISCUSSION

What factors may account for negative attitudes toward the elderly by nurses? Though there is constant turnover for nurses in gerontological settings, what initially attracts nurses to those settings? How can those factors be capitalized upon to induce nurses to remain in gerontological nursing? What inhibiting factors in the setting itself can be minimized? How might they be negated? What type of attitudes toward elderly patients are critical to explore, if it is true that nurses select specific clinical areas because of their interest?

In the study by Gunter, what might account for students expressing more negative attitudes toward elderly patients at the end of a course in geriatrics than in the beginning? What type of creative experiences could be planned for nursing students? If faculties' attitudes are related to the change in attitude of students, what implications does this have for nursing education? How and to what extent can the negative effect indicated by Wilhite and Johnson's study be remedied?

How might the dichotomous findings from studies utilizing Kogan's scale (Futrell and Jones, Taylor and Harned as well as Mercadante's) be explained? To what extent does it appear all of those studies used the same independent variables? How valid and reliable is the Kogan scale? What other variables might account for the different findings? To what extent would you agree that the Kogan's "OP Scale" would be an effective questionnaire in screening nurses for employment in *this* setting?

What are the advantages and disadvantages of utilizing a convenience rather than a randomized sample? How does a convenience sample differ from a "purposeful" sample? What are the implications for validity, reliability, and generalizability of studies utilizing those types of sampling methods?

How appropriate was the use of tetrachoric correlation coefficients for these data? What conditions are necessary to utilize this test? What additional specific statistical analysis might have been performed? How would you justify the use of those statistical methods?

Are there other limitations to this study than Mercandante has indicated? What significance or relationship might there be to the validity of this study in focusing the purpose of the study on use of data to plan continuing education programs in the care of elderly patients?

How do turnover rates in this study compare with findings of other studies? What possibility exists for the length of time for elderly patients to be increased in critical care units? What effect and why might this impact on attitudes of critical care nurses? Are there any explanations of the findings which appear contradictory? If so, what alternative interpretations are possible?

As suggested in this study, why would younger nurses with more educational preparation and less experience working with elderly patients possess more unfavorable attitudes?

How might preservice and in-service education content be designed and implemented to effectively influence the development and maintenance of positive attitudes toward the elderly? What variables and measures need to be utilized to establish direct relationships of the impact of curricula in university and in-service education in the setting?

REFERENCES

American Journal of Nursing
 1979 "Nursing Shortage? Yes!" Special AJN Report. American Journal of Nursing, 79:469–480.

Brief, Arthur P.
 1976 "Turnover Among Hospital Nurses: A Suggested Model." Journal of Nursing Administration, 76(4):55–58.

Brock, Anna M.
 1977 "Improving Nursing Care for the Elderly: An Educational Task." Journal of Gerontological Nursing, 3:26–28.

Brower, H. Terri
 1977 "A Study of Graduate Programs In Gerontological Nursing." Journal of Gerontological Nursing, 3:40–46.

Butler, R. and M. Lewis
 1973 Aging and Mental Health St. Louis: C. V. Mosby Company.

Campbell, Margaret Eleanor
 1971 "Study of Attitudes of Nursing Personnel Toward the Geriatric Patient." Nursing Research, 20:147–151.

DeLora, Jack R. and Dorothy V. Moses
 1969 "Specialty Preferences and Characteristics of Nursing Students in Baccalaureate Programs." Nursing Research, 18:137–144.

Elmore, Marjorie Jane
 1964 "Proposal Relating to the Selection and Organization of Learning Experiences for Nursing Students in the Care of Older Patients." Doctoral Dissertation, Teachers College, Columbia University, New York.

Futrell, Mary and Wyatt Jones
 1977 "Attitudes of Physicians, Nurses, and Social Workers Toward the Elderly and Health Maintenance Services for the Aged: Implications for Health Manpower Policy." Journal of Gerontological Nursing, 3:42–46.

Godfrey, Marjorie A.
 1978a "Job Satisfaction." Part I. Nursing '78 (4):89–102.
 1978b "Job Satisfaction." Part II. Nursing '78 (5):105–120.

Gunter, Laurie
 1971 "Students' Attitudes Toward Geriatric Nursing." Nursing Outlook, 19:466–469.

Hatton, Jean
 1977 "Nurses' Attitude Toward the Aged—Relationship to Nursing Care." Journal of Gerontological Nursing, 3:21–26.

Heller, Barbara R. and Frederick J. Walsh
 1976 "Changing Nursing Students' Attitudes Toward the Aged." Journal of Nursing Education, 15:9–17.

Kogan, Nathan
 1961 "Attitudes Toward Old People: The Development of a Scale and an Examination of Correlates." Journal of Abnormal Social Psychology, 62:44–54.

Lore, Ann
 1979 "Supporting the Hospitalized Elderly Persons." American Journal of Nursing, 79:496–499.

Moses, Dorothy and Carolyn S. Lake
 1971 "Geriatrics in Baccalaureate Nursing Curriculum." Nursing Outlook, 16:41–43.

Solomon, Kenneth and Raymond Vickers
  1979 "Attitudes of Health Workers Toward
         Old People." Journal of the American
         Geriatrics Society 27(4):186–191, April.
Taylor, Kathleen H. and Thomas L. Harned
  1978 "Attitudes Toward Old People: A Study
         of Nurses Who Care for the Elderly."
         Journal of Gerontological Nursing, 4:43–
         47.

White, Caroline M.
  1977 "The Nurse-Patient Encounter: Attitudes
         and Behavior in Action." Journal of Ger-
         ontological Nursing, 3:16–20.
Wilhite, Mary J. and Dale M. Johnson
  1976 "Changes in Nursing Students' Stereo-
         typic Attitudes Toward Old People."
         Nursing Research, 25:6:430–432.

Chapter 22

Psychological Correlates of Pain and Nursing Practice

Rita F. Stein, R.N., Ph.D.
Former Professor and Director of Research
School of Nursing
Indiana University
Indianapolis, Indiana

The pain experience is a significant factor to be taken into account in planning care with the patient. Rita F. Stein attempts to contribute to the understanding of pain by focusing on the person's psychological and verbal responses to pain. She describes a study of 79 patients from 21 to 65 years of age with chronic pain who were admitted to the pain center of a general hospital. The pain center utilizes a holistic, multidisciplinary treatment approach. Therapy and programs for the subjects included: biofeedback, medication control, health education, exercise, and vocational counseling. Stein details the procedures administered on admission, at discharge, and at least 6 months after discharge. The tools used are: a clinical report, the Two-Factor Index of Social Position, the Tennessee Self Concept Scale (TSCS), and the Minnesota Multiphasic Personality Inventory (MMPI) Depression Scale. She indicates that the mean length of stay at the pain center for the study group was 4.72. She reports that only 33 of the initial 79 subjects were able to be studied after discharge. Her major comparisons of the data were made between the group on admission and the group on discharge. The data support Stein's four hypotheses. The demographic data indicated that subjects' mean age was 45 years; there were slightly more females than males; the majority identified with the Protestant faith; over 72 percent were semiskilled to unskilled workers and almost 32 percent of the subjects had six or more siblings.

The major organic problem indicated by 66.2 percent (47) of the subjects was low back disorder. All were on drugs for relief of pain. The 79 patients had a composite index of 123 back surgeries. The findings infer that the subjects on admission had negative feelings toward the various selves measured in the Tennessee Self Concept Scale, which improved significantly on discharge. Likewise, the scores on the MMPI Depression Scale were significantly improved at the time of discharge. Compared to their discharge status, the 33 patients who were followed were not significantly different in most of the self-concept items. However, they indicated significantly higher depressive scores from their status on discharge. It was not feasible to establish direct relationships between the therapy and programs provided for the subject and the produced data.

The psychological phenomena of pain provide the framework for the physiological and medical problems which will be considered in this chapter.[1] This study was initiated in an attempt to contribute to the understanding of pain by focusing on the verbal aspects of the pain experience. It is assumed and recognized that physiological explanations of pain contain psychological manifestations that have an effect on the study and treatment of pain.

Pain is a highly personal experience which is influenced by cultural learning, the meaning of the situation, attention getting, and other factors. Zborowski (1969) observed differences in reaction to pain by different ethnic groups. He found that there were differences in psychological reactions to pain between Irish, Italian, Jewish, and "old American" groups.

Past experiences with others suffering pain have been implicated as determinants of the manner in which pain is expressed (Sternbach, 1978:87). Important psychological processes include: reinforcement of the social consequences of pain; impact of family interactions on consequences of pain; and the use of individuals important to the person in pain to serve as models for the pain experience and its manner of expression (Sternbach, 1978:82). An individual not only perceives pain but reacts to the pain experience (McCafferty, 1979). When a patient speaks of intolerable pain he or she is describing his or her subjective feelings in reaction to it (McCafferty, 1979:15–16; Pawl, 1978:7–8).

Those reaction patterns that stem from subjective life experiences as members of a society require utilization of the concepts and methods from the social and behavioral sciences. Bond feels that there are strong ethnic and racial components which are learned responses to pain (1978:32–33). He also cites personality traits which are important in the potential reactions to the pain experience (1978:32).

Feelings of anxiety, depression, or hostility are expressed in words and actions directly related to the individual's discomfort (McCafferty, 1979). The pain experience acquires a significance as a means of communication in interpersonal relationships between the patient and members of his group (Blendis et al., 1978:185; Pilowsky and Spence, 1976:62).

As long as nurses depend upon a patient's subjective description of his or her pain and suffering, they are mainly concerned with reactions to pain different from those achieved in the laboratory. In evaluating a patient's complaints a doctor or nurse is confronted with verbal representations rather than the actual sensation of pain. Aside from moans, winces, and changes in skin color, the patient's emotions and anxieties are reflected in behavior towards the pain experience (McCafferty, 1979:15–16).

The sole objective of this project is to contribute to the understanding of person's responses to pain. Little is known of the self-concept of persons in pain. Expression of hostility to self and others, existence of depressive syndromes, and psychosomatic problems are discussed in relation to pain phenomena (Applegate, 1980; Sternbach, 1978:203–216; Sternbach and Timmermans, 1975:179).

By focusing on the self-concept and depression as variables in human behavior, one might be able to understand differences in persons as well as similarities in reacting to the pain phenomena. Professionals may also be able to predict and understand future behavior and counsel persons into more effective directions of living.

The Problem

The literature portrays psychological correlates of pain with statements expressing psychological

[1]ACKNOWLEDGMENT This chapter could not be published without acknowledgment to Brenda Astor (R.N.) for her help and cooperation in the development of this study. She was chief nurse on the pain unit and assisted most generously in the collection of the data. She was most patient, kind, and understanding with the subject participants while they responded to the questionnaires. She abstracted from the clinical records the needed information. In short she was an invaluable partner in the collection of data. To her I am indebted for providing the data and help without which this chapter could not have been written.

coping reactions: hostility to self, hostility directed outward to significant others, guilt feelings, assumption of the dependent sick role (Blendis et al., 1978:179-191; Pawl, 1978:2-8; Bond, 1979:93-94).

Nurses need to be aware of psychological dynamics during the pain syndrome because of their frequent encounters with patients who have pain (McCafferty, 1979:7). It is necessary that they plan their assessments and implementations of nursing care to cope with the pain syndrome as this affects the total patient. Giving medication is not enough. The psychological pattern of coping with pain can override the nursing care plan. The pain experience is a significant factor in planning for interpersonal communication between the patient, the patient's family, and the nurse.

Hypotheses

1 Upon admission to the pain center patients with chronic pain had feelings of inadequacy in their social domain, feelings of being inferior to others, had poor self-esteem in the measurement of their self-concept.
2 The self-concept improved after intensive physical and psychological therapy.
3 Those in pain manifested depressive syndromes on admission which could be measured by the Minnesota Multiphasic Personality Inventory (MMPI) Depression Scale.
4 On exit from the program of intensive therapy, depression scores decreased significantly on the MMPI Depression Scale.

Definitions

Pain punishment; a sensation of hurting or strong discomfort in some part of the body, caused by an injury, disease, or functional disorder and transmitted through the nervous system; the distress or suffering, mental or physical, caused by great anxiety, anguish, grief, disappointment, etc. (Webster's Dictionary, 1970).
Depression An emotional illness characterized by feelings of joylessness, hopelessness, low self-esteem, and pessimism. Manifestations of psychomotor retardation are present, social isolation and

self preoccupation, brooding, and irritability (Dahlstrom et al., 1972, 1975a:146; Sternbach, 1974: 42).
Self-Concept The ideas which one has about oneself in relation to others in the environment. A measure of self-esteem and self-acceptance via body image, self-image, and self-evaluation. In the phenomenal world it "is the self as seen, perceived, and experienced by him" (Fitts et al., 1971:3).

Review of the Literature

Throughout history observations exist on what we call "pain." In the sixteenth century, Shakespeare recognized that pain may be influenced by emotion. He stated in his plays that "one pain is lessened by another's anguish," (Shakespeare, 1961a:403) and that "the labor we delight in physics pain" (Shakespeare, 1961b:1053).

In the early part of the twentieth century, Freud (1938:534-535) discussed the phenomena of pain as a common conversion symptom where an unpleasant affect was converted to pain. Pain had a symbolic meaning.

Today, in the twentieth century, there is a continuation in the writings about pain, especially in the interweaving of physical and psychological components as a whole to the pain response. Sternbach (1974:Chap. 2) reported that a person with back pain plays the "loser" in the game of life. He discussed the depressive syndrome as an important part of the pain response.

Sternbach and Timmermans (1975) came to the conclusion that neuroticism associated with chronic pain was the result of pain and was reversible when pain was reduced or abolished. Of 113 patients treated in a 2-year period, 29 patients had surgery for pain relief compared with 84 patients with no surgery. Surgical patients ranked higher on Minnesota Multiphasic Personality Inventory Hysteria and Invalidism Scales and had less pain following surgery, with improvements in personality.

Fear of pain was one of the most acute and realistic of fears. Loneliness was the second fear which had a profound relationship to pain, for fear and pain were found to be most intense when the patient was left alone (Williams, 1976:52).

Pilowsky and Spence (1976:61–71) reported on a study in which 100 patients with pain completed a 52-item Illness Behavior Questionnaire. The patients were divided into six groups on analysis of the data. Group 1 had low scores on all scales and denied that problems existed. Group 2 was sad and anxious about problems. Members of group 3 showed that they were easily angered and complained that pain interfered with relationships. Groups 4 to 6 had greater evidence of abnormal behavior. The syndromes resembled hysteria, conversion reaction, and hypochondriasis.

Blendis et al. (1978:185) stated that among psychiatric patients the most frequent site of pain is the head. Neck and back are the second most frequent sites and pains in the abdomen the third most frequent site. He felt that the influence on the site of pain was through the family and relatives. For the most part children with certain painful sites had mothers so affected.

It was suggested by Sternbach (1978:212) that there was a close link between pain, illness behavior, and the sick role and that this provided a useful framework for viewing the personal, social, and environmental factors as determinants of pain.

Bond (1978:93–94) spoke of changes in emotion occurring among those in pain which resulted from the physical and social consequences of the disorder giving rise to and influencing the personality. He stated that pain led to greater levels of introspection, resulting in anxiety and depression. These conditions sometimes led to alcholism and suicide.

Pawl (1978:2–8) stated that half the misery suffered from painful disorders was psychological. Pain changed the sufferer's personality. He lost the ability to cope with relatives, friends, and business associates. Depression was a common psychological end result of a painful disorder. A person in chronic pain sought help from several

doctors, and consequently fear, anxiety, and depression increased. Consistent worry produced tension in the muscle groups, which heightened the pain experience. The aim of treatment was to relax the muscle groups through medical and psychological means.

McCafferty (1979:11), viewing the pain experience from the perception of the nurse, stated that in evaluating pain, a patient saying he or she had pain for all practical purposes did have pain. Personal and social areas of the subject in pain were important areas of nursing assessment. She felt the anxiety and depression as concomitants to pain could increase pain by increasing muscle tension. Therefore relief from anger, anxiety, and sadness enabled the person to experience less pain (McCafferty, 1979:15). McCafferty continued with a discussion of various technical and interpersonal models to help the patient control pain.

This review cannot appropriately end without reviewing the work of Chapman, Sola, and Bonica (1979:1–7). They compared pain patients from a private practice clinic with those at the University of Washington Pain Center with regard to illness behavior and depression. They found that private patients were significantly less depressed, showed less conviction of disease and less hypochondriasis, and were less somatically focused. However, organic lesions were more easily identified in private practice patients. They did not indicate the length of time patients had pain in the two different settings. Greater time interval of pain in the pain center coupled with finding less organic lesions in this center could lead to the different psychological states.

Applegate (1980:213–216) studied *locus of control* in subjects admitted to a pain center. She reported that nearly all subjects converted from external to internal control on testing after intensive treatment. She further stated that pain control was enhanced when the meaning of pain was confronted at the conscious level. Internally controlled patients experienced less anxiety than externally controlled people.

In summary pain strikes the whole person (physically and psychologically). The word "pain" has intrapsychic, societal, and interpersonal connotations. It is capable of disrupting life by virtue of its function to signal danger.

OVERVIEW OF THE PAIN CENTER TREATMENT PROGRAM

The holistic approach is used at the pain center in which the study was conducted. The theoretical framework related to chronic pain is the theory of *holistic therapy*. Karl Menders, director of the clinic, described the concept of holistic therapy at a speech presentation in 1978.

According to Menders (1978) the holistic approach to the individual recognizes the interaction between the person and his psychosocial environment. This approach reestablishes the emphasis upon the patient rather than medical technology. Thus, any personal disease or disorder is a complex interaction of social factors, physical and psychological stress, the personality of the person subjected to these influences, and the inability of the person to adapt adequately to stress. Thus psychosomatic disease conveys the concept of a fundamental interaction between mind and body. It is a two-way interaction between the brain and the rest of the body.

If illness is viewed as a complex interaction of the above factors, then symptoms can be viewed as an excessive strain upon the mind-body system. An important concept of holistic medicine is that patients and their health practitioners share responsibilities for mind-body interaction (Menders, 1978). In a signed contract the patient and doctor mutually agree to share responsibility for the treatment of pain.

The pain center utilized multidisciplinary personnel which included a wide variety of health professionals. These included physicians, neurosurgeons, registered nurses, social workers, dieticians, an anesthesiologist, a psychologist, and an occupational, a recreational, and a physical therapist. Diagnostic procedures available were x-ray, psychological testing, and electroencephalography. The therapeutic modalities included calisthenics or exercise, biofeedback and relaxation training, medication control, nerve block, recreation training, group therapy, whirlpool baths, swimnastics, health education, and vocational counseling.

Biofeedback was a form of relaxation training. The objective of this relaxation program was to help the patient to relax more effectively, thus reducing pain. The use of this machine helped the patients to control stress and to promote a calm frame of mind and a sense of self-control.

Medication control was established by eliminating the use of addictive drugs and substituting analgesics (such as aspirin, Tylenol, and Darvocet), which were gradually decreased in dosage and time intervals over a period of about a month.

Generally the health education program helped the patients to increase self-knowledge, which resulted in improvements in social interaction, wellness behavior, and pain control. It was felt, additionally, that the patient learned personal control and learned to create the desired life rather than mere reaction to it. This kind of health education was accomplished through assertiveness training, individual counseling, group counseling, and health education classes.

The exercise program consisted of calisthenics, hydrotherapy, swimnastics, body mechanics training, posture training, walking, and cycling. The objective of this program was to promote relaxation and to learn to reduce pain through physical therapy techniques, which, in turn reduces muscle resistance and increases muscle strength and mobility.

Recreation training consisted of community excursions, crafts, art, games, and entertainment. The purpose of this program was to renew interest in recreation and to develop new recreational activities. It was the objective of this program to develop interests and skills, not only new ones, but also at least the prepain activities of daily living.

Vocational counseling had as its objective

to return the patients to vocations practiced previous to pain and if possible help them realize their potentialities in the labor market.

All the above activities stress self-help and the renewal of abilities for personal control, development of musculature, and rehabilitation of personal and social interests. The treatment program was multifaceted in order to obtain an increased satisfaction in life. Instead of eliminating the pain the treatment was aimed at reducing pain by establishing a pattern of wellness which provided self-actualizing experiences.

METHODOLOGY

Sampling

Seventy-nine adults admitted to the pain center with pain and between 21 and 65 years of age were chosen for study. Those above 65 years of age were not included to minimize the complication of geriatric patient needs. All patients who met age stipulations were interviewed and tested on admission and on discharge from the center. The testing procedures and the clinical report are discussed below.

Procedures

I Clinical Report The patient's chart was abstracted for demographic data (age, sex, occupation, education, religion, and diagnosis). The progress reports were scanned for surgery done or anticipated, clinical tests made, drugs taken, symptoms on admission and discharge, length of hospitalization, and previous surgery.

II The Two-Factor Index of Social Position
The Two-Factor Index of Social Position (Hollingshead, 1957:2) was developed "to meet the need for an objective and easily applicable procedure to estimate the positions individuals occupy in the status structure of our society."

Occupation and education are the two factors utilized to determine social position. *Occupation* is given to reflect skill and power as the individuals

perform in the many positions in our society. *Education* reflects knowledge and cultural tastes.

The two-factor index, which measures social economic status (SES), is divided into a range of scores on a continuum and divided into groups of scores as validated by factor analysis. For purposes of this paper, the range of scores for upper, middle, and lower classes will be as follows:

Social class	Range of scores
I, II Upper class	11–27
III Middle class	28–43
IV, V Lower class	44–77

The index attempts to delineate operationally the socially discriminating comparisons people make of each other in their day-to-day behaviors. This scale is premised upon three assumptions: (1) that social stratification exists in the community; (2) that stratification is based upon a few commonly accepted cultural characteristics; (3) that the items which are symbolic of social status may be scaled and grouped by statistical procedures (Hollingshead, 1957).

The rationale for use of the Hollingshead index is provided by Irving Krauss in his book on stratification, class, and conflict (1976). He states that shared understandings and expectations transcend the individual's and guide future interactions. The individual's self-conception is also influenced by group definitions (Krauss, 1976:13).

In selecting criteria it is desirable to select those which are most critical for people's lives. Persons whose occupations are associated with accumulated wealth are compared with those in occupations not requiring skilled labor. There are those who sell mental skills compared with those who do not develop special mental skills. When both occupation and education are considered it can be said that persons' job opportunities are determined by their schooling. Education provides access to social goods and is a necessary condition for entering various occupations (Krauss, 1976:88). In general, the higher a person's occupational role, the better able he or she is to obtain social goods relative to others lower in the hierarchy. In line with upward mobility in a free society, the chance is there for higher education and higher occupational status.

III The Tennessee Self-Concept Scale (TSCS)

The TSCS (referred to above) was originated by William Fitts (1965). He and his coworkers established the validity and reliability of the test and studied the test for its use on different populations (Fitts, 1965; Fitts et al., 1971).

The TSCS represents a construct which is applicable to literate populations and can be completed in 15 to 20 minutes (Fitts, 1965; Fitts et al., 1971). The categories of analysis represent the following (Fitts, 1965):

Self-criticism. These are all mildly derogatory statements that most people admit as being true for them. Individuals who deny most of these statements most often are being defensive and making a deliberate effort to present a favorable picture of themselves. High scores generally indicate a normal, healthy openness and capacity for self-criticism.

The true-false ratio (T-F). These are measures of response set or response bias. These scores indicate whether persons tend to agree or disagree with the items regardless of content.

The distribution scores. These are summary scores of the way persons distribute their answers across the five categories in the scale. It reflects the certainty of how persons see themselves. High scores indicate that patients are very definite in what they say about themselves. Low scores are found in the persons who are defensive and guarded in their self-concepts. These persons "hedge" and avoid commitment by employing "3" responses.

Defensive positive scale (DP). This is a subtle measure of defensiveness. A high DP score indicates a positive self-description stemming from defensive distortion. A significantly low DP score means that the person is lacking in the usual defenses for maintaining even minimal self-esteem.

General maladjustment scale (GM). This serves as a general index of adjustment-maladjustment

but provides no clues as to the nature of the pathology.

Psychosis scale (Psy). This scale differentiates psychotic patients from other groups.

Personality disorder scale (PD). This category pertains to people with basic personality defects and weaknesses in contrast to psychotic states or the various neurotic reactions.

Neurosis scale (N). This measures neurotic perception of self-concept.

Total positive scores. These reflect the overall level of self-esteem. Persons with high scores tend to like themselves, feel that they are persons of value and worth, have confidence in themselves, and act accordingly. People with low scores are doubtful about their own worth; see themselves as undesirable; often feel anxious, depressed, and unhappy; and have little faith or confidence in themselves.

Total net conflict. These scores measure the extent to which an individual's responses to positive items conflict with his or her responses to negative items.

Total conflict scores. It is of interest to determine the total amount of conflict in a subject's self-concept as well as the directional amount of conflict. High scores indicate confusion, contradiction, and general conflict in self-perception. Low scores have the opposite interpretation, but extremely low scores present a self-description so tight and rigid that it becomes suspect as an artificial, defensive stereotype rather than a true self-image.

Variability scores. The variability scores provide a simple measure of the amount of variability, or inconsistency, from one area of self-perception to another. High scores mean that the subject is quite variable in this respect while low scores indicate low variability, which may even approach rigidity if extremely low (below the first percentile).

Row total variability. This is the sum of the variations across rows.

Column total variability. This is the summary of variations with columns.

Physical self. Here individuals are presenting their views of their bodies, state of health, physical appearance, skills, and sexuality.

Moral-ethical self. This score describes the

self from a moral-ethical frame of reference—moral worth, relationship to God, feelings of being a "good" or "bad" person, and satisfaction with one's religion or lack of it.

Personal self. This score reflects the individual's sense of personal worth, feeling of adequacy as a person, and evaluation of his or her personality apart from his or her body or relationships to others.

Family self. This score reflects one's feelings of adequacy, worth, and value as a family member. It refers to the individual's perception of self in reference to his or her closest and most immediate circle of associates.

Social self. This is another "self as perceived in relation to others" category but pertains to "others" in a more general way. It reflects the person's sense of adequacy and worth in social interaction with other people in general.

Identity. These are the "what I am" items. Here individuals are describing their basic identities—what they are as they see themselves.

Self-satisfaction. The individuals describe how they feel about the selves they perceive. In general this score reflects the level of self-satisfaction or self-acceptance.

Behavior. This score measures the individual's perception of his own behavior or the way he or she functions.

Fitts (1965) and Fitts et al. (1971) report that this test was utilized on both normative and psychiatrically ill populations and on other special groups. He shows that these self-concept measures can be quantified and reliably measured. In addition they show validity for the different groups (Fitts, 1965:13–29; Thompson, 1972; Fitts et al., 1971:45–63).

The categorical analyses of the various selves as defined in this section on TSCS were compared in the following manner: the scores in each category of self by the patient group on admission to the pain unit and by that group on discharge from the unit were compared by statistical analysis—a correlated *t*. Statistical analysis with an uncorrelated *t* was made between the group on

admission and TSCS adult group and between the group on discharge and the TSCS adult group. The TSCS adult group scores can be found in the Fitts' manual for the scoring and analysis of groups (1965).

The TSCS adult group from which the norms were developed was a broad sample of 626 people. The sample included people of ages 12 to 60, equal numbers of both sexes, representatives of the black and white races, all socioeconomic and educational levels, and persons from all regions of the country (Fitts, 1965:13).

IV The Minnesota Multiphasic Personality Inventory (MMPI) Depression Scale The depression scale in the clinical profile of the Minnesota Multiphasic Personality Inventory was established to empirically measure the degree of the clinical symptom pattern of depression. The MMPI describes this mood state as being characterized by feelings of hopelessness and worthlessness, pessimism, slowing of thought and behavior, and preoccupation with death (Dahlstrom et al., 1972, 1975:184).

For the Depression Scale of the MMPI there are five clusters: subjective depression, psychomotor retardation, complaints of physical malfunctions, mental dullness, and brooding (Dahlstrom et al., 1972, 1975). These authors state that the items are in several ways in accord with general expectations about clinical manifestations of psychiatric depression.

The majority of the 60 items in the MMPI Depression Scale were selected by comparisons of the depressive state with other psychiatric conditions and "normals" (Dahlstrom et al., 1972, 1975:184).

The validity indicator (Lie Scale) in the MMPI profile is the 15-item scale designed to identify deliberate efforts to evade answering the depression test honestly (Dahlstrom et al., 1972, 1975:109).

In this scale there were a number of statements of personal faults which subjects generally acknowledged were true of themselves. Some subjects denied negative attributes even though these items were true of themselves. The items refer to denial of aggression, bad thoughts, weakness of resolve, poor self-control, and prejudice (Dahlstrom et al., 1972, 1975:109).

Both the 60-item MMPI Depression Scale and the validity indicator (Lie Scale) were administered to the subjects on admission to the pain unit and on discharge from the pain unit.

Comparisons were made between the group on admission and the group on discharge. Subsequent comparisons were made with the MMPI adult group. The t distribution was the statistic of choice.

FINDINGS

The data from the testing instruments and the clinical report are discussed in this section. The information from the clinical report which refers to demography and clinical data (Table 22-1) was computed for analysis by frequency and percent.

DESCRIPTION OF THE SAMPLE

The total sample was 79 patients. Of these patients, 50 ranged in age from 40 to 59 years, the mean being 45 years. There were more females than males (53 and 47 percent, respectively). Married patients accounted for 76 percent and divorced for 15 percent of the sample. The large majority of the patients were white (83.54 percent) and the other 16.46 percent were black. Eleven (13.92 percent) of the subjects were Catholic while 55 (69.62 percent) identified with Protestant denominations. The remaining number of patients were identified as Jewish (1), Apostolic (1), Mormon (2), other faiths (7), and no religion (2). The patients were hospitalized in the pain center for a mean of 4.72 weeks, with the majority of them spending 4 to 5 weeks in the hospital.

While 24 percent of the patients were from middle-class background (small businesses, skilled employees, clerical and sales workers), over 72 percent stemmed from classes IV and V (semiskilled to unskilled workers) of the Hollingshead Index of Social Position. In the midtown Manhattan study by Srole et al. (1962:141) morbidity was inversely related to social class. Mental morbidity was also inversely related to social class. The author of the present study found this same phenomenon taking place, recapitulating the inverse class phenomena of the Srole et al. study (1962). This is particularly so when it can be seen that the patients in the present study experienced depression, conversion reactions, feelings of inferiority, withdrawal, shyness, and inability to work. Thus, the Srole et al. study and the present study are similar in disease characteristics found.

Almost 32 percent of the subjects had six or more siblings, while 20 percent of them had three siblings and 19 percent of them had four or five siblings. Mersky and Spear (1967) found that many patients with persistent pain came from large families with several siblings. The author's present study confirms that observation. The explanation for this is not clear except to hypothesize that the pain experience may go from parent to child in its manifestations, with subsequent competition by the siblings for attention. This attention-getting mechanism may utilize the learned pain response. Thus, this pain response can serve as a form of aggression. In the present study depressive reactions were manifested upon admission.

The fact that pain was a long-standing and chronic complaint for these patients was evidenced by the numerous illnesses which they endured. Thirty-seven percent (29) of the patients suffered from unstable low back. When this was added to the diagnoses of "low back strain" and "low back pain," 66.2 percent (47) of the patients had problems with low back disorder. Sixteen percent (13) of the patients had arachnoiditic conditions. Sixteen percent of the patients presented symptoms of neck pathology (myositis, spondylosis, neuralgia). The

Table 22-1 Demographic Characteristics of Patients at the Pain Center

Age	F	%	Religion	F	%
20–29	7	8.86	Protestant	55	69.62
30–39	15	18.98	Catholic	11	13.92
40–49	25	31.65	Jewish	1	1.27
50–59	25	31.65	Apostolic	1	1.27
60–69	7	8.86	Mormon	2	2.53
			Other	7	8.86
Total	79	100.00	None	2	2.53

$\overline{X} = 45.06$

			Total	79	100.00

Sex	F	%	Race	F	%
Male	37	47.00	Black	13	16.46
Female	42	53.00	White	66	83.54
Total	79	100.00	Total	79	100.00

Marital Status

M $\dfrac{60}{76\%}$	W $\dfrac{1}{1.26\%}$	D $\dfrac{12}{15.18\%}$	Sep $\dfrac{1}{1.26\%}$	Single $\dfrac{5}{6.30\%}$

Total 79
Percent 100.00

No. Siblings	F	%	SES	F	%
0	5	6.33	I, II	3	3.78
1	10	12.66	III	19	24.07
2	9	11.39	IV, V	57	72.15
3	16	20.25			
4	7	8.86	Total	79	100.00
5	7	8.86			
6+	25	31.65			
Total	79	100.00			

$\overline{X} = 4.27$ siblings

Length of hospital stay

Weeks	F	%
2	1	1.27
3	2	2.53
4	39	49.37
5	25	31.65
6	9	11.38
7	3	3.80
Total	79	100.00

$\overline{X} = 4.72$ weeks

rest of the patients suffered from an assortment of ailments listed as: chondromalacia, phantom limb syndrome, arthritis, chest pain, hyperesthesia, sciatica, and general myopathy. Only 10 patients received any kind of surgery during their hospitalization, mostly for caudal epidural block.

In addition to the organic pathology, 37 percent (29) of the subjects suffered from psychological manifestations evidenced by depression, and it was felt by the team of doctors, nurses, and psychologists that 25 percent (20) patients "needed assertive behavior." Thirteen percent (10) of the patients showed withdrawal reactions, 13 percent (10) of them manifested feelings of inferiority, and 13 percent (10) suffered from anxiety. According to Sternbach (1978:61–62) depression and anxiety are part of the "pain experience" and it is difficult to separate pain from depression and anxiety. One must therefore treat the total patient. This total psychological and organic treament base is what the pain center orients the reader to in its description of holistic medicine.

The fact that these patients complained of pain and discomfort over a long period of time is attested to by the long list of previous surgeries in their life histories. The 79 patients had a composite index of 123 surgeries on the back (spinal fusion, laminectomy, ruptured disk removal, caudal epidural block, rhizotomy). The majority of the surgery performed was for ruptured disk and spinal fusion and laminectomy.

Twenty-five, or over one-half, of the women had had hysterectomies performed. Forty percent of the women who had had hysterectomies prior to admission to the pain center also had low back problems. Those with previous hysterectomies had a greater variety of other disorders such as arthritis, myositis, and myopathy. Twelve of the 25 patients who had hysterectomies were on tranquilizer drugs. The relationship between having the hysterectomies and anxieties might be helpful to explore. Further research is indicated to explore this phenomenon.

The Tennessee Self-Concept Scale (TSCS)

Self-Criticism On both admission and discharge the subjects exhibited healthy openness for self-criticism. The means of both admission and discharge are in keeping with the TSCS adult group. They showed conscious efforts to answer the questions honestly and in accord with their known perceptions.

True-False Ratio The admission and discharge scores were significantly different from the TSCS adult group. The subjects achieved self-definition by focusing on what they were rather than on what they were not. They revealed tendencies to agree rather than disagree with the items. The group on discharge was significantly more definitive in its self-perceptions than the group on admission to the pain unit. This could have been a function of self-focusing toward self-actualization, which those personnel at the pain center sought to accomplish while utilizing the holistic approach to patient care.

Distribution Scores The group on discharge was significantly higher in distribution score than on admission. Subjects on admission were not too certain in what they said about themselves. On discharge they were more definite and certain in what they said about themselves. Both on admission and on discharge, the subjects were not significantly different from the TSCS adult group.

Defensive Positive Score On admission the group had a significantly lower score in defensive feelings than on discharge. Their mean score was, however, in keeping with the TSCS adult group. On discharge the group showed a significantly higher mean score than on admission, and this mean score was significantly higher than that of the TSCS adult group. Such a high defensive positive score indicates that on discharge the subjects showed defensive distortion of their positive feelings, which may have helped to give

Table 22-2 Mean Scores on Tennessee Self-Concept Scale (TSCS) and Minnesota Multiphasic Personality Inventory (MMPI) Depression Scale on Admission and Discharge and Comparisons Between Each and the Adult Groups

Factors	Admission group N = 79 $\bar{x}$	S.D.	Discharge group N = 79 $\bar{x}$	S.D.	Admission to discharge group t	p	TSCS adult group N = 626 $\bar{x}$	S.D.	Admission group with TSCS adult group t	p	Discharge group with TSCS adult group t	p
Self criticism	35.97	5.99	34.36	6.35		NS	35.54	6.70		NS		NS
True-false ratio	6.39	5.62	18.73	21.82	4.66	< .001	1.03	.29	8.35	< .001	6.88	< .001
Distribution	115.49	26.92	124.69	29.01	2.02	= .046	120.44	24.19		NS		NS
Defensive positive	53.17	10.77	60.76	10.26	4.42	< .001	54.40	12.38		NS	4.87	< .001
General maladjustment	92.87	10.54	99.71	7.71	4.56	< .008	98.80	9.15	4.75	< .001		NS
Psychosis	47.59	5.98	46.32	6.56		NS	46.10	6.49		NS		NS
Personality disorders	75.31	12.15	81.08	9.87	3.18	< .002	76.39	11.72		NS	3.74	< .001
Neurosis	74.53	12.10	85.75	10.75	5.99	< .001	84.31	11.10	6.79	< .001		NS
Total net conflict	- .11	12.15	- 3.10	15.20		NS	- 4.91	13.01	3.23	< .01		NS
Total positive	333.46	37.67	361.86	31.19	5.01	< .001	345.57	30.70	2.73	< .01	4.20	< .001
Total conflict	33.41	9.56	29.78	9.25	2.33	< .021	30.10	8.21	2.93	< .01		NS
Total variability	51.40	12.26	44.08	12.95	3.55	< .001	48.53	12.42		NS	2.77	< .01
Physical self	59.06	9.86	69.72	8.59	7.03	< .001	71.78	7.67	10.98	< .001		NS
Moral ethical	71.69	8.51	75.40	7.12	2.88	< .005	70.33	8.70		NS	5.58	< .001
Personal self	64.40	8.90	70.66	7.17	4.72	< .001	64.55	7.41		NS	6.82	< .001
Family self	69.95	9.76	73.51	8.73	2.35	< .020	70.83	8.43		NS	2.48	< .05
Social self	68.36	8.62	72.57	7.01	3.26	< .001	68.14	7.86		NS	5.01	< .001
Identity	122.53	11.63	131.17	9.99	4.86	< .001	127.10	9.96	3.32	< .01	3.28	< .01
Self satisfaction	100.68	16.98	113.39	15.34	4.80	< .001	103.67	13.79		NS	5.15	< .001
Behavior	110.26	12.85	117.31	10.85	3.61	= .001	115.01	11.22	3.12	< .01		NS
Row total variability	22.12	6.64	17.56	5.84	4.45	< .001	19.60	5.76		NS		NS
Column total variability	29.28	8.56	26.53	9.71	1.85	< .067	29.03	9.12		NS	2.08	< .05
							MMPI adult group		**MMPI adult with admission group**			
MMPI depression	28.46	6.35	19.36	4.45	9.50	< .001	18.06	4.54	9.30	< .001		NS
MMPI lie scale	11.23	2.20	11.00	3.35			4.16	2.89				NS

higher total positive scores spuriously built upon their own emotional defenses.

General Maladjustment Scores This is an inverse scale, so that lower scores indicate higher maladjustment scores. Indication of maladjustment was evident on admission to the pain center. The score was significantly higher than for the TSCS adult group. The scores decreased on discharge from the unit and were then equivalent to those of the TSCS adult group.

Psychosis There was no evidence of psychosis in this group of subjects, either on admission or on discharge.

Personality Disorders On admission the group mean was in keeping with the TSCS adult group. However, since this is an inverse scale, the group on admission was significantly higher in personality disorder than on discharge from the unit. The group on discharge showed lower scores on personality weakness than on admission and was significantly lower on personality defects than the TSCS adult group.

Neurosis The group on admission showed high-level neurosis, in comparison both with their status on discharge and with the TSCS adult group. This is again an inverse scale.

Total Positive Scores On admission this group had significantly lower overall positive feelings towards various selfhoods than on discharge or when compared with the TSCS adult group. On admission these persons doubted their own worth, had low self-esteem, and felt unhappy. On discharge they had significantly higher positive scores than either on admission or when compared with the TSCS adult group. Higher display of emotional defense may have contributed to significantly higher positive scores spuriously elevated above those of the TSCS group.

Total Net Conflict On admission the scores showed conflict between positive and negative

replies to the items. On discharge these scores achieved equivalence with those of the TSCS normative group.

Total Conflict On admission the subjects showed significantly higher conflict scores than on discharge, at which time the conflict scores achieved the levels of the TSCS group's. On both net and total conflict scores, the persons on admission showed contradiction and general conflict in their self-perceptions.

Total Variability On admission, in contrast to discharge status, the t value showed that the subjects' self-concepts were so variable from one area to another as to reflect little unity or integration. On discharge they significantly improved their scores to even higher levels than that evidenced by the TSCS adult group. This decrease in variability could indicate some rigidity or guarding on answering the items. It could be the product of defensive distortion.

On *row total variability* the subjects on admission showed variability scores significantly greater than on discharge. As above, the featured emphasis was again on less unity between the selves on discharge. *Column total variability* was also higher than on discharge. However, on discharge there was more unity among the several selves than in the TSCS adult group.

Physical Self On admission, the subjects exhibited significantly lower positive feelings with respect to appearance and physique than either on discharge or when compared with the TSCS normative group. On admission the subjects' view of their bodies, state of health, physical appearance, skills, and sexuality were at a low ebb. This improved by the time they were discharged.

Moral-Ethical On admission, the subjects were significantly lower in feelings of moral worth than on discharge, although their scores were in keeping with those of the TSCS adult group. On discharge they were significantly higher than the

TSCS adult group in moral-ethical values. This group went from normative values on admission to higher than normative values on discharge. Their sense of moral worth and of being a good person significantly improved on discharge.

Personal Self Although the subjects on admission showed scores in keeping with the TSCS Adult Group's, these were significatly lower than the scores on discharge. On discharge positive personal feelings were significantly greater than in TSCS adult group. These subjects' sense of personal worth and feelings of adequacy improved during their stay at the pain center.

Family Self On admission the subjects scored significantly lower on positive feelings as family members than they did on discharge. On discharge they scored significantly higher on family self than the TSCS adult group.

Social Self On admission the subjects scored similarly to the TSCS adult group, but they achieved significantly higher positive scores on discharge when compared both with admission status and with the TSCS adult group.

Identity On admission the subjects scored significantly lower than the TSCS adult group and than their discharge scores. They were again significantly higher on identity at the time of discharge.

Self-Satisfaction The subjects' self-acceptance was in line with that of the normative group but significantly rose on discharge.

Behavior On admission their behavior was accepted by them significantly less than on discharge and their scores were significantly lower than those of the TSCS adult group.

MMPI Depression Score

On admission the subjects evidenced significantly higher-level depression scores than on discharge and in comparison with the MMPI Depression Score for adults. The subjects on discharge achieved scores in keeping with those of the MMPI adult group. It can be inferred from the findings that the subjects were depressed on admission and improved significantly on discharge.

Summary

The subjects in the pain center improved from admission to discharge on the various selves in the self-concept and on the depression scale. On admission the subjects showed evidence of conflict and contradiction in their self-perceptions. They showed little unity or integration of the self-concept. The subjects showed significantly less positive feeling toward the various selves. Their various selves (physical, moral ethical, personal, family, social) were expressed on admission with low positive scores, as were identity, self-satisfaction, and behavior. A rise in positive feelings on the various selves was evident on discharge so that the intervening variable of therapy was significant in the residents of the pain center. Some defensive distortion was evident on discharge, affecting the scores to produce spuriously high-level positive feelings, even above those of the TSCS adult group. On discharge, variability scores showed greater unity among the various selves. The persons on discharge showed significantly less conflict in judging their various selves.

On admission the subjects evidenced general maladjustment, personality disorder, and neurosis, which improved significantly on discharge. The subjects evidenced depression on admission, which improved while hospitalized, and on discharge their depressive scores matched those of the TSCS adult group.

In summary, the subjects were admitted with chronic long-term pain to the pain center at a general hospital. On admission they were all on drugs for the relief of pain. They were depressed, had neurotic tendencies, and poor self-concept. Following therapy these scores improved to levels equal to or higher than those of the adult groups.

The pain center stressed holistic medicine, where illness was viewed as an excessive strain upon the mind-body system. The health education program appeared to have helped the patients to increase self-knowledge and self-actualization. This may be reflected in the discharge scores of the subjects. In addition the intensive biofeedback, exercise and vocational counseling programs enabled the subjects to regain control of their bodies and to plan hopefully for a brighter future. Thus the self-concept improved with the atmosphere of self-help as patients shared problems and problem solutions with medical personnel.

Hypotheses 1 to 4 are corroborated. Patients on admission to the pain center had poor positive feelings toward themselves and manifested depression. After intensive physical and psychological therapy they exited from the program as improved.

POSTHOSPITAL GROUP STUDY

As a sequel to the study on the psychological correlates of pain and nursing practice, the posthospital group was tested for self-concept, depression, and clinical report on status of symptomatology.

As a sequel to this study, the subjects were tested 6 months to 1 year after discharge. Those so tested will be hereinafter referred to as the "posthospital group." The same Tennessee Self-Concept Scale was used, as well as the MMPI Depression Scale. A clinical report was completed which attested to the site of duration and intensity of pain, medication, work orientation, and attendance of and visitation to a physician.

All 79 patients of the previous study were contacted at least 6 months after discharge. Of the 79 patients, 10 refused to participate via mail, 22 did not respond to a follow-up letter and postcard, and mailings to 11 were sent to wrong addresses. A total of 36 subjects responded to the follow-up mailing. Three subjects filled out only portions of the questionnaires and these were discarded. Thus, 33 subjects were finally sampled.

Findings of Follow-up Study

Tennessee Self-Concept Scale Compared with discharge status the posthospital group of patients was not significantly different in most of the items on the TSC scale (see Table 22-3). For the follow-up study findings for the posthospital group with discharge status were combined with findings of 40 outpatients in a study described by Dahlstrom (1972–1975). Their defensive positive scores went down from discharge but remained on levels equivalent to the adult group. This means that, compared with their discharge status, there is significantly less emotional defense in arriving at their positive scores. This becomes evident when it is seen that the total positive score (overall positive attitude to self) is lower than on discharge but equivalent to that of the adult group. It was previously suggested that on discharge emotional defense sent the scores to spuriously higher levels. This is not the case in the posthospital group.

Neurosis is measured on an inverse scale so that higher scores indicate less neurosis. As compared with discharge, neurosis scores went up and they also showed a trend to be higher than in the adult group ($1.685, p < .10$). There is more of a neurotic flavor to the posthospital group, which coincides with some return of their symptoms. Accordingly, there is less positive feeling toward their physical selves since discharge, and this is significantly lessened when compared with the adult group.

Self-satisfaction scores deflated significantly from discharge status but were equivalent to those in the adult group. At the same time, identity scores went down from discharge but were also equivalent to the adult group scores. This phenomenon may be a function of two processes. First, emotional defenses are decreased in the posthospital group so that spuriously high scores are no longer an issue. Second, return of symp-

Table 22-3 Comparison of Posthospital Subjects with Discharge Status and with TSCS Adult Group

Factors	Patients on discharge N = 79		Discharge with posthospital		Posthospital patients N = 33		Posthospital with adult		TSCS adult group N = 626	
	x	S.D.	t	p	x	S.D.	t	p	x	S.D.
Self-criticism	34.36	6.35	N.S.		35.67	6.77	N.S.		35.54	6.70
Distribution	124.69	29.01	N.S.		118.21	22.72	N.S.		120.44	24.19
Defensive positive	60.76	10.26	2.016	< .05	55.61	12.870	N.S.		54.40	12.38
General maladjustment	99.71	7.71	N.S.		96.550	11.48	N.S.		98.80	9.15
Psychosis	46.32	6.56	N.S.		47.94	5.61	1.795	< .10	46.10	6.49
Personality deviation	81.08	9.87	N.S.		78.18	11.00	N.S.		76.39	11.72
Neurosis	85.75	10.75	2.05	< .05	79.88	14.66	1.685	< .10	84.31	11.10
Net conflict	- 3.10	15.20	N.S.		- 4.75	15.23	N.S.		- 4.91	13.01
Total positive	361.86	31.19	2.06	< .05	345.52	40.00	N.S.		345.57	30.70
Total conflict	29.78	9.25	N.S.		31.15	10.34	N.S.		30.10	8.21
Total variability	44.08	12.95	N.S.		46.24	12.65	N.S.		48.53	12.42
Physical self	69.72	8.59	3.27	< .01	62.15	11.81	4.56	< .001	71.78	7.67
Moral-ethical	75.40	7.12	N.S.		72.97	8.37	1.73	< .10	70.33	8.70
Personal self	70.66	7.17	N.S.		67.97	10.14	1.88	< .10	64.55	7.41
Family self	73.51	8.73	N.S.		72.12	8.13	N.S.		70.83	8.43
Social	72.57	7.01	N.S.		70.30	9.46	N.S.		68.14	7.86
Identity	131.17	9.99	2.20	< .05	124.70	15.32	N.S.		127.10	9.96
Self-satisfaction	113.39	15.34	2.19	< .05	106.06	16.24	N.S.		103.67	13.79
Behavior	117.31	10.85	N.S.		114.76	12.73	N.S.		115.01	11.22
Row variability	17.56	5.84	1.80	< .10	20.33	7.86	N.S.		19.60	5.76
Column variability	26.53	9.71	N.S.		25.91	7.93	2.15	< .05	29.03	9.12

toms would logically lead to deflated physical self scores with consequently less self-satisfaction. All other scores were not significantly different from those of either the discharge status or the adult group.

MMPI Depression The posthospital group had significantly higher depressive scores from their status on discharge (see Table 22–4). Although they appeared to have become somewhat more depressed when discharged into the community, their scores were still significantly lower than on admission. Their depression scores were above those of the adult group, indicating that they have returned to depression while in the community. This could again be a function of return of symptoms and consequent discomfort, coupled with pressures of job and family.

In conclusion it can be stated that although seven patients (19 percent) had surgery and 9 patients (22 percent) had pain increase, a high percentage (47 percent) of them were on analgesics as prescribed by the pain clinic. Thirty-two subjects (96 percent) continued with exercise and 11 patients (33 percent) continued biofeedback as initiated by the pain center.

Although there was some discouragement and depression associated with the persistence of pain, there was not the overall despondency exhibited on admission to the pain center. More people were functional and working in spite of complaints of pain and their self-concepts were positive. It can be said that although there was discouragement they maintained levels of pain control which were evident on discharge.

Further research is in progress at this time which follows the patients in their homes 1 year after therapy in the pain center. The same instru-

Table 22-4 Pain Study: Posthospital Depression Scores and Comparison with Admission and Discharge Status and with Adult Group (Dahlstrom, 1973)

Admission status N = 79		Discharge status N = 79		Admission N = 79 with posthospital status N = 33		Follow-up posthospital group N = 33		Posthospital group with discharge status N = 33		Dahlstrom adult group N = 40		Posthospital (N = 33) with TSCS outpatient group (N = 40)	
$\bar{x}$	S.D.	$\bar{x}$	S.D.	t	p	$\bar{x}$	S.D.	t	p	$\bar{x}$	S.D.	t	p
28.46	6.35	19.36	3.34	4.858	$< .001$	21.68	6.97	1.792	$< .05$	18.06	4.54	2.997	$< .01$
						21.68	6.97			18.06	4.54		
						21.68	6.974						

ments as in this study are being utilized to study the same sample of subjects. The data are in the process of analysis. (It also is suggested that further research be completed in a manner similar to this study to see if the findings persist.)

In summary, doctors and nurses need to see the pain experience as also a psychological experience which can be very disabling. It can keep an individual from productive employment. Relaxation exercises, recreational therapy, and group therapy are just as important as the physical aspects of therapy for improvement of the pain syndrome.

EDITOR'S QUESTIONS FOR DISCUSSION

What is the research question Stein addresses? What alternatives are there for phrasing the hypotheses? What nursing theoretical framework(s) could be suggested for this study? To what extent are the hypotheses derived from the theoretical framework actually used? Indicate assumptions in this study.

What type of sampling technique is evident? What are the implications for validity and reliability of the study? What is not known concerning the method of sampling and criteria for being a subject? How can that influence the meaningfulness and interpretation of the data?

How valid and reliable is the Two-Factor Index of Social Position? What is the validity and reliability of the Tennessee Self Concept Scale? What are the principal categories of analysis the scale represents? What are the five categories of measurement within the scale? How valid and reliable is the MMPI Depression Scale? How appropriate for this study are the three instruments which were utilized?

What questions can you pose concerning possible relationships in the findings of the demographic data? What questions should be addressed regarding the number of subjects with low-back disorder problems and the amount of surgery previously performed? How, specifically by whom, and to what extent should health professionals intervene with such issues? What preventive measures might be suggested for the phenomena?

Indicate the significance and limitations of this study. To what extent are relationships and findings clearly established? How appropriate were the statistical tests employed for the data? What salient variables are not accounted for in this study? Suggest methods for measuring the effect of therapy and programs on the subjects. What alternative explanations can be offered for the findings? Are there inferences indicated not based on the data? How generalizable are the findings? What alternative research designs and methodologies can be suggested for a study of the same problem? What additional questions can be posed for future research?

REFERENCES

Applegate, Margaret
  1980 Locus of control and educationally based patient care outcomes in a chronic pain center. Doctoral dissertation. Indiana University.
Benedetti, G.
  1974 "Psychologic and psychiatric aspects of pain in recent advances on pain," Chap. X:256–273 in John Bonica, Paola Procacci, and Carlo Pagni (eds.) Springfield, Ill.: Charles C Thomas.
Blendis, Laurence, Oscar Hill, and Harold Mersky
  1978 Abdominal pain and the emotions. Pain 5:179–191.
Bond, Michael
  1978 Pain, its nature, analysis and treatment. New York: Churchill Livingstone.

Bonica, John
  1974 General clinical considerations. "Recent advances on pain," Chap. XI:274–298 in J. Bonica, Paola Procacci, Carlo Pagni (eds.) Springfield, Illinois: Charles C Thomas.
Chapman, Richard C., Anders Sola, and John Bonica
  1979 "Illness behavior and depression compared in pain center and private practice patients." Pain 6:1–7.
Dahlstrom, W. Grant, George Schalger Welsh, and Leona E. Dahlstrom
  1972–75a MMPI Handbook, Vol. I. Minneapolis: Univ. Minnesota.
  1972–75b MMPI Handbook, Vol. II. Minneapolis: Univ. Minnesota.
Fitts, William H.
  1965 Tennessee self concept scale, a manual. Nashville, Tennessee.

Fitts, William, Jennie Adams, Gladys Redford, Wayne Richard, Barbara Thomas, Thomas Murphy, and Warren Thompson
1971 The self concept and self actualization. Research Monograph #3, Nashville, Tennessee: Dede Wallace Center.

Freud, Sigmund
1938 Beyond the pleasure principle. Pp. 534–535 in A. A. Brill (ed.) New York: Modern Library.

Hollingshead, August
1957 Two factor index of social position. Yale Station, New Haven, Conn.

Krauss, Irving
1976 Stratification, class and conflict. New York: Free Press.

McCafferty, Margo
1979 Nursing management of the patient with pain. New York: Lippincott.

Menders, Karl
1978 Speech on holistic medicine, School of Nursing, Indianapolis: Indianapolis University, Purdue University of Indianapolis.

Mersky, H. and F. G. Spear
1967 Pain: psychological and psychiatric aspects. London: Bailliere, Tindall and Cassell.

Mezzich, J. E., F. L. Demarin and J. R. Erickson
1974 "Comparative validity of strategies and indices for differential diagnosis of depressive states from other psychiatry conditions using the MMPI." Journal of Consulting & Clinical Psychology 42: 691–698.

Pawl, Ronald P.
1978 Chronic pain. New York: Yearbook Publishers, pp. 2–8.

Pilowsky, I. and N. D. Spence
1976 "Illness behavior syndromes associated with intractable pain." Pain 2:61–71.

Shakespeare, William
1961a Romeo and Juliet, P. 403 in Complete works of Shakespeare, H. Craig (ed.) Chicago: Scott Foresman.
1961b Macbeth, P. 1053 in Complete Works of Shakespeare, H. Craig (ed.) Chicago: Scott Foresman.

Srole, Leo, Thomas Langner, Stanley Michael, Marvin Opler, and Thomas Rennie
1962 Mental health in the metropolis, Vol. I. New York: McGraw-Hill.

Sternbach, Richard A. (ed.)
1974 Pain Patients. New York: Academic Press.
1978 The Psychology of Pain. New York: Raven Press.

Sternbach, R. A. and Gretchen Timmermans
1975 "Personality changes associated with reduction of pain." Pain 1:177–181.

Thompson, Warren
1972 Correlates of the self concept, a monograph. VI. Nashville, Tenn.: Dede Wallace Center.

Webster's New World Dictionary of the American Language, Second College Edition,
1970 The World Publishing Company.

Williams, Jane
1976 "Understanding the feelings of the dying." Nursing March:52–56.

Zborowski, Mark
1969 People in Pain. San Francisco: Jossey Bass, Inc.

Chapter 23

Nursing Diagnosis: Implementation and Incidence in an Obstetrical-Gynecological Population

Mary Anne Sweeney, R.N., Ph.D.
Associate Professor
Boston College
School of Nursing
Chestnut Hill, Massachusetts
                        and
Marjory Gordon, R.N., Ph.D., F.A.A.N.
Professor
Boston College
School of Nursing
Chestnut Hill, Massachusetts

This study was undertaken by Mary Ann Sweeney and Marjory Gordon to investigate the utilization of nursing diagnoses in a clinical setting. While working in a hospital specializing in the care of obstetrical and gynecological patients, continuing care nurses were taught diagnostic nomenclature to identify actual or potential patient health problems requiring nursing care. A list of 37 nursing diagnoses compiled by the National Conference Group on the Classification of Nursing Diagnoses was used as a guide, and the nurses were encouraged to modify or expand the list as needed in their setting. Data were collected on 163 patients who were referred for follow-up care during the three year period 1975 to 1978. A total of 568 nursing diagnoses were recorded, an average of 3.48 per patient. Sweeney and Gordon particularly call attention to the frequency which nurses added the qualifier term "anticipatory observation." Thus, the nursing diagnoses are listed according to diagnostic categories with and without the inclusion of the label. Medical diagnoses held the rank of third place when the "anticipatory observation" label was used, but fell to rank 12 without it. Intriguing explanations are offered for this dramatic finding. The two diagnoses cited most frequently were: alterations in parenting, and anxiety. When the individual diagnoses were grouped into functional categories describing patient problems, the highest frequencies were found in the following categories: nutritional/metabolic patterns, role patterns, self-perception/conception patterns, and elimination patterns. Other promising areas of investigation on the topic of nursing diagnosis are covered as well. Sweeney and Gordon conclude that there is a need for a holistic nursing assessment of patients' health problems since the data indicate the most prevalent diagnoses for this group of women were not in the expected order or frequency.

INTRODUCTION

Purpose of Using Diagnostic Nomenclature

Diagnostic classification systems enable professionals to organize and systematize information so that it can be utilized effectively in decision making. Category labels within a system are arbitrary word symbols that are useful in communicating a clear message to a professional colleague. They provide a common language which is a form of shorthand for describing a general condition, as well as etiological factors, a selection of possible treatments, and a tentative prognosis. According to Korchin (1976:103), "Diagnostic nomenclature can be viewed simply as descriptive categories characterizing somewhat loosely and incompletely, problems which society or the sufferers themselves bring to professional attention." He adds that the terms not only serve as a guide for description and treatment, but fulfill administrative and legal purposes as well. In clarifying the use of diagnostic nomenclature in the practice of professional nursing, Gordon (1976:1298) defines nursing diagnoses as *actual or potential health problems which nurses by virtue of their education and experience are capable and licensed to treat.*

The progress of creating diagnostic nomenclature in nursing has been fairly similar to the events which led to the development of terminology in other health professions. The process is described by Goldenberg (1973:109) as follows:

This study was funded in part by a Faculty Summer Research Grant from Boston College, Chestnut Hill, Massachusetts 02167.

The authors gratefully acknowledge the participation of Kathleen McKeehan, R.N., M.S., who was the Continuing Care Coordinator at Boston Hospital For Women during the course of the study.

While the taxonomic approach in any science is initially descriptive, relying primarily on phenotypical categorization, such superficial resemblances are discarded as knowledge increases. Classification then proceeds according to genotypical categories, such as grouping by common etiological factors. The 1968 American Psychiatric Association classification system remains for the most part at the phenotypic level, with mental disorders grouped by symptoms rather than etiology.

Utilization of Nursing Diagnoses

The implementation of nursing diagnosis in clinical care has been stimulated by two factors. The initial precipitor was the publication of national standards of practice (American Nurses' Association, 1973) which identify *nursing diagnosis* as a routine step in the delivery of nursing care. The second was the work of the National Conference Group for the Classification of Nursing Diagnoses, which resulted in the identification of diagnostic categories of health problems which nurses felt they were able to treat (Gebbie and Lavin, 1975; Gebbie, 1976; Gebbie, forthcoming). It should be noted that the list of diagnoses resulting from the three meetings of the National Conference Group on the Classification of Nursing Diagnoses was produced by a retrospective pooling of the clinical experiences of nurses who show an interest in this task. Symptoms of patient's problems and suggested labels were discussed and then voted upon in order to be "accepted" as diagnoses. The National Conference list currently consists of 37 areas of nursing diagnoses which were generated in this manner.

Although the generation of a list of nursing diagnoses can be considered as an advancement in the process of specifying nursing care, systematic studies are needed to investigate the validity and clinical usefulness of the diagnostic labels. Numerous articles have been written which suggest varied clinical uses of diagnoses, such as in occupational health nursing (Hornung, 1956), in conjunction with epidemiological approaches (Brown, 1974) and in settings using primary nursing (Mundinger and Jauron, 1975). The next step in the development of diagnostic nomenclature is to subject the proposed list to clinical investigation with different types of clients to determine its relevance to actual patient care situations. Field testing should be carried out to provide empirical evidence to substantiate the utility of such a classification system before attempts are made to standardize the proposed nomenclature.

Thus, the list of 37 nursing diagnoses provided by the National Conference Group, although phenotypical in nature, provided a sound starting point for this research study. Before proceeding to undertake the clinical testing of the National Conference list of nursing diagnoses, two broad questions were posed. First, what would occur when nurses were requested to use the National Conference list of nursing diagnoses in their everyday clinical practice? Second, what would be the result (or the incidence of each label) when these nurses used the National Conference list to identify patient problems?

A large-scale descriptive study was designed to seek information on the utilization of diagnostic nomenclature by experienced nurses in a clinical setting. A health care agency was located which fostered the utilization of diagnostic nomenclature by providing nurses with the staff development, utilization guidelines, ongoing supervision, and record-keeping facilities which are necessary for the implementation of nursing diagnosis.

SETTING

The setting selected for the study was an acute-care hospital specializing in the care of obstetrical and gynecological patients which was located in a large metropolitan area. Boston Hospital for Women, a Harvard University–affiliated teaching hospital, has approximately 300 beds in its Lying-In and Parkway Divisions. During the 3 years prior to the inception of the study, the continuing care department established a policy which made the documentation of a nursing diagnosis a formal part of all discharge nursing referrals and the nursing focus for interdisciplinary conferences. The organization and implementation of this discharge planning process has been previously reported in the literature (La Montague and McKeehan, 1975). Staff education programs regarding nursing diagnosis and the use of diagnostic nomenclature were instituted in 1975. As a part of the extensive training program which has been previously described (McKeehan, 1979), nurses were given the list of accepted nursing diagnoses and their defining signs and symptoms which were generated by the National Conference Group on Classification of Nursing Diagnoses (Gebbie, 1975; Gebbie, 1976).

Instructions for using the National Conference List of Diagnoses included two modifications: nurses could add new diagnoses, and they could qualify existing labels by such terms as *potential* or *high risk*. The use of the qualifiers was explained in the hospital literature (Boston Hospital for Women Nursing Diagnosis Guidelines, 1977:2) as follows:

> Any time a specific nursing intervention is utilized to *prevent* a health problem, simply state your Nursing Diagnosis using the qualifying term "Potential" or "High Risk" for _____ (i.e., Potential Alterations in Parenting, etc.). A Potential Nursing Diagnosis is different from the actual Nursing Diagnosis; therefore, there may be different etiologies and signs and symptoms.

An interdisciplinary health team conference was routinely held on all patients referred for level 1 and level 2 continuing care. The continuing care coordinator, an expert on nursing diagnosis, participated in all team conferences and was available for consultation regarding discharge diagnoses made by the hospital nurses. Her input into the process of making the nursing diagnoses helped to provide some degree of consistency across patients. Pertinent information on patients, including medical and nursing discharge diagnoses, was recorded on departmental continuing care records for 3 years prior to the initiation of this study.

Purpose of the Study

The study was designed to:

1 Investigate the implementation and utilization of nursing diagnoses by nurses planning for the continuing care of patients at the time of hospital discharge.

2 Identify the incidence of nursing diagnoses (by individual label and by functional category) for a group of obstetrical-gynecological patients.

Operational Definitions

The specific meaning of some commonly used terms in this study are as follows:

Nursing diagnosis. This term specified an actual or potential patient health problem which was recorded by nurses in this study on the hospital record and located in a section labeled "nursing diagnosis." Some examples of nursing diagnoses cited on these records are: alterations in parenting, mobility impairment, nutritional deficit.

Continuing care program. All patients who had a formal referral to visiting nurse associations or long-term care facilities were admitted to the Continuing Care Program. (Boston Hospital for Women Nursing Diagnosis Guidelines, 1977).

Level 1 care. This term indicates patients whose conditions were unstable, with complex and/or multiple needs, and warranted immediate and continuous services. (Boston Hospital for Women Nursing Diagnosis Guidelines, 1977).

Level 2 care. This term indicates patients who were periodically in an unstable condition and warranted periodic services to meet their needs.

(Boston Hospital for Women Nursing Diagnosis Guidelines, 1977).

METHOD

Sample

Continuing care records were requested and examined for all obstetrical and gynecological patients who were referred for level 1 or 2 continuing care during the 3-year period 1975–1978. A preliminary screening process was used to determine the actual number of records which fulfilled the overall criteria for inclusion in the study. This screening process was used for two purposes. The first was to eliminate duplication. Some patients were evaluated on more than one occasion and an alteration in the nursing diagnosis often went hand in hand with a change in the health status. Seventeen patients (12 percent of the total sample) were later reevaluated as outpatients with some change in either the number or type of nursing diagnoses. Although this change was noted for future use, only the original diagnoses were utilized for the data analysis in this project.

The screening process was also employed to eliminate patients who would not meet the requirements for becoming subjects or those who would greatly skew the results. A group of neonates who were treated in conjunction with their mothers were eliminated from the sample since they did not meet the overall criteria for becoming subjects. Similarly, obstetrical patients classified as "high-risk family breakdown" were not included in the analysis. They received treatment from a specialized health team owing to the presence of multiple problems such as alcoholism and drug addiction. They were eliminated from this report in an effort to obtain a "typical" sample of level 1 and level 2 obstetrical and gynecological patients.

The sample consisted of 163 patients who were treated for obstetrical or gynecological conditions and referred to the continuing care team for level 1 and level 2 nursing follow-up care. To protect patients' identity, only limited demographic information was recorded, and the code indicating the patient's name and record number was retained by the hospital.

The age range of the 163 female subjects was extremely widespread, as can be noted in Table 23-1. Although the chronological extremes of obstetrical and gynecological age groups were represented by two 14-year-old patients and one 93-year-old patient, it should be noted that the ages of the majority of women fell within the childbearing years.

Classification of subjects according to marital status is presented in Table 23-2 which shows that the total number of subjects who are, or were, married was approximately the same as the number who were single. Almost three-quarters of the subjects (17.3 percent) were assessed as level 2 care while the remainder were considered level 1. It was interesting to note that the vast majority of the subjects (95.1 percent) were referred to visiting nurse associations for follow-up care, while only a small percentage of the patients (4.9 percent) were referred to nursing homes despite the advanced age of some.

Procedure

Demographic data, medical diagnoses, and nursing diagnoses (including etiologies and signs and symtoms) were extracted verbatim from the 163 continuing care records by the investigators and a research assistant. No attempt was made to extra-

Table 23-1   Age Distribution of Subjects

Age	Number of subjects	Percentage
14–19	55	33.74
20–29	45	27.61
30–39	18	11.04
40–49	9	5.52
50–59	5	3.07
60–69	11	6.75
70–79	12	7.36
80–89	7	4.29
90 and up	1	.62
Total	163	100.00

Table 23-2   Marital Status of Subjects

Marital status	Number	Percentage
Single	80	49.08
Married	47	28.83
Divorced	5	3.07
Widowed	19	11.66
Separated	12	7.36
Total	163	100.00

polate or to reclassify this information. In addition, the investigators made numerous checks on the reliability of their data-recording procedures by selecting patient records at random for review. Data were coded, transferred to punched cards, and analyzed in terms of percentage and frequency distributions by the use of SPSS (the Statistical Package for the Social Sciences).

The number and type of medical diagnoses of the subjects were examined to place a rough gauge on the overall complexity of the medical problems of this group of patients. When the number of medical diagnoses was inspected, it was noted that only one diagnosis was listed for 101 (61.6 percent) of the subjects and that the most frequently encountered label was "post-partum." The number of patients having two diagnoses dropped to 37 (22.6 percent) of the sample while the percentage of patients with multiple combinations of diagnoses (varying from three to five) was small, accounting for 9.8, 3.7, and 2.4 percent of the sample, respectively. There was a great amount of qualitative variation in the type of medical label or diagnosis which was applied to this group of individuals. A total of 80 different medical diagnostic labels were documented according to the official listing in the Manual of the International Classification of Diseases, Injuries and Causes of Death (WHO, 1977).

The nursing diagnoses were tabulated and then grouped according to categories within a previously developed functional framework (Gordon, 1975) which was further clarified for this study.

A definition of each of the 13 diagnostic categories appears in Table 23-3. The investi-

Table 23-3 Definitions of Nursing Diagnostic Categories

1 **Nutritional-Metabolic Patterns.** Includes problems or potential problems in the quality or quantity of nutrient and fluid ingestion or retention patterns. Local metabolic disturbances influencing skin integrity and tissue healing are also included.

2 **Exercise-Activity Patterns.** Includes problems or potential problems in activity tolerance or mobility influencing desired or required activity, exercise, and leisure patterns of daily living.

3 **Elimination Patterns.** Includes problems or potential problems in patterns of bowel, bladder, or skin excretion that interfere with daily activities or health maintenance.

4 **Cognitive-Perceptual Patterns.** Includes problems or potential problems in compensating for changes in sensory modes, speech patterns, or cognitive abilities. Also included are problems in managing pain and discomfort.

5 **Sleep-Rest Patterns.** Includes problems or potential problems in the quality and quantity of sleep-rest activities.

6 **Self-Perception–Conception Patterns.** Includes problems or potential problems in subjective states, such as perception of the control and management of life events and subjective reactions to events.

7 **Sexuality-Reproductive Patterns.** Includes individual's perceived problems or potential problems in sexuality or reproductive patterns.

8 **Coping Patterns–Stress Tolerance.** Includes problems or potential problems in the pattern of managing psychological stress. Also included are problems related to the management of decreased immunological capacity.

9 **Health Status Perception–Health Management Patterns.** Includes problems or potential problems in perception of health status, in therapeutic management of disease status, or in using health status information in planning future life activities. Nonproductive health maintenance practices are also included.

10 **Life Patterns–Life-Style.** Includes a composite of cultural, psychological, physical, and environmental patterns of living that place the individual, family, or community at risk for problems in health maintenance.

gators found it necessary to utilize an additional category called *medical diagnosis* to include medical rather than nursing decisions which were recorded by the participants.

RESULTS

The first part of the analysis was focused on the implementation and utilization of nursing diagnoses in planning for the continuing care of patients at the time of hospital discharge. The overall results showed that a total of 568 diagnostic labels were applied to patients. When the 64 medical diagnoses were removed, a total of 504 nursing diagnoses were generated for the 163 patients, an average of 3.09 for each subject. The distribution of actual nursing diagnoses according to the diagnostic categories was variable, as can be seen in Table 23–4.

The data showed that the nurses frequently added the qualifying term "potential" or "high risk" to the National Conference list and also created new labels on their own (such as "loneliness," "isolation," "medication toxicity," and "vision problems"), as suggested in the instructions from hospital administration.

A close inspection of the actual wording used in the diagnostic labels showed that the nurses used qualifying terms for diagnoses with much greater frequency than they generated new labels. In fact, one qualifier which was worded, "anticipatory observation for (followed by a nursing diagnosis)" was used in a great number of instances. The meaning of the phrase, "anticipatory observation for . . . " was not defined, and the differentiation of this label from "potential" or "high risk" which were suggested for use by the nursing administration was unclear. For instance, in the category of *Roles,* it was found that in addition to the two nursing diagnoses related to parenting, "alterations in parenting" ($n = 15$) and "potential alterations in parenting" ($n = 32$), a third diagnosis worded "anticipatory observation for parenting" ($n = 48$) was employed. It appeared that the "anticipatory observation" classification represented a distinctly different

Table 23-4 Classification of Nursing Diagnoses According to Diagnostic Categories

Diagnostic category	Frequency of diagnoses included on the National Conference list without qualifying terms (such as "observe for" or "high risk")	Frequency of diagnoses from National Conference list plus diagnoses generated by Boston Hospital for Women nurses*	
		Without anticipatory observation	With anticipatory observation
Nutritional-metabolic patterns	42	67	84
Exercise-activity patterns	32	30	33
Elimination patterns	28	41	46
Cognitive-perceptual patterns	5	13	18
Sleep-rest patterns	1	0	1
Sexuality-reproductive	1	2	45
Life patterns/life-style	0	5	25
Health status perception–management	2	24	57
Self-perception–conception	39	48	61
Roles	22	56	104
Interpersonal relationship patterns	2	12	19
Coping patterns, stress tolerance	5	5	11
Value-belief systems	0	0	0
(Medical diagnoses)	(0)	(1)	(64)
Total	179	304	568

*Boston Hospital for Women nurses are nurses employed by Boston Hospital for Women who generated nursing diagnoses for continuing care patients.

entity to the nurses, since it was employed in conjunction with these other closely related labels and since it was used so frequently. The use of this "anticipatory observation" designation appeared with decreasing frequency in the most recent patient records. However, it was felt that in analysis it should be examined carefully since it represented a meaningful diagnostic distinction to the nurses providing the data for the study. Therefore, the investigators followed a two-way classification process throughout the remainder of the data analysis. The nursing diagnoses are listed according to diagnostic categories, both with and without the inclusion of the "anticipatory observation" label.

The first column of Table 23-4 lists the frequency of nursing diagnoses with those removed that were qualified as "anticipatory observation." The actual number of nursing diagnoses drops to 303 with an average of 1.8 for each patient. The greatest single variation in the diagnostic categories between columns 1 and 2 in Table 23-4 is in the medical diagnosis list. The number of medical diagnoses increased from 1 to 64 when

"anticipatory observation" was utilized. The investigators tabulated a total of 179 nursing diagnoses that were cited in wording identical to the National Conference list without the use of any qualifying terms such as "potential," "observation for," or "anticipatory observation for" preceding the label itself.

The second purpose of the study entailed a detailed analysis of the incidence of nursing diagnoses recorded for the sample group. The diagnostic categories have been separated into two groups according to the presence of the "anticipatory observation" label, and the individual categories have been rank-ordered within the two lists as can be noted in Table 23-5.

There are several notable differences in the two lists. The most dramatic alteration in the ranking of diagnostic categories is in the position of the medical diagnosis category. Medical diagnosis holds the prominent rank of third place when the "anticipatory observation" label is used, but falls to rank 12 without it. Two other sizable differences in the rank order were noted. Cognitive-perceptual patterns rank higher without

Table 23-5   Ranking of Diagnostic Categories

Without anticipatory observation	With anticipatory observation
1 Nutritional–metabolic patterns	1 Roles–relationship patterns
2 Roles–relationship patterns	2 Nutritional–metabolic patterns
3 Self-perception–conception patterns	3 Medical diagnoses
4 Elimination patterns	4 Self-perception–conception patterns
5 Exercise–activity patterns	5 Health status–management patterns
6 Health status–management patterns	6 Elimination patterns
7 Cognitive-perceptual patterns	7 Sexuality–reproductive patterns
8 Interpersonal relationship pattern	8 Exercise–activity patterns
9 Life patterns–life-style	9 Life patterns–life-style
10 Coping patterns–stress tolerance	10 Interpersonal relationship pattern
11 Sexuality–reproductive patterns	11 Cognitive–perceptual patterns
12 Medical diagnoses	12 Coping patterns–stress tolerance
13 Sleep–rest patterns	13 Sleep–rest patterns
14 Value–belief patterns	14 Value–belief patterns

"anticipatory observation" while the sexuality-reproductive patterns category ranks lower. The remainder of the categories showed little variation between the two lists.

The most frequently utilized category of nursing diagnosis in list 1 was "disturbances in nutritional-metabolic patterns." An inspection of the nursing diagnoses yielded a varied pattern which includes such items as problems in: adherence to special diets, deficits in nutritional intake, excess body fluids, and obesity. The predominance of this category on list 1 and its second place ranking on list 2 in a group of patients who were being treated medically for obstetrical and gynecological problems was not anticipated.

The second most prevalent category of nursing diagnoses in list 1 was disturbances in role patterns. [This was an expected finding with this population since the single most prevalent nursing diagnosis for the sample, "alteration in parenting" ($n = 95$), was contained in this category.] It should be noted that other diagnoses in this section reflected other types of problems with fulfilling roles such as the attainment of independence, dependence, and the handling of the grieving process.

The diagnostic category "self-perception-conception patterns" was ranked third on list 1. It contained the second most frequently cited nursing diagnosis, which was the label "anxiety" ($n = 20$). Pain, discomfort, and alteration in body image were labels utilized in this category as well. The fourth-ranking category of list 1, elimination patterns, was almost evenly divided between problems with bowel and problems with bladder elimination and control. The exercise-activity patterns category contained the frequently mentioned nursing diagnosis of mobility impairment ($n = 16$) and included labels such as interruption of circulation and respiratory dysfunction. Nursing diagnoses mentioned within the cognitive-perceptual pattern category included things such as knowledge deficits as well as vision and hearing problems. The remainder of the diagnostic categories contained a scattering of nursing diagnoses with extremely low frequencies.

DISCUSSION

The results indicate that the National Conference list of nursing diagnoses contains labels describing patient's health problems which can be applied to a group of patients in a natural setting. However, the study pointed out the necessity of allowing for expansion of the list to include descriptions of other types of problems. A cautionary note should be added for those involved in implementing nursing diagnoses in clinical settings. The options for adding new terminology should be clearly explained and the new labels should be specifically defined. The process should include monitoring to maintain the decision-making focus on nursing problems, since the nurses in this study showed a tendency to also label medical symptoms and problems.

The investigation into the utilization of nursing diagnoses provided several interesting observations. The use of the phrase "anticipatory observation" was widespread among the nurses providing the data for this study. One explanation may be that the nurses experienced some reluctance in making a firm decision about a nursing diagnosis and were not willing to put it on the patient's record without a great degree of qualification. Another explanation could be connected with the use of medical information, since the most prominent difference between lists 1 and 2 (Table 23-4) was the medical diagnosis category. This may indicate that the nurse participants wanted to get involved with making medical decisions or that they viewed the observation and identification of medical problems as a part of their nursing role. They were willing to do so, however, only when they used the "anticipatory observation" label to cite medical symptoms. The notable drop in the utilization of nursing diagnoses for labeling medical problems in list 1 indicated that nurses need to be especially careful in assessing patient problems within their own province of nursing expertise. The utilization of a list of nursing diagnostic categories in combination with an educational program for nurse diagnosticians may not provide sufficient safeguards to ensure a nursing rather than a medical focus.

The use of the "anticipatory observation" label may be connected with another diagnostic issue. It is possible that the type of information or "cues" deemed necessary for establishing a diagnosis could have brought about the use of this phase. Some of the differences between the rank order of the diagnostic categories in Table 23–4 may be attributed to the fact that nurses may utilize objective information in different ways in applying diagnostic labels.

A drop in the rank order occurs in list 1 in the placement of the diagnostic category of sexual and reproductive patterns. The drop in the proportionate frequency of use in list 1 may be due to the lack of objective, identifiable data upon which a nurse can feel safe in making such a decision. The availability of objective information on which a nurse can assess cognitive and perceptual patterns (such as lack of understanding about medications or treatments) may account for the rise in frequency of this label in list 1 when the "anticipatory observation" label is removed. Some of the differences between the two lists in Table 23–4 point out interesting areas for further research in regard to the use of cues in the decision-making process.

The incidence of the use of nursing diagnoses for the patients in this obstetrical-gynecological population resulted in some unexpected findings. One of the two most frequently identified nursing problem categories in this group of patients was difficulties in nutritional-metabolic patterns. Although the inspection of the individual nursing diagnoses yielded a varied pattern that included such items as problems with adherence to special diets and deficits in nutritional intake, the finding was unanticipated. Much of the literature in the maternal-child area points out the varied feeding

difficulties with newborns as opposed to postpartum maternal nutrition. It should be noted once again that this particular group of subjects excluded neonates. However, these results highlight an area of increasing concern to nurses and clearly point out a need for comprehensive nursing assessment on patients regardless of the presenting medical diagnosis or the primary reason for hospitalization. In fact, the wide-ranging incidence of different nursing diagnoses in numerous categories was reflective of the gamut of problems which nurses need to be able to identify as a routine part of their clinical work.

The other predominant group of nursing diagnoses were in the category of role patterns. This was expected in this specialized population and the majority of the diagnostic labels centered around parenting issues, which is consistent with the literature in this specialty which chronicles problems involved with bonding as well as those involved with assuming a parental role. However, it should be noted that labels indicating problems with role independence and dependence were utilized as well.

The relatively low frequency of nursing diagnoses in the category sexuality-reproductive patterns was unexpected in light of the fact that this patient population was thought to be a prime group for displaying these types of health problems. The low incidence of other types of anticipated problems, such as those in the categories of coping patterns-stress tolerance, or sleep-rest patterns may indicate that these nursing diagnoses require cues which may be more difficult to observe or may require a longer time period to substantiate.

In summary, nursing diagnoses were applied to a group of obstetrical and gynecological patients in a naturalistic setting. The nurses utilized the National Conference List of Nursing Diagnoses with some additions and modifications. Predominating among the diagnoses were labels in the categories dealing with problems of nutritional-metabolic patterns and role patterns. The two individual nursing diagnoses utilized most frequently were "alterations in parenting" and "anxiety." The study indicated the need for a holistic nursing assessment of patient's health problems since the most prevalent diagnoses for this group of women admitted to a specialty service were not in the expected order or frequency.

EDITOR'S QUESTIONS FOR DISCUSSION

What suggestions do you have for research designs to further investigate the validity and clinical usefulness of nursing diagnostic labels? How can categories of nursing diagnoses be utilized for defining the type of nursing care, the appropriate provider for the care, and implementation of reimbursement to the department of nursing service for the provision of care? What implications might this have for the quality of care, nurse staffing and assignments, third-party payers, and the evolution of legal questions? What positive and negative factors may be inherent in utilizing labels and classification systems for patients?

What methods were used by the investigators to increase the validity and reliability of their study? How appropriate was their sampling procedures?

What are the implications in collaborative relationships with medicine in patient care, regarding the differences in type and qualitative variation of labels or diagnoses utilized by nursing and medicine? What are the advantages and disadvantages for including the medical diagnoses category in the classification system? To what extent did the nurses tend to use qualifying terms for nursing diagnoses when compared with the number and type indicated for medical diagnoses? Would you expect the increased use of qualifying terms to develop as a trend in nursing diagnoses?

How might you account for the nurses' tendency in this study to also label medical symptoms and problems? What are the implications for the role of nurses in the findings concerning the use of the label "anticipatory observation"? Is there evidence of "traditional" role behavior and expectations for and by nurses in this study? What are the pros and cons of retaining the "anticipatory observation" label? What type of "cues" could have brought about the use of the phrase? What methods can be utilized to ensure a nursing focus rather than a medical focus? What alternative explanations might be offered for Sweeney and Gordon's findings?

Compare relationships in this study with Clayton's (Chap. 10). How would you account for the different findings regarding the assessment of nutritional status by nurses?

REFERENCES

American Nurses Association
1973 Standards of Nursing Practice. Kansas City, Mo.: American Nurses Association.
Boston Hospital for Women Nursing Diagnosis Guidelines
1977 Unpublished.
Brown, M.
1974 "The epidemiologic approach to the study of clinical nursing diagnosis." Nursing Forum 13:346–359.

Gebbie, K. (ed.)
1976 Summary of the Second National Conference: Classification of Nursing Diagnoses. St. Louis: Clearinghouse, National Group for Classification of Nursing Diagnoses.
Gebbie, K. (ed.)
Forthcoming Proceedings of the Third National Conference: Classification of Nursing Diagnoses.
Gebbie, K. and M. A. Lavin (eds.)
1975 Proceedings of the First National Confer-

ence: Classification of Nursing Diagnoses. St. Louis: Mosby.

Goldenberg, H.
1973 Contemporary Clinical Psychology. Monterey, Calif.: Brooks/Cole.

Gordon, M.
1976 "Nursing diagnoses and the diagnostic process." American Journal of Nursing 1976:1298–1300.
1975 Functional Health Problems Typology. Unpublished course materials. Chestnut Hill, Mass.: Boston College School of Nursing.

Hornung, G.
1956 "The nursing diagnosis—an exercise in judgment." Nursing Outlook 4:29–30.

Korchin, S.
1976 Modern Clinical Psychology. New York: Basic Books.

La Montague, M. and K. McKeehan
1975 "Profile of a continuing care program emphasizing discharge planning." Journal of Nursing Administration 5:22–23.

McKeehan, K.
1979 "Use of nursing diagnoses in a continuing care program." Nursing Clinics of North America 14:517–524.

Mundinger, M. and G. Jauron
1975 "Developing a nursing diagnosis." Nursing Outlook 23:94–98.

World Health Organization
1977 Manual of the International Statistical Classification of Diseases, Injuries and Causes of Death. Vols. I and II. Geneva: World Health Organization.

Chapter 24

Role Differentiation with Specialization and its Effects on Quality Patient Care

Margaret Hardy, R.N., Ph.D., F.A.A.N.
Associate Professor
School of Nursing
Boston University
Boston, Massachusetts

Research related to nursing roles and the quality of care provided is emphasized in this chapter, followed by studies describing emerging roles in the chapters by Williams and Brown.

Since a hospital's major goal is quality patient care, the effectiveness of a hospital needs to take into account the system of roles in providing care. Margaret Hardy investigates the effect that implementing clinical nurse specialists and unit managers has on the organizational goal of quality patient care. She examines the wards from two medical-surgical units of a 380-bed urban university medical-center hospital 6 months after clinical nurse specialists and unit managers were established.

A sample of 40 patients was randomly selected each from the wards that had both unit managers and clinical nurse specialists and from wards without those roles. The patients were chosen from a list of patients being discharged who had been hospitalized four days or more. Three simultaneous surveys were conducted during a 3-month period. Patients, nursing staff, and nurse-interviewers were queried for their perceptions of the care received by patients. A Likert-type tool was constructed used by the nurse-interviewers, to measure patient perceptions of general hospital care, nursing care, and problems patients identified as associated with hospitalization. Demographic questions were also included. A similar Likert-type questionnaire was distributed to the hospital nurses.

The data indicate that the quality of care was generally perceived as similar by patients and hospital nurses on wards with and without ward managers and clinical nurse specialists. Only the nurse-interviewers reported a statistically significant difference between the experimental and control groups. The nursing care aspects of socioemotional care, planning for discharge, and provision of information were perceived more favorably on the experimental wards. Hardy presents concerns regarding the extent to which patients' evaluation of nursing care is a valid measure of that care. She concludes the question of the effect of unit managers and clinical nurse specialists on care received by patients has not been clearly answered. Hardy suggests that future studies may indicate changes in the social structure of hospitals and may be more effective in meeting organizational goals than improving quality of direct nursing care.

A social organization such as a hospital may be defined as a system of roles. Katz and Kahn (1966), in using this perspective, emphasized two facts about organizations, namely, their contrived nature and their unique property as a structure consisting of acts or events. Organizations, as contrived entities designed to achieve specific organizational goals, are subject to relatively rational and purposeful change. Part of the existing social structure may be changed, for example, to accommodate expanding organizational goals or to facilitate the achievement of existing goals. Although such changes may be made purposefully, their actual effect on other units within the organization and on specific organizational goals is often unclear and difficult to determine. Since a hospital's major goal is quality patient care, any study of the effectiveness of a hospital, or of a hospital subsystem such as nursing, must focus on assessing care.

This study was undertaken to examine the effect that modification of the role system in an acute care hospital has on the organizational goal of quality patient care. A comparative analysis is made of the perceived quality of patient care in an acute care hospital in which role differentiation with specialization was implemented. The changes on selected wards included employment of unit managers to perform nonnursing administrative functions and clinical nurse specialists to provide expert nursing care.

The social structure of role behavior was the

This study was supported in part by funds from Boston University School of Nursing. The author wishes to thank Myra Kerr and Joan Gallagher for assistance in data analysis, W. L. Hardy for computer and editorial assistance, and Mary Conway for additional assistance. Special recognition goes to the graduate nurse students who helped in pretesting and data collection.

focus of this study. Patient care is a major role behavior of nonadministrative hospital nurses. Role behaviors in this study were primarily examined from the perspective of patients; comparative perceptions by staff nurses and designated nurse-interviewers were reported to clarify and validate interpretations.

It is assumed that an organization is an open social system whose structure may be examined in terms of social positions, norms, roles, and role behavior. Each position has associated with it norms, beliefs, standards, and expectations which prescribe and proscribe behavior. Role differentiation with specialization occurs when an existing role, such as that of staff nurse, is divided into several roles, such as head nurse, staff nurse, and clinical specialist. Such specialization occurs as increased expertise and skill are demanded. The head nurse is expected to be skilled in nursing management and administration; staff nurses may specialize in intensive care, dialysis, or primary care.

As organizational growth takes place, differentiation with specialization occurs. Changes in the complementary characteristics of a system of roles are stimulated by technology, increased organizational complexity, and new output demands. Role differentiation involves the reallocation of existing role expectations to new positions to meet organizational expectations. Specialization refers to the increased expertise and complexity of activities required of role incumbents to fulfill the role requirements of emerging positions. These definitions of role concepts are consistent with those used by a number of theorists (Biddle and Thomas, 1966; Hardy and Conway, 1978; Katz and Kahn, 1966).

Within the hospital system there has been a continuous concern for establishing an effective balance between the clinical and coordinating activities of professionals. The concept of unit manager was first introduced over 30 years ago to reduce the number of nonnursing activities performed by nurses. Theoretically, implementation of unit management should lessen the need for nonnursing activities performed by nurses and thus should make more time available for nurses to carry out their primary function, that of providing patient care.

While the institution of unit management has indeed been shown to reduce the role overload of nurses, the direct impact of unit management on patient care, especially that given by nurses, is unclear (Jelinek et al., 1971). Some studies report that nurses freed of nonnursing duties do spend more time with patients (Mckenna, 1968; Regan, 1969; Underwood, 1967); some studies report a slight improvement in selected aspects of patient care (Jelinek et al., 1971; Palmer, 1969; Yankauer and Levine, 1954); some studies report no change in time spent with patients (Hotz, 1962; Jelinek et al., 1971; Schmeiding, 1966); and others find no impact at all on patient welfare (Brandt and Anderson, 1967; Mckenna, 1968). None of these studies, it should be noted, reports statistically significant findings nor gives measures of statistical significance.

The inconsistency of the findings may be due to the variety of variables examined, insufficient control of variables, or differences in the settings themselves. The failure to detect significant improvement of patient care in these studies may simply be an indication of lack of sufficiently sensitive tools for measurement of patient care, but it may also indicate that the quality of patient care has actually not been significantly improved by structural changes intended to free nurses from nonnursing activities and responsibilities.

It would seem logical that the addition of specially trained unit managers to the hospital ward structure to perform many of the administrative and managerial tasks formerly performed by nurses should increase the efficiency of ward activities and should result in more time available to nurses for direct patient care. One reason for the limited impact of unit managers on the quality of nursing care may be that, to a great extent, hospitals both directly and indirectly reward the administrative activities of nurses rather than their patient-care activities. Thus, the nurse-administrator is more likely to be rewarded than the nurse-clinician. Many administrative functions traditionally undertaken by nurses are highly visible and subject to sanctions; record keeping is a prime example. Many direct care activities, on the other hand, involve complex interactions with patients, interactions which go unrecorded, are not highly visible, are not subject to others' evaluations, and are relatively free of either positive or negative sanctions. In addition, administrative role behaviors on the part of the nurse have traditionally been rewarded by the hospital system; usually the only promotion possible for a staff nurse in a traditional setting is to a head nurse or supervisory position, one which entails less direct patient care and more administrative responsibility.

The simultaneous implementation of two specialized positions—unit manager and clinical nurse specialist—should reduce nonnursing demands on nurses, while reinforcing, at least for the nurses, the value of quality patient care. Although it is extremely difficult to change role behaviors and social norms, ultimately the formal recognition of the importance of clinical skill should encourage hospital personnel, both nursing and nonnursing, to place increased value on patient care.

Thus the differentiation of the role of the clinical specialist from that of the nurse-manager should contribute to more optimal overall care. Specifically, the creation of the positions of clinical nurse specialist and of unit manager should facilitate the provision of more sustained nursing care and increase the quality of that care. If these changes in care do occur, then patients on these more differentiated wards would be likely to perceive their care as being of higher quality than would patients on more traditionally structured wards.

The specific hypothesis tested in this study was:

Patients on wards in which there are both clinical-nurse specialists and unit managers will perceive a higher quality of general care, nursing care, and patient care than will patients on wards having neither clinical-nurse specialists nor unit managers.

METHODOLOGY

Six months prior to this investigation, the 380-bed urban university medical-center hospital to be studied had carefully planned and established unit managers and clinical nurse specialists on two medical-surgical units. The changes were implemented on a trial basis only. If the changes were judged to be effective, similar changes were to be made throughout the hospital.

To assess the effectiveness of the implementation of unit managers and clinical nurse specialists, three simultaneous surveys were conducted during a 3-month period. Patients, nursing staff, and nurse-interviewers were asked to give their perceptions of the care received by patients. Since these three surveys were to complement each other, care was taken to include in the questionnaire distributed to the hospital nurses questions similar to those to be included in the interview schedule developed for patients. Although this report will focus primarily on the patients' perceptions of their care, some of the data obtained from the nurse-respondents will be included in order to examine alternative explanations of the findings.

Although the 6-month postimplementation time lapse made it possible to avoid distortions directly associated with the transition process, that lapse also meant that it was not possible to obtain direct "before" and "after" measures. Thus, the conclusion that the differences found occurred as a direct result of role differentiation in the social structure could not be drawn. However, comparisons could be made between patients on the basis of their perceptions of the care they received in each type of ward. If the perceived care in the two types of settings differed and if the two types were observed to be similar in all respects

other than the presence or absence of unit manager and clinical nurse specialist, then it could be inferred that the differences were due to the altered social structure.

In order to examine extraneous variables which might influence the findings, data related to possible differences in the two settings were obtained. These data included demographic information on patients, rate of staff turnover, educational preparation of nurses, number of nurses per patient, bed count, typical diagnoses of patients, previous patient hospitalizations, length of stay on the ward under study, and patient perception of health status.

Study Design

A sample of 40 patients from the wards which had both unit managers and clinical-nurse specialists was selected for study along with a comparable sample of 40 patients from wards without unit managers and clinical nurse specialists. The sample was a systematic probability sample in that patients interviewed were randomly selected from a list of patients to be discharged. Following the initial contact, all patients who had been hospitalized 4 days or more were solicited as subjects until data were obtained from a total of 40 patients in each setting. The criterion of a minimum hospital stay was utilized to provide adequate time for patients to develop a reasonable impression of general hospital care and nursing care. Of all the patients approached, only one declined to participate. This patient was on a ward having the traditional structure.

Variables

The independent variable, role differentiation with specialization, was defined in terms of the social structure. Role differentiation was operationally defined as the presence or absence of unit managers and clinical nurse specialists. High role differentiation with specialization describes the organization of specialized wards, wards characterized by a management team composed of a unit coordinator, a unit manager, a secretary, a coordinator-assistant, and a nursing team composed of an area nursing director, a clinical nurse specialist, a nurse-clinician and a normal complement of staff nurses. The unit coordinators were responsible to the administrator for inpatient services, whereas the clinical nurse specialists were responsible to the director of nursing service. Units without specialization, or traditional wards, had the traditional organizational positions of nurse-supervisor, head nurse, and staff nurses.

The dependent variable, patient care, included patient perception of (1) general hospital care, (2) nursing care, and (3) problems that subjects identified as associated with hospitalization. These aspects of patient care were used as measurements in order to obtain a relatively complete assessment—from the patient's point of view—of care received while in the hospital.

   1 *General care.* Patients were asked to rate (a) the general quality of care they received within the hospital, (b) the extent to which services provided to them were well coordinated, and (c) the extent to which the personnel concerned with patient care worked together harmoniously.
   2 *Nursing care.* Patients were asked to rate (a) the overall nursing care given to others; (b) five specific aspects of direct nursing care: physical comfort, socioemotional needs fulfillment, information giving, coordination of inpatient care, and assistance to the patient in planning for care after discharge; and (c) general perceptions of such elements of nursing care as the number of nurses available, the importance of nurses to patient care, the judgment demonstrated by nurses in giving patient care, the knowledge shown by nurses in regard to diseases, medications, and treatments, and the degree of skill exhibited by nurses.
   3 *Problems associated with hospitalization.* Patients were asked to rate the extent to which potential problems—problems such as hospital routine, lack of privacy, separation from family, changes in diet, lack of normal leisure activities, noisy surroundings, variety of medications and treatment, number of persons involved in care, decisions being made for patient by other people,

confinement, uncertainty of health, and hospital-related health complications—were viewed as actual problems.

Problems associated with hospitalization were included because it was thought that potential problems might be perceived by patients as being related to nursing care, whether in fact they were or not.

Development of the Tool

To determine patients' perceptions of their care, an interview schedule calling for Likert-type responses was constructed. Face and construct validity were established, and three pretests were conducted. Scaling was developed before the interview schedule was finalized. Demographic questions were also included in the instrument.[1]

Data Collection

Two senior baccalaureate students and 13 graduate nursing students were hired and trained as interviewers. All wore street clothes and identified themselves as university students assisting in a study of care received by hospitalized patients. Interviewers were not informed of the purpose of the study. They were instructed to assure patients of the anonymity and the confidentiality of information provided, to ensure that the patients understood that their participation was voluntary, and to terminate the interview at any time if the patient requested it or the patient's health status appeared to warrant such termination.

FINDINGS

The sociodemographic characteristics of patients were remarkably similar for the specialized and the

---

[1] More extensive discussion of the tool development is reported by Hardy in "Implementation of Unit Management and Clinical Nurse Specialists: Patients' Perception of the Quality of General Hospital Care and Nursing Care," in M. Batey (ed.) *Communication Nursing Research*, vol. 8 (Boulder, Colo.: Western Interstate Commission for Higher Education, 1977), pp. 325–335.

traditional wards. Patient ages in the sample ranged from 14 to 87. Mean ages on the specialized and traditional wards were 54 and 50, respectively. In each sample of 40 patients, 21 were female; 35 patients from the specialized wards designated themselves Caucasian as did 36 from the traditional wards; three of each sample were black. Religious affiliation of patients on the specialized wards was distributed as follows: 8 were Protestant, 17 Catholic, and 10 Jewish. On the traditional wards the figures were 11, 12, and 4, respectively.

The typical patient in the total sample was from the lower-middle class (as measured by occupation), had had 2 years of high school, lived with his or her immediate family, was advised to enter the hospital by a medical specialist rather than by a family physician, had medical insurance, and knew his or her diagnosis.

The patients' diagnoses, classified according to the primary physiological system involved, differed for the two types of wards. The major difference related to cardiovascular problems; there were 22 patients with such problems on the specialized wards and only nine on the traditional wards. There were four patients having orthopedic problems on the specialized wards, and 12 on the traditional wards. The specialized wards were treating no patients with reproductive system problems, while the traditional wards had four such patients. There were four patients with renal problems on the specialized wards, and none on the traditional.

General Care and Coordination of Care

Most patients evaluated their general care very favorably. Of the patients interviewed, 82 percent described the care as very good or excellent. Patients generally perceived the hospital personnel as being quite concerned with patient care and perceived general health care services as being very well coordinated.

It had been expected that patients would perceive a higher level of organization and improved management of their general care where unit managers and clinical nurse specialists were established

Yet the data presented in Table 24-1 make it apparent that patients rated their general care and the coordination of this care very favorably in both settings, with little difference measured between the types of wards.

Nursing Care

As with their assessment of the general care within the hospital, patients assessed the overall nursing care very favorably. Of the total patient sample, 83 percent rated nursing care as good to excellent. The proportion was 88 percent on those wards having unit managers and clinical nurse specialists and 78 percent on the traditional wards. The difference is not statistically significant.

Patients generally gave a favorable assessment of the quality of direct nursing care they received, and their assessment was relatively unaffected by the ward structure. Over 90 percent of all patients rated their personal nursing care as good to excellent. Sixty percent of the patients on the specialized wards and 88 percent of those on the traditional wards rated the care excellent. Again this difference is not statistically significant.

Specific Aspects of Nursing Care Patients were asked to evaluate both the importance and the quality of specific aspects of the nursing care they received while taking into consideration their own health needs and condition. They were then asked to rate both the importance to them of a nursing care activity, and how well nurses carried out this care (see Table 24-2). Patients rated 14 nursing care activities. These activities were combined at the data analysis stage of the study into five specific aspects of nursing care. Such activities were generally rated as being very important, and the care was evaluated as being very good. Ratings did not seem to depend on the ward type. Of the patients who rated the components of nursing care as important, it was found that about 70 percent of the patients assessed physical care, socioemotional care, provision of information, and continuity of care as important or very important. However, just under 60 percent of the patients assigned this

Table 24-1   Patients Rating the Quality of Selected Aspects of Nursing Care as Very Good*

	Unit management and clinical nurse specialist			
	Present (Specialized wards)		Absent (Traditional wards)	
Care variables	N[†]	%	N[†]	%
General care and coordination of care				
General care	34	85	32	80
Organization of patient services	32	80	32	80
Harmony with which personnel functioned	32	80	30	75
Nursing care				
Overall nursing care:				
Nursing care in general	35	88	31	78
Nursing care patient received	37	93	35	88
Specific aspects[‡]				
Physical comfort	31	78	29	73
Socioemotional care	33	83	30	75
Information provision	25	63	25	63
Continuity of care	25	63	30	75
Assistance in planning care				
after discharge	13	33	11	28
General aspects				
Number of nurses on ward[§]	29	73	24	60
Importance of nurses to care	36	90	38	95
Judgment shown in patient care	36	90	35	88
Knowledge of diseases, treatments	29	73	30	75
Skill shown in patient care	37	93	35	88

*Includes patients giving only the rating of "excellent" and "very good" or those choosing categories 1 and 2 at the favorable end of a 5-point scale. Chi-square values were computed for the unit management/clinical nurse specialist variable cross-tabulated with each of the nursing care variables (2 × 2 tables). t-Tests were also computed. The critical level was set at .05; none of these values was statistically significant.

[†]Forty patients were in each sample group.

[‡]Mean value of these five components is 64% for specialized wards and 63% for traditional.

[§]Indicates patients who perceived enough or more than enough nurses on the ward.

same importance to assisting with plans for health-related care after discharge from the hospital. The assessment of importance was unaffected by ward type.

The assessment of how well these 14 nursing activities were carried out also did not vary with type of ward. The proportion of the patients assessing the quality of their nursing care as very good to excellent is illustrated in Tables 24-1 and 24-2. It should be noted that the proportion of patients giving a favorable rating to the planning of their care after discharge is relatively low. Half

of the patients indicated that this nursing care activity was not important for them. As might be expected, an independent evaluation of nursing care by the nurse-interviewers differed from the patients' assessment of the relative importance of this aspect of care. The nurse-interviewers rated planning of care after discharge as very important.

Whether staff nurses failed to discuss discharge plans with patients or whether the majority of patients failed to recall the nurses having provided such information is unclear. Regardless of the reason, it is a fact that only a minority of patients

Table 24-2 Percentage of Patients, Hospital Nurses, and Nurse-Interviewers Favorably Rating the Quality of Nursing Care For Both Settings

Nursing care	Percentage assessing care as "very good" or "excellent"					
	Ward nurses (N = 68)	Patients (N = 80)	Nurse-Interviewers (N = 60)	Patients (N = 80)	Nurse-Interviewer (N = 60)	Ward nurses (N = 68)
Physical comfort						
Provides physical care (bath, skin care, etc.)	72*	66	45*	66	45*	72
Provides pleasant environment	65*	84	58*	84	58	65
Socioemotional care						
Treats as individual	85	88	62*	88	62*	85
Aware of worries and concerns	76*	64	32*	64	32*	76
Helps with worries and tension	71	66	42*	66	42*	71
Easy and comfortable to talk with	7*	93	63*	93	63	7
Information provision						
Provides information on disease	76	69	43*	69	43*	76
Provides information on procedures, treatments, and medications	62*	51	27*	51	27*	62
Provides honest information when wanted	80*	64	43*	64	43*	80
Continuity of care						
Ensures continuity of care on the ward (passes information on to other nurses and doctors)	82	75	58*	75	58*	82
Works with other nurses to solve problems and difficulties in nursing care	79	63	47*	63	47*	79
Works with other health care workers (doctors, dietitian, etc.)	79	68	43*	68	43*	79
Assistance in planning care after discharge						
Works with patient and family on care after discharge	48*	30	17	30	17*	48
Makes plans with patient for care after discharge	42	29	17	29	17*	42

*Score calculated for difference in proportions was significant at .05 level.

who were at the point of discharge from the hospital, whether from a specialized or a traditional ward, recalled or valued the nurses' discussion relating to posthospital care.

In this study, nursing care was seldom evaluated as being either poorly or very poorly carried out, but patients frequently identified nursing care as "not applying." This category was available to patients when they were asked to judge either the importance of care or the adequacy with which

care was performed. The data suggest that some activities considered part of traditional nursing care are not seen by all patients as nursing tasks. For example, almost one-third (30 percent) of the patients responded to the importance of nurse involvement in planning of their postdischarge care by indicating that this activity did not apply, 25 percent of the patients indicated that providing information did not apply, and 20 percent indicated that providing continuity of care did not apply.

These proportions do not differ significantly for the two ward types. An assessment by nurse-interviewers as independent observers differed from the assessments made by patients.

In summary, there were no statistically significant differences in patients' perceptions of nursing care on wards with unit managers and clinical nurse specialists and on wards without these positions. On examining the hospital nurses' perceptions of the nursing care received by patients in the two settings, one finds a similar lack of significant differences. However, the assessment of the nurse-interviewers suggests that the nursing care was indeed different. Patients on the wards with unit managers and clinical-nurse specialists were perceived by the nurse-interviewers as receiving better socioemotional care, and the differences were statistically significant for the four questions related to socioemotional care. Patients on the newly organized wards were also perceived as more likely to receive information when it was wanted and to receive help with discharge plans. The nurse-interviewers perceived patients on the wards having unit managers and nurse-clinicians as receiving better nursing care for seven of the 14 nursing care questions. These differences are statistically significant at the .05 level.

General Aspects of Nursing Care. Patients were requested to assess nurses and nursing care on several additional dimensions. As seen in Table 24–1 responses by patients to a number of questions pertaining to the time pressures exerted on nurses indicated that the perceptions of patients were unaffected by the ward structure. Patients' perceptions of the number of nurses on the ward, of the importance of nurses to patient care, and of the nurses' knowledge, judgment, and skill were likewise unaffected by ward structure.

It should be noted that nurses were generally rated very highly on these latter behaviors, with 96 percent of the patients perceiving nurses as very important to their care, and 89 percent of the patients assessing the nurses as being highly skilled. These ratings tended to be slightly higher for wards

having unit managers and clinical nurse specialists than for wards without such specialists, but the differences are not statistically significant.

Problems Associated with Hospitalization

Patients were asked to rate on a Likert scale the extent to which 12 specific hospital-related experiences were problems for them. These potential problems were included since patients might perceive these experiences as being related to nursing care and an assessment would be an indirect assessment of nursing care. In general, either no difficulty or minimal difficulty was perceived by patients as being associated with the hospital routine, lack of privacy, separation from friends and family, decisions controlled by others, the variety of procedures, medications, and treatments, the large number of persons involved in caring for patient, noisy surroundings, lack of normal leisure activities, confinement, and hospital-related health complications. (See Table 24–3.) Changes in diet and in availability of food and uncertainty of health status were viewed by more patients as creating problems, but these ratings were relatively unaffected by the ward structure. Chi-square tests were not statistically significant, and a *t*-test indicated statistically significant differences in only two of the 11 ratings—perceptions of the variety of procedures, medications, and treatments and of hospital-related health complications. Patients on wards with unit managers and clinical nurse specialists tended to perceive the variety of procedures, medications, and treatments as more of a problem and hospital-related health complications as less of a problem than did patients on the traditional wards.

Health Status[2]

Patients in each of the two settings were asked to rank their health status as an indicator of the ex-

---

[2] The perceived health status of patients was assessed to determine if the two medical-surgical groups of patients were similar in their health care needs. It was expected that they would be.

Table 24-3 Patients Rating the Extent to Which Selected Hospital Experiences Presented No Problem or a Slight Problem*

| Problem areas associated with hospitalization | Unit coordination and clinical nurse specialist | | | |
| | Present (Specialized ward) | | Absent (Traditional ward) | |
	$N^\dagger$	%	$N^\dagger$	%
Hospital routine	31	78	32	80
Lack of privacy	26	65	28	70
Separation from friends and family	26	65	28	70
Changes in diet and in availability of food	14	35	19	48
Lack of normal leisure activities	27	68	21	53
Noisy surroundings	25	63	23	58
Decisions controlled by others (physicians, nurses)	32	80	33	83
The variety of procedures, medications, and treatments	32	80	35‡	88
Large number of persons involved in caring for patient	30	75	35	88
Being confined	25	63	24	60
Uncertainty of health	14	35	18	45
Hospital-related health complications	37	93	31‡	78

*Patients rated each problem area on a scale of 1 ("no problem") to 5 ("major problem"). Chi-square values were computed for the unit management clinical nurse specialist variables (present or absent) cross-tabulated with each of the hospital problems. The critical level was set at .05; none of these values was statistically significant.

‡t-Test was computed and values were significant at the .05 level. For the t-test, the Likert scale of 1 to 5 for the hospital experiences was not collapsed into two categories as it was for the chi-square.

†Forty patients were in each sample group.

tent of loss of health that they felt was associated with illness. Patients were presented with a 0-to-100 scale and asked to identify a minor illness and rank it "0" and then to identify the most serious illness they could think of and rank it "100." Patients were asked to use this scale to rate their normal state of health, their health status the year prior to hospitalization, during hospitalization, and at the end of their hospitalization, and then to predict their expected status 5 years hence. *T*-tests were computed for these ratings. It was expected that results in the two settings would be comparable, but the mean differences between groups were statistically significant at the .05 level for four of these five patient-ratings. Patients on the wards with unit managers and clinical nurse specialists saw themselves as normally being more ill, being sicker during their hospitalization, being sicker at the end of their hospitalization, and being less well 5 years in the future than did patients who were on traditional wards. The only area where

no difference between groups was observed was in their rating of their health status for the year prior to hospitalization.

VALIDITY OF PATIENTS' EVALUATION OF NURSING CARE

Of concern in this study is the extent to which patient evaluation of nursing care is a valid measure of that care. It can be argued that nursing care is often nonvisible to patients and is too highly specialized to permit lay persons—the patients themselves—to make judgments about quality. Certainly a highly specialized body of knowledge is one of the major characteristics of professions (Greenwood, 1957; Moore, 1970). On the other hand, a point can be made for asking the consumers themselves—the patients—to take an active part in their health care, and an active role would naturally include making judgments as to the care received.

An assessment of patients' perceptions of nursing care as a valid evaluation of such care can be made using data from this research. A comparison of the perceptions reported by patients, nurses on the wards of those patients, and nurse-interviewers was made. A comparison of nursing care assessed as very good and excellent (the two top categories on a 5-point Likert scale) by patients, hospital nurses, and nurse-interviewers is presented in Table 24-2. On six of the 14 items, the patients' assessments do not differ significantly from those of the hospital nurses. The results of assessments by the nurse-interviewers yield rather different findings. In 12 of the 14 nursing care items a significantly higher proportion of patients judged the nursing care more favorably than did the nurse-interviewers. Even greater disparity is seen between the evaluations of hospital nurses and those of nurse-interviewers; a significantly higher proportion of hospital nurses judged their nursing care more positively than did the nurse-interviewers. A relatively larger proportion of patients and hospital nurses assessed nursing care more favorably than did nurse-interviewers. These findings on the validity of patient perception of nursing care as an accurate measure of that care must be taken into account in interpreting the results reported here.

DISCUSSION

The principal thesis developed at the beginning of this paper was that the simultaneous implementation of unit coordination and clinical nurse specialists should produce an improvement in the quality of patient care. On the basis of patients' evaluation of their general care and their personal nursing care, it appears that implementation of unit management and the clinical nurse specialist role does not produce the intended improvement in quality of patient care, at least as that care is perceived by patients. However, drawing such a specific conclusion from the data in this study may not be warranted.

In reexamining the details of implementation of these positions, it becomes apparent that unit coordination was implemented by introducing three

managerial-supervisory positions—unit managers similar to department heads, coordinators who supervised and managed areas within the hospital, and coordinator-assistants on each ward. Also, ward secretaries were moved into this coordination system. On the other hand, far fewer role changes were implemented in nursing care. Here, the only role change imposed was the creation of the clinical nurse specialist position.

Clinical nurse specialists were given the position of clinical coordinators and were made responsible for direct patient care and coordination of patient care on several wards. Name changes, such as that of assistant director to area director and head nurse to nurse-clinician, occurred, but actual additions and changes made in nursing structure were far fewer than those made in unit management. In effect, the manipulation of the independent variable was not as strong in the area of nursing as in the area of management. These changes in the hospital structure appear to have primarily effected an efficient ward management system rather than an improvement in direct patient care.

The data indicate that the quality of patient care was generally perceived as similar by patients on wards with and without ward managers and clinical nurse specialists. It was also perceived as similar across the settings by the hospital-nurse subjects in the study. This may be interpreted to mean that administrative efficiency and improved delivery of nursing care did not occur, or, if such improvements did occur, they were not perceived by the patients. On the other hand, the data may be interpreted to mean that either administrative efficiency or improved delivery of nursing care did not result, and thus the quality of patient care was similar in the two settings. Unfortunately, both of these interpretations are based on two assumptions which may be faulty.

The first assumption was that patients can discriminate between "good" and "not so good" nursing care. While the data indicate that patients can and do evaluate the quality of the care they receive, such evaluations are relatively nondiscriminatory and tend to be very favorable. Patients assessed the quality of their nursing care as excellent, even though they indicated that many aspects of patient care generally considered by nurse-interviewers as being important were not given or "did not apply." In particular, important aspects of patient teaching apparently were either completely omitted or, if given, did not have sufficient impact to be recognized as such by patients. In addition, some components of nursing care usually considered part of good nursing care by nurses were seen as being inapplicable by 30 to 50 percent of the patients.

It was also assumed that patients would be able to identify the domain of nursing care and make judgments about such care. Although this assumption has been discussed earlier, it should be noted that a discrepancy between patient identification of the domain of nursing care and that domain as identified by nurses has also been found in a study conducted by Ryan (1974) which focused on patient teaching. Ryan's data indicate that traditional major types of nursing care are frequently not viewed as nursing functions by patients. Ryan found that patients seldom identified health teaching as being initiated by health professionals or as being the responsibility of nurses. If such teaching was initiated at all, patients generally perceived the initiator as being a physician (Ryan, 1974).

It is therefore difficult to know whether patients truly received the excellent nursing care that they reported receiving or whether the care was less than excellent. The ability of the patient to judge accurately quality of nursing care is open to question. In the ratings of the 14 nursing care questions reported here, 11 aspects were rated slightly more favorably by patients on the wards with unit managers and clinical nurse specialists wards than on the traditional wards. Although the individual differences are not statistically significant, the trend is more persistent than one would expect on the basis of chance alone.

The question of the effect of unit managers and clinical nurse specialists on care received by patients has not been clearly answered in this study.

Patients and hospital nurses perceived similar nursing care on both the experimental and traditional wards. Only the nurse-interviewers reported a significant difference in the nursing care. The nurse-interviewers reported statistically significant differences on seven of the 14 nursing care items. They perceived that patients on the experimental wards received more favorable socioemotional care, better planning for discharge, and more provision of information than did other patients. Their evaluation suggests that, in the realm of nursing care, nurses and patients on the nontraditional wards communicated relatively more frequently.

If variables other than patient care are examined, a statistically significant difference between the two wards can be detected. Patients on the experimental wards perceived the variety of treatments, medications, and procedures as more of a problem than did patients on the traditional wards. They also were less concerned about hospital-related health complications. Both of these perceptions could reflect a high quality of care on the experimental wards. However, patients on these wards did perceive themselves generally as being sicker than did patients on the traditional wards. It is possible that the patients on the experimental wards were indeed sicker. However, even though there were more cardiac patients on these wards, the difference was not statistically significant, nor was the length of patient hospitalization significantly longer on the experimental wards.

Perhaps the patients on the experimental wards perceived themselves as being in relatively poorer health because these patients were more aware of their health status as a result of the relatively open communication between nurses and patients on these wards. If this reasoning is correct, it is possible that increased patient awareness could have resulted in a less favorable, but perhaps more realistic, appraisal of health status.

SUMMARY

In this study it was hypothesized that role differentiation with specialization on medical-surgical wards in an acute care hospital would result in patient perception of higher quality of care. Forty patients from traditional settings and 40 patients from newly organized wards with unit management and clinical-nurse specialists were systematically interviewed. Statistical analysis showed that the prediction of a perception of higher quality of care on the nontraditional wards was not directly supported. However, independent nurse-interviewers did perceive higher quality in some aspects of nursing care provided to patients on the nontraditional wards. Some possible explanations for the findings have been proposed in this paper.

The lack of a strong, clear impact on patients' perceptions of the quality of care they receive may be an indication of a failure to create a major alteration in the social structure relative to direct patient care. An alternative explanation, which is beyond the scope of this study but which may warrant future investigation, is that such changes in the social structure as occurred in the hospital under study may, in fact, be more effective in meeting other organizational goals than in improving the quality of direct nursing care.

EDITOR'S QUESTIONS FOR DISCUSSION

What other variables might account for the hypothesis of this study not being supported by the data? Are there alternative methods to determine whether structural changes can be directly related to the quality of patient care? To what extent can it be inferred in this study that the differences were due to the altered social structure?

What suggestions do you have for encouraging change in role behaviors, social norms, and reward systems for nurses in hospitals? How likely is there to be difficulty for a nurse to relinquish "administrative" duties to a nonnurse unit manager? What methods can be utilized for role transitions? What status and authority issues may arise in settings where there are clinical nurse specialists and nonnurse unit managers? How can these be resolved?

What type of research design is utilized? What assumptions exist in this study? What are the limitations of the study and implications for interpretation of the findings? What were the criteria for the sample? Discuss the validity and reliability of the tool and data collection methods. What differences might exist between the interviewers and nurses in the wards to suggest other explanations for their disparate perceptions?

What effect did the sociodemographic variables and patients' diagnosis and acuity have on the perceptions measured?

What relationships might exist between the number and type of roles simultaneously being implemented and patients' perceptions of their health status and quality of care provided? What are the implications for nursing care in the fact that half of the patients did not view discharge planning as an important nursing activity? How do you account for data suggesting some activities considered part of traditional nursing care are not seen by all patients as nursing tasks? What alternative explanations might be offered for the findings of this study?

What implications are there for the profession and quality of care provided in discrepancies between patients' identification of the domain of nursing care and the domain identified by nurses? Compare the discrepancies in this study with Monnig's (Chap. 3) findings and Clayton's study (Chap. 10). Identify the extent that there is congruence in defining the domain of nursing by patients, nurses, and physicians. Should congruence be expected? How might studies be designed for measuring quality of care, to effectively identify and correlate findings of the critical variables identified by patients, nurses, and physicians? What methodological problems need to be considered and resolved?

REFERENCES

Biddle, B. and E. Thomas
1966 Role Theory Concepts and Research. New York: Wiley.
Brandt, D. and E. Anderson
1967 "Validation of a patient welfare evaluation instrument." Nursing Research 16: 169–173.
Greenwood, E.
1957 "The elements of professionalization." Social Work 2:44–55.
Hardy, M. and M. Conway (eds.)
1978 Role Theory: Perspectives for Health Professionals. New York: Appleton-Century-Crofts.
Hotz, D.
1962 "Unit manager plan provides administrative control of wards." Modern Hospital 99:75–76.
Jelinek, R., F. Munson, and R. L. Smith
1971 Service unit management. Battle Creek, Michigan: W. K. Kellogg Foundation.
Katz, R. L. and R. Khan
1966 The Social Psychology of Organizations. New York: Wiley.
McKenna, J. V.
1968 "Final project report: The service manager system: Nurse efficiency and cost." Ann Arbor, Michigan: University Microfilms Inc.
Moore, W.
1970 The Professions: Roles and Rules. New York: Russell Sage Foundation.
Palmer, H.
1969 "Nurses for nursing." Canadian Nurse 65:36–39.
Regan, P. A.
1969 "Measuring the effectiveness of a unit management program." Hospital Progress 50:28–33.
Ryan, N.
1974 "Evaluation of the hospitalized patients' perception of health teaching." Unpublished master's thesis. Boston University.
Schmeiding, N.
1966 "Study of nurse activity after removal of management functions." Journal of Psychiatric Nursing 4:534–536.
Underwood, C. B.
1967 "Comparison of nursing activities before and after implementation of the patient unit management." No. 1103 Ann Arbor, Michigan: University Microfilms.
Yankauer, R. and E. Levine
1954 "The floor-manager position—does it help the nursing unit?" Nursing Research 3:4–10.

Chapter 25

The Nurse-Practitioner Role and Primary Care Research

Carolyn A. Williams, R.N., Ph.D., F.A.A.N.
Associate Professor
School of Nursing
        and
Department of Epidemiology
School of Public Health
University of North Carolina
Chapel Hill, North Carolina

Although nurses have long been involved in the nurse-practitioner movement, primary care research is in its infancy. Carolyn Williams examines the numerous perspectives of the nurse-practitioner role. She uses the term generally to refer to nurses who, after receiving preparation beyond their basic nursing education, have increased the scope of their services to include selected assessment and management decisions formerly made only by physicians. Williams portrays the difficulties in finding appropriate groups for data comparisons. She examines predominantly studies concerning the extent to which nurse practitioners are employed in rural or underserved areas, acceptability by the physician, and cost effectiveness. Emphasis is on data generated in Phase 2 of the Longitudinal Study of Nurse Practitioners and a study conducted by System Sciences. She notes the majority of graduates located in rural areas indicated by the Phase 2 study, the lower proportion of Medex graduates, and the preponderance of graduates from the Chapel Hill program who are employed in rural areas.

Williams' review suggests that in general nurse practitioners are accepted by patients and physician colleagues; services provided by nurse practitioners compare favorably with physicians on both process and outcome measures; and there is evidence that utilization of the full potential of this group may result in a more favorable cost picture.

She cautions against facile interpretation of data from all the studies reviewed due to numerous factors such as philosophical and political perspective of the investigators, the audience to which their findings were directed, measures utilized, lack of stratification of patients' problems, and selective samples.

Williams defines the role as a copractitioner complementary to the physician with the critical difference between the two disciplinary orientations being their frame of reference for problem definition and resolution. Williams concludes with an agenda of four vital areas for primary care research.

To date involvement of nurses in primary care research has been confined largely to studies of the nurse-practitioner role, and most of this participation has been as the phenomena under study. Only a few nurses have been involved as investigators. While this is understandable from a developmental perspective, the quality of primary care rendered in the future and the realization of nursing's potential for leadership in that arena will be influenced by the extent to which we assume leadership in primary care research and by the type of questions we address.

This chapter presents evidence from a variety of perspectives in support of the nurse-practitioner role, comments on the distinction between the role of physician substitute and the role of copractitioner, and then looks at the necessity for nurses to become more active in primary care research. Finally, some potentially fruitful areas of inquiry are suggested.

Emergence of the nurse-practitioner movement can be traced to a number of factors, not the least in importance of which was the felt need on the part of many practicing nurses in ambulatory settings for more meaningful roles in patient care—roles which would provide for increased autonomy and responsibility in decision making, would enhance patient care, and would legitimize the practice by significant groups. Such aspirations on the part of some nurses were a necessary condition for the development of the present pool of approximately 20,300 graduate nurse practitioners, including nurse midwives. However, since these aspirations predated the development of the first formalized program to prepare nurse practitioners, it can be argued that, though they were a necessary condition, they were not sufficient in themselves to explain the momentum and vitality of the nurse-practitioner movement. It will be the task of future historians to put the various determinants of the nurse-practitioner movement into perspective.

For those of us who were participants in the movement, factors other than those early aspirations, factors frequently commented on by colleagues involved in the early educational programs, included: an increased awareness of the importance of primary care on the part of the public and of policy makers; a concomitant awareness of gaps in accessibility to, and quality of, primary care services, gaps due in part to geographic and specialty maldistribution of personnel; national interest in making primary care accessible to all segments of the population; the potential the movement held for contributing to cost containment; and the interest of segments of the medical community in exploring the development of new nonphysician primary care roles, those of the physician's assistant and the nurse practitioner.

Despite initial resistance on the part of a number of nursing leaders who counseled caution and who argued that participation with medicine represented capitulation to the physician, preparation for nurse-practitioner roles has moved from its initial location in short-term continuing education programs into the mainstream of nursing education, where it is being institutionalized in academic settings. And, as will be discussed in the next section of this paper, there is evidence that the nurse-practitioner role is at last perceived as a viable role in the present world of practice.

There should be some clarification of the terminology used in this chapter.

In one sense it is simplistic to use the term "nurse-practitioner role," since a variety of practitioner roles have developed, ranging from those which focus on care for individuals in specific age groups (pediatric nurse practitioners, adult nurse practitioners, geriatric nurse practitioners) or for patients presenting particular needs (family planning nurse practitioners, ob-gyn nurse practitioners) to the generalized family nurse practitioner whose concerns cut across groupings by age and care problems. However, the term "nurse practitioner" is used here in its general sense to refer to nurses who, in addition to basic nursing education, have received additional preparation which enables them to increase the scope of their services to include selected assessment and management decisions formerly made only by physicians. Thus, the term "nurse practitioner" will be used here to refer to all of the many types of nurse practitioners.

EFFICACY OF THE NURSE-PRACTITIONER ROLE

The efficacy of the nurse-practitioner role, that is, the degree to which the intended effect is achieved, can be examined from a number of perspectives:

- the extent to which the envisioned role is practiced, i.e., do graduates of educational programs actually practice in a primary care role,—more specifically, the role for which they were prepared?
- the extent to which nurse practitioners contribute to reducing the maldistribution of health care personnel by providing care in rural or other underserved areas;
- the extent to which nurse practitioners are accepted by patients, physicians, and other target groups;
- the extent to which the role of nurse practitioners is economically viable;
- the extent to which quality of care is maintained or improved.

In the following paragraphs evidence pertaining to each of these perspectives will be briefly reviewed. Insofar as possible, national-level data will be emphasized.

Nurse Practitioners in Primary Care Roles

The most complete data set which provides information on this question was generated in Phase 2 of the Longitudinal Study of Nurse Practitioners, based at the State University of New York (SUNY) at Buffalo, funded by the Division of Nursing, Health and Human Services (HHS) (hereafter referred to as the SUNY Study, Phase 2) (Sultz et al., 1977). This study generated follow-up data on the cohort of nurse-practitioner students (1) who were enrolled in programs based in educational institutions in operation on January 1, 1974, and (2) who were graduated from the practitioner program

between May, 1974, and June, 1975. This follow-up survey of graduates, carried out approximately 1 year following graduation, utilized a self-administered questionnaire. Besides gathering data from nurse-practitioner program graduates, the study also surveyed employers of those engaged in primary care (Sultz et al., 1979a).

Of the graduates who responded,[1] 73.4 percent (724) were employed either full-time or part-time as nurse practitioners, and the vast majority (69.1 percent) were providing primary care, as opposed to being engaged in roles limited to teaching or consultation. About 17 percent were employed in nonpractitioner roles; only 9.7 percent were not employed (Sultz et al., 1979b). Reasons cited for being unemployed were personal, such as "marriage, pregnancy, or family relocation" (Sultz et al., 1979b:11).

In considering these data, questions that are difficult to address are (1) What constitutes an appropriate comparison group? (2) What represents successful attainment? However, Scheffler (1979) commented that the data compared favorably with information he collected in a national cohort study of almost 2000 physicians' assistants and MEDEX graduates, in which he found that 80 percent of those who responded reported that they practiced with a primary care physician.[2]

Nurse Practitioners in Underserved Areas

A question of considerable importance is: to what extent are graduates of nurse-practitioner programs practicing in locations traditionally plagued by problems of access to primary care, specifically inner-city and rural areas? The SUNY Study, Phase 2, showed that of the graduates responding,

---

[1] A 68 percent response rate was reported. Further inquiry was made to determine if nonrespondents had lower rates of employment, since that would suggest a bias. However, the data showed that the nonrespondents had a higher employment rate, suggesting that the figures reported here may be conservative.

[2] MEDEX is a particular type of physician's assistant program funded by the National Center for Health Services Research.

approximately 34 percent of those employed in direct care roles were in inner-city locations and 17 percent were in rural settings (Sultz et al., 1977). Thus, over half the respondents who were engaged in practice were in one or another of the geographical settings with high potential for being underserved.

Since the initiation of federal support for nurse-practitioner, physician's assistant, and MEDEX programs, a central policy objective has been that graduates should ease the maldistribution of health personnel by practicing in rural areas. How do data on nurse practitioners compare with those for physicians' assistants and MEDEX graduates? In a study of 277 graduates from eight MEDEX programs between 1969 and 1974, Lawrence et al. (1975) reported that 56 percent of the MEDEX graduates were located in towns of 10,000 or less. However, more recent data from a study conducted by System Sciences and published in the Research Digest Series of the National Center for Health Services Research (1977) showed a much lower percent in rural areas—only 37.1 percent in non-SMSAs (Standardized Metropolitan Statistical Areas) of less than 50,000. Of the four provider groups involved in the System Sciences analysis (i.e., graduates of master's-level nurse-practitioner programs, certificate-level nurse-practitioner programs, MEDEX programs, and physician's assistant programs), the MEDEX graduates had the highest percentage in the most rural category, the nurse practitioners with master's degrees had the lowest (5.5 percent), and the other two groups were about equal at 17.7 percent and 17.8 percent, respectively.

A much higher concentration of nurse-practitioner graduates in rural areas was found in a follow-up study of those completing their academic preparation at the University of North Carolina at Chapel Hill, an institution which attempted to address systematically the problem of access to primary care within the state. Those data show that 54 percent of the graduates (52 out of a population of 96) from the first eight classes who were practicing in North Carolina were in rural areas (towns or places with a population less than 10,000). Further longitudinal analyses based on from 1 to 5 years of exposure showed that, once placed in rural areas, there was not the urban drift anticipated by some (Williams et al., 1977). The preponderance of graduates in rural areas from the early Chapel Hill program was not expected, since during the time studied the training program deliberately attempted to place graduates in settings which would serve traditionally underserved populations. In that it engaged in deployment activities similar to those associated with MEDEX programs as described by Lawrence et al. (1975), the Chapel Hill program was distinctive from many programs for nurses.

Nurse Practitioners and Patient and Physician Acceptance/Satisfaction

The vast majority of published data dealing with the acceptance of nurse practitioners and physicians' assistants by patients and consumer groups show positive findings; that is, satisfaction with services provided by nurse practitioners is found to be equal to or greater than satisfaction with physician care. To some extent the results may be influenced by a methodological problem inherent in most studies of patient satisfaction—the selective nature of the population surveyed. Such studies are conducted in practice settings in which patients who are surveyed are those who are willing to see nurse practitioners and physicians. Patients who have doubts may choose not to go to those settings, and the dissatisfied may choose not to return. Thus this population is less likely to be included in the surveys. Another limitation is the potential for bias on the part of the investigators, many of whom have been associated with training programs. Despite these potential limitations, the consistently positive nature of the data gathered from many groups and in a wide variety of settings must be acknowledged.

In a review of studies on patient satisfaction prepared as a background paper for the Institute of Medicine's Primary Care Study, Ruby noted that "high acceptance is reported for nurse practitioners and physician assistants functioning at all levels of independence, delivering many types of care (well baby care, care for chronic disease, care for broad range problems), functioning in all settings and performing varied activities" (1977: 23). However, she further observed that the limits of patient satisfaction have yet to be established: that is, there are no published data on consumer satisfaction with nurse practitioners or physicians' assistants functioning independently in their own practice and delivering a broad range of services.

System Sciences investigators (1980a) have pointed out that direct questioning of patients about their satisfaction with providers and care received invariably results in positive responses. Thus, it would be desirable to have complementary data on patient satisfaction from other sources, such as the employer or the physician colleague of the nurse practitioner. System Sciences did an analysis of nine national studies which dealt with either nurse practitioners or physicians' assistants. Six of the nine studies had involved nurse practitioners, and two of these six had dealt exclusively with nurse practitioners, the SUNY Study, Phase 2, being one of them. In their reanalysis of the SUNY Study, Phase 2, data set System Sciences found that 90 percent (414) of the responding employers—some of them physicians—reported that nurse practitioners were well or fairly well accepted by patients. The System Sciences study concluded that

> patient satisfaction with physician extender [a term used to refer to both nurse practitioners and physicians' assistants] service was not directly addressed by any of the nine studies included in this evaluation analysis. However, several of the nine studies inquired about patient satisfaction from responding providers. Physicians and physician extenders had the same positive view of patient satisfaction, i.e., that patients were satisfied with and accepted the physician extender. (System Sciences, 1980a:60-61.)

In considering the issue of physician acceptance

of/and satisfaction with nurse practitioners, three questions can be asked:

1 To what extent are physicians willing to employ the nurse practitioner?
2 When a nurse practitioner has been employed, how satisfied are physicians in working with this colleague?
3 When a nurse practitioner has been employed, what types of responsibility are physicians willing to share with this colleague?

A number of factors affect the response to the first and third questions above, and a discussion of these issues is clearly beyond the intended scope of this paper. Thus, only the second question will be considered. Here we turn again to the System Sciences (1980b) reanalysis of the SUNY Study, Phase 2, data set in which it was reported that the employers (who included physicians) of nurse practitioners expressed high overall satisfaction—96 percent for master's-level graduates and 99 percent for certificate-level graduates. Further, it was reported that employers were equally satisfied with the integration of the nurse-practitioner role in the practice. These data are quite positive. However, it should be noted that the employers' responses may have some bias in that they reflect the perception of employers presently working with nurse practitioners— employers who were disenchanted or unhappy with the situation may have left the practice setting and would not be included in the data.

Economic Viability of the Nurse-Practitioner Role

In 1977, Jane Record, an economist, headed a team of investigators funded by the Division of Medicine, Bureau of Health Manpower, D.H.E.W. to undertake an analysis of the literature on the issues of delegation, productivity, and cost of primary care by nonphysician personnel (nurse practitioners and physicians' assistants). Their search of the literature on these three topics yielded over 1000 items, including monographs, journal articles, and research reports. About 400 of these documents were considered to merit intensive analysis, and they formed the basis of the report submitted to the Division of Medicine (Record, 1979). One of the major conclusions which emerged from the analysis was:

It seems reasonably clear from the empirical record that non-physician health personnel, when well used, tend to substitute adequately for physicians in a high percentage of primary care services, and that, given supportive market conditions non-physician providers can achieve the activity level that will assure their cost effectiveness; certainly the latter is true if the present differential in the cost of M.D.s and non-physician health providers is maintained. (Record, 1979:10)

The System Sciences study mentioned above also addressed several economic issues. The overall conclusions, based primarily on information from four of the nine studies, three of which involved nurse practitioners, were:

Supervising physician/employers were very satisfied with physician extender productivity and cost effectiveness; physician extenders increased the volume of patients seen at a lower cost increment than adding an equivalent half time position; and some of this cost saving was passed on to the consumer or the third-party payer. (System Sciences 1980c:90.)

The investigators cautioned, however, that generalized cost-of-care conclusions cannot be drawn from these data without additional information on hospitalization rates, laboratory costs, referrals, etc. Further, it should be noted that a convention in presenting data and conclusions developed by the System Sciences team was to summarize data without separating nurse practitioners and physicians' assistants unless the data differed in meaningful ways.

The Nurse Practitioner's Impact on the Quality of Care

Since 1974, there have been five comprehensive reviews of studies of the quality of care provided by nurse practitioners (Cohen, 1974; Health Resources Administration, 1977; Lawrence, 1978; Sox, 1979; Prescott and Driscoll, 1980). Cohen reported that numerous small studies supported the conclusion that nurse practitioners and physicians' assistants "performed as well as physicians, judged by standards developed within practice settings" (1974:128). After reviewing a variety of studies available by 1977, the authors of the Health Resources Administration's Physician Extender Work Group Report concluded that, within the limits of current methods for measuring quality of care, "the performance of the nurse practitioner/physician's assistant has compared favorably with that of the physician on both process and outcome measures." They went on to say, "Therefore until better methods are developed to measure quality of care, this issue needs no further research" (H.R.A., 1977:51). Lawrence (1978) suggested that there is little evidence that quality declines when nonphysician health providers are used to render routine services. In fact, he pointed to indications that nonphysician health providers in certain cases may obtain somewhat better outcomes—for example, in the level of patient compliance and in behavioral outcomes for patients suffering from selected chronic diseases.

Sox (1979) analyzed 21 studies published between 1967 and 1977 in which care provided by nurse practitioners or physicians' assistants was compared with that given by physicians. After careful consideration of these studies, Sox concluded that "this review has shown that in these studies the quality of primary ambulatory care given by nurse practitioners and physician's assistants was indistinguishable from that given by physicians" (1979:465). However, he pointed out a number of limitations in the studies. For example, only a few investigators used detailed quality of care measures or surveyed patient groups that had been adequately characterized or that appeared comparable. And a number of the studies dealt with a very narrow range of patient groups or measures of performance. Additional criticisms by Sox included the scarcity of information on care given in emergency rooms and nursing homes and the lack of stratification for difficulty of patient problems. Thus, the care of patients with serious medical problems may have been overlooked. Finally, Sox correctly pointed out that those who participated in such studies might have been unusually cooperative and above average in quality of care given in their practice, and some caution should therefore be used in generalizing the findings to cover the broader practice community. Despite these limitations, Sox stated:

> the primary care physician has enough information to predict the impact of a nurse practitioner or physician's assistant on the quality of care in a practice. A nurse practitioner or physician's assistant should be well accepted by patients, and provide the average office patient with primary care that compares very favorably with care given by the physician. (1979:467)

In a published review of 26 studies comparing nurse-practitioner performance to that of the physician, Prescott and Driscoll (1980) reported "no difference" between the two provider groups as the predominant finding. However, they further noted that some findings were frequently overlooked; findings not taken into account indicated nurse practitioners had better scores than physicians in some areas: the amount and depth of discussion regarding child care, therapeutic listening, support offered the patient, preventive care, completeness of history, physical exams, and patient knowledge of management plans. In addition to questioning the lack of attention paid to the positive differences between nurses and physicians, Prescott and Driscoll raised the basic issue of the appropriateness of a comparison between nurse practitioners and physicians.

It may be useful to ask some further questions:

• From what philosophical framework and political perspective did most of these studies evolve?
• To what audience were their findings directed?

The overwhelming majority of the primary authors of the studies comparing nurse practitioners and physicians were physicians. Further, many of the investigations and review papers such as Sox's (1979), which was published in the *Annals of Internal Medicine*, were directed to physician audiences or other groups, including nonphysician administrators who must negotiate with physicians regarding the employment of personnel such as nurse practitioners.

The majority of studies pertaining to the nurse-practitioner role do provide information to be used in making administrative decisions related to the employment of nurses in such roles and to the development and maintenance of educational programs. These studies, some of which have been cited above, have suggested that the graduates of practitioner programs are indeed functioning in the primary care role; that their practice is acceptable to patients and physician colleagues; that, whether measured in terms of the process or of the outcome of medical care, services provided by nurses are deemed as good as those provided by physicians to similar groups of patients; and that full utilization of the potential of this group can result in a more favorable cost picture. Although such studies do not ask all the important questions, particularly those of most interest to many nurses, they are important first steps in dealing with what has come to be understood as an innovation in health care delivery. As such, these studies have probably been extremely influential in fostering opportunities for nurses to be more meaningfully involved in the health care delivery system.

THE NURSE-PRACTITIONER ROLE— PHYSICIAN SUBSTITUTE OR COPRACTITIONER?

Since the beginning of the nurse-practitioner movement, there has been an underlying conflict as to whether the nurse practitioner is or should be in a physician-substitute role or in a role complementary to that of the physician. At a national policy level the notion of substitutability has gained considerable prominence. This is evident in the very language used in national reports and studies. First, there is a tendency to group nurse practitioners together with physicians' assistants, a provider group clearly created by physicians to extend their coverage of patient care. Second, there is a tendency to refer to both nurse practitioners and physicians' assistants as physician extenders or as nonphysician health providers, again emphasizing the notion of substitutability. An underlying assumption in such usage is that it is doctoring (medical care) which is the only really important component of primary care. Such a view is, of course, unacceptable to the nursing community. More importantly, such a view may fail to deal adequately with some of the most prevalent primary care problems.

If we accept the proposition that a very high proportion of contacts in primary care involve patients needing services other than sophisticated medical management, then it follows that someone other than a physician substitute should be capable of dealing with the situation. However, it does not follow that what is needed is inherently less sophisticated management. The care needed may not be highly sophisticated in a medical-technician sense, but it may be very sophisticated in other ways—for example, in dealing with psychosocial concerns and particularly in providing selected medical-technical services to meet such concerns.

It was the belief that an alternative to physician-only primary providers was important that motivated many nurses to join with physician colleagues in an attempt to evolve a role which would integrate some aspects of medicine with traditional components of nursing. It may be argued that the increased participation of nurses in primary care since the beginning of the nurse-practitioner movement is only for the short term, a condition accepted while the training and deployment of primary care physicians is stepped up. Here it should be noted that there is concern about a possible oversupply of physicians within the decade. In fact, in a discussion of factors which represent impediments to full use of nurse practitioners and physicians' assistants, Record said that "the most serious constraint may be an oversupply of primary care physicians by 1990" (1979:27). From a supply-and-demand perspective and in view of the relative positions of nursing and medicine in the politics of health care delivery, it is reasonable to ask the question: Will the nurse practitioner fade from the scene if the problem of physician distribution is resolved? The answer may depend in large part on whether the nurse-practitioner role is conceptualized, prepared for, and, most importantly, practiced merely as a physician-substitute role, or whether it is seen as a primary care role, one complementary to that of the physician.

What does a complementary role entail? The distinction between the role as physician substitute and the role as coopractitioner is not to be found either in the type of patient seen by each provider or in the type of consultation between physician and nurse. Rather, the critical distinction is in the particular frame of reference for problem definition and resolution. The basic orientation of the nurse is toward promoting preventive behaviors and health maintenance, toward patient education, and toward facilitating effective coping with an illness state. In contrast, the prevalent philosophical orientation of medicine is one in which the major emphasis is on identifying problems, predominantly in biological terms, and on prescribing solutions at that level. Thus, a basic difference between the two orientations is in their relative positions on a continuum, with emphasis on ongoing health maintenance care at one end and emphasis on sickness care at the other. Of course, not all nurse practitioners act upon this health maintenance philosophy, nor do all physicians practice with a sickness orientation.

Today there is little question about the appropriateness of preparing nurse practitioners to make selected medically oriented assessment and management decisions, that is, decisions formerly limited to the practice of medicine. However, a clear expectation is that such decisions will be made in the context of health-oriented practice. Operationally, this means that in the assessment and management of patients, nurse practitioners are expected to have a broad approach to practice. As suggested by Williams in an earlier paper, in such an approach to practice:

> . . .the patient's biological status is considered along with and in relation to other patient data, including affective and cognitive factors, family level data, and information regarding the patient's broader social network, that is, his social support system and work role. The argument for supporting such a health oriented approach in primary care rests on the view that primary care problems represent a broad spectrum and the assumption (not yet adequately tested) that, over time, patient outcomes will be best when such care is provided. (1978:209)

Unless nurses give more attention to research activities, however, this will remain only an assumption and one which may not be supported by health care dollars.

PRIMARY CARE RESEARCH

To date most studies of the nurse-practitioner role address the issue of acceptability—acceptability by patients and physicians and acceptability in terms of costs and quality of performance. Necessary and useful as such efforts may have been in providing data on which to base decisions regarding the utilization of nurse practitioners, these studies have not generated information on which clinical decisions can be based, that is, decisions regarding the assessment and management of specific subgroups of patients. While the finding of "no differences" in outcomes of medical management by nurse and physician primary care providers has been viewed by some in the medical community as a measure of success, many nurses are not content. One reason for this is the realization that "the particular contributions which nurses bring

to primary care were not assessed and studied" (Williams, 1975:176). Thus, whether the conclusion is "no differences" or "some differences" in favor of nurse management (e.g., Lewis et al., 1969; Bessman, 1974; Runyan, 1975), processes of care other than the medical-technical are either not made explicit or are not directly assessed. It is, therefore, not possible to know what, if anything, is different in the nurse-provided care from that given by physicians. Tenable hypotheses exist and should be tested. These hypotheses postulate, among other things, differences in continuity over a series of patient encounters; differences in problem definitions as a function of a broader approach to patient assessment; differences in management style, such as facilitating active involvement of the patient; and differences in the effectiveness of teaching and counseling. Research programs designed to develop the necessary methods to test these hypotheses could constitute a fruitful agenda for nurse-initiated studies in primary care.

An essential component of such a research would be to give more priority than has been given to date to conceptualizing and operationalizing relevant patient characteristics (e.g., potential for self-care) and relevant aspects of the patient-provider transaction. Primary care research is in its infancy and one of the most serious needs in the field is for stronger and more useful theoretical formulations. Studies which have the theoretical strength represented by the work of Johnson (1972; Johnson and Rice, 1974; Johnson et al., 1975) are clearly in order. Such work is essential to the development of a scientific basis for primary care nursing and to providing the best possible patient care. And, the results of such inquiry have the potential to determine whether the role of the nurse practitioner is to be one of physician substitute or one of copractitioner and colleague in the fullest sense.

EDITOR'S QUESTIONS FOR DISCUSSION

What factors may determine the future of the nurse-practitioner movement? To what extent is there contradictory evidence of the viability of the nurse-practitioner role? What accounts for disposition evident in current research findings? How likely is it that the maldistribution of health care personnel in rural or underserved areas will be corrected? Identify issues of concern to nurse practitioners that may be similar and different from those of physicians that pertain to attracting and maintaining health care personnel in underserved areas? What are implications for nurse-practitioner programs whose graduates choose to locate in an urban area?

What methodological procedures can be utilized to deal with the issue of response set bias in studies of patient satisfaction and employers of nurse practitioners? What implications does an investigator's philosophy and political perspective have for interpretation of data and valid research?

What are the limitations in comparing the data of the Phase 2 SUNY Study and System Science Study? How appropriate is it to compare data among nurse practitioners, physician assistants, and physicians? What factors are essential for valid comparisons and interpretations of studies? To the extent those factors do not exist, under what conditions might comparisons be made?

What are the implications for the nursing profession and society of the tendency to view the nurse-practitioner role as a physician substitute role? How do you conceptualize the role? Williams provides a general definition of the term "nurse practitioner" early in this chapter. Later, she presents critical distinctions between the nurse practitioner as a complementary role and a physician substitute role. What type of selected assessment and management decisions formerly made only by physicians appropriately qualify for Williams' criteria of a complementary role? Should aspects of physicians traditional practice of medicine be integrated into the nurse-practitioner role? How would the varying views of the nurse-practitioner role reconcile with beliefs presented by Monnig (Chap. 3), Williamson (Chap. 5), and Peterson (Chap. 7)?

Suggest research designs for implementing studies in the areas of primary care indicated by Williams. How can differences in the processes of care be explicitly assessed? Justify a theoretical base for each proposed study? What nursing theoretical or conceptual base would be appropriate?

REFERENCES

Bessman, Alice
  1974 "Comparison of medical care in nurse clinician and physician clinics in medical school affiliated hospitals." Journal of Chronic Diseases 27:115–125.
Cohen, Eva D.
  1974 "An Evaluation of Policy Related Research on New and Expanded Roles of Health Workers." New Haven: Office of Regional Activities and Continuing Education, Yale University School of Medicine.

Health Resources Administration
  1977 Report of the Physician Extender Work Group to the Health Resources Administration's Policy Board. Department of Health and Human Resources No. 017–022–00555–6. Washington, D.C.: U.S. Government Printing Office.
Johnson, Jean E.
  1972 "Effects of structuring patient's expectations or their reactions to threatening events." Nursing Research 21:499–504.
Johnson, Jean E. and Virginia H. Rice
  1974 "Sensory and distress components of pain." Nursing Research 23:203–209.

Johnson, Jean E., Karen T. Circhoff, and Patricia M. Endress
1975 "Altering children's distress behavior during orthopedic cast removal." Nursing Research 24:404–410.

Lawrence, David
1978 "The impact of physician assistants and nurse practitioners on health care access, costs, and quality: A review of the literature." Health and Medical Care Services Review 1:1–12.

Lawrence, David, William M. Wilson, and C. Hilmon Castle
1975 "Employment of MEDEX graduates and trainees." Journal of The American Medical Association 234(2):174–177.

Lewis, Charles E., Barbara A. Resnick, Glenda Schmidt, and David Waxman
1969 "Activities, events and outcomes in ambulatory patient care." New England Journal of Medicine 280:645–649.

National Center for Health Services Research
1977 Nurse Practitioner and Physician Assistant Training and Deployment. Research Digest Series. Health and Human Resources Publication No. (HRA) 77–3173. Washington, D.C.: U.S. Government Printing Office.

Prescott, Patricia A. and Laura Driscoll
1980 "Evaluating nurse practitioner performance." Nurse Practitioner 5:28–32.

Record, Jane
1979 "An overview." In Jane C. Record (ed.), Final Report on Provider Requirements, Cost Savings, and the New Health Practitioner in Primary Care: National Estimates for 1990. Unpublished. Prepared for the Division of Medicine, Bureau of Health Manpower, Washington, D.C.: Department of Health and Human Resources, Contract No. 231–77–0077.

Ruby, Gloria
1977 "Consumer acceptance of nurse practitioners and physician assistants." Washington D.C.: National Academy of Sciences, Institute of Medicine. Unpublished staff paper.

Runyan, John W.
1975 "The Memphis chronic disease program: Comparisons in outcome and the nurse's extended role." Journal of the American Medical Association 231:264–267.

Scheffler, Richard M.
1979 "Discussion of nurse practitioner employment." Pp. 23–24 in H. A. Sultz, O. M. Henry, and J. A. Sullivan (eds.), Nurse Practitioners U.S.A. Lexington, Mass.: Lexington Books.

Sox, Harold C.
1979 "Quality of patient care by nurse practitioners and physician's assistants: A ten-year perspective." Annals of Internal Medicine 91:459–468.

Sultz, Harry A., Marie Zielezny, and Jane Mathews
1977 The Longitudinal Study to Evaluate the Education, Functions and Utilization of Nurses in Extended Roles, Phase Two. Buffalo, New York: Department of Social and Preventive Medicine, School of Medicine, State University of New York at Buffalo. Unpublished data.

Sultz, Harry A., Louis Kinyon, and O. Marie Henry
1979a "Introduction and method." Pp. 3–9 in H. A. Sultz, O. M. Henry, and J. A. Sullivan (eds.), Nurse Practitioners: U.S.A. Lexington, Mass.: Lexington Books.

Sultz, Harry A., Jane Mathews, Marie Zielezny, and O. Marie Henry
1979b "Nurse practitioner employment." Pp. 11–24 in H. A. Sultz, O. M. Henry, and J. A. Sullivan (eds.), Nurse Practitioners: U.S.A. Lexington, Mass.: Lexington Books.

System Sciences, Inc.
1980a "Major issues: Issue 1—patient satisfaction." Pp. 59–61 in Final Report on Evaluation of Findings from Nurse Practitioner and Physician Assistant Studies. Unpublished. Prepared for the National Center for Health Services Research. Washington, D.C. Department of Health and Human Resources, Contract No. 233–78–3015.

1980b "Major issues: Issue 2—physician/employer acceptance." Pp. 63–66 in Final Report on Evaluation of Findings from Nurse Practitioner and Physician Assistant. Unpublished. Prepared for the National Center for Health Services Research. Washington, D.C.: Department of Health and Human Resources, Contract No. 233–78–3015.

1980c "Major issues: Issue 6–practice site productivity and income." Pp. 87–91 in Final Report on Evaluation of Findings from Nurse Practitioner and Physician Assistant. Unpublished. Prepared for the National Center for Health Services Research. Washington, D.C.: Department of Health and Human Resources, Contract No. 233–78–3015.

Williams, Carolyn A.
1975 "Nurse practitioner research: Some neglected issues." Nursing Outlook 23: 172–177.

1978 "Primary care: contributions of nursing personnel." Annals of the New York Academy of Sciences 310:207–211.

Williams, Carolyn A., Jean T. Warren, Priscilla A. Rigby, and Ann R. Woodward.
1977 Practice-Based Evaluation, Part 3. Final Progress Report on the Family Nurse Practitioners in North Carolina–Primex. Unpublished. Chapel Hill: School of Nursing, University of North Carolina at Chapel Hill.

1978 "Primary care: Contributions of nursing personnel." Annals of the New York Academy of Sciences 310:207–211.

Chapter 26

Nurse Practitioners Guide Change in Primary Health Care

Myrtle Irene Brown, R.N., Ph.D., F.A.A.N.
Professor Emeritus
College of Nursing
University of South Carolina
Columbia, South Carolina

Myrtle Irene Brown's chapter is in order in that it provides evidence that the potential Williams indicates for the role of the nurse practitioner is beginning to be realized. She describes the essential nursing components in primary care which nurse practitioners utilize. Emphasis is on a broad base of family and community nursing. The goal is healthful development and effective functioning of the client.

Brown traces some of the confusion regarding the role for nurse practitioners. Indiscriminate use of the term, applied to nurses prepared in educational programs of various length and levels, that centered on abilities to take health histories and perform physical examinations appears to have misled many persons as to the appropriate potential role of the nurse practitioner. Brown uses the term to refer only to professional nurses prepared at the master's level to function in a great variety of emerging roles due to changes in nursing, in society, and in the primary health care system.

Brown identifies changes in society, family units, and health problems and needs which directed a need for extensive primary care services. She summarizes some of the primary health care deficiencies that provide opportunities for nurse practitioners to fully develop their emerging role. She aptly clarifies the ambiguity about the role by exploring the great diversity of practice content in the transitional roles of nurse practitioners in primary health care.

Brown's chapter is based on a small sample of 26 ($N = 58$) graduates who responded to a questionnaire that focused on the components of practice and interviews reported by these nurses as they described their practice. She identifies the variability and commonalities in beliefs, values, and goals in the evolving practice of professional nurses prepared for primary health care. It is apparent that a firm foundation in nursing theory and skills exists. Long-term goals are usually established with clients through the nursing process. Brown justifies the extremely broad knowledge base utilized by the nurse practitioner, including the application of nursing theories in practice.

Brown explicates two broad categories of practice—the nursing process and functional change processes. She views the medical processes of diagnosis and treatment as subsumed in utilizing the nursing process under problem identification, formulation, and implementation of plan of action. Skills for each phase of the nursing process are identified. Brown discusses the use of protocols that direct immediate referral of a patient to a physician. She further cites three conditions that must exist whenever nurse practitioners carry out medically delegated responsibilities. The criteria are: the nurse has the competence, the laws under which he or she practices so permit, and adequate medical consultation and/or supervision are readily available.

Through the interviews she presents, Brown demonstrates the effectiveness of cooperative patient management relationships with physicians, the relationship of individual and family care in practice, the variety of functional skills used to effect change in primary care, and the development and implementation of new roles in health promotion with the well, elderly, and chronically ill. The use of nursing process is clearly illustrated in the interviews. Brown's portrayal provides evidence for the characteristics, contributions, and domain of nursing practice in primary care.

Nurse practitioners who are functioning as health nursing specialists are effecting change in both the content and the delivery methods of primary health care. Freeman recognized this potential when she forecast:

> The family health nurse practitioner, the nurse midwife, the pediatric nurse practitioner, and a score of other "extended role" categories have been hailed as an economic source of relief for the hard pressed physician. Nurses find the practitioner role challenging and satisfying. But even more important, planners see the nurse practitioner as offering to the public a kind of care that goes beyond the combination of traditional medical and nursing skills, and is characterized by high impact, broad range and personalized application. (1974:21)

This paper provides evidence that this potential is beginning to be realized.

THE CHANGING MEANING OF PRIMARY HEALTH CARE

Because nursing in primary care settings has its roots in public health nursing, it has readily identifiable characteristics that affect the content of

Report based in part on information from graduates of a Master of Nursing program developed with the support of Division of Nursing DHEW grant No. 5–D24–NU00034–02.

primary care. The central goal of such practice is healthful development and effective functioning of the client. Primary care nurses assist individuals, families, small groups, and communities to set health goals, make decisions, develop plans, and act to promote health. The recipients of such care learn to effectively cope with and utilize stressful experiences and situations.

Because clients are often experiencing problems of disease and chronic disability, such practice has a large component of data collection, preliminary diagnosis, conjoint planning of corrective action, and collaboration with physicians and other therapists. It is in this component of nursing in primary care that nurse practitioners utilize knowledge drawn from the medical sciences and practice skills that traditionally and legally are in the domain of medical practitioners.

Nurse practitioners are also bringing change to methods by which primary care is delivered. They demonstrate little hesitation to reach out to underserved populations, to render service in the clients' own territory of homes, schools, and places of work, and to assume the role of patient advocate whenever there is need. This relation to potential clients arises historically from practice in official public health agencies, which by law have responsibility for the health and welfare of the public. Multidisciplinary team practice and coordination and collaboration with physicians and other health care givers come readily to this group of professionals whose practice is expected to include competence in case finding, referral to physicians and a multiplicity of health and social service agencies, and community planning and implementation of health services.

Continuity of care for individuals and families is the accepted method of practice in a profession that has nursed generations of reproductive families, has maintained surveillance of the health and development of infants and children, and has provided direct patient care in their homes to chronically ill and dependent persons and their families.

Nurse practitioners who incorporate this broad base of public health nursing into their practice are adding dimensions to the frequently quoted definition of primary care stated in *Extending the Scope of Nursing Practice*, the report of the committee to study extended roles for nurses.

> The term Primary Care. . . has two dimensions: (a) a person's first contact in a given episode of illness with the health care system that leads to a decision of what must be done to help resolve his problem; and (b) the responsibility for the continuum of care, i.e., maintenance of health, evaluation and management of symptoms, and appropriate referrals. (U.S.D.H.E.W., 1971:8.)

This definition arose out of the traditional practice of private physicians for whom physician extenders were sought. Scant recognition of the content of public health nursing was granted by the inclusion of the phrases "maintenance of health" and "appropriate referrals," two emphases rarely seen in private medical practice at that time.

More recent definitions of primary care challenge this limited focus. Recognizing the neglect of specific population groups and the changing expectations of the public, deTornyay (1977) states the need for reduction of overreliance on physicians in primary health care, for recognition of the rebirth of self-care and consumer group action, and for acknowledgment of the family as the basic unit in health and health care.

No attempt will be made in this paper to present a fully developed definition of primary care.

Rather, the changes being made by professional nurses functioning on the broad base of family and community nursing in their practitioner roles will be described.

WHO IS A PROFESSIONAL NURSE PRACTITIONER?

In the years since the title of "nurse practitioner" first appeared in 1965 (Ford and Silver, 1967), it has been applied indiscriminately to nurses prepared in educational programs of various lengths and levels for a variety of primary care activities. In the most limited definitions, emphasis has been placed on the ability of nurse practitioners to perform physical examinations and take health histories of persons presenting themselves for medical or health care and to utilize the data, so collected, in preparing and implementing a plan of care.

In this paper the term "nurse practitioner" will refer only to professional nurses prepared at the master's level to function in the great variety of expanded nursing roles emerging through changes in nursing, in society, and in the primary health care system. Because these emerging roles are highly variable in their demands upon professional nurse practitioners, the diversity of content of practice demands description and analysis.

In contrast to quantitative surveys of large samples of graduates of all kinds of nurse-practitioner programs (Jelinek, 1978; Sultz et al., 1980), surveys which have focused on commonalities and limited classes of variability, this chapter seeks to begin to explore the great diversity of practice content in the transitional roles of nurse practitioners in primary health care.

Content of the paper is partially based on questionnaire responses of Master of Nursing graduates who pursued a program with a major in health nursing at the University of South Carolina. Between September, 1974, and December, 1979, 58 nurses completed a curriculum designed to prepare professional practitioners of nursing as specialists in primary health care of families and selected populations in the community. Academic minors provided beginning specializations in either (a) primary care to a selected population or group, such as infants and young children, school-age children and youths, reproductive families, and the aged or (b) the functional areas of teaching or administration.

Of the 58 graduates, 12 had completed a longer variant of the health-nursing program for which they were awarded both the degree of master of nursing and a certificate of graduate study in family nursing practice. The development of the family nurse-practitioner variant was supported by a 3 year grant awarded July 1, 1976, through June 30, 1979, by the Division of Nursing, D.H.E.W.

Of the 26 who responded to a questionnaire which focused on the components of practice, 23 reported on direct practice with individuals or families. Seven were graduates of the longer family nurse-practitioner variant. The 32 nonrespondents included 21 graduates who are known to be on faculties of schools of nursing or in administrative positions in health agencies.

A paper based on the study of such a small sample is justified only by the use of case materials reported by these nurses as they described their practice. Rather than proposing that nurse practitioners have already made a great impact on primary care, it is the position of this report that individuals are demonstrating a great diversity of expanded roles and functions in primary care. The potential for a significant and long-term impact of nurse practitioners on primary care will be realized only if the numbers of such professional nurses are greatly augmented and their preparation and employment supported by the public, by nurses and other health professions, by institutions of higher education, by third-party payers for health care, and by governmental agencies.

CHANGING SOCIAL LIFE PROVIDES OPPORTUNITY FOR THE EXPANDED ROLE IN PRACTICE

There is a time in a society when new roles may develop. Changes in social life, health and illness, and patterns of health care are providing the op-

portunity for nurse practitioners to play a broader role in primary health care than that of physician extender.

Social Change

Since the Second World War, society has experienced escalating changes. Economic expansion and prosperity set the stage for rising expectations. Higher levels of technical productivity created a margin of wealth which supported greater material affluence, greater leisure for adult play, and greater individual choice than were ever before enjoyed by the average person. Possession of these benefits was quickly translated into "rights." The mass media made "the good life" the norm of expectation. The demands of minority groups for their share of the wealth and freedoms were answered by recognition of cultural pluralism, initiation of vast social welfare programs, and increased national centralization of government.

These changes had a great effect on the basic social unit, the family (Duvall, 1977; Reinhardt and Quinn, 1980). Mobility, urbanization followed by suburbanization, and ready accessibility to housing resulted in a sharp increase in the two-generation nuclear family. Loss of help from extended families and neighbors placed stress on families involved in bearing and rearing children and on elderly families. The women's movement, with increased employment of wives and mothers, resulted in fewer children and more demands for community child care.

Sexual freedom and divorce became new social norms. Divorce, together with an epidemic of pregnancies among unwed teenagers, resulted in one-parent families, placing additional stress on the family as a social unit and on its members. Child neglect and abuse, runaway children, early misuse of chemicals, learning failures, and school dropouts reflect the ineffectiveness of many families to nurture and socialize their children for successful functioning in society.

At the present time there appears to be a demand for a return to earlier American traditions—a demand voiced by those who believe a woman's place is in the home and who advocate outlawing abortions, reducing government spending, and returning the control of government to local and state authorities. This trend is reflected in the growing strength of conservative politics, organized demonstrations against ERA and legalized abortion, and the extensive political use of the mass media by fundamentalistic religious groups. The extent and longevity of this trend are uncertain; however, these phenomena provide evidence of the continued variability and change that will influence health demands and the patterns of service within which nurses will practice. Flexibility is and will continue to be a requirement for nurse practitioners.

CHANGE IN HEALTH PROBLEMS AND NEEDS

The patterns of illnesses and health problems have changed with the transformation of social and family life. Improved infant care and nutrition, control of many infectious and communicable diseases, and smaller families have increased the proportion of adults and older persons in the United States. Age-related chronic diseases, such as degenerative conditions of the heart, malignant neoplasms, diabetes, arthritis, chronic obstructive pulmonary disease, stroke, hypertension, and arteriosclerosis, create demand not only for temporary diagnostic and treatment services in hospitals but also for informed patients, for the control and management of disease depends on patient behavior during long-term direct nursing care at home and in nursing homes. Treatment of these diseases also calls for mobilization and coordination of complex medical, social, and economic services to support the patient and family care givers.

A society whose mobility is based on high-speed automoblies, airplanes, and motor-driven boats and cycles and whose industry is automated experiences many accidents requiring highly accessible emergency facilities and care, expert surgical skills, and medical and technical support of essential body functions. The high accident rate also demands preventive measures, effective rehabilitative services, and long-term family and nursing care of the severely disabled.

Further listing of current health problems would serve only to add to the evidence that a well-developed system of health care must provide for extensive primary care services as well as the highly technical and scientific diagnostic and therapeutic services provided at great expense in hospitals.

Already, national health policies are showing a shift to preventive health emphases, early detection of health problems, and improvements in long-term care. This shift of emphasis was enunciated in 1975 in the national health priorities listed by Congress in the National Health Planning and Development Act.

The Congress finds the following deserve priority consideration in the formulation of national health planning goals and in the development and operation of Federal, State, and area health planning and resources development programs:

(1) The provision of primary care services for medically underserved populations, especially those which are located in rural and economically depressed areas. . . .

(4) The training and increased utilization of physician assistants, especially nurse clinicians. . . .

(8) The promotion of activities for the prevention of disease. . . . (U.S. Congress, 1975)

The central theme of the *1977–1981 Forward Plan for Health* of the U.S. Department of Health, Education, and Welfare was described by Abdellah (1976) as "preventive health care." Further, this chief nurse officer of the Public Health Service described the great need for nurses to provide the unmet care component of primary care.

Though the original need for the nurse practitioner was seen as embodied in the role of the physician extender, that aspect of the role will decrease as the supply of physicians is increased. In an early 1980 DHHS news release, it was projected that "By 1990 physician requirements are predicted to range from 553,000 to 596,000 compared to an anticipated supply of 600,000." In the 10-year interim, nurse practitioners have the opportunity to demonstrate the broader personalized, individualized, and family-oriented contribution they can make and are making to primary health care.

In summary, some of the primary health care deficiencies that provide opportunities for nurse practitioners to develop fully their expanding roles are needs for:

1 wholeness care that promotes health, development, and self-care competence;

2 client-professional interaction that effects change in client health behaviors;

3 long-term care that optimizes freedom and independence of action, yet gives comfort and support in irreversible conditions;

4 promotion of human development that strengthens the functioning of individuals and the effectiveness of families;

5 clinical research and studies for knowledge and skills to meet the challenge of unresolved health problems and of new ones that emerge with continuing social and technological change;

6 coordination and collaboration that increase the efficiency and effectiveness of the efforts of clients and health personnel;

7 Evaluative research to determine the effectiveness of the modalities of practice.

Nurse practitioners prepared in the principles of change theory are not dismayed by the disequilibrium of the health care system but rather are challenged by its resultant openness to intervention. They anticipate working to reduce negative and traditional forces and to strengthen positive and creative innovations. From efforts to guide change come enhanced and satisfying roles and functions of clients, nurses, and other health workers.

CHARACTERISTICS OF EXPANDED ROLE FUNCTIONING OF NURSE PRACTITIONERS IN PRIMARY CARE

Variability, as well as commonalities, characterizes the emerging practice of professional nurses prepared for primary health care. Their philosophy

has its roots in nursing and incorporates a set of strong values related to their clients, to themselves as professional practitioners, to nursing, and to their relationships with physicians and other health practitioners. Their goals, which arise out of their philosophy, have a firm foundation in nursing theory and skills. The content of practice also is greatly affected by the particular position in which a practitioner functions and by the clients for whom the service is offered.

Beliefs and Values

Though each nurse may enunciate a different emphasis in his or her philosophy, most have been socialized through academic study and professional practice to place value on the following beliefs.

1 Each client is a unique individual with the right and potential for development achieved through dynamic interaction with his or her internal stimuli and external environment. Rogers's (1970) enunciation of the tenet that the proper study of nursing is the whole man was a benchmark in nursing education that is now generally accepted by nurses.

2 As man is a social being, clients may be individuals, families, groups with shared interests, or whole communities who seek assistance in solving a health-illness-related problem.

3 Nursing is a profession that can provide comprehensive care with continuity to persons with concerns of disease and health, disequilibrium and adaptation, and dependence and independence of functioning.

4 Prepared nurse practitioners have the right and the responsibility to develop and demonstrate helping roles wherever people seek or accept primary health care.

5 As nursing is practiced in close proximity to medicine, which is a highly valued profession with broad scientific and technological content and a social position of great power, it is critical for all concerned to coordinate their complementary practices.

Dunn, in his plea for the goal of "high-level wellness," spoke to the wholeness of man and to the need for a coordinated approach by the health professions. "Harmony [between the professional jurisdictions] will result when the fact is faced that man is a physical, mental and spiritual unity—a unity which is constantly undergoing a process of growth and adjustment within a continually changing physical, biological, social, and cultural environment." (1959:789).

6 Each nurse believes that she or he is an able practitioner who will grow in competence through continued study and practice.

Goals of Practice

From such values the professional perceives long-term goals for clients that are more far-reaching than the short-termed, problem-oriented goals that are usually jointly developed through the nurse-client interaction which characterizes the nursing process. Among the more inclusive goals that guide practice are these:

1 Through participation with the nurse in solving problems, clients will increase their ability to clarify complex situations, set goals, make decisions, use resources, and take action, thus increasing their competence to adapt to stress and meet other needs.

2 Through nursing, clients will achieve a better quality of life, whether this be a higher level of health or increased comfort and self-fulfillment in the presence of permanent disability or terminal disease.

3 Through nursing, families and other primary groups will increase in their integrity and effectiveness to function and to exhibit behaviors directed at promotion of the health of their members.

4 Comprehensive health care will become increasingly available to and utilized by high-risk populations, disorganized and troubled families, and underserved populations.

The Knowledge Base of Practice

The knowledge base of the nurse practitioner is extremely broad and expands exponentially. It is drawn from the natural and behavioral sciences and from the applied sciences of nursing, medicine,

public health, social work, and health education. A wealth of theory, learned at least to the level of application, is critical to effective practice. Helpful tools needed and used by practitioners in organizing and mobilizing this vast store of knowledge include general systems theory, comprehensive and orderly taxonomies, collations of useful nominative and process concepts, and emerging nursing models and theories.

General systems theory has been so widely used by the several professions that it serves as a communication bridge between persons of different disciplines and among nursing specialists. Systems theory concepts are readily employed in describing both structure of reality and processes underlying human behavior. The study of *Distributive Nursing Practice: A Systems Approach to Community Health*, edited by Hall and Weaver (1977), greatly clarifies the nature of man, the processes and interventions used by nurses in primary care, and the unique and common characteristics of a variety of family and group clients and settings of practice.

Listing and classifying of similar phenomena is a new-found skill which delights the school-age child; it remains a tool of the scholar, the researcher, the teacher, and the practitioner. The practitioner uses classified lists to retain knowledge of anatomy, pharmacology, kinds of diseases, stages of development, family patterns, personality adaptative mechanisms, and nursing interventions. Classification is utilized also in analyzing and synthesizing information for diagnosis of health and nursing problems and resources for adaptation.

As a basic student, the nurse becomes familiar with many concepts needed to understand clients and patients, concepts such as health, illness, development, nursing, role, territoriality, loss, crisis, adaptation, health service delivery, and pain. Graduate students refine the meanings of and operationalize familiar concepts and expand their repertoire of new ones. Conscious use of concepts in analyzing data increases with study and experience.

The past decade has seen the emergence of nursing theory past the initial level of concept formation and simple taxonomies. An understanding of the writings of Orem (1971), Auger (1976), Roy (1970; 1971), Peplau (1952), Rogers (1970), and other nurse-theorists provides the practitioner with optional models for organizing and conceptualizing phenomena, for describing structure and process, and for small steps in prediction of behavior. Texts such as Riehl and Roy (1980) assist the practitioner in the application of these theories to practice.

Maintaining current knowledge of human health affairs is equally critical to the practitioner. Quick overviews of lay magazines, newspaper feature articles, and other mass media provide insight into the dietary, exercise, sexual, and other health practices and beliefs of the public. Professional health journals update awareness of governmental policies, research findings, service emphases, and trends in health care. Selected nursing journals provide a channel of exchange for pertinent information among practitioners.

Skills of Practice

So much emphasis has been placed upon the data-gathering skills of giving physical examinations and taking health histories by those who see nurse practitioners primarily as physician extenders that scant attention has been paid to the many nursing, psychomotor, communication, and sociocultural skills of the professional nurse in the specialized practice of primary care. Many of these skills are subsumed under two broad categories of practice, namely, the nursing process and functional change processes.

Nursing Process The nursing process continues to be the method of practice of the nurse practitioner; the medical processes of diagnosis and treatment are subsumed under two of the steps, namely, problem identification and formulation and implementation of a plan of action.

Each phase of the nursing process demands many skills. Initiating a nurse-client relationship includes outreach, case finding, communication,

establishing trust, and negotiating a verbal contract of relevant responsibilities and rights. Data collection about the client and his or her environment requires skills in observation; in interviewing; in giving physical examinations; in administering selected tests of pathophysiology, development, functioning, health knowledge and health practices; and sometimes in surveying the environment. The identification of the health problem(s) and resources emerges from the analysis and synthesis of these data, using various theoretical frameworks and the comparison of findings with established norms and standards.

Though client involvement is essential throughout this interactional process, it is critical that the client actively set the short-term goals and objectives and help formulate the plan of action by which the desired end is sought. Throughout the nursing process, the nurse must utilize communication skills that can effect a helping, problem-solving interaction, a model of which is well described by Egan (1975).

Implementation of the plan requires a vast repertoire of nursing interventions or helping modalities. The more common nursing actions are direct personal care, support of healthful physiologic functioning, clarifying and informing, teaching, individual and group counseling, referral and advocacy, mobilization of resources, and promoting coordination, collaboration, and liaison with other helping persons and agencies.

Evaluation, the final step, determines the effectiveness of the process by assessing the extent of achievement of goals and of satisfaction of both client and nurse with the process and the outcome. Though termination of the immediate contract may occur at this point, plans are often made for reassessment at a later time. Minimally, the availability of the nurse to the client, or some other known gatekeeper, for reentry into primary health care is made known to the client.

The nurse practitioner's skill in carrying out the nursing process differs from the skill demanded of most nurses because the nurse practitioner has been prepared for and has been delegated the

authority to recognize and intervene in more problems of pathophysiology. Because of traditional
patterns in the United States, clients usually seek
primary care only when they believe they are
sick; therefore, nurse practitioners in physicians'
offices, clinics, and family practice centers frequently begin the process of differential diagnosis
of disease. They often use protocols that direct
immediate referral to a physician when there is
present a constellation of symptoms that suggest
an emergency or high-risk condition.

Management of symptoms of minor and self-
limiting disease is often carried out by nurse practitioners using medical standing orders, nursing
interventions, or practices considered safe for the
public to use. Continued surveillance and minor
adjustments in medical regimens of persons with
chronic diseases, such as hypertension, arthritis,
and diabetes, are frequently practiced, as is chronic-
disease nursing in the home, in clinics, and nursing
homes. Whenever nurse practitioners carry out
these medically delegated responsibilities, three
conditions should obtain: (1) the nurse has the
competence; (2) the laws under which the nurse
practices so permit; and (3) adequate medical
consultation or supervision is readily available.

Nurse practitioners and physicians who work
together gain respect for each other's competence.
The nurse truly appreciates the physician's skill of
differential diagnosis and the rich base of knowledge underlying the medical management of
disease processes in persons with complex path-
ologies. In turn, the physician respects the nurse's
interpersonal skills, knowledge of resources and
creativity in their use, and ability to solve complex
human situations. An example of the effectiveness
of such cooperation is described by B. G., a
master's-prepared nurse practitioner with long experience as a public health nurse with a particular
lower socioeconomic, rural, ethnic group.[1]

Clara, a 15-year-old girl, was brought by an
aunt to the private physician with whom I was

[1] Written permission was obtained for publication of
the interviews which follow.

practicing to verify a suspected pregnancy.
When the physician tried to examine her, Clara
became loud, angry, and almost combative,
shouting: "Get your damn hands off me! Ain't
no man gonna touch me. Let me out of here.
I'll get rid of this thing somehow." The physician told the aunt that he would not take her
as a patient until she calmed down and he could
examine her.

Having overheard, I approached the physician as he left the examining room and suggested that I spend some time with Clara. He
readily agreed. I knew the reluctance of a girl
of this culture to have a male physician examine her "privates." I also feared that without
a successful referral, she would bring about a
self-induced abortion with primitive and hazardous methods, thus risking her life.

I went in, sat down, and talked quietly with
her, asking open-ended questions about school,
sports, and friends. I found Clara had no parents
and was being reared primarily by a cousin,
Mary, whom I knew. Mary was presently in an
intensive care unit in a nearby city following an
auto accident that had taken the life of her
passenger.

Now everything fell into place. I knew why
the young girl was hostile and afraid. Her only
support person in this entire world was gone
and might not be back. Clara continued to express annoyance at being pregnant, refused to
talk about placing the baby for adoption, and
threatened, "I'll do something, you'll see."

I directed the conversation to Mary and her
need to have Clara healthy and strong when she
returned home. This pleased Clara and she
warmed up to me. She agreed to let a woman
examine her. Having estimated that she was 8
to 10 weeks pregnant, I knew a plan must be
executed at once. I called a nurse practitioner
in the local family planning clinic and asked
her to see the girl as an emergency and to set
up a pregnancy test to confirm my findings
before referring her out of town to an abortion clinic. I shared the plan with the physician
who was delighted with the progress and plan.

Clara left the office calm and smiling, determined to carry out the plan which was acceptable to her and which would protect her

health. Rapport had been established so that she might return if she felt the need.

As seen in the episode described by B. G., primary care can rarely be effective unless the family of the client is incorporated. Often the whole family is the client. The nursing process is conducted not only with each member but with the total unit so that the family is strengthened by the process. A. C., prepared as a family nurse practitioner, is employed as a specialist in family health nursing. Her description demonstrates the relationship of individual and family care in practice.

At the time of the first encounter there were four members in the household: The husband-father, the wife-mother, one teenaged son, and the invalid mother of the wife-mother. The husband was terminally ill with cancer of the lungs, complicated by asthma and COPD. The invalid mother-in-law was totally dependent in all care areas. The teenaged son was having extreme difficulty in school, and the wife was bearing the burden of this family and its problems.

Personal nursing care was provided to the husband and mother-in-law. During these interactions a variety of management methods were discussed including nursing home care for the mother-in-law and more involvement by the husband in his care. Although he was attending to the needs of daily living, he was not following the plan of care outlined by his physician as this plan related to health maintenance and promotion.

The family participated in defining their individual and collective needs and began to verbalize problems and ways to solve or modify these problems. Specific health care needs were spoken to, such as management of the medication regimen to include the use of oxygen and the signs and symptoms to report to the physician. The husband, wife, and son were to work cooperatively to achieve what they determined would be optimum for them. The wife had to decide what was the best level of care for her mother.

Alternatives and the consequences of choices were discussed with each of the family members. I provided assistance to the family by identifiying resources and making initial contacts or providing such information as was necessary to make the contacts. Because the mother was capable of making rational decisions in the presence of supportive objectivity she became the primary resource of the family for a time.

There were four major outcomes. (1) The mother-in-law was placed in a nursing home and arrangements and schedules were made for visiting. (2) The father, with greater understanding of his illness and its treatment, began to participate in his care and look forward to new treatment modalities such as pulmonary toilet. (3) He also began to be interested in sharing the responsibilities of his wife and son and was returning to his head of household status. (4) The change in the psychosocial status of this family made it possible for the husband and wife to work together on the problem of the teenaged son. These are not resolved at this time but appropriate resources for assistance have been identified and steps have been taken to utilize these resources.

In addition to a high level of competence in using the nursing process to help individuals and families to solve problems relative to health and disease, nurse practitioners are utilizing a variety of functional skills to effect change in primary care.

Functional Skills Because nurses prepared as specialists in primary care function in such diverse roles, it is critical that they be prepared in skills needed for personnel development, goal-directed program planning and implementation, consultation to agencies undergoing change, conduct of research and studies, mobilization of financial and authority bases for action, and new role development and implementation. As they use these skills they demonstrate different methods of leadership and directly influence the services offered to persons using primary care. The environments in which they function are as diverse as colleges, nursing homes, housing complexes for the elderly, industries, health departments, and long-term care institutions, as well as the more usual primary care settings of clinics, family practice centers, and physicians' offices.

The largest proportion of the master's graduates of the South Carolina program are teaching in schools of nursing or in in-service educational programs of service agencies or are administering health service programs in health departments. Their traditional functions—production of personnel and administration of public service—provide opportunity for innovation. Of particular note are the faculty members who continue direct practice by joint appointments on faculties and service agencies, by the maintenance of independent practices, or by summer employment in primary care settings. The administrators create opportunities and support for new nurse-practitioner roles and improve the quality of care by staff development, demonstration projects, and use of consultants.

The extent of the potential for changing primary care is best illustrated by L. M. and E. H., two practitioners who report their development and implementation of new roles.

L. M. developed a health promotional role in a university student-health service during her practicum in a community nursing course, a role which was so productive that a position was created 2 years ago for her full-time employment. She describes her present role.

As part of the admission procedure to the university, all new students are required to complete a comprehensive health questionnaire that deals with personal and family medical history, as well as life-style practices. By computer analysis, individuals are compared and a Health Risk Index (HRI) is formulated, which points out detrimental life-style habits and the number of years these habits may subtract from the total life span.

As coordinator of this program, I review all computer printouts, identifying those students who have chronic diseases and disorders and those at high risk. I contact these students by mail or phone and ask them to come see me so I can share this information with them. Response to this contact has been very positive.

Students are interested in knowing more about their health, and I capitalize on this during our interviews. Together we go over the condensed medical report and the HRI. While total life span and the number of years subtracted due to detrimental life-style habits are the focus of the HRI, I gear the conference toward where that individual is on the continum from illness to wellness, and how he or she can feel better (emotionally and physically), look better, and feel better about himself or herself as a person. In short, I strive to plant the idea of adding "life to years" in addition to adding "years to life" by students becoming active participants in their health care.

I make referrals to the walk-in clinic, counseling services, financial aid, student affairs, health education groups in exercise and smoking cessation, and any other appropriate university or community resource.

With the help of graduate nursing students, support/self-help groups have been established for students with diabetes, sickle-cell-anemia trait, hypertension, and physical disabilities. Some of these groups have continued with me serving as group facilitator. Group members discuss needs and problems, and share feelings and strategies for coping with university life.

I am also a health consultant for some 20 university employees in a Faculty/Staff Wellness Project. After a battery of psychophysiological tests, I meet with each participant for an intensive consultation, interpreting test results, discussing health needs, problems, and finally assisting each individual in formulating his or her wellness goals and the strategies for reaching these goals. Close individual contact is maintained throughout the year, during which I check on progress, send informative health related articles, set up exercise programs, and serve as a role model and a resource/support person.

In contrast to L. M., who works primarily with relatively well young persons, E. H. has created a role with elderly, chronically-ill patients in a large governmental hospital.

With the encouragement of my chief nursing administrator and the support of the hospital director and chief of medical services, I assumed 2 years ago the responsibility of primary care giver in a discharge unit of 20–40 beds. This newly created position for a clinical nurse specialist provided for clinical privileges consistent with the expanded and extended scope of nursing practice, which were incorporated into the medical staff bylaws. A physician was designated as my consultant and medical support. I was selected for this position because of 2 decades of effective nursing practice in medical, surgical, and psychiatric inpatient units and all ambulatory care clinics of this hospital; my skill in facilitating continuity of services by work with patients, families, staff and community resources; my graduate education; and my near-passionate commitment to nursing.

My functions of primary care giver involve many activities of both an expanded and extended nursing role. I screen and select for the unit hard-to-discharge patients referred by their physicians when their medical conditions are stable and for whom a medical summary is complete. On the unit I reassess their status and needs and prepare a plan of care. Monitoring the patients closely, I maintain and modify their plan of care as needed, carrying out activities permitted by protocol and medical standing orders, including ordering, interpreting, and following up on diagnostic tests; modifying diet and modes of nutrition; ordering medicines, equipment, and supplies; and adjusting prescribed medications. With this aged, chronically ill population most of the emergent problems are nursing ones which can be met by the nurses guided and assisted by me and/or the head nurse. As needed, the medical consultant has been readily available and supportive.

Activities that have led to a highly successful discharge record include conducting regularly scheduled interdisciplinary discharge planning with direct involvement of patients and families; writing and signing communications for patients referred to public health nursing services, local physicians, and community agencies; preparing patients and families for home care; granting passes for authorized absences and determining when patients are ready for discharge; preparing prescriptions for physician's signature for medication to use after discharge; and preparing and co-signing an addendum to the medical summary at the time of discharge.

In 2 years the unit has gained a good reputation of individualized care and effective discharges. I am challenged and fulfilled by the work and gratified that the expanded role is now well established. I know that I am providing better care to our patients, reducing costs by earlier discharge, adding to knowledge through clinical research, and sharing with other practitioners my experiences by direct contact and publications.

These few reports, and many more sent in response to the survey, provide rich evidence of how these master's-prepared nurses are demonstrating expanded roles in primary care. They are fully utilizing their knowledge and skills as they seek to achieve broad outcome goals for clients and patients they nurse in a variety of primary care settings. Though each one is making highly significant contributions to both clients and colleagues, a lasting improvement in primary health care will be achieved only if their numbers are greatly increased and the valuable nature of their practice is made known.

EDITOR'S QUESTIONS FOR DISCUSSION

What uncertainties regarding the role of the nurse practitioner have been clarified for you in Brown's chapter? What concerns might have been raised? What potential controversy and/or conflict may arise as the role further emerges for clients, nurses, and the profession? What means can be utilized to prevent and/or resolve those issues?

What guidelines are suggested in this chapter to maintain clarity as to the definition and domain of nursing practice and medical practice in primary care? What is the value of studies in primary care which focus on commonalities and classes of variability?

To what extent is the nurse practitioner an extended role from traditional public health nursing? How do nurse-practitioner graduate programs differ from community health graduate programs? Are there contradictions in the philosophy of graduate education and nurse- or family-practitioner programs? How can differences be reconciled? What are the pros and cons of "two tracks" being offered in community health graduate programs? If family nursing were offered as a program in graduate curricula, what suggestions would you have for goals, content, and the population to be served?

How true might it be that terms used for the role of the nurse practitioner have resulted in confusion and conflict rather than the role itself actualized in practice? Are there any differences in Brown's description of the role and Williams' conceptualization in Chap. 25? What factors contributed to a reconceptualization of the nurse practitioner role from when it initially was seen as a need? How do you account for the variability in practice that has emerged? What conditions may exist for the role of the nurse practitioner which contribute to inherent difficulties in clarifying the role? What negotiations need to be made with physicians in collaborating for the management of well and ill clients? To what extent can and/or should a nurse practitioner be autonomous in practice?

How can a nursing focus be ensured in practice? What nursing theories or conceptual frameworks are most appropriate for development of the nursing knowledge base and application in practice? Can the nursing process as described by Brown be reconceptualized as a nursing theory or conceptual framework for nurse practitioners? What is the difference between nursing process per se and nursing theory?

What are the advantages and disadvantages of qualitative and quantitative data? For what type of research question(s) might one type of data be more appropriate than another? How representative and generalizable are the findings of this survey? Complete a content analysis on the interviews included in Brown's chapter. What other findings are evident? To what extent do you agree with the interpretation of the interviews?

REFERENCES

Abdellah, Faye
1976 "Nursing's role in future health care." AORN Journal 24:236–240.

Auger, Jeanine Roose
1976 Behavioral Systems and Nursing. Englewood Cliffs, N.J.: Prentice-Hall.

deTornyay, Rheba
1977 "Primary care in a pluralistic society: Impediments to health care delivery." Pp. 1–22 in Primary Care in a Pluralistic Society. American Academy of Nursing Scientific Session, September 19, 1977. Kansas City, Mo.: ANA.

Dunn, Halbert L.
1959 "High-level wellness for man and society." American Journal of Public Health 49(6): 786–792.

Duvall, Evelyn Millis
1977 Marriage and Family Development. Pp. 23–67 in 5th ed. New York: Lippincott.

Egan, Girard
1975 The Skilled Helper: A Model for Systematic Helping and Interpersonal Relating. Monterey, Calif.: Brooks/Cole.

Ford, Loretta C. and Henry K. Silver
1967 "The expanded role of the nurse in child care." Nursing Outlook 15:43–45.

Freeman, Ruth
1974 "Nurse practitioners in the community health agency." Journal of Nursing Administration 4:21–24.

Hall, Joanne and Barbara R. Weaver (eds.)
1977 Distributive Nursing Practice: A Systems

Approach to Community Nursing. Philadelphia: Lippincott.

Jelinek, Darlene
1978 "The longitudinal study of nurse practitioners: Report of phase II." Nurse Practitioner 3:17–19.

Orem, Dorothea E.
1971 Concepts of Practice. New York: McGraw-Hill.

Peplau, Hildegarde E.
1952 Interpersonal Relations in Nursing. New York: Putnam.

Reinhardt, Adina M. and Mildred D. Quinn (eds.)
1980 "Family life styles today, Part Two." Pp. 39–110 in Family-Centered Community Nursing. Vol. 2. St. Louis: Mosby.

Riehl, Joan and Sister Callista Roy
1980 Conceptual Models for Nursing Practice. 2d ed. New York: Appleton-Century-Crofts.

Rogers, Martha E.
1970 An Introduction to the Theoretical Basis of Nursing. Philadelphia: Davis.

Roy, Sister Callista
1970 "Adaptation, a conceptual framework for nursing." Nursing Outlook 18(3):42–45.

1971 Adaptation: A basis for nursing practice." Nursing Outlook 19(4):254–257.

Sultz, Harry, Maria Zielezny, and Jane M. Gentry
1980 Longitudinal Study of Nurse Practitioners, Phase III. DHHS Publication No. HRA 80–2. Washington, D.C.: U.S. Government Printing Office.

U.S. Congress
1975 Public Law 93–641. P. vii in DHEW, Papers on the National Health Guidelines for Setting Health Goals and Standards. Washington, D.C.: U.S. Government Printing Office.

U.S. Department of Health, Education, and Welfare
1971 Extending the Scope of Nursing Practice: A Report of the Secretary's Committee to Study Extended Roles for Nurses. Washington, D.C.: U.S. Government Printing Office.

1980 "Substantial increases in nation's health professionals." Based on A Report to the President and Congress on the Status of Health Professions Personnel in the United States. DHHS News.

Chapter 27

Factors Influencing Job Satisfaction in Nursing Practice

Rita Braito, R.N., Ph.D.
Associate Professor
Department of Sociology
University of Denver
Denver, Colorado
        and
Richard Caston, Ph.D.
Assistant Professor
Department of Sociology
University of Denver
Denver, Colorado

After examining investigations addressing the relevance, nature, modes of nursing research, specific studies focusing on ethical and clinical problems, and quality of care and emerging nursing roles, this section concludes with a significant study of the satisfaction of nursing care providers themselves. Job satisfaction, dissatisfaction, and turnover of nurses are constant perplexing concerns for the profession. Not only is job satisfaction relevant to the productivity of providers of care but it may have a direct impact on the quality of care. Recognizing the increasing demands and shortage of nurses, Rita Braito and Richard Caston adroitly explicate critical variables of job satisfaction in this comprehensive study of practicing nurses.

First, they present an extensive literature review of basic issues and research pertaining to job satisfaction and nursing. General factors discussed are: unknowns concerning desired rewards; value discrepancies; patient care orientation; staffing, promotion, autonomy, and stress issues; and problems related to different education programs for entry levels into nursing. Controversies about job satisfaction are cited as stemming from differing theoretical perspectives and the measurement of job satisfaction. Consequently, they focus their study on three job facets: hospital satisfaction, activity satisfaction, and total job satisfaction. They utilize both facet-free and facet-specific measures.

Their original sample consisted of the total population (719) of nurses in three metropolitan hospitals that differ in size and sponsorship. The results of their constructed mailed questionnaire yielded a final sample of 467, for a response rate of 64 percent.

This research was supported in part by the American Nurses' Foundation.

Besides the basic demographic variables, numerous other independent variables are included in the investigation. Some of the organizational variables are: position of the nurse, part or full-time employment, and shift. Contextual variables include hospital and ward type and unit or ward consensus. Activity related facets of nursing were developed into scales measuring four dimensions: enjoyment of routine physical and routine social activities of nursing and the intrinsic and extrinsic rewards of nursing. Braito and Caston also correlate their measures of job satisfaction with statements as to whether the nurse would be pleased to have a child choose nursing and whether the nurse would choose to work if not necessary.

Extensive data analysis is presented. The initial findings indicate that nurses are somewhat satisfied with the activities of their work, very satisfied with the hospitals in which they work, and on the whole highly satisfied. Some of the other major findings are: Satisfaction tended to increase with age, as well as for those who were divorced, widowed, or separated; increased level of education was associated with decreased levels of job satisfaction; the longer the nurse was employed the higher the satisfaction score; the hierarchical position of the nurse was not significantly related to satisfaction; assistant head nurses tended to be the least satisfied, while assistant directors of nursing were the most satisfied; the type of work significantly affected satisfaction with nurses employed in obstetrics having the highest satisfaction while those in outpatient departments and emergency rooms rated the lowest; the type of sponsorship of the hospital appeared to be influential. There were discrepant findings concerning the effects of ward consensus on aspects of satisfaction. In addition, only perceived hospital influence significantly affected one of the satisfaction measures. The effects of the scaled measures for the activity related facets of nursing were statistically significant and positive in all four dimensions. The only exception, for a nonsignificant relationship, was that between enjoyment of social activities and satisfaction with one's routine physical activities.

To observe and compare the effects of a variable in producing variations in another variable, Braito and Caston used multivariate regression analysis. The results of their final analysis indicate that age was the only significant demographic variable. No organizational position variables made a significant net contribution in any of the satisfaction variables. The hospital in which one is employed had a significant net effect on satisfaction with the hospital. The significance of the religious sponsorship of the hospital was negated. There were no differences among the type of wards in their net effects. Consensus of satisfaction on the ward continued to have a strong impact on the satisfaction a nurse feels. A lack of agreement decreases one's satisfaction. No "setting" influence has a significant effect.

Concerning the facet activity scales, the final analysis indicates that the net relationship between enjoyment of social activities and satisfaction with routine physical activities was significantly negative. For overall job satisfaction, only enjoyment of the physical activities of nursing made a significant net contribution to variance in job satisfaction. Turning to intrinsic and extrinsic rewards the data show that nurses who find their work self-fulfilling (intrinsic) are in general more satisfied. It is evident in this sample that the contributions of extrinsic rewards, such as salary increases, do not increase satisfaction.

Braito and Caston conclude that the two strongest contributors to nurses' satisfaction with the *hospital* are the intrinsic rewards of the work and the degree to which the ward is cohesive. Next in importance is age. Again, the largest contributor to satisfaction with *activities* is the degree to which the nurse finds the work intrinsically rewarding. In the final analysis for *overall* job satisfaction, intrinsic reward is the most important contributor.

As a result of the outcome measures, Braito and Caston infer that as job satisfaction increases, so do positive responses in having a child choose nursing and one's commitment to work. Job satisfaction findings in this investigation of nurses have multiple implications for the recruitment and retention of employees for employers of nurses, nursing education, and the profession.

There has been a preoccupation on the part of American social scientists with the concept of job satisfaction. Much concern has been shown for the relation that has been found between job satisfaction and such phenomena as turnover, absenteeism, job performance, health and stress, and quality of life, to mention only a few. There is no question but that the quality of work is a central concern in the lives of most employed people, and that the nature of work has consequences for both lifestyle and life chances.

While the literature on job satisfaction is extensive and covers most occupational groups, the focus in this review of literature will be on nurses and what is known about their satisfaction and dissatisfaction with work. For purposes of general understanding, we shall indicate when findings about nurses are similar to those known about other occupational groups. While this section reviews basic issues of job satisfaction and nursing in general, the methods section will review basic research related to particular variables we shall be considering in our analysis.

Owing to several factors, a personnel shortage is predicted for nursing in the future: an increasing affluence in society is leading to increased health care demands; increased coverage is being provided through various types of insurance programs; usage of Medicare and Medicaid is becoming more widespread; there is an increased growth in the proportion of Americans who are elderly; and various types of health care possibilities, such as organ transplants and cardiac surgery, are becoming more available. Yet another contribution to the nursing shortage is related to the changing role of women in the U.S. labor force and elsewhere.

Whereas the two main professions considered appropriate for women in the past were elementary school teaching and nursing, today many women are turning as well to such diverse fields as law, medicine, accounting, and public and business administration. Thus the demand for nurses is increasing while the supply of applicants is staying the same or decreasing. The increasing movement of women into the labor force does not seem to be alleviating this situation substantially. (This is not to suggest that schools of nursing are experiencing problems attracting candidates—they are not, but they are not able to produce as many nurses as are in demand.) Nursing also has experienced a diminishing pool in that many educated nurses are leaving the field in pursuit of other work activities (Reeder and Mausch, 1979). Although there are many different conditions that could give rise to these job changes, such as inadequate salary and sexism in the health delivery system (Bullough and Bullough, 1975), the conditions of work and job satisfaction are no doubt important factors.

Our research focuses on a number of job facets that could contribute to job satisfaction, which itself is made operational several different ways—job satisfaction in general, satisfaction with the hospital in which one is employed, and satisfaction with the activities that occupy most of one's time. The independent variables, to be discussed in more detail in the methods section, are as follows: enjoyment of the physically oriented activities of nursing; enjoyment of the socially oriented activities of nursing; extrinsic rewards (economic considerations of work); intrinsic rewards (self-actualizing characteristics of work); major sources of reference group influences on one's job; hospital and ward type in which one is employed; unit or ward consensus; basic demographic variables, including age, religion, marital status, amount of nursing education, and father's socioeconomic status (SES); and organizationally based statuses—staff position in the hospital hierarchy, years of employment, shift, and full- and part-time employment. Finally, our measures of job satisfaction have been correlated with an expression of agreement or disagreement with statements indicating whether one would desire to continue to work and whether one would be happy to have a daughter choose to become a nurse.[1]

JOB SATISFACTION AND DISSATISFACTION

Research related to job satisfaction and dissatisfaction in nursing indicates that there are a number of general issues that create conflict for nurses and could result in job satisfaction or dissatisfaction.

Ideal versus Actual Situations

In a study of nurses in an outpatient department (OPD), Benne and Bennis (1959) suggested that nurses hold an idealized vision of what nurses should do. They argued that nurses often regarded some common nursing demands as illegitimate—such as work a physician could do alone or that less qualified people could do. The investigators believed that such discrepancies between actual task assignments and what a nurse identifies as "real" nursing may be a source of frustration. These same investigators also found no relationship between what nurses hoped for and what they predicted would occur as a consequence of doing a

[1] This was not intended to be sexist, but there is no question if one looks at occupational density that nursing is an occupation composed primarily of women. Therefore, we did not want to distort the meaning of the question in terms of its relevance for respondents by generalizing the question to include "son" as well as "daughter." On the other hand, the desire to have sons become nurses should be explored, since men represent a population that is relevant to nursing in that they make up a large percent of the client population and need to be better represented as nurses in health delivery systems.

good job. The investigators thought the supervisors might be unaware, therefore, of what rewards the OPD nurses desired. In addition, the actual rewards the OPD nurses desired were not within the control of the supervisor.

In terms of loyalty, the nurses expressed highest commitment to the nursing profession and lowest to nursing service. Of course these two phenomena are not inherently mutually exclusive. Where conflicts might exist between them, however, it would seem likely that nursing administration would use organizational prerogatives to ensure that nursing services would come first. Thus nurses might be required to provide patient care that they did not agree with. In support of this latter conjecture, Godfrey (1978a) found widespread dissatisfaction with staffing—many nurses believed that understaffing was a serious threat to the patient and put the nurses in an untenable position. Furthermore, Georgopoulos and Mann (1962), in their evaluation of nursing care, found that registered nurses, in comparison with the medical staff, laboratory and x-ray technicians, and administrators, gave the least favorable evaluation of the nursing care provided. In another study of job satisfaction among hospital personnel, Palola and Larson (1965) noted that nurses had the lowest job satisfaction scores of the groups they studied: paramedics, office workers, unskilled workers (mainly laundry and kitchen), and nursing auxiliaries. As was true of the groups studied by Georgopoulos and Mann (1962), these findings reflect differences among groups that would be in contact with each other within a given hospital and would share collective responsibility for health care of patients or conditions related to their health care. Godfrey (1978b) reported that only 43 percent of her nurse respondents seldom or never compromised professional standards, while 35 percent did so occasionally and 22 percent frequently. It may be that understaffing contributes to such compromising of standards and, in turn, to job dissatisfaction, or at least to lower satisfaction with the quality of the patient care provided.

Smith (1965) suggested that value discrepancies

between nurse-educators and head nurses over issues of autonomy and conceptions of desirable patient care are sources of conflict for nurses. She showed that the two groups valued and rewarded different kinds of behavior of student nurses. To the degree that promotion in industry tends to be achieved by those who agree with management, values inculcated in the educational experience that conflict with those of nursing administrators may be an intermittent source of frustration and dissatisfaction throughout the careers of the nurses. Smith, herself a nurse-educator, suggests:

> "If students are not to be alienated from nursing as a career as a result of exposure to conflicting values and expectations, nursing service administrators should reexamine the bureaucratic and administrative policies of the hospital as they influence professional practice and nursing education." (1965:202)

Much data indicate that a *patient care orientation* prevails among nurses, i.e., an orientation to the caring and curing of patients versus an orientation to promotion, to hospital administration, or to the cure aspects of nursing only. Godfrey's data (1978a), for example, show that 70 percent of the nurses reported positive feedback from patients and families; this would, of course, reinforce the orientation of nurses toward client care. Feedback from administration, on the other hand, was rated excellent by only 8 percent of the diverse groups of nurses represented in her sample (students, licensed practical nurses, diploma and baccalaureate nurses, and nurses having master's and doctorate degrees). While 31 percent stated that the administration was good, 61 percent suggested that the administration was fair or worse. Godfrey (1978a) also found that only 51 percent of her respondents believed that the nursing administration would support them if they ran into problems; this situation would further orient nurses more to the patient than to the administration. Most theoretical perspectives—e.g., exchange theory, behaviorism—would find such a patient orientation understandable in the light of these nurses' on-the-

job experiences. We must also keep in mind that mobility in a hospital is limited. The hierarchy of an organization narrows in numbers of positions as one moves up. Consequently, many nurses will be at a staff level during most or all of their careers. Since patients reward nurses verbally more than do administrators and payday is not a daily activity, a patient orientation would serve as an enduring source of reinforcement.

Meyer and Hoffman (1964), quoting other sources, suggest that the typical image of the nurse in the past has been the nurse with the patient, while the present image is of the nurse with a colleague. The data, however, indicate that nurses continue to spend more time with patients than with colleagues. As constraints on collegiality conflict with the new image of the nurse, dissatisfaction may grow.

Similarly, to the degree that there is conflict between the care and cure aspects of nursing, job dissatisfaction may increase. Nurses might be spending more time with the patient providing cure aspects, e.g., being an IV (intravenous) nurse, and yet have the desire to provide more social, emotional, or total care.

Promotion

The positions of team leader, head nurse, and other supervisory levels are bureaucratic, administrative routes of organizational mobility. Their patient contact is more indirect and, consequently, they involve more indirect cure and caring aspects than are otherwise idealized in the patient care orientation. Many people who choose nursing, however, do not do so out of interest in power, politics, and administrative problems. Thus the major channel of promotion for nurses involves types of behavior not congruent with the ideal image of nursing they hold upon entrance into the profession. The ideal image of nursing, then, as being more directly involved in patient care, could limit opportunities for advancement and frustrate those who choose promotion as a route of upward mobility.

Some of Godfrey's (1978c) respondents, for

example, mentioned as reasons for leaving administrative positions desire to return to more direct patient contact. Bennis and others (1959) suggested that nursing at the bedside did not result in promotion because no clinical promotion ladder is available. This is yet an unresolved issue; a clinical track for the promotion of registered nurses still has not been well formalized within the hospital context. (We are not here ignoring the clinical expert position in nursing; such a position is emerging, but basically is still limited in number as compared with other positions, such as team leader, assistant and head nurse, and other administrative and supervisory levels.) Alt et al. (1980), although focusing on cost-effectiveness issues, notes the same problems and suggests not only that a clinical track is something to be seriously considered because of its potential for cost effectiveness, but also that such a track is necessary as the total direct patient care by registered nurses becomes a more viable form of health delivery.

Not only are the above aspects relevant to promotion and nurses' image of nursing, but Godfrey (1978c) reports that only 8 percent of the nurses of all types (as noted above) believed promotion depended upon performance, 27 percent thought promotion was dependent upon performance somewhat, 14 percent thought promotion was dependent upon performance very little, and 2 percent felt promotion was unrelated to performance. Many commented that promotion was a matter of politics, favoritism, seniority, and having a baccalaureate degree—not performance.

Autonomy

Benne and Bennis (1959) noted that conflict exists between nurses and physicians. Alt et al. (1980) suggests that this conflict exists over issues of the dependability and "servility" of nurses versus their professional dignity and autonomy and serves as a source of dissatisfaction. Reeder and Mauksch (1979) suggest as well that conflict between physicians and nurses continues to persist with respect to autonomy and professional responsibility and

decision making. While Benne and Bennis (1959) might not use the term "servility" today, the issue of autonomy is still a source of problems within nursing practice—whether that be in the area of hospital practice in a ward situation or as a nurse practitioner. Constant disputes have arisen because changing the nurse practice laws to permit more autonomy for nurses has constantly been opposed by many medical doctors.

Bullough (1975) thinks there is sexism in the entire health delivery system. The relationship between nurses and doctors is but one aspect of it. They believe that the unequal relationships between men and women are reflected in the differences in monetary rewards, power, prestige, and autonomy in the practice of health care. Such discrimination has been found as well in the presence of sexist statements in medical textbooks (Scully and Bart, 1973) and in the treatment of women with excessive medications and surgery. Thus the conflict between nurses and doctors over autonomy mirrors the larger social system of which health delivery is a part. It creates particular problems, however, owing to the overrepresentation of men as medical doctors and women as nurses. In addition, Stamps, Piedmont, Slavitt, and Haase (1978) indicate that autonomy is ranked as most important by nurses from three different samples. For a paid employee, even a professional, autonomy is going to be limited not only by sex but also by organizational concerns. In addition, the majority of medical doctors are not in health maintenance organizations and consequently are less subject to organizational constraints. Godfrey (1978a) noted that although 76 percent of her sample reported professional relationships with doctors as satisfactory, 29 percent reported some respect from doctors, while 9 percent felt they got little or no respect from them.

Tension and Stress

Menzies (1960) in her study of nurses in London focused on the effect of social systems on nursing anxiety. She suggested that the nature of nursing tasks and working with patients and relatives of patients involved demands which increased the experience of stress. She also found colleagues and their demands to be sources of stress. Defenses against such stress took the form of such checks and counterchecks as exaggerated concerns over coworker competence, idealizing one's own personal qualities as though they were organizational requirements, and avoiding change. She further suggested that high levels of tension, stress, and anxiety lead to withdrawal from duty, student dropout, high position turnover, and increased postgraduate training. Bullough and Bullough (1975) suggest in addition that moves into administration and higher education provide mechanisms for reducing stress and discrimination. Some of Godfrey's (1978a) respondents made comments supportive of the Bulloughs' contention. Given the increased number of cardiac care units, number of intensive care units, incidence of chronic disease among the growing elderly population, and forms of surgery that are now technologically possible, increased demands are placed upon patients, families, and health deliverers. It is likely, therefore, that tension levels in hospitals have increased since Godfrey's study and will continue to do so, rather than to decrease.

Education

Education has frequently been associated with job satisfaction. In regard to nurses, Corwin (1961) reported that type of education received—diploma versus degree—made a difference in type and nature of role conflict experienced. He suggested that degree graduates with professional orientations experienced increased conflicts after graduation due to an attempt to combine both the bureaucratic and professional orientations. For them the discrepancy between the real and ideal perceptions of nursing increased after graduation, suggesting greater frustration or dissatisfaction with increased education.

The very presence of the different types of education leading to the registered nurse position

in itself may create problems in nursing—e.g., the term technical nurse has been suggested as appropriate for nurses with an associate of arts (A.A.) degree but was rejected by them. The fact that differential recruitment occurs for the various programs which provide eligibility for a student to be licensed as a registered nurse must also increase problems in the field. A.A. students, for example, are older and have the lowest high school grade-point averages of all three major groups (diploma, A.A. and B.S.). B.S. graduates, by contrast, have the highest high school grade-point average and are recruited from higher socioeconomic positions in terms of father's occupation, education, and income. Interestingly, the mothers of the students from B.S. programs were more apt to have been nurses than were mothers of either the diploma or A.A. programs. A higher percentage of students in the diploma programs was apt to be Catholic than in either of the other programs, while more black students were in the A.A. programs.

Not only is there differential participation in the three programs by race, SES, and religion, which in itself would create problems, but there is also a different educational emphasis in each program which would increase the differences among these groups as they move from school into the work situation (McLemore and Hill, 1966). Godfrey (1978a) found that as education increased, so did critical attitudes toward nursing—97 percent of the students rated nursing as a profession as positive, as did 92 percent of the A.A. and diploma nurses, 88 percent of the B.S. nurses, and 50 percent of nurses with Ph.D.s.

Role Consensus

Larsen (1968) investigated role consensus among nurses, doctors, and patients in a hospital. He found that the greatest disagreement occurs in the areas of task performance, decision making, and nurse-patient relationships. There were also differences between nurses and doctors over their rights and obligations. A greater consensus was found in the area of rights than in that of obligations. All the groups had greater consensus on pre-scriptions than on proscriptions. Factors related to higher consensus were formal training of group members, homogeneity of formal training, and length of exposure to socialization in the health field. In the area of satisfaction with work, it was found that satisfaction was directly related to the degree of consensus with others on definitions of role. Thus, though satisfaction was present in some domains, there were also domains where low consensus was related to low satisfaction.

Devereaux and Weiner (1950) have suggested that the average nurse is doomed to a great deal of frustration owing to the ill-defined professional hierarchy and social position a nurse occupies. Some of Godfrey's (1978a) respondents felt that the term "professional" was used against them every time they made remuneration demands and was called upon when overtime and other hospital demands were made. Devereaux and Weiner (1950) also felt that nurses did not have adequate oppor-tunities to replenish ego resources and expressed surprise that so many nurses were able to be so creative and professionally expert despite the do-main in which they functioned.

Turnover

Turnover among employees has been used as an indicator of low job satisfaction. More recent data have challenged such a direct relationship and found job turnover was related more to commit-ment to leave, which itself is not directly related to job dissatisfaction. Other factors of importance related to turnover include job opportunities else-where and the social and economic costs related to making a job change. Low personal cost of leaving a job in terms of salary loss, promotion loss, or changed housing arrangements would contribute to high turnover, even with job satisfaction held constant. Levine found that

> professional staff nurses have the greatest insta-bility of all other groups of personnel. Within a twelve month period covered by the study, res-

> ignations occurred in nearly half of all the staff nurse positions. . . . (1957:53)

He noted that the turnover rate for nursing per-sonnel is higher than for female factory workers. Price (1973) noted that turnover among nurses was greatest among the new employees and lowest at the higher levels of nursing positions in hospitals.

The degree of stability of any group in a given organization is related to supply and demand. In view of the continuing shortages of nurses, nursing turnover could well be related to other job oppor-tunities. The exodus of nurses from nursing would suggest, as well, that something in the work situa-tions in which nurses find themselves is unsatis-factory. These two factors will create a push-pull situation (something in the job situation pushes nurses out—the push phenomenon; increased job opportunities elsewhere pull nurses away— the pull phenomenon). McCloskey (1975) for example, found that nurses who left their jobs for family reasons would have remained if they had been of-fered more rewards, the most important being:

> (1) more opportunities to attend educational programs; (2) more opportunity to continue course work that could earn credits for the next degree; (3) more opportunity for career ad-vancement other than as assistant head nurse or head nurse; and (4) more recognition for their work from peers and supervisors. A salary raise of $150.00 per month was rated only fifth.

Leaving for family reasons in the future could be a decreasing pull phenomenon as having two wage earners in the family is increasingly seen as essen-tial for most families and has been one of the major changes in work behavior of women from the six-ties onward. If the job market were to become tighter, it might also reduce turnover, as the pull phenomenon would cease to operate to the same degree.

Yet another source of turnover is suggested by Kramer (1974), who proposed that nurses leave nursing because of the lack of congruence between the public image of nursing and actual work realities. She uses the term *reality shock* to refer to the experience of nurses after graduation. In addition she suggests that not only do nurses drop out, but that they may respond with dissatisfaction and nonparticipation. Most authors discussing the reality shock phenomenon, although using different terms, generally agree that it is a source of stress and dissatisfaction.

Summary

As can be seen from the review of literature related to job satisfaction and nursing, job satisfaction has been an issue of varying degrees of salience over time. It is important to note that the factors contributing to job dissatisfaction have received more attention in the literature than sources contributing to job satisfaction. In spite of the multiple assertions suggesting widespread job dissatisfaction, Godfrey (1978a) reported that the majority of nurses, regardless of which categories (registered nurses, licensed practical nurses, or students) considered themselves satisfied with their jobs. The most important sources of satisfaction were helping people (almost 50 percent), the worthwhile, intellectually challenging, or interesting nature of work (46 percent), financial security (2 percent), and prestige accorded nurses (1 percent). Seventy-five percent of Godfrey's respondents enjoyed their work most of the time. Nurses, like other professionals and workers in the United States, are generally satisfied with their jobs (Andrisani et al., 1978).

CONTROVERSIES ABOUT JOB SATISFACTION IN GENERAL

Mortimer (1979) in a review of literature and summary statement related to job satisfaction, suggests that controversy about job satisfaction is widespread and largely unresolved. Locke (1976) notes that more than 33,000 articles, books, and dissertations have been written on job satisfaction. A computer search we undertook of related literature suggests that there has been little alteration or abatement in the literature on job satisfaction since Locke's estimate as of 1976. According to Mortimer (1979), the controversy about job satisfaction stems from different theoretical perspectives, i.e., the physical economic school versus the human relations school. In addition, these schools of thought have given rise to controversy over the alleged sources of satisfaction, such as the questions of intrinsic versus extrinsic sources and whether job satisfaction is and should be measured as facet-free versus facet-specific. Each of these issues will be briefly discussed.

The Economic School

Taylor has been considered to be the father of scientific management. His school of thought was developed during the 1920s when he and his followers were concerned with rationalizing the flow of work. A *rationalized* work flow would maintain the highest levels of work efficiency through pay incentives, which Taylor and his followers believed would encourage the greatest amount of productivity on the part of the worker. The Taylor economic school gave rise as well to the notion of rationalizing decision making, to time and motion studies, to issues and models related to span of control, and to an emphasis on the formal structure of organizations (Haas and Drabek, 1973). While the happiness of workers was not at issue in this school of thought, we could infer that workers who would be concerned primarily with having an organized process for getting and boosting their pay would be most content with a rationalized work setting.

The Human Relations School

By contrast, the human relations school, developed in the 1930s, focused on the needs of the workers as human beings, such as the needs for appreciation, recognition, influence, and a feeling of accomplishment. Workers, according to this perspective, have ego motives, security motives, curiosity, creativity, and economic motives. Of central concern was the function of the work group in meeting these worker needs and the importance of style of supervision and worker-supervisor relations in producing worker satisfaction or dissatisfaction. In the human relations school, worker needs are regarded not only as extrinsically motivated (e.g., by pay) but also as intrinsically motivated as well (e.g., by self-fullfillment). A happy worker then is a product of a happy work group and a good supervisor-subordinate relationship. Such conditions should give rise to greater productivity (Argyris, 1964).

Fein (1976) has suggested that the nature of the work and the importance and challenge of work are central to understanding worker behavior. Herzberg et al. (1959) argued that the intrinsic features of work itself, such as achievement, personal growth, responsibility, and recognition are integral parts of the work experience, giving rise to job satisfaction. They suggested that extrinsic features such as salary, supervision, interpersonal relations, and working conditions will give rise to job dissatisfaction if absent, but do not give rise to satisfaction. The variables that derived from Herzberg's early work have been subject to much controversy [Russell, (1975) and Mortimer (1979) cite some of the literature relevant to the controversy].

Other theoretical schools of thought have developed in which job satisfaction is an important variable, especially as related to productivity. These schools of thought have been influenced by the economic school and the human relations school. Because of the concern with satisfaction and productivity, job satisfaction and dissatisfaction have consistently been studied regardless of which school has been utilized in attempting to understand worker behavior.

Intrinsic versus Extrinsic Sources of Job Satisfaction

Although the major schools of thought can be seen as contributing to an elaboration of dimensions of work as sources of job satisfaction, other perspectives have also impacted the theoretical development of the argument. Maslow (1954) has suggested that there is a hierarchy of needs from lower order, biological needs (e.g., for food) to higher-order needs (e.g., for love) that culminate with a need for self-actualization. The lower order, extrinsic needs must be met before higher order needs can emerge. Worker needs, consequently, must be considered in the context of the overall hierarchy of needs. Both intrinsic and extrinsic needs have been found to be associated with job satisfaction.

Voydanoff (1978) showed that both intrinsic and extrinsic factors were important and the degree of importance depended upon the occupational group. She recommended, however, that job changes in the area of self-expression, role-strain, and improvements in promotions and financial rewards would increase satisfaction in all work groups, from professionals to laborers. The effect of quality and amount of supervision, although apparent in zero-order relationships, did not contribute to explained variance in her regression equations. The controversy over the contribution of extrinsic and intrinsic rewards to job satisfaction remains unsettled.

Facet-free Versus Facet-Specific

Literature on the measurement of job satisfaction has been concerned with whether it should be indexed through a facet-free or facet-specific approach. Seashore and Taber (1975) have summarized the differences between these two types of approach very well. Facet-free data are obtained when respondents are asked to indicate global satisfaction with a job. Such an approach does not require a respondent to specify the particular aspects of a job or how they are to be combined in assessing satisfaction. Each respondent thus considers his or her own fit to the job utilizing his or her own cognitions and perceptions. The questions are usually asked with an intent to impose the fewest possible constraints on the response. For example, a question that asks, "How satisfied are you with your pay?" permits the respondent to consider and weigh, as he or she is inclined, such factors as fringe benefits, adequacy to meet living requirements, amount of pay, types of paying schedules, this year's pay as compared with last year's, and how the pay may compare with a friend's in a similar position, to mention only a few possibilities. It is possible for a number of these facet-free items to be combined into a more global measure.

Facet-specific data permit the investigator to determine just what facets the respondent will consider in answering the question. An example would be, "How much enjoyment do you get at work from visiting with patients, charting, or talking with patients?" No matter how specific the facet, it is never exhaustive, as it is not possible, in most instances, to identify and ask about every specific aspect of work. The difference between the two types of measurement (facet-free and facet-specific) is one of degree. In our research we have utilized both facet-free and facet-specific measures. Our facet-free indexes tap overall job satisfaction, satisfaction with activities in general, and satisfaction with the hospital in which one is working. Our facet-specific indicators tap such specific tasks as charting, talking with patients, and similar activities.

IMPORTANCE OF THE PRESENT RESEARCH

Although there have been many studies of job satisfaction in general and a few of job satisfaction of nurses in particular, few studies, either nationally or occupationally specific, have been able to investigate as many of the numerous factors that may impact job satisfaction as we included in the present investigation. We included unique, organizationally based variables by controlling organizational context. It is possible, therefore, to consider the contributions to job satisfaction of nurses' particular hospitals, the types of unit in which they work, and coworker consensus as it contributed to presence or absence of satisfaction. In addition, our respondents were asked to identify and rank specific sources of reference group in-

fluence as they affected them in the work setting. It was thus possible to compare worker perceptions of influence with the actual influence exerted by some of these contextual sources. In addition, demographic variables and other background factors were included.

It was not possible to include all variables which further investigators should be concerned with. Variables for role-strain (Voydanoff, 1978), for example were not included. Likewise, variables for organizational climate (Lyon and Ivancevich, 1974) and role accuracy (Green and Organ, 1973) are much needed. On the other hand, we do have variables relevant to issues of autonomy, achievement, recognition, and security, as well as extensive measures of the enjoyment of routine physical and social activities of nurses.

RESEARCH DESIGN AND PROCEDURE

The contribution of various factors toward job satisfaction could be examined with many different sampling designs of workers. Because of our interest in nursing and in organizationally based contributions to job satisfaction, it was necessary to examine *total populations* of nurses within hospitals, rather than to draw a random sample of nurses across a great many hospitals.[1] The three hospitals that were selected were located in a metropolitan area in the Northwest and differed by size and sponsorship, making our hospital-based registered nurse sample somewhat more representative of basic types of hospitals.

The hospitals included a county hospital, a Catholic-sponsored hospital, and a private, non-

---

[1] This research was a part of a larger study of registered nurses concerned with their conflicts, legitimations, forms of protest, salary demands, and factors that would affect such demands. Consequently it was necessary to select hospitals that were currently in the process of negotiating salary demands and other issues through the appropriate state nurses' association. In the metropolitan area studied, the three largest hospitals were selected which met the criteria of the larger study and permitted research access.

denominational hospital. Arrangements were made to mail the questionnaires to the home addresses of the nurses at two of the hospitals; the third hospital required the direct delivery of the questionnaires to the nurses within the hospital by the area supervisors. In this latter situation, the envelope containing the questionnaire was stamped on the outside with the request that it not be opened until the person arrived home.[1] A cover letter from each director of nursing accompanied the investigator's cover letter and questionnaire. In order to assure anonymity and hopefully to increase the response rate, a stamped postcard was enclosed for the respondent to sign and mail to the investigator upon completion and mailing of the questionnaire. Upon receipt of the signed, returned card, the name of the respondent was crossed off a list. It was therefore not possible to associate any signed card with any questionnaire. In addition, the questionnaires had been coded for each hospital, making it possible to estimate the number of nonrespondents by hospital. Two weeks later a letter was mailed or delivered to all those whose signed postcard was not returned. Two weeks after this follow-up a third letter and questionnaire together with a postcard were again mailed or delivered according to the original pattern.

The response by hospitals (classified on the basis of size of hospital) was as follows:

Since no data were obtained on the nonrespondents (to protect confidentiality of all employees), it was not possible to determine if there were any potentially biasing characteristics of respondents versus nonrespondents. Questionnaires that were returned with a great deal of information missing were discarded. Not counting these latter cases, the overall response was 64 percent.

Measurement of Dependent Variables—Hospital Satisfaction, Activity Satisfaction, and Total Job Satisfaction

Literature from the human relations school of organizational behavior has noted the importance of particular types of organizational affiliation as contributions to job satisfaction. The organization provides individuals not only with prestige, but, by implication, would also influence leadership style, organizational climate, and patterns of interaction; all these may increase or decrease job satisfaction through their impact upon workers' ego needs, security needs, curiosity needs, and economic motives. The question asked to ascertain satisfaction as it relates to organizational affiliation was "How do you like working in the hospital in which you are currently working?" The response "not at all" was represented by 1 and "very much" was represented by 6. The nurse respondents were asked to

Hospitals	Total	Percent	Number (*N*) responding
Small	160	67	(*N* = 107)
Medium	201	55	(*N* = 111)
Large	358	74	(*N* = 249)
		Total	*N* = 467

[1] Of course, standardization of administration is desirable in survey research. In view of the difficulty of access to the hospitals due to the nature and salience of the issues and concern with the protection of the staff lists, it was decided that it would be better to alter the delivery of the questionnaire in the third hospital rather than lose that particular population of registered nurses from the sample. Any biases that may have been introduced by this alteration remain unknown.

circle the number from 1 to 6 which represented their view as it related to the current work situation.

In literature on job satisfaction, general satisfaction with routine work activities has been considered of obvious importance. Godfrey (1978a), for example, has asked nurses what activities they like doing most and least. Then too, satisfaction with work activities is a part of the commonly used Job Description Inventory developed by Smith, Kendall, and Hulin (1969). Other frequently used measures also incorporate this component of job satisfaction (Cherniss and Egnatios, 1978). Our question related to satisfaction with activities was: "In general I would say that I am satisfied with the activities which involve most of my time." The respondents were asked to circle the number from 1 to 10 that best represented their point of view. A response of 1 represented "strongly agree" and 10 represented "strongly disagree." The coding was then reversed so that a high number reflected high satisfaction. A composite index from both of these items was then developed (see Appendix A) to measure total satisfaction.

Demographic and Background Variables (Father's SES)

Basic demographic data were collected as follows:

What is your age to your nearest birthday? _____years
What is your marital status? _____Single; _____Married; _____Separated; _____Widowed; _____Divorced (Owing to small numbers, the last three categories were collapsed in a part of the analysis—all shared the similarity of spouse absence.)
What type of formal educational preparation have you received? _____2-year associate degree; _____3-year diploma school of nursing program; _____3-year diploma school of nursing plus a bachelors degree; _____4- or 5-year collegiate school of nursing? _____M.A. or M.S. _____Ph.D.

Religion was indexed as follows:

My religion is _____Catholic; _____Jewish; _____Protestant; _____other (specify)

Since very few cases occurred of non-Catholic, non-Protestant nurses in the sample, those cases were deleted in the analysis. Also, although race

and sex were determined, variations in their distributions were not sufficient for analysis.

Among traditional organizational variables, staff positions were indicated as follows:

What position do you currently hold in the hospital? _____staff nurse; _____assistant head nurse; _____head nurse; _____supervisor; _____assistant director of nursing

Age and marital status have frequently been found to be related to job satisfaction. In particular, younger workers are usually found to be less satisfied than older workers (Glenn, Taylor, and Weaver, 1977). Differences also have been found between graduates versus collegiate graduates in their traditional-professional orientations. In addition, other value differences have been found when different types of degree programs have been compared (Habenstein and Christ, 1963).

The father's socioeconomic status was determined as was that of the spouse. The spouse's status was not used in this analysis since it would have eliminated all currently unmarried nurses from our multivariate analysis. The occupation of the father and his education were obtained and combined into a Hollingshead two-factor index. We anticipated that nurses who were upwardly mobile as compared with their fathers would be more satisfied with their activities, their hospital, and their job in general.

Directors of nursing were nor surveyed as it was necessary to make arrangements through them to obtain organization access.[1] Organizational research has consistently demonstrated that the higher one is in a hierarchy, the greater is one's job satisfaction. Most of this research, however, has involved random samples of persons across occupations; little research has investigated single occupations within their organizational contexts. Wood (1971) studied engineers and found that work value and background characteristics distin-

---

[1] This involved their reading of the questionnaire in its preliminary form plus discussion.

guished different engineering groups. Similar results have been found for psychologists, where satisfaction differed by work setting (Garfield and Kuntz, 1975). Work satisfaction research also has compared managers and assistant managers. Position and type of organizational affiliation have been shown to affect job satisfaction.

We were interested in the effect of part-time employment as compared with full-time employment. This information was obtained as follows:

Do you work ____part time? ____full time?

Little research has been done including this variable. Since part-time workers need not feel as involved in their jobs as full-time workers, they may have less cause for dissatisfaction.

The shift one works has been shown to be related to job satisfaction. Respondents could indicate that they worked "day," "evening," "night," or "rotating" shifts. Godfrey (1978b) indicated that while most nurses liked the shift that they worked, nurses on the day shift liked theirs best of all. Most did not think that their job and hours interfered with their families. Since people may choose to work particular shifts in order to meet family, educational, or social demands, the nature of its contribution to job satisfaction is uncertain. The general comments by nurses responding to Godfrey's survey (1978a) would suggest that further exploration of this issue is in order.

Contextual Variables

The hospital at which the respondent was employed was determined by paper coding the questionnaire by hospital.[1] The human relations school has suggested that organizational affiliation would have an impact on perceptions of the job. Lyon and Ivancevich have shown that the organizational climate of a teaching-referral hospital has different impacts on the satisfaction of nurses and administrators. They reported "in general that organiza-

tional climate for both occupational groups studied has the most significant impact upon self-actualization (personal growth, sense of accomplishment, advancement opportunity, and challenging work), a lesser impact on autonomy . . ." (1974:646). The concept of organizational climate refers to the observation that each type of organization, owing to its function and history, will develop norms and values about defense and acquisition, exchange and reciprocity which are reflected in the norms and values of an organization (Katz and Kahn, 1978). Schools as compared with hospitals will have a climate that is less stressful. A prison under siege by inmates and law enforcement personnel will have a different climate from a prison where administrative control is firmly exercised.

We did not study organizational climate directly, but assume that there may be different perceptions by ward. We have, therefore, tapped organizational impact through hospital, ward type, and ward consensus. Unfortunately, hospital sponsorship and hospital size are identically arrayed in our sample. Hence the effects of these factors cannot be separated. A further study including many more organizations and their total nurse populations and varying by size, sponsorship, and climate would be necessary to separate out the effects. Prestige rankings of the hospitals would also be useful in assessing the effect of status affiliation.

The effect of ward specialty has frequently been alluded to. Yet few studies have been done which compared the different types of units. Studies have more often been of single units, such as outpatient departments (Benne and Bennis, 1959) or intensive care units. Godfrey's sample indicated that most nurses (79 percent) report high job satisfaction (1978a:107). She noted that work setting made a difference in that industrial nurses were most satisfied (92 percent), while fewer hospital and ECF nurses were as satisfied (78 percent). With regard to specialty, over 80 percent of the nurses in emergency room, administration, and education reported being very satisfied. Eighty percent of the nurses in pediatrics, intensive care units, and coronary care units were

[1] A different grain of paper was used for each hospital.

very satisfied, while 73 to 78 percent of geriatric, psychiatric, obstetrics-gynecology, and medical-surgical nurses reported high job satisfaction. While specialty was shown to make a difference in job satisfaction in her study, its contribution to job satisfaction in a multivariate controlled analysis remains unknown. Our data analysis will shed light on this issue.

Ward consensus on satisfaction with hospital and satisfaction with routine activities was developed from the earlier mentioned measures of general satisfaction with activities and with one's hospital. The two consensus variables we constructed indicate the standard deviations of scores around the means of each of the satisfaction measures calculated within wards of five or more responding nurses. Thus, nurses from wards with fewer than four responding colleagues were not assigned consensus scores. The resulting scores indicate that nurses with high scores come from wards with greater "dissensus" in common job satisfaction; reciprocally, nurses receiving low scores come from wards with much consensus. Small group research frequently has shown the importance of such consensus in regulating group behavior. Deviants are excluded or treated as marginal when they do not meet group norms.

Work group influence has also been shown to be important. Benne and Bennis (1959) were concerned with the influence of work groups, hospitals, and doctors on nurses' responses to ideal and actual situations. One of their recommendations was that future research include the school of nursing the person graduated from and his or her professional association among such sources of influence. They believed that the inclusion of such additional reference groups would have provided a better understanding of the responses of (outpatient department) nurses in their sample. Because we were interested in the influence of reference groups upon nurses' job satisfaction, those included in the Benne and Bennis study, as well as those recommended, were included in this investigation. This information was indexed by having respondents rank each of the following sources in order of their importance in influencing their work activities: professional association, school of nursing, work group, spouse, hospital, and doctors. The category for spouses was not included in the analysis since all nurses presently not married would have had to be excluded in order to do so. High numbers on any of the resultant scales for sources of influence, then, indicate low perceived importance for that particular source.

Facets of Activities

Many indicators of activity-related facets of nursing were included in the questionnaire to represent the following four basic dimensions: enjoyment of routine physical activities of nursing, enjoyment of routine social activities of nursing, satisfaction with the intrinsic rewards of nursing, and satisfaction with the extrinsic rewards of nursing. Scales were developed from these indicators to represent each of the four dimensions. A description of these items and their summated scales are given in Appendix A.

RESULTS AND DISCUSSION

The Univariate Distribution

As can be seen from Table 27–1 the nurses were, on the whole, very satisfied with the hospitals they worked in and somewhat satisfied with the routine activities that occupied most of their time. On a scale from 1 to 6, with 6 being the highest score, the mean score for satisfaction with hospital was 5.4. Likewise, with 10 as the highest score on a 10-point scale, mean satisfaction with activities was 7.4. Both distributions, then, are highly skewed, with the preponderant number of cases piling up at the very satisfied end of each scale. The correlation between the two satisfaction measures is .29. When a linear, standardized job satisfaction scale was constructed from these variables (see Appendix A), it retained the same skewed distribution.

From examining these intitial results we see the same pattern of the "happy worker" that is almost universally found in other job satisfaction studies.

Table 27-1   Means, Standard Deviations, Medians, and Skews of Facet-Free Satisfaction Measures

	Satisfaction with hospitals	Satisfaction with activities	Total job satisfaction scale
Means	5.4	7.4	0.0
Standard deviations	1.1	2.4	.8
Medians	5.7	8.0	.2
Skew	−1.9	−.9	−1.1
Sample size	465	445	444

Nurses, on the whole, are highly satisfied with their work and with the hospitals in which they work. This is true despite the fact that at the time of the survey our sample was considering a strike in favor of higher pay. Our data, therefore, would not support any suggestions that nurses who want more salary or who are fomenters of organizational problems are also dissatisfied with their jobs. Crozier (1964) also found this to be true in his study of bureaucracies, where the productive, satisfied workers were willing to stay out on strike the longest.

Given the way the cases pile up at the satisfied end of the distributions, we would suspect that persons who would have been dissatisfied with a particular hospital either took jobs at other hospitals they found more satisfying or left the profession. Likewise, persons who would have been dissatisfied with some or all the standard nursing activities either were unlikely to have entered the profession or were highly likely to have left. It is likely that an additional factor is that people tend to learn to adapt to their working conditions and thereby become satisfied with them over time. As we shall show momentarily, a mean breakdown of the satisfaction measures on length of employment is consistent with these possible explanations.

Mean Breakdowns

While Table 27-1 indicates a high degree of job satisfaction among nurses, we would want to know what variables would account for the distribution of scores on the satisfaction measures. Therefore in Table 27-2, mean breakdowns are provided for each of the satisfaction measures across the major demographic, organizational, setting, and activities variables described earlier. We shall first explore the relationships of the basic demographic variables with the satisfaction measures.

Demographic Variables

Age is significantly related to satisfaction with hospital and with activities, accounting for 7 and 5 percent of the variation of each, respectively. The trends include fairly straightforward monotonic distributions of increasing satisfaction with the hospital in which respondents were working and the activities they engaged in as their age ranges increased. The greatest exception to this monotonicity in the distributions is a drop in the mean satisfaction with activities between ages of 50 and 54. The distribution for overall job satisfaction, while containing more slight deviations from monotonicity also suggest a positive relation between age and satisfaction. Of course our cross-sectional data would not allow us to conclude that increasing age and its correlates *lead to* increasing job satisfaction; still, such a conclusion is tempting and consistent with our findings to this point (see Glenn, Taylor, and Weaver, 1977).

Nurses who are divorced, widowed, or separated tend to be happier with the hospital in which they work than are nurses who are single or married. Singles and marrieds are virtually indistinguishable in their levels of satisfaction. The difference between the widowed, divorced, and separated on

Table 27-2 Mean Breakdowns of Demographic Variables, Organizational Position Variables, Contextual Variables, and Facet of Nursing Activities Variables on the Satisfaction Measures

	Hospital satisfaction scale	Activities satisfaction scale	Job satisfaction scale
Age			
Sig. of F	.00‡	.00‡	.00‡
ETA squared	.07	.05	.06
Grand mean	5.4	7.4	0.0
20–24	5.0	6.8	−.3
25–29	5.1	7.1	−.2
30–34	5.1	7.6	−.0
35–39	5.1	7.4	−.1
40–44	5.5	7.8	.2
45–49	5.6	7.5	.1
50–54	5.6	7.7	.2
55–59	5.8	6.3	.0
60–64	5.8	8.4	.4
65 +	5.7	8.6*	.4*
Marital status			
Sig. of F	.06	.46	.16
ETA squared	.02	.00	.01
Grand mean	5.4	7.4	0.0
Single	5.2	7.3	−.1
Married	5.3	7.4	.0
Separated	6.0†	8.8†	.6†
Widowed	5.7	8.0	.3
Divorced	5.7	6.9	.0
Highest education			
Sig. of F	.09	.27	.05¶
ETA squared	.02	.01	.02
Grand mean	5.4	7.4	0.0
2-yr assoc. degree	5.6*	6.8*	0.0*
3-yr diploma	5.4	7.5	0.0
3-yr diploma plus bachelor's degree	5.5	7.7	.1
4–5 yr college	5.2	7.1	−.1
M.A. or M.S.	5.0	6.7	−.3

* Fewer than 5 cases.
† Fewer than 10 cases.
‡ Significant at ≤ .01 level.
¶ Significant at ≤ .05 level.

Table 27-2 Continued

	Hospital satisfaction scale	Activities satisfaction scale	Job satisfaction scale
Social class of father			
Sig. of F	.88	.23	.51
ETA squared	.00	.01	.01
Grand mean	5.3	7.4	0.0
Low	5.3	8.1	.1
	5.3	7.4	0.0
	5.3	7.2	0.0
	5.4	7.4	0.0
High	5.2	6.7	−.2
Religion			
Sig. of F	.03 ¶	.55 ¶	.05
ETA squared	.01	.00	.01
Grand mean	5.3	7.4	0.0
Catholic	5.2	7.2	−.1
Protestant	5.4	7.4	.0
Employed time			
Sig. of F	.00 ‡	.08 ‡	.00
ETA squared	.07	.04	.07
Grand mean	5.3	7.4	.0
< 3 months	5.3	7.3	.0
3–12 months	4.8	6.8	−.3
1–3 years	5.3	7.2	.1
3–6 years	5.4	7.3	.0
6–9 years	5.7	8.0	.4
9–12 years	5.7	8.0	.3
12–15 years	5.5	7.9	.2
15–18 years	5.5	7.8	.2
18 + years	5.7	7.9	.3
Staff position			
Sig. of F	.88	.43	.49
ETA squared	.00	.01	.01
Grand mean	5.3	7.4	.0
Staff nurse	5.3	7.4	.0
Assist. head nurse	5.1	6.2	−.4
Head nurse	5.4	7.3	.0
Supervisor	5.4	7.3	.0
Asst. director of nurses	5.0 †	8.3 †	.0 †

* Fewer than 5 cases.
† Fewer than 10 cases.
‡ Significant at ≤ .01 level.
¶ Significant at ≤ .05 level.

Table 27-2 Continued

	Hospital satisfaction scale	Activities satisfaction scale	Job satisfaction scale
Part time–full time			
Sig. of F	.66	.25	.66
ETA squared	.00	.00	.00
Grand mean	5.3	7.4	.0
Part time	5.3	7.6	.0
Full time	5.4	7.3	.0
Work shift			
Sig. of F	.63	.66	.76
ETA squared	.00	.00	.00
Grand mean	5.4	7.4	.0
Day	5.4	7.3	.0
Evening	5.3	7.3	−.1
Night	5.3	7.7	.0
Rotating	5.2	7.4	−.1
Hospital			
Sig. of F	.00[‡]	.16	.00[‡]
ETA squared	.07	.01	.04
Grand mean	5.4	7.4	.0
A	5.3	7.0	−.1
B	4.9	7.4	−.2
C	5.6	7.5	.1
Perceived professional association influence			
Sig. of F	.15	.27	.10
ETA squared	.02	.02	.02
Grand mean	5.3	7.3	.0
High	5.6	7.5	.2
	5.2	7.1	−.1
	5.2	6.9	−.2
	5.4	7.6	.1
	5.3	7.6	.0
	5.1	6.9	−.2
Low	5.2	7.5	.0
Perceived school of nursing influence			
Sig. of F	.36	.52	.55
ETA squared	.02	.01	.01
Grand mean	5.3	7.3	.0
High	5.5	7.2	.0
	5.6	7.4	.1
	5.2	7.8	.0
	5.2	7.6	.0
	5.2	7.1	−.1
	5.4	7.4	.0
Low	5.2	6.6	−.2

Table 27-2 Continued

	Hospital satisfaction scale	Activities satisfaction scale	Job satisfaction scale
Perceived work group influence			
Sig. of F	.59	.46	.32
ETA squared	.01	.01	.01
Grand mean	5.3	7.4	.0
High	5.3	7.5	.0
	5.3	7.4	.0
	5.4	7.3	.0
	5.2	6.9	−.2
	5.6	8.0	.2
Low	5.7*	7.2	.2*
Perceived hospital influence			
Sig. of F	.01‡	.63	.07
ETA squared	.04	.01	.03
Grand mean	5.3	7.4	.00
High	5.5	7.6	.1
	5.5	7.5	.1
	5.4	7.3	.0
	5.2	7.4	−.1
	5.1	6.7	−.3
	5.4	6.7	−.1
Low	4.0*	6.8*	−.8*
Perceived doctors influence			
Sig. of F	.82	.66	.90
ETA squared	.01	.01	.00
Grand mean	5.3	7.3	.0
High	5.2	7.9	.0
	5.3	7.2	−.1
	5.3	7.4	.0
	5.4	7.0	.0
	5.4	7.5	.0
	5.2	7.4	−.1
Low	5.2*	6.4*	−.3
Ward consensus on satisfaction with hospital			
Sig. of F	.00‡	.70	.00‡
ETA squared	.11	.00	.05
Grand mean	5.3	7.4	.0
High	5.8	7.5	.2
	5.6	7.4	.1
	5.0	7.2	−.2
Low	4.9	7.5	−.2

* Fewer than 5 cases.
† Fewer than 10 cases.
‡ Significant at ≤ .01 level.
¶ Significant at ≤ .05 level.

Table 27-2 Continued

	Hospital satisfaction scale	Activities satisfaction scale	Job satisfaction scale
Ward consensus on satisfaction with routine activities			
Sig. of F	.01 ‡	.00 ‡	.00 ‡
ETA squared	.03	.06	.04
Grand mean	5.3	7.4	.0
High	5.6	8.1	.2
	5.1	7.8	.0
	5.2	7.3	-.1
Low	5.4	6.5	-.2
Ward type			
Sig. of F	.54	.03 ¶	.05 ¶
ETA squared	.01	.03	.03
Grand mean	5.4	7.4	.0
Medical	5.4	7.3	.0
Surgical	5.3	7.2	-.1
Labor, del., obst., nursery	5.6	8.2	.2
OPD/ER	5.3	6.8	-.2
Pediatrics	5.2	7.1	-.1
Enjoyment of physical activities of nursing scale			
Sig. of F	.00 ‡	.00 ‡	.00 ¶
ETA squared	.07	.09	.12
Grand mean	5.4	7.3	.0
Low	5.0	6.2	-.4
	5.2	7.1	-.1
	5.5	8.1	.2
High	5.7	7.9	.2
Enjoyment of social activities of nursing scale			
Sig. of F	.00 ‡	.66	.02 ¶
ETA squared	.04	.00	.02
Grand mean	5.4	7.4	.0
Low	5.1	7.3	-.1
	5.3	7.3	-.1
	5.4	7.3	.0
High	5.6	7.6	.2
Satisfaction with intrinsic reward scale			
Sig. of F	.00 ‡	.00 ¶	.00 ‡
ETA squared	.16	.19	.26
Grand mean	5.4	7.4	.0
Low	4.7	5.8	-.7
	5.3	7.2	-.1
	5.7	7.9	.3
High	5.7	8.7	.4

Table 27-2 Continued

	Hospital satisfaction scale	Activities satisfaction scale	Job satisfaction scale
	Satisfaction with extrinsic reward scale		
Sig. of F	.00‡	.00‡	.00‡
ETA squared	.09	.05	.11
Grand mean	5.4	7.4	.0
Low	4.9	6.5	-.4
	5.3	7.6	.0
	5.5	7.4	.1
High	5.7	8.0	.3

* Fewer than 5 cases.
† Fewer than 10 cases.
‡ Significant at ≤ .01 level.
¶ Significant at ≤ .05 level.

the one hand and the singles and married on the other are close to significance at the .05 level only with regard to satisfaction with the hospital. No significant differences in satisfaction with activities or overall job satisfaction appear among the marital statuses. It is possibly the case that separated, widowed, and divorced nurses look more to their jobs to give them their basic satisfactions in life and are more dependent on their jobs for survival since mean satisfaction levels for these marital statuses tend to be the highest in each satisfaction distribution (with the exception of divorced nurses, who have the lowest satisfaction with their activities). We cannot fully account for this state of affairs, however.

The effect of nursing education is fairly linear and negative on the satisfaction expressed for working in the hospital and for total job satisfaction. This relationship is significant at the .05 level, however, only for the composite job satisfaction measure. A nonsignificant curvilinear trend was found for satisfaction with activities such that those with the lowest and those with the highest educations were least satisfied. It is ironic that increasing levels of education should be associated with decreasing levels of job satisfaction, given the prevailing emphasis on enhancing the amount of nursing education. This negative relationship has also been noted by other researchers (Bruce, Bonjean, and Williams, 1968; Vollmer and Kinney,

1955). It is possible that nurses who are more highly educated hold higher standards and expectations for their conditions of employment and are more professionally committed; they could therefore be more dissatisfied with the actual conditions of their work. Though the curvilinear trend is nonsignificant, it is also possible that nurses with lower numbers of years of education could also be somewhat dissatisfied owing to the restricted mobility into head nurse and supervisor positions. People with restricted mobility options have been shown to be less committed to their organizations and to focus their attentions on other types of nonorganizational activities (Kanter, 1977).

The social class of nurses' fathers did not significantly affect the satisfaction the nurses felt on any of the three measures. The nonsignificant trends suggest increasing satisfaction with nursing activities as background socioeconomic status (SES) decreased; this would imply that being upwardly mobile could make a minor contribution to job satisfaction, with the downwardly mobile, vis-à-vis the fathers' SES, being least satisfied.

A significant difference on satisfaction with hospital and overall job satisfaction was found by religion, with Protestants being more satisfied than Catholics. While there might be some temptation here to invoke the Protestant work ethic to account for this difference, we must keep in mind that no significant difference between religions is found with regard to satisfaction with work activities. As we shall indicate below we believe that the observed differences in satisfaction by religion are an artifact of the effect of hospitals.

Organizational Variables

We turn now to organizational variables. Length of employment significantly accounted for 7 percent of the variance in nurses' satisfaction with their hospitals. This distribution is roughly positive, with nurses longer employed at the hospital tending to be more satisfied. A drop in satisfaction is noted among those nurses who have been at their hospital for 3 to 12 months. It is perhaps at this time that the least satisfied are more likely to look for other work, leaving behind the more satisfied to contribute to the higher observed mean levels in groups who stay longer, or some form of situational adaptation may also occur. Thus, as nurses develop more friends and greater colleagueship, their satisfaction level may increase. This may also be the period when there is highest turnover, a point which needs to be explored in further research because of its relevance for professional attrition as well as turnover. While nonsignificant, this pattern is roughly the same for satisfaction with activities, accounting for 4 percent of the variance in this latter variable.

Nursing position in the organization does not significantly account for variation in any of the satisfaction measures. While no overall significant trend is apparent, assistant head nurses tend to be the least satisfied. In contrast, assistant directors of nurses (a small but fully represented population) tend to be most satisfied with their activities and most dissatisfied with their hospital; this latter finding might reflect their current reaction to the intrainstitutional pressures related to salary demands by nurses. Neither of the remaining variables of working *part-time or full-time* or of *shift worked* has a significant effect on job satisfaction.

Contextual Variables

Turning to contextual variables, the hospital in which one works does not significantly affect satisfaction with routine activities, but does significantly affect one's satisfaction with the hospital itself and with overall job satisfaction (with 7 percent of the variance accounted for in the first case and 4 percent in the latter). Keeping in mind that one of the three hospitals was Catholic-affiliated, it is no surprise, as is shown in Table 27-3, that religious preference is highly associated with the hospital in which one works. Thus there is good reason to believe that the earlier noted effect of religion on job satisfaction is unduly inflated. We shall demonstrate this more conclusively in our subsequent multivariate analysis.

Ward type significantly affects satisfaction with routine nurses' activities and with overall job satisfaction. In both cases, labor, delivery, obstetrics, and nursery wards have highest satisfaction while outpatient department (OPD) and emergency room lead the rest of the wards for having the lowest satisfaction. We would speculate that obstetrical-related units tend to deal with "healthy", "normal" processes (e.g., birth) rather than pathological processes and thus may result in less stress and anxiety than might be present in other units. Emergency units are generally recognized as stress-producing. It is also in such units as emergency and OPD that health professionals are in greater "organizational boundary positions," which are constrained by greater and more immediate public visibility and demands; such conditions have been found to be stress-producing in other types of organizations (Kahn et al., 1964).

Of the major perceived sources of influence on

Table 27-3 Percentages of Religious Affiliation by Hospital

	Catholic	Protestant	N
Hospital A	20.7%	79.3%	92
Hospital B	73.2%	26.8%	97
Hospital C	22.8%	77.2%	228

nursing practice (professional association, school of nursing, work group, hospital, and doctors), only perceived hospital influence significantly affected one of the satisfaction measures at the .05 level. The single significant effect indicates that those who tend to see the hospital as most influential in its effects on their work tend also to be more satisfied working at the hospital. (The aberrant jump in satisfaction toward that end of the scale that indicated less influence by the hospital is based on only 11 cases and hence does not represent a significant departure from monotonicity.) The human relations school suggests that people who derive their status from an organization are more satisfied with that organization. If such is the case, an endorsement of a hospital as a source of influence might legitimate that organizational influence. On the other hand, it might also reflect the reality of the policies and organizational structure of the hospital in its direct influence on what nurses do and how it is done.

The degree of impact is fairly substantial for the way in which a ward's consensus in the satisfaction of its members will affect the satisfaction of each individual nurse. Where ward consensus is high on satisfaction or dissatisfaction with the hospital, nurses will tend to have significantly more satisfaction with the hospital they work in and with the overall job. As much as 11 percent of the variation in hospital satisfaction is accounted for by this effect.

There is no effect, however, of ward consensus with regard to hospital satisfaction on nurses' satisfaction with the activities they perform. Ward consensus on satisfaction or dissatisfaction with routine ward activities, by contrast, related significantly to individual nurses' responses to all three satisfaction measures. The relationship is linear in two cases, with higher consensus leading to higher satisfaction with activities and overall job satisfaction. It is, however, curvilinear for satisfaction with hospital, with high satisfaction for both high and low consensus. We cannot offer an interpretation for this latter, unexpected result,

but the strength of the other linear relations between consensus and satisfaction suggests that nurses are much affected by the harmony in views held by their work groups. Discord in coworkers views will serve to decrease a nurse's job satisfaction. Much small-group research would suggest that consensus is important and that people who do not conform become marginal to the group.

Facets of Nursing Activities

Finally, we shall examine the effects of the scaled measures (descriptions of the scales are included in Appendix A). Enjoyment of physical activities of nursing significantly affects all three satisfaction measures, accounting for as much as 12 percent of the variance in total job satisfaction. These effects are all monotonically positive. The same pattern of effects is seen for the enjoyment of social activities of nursing scale, though the effects are nowhere near as strong and are nonsignificant for satisfaction with routine activities. The intrinsic rewards scale accounts for a huge 26 percent of the variance in total job satisfaction; its relation to all three satisfaction measures is significant and positive. Finally, the extrinsic reward scale yields significant, positive, monotonic relations to all satisfaction measures and accounts for as much as 11 percent of the variance in total job satisfaction. In sum, all four scales are significant and positively related to all the satisfaction measures at the zero order, with the exception of a nonsignificant relation between enjoyment of social activities and satisfaction with one's routine activities.

Multivariate Regression Analysis

The whole story of the effect of a variable in producing variation in another variable is not always fully revealed in analyses of such simple zero-order relations as have thus far been represented in mean breakdowns. To observe and compare the effects of all variables simultaneously, we need to utilize multivariate statistical techniques. We shall do so using multivariate regressions. When the above

described variables are entered into three prediction equations, one for each of the satisfaction
measures, the resulting net standardized effects
of each variable are as given in Table 27-4.

When correction is made for the degrees of

freedom constrained by the number of variables
entering each equation, we find that about a third
of the variance in nurses' satisfaction with hospital
and overall job satisfaction can be explained with
the variables entered into the equations, while

Table 27-4   Multiple Regressions of All Variables on the Three-Satisfaction Measures[†]

Independent variables	Satisfaction with hospital	Satisfaction with activities	Total job satisfaction
Adjusted R^2	.34	.26	.38
A Demographic variables			
1 Religion	-.02	.09	.05
2 Age	.19*	.00	.11
3 Marital status	NS[†]	NS	NS
4 Education	-.01	0.0	-.02
5 Father's SES	.02	-.07	-.02
B Organizational position variables			
6 Time employed by hospital	.02	.06	.04
7 Staff position	NS	NS	NS
8 Full time–part time	-.03	-.07	-.06
9 Work shift	NS	NS	NS
C Contextual variables			
10 Hospital employed at	SIG[‡]	NS	NS
11 Ward type	NS	NS	NS
12 Ward consensus on satisfaction with the hospital	-.28*	.11	.10
13 Ward consensus on satisfaction with routine activities	-.02	-.20*	-.14*
14 Influence by professional	-.04	.08	.02
15 Influence by school of nursing	0.0	-.02	-.01
16 Influence by work groups	-.01	-.06	-.04
17 Influence by hospital	-.08	0.0	-.06
18 Influence by doctors	0.0	.00	.01
D Facets of nursing activities			
19 Enjoyment of physical work activities scale	.07	.25*	.20*
20 Enjoyment of social work activities scale	.05	-.16*	-.06
21 Intrinsic rewards scale	.28*	.36*	.40*
22 Extrinsic rewards scale	.14*	.05*	.12*

Dependent measures (N = 316)

*Significant at the ≤ .05 level, one-tail test.
[†]NS means combined effect of the categorical variable is not significant.
[‡]SIG means the difference between means for hospital B and C is significant at the ≤ .05 level.
[†]A pairwise present correlation matrix is used with a *minimum subsample size of 316 cases*.
Results are given in standardized coefficients with the categorical variables of marital status, staff
position, work shift and wardtype pooled as either not significant (NS) at the .05 level, two-tailed
test, or significant (SIG). R² is adjusted for the degrees of freedom within the equations.

about a fourth of the variance in satisfaction with nursing activities is similarly explained. Though ideally we would like to account for all the variance in these three satisfaction measures and thereby perfectly specify all the conditions that are needed to account for nursing satisfaction, it is very unusual in the social sciences to account for as much variance as we have here.

Demographic Variables

Looking first at the demographic variables, one sees that only age has a significant effect on a satisfaction measure. Net of all other variables, older nurses are more likely to be satisfied with the hospital in which they work than are younger nurses. Marital status, education, father's background, SES, and religion have no significant net effects on nurses' satisfaction. Thus the earlier described zero-order effects of education and religion on job satisfaction are eliminated in this multivariate analysis, as are the effects of age on satisfaction with activities and total job satisfaction. Net of the other variables in the analysis, education and religion do not directly affect job satisfaction. Age continues its direct effect only for satisfaction with the hospital.

Organizational Position Variables

No organizational position variable makes a significant net contribution to explaining variance in any of the satisfaction variables. The significant zero-order effect of employment time has now been totally controlled. It is likely that employment time is a mediator for the effects of age on job satisfaction since employment time and age are correlated at .62, but the effect of employment time must itself be mediated by unknown factors.

Contextual Variables

Among the contextual variables, the hospital in which one is employed has a significant net effect on satisfaction with the hospital. An increment of R^2 test indicates that, net of all other variables, nurses at hospital A are significantly more satisfied with their hospital than are those at hospital B. (Hospital A and C have almost identical estimated means levels of satisfaction net of all other variables.) Hospital B is the Catholic-sponsored hospital, with 73.2 percent of its nurses declaring themselves to be Catholic. Hospital A, by contrast, is nonreligiously sponsored, with 79.3 percent of its nurses declaring themselves to be Protestant. Thus, while our zero-order analysis has suggested that Protestant nurses are more satisfied with their hospital than are Catholic nurses, we can now see that the hospital in which one works is the more important net contributor and has inflated the zero-order relation between religion and satisfaction.

There are no net differences among wards in their effects on the three satisfaction measures. The earlier observed zero-order differences do not appear here and are probably mediated by enjoyment-of-nursing-activities measures.

Some significant effects of ward consensus, however, did occur. Increasing consensus of ward satisfaction or dissatisfaction with the hospital significantly increases nurses satisfaction with hospital net of all other variables, but does not affect satisfaction with activities or overall satisfaction. Increasing consensus of ward satisfaction or dissatisfaction with routine activities, on the other hand, does significantly increase nurses' satisfaction with their activities and their overall satisfaction. We can see in this multivariate analysis, then, that consensus of satisfaction on the ward continues to have a strong impact on the satisfaction a nurse feels. A lack of ward agreement on satisfaction or dissatisfaction decreases one's satisfaction at work.

While, as we saw earlier, the perceived influence of the hospital on nurses' activities had a significant zero-order effect on satisfaction with their hospital, no setting influence source (professional association, school of nursing, work group, hospital, or doctors) now has a significant effect on nursing satisfaction. It is interesting that neither the perception of hospital influence nor the perception of work group influence yields a net effect on any satisfaction measure, while we have shown that the actual fact is that the total milieu of the hospital in which a nurse works and the consensus of the ward does affect job satisfaction. These findings are consistent with social scientific literature that suggests that we are often unaware of the influence exerted upon us by our environment.

Facets of Nursing Activities

Turning to the facets of activities scales, we note that neither enjoyment of the physical activities of nursing nor enjoyment of the social activities contributes to satisfaction with the hospital. Thus a nurse's satisfaction in working at a hospital is not directly dependent on whether the nurse finds routine nursing activities are enjoyable. These net findings mitigate the earlier reported zero-order findings and suggest that the effects of enjoyment of nursing activities on satisfaction with one's hospital are mediated by some as yet unidentified factors.

Both the scales for enjoyment of physical activities and that for enjoyment of social activities, however, make significant net contributions to explaining variance in satisfaction with those nursing activities that occupy most of one's time. The more nurses enjoy routine physical activities, the more likely it is that they will report satisfaction with the routine activities they generally perform. While no significant zero-order relationship appeared between enjoyment of social activities and satisfaction with routine nursing activities, the net relation between these two variables is now *significantly negative*! Nurses who enjoy social activities on the job tend to express less satisfaction with the activities that occupy most of their time. We should not be misled by this finding. Our data do not suggest that nurses are antisocial. On a scale from 1 to 7, with 7 as a high score, the average enjoyment by all nurses of the various social activities included in the composite social activities scale ranged from a low of 5.5 to a high of 6.3. Most of these averages hovered about 6.0. By contrast, their enjoyment of the various physical activities ranged from 4.5 to 6.3, with many scores hovering about 5.5. Furthermore, we found that the degree of enjoyment nurses expressed for the various physical and social activities exceeded the frequency with which they were able to engage in those activities, and the magnitude of these discrepancies was on the average about a third larger for social activities than for physical activities.

One could interpret these results as indicating that nurses who enjoy socializing on the job find less opportunity to do so than they desire; hence they are less satisfied with those activities that do in fact occupy most of their time. By contrast, nurses who enjoy physical activities find the amount of physical activities required of them relatively adequate to keep them satisfied. The correlation between the two enjoyment-of-activities scales is moderately strong and positive at .46. Many nurses, then, might face the conflicting pressures of satisfaction derived from their work because of their enjoyment of its required physical activities and dissatisfactions due to limitations on its social activities, which they also otherwise enjoy.[1]

For overall job satisfaction, only enjoyment of the physical activities of nursing now makes a significant net contribution to variance explained. This relationship is positive and emphasizes the importance for nursing satisfaction of enjoying such activities as giving medications, giving treatments, charting, noting orders, collecting specimens, providing direct physical care to patients, and working with instruments, trays, and other equipment. Net of all other variables, persons who do not enjoy these activities tend to be the least satisfied in the nursing profession.

Turning finally to the intrinsic and extrinsic rewards of work, we see that the composite scale for intrinsic rewards provides a strong, positive, net effect on all the satisfaction measures. Our data indicate that nurses who find their work

---

[1] In a paper in preparation, we show that this interpretation is not supported by further analyses. Consequently the finding remains puzzling and may be a fluke. A research replication is much needed.

self-fulfilling are more satisfied in general with their jobs and in particular with the hospital they work in and the activities that occupy most of their time. The contribution of extrinsic rewards to nursing satisfaction is smaller and does not affect satisfaction with nursing activities. The extrinsic reward scale, which consists of variables for satisfaction with salary, nurses' perception of the concern for their welfare by people for whom they work, and anticipated opportunity for promotion, significantly contributes to variance explained in satisfaction with the hospital in which the nurse works and overall job satisfaction. These effects are such that nurses who perceive higher extrinsic rewards in their work are more satisfied on these two dimensions. Nurses who perceive either high or low extrinsic rewards, however, are not necessarily more or less satisfied with the activities that occupy most of their time. Thus while a policy of increasing extrinsic rewards for nurses may result in their being more satisfied overall with their jobs and more satisfied with the hospitals in which they work, it will not significantly increase their satisfaction with their routine activities.

A Standardized Comparison and Summary

Looking across the standardized coefficients, we note that the two strongest contributors to nurses' satisfaction with their hospital are the intrinsic rewards of their work (i.e., the degree to which they find the work self-fulfilling) and the degree to which their ward is cohesive in its view of the satisfactory character of the hospital. Next in importance is age and finally come the extrinsic rewards they perceived as being offered at the hospital and the total milieu of the hospital itself. Other variables that might be expected to contribute to satisfaction, such as enjoyment of nursing duties and organizational position, have no significant influence.

The single largest contributor to satisfaction with the activities that occupy most of nurses' time is the degree to which they find their work

intrinsically rewarding. Next in importance is their enjoyment of physical activities, and then the consensus of satisfaction and dissatisfaction among their colleagues on the same ward with the routine activities of that ward. Last, is enjoyment of the social activities associated with the nursing practice. No other variable in the regression, such as the demographic variables or organizational position variables, yields a significant net effect on satisfaction with routine activities. It is particularly interesting that organizational position variables would not directly affect satisfaction with routine nursing activities since the nature of those activities should vary by organizational position. Our data would suggest therefore, that changes in one's staff position will not increase one's satisfaction with one's work.

In accounting for overall job satisfaction, intrinsic rewards are again the most important contributor. These are followed in importance by enjoyment of physical activities and then by ward consensus on satisfaction or dissatisfaction with routine activities and by extrinsic rewards. Net of these variables, the hospital these nurses worked in, the ward type they were associated with, the perceived sources of influence on their routine work, their basic demographic characteristics and organizational positions, and their enjoyment of social activities at work had no significant net effect on their overall job satisfaction.

OUTCOME MEASURES

Although, the primary purpose of the study was to identify the variables that contributed to job satisfaction for a total sample of nurses from three different types of hospitals, we were also concerned with the consequences of job satisfaction for this particular group. Attempts to find the exact causal relationship between independent and dependent measures of most of the job satisfaction investigations have assumed that certain aspects of work give rise to job satisfaction. It is also possible that being satisfied in general with your work will make you more satisfied with certain aspects of your job. As outcome measures of job satisfaction we selected two variables—"I would be pleased to have a daughter of mine choose to be a nurse"; and, commitment to work in general—"I would choose to work even if it were not economically necessary." We doubt that a nurse who is not satisfied with nursing would be pleased to have a daughter choose that profession. The second question, though not directly related to commitment to working as a nurse, should indicate the intrinsic value of nursing to the respondents. The correlations between these two items and the measures of satisfaction are as follows:

dent variables. Additional comments about job satisfaction and outcome measures used in other studies are indicated. Wanous (1974) in studying telephone operators reported a relationship between job satisfaction and performance; the direction of causality in the relationship, however, was unclear. Additional research shows that performance is most highly related to job satisfaction and job involvement of high-need achievers. McDonald (1972) in a study of navy personnel noted relationships between job satisfaction, the health opinion survey, and the number of dispensary visits. He suggested that increased illnesses in military settings were related to job dissatisfaction.

	Hospital satisfaction (n = 465)	Activity satisfaction (n = 445)	Total satisfaction (n = 444)
Pleased to have daughter choose nursing	.15	.22	.23
Choose to work even if not economically necessary	.26	.29	.34

It can be seen that at the zero-order level the two outcome measures are moderately related to the three satisfaction measures, with hospital satisfaction being least relevant to pleasure at having a daughter choose nursing. From these findings one could tentatively infer that as job satisfaction increased, so would positive responses to having a daughter choose nursing and to one's commitment to work. We have found that, among all variables entered into the previous regressions, the intrinsic rewards of work are the most highly related to these two outcome measures, as well as to job satisfaction itself. Thus, for continued recruitment through current practicing nurses, job redesign which would increase the intrinsic measures would increase not only job satisfaction but recruitment and retention of nurses as well.

We have in the analysis section suggested the implications for nursing of the various indepen-

There is also research that indicates that higher job satisfaction is associated with less job anxiety (Srivastava and Sinha, 1972). Steers (1975) and Gechman (1975) have reported as well that mental health is positively related to job satisfaction, but unrelated to job involvement. Daubs (1973) has also reported a relationship between occupational health (absenteeism, injury, longevity, mobility, and occupational mortality rates) and suggested that suicide is related to job dissatisfaction; he discussed the implications of these variables for optometrists in increasing their job satisfaction and thus reducing their suicide incidence. Though there were methodological problems associated with his study, such as an ecological fallacy, his suggestions should not be overlooked and mental health measures should receive more attention. Schar, Reeder, and Dirken (1973) have suggested that the most important predictor of cardiovascular disease is the work satisfaction scale—low work satisfaction is accompanied by high stress. To summarize, job satisfaction not only has implications for the recruitment and retention of employees in an occupational group, but for the health of the members as well.

We did not collect data on anxiety, quality of performance, or mental health, and in retrospect think that these dimensions might have contributed to the understanding of job satisfaction either as outcome variables or as independent variables. If there is a causal relationship between job satisfaction and the outcome measures noted above, then job satisfaction is important for nurses not only in terms of recruitment and retention but also for their mental health and job performance—and ultimately for patient care either directly or indirectly; such effects would be of obvious concern not only to professional nurses, but to the entire health delivery establishment and the consumers as well.

APPENDIX A

In any single measure of a characteristic there is some, usually unknown, proportion of error. The magnitude of this error represents the *unreliability* of the measure. The measurement of a characteristic can be made more *reliable*, however, if several independent measures of the characteristic are combined together into a composite *scale*. It is this strategy that we followed in constructing scaled measures of *total job satisfaction, enjoyment of routine physical job activities, enjoyment of routine social activities*, self-fulfilling or *intrinsic rewards of work*, and economic or *extrinsic rewards of work*. In each case, the composite scale was formed by calculating an unweighted sum of the standardized scores for all variables considered relevant to each characteristic of interest. In the case of total job satisfaction, the individual con-

stituent measures of satisfaction with the hospital and with one's routine activities were correlated at .29 and were added together in this fashion to form a composite scale. The variables used in the construction of each of the other composite scales are given in Table 27-A1. The patterns of zero-order correlations of each of the composite variables with the satisfaction measures are also given in the table, as are the reliabilities of each scale.

Since reliabilities run from 0.0 to 1.0, one would hope to have reliabilities as close to 1.0 as possible. Reliabilities of .6 or better, however, are generally considered acceptable for social measures. Of the four scales described in Table 27-A1, only the one for extrinsic rewards possesses a reliability as low as .48. In no way were we able to adjust this scale to improve its reliability. Still, its current formulation exceeds the estimated reliability of any of its composite measures and is our best indicator of extrinsic rewards.

The trends in the zero-order correlations of the variables with the satisfaction measures are generally positive and significant, except for those included in the scale for enjoyment of *social activities*. Interestingly, enjoyment of none of the listed social activities affects nurses' satisfaction with their routine tasks. Furthermore, nurses' satisfaction with hospital and overall job satisfaction are almost entirely unaffected by their enjoyment of social interaction with patients or visitors (an exception is that enjoyment of talking to visitors is somewhat positively associated with overall job satisfaction). Rather, enjoyment of interaction with colleagues on the job includes almost the only significant (positive) effects on these latter satisfaction measures. Working with things or interacting with colleagues may involve more certainty and control, and hence less negotiation than does talking with patients and visitors, when what is said must be more carefully monitored because of the implications for the image of health care.

Table 27-A1 Zero-Order Correlation of All Scale Items with the Three Satisfaction Measures: 1) Satisfaction with Hospital; 2) Satisfaction with Activities that Occupy Most of One's Time; 3) Total Job Satisfaction.

Enjoyment of physical activities scale

Variables in scale	Satisfaction measures		
	1	2	3
1. Enjoy giving medications	.22*	.17*	.25*
2. Enjoy giving treatments	.15*	.15*	.19*
3. Enjoy charting	.21*	.20*	.25*
4. Enjoy noting orders	.24*	.21*	.29*
5. Enjoy collecting specimens	.16*	.21*	.23*
6. Enjoy providing direct physical care to patients	.07*	.17*	.16*
7. Enjoy working with instruments trays and things	.14*	.16*	.19*
Scale reliabilities (Standardized Cronbach's alpha)		.80	

Enjoyment of social activities scale

Variables in scale	Satisfaction measures		
	1	2	3
1. Enjoy talking with patients	.07	.06	.10*
2. Enjoy talking with visitors	-.01	.01	.00
3. Enjoy social chitchat with nurses and other personnel in this area			
4. Enjoy discussing work-related business with other nurses and other personnel in the area.	.15*	.08	.15*
5. Enjoy working with interns, residents, and doctors	.19*	.06	.17*
6. Enjoy supervising others in the provision of patient care	.13*	.07	.14*
7. Enjoy teaching patients	.06	.04	.07
8. Enjoy providing information for patients	.04	-.07	-.01
	.04	-.06	-.01
Scale reliability (Standardized Cronbach's alpha)		.81	

	Satisfaction with intrinsic rewards of work		
1. Chance to do things you do best	.39*	.40*	.48*
2. Feeling of accomplishment from the work you are doing	.44*	.40*	.52*
3. Opportunity to give the type and quality of nursing care which you are capable of giving	.30*	.35*	.40*
4. Opportunity to give the type and quality of nursing care which you think should be given	.28*	.32*	.38*
5. Opportunity to give the type and quality of supervision which you are capable of giving	.24*	.20*	.28*
6. Opportunity to give the type of quality of supervision which you think should be given	.22*	.24*	.29*
7. Feel that the work that you do is important	.28*	.29*	.36*
8. Feel that you are an important member of the health team	.30*	.31*	.33*
9. Feel that you are recognized as an important member of the health team	.31*	.31*	.38*
10. Feel that learning experiences are provided for you within your job	.29*	.22*	.32*
Scale reliability	.87		

	Satisfaction with extrinsic rewards of work		
1. Satisfaction with salary	.21*	.16*	.22*
2. Feel that the people for whom you work are concerned about your welfare	.36*	.26*	.39*
3. Think that you have an opportunity for promotion	.14*	.03	.11*

*Significant at the ≤ .05 level, two-tail.

EDITOR'S QUESTIONS FOR DISCUSSION

What other factors are contributing to a nursing shortage? What emerging problems are schools of nursing experiencing in attracting applicants? In Braito's and Caston's discussion of loyalty conflicts of nurses between professional ideals and nursing service, what other factors and issues need to be considered?

What evidence is there for the implication suggested by Braito and Caston concerning a relationship between understaffing and requirements in providing nursing care? What effects might there be on patient care orientation when nursing theoretical and conceptual frameworks have been implemented into practice settings? In the review of literature concerning issues and research pertaining to job satisfaction and nursing, cite additional research or trends occurring to support or refute the presentation and discussion of findings. What relationships exist between the findings of Mercadante's study (Chap. 21) and Braito and Caston's research? What implications are there in Chap. 3 (Monnig), Chap. 5 (Williamson), Chap. 7 (Peterson), Chap. 8 (Santora), Chap. 9 (Sargis), and Chap. 11 (Dalme) for the issues identified by Braito and Caston as being related to job dissatisfaction?

What are the advantages and disadvantages of facet-free and facet-specific approaches to measurement in research? What advantages and disadvantages are there to examining total populations of nurses within hospitals? Regarding mailed questionnaires, what are the possibilities for bias in the various methods which can be utilized? How can the possibilities for a self-selected sample be minimized? Discuss the validity and reliability of the measures developed for this study?

Are there any other organizational or contextual variables that might have been included in this study? Would the inclusion of nursing process activities and/or activities related to the application of nursing theoretical or conceptual frameworks be an appropriate additional dimension for the scales measuring activity related facets of nursing? How might the inclusion of those activities affect the findings? How might job satisfaction impact on the quality of care provided?

What implications are there for the profession if widowed, divorced, and separated nurses look more to their jobs for survival and basic satisfactions in life than single or married nurses? How do the explanations provided in this study, for the finding that increased levels of education are associated with decreased levels of job satisfaction, correlate with Mercadante's (Chap. 21) findings and interpretation? How does this increased evidence indicate serious implications for nursing education? How can nursing administration effectively deal with the drop in satisfaction that was noted among nurses who have been at their hospital 3 to 12 months? How might you account for assistant directors of nursing being the most satisfied with their activities and assistant head nurses the least satisfied? What other explanations can you offer regarding the strength of the relations between consensus and satisfaction? What unknown factors might mediate the effect of employment time on satisfaction? What unidentified factors might mediate the effects of enjoyment of nursing activities on satisfaction? How might intrinsic rewards be further developed and promoted in the employment of nurses? Are there alternative explanations for the significant findings?

Identify the statistical tests and analysis conducted in this study? What are the criteria for utilizing these tests? What are the advantages and disadvantages of using mean scores in data analysis? If data are highly skewed, is there a test that may appropriately be used? How do you explain the investigator's ability in this study to account for as much variance in the measures as they did? Are there methodological issues resolved in this study? What alternative methods of statistical analysis might be applied to Braito's data?

What suggestions do you have in further research regarding job satisfaction of nurses? What are the implications of this study for nursing practice, nursing administration, nursing education, and the profession?

REFERENCES

Alt, Joyce M., Mary D. Bates, Mary Ann Gilmore, Gary R. Houston, and Robbie S. Stoner
1980   "New hope for 'hands-on' nurses: Clinical promotions." RN 43(6):48–51.
Andrisani, Paul J., Eileen Applebaum, Ross Koppel, and Robert C. Miljus
1978   Work Attitudes and Labor Market Experience: Evidence from the National Longitudinal Surveys. New York: Praeger Publishers.
Argyris, Chris
1964   Integrating the Individual and the Organization. New York: Wiley.
Benne, Kenneth D. and Warren Bennis
1959   "Role confusion and conflict in nursing: The role of the hospital nurse." American Journal of Nursing 59(2):196–198.
Bennis, W. G., N. Berkowitz, M. Affinito, and M. Malone
1959   "Reference groups and loyalties in the out-patient department." Administrative Service Quarterly II 9:481–500.
Bruce, G. D., C. M. Bonjean, and J. A. Williams, Jr.
1968   "Job satisfaction among independent businessmen: A correlative study." Sociology and Social Research 52:195–202.
Bullough, Bonnie and Vern Bullough
1971   "Career ladder in nursing: Problems and prospects." American Journal of Nursing 71(10):1938–43.
1975   "Sex discrimination in health care." Nursing Outlook 23, 1:40–45.
Cherniss, Gary, and Edward Egnatios
1978   "Is there job satisfaction in community mental health?" Community Mental Health Journal 14(4):309–18.
Corwin, Ronald G.
1961   "The professional employee: A study of conflict in nursing roles." The American Journal of Sociology 66:604–615.
Crozier, Michel
1964   Bureaucratic Phenomena. Chicago: University of Chicago Press.

Cummings, L. L., and Chris J. Berger
1976   "Organization structure: How does it influence attitudes and performance." Organization Dynamics 5(2):34–39.
Daubs, J.
1973   "The mental health crisis in ophthalmology." American Journal of Optometry and Archives of American Academy of Optometry 50(10):816–822.
Devereux, George and F. R. Weiner
1950   "The conceptual status of nurses." American Sociological Review 15(5):628–634.
Fein, Mitchell
1976   "Motivation for work." Pp. 465–530 in Robert Dubin (ed.), Handbook of Work, Organization and Society. Chicago: Rand McNally.
Ferree, Myra M.
1976   "Working-class jobs: Housework and paid work as sources of satisfaction." Social Problems 23,4:431–441.
Forster, John F.
1978   "The dollars and sense of an all R.N. staff." Nursing Administration Quarterly 3(1):41–47.
Garfield, Sol L., and Richard M. Kuntz
1975   "Training and career satisfaction among clinical psychologists." Clinical Psychologist 28,2:6–9.
Gechman, Arthur S., and Yoash Wiener
1975   "Job involvement and satisfaction as related to mental health and personal time devoted to work." Journal of Applied Psychology 60(4):521–523.
Georgopoulos, Basil S., and Floyd C. Mann
1962   The Community General Hospital. New York: Macmillan.
Glenn, Norval D., Patricia A. Taylor, and Charles N. Weaver
1977   "Age and job satisfaction among males and females: A multivariate, multi-survey study." Journal of Applied Psychology 62(2):189–193.

Godfrey, Marjorie A.
1978a "Job satisfaction or should that be dissatisfaction?: How nurses feel about nursing. Part one." Nursing 8(4):89–102.
1978b "Job satisfaction or should that be dissatisfaction?: How nurses feel about nursing. Part two." Nursing 8(5):105–120.
1978c "Job satisfaction or should that be dissatisfaction?: How nurses feel about nursing. Part three." Nursing 8(6):81–95.
Green, Charles N. and Dennis W. Organ
1973 "An evaluation of causal models linking the received role with job satisfaction." Administrative Science Quarterly 18(1): 95–103.
Haas, J. Eugene and Thomas E. Drabek
1973 Complex Organizations: A Sociological Perspective. New York: Macmillan.
Habenstein, Robert W., and Edwin A. Christ
1963 Professionalizer, Traditionalizer and Utilizer. Columbia, Missouri: University of Missouri Press.
Herzberg, Frederick, Bernard Mausner, and Barbara B. Snyderman.
1959 The Motivation to Work, 2d ed. New York: Wiley.
Kahn, Robert L., Donald M. Wolfe, Robert P. Quinn, J. Diedrick Snoek, in collaboration with Robert A. Rosenthal
1964 Organizational Stress Studies in Role Conflict and Ambiguity. New York: Wiley.
Kanter, Rosabeth Moss
1977 Men and Women of the Corporation. New York: Basic Books, Inc.
Katz, Daniel and Robert L. Kahn
1978 The Social Psychology of Organizations. New York: Wiley.
Kerlinger, Fred N., and Elazar J. Pedhazur
1973 Multiple Regression in Behavioral Research. New York: Holt, Rinehart and Winston, Inc.
Kesselman, Gerald A., Eileen L. Hagen, and Robert J. Wherry
1974 "A factor analytic test of the Porter-Lawler expectancy model of work motivation." Personnel Psychology 27(4):569–579.

Kesselman, Gerald A., Michael T. Wood, and Eileen L. Hagen
1974 "Relationships between performance and satisfaction under contingent and noncontingent reward systems." Journal of Applied Psychology 59(3):374–376.
Kralewski, John Edward
1969 The Professional Nurse in the Hospital Organization: A Study of Conflict Resolution. University of Minnesota (unpublished doctoral dissertation).
Kramer, M.
1969 "Collegiate graduate nurses in Medical Center Hospital: Mutual challenge or duels." Nursing Research:196–210.
Kramer, Marlene
1974 Reality Shock: Why Nurses Leave Nursing. St. Louis: C. V. Mosby.
Kramer, M., et al.
1972 "Self actualization and role adaptation of baccalaureate degree nurses." Nursing Research 21:111–112.
Kuhn, Robert L., et al.
1964 Organizational Stress: Studies in Role Conflict and Ambiguity. New York: Wiley.
Larsen, Donald E.
1968 "A study of consensus on the role of the psychiatric nurse" (dissertation abstract). Human and Social Sciences 38,10.
Larsen, Otto N.
1964 "Social effects of mass communication," in Robert E. L. Farris (ed.), Handbook of Modern Sociology. Chicago: Rand McNally.
Levine, Eugene
1957 "Turn-over among nursing personnel in in general hospitals." Hospitals, Journal of the American Hospital Association, 31,2:38–42.
Locke, Edwin A.
1976 "The nature and causes of job satisfaction." Pp. 1297–1349 in Marvin D. Dunnette (ed.), Handbook of Industrial and Organizational Psychology. Chicago: Rand McNally.
Lyon, Herbert L., and John M. Ivancevich
1974 "An exploratory investigation of organiza-

tional climate and job satisfaction in a hospital." Academy of Management Journal 17(4):635–648.

Maslow, Abraham H.
1954 Motivation and Personality. New York: Harper & Row.

McCloskey, Joanne Comi
1975 "What rewards will keep nurses on the job?" American Journal of Nursing, 75(4):600–602.

McDonald, Blair W.
1972 Correlates of Job Satisfaction Aboard Navy Ships. Proceedings of the Annual Convention of the American Psychological Association Vol. 7, part 2:635–636.

McLemore, S. Dale and Richard J. Hill
1966 "Role change and socialization in nursing." Pp. 111–122 in Jeanette R. Folta and Edith S. Deck (eds.), Sociological Framework for Patient Care. New York: Wiley.

Menzies, Isabel E. P.
1960 "A case study in the functioning of social systems as a defense against and anxiety." Human Relations, A Journal of Studies Towards the Integration of the Social Sciences 13(2):95–121.

Meyer, Genevieve R., and Mable J. Hoffman
1964 "Nurses' inner values and their behavior at work: A comparison of an expressed preference with observed behavior." Nursing Research 13(3):244–248.

Mortimer, Jaylan T.
1979 Highlights of the Literature: Changing Attitudes Toward Work. Work in America Institute Studies in Productivity. Scarsdale, New York: Work in America Institute, Inc.

Moss, Rosabeth Kanter
1977 Men and Women of the Corporation. New York: Basic Books, Inc.

Palola, Ernest G., and William R. Larson
1965 "Some dimensions of job satisfaction among hospital personnel." Sociology and Research 49:203–213.

Pavalko, Jean Hayter
1971 "Follow-up study of graduates of the University of Kentucky College of Nurs-

ing, 1964–1969." Nursing Research 20: 55–60.

Porter, Lyman W., Richard M. Steers, Richard T. Mowday, and Paul V. Boulian
1974 "Organizational commitment, job satisfaction, and turnover among psychiatric technicians." Journal of Applied Psychology 59(5):603–609.

Price, James L.
1973 "The correlates of turnover." Sociology Working Paper Series #73-1. Iowa City, Iowa: University of Iowa.

Profhansky, Harold, and Bernard Seidenberg (eds.)
1965 Basic Studies in Social Psychology. New York: Holt, Rinehart and Winston.

Reeder, Sharon J. and Hans Mauksch
1979 "Nursing: Continuing change," in Howard E. Freeman, Sol Levine and Leo G. Reeder (eds.), Handbook of Medical Sociology. Englewood Cliffs, New Jersey: Prentice-Hall.

Roberts, Karlene H., Gordon A. Walter, and Raymond E. Miles
1971 "Analytic study of job satisfaction items designed to measure Maslow need categories." Personnel Psychology 24(2): 205–220.

Rose, Mary Ann
1979 "Organization in the hospital: Some strategies for nurses." Nursing Administration Quarterly 3(2):89–93.

Russell, Kevin J.
1975 "Variations in orientation to work and job satisfaction." Sociology of Work and Occupations 2(4):299–322.

Schar, M, L. G. Reeder, and J. M. Dirken
1973 "Stress and cardiovascular health: An international cooperative study: II. The male population of a factory at Zurich." Social Science and Medicine 7(8) (August):585–603.

Scully, D., and P. Bart
1973 "A funny thing happened on the way to the office: Women gynecology textbooks." American Journal of Sociology 79 (January): 1045–1050.

Seashore, Stanley E., and Thomas D. Taber
1975 "Job satisfaction indicators and their

correlates." American Behavioral Scientist 18(3):333–369.

Sharma, Motilan
1975   "Social climate and its relationship with principal effectiveness and teacher satisfaction." Journal of Psychological Research 21(3) (September):105–107.

Siassi, Iradj, Guido Crocetti, and R. Spiro-Herzl
1975   "Emotional health, life and job satisfaction in aging workers." Industrial Gerontology 2(4):289–296.

Smith, Kathryn M.
1965   "Discrepancies in the role-specific values of head nurses and nursing educators." Nursing Research 14:196–202.

Smith, P. C., L. M. Kendall, and C. L. Hulin
1969   The Measurement of Job Satisfaction in Work and Retirement. Chicago: Rand McNally.

Srivastava, A.K., and M.M. Sinha
1972   "An inquiry into the relationship between job satisfaction and job anxiety." Journal of The Indian Academy of Applied Psychology 19(2):39–44.

Stamps, Paula L., Eugene B. Piedmont, Dinah B. Slavitt, and Marie Haase
1978   "Measurement of work satisfaction among health professionals." Medical Care 16(4):337–352.

Steers, Richard M.
1975   "Effects of need for achievement on the job performance–job attitude relation-

ship." Journal of Applied Psychology 60(6):678–682.

Taylor, Kenneth E., and D. J. Weiss
1969   "Prediction of individual job termination from measured job satisfaction and biographical data." Research report No. 30, Work Adjustment Project, University of Minnesota.

Vollmer, M. H., and J. A. Kinney
1955   "Age, education, and job satisfaction." Personnel 32:38–43.

Voydanoff, Patricia
1978   "The relationship between perceived job characteristics and job satisfaction among occupational status groups." Sociology of Work and Occupations 5(2):179–192.

Wanous, John P.
1974   "A causal-correlational analysis of the job satisfaction and performance relationship." Journal of Applied Psychology 59(2):139–144.

Wood, Donald A.
1971   "Background characteristics and work values distinguishing satisfaction levels among engineers." Journal of Applied Psychology 55(6):537–542.

Yett, Donald E.
1965   "The supply of nurses: An economist's view." Hospital Progress 46:88–92, 94, 96–99,102.

Part Four

Nursing Theory

A time for giving birth, . . .
a time for knocking down,
a time for building

Perhaps no area of nursing has advanced as much in the last five years as in nursing theory. Nursing is giving birth to a scientific knowledge base for the profession and the professional practice of nursing. The knocking down of theories or partial theories is essential through testing in nursing research. The building of the knowledge base for practice occurs through repeated testing of theories or partial theories in multiple settings and situations. Building also occurs through sharing and dialogue with others.

United efforts of nurse scholars and practitioners of nursing are identifying the knowledge base for nursing and formulating theory to substantiate professional practice. There are disparate views regarding the status, development, and application of nursing knowledge. However, there is unity in purpose. Though the value of nursing theory has been a question to be resolved, the awareness of its necessity has increased among practitioners and scholars in nursing. The progress that has been made, various approaches in formulating nursing theory, and directions for the future are obvious in the contributions to this section.

Chapter 28

The Continuing Revolution: A History of Nursing Science

Margaret A. Newman, R.N., Ph.D., F.A.A.N.
Professor
Department of Nursing
Pennsylvania State University
University Park, Pennsylvania

Nursing is being recognized as a legitimate science in this decade. The past and present endeavors to promote nursing as a science could not have been actualized if it were not for the continuing efforts of numerous nursing theorists. Margaret A. Newman's chapter is a succinct introduction to the history of nursing science and theory development in nursing. The following six chapters are extensive treatises concerning the maturation of nursing theory.

Newman traces the evolution of nursing as a science from Nightingale's explication of the phenomena of nursing to the present. Drawing from Popper and Kahn, she defines science as a process of knowing, challenging, and continuing revolution. The ability to view phenomena and experiential data from *different* perspectives is emphasized as being critical for progress. Newman reviews the process of knowing by citing the examples of Columbus, Copernicus, Newton, and Einstein. She notes a paradigm (model of reality) shift as it occurred among the thinkers. The same process is identified in nursing.

Newman credits Nightingale with delineating the domain of nursing as the nurse, the patient, the situation in which they find themselves, and the purpose of their being together—the health of the patient. Translating these concepts into the formal jargon of today, Newman defines the components of the nursing paradigm to be: nursing, client, environment, and health. She points out that differences among theoreticians lie in varying emphases and view of the relationship of the concepts.

Historically, environmental factors were a prime focus for Nightingale. Attention to controlling the environment continued well into the twentieth century. A shift occurred in the 1950s to the nature and processes of the nurse-client relationship, influenced by the works of Peplau, Orlando, and King. At the same time other theorists, e.g., Henderson, Orem, Johnson, and Roy, were concerned with defining the purpose of nursing and nature of nursing practice. Attention was directed to the client and his or her adjustment to changes in self or environment. Rogers offered another course by insisting on the inseparability of "man-environment," interaction of the two, and concentration principally on understanding the person—the client. Currently the concept of health is being examined as an essential component of all the previous frameworks.

Newman asserts that the science of nursing must take into account all the relevant phenomena of the nursing paradigm. She predicts that, if shifts continue to develop in the way of viewing the phenomena, a unified model may eventually evolve. Newman concludes that once a particular view of the phenomena prevails, the first scientific stage of nursing's development as a science has occurred. There is evidence that nursing as a science has reached that stage.

The development of a science, contrary to what one might assume, is not a smooth, orderly process. The beginnings center around a vague discontent regarding phenomena for which there are no available explanations. Moreover, the identity and nature of the phenomena themselves are not very clear. Nevertheless, there is the conviction that there is something there which needs to be identified, described, and explained, and persons concerned with the same phenomena begin to examine them in some sort of systematic manner.

The process of the development of a science for a profession has some inherent advantages and disadvantages. One of the advantages is the great body of experiential data which provide a wealth of tacit knowledge (Polanyi, 1962) regarding the phenomena of inquiry. One of the disadvantages is the tendency of practitioners to view this phenomenon in a limited way, thereby decreasing the possibility of gaining new insights. It is this latter ability, the ability to view phenomena from different perspectives, that marks progress in the development of a science or, as Kuhn (1970) phrases it, revolutions in scientific thinking.

Nursing has had its share of revolutions in the way in which the scientific base of practice is viewed. Nightingale's explication of the phenomena of nursing's concern perhaps marks the beginning of the systematic inquiry and the identification of these phenomena. The purpose of this paper is to trace the major emphases of nursing's thinkers from Nightingale to the present and to illustrate how the shifts in thinking mark progress in the development of nursing science.

Before looking specifically at nursing science,

however, I would like to begin by examining the development of science in general.

A preliminary definition of science could be "the process of knowing." There are, however, many ways of knowing: by faith, by authority, by experience—or by systematic, controlled investigation, which some call the scientific method. Most would agree that science is not developed by faith, authority, or experience alone, but even the scientific method, which is more acceptable in scientific circles as a way of knowing, is fallible. We find, to a large extent, what we are looking for; we are limited by the ability to see; and we are limited by the inability to think beyond the prevailing perspective of the day. For these reasons, Popper (1965) would add to this definition of science that the process of knowing is developed by the processes of challenging and questioning. Popper says one can have confidence only in those theories that cannot be overthrown or rejected, and, therefore, the most important contribution that one can make to a theory is to try to refute it, to devise the most stringent test possible, so that if the theory stands up under that kind of testing, greater confidence in its validity may be assumed (1965:3-65, 215-250). Further, Kuhn, in his analysis of the great discoveries throughout the history of science, sees them as points of radical shifts in the way of viewing things:

> . . . a new theory . . . is seldom or never just an increment to what is already known. Its assimilation requires the reconstruction of prior theory and the re-evaluation of prior fact, an intrinsically revolutionary process that is

seldom completed by a single man [sic] and never overnight. (1970:7)

The preliminary definition of science then may be expanded: it is a process of knowing, a process of challenging, and a continuing revolution. A familiar example serves to show how this process works. There was a time when people thought the world was flat. (Considering how long the world has been around that was not very long ago—approximately 500 years; most of what we know about the world has been developed in that short period of time.) The theory that the world is flat was based on very limited observations. But as the science of mathematics began to be developed, or redeveloped, someone came along and speculated that the world was round. Columbus and his associates checked the theory out and found that it is so, and after a while, it became common knowledge that the planet we live on is a finite sphere. But even so, people of that day were convinced, primarily because of their religion (knowing by faith), that they were the center of the world and that everything revolved around them. Therefore, the world had to be the center of the universe, with the sun and other planets revolving around this planet—again, a limited view of things. Then Copernicus came along and projected the theory that the sun is the center of this universe and that this and all the other planets revolve around the sun. This is a good example of a paradigm shift.[1] Copernicus was looking at the same sun and planets but seeing them differently. Of course, nobody listened to him for a long time, but eventually, on the basis of the calculations of other astronomers, this new view of relationships was accepted. Toward the end of the seventeenth century, Newton put forth this theory of force, or the law of gravity, which was thought to be the ultimate in explaining the laws of the physical world. With the advent of better telescopes, however, people found that some of the predictions of Newton's theory were not true. Then in the early twentieth century, Einstein was able to explain things that Newton's theory could not explain. At this point, Newton's theory became a special case in a broader, more comprehensive theory.

A new theory disposes of the mistakes of the old theory. In order to devise a new theory, the scientist must be able to perceive that something is amiss, that something does not quite fit, and then, rather than explain it away within the limits of the old theory, be prepared to look at things in an entirely new way.

In science in general and in nursing in particular, the question keeps coming up: "Are we moving toward one big theory?" In view of the way science has progressed thus far, the answer appears to be "no." One theory contradicts and, in some instances, replaces the other. Einstein's theory contradicts Newton's. Newton's had previously contradicted Galileo's. Agassi describes it this way:

. . . Galileo's theory said that gravity is the same everywhere. Newton said that this is not quite true; gravity decreases the farther away you go from the earth. In Newton's theory, gravity acts at a distance. Einstein said that this is not quite true; the force of gravity moves outward from a body with the speed of light.

We can say that Galileo's theory or Kepler's theory is a good approximation to Newton's theory, and Newton's theory is a good approximation to Einstein's theory. That is to say, the results we get from Newton's theory are nearly the same as the results we get from Einstein's theory under normal conditions. And Galileo's theory gives results which are nearly the same as the resutls we get from Newton's theory under normal conditions. But for astronauts, Newton's theory holds good while Galileo's does not. And with high-speed rockets,

---

[1] According to Pelletier: "Paradigms impose order upon basically random phenomena. A paradigm is a model of reality, and it gives rise to a philosophical predisposition that directs and interprets the scientific activity of its adherents. Its implicit judgments about the nature of reality include some and exclude other phenomena from scientific inquiry" (1978:37).

Newton's theory does not hold good at all, while Einstein's theory is fine. (1968:147)

The old theories are approximations of the new ones and, as illustrated, are still useful in certain situations. The new theories go beyond the old theories and explain things the old theories could not explain. The process is one of evolution and accretion rather than accumulation.

So, too, the process has evolved in the shifting of theories throughout the history of nursing. A theory can be thought of as "one, powerful idea" (Popper, 1965:58). From this standpoint, the progress of science can be viewed as a history of ideas; therefore the purpose here is to highlight the predominant ideas, or theories, which have influenced nursing since the time of Florence Nightingale.

The domain of nursing has always included the nurse, the patient, the situation in which they find themselves, and, the purpose of their being together, or the health of the patient. In more formalized terms, or in the jargon of the day, the phenomena of our concern—the major components of the nursing paradigm—are *nursing* (as an action), *client* (human being), *environment* (of the client and of the nurse-client), and *health*. The *nurse* interacts with the *client* and the *environment* for the purpose of facilitating the *health* of the client. It is within the context of these four major components and their interrelationships that theory development in nursing has proceeded. Theoretical differences relate to the emphasis placed on one or more of the components and to the way in which their relationships are viewed.

The first major emphasis in the development of nursing science, based on Nightingale's work,

was given to *environment*. Nightingale (1859) viewed disease as a reparative process, the effort of nature to remedy a process "of poisoning or of decay," and she viewed the suffering which accompanied disease as being the result of deficiencies in the environment (1946:5). In her own words, nursing "ought to signify the proper use of fresh air, light, warmth, cleanliness, quiet, and the proper selection and administration of diet . . ." (1946:6). The objective of these activities was the health of the patient. Nightingale's approach might be diagramed as in Fig. 28-2.

Nightingale equated the science of health with the science of nursing, and based on the most pressing problems confronting her in the Crimea, she focused her efforts on the development of knowledge of the environmental factors she considered essential to health. She also included three other categories of nursing knowledge: observation of the patient, personal hygiene of the patient, and communication skills; but her major emphasis by far was that of controlling the environment.

This emphasis on environmental factors continued well into the twentieth century. Nursing practice was associated with the care of the ill. Medical science had little to offer in terms of curative treatment. The knowledge of nursing practice, therefore, emphasized altering the environment to render it conducive to healing. As important as this factor is, it was not sufficient.

The next impetus to the development of nursing science does not appear to emerge until the middle of this century. Recognizing that I have done only

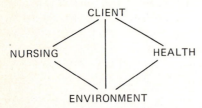

Figure 28-1   The nursing paradigm.

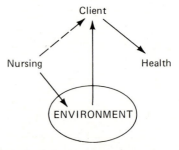

Figure 28-2   Schematic of Nightingale's approach to nursing.

a superficial review of the nursing literature of the first half of this century, I do not find much activity during that period aimed at the advancement and testing of new ideas. It is reasonable to assume that nursing leaders were preoccupied with improving nursing education and were convinced that, by so doing, the way would be cleared for the advancement of nursing science. At the same time, the demands of two world wars took priority in terms of accelerated education and practice within acute care centers, with little time for the scholarly activities of contemplation and analysis.

At the end of this period, however, in 1948, Esther Lucille Brown's report on nursing education was published, and first among her recommendations was the "need for nurses to study and analyze nursing functions" (Dolan, 1973:277). Shortly thereafter, in 1952, the first research journal in nursing, *Nursing Research*, was published, and the die was cast for establishing a scientific basis for nursing practice. Even so, the research efforts of the next decade revealed a great deal of uncertainty as to what to study and analyze, and, as a matter of fact, Brown's recommendation may have contributed to the confusion. Many fledgling researchers took her literally and focused their studies on the more obvious functions of nursing, i.e., the techniques employed by nurses in the performance of their responsibilities. After a decade or so of this type of research, it became clear that the accumulation of such studies was not contributing in a noticeable way to the understanding of nursing practice.

An era of concerted effort toward the development of nursing science emerged in the fifties and early sixties. The emphasis shifted from environmental factors to the nature and purpose of the *nurse-client relationship*. (See Fig. 28-3.) Recognizing that nursing was concerned not merely with doing things for patients in relation to their discomfort or disability, but also, and perhaps primarily, with the nature of the ongoing interpersonal processes, a number of nursing theorists began to identify these processes more specifically. Peplau (1952) brought the interper-

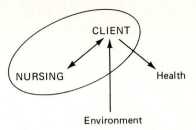

Figure 28-3 Schematic of emphasis during the 1950s and early 1960s.

sonal theories from psychiatry into the realm of nursing and provided a basis for nurses to begin to analyze the process of their interaction with patients in terms of its therapeutic quality. Similarly, Orlando (1961) utilized communications theory in describing what she termed "a deliberate nursing approach." Later, but in the same context, King (1971) began to explicate the complex transactional process occurring between nurse and patient.

Other theorists during this period emphasized the purpose of the nurse-client relationship. In seeking licensure for professional nursing, the profession became preoccupied with defining nursing and trying to differentiate the nature of nursing practice from that of medical practice. Henderson's (1966) definition of nursing is perhaps the most frequently noted—doing for the patient what he cannot do for himself with the intent of promoting independence. Similarly, Orem (1971) conceptualized nursing as the promotion of self-care in the patient. Johnson (1961) identified equilibrium, or dynamic stability, as the goal of nursing care. Roy's (1970) adaptation theory states that nursing's role is that of facilitating the adaptive potential of the patient.

All of these theorists have concentrated on situations in which clients are incapacitated in some way and require the assistance of someone else to supplement their own resources until they can again be independent, maintain self-care, establish equilibrium, or adapt to the situation. Most of these theorists view health and illness on a continuum, with the purpose of nursing being

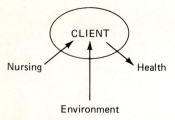

Figure 28-4 Schematic showing shift of emphasis to client.

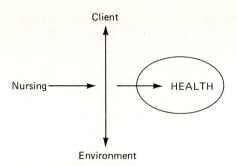

Figure 28-6 Schematic of current emphasis.

to move the client toward health. Here the emphasis is clearly on the *client*, the person adjusting to changes in himself or herself or in the environment.

Rogers's (1970) conceptualization provides another shift and emphasizes the unitary nature of man and the inseparability of man-environment. She sees the purpose of nursing as the promotion of symphonic interaction between man and environment and views health and illness as simply expressions of the life process. This view differs considerably from that which is based on man's adaptation to the environment. In Rogers's view, both man and environment are exerting their influences simultaneously, and the process is one of mutual evolutionary change. Even so, the emphasis in Rogers' framework (Fig. 28-5) is on an understanding of the man, the client, within his or her environment. This she sees as the focus of nursing's concern.

Currently there is increasing emphasis on the concept of *health* (Beckstrand, 1978; Smith, 1979;

Newman, 1979). Health has been seen as an essential component of all nursing frameworks from the time of Nightingale to the present. Each of the earlier explications of health has moved us a little closer to the views set forth today. Nightingale equated health with nursing and admitted that it was an unknown entity. We have moved from a conceptualization of health that depicts it as absence of disease to increasingly dynamic concepts: health and illness as a continuum (Roy, 1970), health and illness as expressions of the life process (Rogers, 1970), health as a process of human growth and development (King, 1971), health as the expansion of consciousness (Newman, 1979). Much work is needed in the elaboration and exploration of factors in the client-environment relationship which relate to health. Beyond that, theory must be developed to direct nursing action toward facilitating the process of health.

As the earlier discussion of the development of the science of physics demonstrated, we see that each theory contributed was an approximation of the next theory. No one theory said it all. One theorist picked up where another left off. Each new theory came about when someone saw that something was missing in the old theory. As we look at the various emphases in nursing theory through the years, we can begin to see that what the theorist chose to examine reflected the needs of that particular time, whether it was the lack of proper sanitation and the lack of medical treatment for infectious disease in the late nineteenth century or the increasing numbers of people surviving traumatic injuries and developing

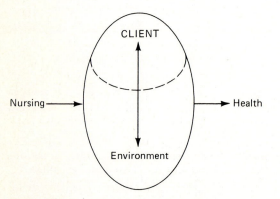

Figure 28-5 Schematic of Roger's emphasis.

chronic, debilitating diseases in the mid-twentieth century. The emphasis on controlling environment shifted to an emphasis on rehabilitation, which in turn gave way to an emphasis on prevention and finally to an emphasis on facilitation of health. Some theorists looked primarily at the nurse-client interpersonal process, others concentrated on understanding the complex processes of the human being as a unit, and others extended that thinking to include interaction with the environment. Finally, health, an integral component of all these interactions, is being examined as a dynamic process fluctuating across the life span.

As already pointed out, some of the theories contradict each other. This however, does not negate the usefulness of the various approaches in certain situations. It does mean that one has to determine under what conditions the theory applies. I would suggest that one of the factors determining the applicability of a theory is the temporal frame of reference. For example, if one is viewing a relatively short time frame, the adaptation model might apply, whereas in a longer time frame, phenomena would be apparent that could not be explained by adaptation alone.

In the early stages of the elaboration of various conceptual models in nursing, there was a tendency to view the models set forth by theorists as competitive or to place relative values on them. This situation is consistent with Hardy's assertion that nursing is in the preparadigm stage of scientific development, a stage "characterized by divergent schools of thought which, although addressing the same range of phenomena, usually describe and interpret these phenomena in different ways" (1978: 75). Whereas in the past emphasis has been placed on the aspect of the nursing phenomena most relevant to that particular time and situation, it is apparent from this review of the development of nursing theory that the science of nursing must now take into consideration *all* of the relevant phenomena.

Riehl and Roy take the position that many of the current nursing models present a similar view of the human and the environment, and they

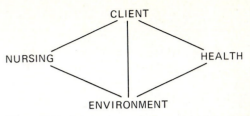

Figure 28-7 Schematic predicting emphasis in the future.

propose that nursing move toward "a single view of the person and of the goal of nursing," or a unified model (1980:399). If a particular view of the phenomena of nursing science prevails —and I think the work of the nurse-theorist group associated with the National Conference on Classification of Nursing Diagnosis indicates that we are approaching some unity in our way of viewing these major concepts—then we may be entering the first scientific stage of our development.[2] If indeed the development of science proceeds by shifts in the way of viewing phenomena, a unified model will exist for a period of time during which it is useful and eventually will be overthrown by a model which explains the phenomena more completely. What we are looking for are the ideas, or theories, that best fit our observations, but again, we must be cautious and not be limited by observations alone. Remember, that though Copernicus saw the same stars and planets in the sky, he saw them differently from other people. As nursing science develops, we will continue to look at the same major concepts, but at times certain persons among us will see them differently. Theory development in nursing is a continuing revolution.

[2] The concepts of unitary man, health, and nursing have been addressed by this group which consists of Chairperson Sister Callista Roy, Andrea A. Bircher, Rosemary Ellis, Joyce J. Fitzpatrick, Margaret Hardy, Imogene King, Rose McKay, Margaret A. Newman, Dorothea Orem, Rose Marie Parse, Martha Rogers, Mary Jane Smith, and Gertrude Torres. A report of these proceedings may be found in M. J. Kim and D. A. Moritz (eds.), *Classification of Nursing Diagnosis: Proceedings of the Third and Fourth National Conferences*, April 1978 and 1980 (New York: McGraw-Hill, 1982), p. 220.

EDITOR'S QUESTIONS FOR DISCUSSION

Compare the influence of Nightingale in the development of nursing as a science as described in Newman's chapter with the original notes and writings of Nightingale as portrayed in Palmer's chapter (Chap. 1). Is there evidence that Nightingale emphasized one component of the nursing paradigm more than another? To what extent is there evidence that Nightingale integrated all the components? Has the use of jargon today in defining components of the nursing paradigm influenced a different meaning or misinterpretation of the original domain of nursing, which Newman indicates has existed since the time of Nightingale? For example, to what extent is the current use and definition of the term "environment" inclusive of concepts which might be included in "the situation in which they find themselves?" Does the component "health" in the nursing paradigm isolate something different from the *total* "purpose of their being together" as originally included in the domain of nursing?

Could it be possible that part of the reason for the varying shifts in the focus of theory development and confusion that exists regarding the relevance of theory for knowledge and practice of nursing is related to inherent difficulties in establishing systematic linkages between concepts and the purpose of nursing? What evidence is there that nursing was beginning to be considered as a science in the 1950s? What evidence exists from curricula and practice that the *purpose* of nursing was indirectly being defined differently in the 1950s and early 1960s than at present? To what extent did focusing on nursing as an art inhibit the development of nursing as a science? Is there evidence in Nightingale's writings (review Palmer's Chap. 1) that nursing was conceived of as both an art and a science? What historical forces and factors have contributed to one aspect being given the primary attention more than another, rather than an integration of the two? How did Brown's recommendations contribute to the confusion? What forces led to a shift from emphasis on the interpersonal processes of nursing to explicit explorations of the nature and purpose of nursing practice? What old theories, as suggested by Newman, are approximations of new ones and still useful in certain situations?

Review Santora's chapter (Chap. 8) for definition of terms and explicate similarities and differences between theorists as presented in this and the following chapters. Are there semantic differences or essential contradictions?

What is the difference between accretion, accumulation, and concentration in theory development as inferred in Newman's chapter? Justify other criteria for determining the applicability of a theory besides the temporal frame of reference. Is it possible to apply the adaptation model as a continuous process? Do you agree with the assertion that nursing is in the preparadigm stage of scientific development? What is the evidence that nursing has moved toward an integrated view of the phenomena of nursing? Does that imply that nursing is moving toward one massive theory? Is it possible that numerous theoretical postures proffered today are integral parts of Roger's theory or would Roger's conceptualization be one perspective to be integrated into a unified theory of nursing science? How does the work of the nurse-theorist group associated with the classification of nursing diagnoses indicate some unity in viewing major theoretical concepts? Utilizing an inductive method, should nursing as a science develop one eminent theory from the selective integration of concepts, proposiitons, and/or theories from all the current competing frameworks? What is the relationship between the evolution of nursing theory as described by Newman and the proposed model for the development of nursing's knowledge base by Conway in Chap. 2? What discussion and questions posed by the editor in Chap. 8 (Santora) and Chap. 14 (Fawcett) also relate to Newman's presentation?

REFERENCES

Agassi, Joseph
1968 The Continuing Revolution. New York: McGraw-Hill.

Beckstrand, Janis Kay
1978 "A conceptual and logical analysis of selected health indicators." Unpublished Ph.D. dissertation, University of Texas.

Dolan, Josephine A.
1973 Nursing in Society: A Historical Perspective. Philadelphia: Saunders.

Hardy, Margaret E.
1978 "Evaluating nursing theory." Pp. 75–86 in Theory Development: What, Why, How? New York: NLN.

Henderson, V.
1966 The Nature of Nursing. New York: Macmillan.

Johnson, Dorothy
1961 "The significance of nursing care." American Journal of Nursing 61(11):63–66.

King, Imogene M.
1971 Toward a Theory for Nursing. New York: Wiley.

Kuhn, Thomas
1970 The Structure of Scientific Revolutions. Chicago: University of Chicago Press.

Newman, Margaret
1979 "Toward a theory of health." Pp. 55–67 in Margaret A. Newman (ed.), Theory Development in Nursing. Philadelphia: Davis.

Nightingale, Florence
1946 Notes on Nursing. Facsimile of 1st edition printed in London, 1859. Philadelphia: Lippincott.

Orem, Dorothea
1971 Nursing: Concepts of Practice. New York: McGraw-Hill.

Orlando, Ida J.
1961 The Dynamic Nurse-Patient Relationship: Function, Process, and Principles. New York: Putnam.

Pelletier, Kenneth R.
1978 Toward a Science of Consciousness. New York: Dell.

Peplau, Hildegarde
1952 Interpersonal Relations in Nursing. New York: Putnam.

Polanyi, Michael
1962 Personal Knowledge. New York: Harper Torchbooks.

Popper, Karl R.
1965 Conjectures and Refutations. New York: Harper & Row.

Riehl, Joan P. and Sister Callista Roy
1980 "A unified model of nursing." Pp. 399–403 in Joan P. Riehl and Sister Callista Roy (eds.), Conceptual Models for Nursing Practice. New York: Appleton-Century-Crofts.

Rogers, Martha E.
1970 An Introduction to the Theoretical Basis of Nursing. Philadelphia: Davis.

Roy, Sister Callista
1970 "Adaptation: A conceptual framework for nursing." Nursing Outlook 18:42–45.

Smith, Judy
1979 "The idea of health." Unpublished Ph.D. dissertation, New York University.

Chapter 29

Nursing Theory Development: Where We Have Been and Where We Are Going

Peggy L. Chinn, R.N., Ph,D., F.A.A.N.
Editor
Advances in Nursing Science
and
Professor
School of Nursing
State University of New York at Buffalo
Buffalo, New York

Certain philosophical perspectives held in common by the majority of the members of a discipline are the basis for the development of any science. Peggy L. Chinn aptly clarifies the predominant concepts which reveal the nature of nursing as a distinct discipline, and indicates direction for the continuing evolution of nursing knowledge. She attributes the impetus for establishing nursing as a discipline to Florence Nightingale. Nightingale's writings indicate that the nature of nursing as a profession required knowledge distinct from medicine. Chinn cites intervening influences which have inhibited Nightingale's mandate, as well as factors which promoted a commitment to follow through from the initial command.

Enlarging the discussion in Newman's chapter (Chap. 28), each of the key concepts— the nature of nursing, the individual who receives care, society/environment, and health—is examined. It is important to note the commonalities and differences in the way the concepts are viewed by the authors in this section of the text. Variation is typical in the discipline as a whole, as well as consensus as to which concepts comprise the entity of nursing. Chinn describes the principal focus of the *nature of nursing* as being interpersonal interactions. She believes it to be the basis for forming theoretical propositions regarding nursing actions and knowledge. She shows that one essential difference between nursing and medicine is that interpersonal interactions are the primary focus in nursing with technical interventions as secondary. Chinn notes that the prevailing views regarding the nature of nursing differ philosophically between academicians and practitioners. This is illustrated in comparing articles from the October, 1980, issues of the *American Journal of Nursing* and *Advances in Nursing Science.* She proposes, with the central focus being on a disease state in the *AJN* issue and in medicine, that in practice nursing is not as clearly distinct from medicine as it is portrayed in academic nursing literature. The same divergence is noted in the journals regarding the concept of *health.* For most health is visualized as a health-illness continuum, whereas some nursing scholars conceptualize health as a phenomenon in itself.

In general, the most consistent philosophical component of the *individual* is the dimension of wholeness—a holistic view. Alternative views of the third concept, society and environment, have not become clearly evident.

Chinn further describes the relationship between the ways of knowing, judging the adequacy of knowledge, and the limitations of empirical approaches to validate the importance of phenomena in nursing. She indicates that although a clear philosophic trend is evident regarding the key concepts, there remains a lack of clarity as to nursing as a distinct discipline. Chinn projects a three-pronged approach to the problem through the combined efforts of nursing education, nursing practice, and nursing research.

Chinn advocates orientation to nursing theory in baccalaureate curricula; master's level programs designed to enable students to analyze, critique, and test existing model and theoretical conceptualizations; and nursing doctoral programs designed to further develop and test existing and new theories and approaches to obtaining knowledge. She sees the practicing community as the primary arena in which theories are tested and where knowledge is applied. A shift is indicated in that the differences between practitioners and scholars is decreasing. Research is essential to address the major propositions posed by the nursing theories and problems in practice. Chinn concludes that the most significant developments, that nursing as a total discipline is moving toward increasing competence in construction of nursing theory, are: first, the initiation of doctoral programs in nursing and, second, the increasing awareness by the practicing community of their great potential for contributing to theory development, nursing knowledge as well as the practice of nursing.

INTRODUCTION

In establishing the discipline of nursing, Florence Nightingale spoke with firm conviction about the nature of nursing as a profession requiring knowledge distinct from medical knowledge (Nightingale, 1969:3). The development of a knowledge base for nursing has been an extremely slow process since the original 1860 publication of Nightingale's *Notes on Nursing.* Indeed, for most of the intervening time period, nursing's knowledge base has not been viewed as distinct from that of medicine, and it has only been recently that serious efforts have been made to articulate, develop, and test nursing knowledge. The intervening influences which have guided the development of nursing as a discipline have themselves been the object of

scholarly investigation in recent years (Ashley, 1976, 1980; Hughes, 1980; Kjervik and Martinson, 1979; Lovell, 1980). It is evident that forces both within and outside of the discipline of nursing have operated to create an anti-intellectual, anti-scholarly climate that prevailed until the 1950s and remains in evidence today (Flaskerud and Halloran, 1980; Ashley, 1976).

The shift toward actively engaging in serious development of nursing's knowledge was stimulated primarily by the emergence of nursing education based in institutions of higher learning rather than in hospitals, along with the requirements of academic institutions for faculty holding advanced degrees in the discipline and the need to meet standards of higher education for the curriculum. In addition, nursing philosophy and ideology have remained committed, throughout the intervening century, to the notion that nursing does indeed require a distinct body of knowledge (Abdellah, 1969; Hall, 1964; Henderson, 1964; Krueter, 1957). This commitment grew from the consistently observed fact that while the goals of nursing and medicine may in some instances be similar or related, the essential goals and functions of nursing often require a body of knowledge that is not provided by medical knowledge or by the knowledge of any other single discipline outside of nursing. During the period since nursing was established as a profession, nursing has been practiced primarily on an intuitive basis and viewed primarily as a nurturing and technical art requiring apprenticeship learning and innate personality traits congruent with the art (Ashley, 1976; Hughes, 1980). Once the abilities to develop nursing knowledge were acquired by a small but significant number of nurse scholars, activities to develop nursing knowledge and theory began to emerge. The purpose of this chapter is to provide a perspective on the prevailing philosophic and related methodological approaches evident in this development and to project directions for future development based on the foundation that has been laid.

PHILOSOPHIC DIRECTIONS

The development of any science is grounded in certain philosophic views that are held by the majority of the members of the discipline. Varying schools of thought emerge within each discipline and sometimes compete for primary attention, a process that is essential to the continuing development of the body of knowledge in the discipline. However, each discipline holds certain common ideas regarding the nature of the discipline and criteria by which new theories and methods are judged as adequate for the discipline. If a certain segment of the discipline develops alternative philosophic views and methods or approaches that are not consistent with that of the discipline, a new discipline emerges (Hardy, 1978).

As Hardy (1978:39) observes, nursing has been in a stage of searching to determine what entities are of particular concern to the discipline, where to locate these entities, and how to study them. Since the first efforts to develop nursing theory and knowledge, there has been a tendency to concentrate on differences between various approaches to nursing knowledge. As Flaskerud and Halloran (1980) point out, this internal dissent may have been detrimental to the development of nursing knowledge and the disagreements may be more imagined than real. On the most general level of abstraction regarding the nature of nursing, there does appear to be general academic concensus regarding those concepts that are central to the discipline. However, when more specific and concrete concepts are identified, there continue to exist alternative views serving either to stimulate or to inhibit further development. Given the progressively advancing collective abilities of nurse-scholars, these alternative views hold more potential for stimulation rather than inhibition, because there seems to be a growing awareness of the common key concepts of the discipline. The following sections describing similarities and differences in philosophic approaches will provide specific examples.

Views of Nursing

There is general agreement that the central concepts of the discipline of nursing are the *nature of nursing*, the *individual* who receives nursing care, *society-environment*, and *health* (Yura and Torres, 1975; Fawcett, 1978). It is the way in which each of these concepts is viewed that reveals the nature of nursing as a distinct discipline, and that provides a direction for the development of nursing knowledge.

The *nature of nursing*, as reflected in the literature, is generally viewed as that of a helping discipline, with the primary focus being on interpersonal interactions that occur between the nurse and the client. While this general description does not clearly distinguish nursing from other helping disciplines, it does provide a focal point for delineating theoretical propositions regarding nursing actions and the knowledge needed in order to develop and improve nursing practice. This focus does make one clear distinction between nursing and medicine in that medicine focuses on surgical and pharmacologic interventions, with interpersonal interactions being an adjunct to these interventions. In contrast, technical interventions are viewed in nursing as being an adjunct to the primary interpersonal interactions. Examination of the views prevailing concerning the other key concepts of health, environment, and the individual provides further distinction between nursing, medicine, and other related disciplines, as will be evident in the following discussions of these concepts.

The prevailing views of the nature of nursing are generated primarily by nurse-scholars and academicians, and while attempts are made to provide evidence of the consistency of these views in the larger arena of nursing practice, prevailing views regarding the nature of nursing coming from the realm of nursing practice is not clear. This view can be inferred, however, from the implied views communicated in literature that is published for practicing nurses. In the October 1980 issue of the American Journal of Nursing, the implied view of the nature of nursing appears to be only partially congruent with the view published in academically oriented literature, and there appears to be little distinction between the nature of nursing and medicine. None of the 14 articles published in this issue reflect consideration or use of the prevailing theories or models of nursing. Only one article, which was a personal experience account, presented a view of nursing as primarily an interpersonal encounter (Greishaw, 1980). An article on assertiveness training for nurses focused on the skill of assertiveness in relating to other health care workers on the job rather than as an interpersonal skill fundamental to nursing practice (Numerof, 1980). An article reporting a nurse practitioner program for women's health was described as providing learning opportunities about "obstetric and gynecological health care" (Ed-mundson, Jennings, and Kowalski, 1980). The list of seven learning objectives given in the article for students who complete the program includes only one that refers in any manner to the potential use of interpersonal processes as a component of the role being taught. In describing teaching methods used, approaches to be used in relating to the patient are secondary and supplementary to the performance of assessment techniques, and the assessment parameters reflect a predominantly medical view of women's health (Edmundson, Jennings, and Kowalski, 1980).

Literature that is oriented to an academic nursing audience does reflect a growing application in practice of the academically espoused view of the nature of nursing. In the October 1980 issue of *Advances in Nursing Science*, three practicing nurses present a model developed for research and practice in an acute care cancer center (Scott et al., 1980). Other articles in the same issue reflect an implied assumption of the nature of nursing as essentially an interpersonal process and an attempt to implement research, analysis, and practice based on this view.

The central concept of the *individual* is also viewed with general consistency among existing nursing models and theories. The most consistent philosophic component of this concept is the dimension of wholeness, or a holistic view of individuals. The nature of holism as a concept is subject to some debate, arising partially from the cognitive, methodological, and practical problems of generating knowledge in a manner that is consistent with the concept of holism in its purest sense. When a person is viewed as a system of biological, psychological, and sociocultural parts (an approach generally not consistent with the concept of holism), there is still a strong commitment to the notion that no sphere or dimension of the individual can be viewed in isolation or take precedence over another (Flaskerud and Halloran, 1980).

The concept of *society and environment* is consistently viewed as a central concept to the discipline, although it is not as clearly articulated, and therefore alternative views of this concept have not become clearly evident. The primary role of society-environment is viewed as a critical interacting factor with the individual, and this interaction is viewed alternatively by different nurse scholars. For some, the person-environment interaction is one of several important interactions. For others, the person-environment interaction is central to the model or concept of nursing (Flaskerud and Halloran, 1980).

The concept of *health* is most often viewed as a health-illness continuum, although some nursing scholars are presenting views of health that reject the health-illness conceptualization and view health as a phenomenon existing regardless of the presence or absence of illness. Carper[1] states:

> What seems to be of paramount importance, at least at this stage in the development of nursing science, is that these preparadigm conceptual structures and theoretical models present new perspectives for considering the familiar phenomena of health and illness in relation to the human life process; as such they can and should be legitimately counted as discoveries in the discipline. The representation of health permits health to be thought of as a dynamic state or process which changes over a given period of time and varies according to circumstances rather than a static either/or entity. The conceptual change in turn makes it possible to raise questions that previously would have been literally unintelligible (1978: 14–15).

As with the concept of the nature of nursing, there appears to exist a significant diverson of views concerning health coming from the academic community in nursing and the practitioner community. Again, the October 1980 issue of the *American Journal of Nursing* (1980) reflects this divergence. Of the 14 articles appearing in the issue, eight had a disease named in the title of

[1] Reprinted from "Fundamental patterns of knowing in nursing," by Barbara Carper, by permission of Aspen Systems Corporation.

the article, and all but two focused on a disease state. Given the fact that illness is a central concept to the discipline of medicine, this suggests that in practice nursing is not as clearly distinguished from medicine as it is in academic nursing literature.

Philosophy of the Development of Nursing as a Science

As stated earlier, until recently there was a prevailing resistance or refusal to acknowledge the value or need for developing nursing as a science. Given the evidence that still exists regarding the differences in the prevailing views of nursing concepts by nurse-scholars and the practicing community, there remains a lack of clarity in the discipline regarding nursing as a distinct discipline. Since a distinct discipline in any field does not simply exist, but rather is created by the development of knowledge, then the gains made in the development of nursing knowledge over the past two decades have been remarkably significant, even if this development is not yet reflected in current nursing practice and practice-oriented literature.

As the discussion of the views of nursing indicates, there is general agreement in nursing regarding the global, most general concepts that are critical for nursing science. Thus, while there are variations in the manner of viewing these general concepts, there is general concensus regarding what entities are of particular concern to the discipline. As Hardy (1978) points out, the scientists of a discipline must also develop approaches in locating these entities and ways to study them. The philosophic foundations upon which these endeavors are based are critical to the development of the discipline, and nursing science has not yet resolved some of the primary philosophic problems involved in the process of developing theory and knowledge.

The philosophic dilemma of how to know and how to judge the adequacy of knowledge is closely related to the nature of the key concepts of the discipline of nursing. For example, the concept of the individual as holistic presents a basic contradiction between the traditional views of science and of holism. Science is commonly understood to be a body of knowledge or a process based on observed facts and tested truth according to precise and exact methods of measurement. Given this view of science, the approach to knowledge requires the systematic examination of discrete events, phenomena, or objects in terms of narrowly defined problems and variables. The concept of holism, on the other hand, is philosophically opposed to this approach to knowledge in that no phenomenon can be analyzed without residue into the sum of its parts or reduced to discrete elements (Newman, 1979[2]; Francis and Munjas, 1979; Winstead-Fry, 1980). Newman, in addressing this problem states:

> A holistic approach is not to be confused with, or construed to mean, a multivariate approach. It is not the summing up of many factors (psychological, social, physiological and so on) to make a whole. It is the identification of patterns which are reflective of the whole. What these parameters are will vary according to one's ability to see the whole. For some, the universe can be seen in a grain of sand. For others, characteristics which present identifiable patterns of the individual, e.g. the way a person walks or the way he [sic] talks, are a good place to start. The task is not easy. When one has grasped the meaning of holism and identified the phenomenon of inquiry, the next step is to find valid ways of measuring it (1979:70).

Carper (1978) has described the fundamental problems inherent in what it means to know and in determining what kinds of knowledge are held to be of most value for the discipline of nursing. In most other sciences and in nursing, the most valued means of establishing new knowledge has been the demonstration of reliable and valid empirical evidence. The adequacy of theories in the discipline is generally measured in part by the ability of the theory to stimulate the gathering of empirical evidence that supports the theoretical propositions. In accord with changes emerging in other scientific disciplines, the limitations of the empirical approaches to knowledge as the only way to know has become increasingly evident. Given the views concerning the nature of nursing and other key concepts of the discipline, there are severe limitations in known approaches or tools that can be used to generate empirical evidence relating to these concepts. While the value of the empirical approach to knowledge is evident and not to be discounted, Carper proposes that the views of what is legitimate knowledge in the discipline of nursing can be extended to include aesthetic, personal, and ethical ways of knowing. Each of these patterns of knowing has potential for future empirical validation, but the fact that empirical evidence as we now conceive it cannot be fully relied upon or validated has presented a major obstacle to acknowledging the importance of certain phenomena in nursing. In describing the personal component of knowledge, Carper states:

> Certainly empirical knowledge is essential to the purposes of nursing. But nursing also requires that we be alert to the fact that models of human nature and their abstract and generalized categories refer to and describe behaviors and traits that groups have in common. However, none of these categories can ever encompass or express the uniqueness of the individual encountered as a person, as a "self." These and many other similar considerations are involved in the realm of personal knowledge, which can be broadly characterized as subjective, concrete and existential. It is concerned with the kind of knowing that promotes wholeness and integrity in the personal encounter, the achievement of engagement rather than detachment; and it denies the manipulative, impersonal orientation (1978:19–20).

In summary, while there is considerable diversity in the specific construction of the current

[2] Reprinted from Theory Development in Nursing, by Margaret Newman. Philadelphia: F. A. Davis, 1979.

nursing theoretical conceptualizations, a clear philosophic trend is evident concerning the key concepts of the discipline. Since theories serve to provide ways of viewing reality and subsequently a stimulus for testing those views, the emerging nursing theories hold great promise for generating new knowledge. The approach to theory construction that has predominated to date has been largely deductive in that scholars have formulated theoretical descriptions of reality based on intuitive knowledge and casual observation, grounded in a philosophy that is becoming clearly evident. Given the common philosophic commitments, the current diversity of construction of different conceptualizations serves as an impetus for further development. As research methods emerge to provide more adequate ways to test nursing's early theories, current formulations will be revised, extended, and improved, and new nursing theory will emerge.

PROJECTIONS FOR FUTURE DEVELOPMENT

The development of theory and knowledge in a practice discipline is three-pronged. First, educational programs are required that provide orientation to the prevailing views of the discipline for future practitioners and scholars. As such, educational programs provide an important stimulus for the future directions taken in the discipline as well as the atmosphere in which new ideas and knowledge can be freely explored and developed. Second, the practicing community provides the primary arena in which theories are tested and in which knowledge that is generated is applied. The practice of the discipline also provides a major stimulus for the generation of new problems, necessitating the continuing development of theories and knowledge that can be applied to these problems. Finally, research is required that addresses the major propositions posed by the theories of the discipline and by the problems in practice.

Nursing Education

The standards and criteria for accreditation of baccalaureate and higher degree programs in nursing have clearly articulated a commitment to the development of nursing as a distinct discipline (National League for Nursing, 1977). However, the curricula of many basic programs in nursing at the baccaluareate level and master's level specialty programs are currently formulated in such a way that these programs have not yet made a significant contribution to the development of nursing theory. While the criteria for accreditation require that nursing faculty holds at least a master's degree in nursing, many faculty members holding this credential have not been introduced to the current models and theories that have been developed in the discipline of nursing. Baccalaureate curricula, in turn, are generally lacking in their orientation to nursing theory. Where curricula are designed which use an existing model of nursing or are based on a clear conceptualization of the key concepts of the discipline, chances are increased that beginning practitioners will have been exposed to the predominant conceptualizations developed in the discipline and will be able to design their approaches to nursing practice in accordance with these conceptualizations. As nursing education programs begin to be more clearly designed to fulfill a specific function in relation to theory development, the future development of nursing theory and knowledge will certainly be enhanced.

Development of an individual's ideas and thinking requires several years of maturity, and there is an urgent need to assess and revise curricula of the first professional degree programs in nursing in light of the prevailing views of the key concepts of the discipline. Such approaches to curricula will nurture the probability of future practitioners and scholars to make a contribution to the development of nursing science.

Master's level programs, instead of introducing current theories and models of the discipline, should be designed to enable the student to analyze, critique, and test existing models and theoretical conceptualizations in nursing. The nature of specialization and advanced practice of nursing also needs to be critically addressed in light of the nature of the key concepts of the discipline, and revisions need to be made in master's curricula that are consistent with these concepts.

Nursing doctoral programs, whether granting professional or academic degrees, need to be designed to enable students to further develop and test existing theories as well as to develop new theories and approaches in acquiring knowledge. Given the fact that the majority of nurse-scholars to date have received their doctoral degrees in widely diverse fields other than nursing and have learned the views of science predominant in other fields, there remains diversity of view concerning the proper approaches and methods to be used in generating nursing knowledge. Further, while nurse-conceived research has steadily increased over the past two decades, there is generally a lack of maturity in the collective efforts of applying the diverse approaches of other sciences directly to nursing problems. Further, the theoretical base for nursing research has been predominantly borrowed from other disciplines, which compromises the potential of the existing research to contribute to the development of nursing theory. In addition, there has been a relative absence of sufficiently developed theory within the discipline of nursing on which to base research (Feldman, 1980). The philosophic diversity as to which approaches will be most fruitful in the development of nursing knowledge is evident at present, and future development will be critically influenced by the directions established in nursing doctoral programs. Thus, the proliferation of doctoral study in nursing and its growing accessibility for increasing numbers of nurses is probably one of the most important steps in the development of nursing science.

Nursing Practice

As noted earlier in this chapter, there continue to exist significant differences between views held by nursing practice and by nursing scholars. There are important indications that shifts are occurring that will lessen these differences and make it possible for the interaction between these two communities within the discipline to function more effectively to mutually contribute to the development of theory in nursing. There is consistent evidence in literature generated by nurse-scholars that application of their thinking in practice is used to test and verify theoretical ideas (Henderson, 1978; Jacobs and Huether, 1978; Chang, 1980; Arakelian, 1980; Langner and Innes, 1980).

The Fourth National Conference on Nursing Diagnosis (1980) represented a significant event in efforts to reduce the damaging types of barriers that have existed between nursing scholars and nurse practitioners. A group of nurse-theorists was organized as an outcome of previous conferences and developed a nursing theoretical model that was presented at the Fourth Conference in order to stimulate formulation and testing of nursing diagnoses consistent with the prevailing views of the discipline. The theorist group was composed of such widely diverse scholars as Martha Rogers, Sister Callista Roy, Margaret Hardy, Margaret Newman, Gertrude Torres, Imogene King, and several others. Their proposal did not reflect the singular thinking or approach of any one of the members of the group but rather reflected the concensus regarding the key concepts of the discipline. The model was fluid and open, allowing any number of specific approaches and subconcepts to be used in conjunction with it. It was intended to serve primarily as a way of viewing nursing phenomena and of labeling and classifying these phenomena.

After presentation of the model, the participants of the conference, a significant proportion of whom were practicing nurses, discussed the utility of the model in formulating nursing diagnoses in their practice and mentally tested the results that might occur if they were to apply the model in formulating diagnoses and projecting interactions. The discussion resulted in minor modifications in the theoretical conceptualization, but the conference ended with an enthusiastic support for the potential of using a nursing model in practice and a generally expressed desire to begin to conceptualize nursing diagnoses consistent with a nursing model.

This event provided evidence of the readiness and ability of nurse-scholars and practicing nurses to pursue fruitful collaboration in the development of nursing theory. As other similar groups emerge locally and nationally, the effect will be seen both in nursing practice and in nursing scholarship.

Nursing Research

Two events of significance to nursing research have occurred over the past few years: the emergence of nursing doctoral programs and the establishment of new journals in the discipline designed for the purpose of reporting nursing research and theory development. Each of these events attest to the growing strength of nursing research but also provide important stimuli for the further development of nursing research. While limitations in funding for nursing research continue to exist, and the fact remains that much of nursing research is in an embryonic stage of development, gains have been made in research. In the future there needs to be an increasingly clear commitment to the development of knowledge that reflects prevailing views of the discipline and to the testing of nursing concepts and theoretical formulations. The need to conceive and implement new approaches for the testing

of nursing knowledge is critical; the nature of the concepts of the discipline and the lack of existing means to verify or validate phenomena that are important to the practice of nursing are a major challenge for the community of nurse-researchers (Deets, 1980; Field, 1979).

CONCLUSION

The development of nursing theory to the present demonstrates the vitality of nursing as a discipline. Nursing has demonstrated a concern with phenomena that are important to the health of individuals and society and the commitment and ability to view these phenomena in ways that are stimuli for the investigation of new knowledge. There are significant signs that education, practice, and research have reached a point of readiness to move with increasing competence toward the development of nursing theory. In education, the most significant development has been the initiation of doctoral programs in nursing, which holds the promise to stimulate the development of new theories and new methods for testing nursing theories. Members of the practicing community are increasingly aware of the potential for making a contribution to the development of nursing theory and of the value of nursing knowledge in the practice of nursing. Nurse-researchers are increasing in numbers, and the scope and quality of nursing research have shown dramatic improvements. The future development of nursing as a discipline now hinges on the directions that evolve in education, practice, and research in relation to theory development.

EDITOR'S QUESTIONS FOR DISCUSSION

What forces and factors within and outside the discipline of nursing have operated to create an anti-intellectual climate that Chinn indicates still is evident? What strategies can be offered to constructively and effectively diminish those forces? What forces or factors influenced and nurtured nursing to be practiced on an "intuitive basis"? How would you respond to arguments for and against the basis of nursing practice and the quality of care provided in the era of the 1950s and 1960s compared with the 1970s and 1980s? Was the early tendency to concentrate on differences between approaches to nursing knowledge a reflection of dissent in nursing as a whole? Indicate through examples of the process in developing nursing knowledge the positive aspects of conflict for nursing as a profession. What are the significant gains in the development of nursing knowledge the past two decades? What accounts for a lag between the development of knowledge and implementation into practice? What forces contribute to the lag? What strategies can be proposed to alter those forces?

Trace the change in focus in interpersonal interactions between the nurse and client from the earliest writings (Chap. 28) to the present. What is the relationship between the essential distinction made by Chinn between nursing and medicine and the critical differences conceptualized by Williams (Chap. 25) and examined by Brown (Chap. 26)? Which scholar(s) would consider the person-environment interaction as one of several important interactions, and which scholar(s) would consider it central to the concept of nursing? Why have not alternative views of the concepts society and environment become clearly evident? What implication is there for reconceptualizing health as an entity in itself rather than as part of a health-illness continuum?

What are the advantages and disadvantages for the profession when philosophical differences concerning the nature of nursing are reflected in professional journals? What strategies might be suggested to utilize those occurrences as a means to unify the profession? What variables exist in practice which may influence the degree which one is able to clearly distinguish nursing from medicine? What factors in academia, and in academic literature, might make it easier to define clear distinctions?

What relationship exists between Newman's definition of science (Chap. 27) and the way it is commonly understood in this chapter? What problems are inherent in what it means to know? What measures can be suggested to indicate the adequacy of knowledge? What are the limitations in known approaches or tools to generate empirical evidence for validating concepts? What other methods can be utilized to identify, measure, and validate nebulous concepts, such as "holism"? What application is there in Ketefian's chapter (Chap. 19) to the extension of knowledge in nursing proposed by Carper? To what extent and for what purpose should attempts be made to categorize the uniqueness of the individual? What are the advantages and disadvantages of deductive and inductive approaches to theory construction? What approaches and methods are appropriate to generate nursing knowledge?

What considerations are essential in conveying prevailing views of a discipline to nursing students? What questions previously raised for discussion in Santora's chapter (Chap. 8) and Peterson's chapter (Chap. 7) also can be addressed to Chinn's chapter? How do the findings of Santora's study (Chap. 8) relate to Chinn's statements regarding a lack of orientation to nursing theory in baccalaureate curricula and its importance in master's programs? What commonalities and differences exist in views concerning education programs among Chinn, Williamson (Chap. 5), and Grace (Chap. 12)? What findings of O'Connell's study (Chap. 15) and in Fawcett's chapter (Chap.14) lend support or raise other questions regarding Chinn's observations concerning collaborative research and the theoretical base of nursing research? What are the pros and cons of philosophical and theoretical diversity in the research base for the development of nursing knowledge?

What evidence exists that the differences between nursing practitioners and scholars are decreasing? What differences in concepts of nursing continue to exist between practitioners and scholars? At what stage in the development of the model for nursing diagnosis was there collaboration of nurse-scholars with practitioners? What type of contribution was elicited from practitioners before the presentation of the model at the Fourth National Conference on Nursing Diagnosis? What strategies can be offered to increase this initial collaboration with practitioners and promote collaboration in all areas of nursing?

REFERENCES

Abdellah, Fay G.
  1969 "The nature of nursing science" Nursing Research 18(5):39.
American Journal of Nursing
  1980 10:entire issue.
Arakelian, Maureen
  1980 "An assessment and nursing application of the concept of locus of control." Advances in Nursing Science 3(1):25–42.
Ashley, Jo Ann
  1976 Hospitals, Paternalism, and the Role of the Nurse. New York: Teacher's College Press.
  1980 "Power in structured misogyny: Implications for the politics of care." Advances in Nursing Science 2(3):3–22.
Carper, Barbara
  1978 "Fundamental patterns of knowing in nursing." Advances in Nursing Science 1(1):13–24.
Chang, Betty L.
  1980 "Evaluation of health care professionals in facilitating self-care: Review of the literature and a conceptual model." Advances in Nursing Science 3(1):43–58.
Deets, Carol A.
  1980 "Methodological concerns in the testing of nursing interventions." Advances in Nursing Science 2(2):1–12.
Edmundson, Margaret A., Betty J. Jennings, and Karren Kowalski
  1980 "A nurse practitioner program for women's health care." American Journal of Nursing 80:1784–1785.
Fawcett, Jacquelyn
  1978 "The what of theory development." Pp. 17–53 in Theory Development: What, Why and How. New York: National League for Nursing.
Feldman, Harriet R.
  1980 "Nursing research in the 1980's: Issues and implications." Advances in Nursing Science 3(1):85–92.
Field, Mildred
  1979 "Casual inferences in behavioral research." Advances in Nursing Science 2(1):81–94.
Flaskerud, Jacquelyn H. and Edward J. Halloran
  1980 "Areas of agreement in nursing theory development." Advances in Nursing Science 3(1):1–7.
Francis, Gloria and Barbara A. Munjas
  1979 Promoting Psychological Comfort, 3d ed. Dubuque: William C. Brown.
Fourth National Conference on Nursing Diagnosis
  1980 National Clearinghouse for Nursing Diagnosis, St. Louis: St. Louis University.
Greishaw, Susan
  1980 "My, these are beautiful flowers." American Journal of Nursing 80:1782–1783.
Hall, Lydia
  1964 "Nursing: What is it?" Canadian Nurse 60(2):150–154.
Hardy, Margaret E.
  1978 "Perspectives on nursing theory." Advances in Nursing Science 1,1:37–48.
Henderson, Betty
  1978 "Nursing diagnosis: Theory and practice." Advances in Nursing Science 1(1):75–84.
Henderson, Virginia
  1964 "The nature of nursing." American Journal of Nursing 64(8):62–68.
Hughes, Linda
  1980 "The public image of the nurse." Advances in Nursing Science 2(3):55–72.
Jacobs, Maeona K., and Sue E. Huether
  1978 "Nursing science: The theory-practice linkage." Advances in Nursing Science 1(1):63–74.
Kjervik, Diane K., and Ida M. Martinson (eds.)
  1979 Women in Stress: A Nursing Perspective. New York: Appleton-Century-Crofts.
Krueter, Francis Reiter
  1957 "What is good nursing?" Nursing Outlook 5(5):302–304.

Langner, Suzanne R. and Carolyn Innes
  1980 "Breathing, holism and health." Topics in Clinical Nursing 2(3):1–10.
Lovell, Mariann
  1980 "The politics of medical deception: Challenging the trajectory of history." Advances in Nursing Science 2(3):73–86.
National League for Nursing
  1977 Criteria for the Appraisal of Baccalaureate and Higher Degree Programs, 4th ed. NLN Publication #15–1251. New York: National League for Nursing.
Newman, Margaret
  1979 Theory Development in Nursing. Philadelphia: F. A. Davis.
Nightingale, Florence
  (1860)
  1969 Notes on Nursing: What It Is, What It Is Not. New York: Dover.

Numerof, Rita E.
  1980 "Assertiveness training." American Journal of Nursing 80:1796–1799.
Scott, Diane W., Marilyn T. Oberst, and Mary Jo Dropkin
  1980 "A stress-coping model." Advances in Nursing Science 3(1):9–24.
Winstead-Fry, Patricia
  1980 "The scientific method and its impact on holistic health." Advances in Nursing Science 2(4):1–8.
Yura, Helen and Gertrude Torres
  1975 Today's Conceptual Frameworks within Baccalaureate Nursing Programs. NLN Publication #15–1558. New York: National League for Nursing.

Chapter 30

Theory and Research in the Development of Nursing as a Discipline: Retrospect and Prospect

Lorraine Olszewski Walker, R.N., Ed.D. F.A.A.N.
Professor
School of Nursing
University of Texas at Austin
Austin, Texas

The focus in this chapter is on three movements which, according to Lorraine Walker, were the basis of nursing's evolution as a science. The three movements are: metatheoretical, theoretical, and practice theory. In defining the first two terms, Walker refers to different levels of analysis. The metatheoretical level focuses on methods and issues encountered in the theoretical level, while the theoretical level includes statements about states of affairs or events. Lorraine Walker examines aspects of each movement as to their contributions and limitations.

In elucidating the three movements, Walker addresses primarily the metatheoretical movement. She considers the theory of theories work of Dickoff and James as metatheoretical. While she acknowledges their contribution of a proposed four-level model of theory for practice, Walker cites as a criticism the dearth of outcomes the theory of theories has produced. However, she recognizes them for the explicit delineation of values and normative decisions in the theory and practice of nursing. Walker credits Dickoff and James for explicating the concept of practice theory via their fourth level of theory development.

The fourth level of theory development (situation-producing theory), proposed by Dickoff and James, is not to be confused with Walker's discussion of the third movement—practice theory. Situation-producing theory, prescriptive theory, and practice theory are terms that at times have been used interchangeably in the literature. It should be noted that the practice theory movement in itself was heralded before the time of Dickoff and James. Walker indicates that the failure of the movement is related to the need for a practice theory to be both general and contextual.

Within the metatheoretical movement, Walker describes two perspectives, applied and basic science, as reflected in the writings of Dorothy Johnson and Martha Rogers.

According to Walker, both Johnson and Rogers emphasize drawing from the applied and basic sciences in developing the knowledge base for nursing science. The stress on basic research in nursing is more evident in Rogers' writings, while Johnson emphasizes redefining concepts for application in nursing to provide causal accounts of nursing phenomena.

In addressing the theoretical movement, Walker advocates theory evaluation and theory synthesis in order to accelerate development of the movement. She suggests that critical review and scholarly open debate are in order. Walker recommends the integration of two or more theories into one or more complete theories and linkage of theoretical works to measureable outcomes. She offers criteria for doing theory synthesis.

In conclusion, Walker states and argues for three positions to be taken in regard to the integration of basic research, theory, and practice. Essentially the prospectus is: that innovation in nursing practice will be enhanced by basic research addressing fundamental processes pertinent to nursing situations; that true innovations in practice are made greater through using a theoretical perspective which initially may appear obscure; and that application of basic research and theory to practice is in itself a form of art. In presenting her beliefs, Walker contends that shyness is an impediment to a practice discipline in some ways. She affirms that requiring direct clinical relevance is too restricting a criterion for all research in nursing, that challenging speculative theoretical approaches may provide the basis for major innovations in practice, and that creativity is needed in applying research and theory to practice as a distinct act.

In this chapter three movements which have heavily influenced the nursing profession are reviewed retrospectively and then prospectively. These movements, the *metatheoretical*, the *theoretical*, and the *practice theory*, were foundational to the development of recent thought about nursing as a scholarly discipline.[1]

During the late 1960s and early 1970s the nursing profession underwent an intense consideration of the theory and science of nursing (e.g., Norris, 1969, 1970, 1971; Wooldridge, Skipper, and Leonard, 1968; Conference on the Nature of Science and Nursing, 1968; Conference on the Nature of Science in Nursing, 1969; Symposium on Approaches to the Study of Nursing Questions and the Development of Nursing Science, 1972; Symposium of Theory Development in Nursing, 1968). The largely *metatheoretical* focus of these discussions included consideration of the nature and purpose of theory in nursing, criteria for evaluating theories, and sources of theory.

At approximately the same time as the metatheoretical movement was flourishing, a second movement which was *theoretically* focused occurred. The second movement consisted of primarily individual nurse-authors who published substantive theoretical works. In chronological order the second movement consisted of authors such as: Orlando (1961), Wiedenbach (1964), Henderson (1966), Ujhely (1968), Rogers (1970), King (1971), Orem (1971), Rickelman (1971), Travelbee (1971), The Nursing Development Conference Group (1973), Roy (1976), and Auger[2] (1976). These works described nursing at various

---

[1] The terms *meta-theoretical* and *theoretical* refer to different levels of analysis. The theoretical level includes statements about states of affairs of events. For example, the statement, "empathy from nurses increases patients' compliance," is at the theoretical level. The metatheoretical level focuses on methods and issues encountered in the theoretical level. For example, debate about the purposes and criteria for theory in nursing would be content at the metatheoretical level.

[2] Auger's work is largely built on the unpublished work of Dorothy Johnson.

levels: a communication network, a goal-directed service, and/or a professional discipline with "man," in the larger sense, as an object of analysis.

Amidst the metatheoretical and theoretical movements, a third movement occurred which focused on *practice theory*. The third movement may be seen as methodological and was centered in the practice theory or theory of theories concepts of Dickoff and James (1968; Dickoff, James, and Wiedenbach, 1968). This movement focused on an explication of the purpose and structural components of theory in an applied practice field. The theory of theories work of Dickoff and James may rightly be called metatheoretical. It is more than that, however, in that a structure and format for theory development was not only described and analyzed but also proposed.

While these three movements occurred at overlapping time periods, they were surprisingly insulated from each other. For example, except for occasional pieces such as McCarthy (1972) and Grew (1976), the practice theory movement did little to advance the theoretical movement. The metatheoretical movement, in turn, produced only a small body of analytic literature pertinent to the theoretical (e.g., Duffy and Muhlenkamp, 1974) or practice theory (e.g., Walker, 1971) movements.

In this chapter, I will critically examine aspects of each of these three movements in terms of what they have yielded and what their limitations have been. The analysis will be followed by an attempt to construct some bridges to the future. The prospect will aim at building on what has been learned from the past and using that knowledge to formulate more seasoned, and hopefully more integrative, perspectives for the future.

RETROSPECT

Practice Theory: The Limitations and Contributions

The practice theory movement was heralded in nursing by Wald and Leonard's call for nursing practice theory which they described as the study of "ways to achieve change" (1964:311). The concept of practice theory reached its most elaborate explication in the writings of Dickoff and James in 1968.[3] With Wiedenbach, Dickoff and James proposed a four-level model of theory in a practice discipline: (1) factor-isolating, (2) factor-relating, (3) situation-relating, and (4) situation-producing theories. In their proposal, the fourth level of theory, situation-producing or practice theory, represented the quintessence of theory in practice in that means, "prescriptions for activity," and ends, "goal-content," were specified (Dickoff, James, and Wiedenbach, 1968:421).

Now, some 12 years later, it is possible to disregard the rhetoric and zeal that surrounded the Dickoff-James proposal and evaluate it on its own merits. Probably the most concrete criticism of the Dickoff-James theory of theories proposal is found in the dearth of outcomes it has produced. The proposal did not lead to a proliferation of practice theories that can be readily identified. A more conceptual criticism may also be made. While Dickoff and James delineated levels of theory for practice, the methods to be used in progressing from one level to the next remained obscure. The later Dickoff-James paper (1975) notwithstanding, the theory of theories proposal became the kind of ivory-tower work that they found so repugnant in nursing. Extensions of the Dickoff-James proposal (Diers, 1979; Kritek, 1978) may provide more serviceable interpretations of that work. It remains to be seen if the structure for theory proposed by Dickoff and James can be made operational by others. To date, it appears appropriate to judge the theory of theories concept as one whose time has passed.

The fourth level of theory, called *practice theory* here, appeared to offer promise in integrating theory with practice (Harris, 1971; Jacox, 1974). However, it suffers from its own difficul-

[3] A similar, but less definitive explication of practice theory was also made by Wooldridge, Skipper, and Leonard (1968).

ties. In order to be applicable to a wide variety of nursing situations, practice theory must be general, i.e., not bound by time and place. However, to be readily usable in a specific situation, practice theory must be contextual, i.e., time- and place-bound. No matter in which direction practice theory is developed, general or specific, it loses its potency. In the former case, it may at best serve as a guide; in the latter, transferring the theory from one situation to another without regard for situational variations is imprudent. This author argues here that the concept of practice theory is simply an appealing device that has been used to hide the real and genuine complexities of relating theory—the general model—to practice —the specific situation. Let us be reminded again that there are no simple shortcuts to this complex process (Kerlinger, 1977; Walker, 1973).

Any consideration of Dickoff and James' work must also acknowledge its positive contributions. What are these? This author would underscore one: the explicit delineation of values and normative decisions in the theory and practice of nursing. Value judgments are implicit in any rationalization of practice. Dickoff and James have helped to make this clear.

The Elusive Link of Theory to Practice

If the practice theory movement failed to result in a fruitful perspective for theory in a practice discipline, what other perspectives were proposed within the metatheoretical movement? Two will be considered here: *applied science* and *basic science* perspectives as reflected in the writings of Dorothy Johnson and Martha Rogers, respectively. These accounts will not attempt to be exhaustive reviews of Johnson and Rogers, but rather sketches presenting a sense of the perspectives of these two influential nursing leaders.[4]

Johnson (1959) began her perspective on

---

[4] The views of Rogers and Johnson reported here were important historical anchors in the development of nursing thought. These views may not represent the current or future positions of these two nursing leaders.

nursing as an applied science by noting that the continued existence of a profession was contingent upon having an explicit theoretical base for its practice. Calling the theoretical base for nursing "nursing science," Johnson proceeded to differentiate between basic and applied sciences: the former are concerned with explanation of natural phenomena and the systematization of scientific knowledge, while the latter derive their knowledge base largely from the basic sciences and focus on application of that knowledge to socially defined ends. Johnson qualified the distinction between basic and applied science by noting that, beyond a difference in purpose, many similarities in fact exist between these two branches of science. Johnson saw professional disciplines as applied sciences "which draw heavily upon the basic sciences to derive their bodies of knowledge (1959:292)." Johnson then characterized nursing science as "a synthesis, reorganization, or extension of concepts drawn from the basic or other applied sciences which in their reformulation tend to become 'new' concepts (1959:292)." For Johnson, the "new" concepts provided causal accounts of nursing phenomena which ultimately led to development of diagnostic categories and theories of intervention. The latter were to "yield predictable (and desirable) responses in patients when implemented in nursing care (1959:292)."

Nursing science was linked to practice in two ways: (1) by use of diagnostic labels which were enmeshed in causal models of practice phenomena and (2) by use of knowledge of interventions which matched diagnostic conditions to predictable desired outcomes. Fundamental to Johnson's position was the idea that nursing science as applied science was dependent on other disciplines for the "stuff" from which nursing science was then reconstructed. While nursing concepts might be called new, they would not necessarily be novel or surprising, but rather realigned or redefined concepts from other disciplines.

Martha Rogers (1967b) argued that nursing was a "learned profession." A key ingredient of a learned profession was an abstract knowledge base. Rogers called the knowledge base for nursing "nursing science" and described it as a "body of scientific knowledge characterized by descriptive, explanatory, and predictive principles about the life process of man" (1963,1:11). Further, nursing science was developed "through synthesis and re-synthesis of selected knowledges from the human-ities and the biological, physical, and social sciences for new concepts and understandings about man and his evironment" (1963,1:11). Rogers under-scored the novel aspects of nursing science further by saying, "Nursing science is *not* a summation of facts and principles drawn from the basic sciences and other disciplines. It is a new product" (1967b: 8). Rogers further tempered the derivative nature of nursing science by arguing that basic research in nursing was crucial to development of nursing science (1967a). While acknowledging the impor-tance of applied research to nursing, Rogers also affirmed the basic science perspective: "The over-riding need in nursing today is for basic research in the science of nursing" (1967a:5). For Rogers the linkage of nursing science and practice is less clear than in Johnson's account. Through basic research, Rogers saw knowledge developed and then utilized in nursing practice through (1) evaluative and diagnostic and (2) interventive processes (1964).

Both these important writers, while differing in their fundamental basic or applied perspectives of nursing science, shared a view of that science as derivative from other disciplines. In a sense, both limited the scope of nursing as an independent discipline by viewing nursing science as a deriva-tive product. While Johnson's perspective more clearly linked nursing science to practice than Roger's, even here the perspective was incomplete and followed the medical perspective of diagnosis and intervention.

In closing, this review must be tempered, how-ever, by recognition of the historical importance of Johnson's and Roger's accounts of nursing science. Both contributed to a vision of nursing which went beyond unquestioned procedures and techniques.

Nursing Theories: Pro and Con on the Big Picture Approach

The quest for a conceptual and theoretical base for practice in nursing has been admirably provided by those "nursing theories" produced within the theoretical movement. (See the introduction for a representative listing of nursing theorists.) The content of these "nursing theories" embodied events and processes inherent in the practice of nursing. In that the "nursing theories" filled a void in the nursing profession for theoretical material, their value was absolute. However, from the stand-point of more extrinsic criteria, e.g., their scientific adequacy, questions about their value may indeed be raised. This issue will be discussed further in the next section.

If the appearance of nursing theories has pro-vided professional respectability for nursing, that respectability may also have its limitations. While nursing may have acquired the surface character-istics of a scholarly profession or discipline, it still may not have achieved its substance, i.e., a conceptual base that truly provides a depth of understanding commensurate with professional or scholarly status.

Growth requires reflection, sometimes painful, upon what one is about. In contrast, nursing theories have often been accepted or adopted in uncritical ways. The careful and critical scrutiny of ideas that one would hope would apply within a scholarly community has largely been bypassed in incorporating nursing theories as frameworks for research, practice, and curricula in nursing. What is needed next are thoughtful and enlightened critiques of major nursing theories.

PROSPECT

Nursing Theories: Sampling the Fruit Before You Buy

Hardy suggested that nursing was in a "prepara-digm" stage in the development of theoretical as-pects of the discipline. In a preparadigm stage, a discipline has not yet reached consensus about "what entities are of particular concern, where to locate these entities or how to study them." (1978:39) How may progress toward the stage of paradigmatic consensus be accelerated? Two ways are proposed here: (1) theory evaluation and (2) theory synthesis.

At its simplest level, evaluation of nursing theories may be done by using extant criteria (e.g., Ellis, 1968; Hardy, 1978) as part of a critical and systematic assessment of theories.[5] For a deeper level of analysis, clarification of the multiple purposes of theories in nursing, development of standards consistent with these purposes, and then application of these standards to theoretical works in nursing are needed. For example, delineation of valuational versus descriptive purposes of theories may lead to significant and peculiar constraints on the standards for evaluating nursing theories. Theories that are understood to deal with valuational aspects of nursing may be judged by quite different standards or canons than descriptive theories. Nursing theories that attempt to combine both valuational and descriptive purposes may warrant still different criteria for evaluation. Theories that are descriptive, i.e., scientific, may appear to be the easiest to evaluate in that standards, e.g., internal consistency and testability, are more accessible. But even here, the task of critical review requires great sensitivity to the complexity of making scientific evaluations (Hempel, 1966:70–84).

Undertaking the critical review of nursing theories requires more than technical analytic skills, however. It also requires a scholarly community that supports and expects open debate and a community whose members take on the tedious responsibility for critical review of each other's works. These are the more subtle and refined marks of a mature profession and discipline. These characteristics are only beginning to appear with regularity in the nursing community.

Through the process of critical review, both

strengths and weaknesses of theories may be identified. This information may then serve as signposts for: (1) where further productive work needs to be done to improve theories; (2) dead-end directions to be avoided; and (3) selection of promising theoretical paradigms.

Theory synthesis is the second approach recommended to accelerate theoretical development in nursing. By theory synthesis this author means at least two things: (1) the thoughtful conceptual integration of two or more theories into one more adequate and complete theory, and (2) the linkage of theoretical works to operational or measurable outcomes. Both of these are complex. Where it can be shown that theoretical works cover essentially the same phenomena and use only slightly different language, or where two or more theoretical works cover different phases or aspects of the same process and the combining of these gives a more complete view of the process, then theory synthesis should be considered. Successful theory synthesis should result in a more conceptually integrated and complete perspective of the phenomena or events than any theory taken alone. [See Burr (1972) and Robinson (1977:11–30) for examples of theory synthesis.]

The second aspect of theory synthesis, linkages between theoretical works and operational or measurable outcomes, is especially needed where a theory has not yet been empirically tested and the method for testing is obscure. Let us call the second approach *operational theory synthesis*. In order to do operational theory synthesis, two things are required: (1) construction of operational definitions of theoretical terms that one may expect to measure rather directly and/or (2) formulation of bridge principles (Hempel, 1966:72–75) for theoretical terms that one expects to measure only through linkage with additional mediating terms which are themselves measurable. Operational theory synthesis may prove to be especially problematic in nursing in that the growth of theories here has preceded the development of a large stock of sound, data-based generalizations (or laws) about nursing situations.

---

[5] A beginning step toward theory evaluation is contained in the Nursing Theories Conference Group book, *Nursing Theories* (1980).

Typically, in the natural or physical sciences laws or data-based generalizations have preceded theories. Laws and generalizations by providing both the language and methods needed to link abstract theories to empirical events have facilitated operational theory synthesis. Since nursing lacks a body of well-supported generalizations, it would appear that development of data-based generalizations about nursing situations and the theories themselves may have to occur simultaneously. This situation would further seem to challenge theorists in nursing and researchers to work together closely in order that each might benefit from the other's ongoing work.

Basic Research and Theory as Perspective for Innovation

This author argues for a perhaps unpopular set of positions: (1) that innovation in nursing practice will be enhanced by basic research which addresses fundamental processes pertinent to nursing situations (though the nursing connection may not always be obvious at first); (2) that true innovations in practice are enhanced by use of a theoretical perspective which may appear obscure or irrelevant at first glance; and (3) that application of basic research and theory to practice is an art form in its own right, not a reflex action of either the researcher or practitioner.

The positions put forth here argue against timidity in a practice discipline in several ways. First, promotion of basic research focused on fundamental processes of only potential pertinence to nursing removes the supportive prop of direct clinical relevance to which the timid may cling. By its very nature, basic research may not have direct relevance to practice (Kerlinger, 1977:5-7). Requiring direct clinical relevance is too short-sighted a criterion for all research in nursing: the criterion assumes that one knows the results of the research before it is conducted and, further, that the manner of applying that knowledge is also similarly clear. While not discounting the importance of the clinical relevance criterion in an applied nursing research context, the criterion is too stringent, this author believes, for basic research in nursing. Further, limiting nursing research to only applied research, where clinical relevance is more apparent, continues to place nursing in a dependent position relative to other disciplines for the basic knowledge needed to advance practice. In one medical specialty area, Comroe and Dripps (1976) have shown the crucial role of research directed at fundamental processes in advancing practice. While one such example does not make a definitive case for basic research, it certainly is suggestive of the interplay and importance of both basic and applied research in an emerging discipline and profession.

Second, this author argues against timidity in creating and selecting the perspectives or visions from which innovations in practice evolve. Daring, "irrelevant," and speculative theoretical perspectives may in the long run provide the basis for major innovations in practice. Where innovations in practice are only variations of prevailing practices, the likelihood of startling new results is small. New theoretical perspectives may, however, provide new ways of looking at practice phenomena and conceptualizing approaches used in practice. (There is, of course, no guarantee that new theoretical perspectives will always be fruitful or successful in advancing practice.) Problems of concern to the researcher and practitioner, e.g., patient noncompliance and adolescent pregnancy, may remain generally refractory to conventional approaches until new theoretical perspectives on these problem areas are conceptualized.

Bromwich's work (1976; Bromwich and Parmalee, 1979) provides an intriguing example of how new theoretical perspectives may lead to innovations in practice.[6] In constructing an intervention program for high-risk infants, Bromwich focused the program on enhancing "parents' enjoyment of and sensitivity and responsiveness

---

[6]Since Bromwich's theoretical model has been tested in only one clinical study to date, her research is reported more for its illustrative than substantive import.

to their infants" (Bromwich and Parmalee, 1979: 390). This focus grew out of a model of the parental behavior progression needed "for the kind of care giver–infant interactions which lay the foundation for optimal infant development" (Bromwich and Parmalee, 1979:396). Bromwich's program, which begins with parental enjoyment of the infant, broke from the tradition of other infant programs which stressed an infant developmental curriculum (1976). The theoretical model provided the perspective for this departure from traditional programs.

Third, this author argues here against timid ways of thinking about the act of applying research and theory to practice. While the prevailing paradigm might dictate that researchers include implications for practice as the "last act" of the research report, or that practitioners read research reports so they may update their practice, this view underestimates the complexity and creativity needed to apply research to practice. Further, Ellis (1969) has outlined the complex process of the practitioner using theories in practice. Following E. S. Maccia, this author has argued elsewhere for the concept of practice development as a bridging activity between theory and research on the one hand and practice on the other (Walker, 1973:3–4). While recognizing the perspective and knowledge that arise from theory and research, these do not logically entail the exact form, sequence, materials, personnel, or client conditions under which application is to occur. The transformation of theory and research findings into a clear and useful form for the practitioner is a distinct act. Practice development involves integrating theory and research-based knowledge with practice constraints and goals. Thus, concerns such as cost, relative effectiveness, risk, feasibility, and ethical desirability would all be considered in fully developing new approaches to practice. While distinct from research and theory, practice development is of necessity closely tied to each of these. The concept of practice development, while not widespread in nursing, is reflected in nursing projects such as that reported by Haller, Reynolds, and Horsley (1979). Practice development as here envisioned is not an ancillary task of the researcher or practitioner but a distinct process warranting the time, effort, and creativity of the best minds in the profession.

This author would like to close this "prospect" with a "retrospective" comment. A vision for the future is always facilitated by the clarity of thought that preceded it. Regardless of the ultimate value of the prospect presented here, attempting to construct it has been facilitated by the important and clear thought on which it builds. Thus, in closing this chapter, this author would like to acknowledge her debt to Dorothy Johnson and Martha Rogers for the illumination their work has personally provided for her.

EDITOR'S QUESTIONS FOR DISCUSSION

What is the difference between situation-producing, prescriptive and practice theory? What is the difference between a metatheoretical focus and a preparadigm stage in the development of theory? What are the difficulties inherent in developing practice theory? How can linkages be established between nursing theoretical perspectives and the concept of practice development? What are the potential risks in practice development in making it distinct from research and theory? How might Fawcett (Chap. 14) view practice development? To what extent is there agreement between Walker and Fawcett regarding practice development?

What is the difference between Johnson's and Rogers's approach to drawing from the basic and applied sciences and the outcome for developing nursing science? How do the "new concepts" referred to by Johnson differ from "a new product" according to Rogers's view? According to Walker, how is Rogers's linkage of nursing science and practice less clear than Johnson's? Would you agree with Walker that Johnson's perspective follows the medical frame of reference of diagnosis and intervention?

To what extent would you agree that nursing is in a "preparadigm" stage in the development of theory? Is there evidence for your view? What criteria may be suggested for a critical and systematic assessment of theories? Are there criteria that might be more appropriate for one type of theory versus another, i.e., descriptive, valuational as suggested by Walker? If a theory is a theory, should it not be judged by one set of criteria?

REFERENCES

Auger, Jeanine Rose
  1976 Behavioral Systems and Nursing. Englewood Cliffs, N.J.: Prentice-Hall.
Bromwich, R. M.
  1976 "Focus on maternal behavior in infant intervention." American Journal of Orthopsychiatry 46:439–46.
Bromwich, R. M. and A. H. Parmalee
  1979 "An intervention program for pre-term infants," Pp. 389–411 in T. M. Field (ed.), Infants Born at Risk: Behavior and Development. New York: SP Medical and Scientific Books.
Burr, Wesley R.
  1972 "Role transitions: A reformulation of theory." Journal of Marriage and the Family 34:407–16.
Comroe, Julius H. and Robert D. Dripps
  1976 "Scientific basis for the support of biomedical science." Science 192(2435): 105–111.
Conference on the Nature of Science and Nursing
  1968 "Conference on the nature of science and nursing." Nursing Research 17:484–512.
Conference on the Nature of Science in Nursing
  1969 "Conference on the nature of science in nursing." Nursing Research 18:388–411.
Dickoff, J and P. James
  1968 "A theory of theories: A position paper." Nursing Research 17:197–203.
  1975 "Theory development in nursing," Pp. 45–92 in P. J. Verhonick (ed.), Nursing Research I. Boston: Little, Brown.
Dickoff, James, Patricia James, and Ernestine Wiedenbach
  1968 "Theory in a practice discipline, part I." Nursing Research 17:415–35.

Diers, D.
  1979 Research in Nursing Practice. Philadelphia: Lippincott.
Duffy, Margery and Anne F. Muhlenkamp
  1974 "A framework for theory analysis." Nursing Outlook 22:570–4.
Ellis, Rosemary
  1968 "Characteristics of significant theories." Nursing Research 17:217–22.
  1969 "The practitioner as theorist." American Journal of Nursing 69:1434–38.
Grew, E.
  1976 "A prescriptive theory of maternity nursing." Pp. 3–15 in L. K. McNall and J. T. Galeener (eds.), Current Practice in Obstetrics and Gynecologic Nursing. St. Louis: C. V. Mosby.
Haller, Karen B., M. A. Reynolds, and J. A. Horsley
  1979 "Developing research-based innovation protocols: Process, criteria, and issues." Research in Nursing and Health 2:45–51.
Hardy, Margaret E.
  1978 "Perspectives on nursing theory." Advances in Nursing Science 1:37–48.
Harris, M. Isabel
  1971 "Theory building in nursing: A review of literature." Image 4:6–10.
Hempel, Carl G.
  1966 Philosophy of Natural Science. Englewood Cliffs, N.J.: Prentice-Hall.
Henderson, Virginia
  1966 The Nature of Nursing. New York: Macmillan.
Jacox, Ada
  1974 "Theory construction in nursing: An overview." Nursing Research 23:4–13.
Johnson, Dorothy E.
  1959 "The nature of a science of nursing." Nursing Outlook 7:291–94.

Kerlinger, Fred N.
1977 "The influence of research on educational practice." Educational Researcher 6:5-12.

King, Imogene
1971 Toward a Theory of Nursing. New York: Wiley.

Kritek, P.
1978 "The generation of classification of nursing diagnoses: Toward a theory of nursing." Image 10:33-40.

McCarthy, Rosemary
1972 "A practice theory of nursing care." Nursing Research 21:405-10.

Norris, Catherine M. (ed.)
1969 Proceedings. First Nursing Theory Conference. Kansas City: University of Kansas Medical Center Department of Nursing.
1970 Proceedings. Second Nursing Theory Conference. Kansas City: University of Kansas Medical Center Department of Nursing.
1971 Proceedings. Third Nursing Theory Conference. Kansas City: University of Kansas Medical Center Department of Nursing.

Nursing Development Conference Group
1973 Concept Formalization in Nursing. Boston: Little, Brown.

Nursing Theories Conference Group
1980 Nursing Theories. Englewood Cliffs, N.J.: Prentice-Hall.

Orem, Dorothea
1971 Nursing: Concepts of Practice. New York: McGraw-Hill.

Orlando, Ida Jean
1961 The Dynamic Nurse-Patient Relationship. New York: Putnam's.

Rickelman, Bonnie
1971 "Bio-psycho-social linguistics: A conceptual approach to nurse-patient interactions." Nursing Research 20:398-403.

Robinson, Beverlyanne
1977 The Service of Nursing: Theory Development Using Marketing Research. Unpublished Ph.D. dissertation, The University of Texas at Austin.

Rogers, Martha E.
1963 "Some comments on the theoretical basis of nursing practice." Nursing Science 1:11-13 and 60-61.
1964 Reveille in Nursing. Philadelphia: Davis.
1967a "Nursing science: Research and researchers." Unpublished paper presented at the Annual Conference of Research and Nursing, Division of Nursing Education, Teachers College, Columbia University, February 3, 1967.
1967b "Nursing: Today's happening." Unpublished paper presented at Annual Alumnae Day, University of North Carolina, School of Nursing, June 2, 1967.
1970 An Introduction to the Theoretical Basis of Nursing. Philadelphia: Davis.

Roy, Sister Callista
1976 Introduction to Nursing: An Adaptation Model. Englewood Cliffs, N.J.: Prentice-Hall.

Symposium on Approaches to the Study of Nursing Questions and the Development of Nursing Science
1972 "Symposium of approaches to the study of nursing questions and the development of nursing science." Nursing Research 21:484-517.

Symposium of Theory Development in Nursing
1968 "Symposium of theory development in nursing." Nursing Research 17:196-227.

Travelbee, Joyce
1971 Interpersonal Aspects of Nursing. Philadelphia: Davis.

Ujhely, Gertrude
1968 Determinants of the Nurse-Patient Relationship. New York: Springer.

Wald, Florence S. and Robert C. Leonard
1964 "Towards development of nursing practice theory." Nursing Research 13:309-313.

Walker, Lorraine Olszewski
1971 "Toward a clearer understanding of the concept of nursing theory." Nursing Research 20:428-435.
1973 "Theory, practice and research in perspective." Proceedings of the Ninth American Nurses' Association Nursing Research Conference, March 21, 1973, San Antonio, Texas.

Wiedenbach, Ernestine
1964 Clinical Nursing. New York: Springer.

Wooldridge, Pohaton, James K. Skipper, Jr., and Robert C. Leonard
1968 Behavioral Science, Social Practice, and the Nursing Profession. Cleveland: Case Western Reserve.

Chapter 31

Critical Analysis of Theory Development in Nursing

Edna M. Menke, R.N., Ph.D.
Associate Professor
School of Nursing
Graduate Department
Ohio State University
Columbus, Ohio

The plea for more collaboration and colleagueship among nurse-scholars in the development of nursing science is evident throughout the presentation by Edna M. Menke. She believes there is consensus that the purpose of nursing is health promotion and the focus of nursing science is the "phenomenon of man." In her analysis Menke perceives nursing science to be primarily at the conceptual framework stage in its theory development. At the same time she indicates that the state of knowledge in nursing evolved in the 1970s to the point where it could be labeled scientific. Menke reviews the terminology associated with theory.

Somewhat different from the previous chapters in this section, this chapter discusses five approaches to theory development. The use of inductive or deductive reasoning is offered as one alternative. Another is to link theory development with inquiry, by either making observations and developing theory or formulating theory and empirically testing it. Menke describes Jacox's three stages of theory development as a third approach. The stages include: concept specification, definition, and classification; statements proposing the relationship of concepts; and systematic designation of the propositions. The model constructed by Chinn and Jacobs is offered as another guide. According to Menke, this model comprises: concept examination and analysis, formulation and validation of relational statements, actual theory construction, and practical application of the theory. Chinn and Jacobs advocate the importance of developing theory regarding any phenomenon that is perceived to be within the domain of nursing. The final approach outlined by Menke is that of selecting an existing conceptual model to derive theory utilizing Dickoff, James, and Widenbach's four levels of theory.

Menke briefly reviews the historical development of theory in nursing. With the exception of Nightingale's efforts and a few others, Menke cites the era before 1960 as prescientific. With the identification of nurse-scholars as pioneers in conceptualizing nursing knowledge around 1960, Menke perceives the launching of the scientific era. Defining a metatheorist as an individual who analyzes the status of theory development in nursing, she notes the number that have increased.

Menke devotes considerable analysis to the work of Dickoff, James, and Widenbach. In her view, they advocate varied approaches to the development of theory, not a theory of nursing, and ultimately a theory that is prescriptive for practice. Menke further compares their work with Beckstrand's. In so doing the terms *practice, prescriptive theory,* and *predictive theory* at times appear to be used interchangeably.

According to Menke, Beckstrand argues logically that practice theory in itself is not useful to the progress of nursing science. However, she perceives Beckstrand as contributing to a base for developing predictive theory in nursing. The point is made that "practice or prescriptive" theory can be considered one type of scientific theory if it is derived from valid deductive arguments. Menke further takes issue with Beckstrand's interpretation of Jacox's set of rules practice theory. According to Menke, practitioners would use the theory only if it were congruent with their belief system. Menke indicates Beckstrand's three parameters of knowledge for it to be useful in practice. She contends that Beckstrand is using the term "practice theory" as a framework for guiding one's practice not as meaning a scientific theory.

Menke addresses Hardy's argument that nursing science is at the preparadigm stage, characterized by ambiguity and divergent schools of thought regarding phenomena. She appears to agree with Hardy, specifying that none of the competing models could be labeled a scientific paradigm according to Kuhn's classification. She advocates scholars to use existing conceptual frameworks to derive theories and concludes nursing has the base for a paradigm.

In conclusion, Menke cites three impediments to the development of nursing theory: lack of consensus among nurses that nursing science exists or has value for practice; the idea that there needs to be the theory of nursing, a grand theory or unification model accepted by the majority of the scientific community; and a laissez-faire approach to theory development. She strongly argues and offers concrete strategies for cooperative endeavors. Menke projects the ultimate goal to be to create predictive or prescriptive theory. She urges nurse scholars to make a long-term commitment to advance knowledge.

Theory development has a direct relationship to the growth of a discipline as a science. During the past decade theory development in nursing has progressed a great deal; the profession has entered a new era in developing a scientific body of knowledge. Nursing can only become a legitimate science if nurse-scholars develop a highly organized, cumulative, specialized field of knowledge and concomitantly continue to be seekers of knowledge. Nurse-scholars concur that there has been advancement in the development of nursing science (Andreoli and Thompson, 1977; Donaldson and Crowley, 1978; Downs, 1979; Gortner, 1980). There have been new books published regarding theory development in nursing (Newman, 1979; Riehl and Roy, 1980; Stevens, 1979), and there are new journals, such as *Advances in Nursing Science* and *Research in Nursing and Health*.

The advancement in the development of nursing science can be attributed to a change in thinking among nurse-scholars. There is consensus that the purpose of nursing is health promotion and that the focus of nursing science is the phenomenon of man (Newman, 1979; Rogers, 1970; Stevens, 1979). Thus, theory development has a delineated focus. According to Fawcett, nursing theory is "a set of interrelated propositions and definitions which present a systematic view of one or more of the essential units of nursing—person, environment, health, nursing—by specifying relations among relevant variables" (1978b:26). Similarly, the cadre of nurse-scholars has increased, and many of the new scholars are a different breed. The development of more doctoral programs in nursing facilitated an increase in the number of scholars studying and developing nursing science. It is an exciting area for nursing science.

The purpose of this paper is to present an overview and a critical analysis of theory development in nursing. The analysis will include a historical review of past endeavors and discussions of the current status of and the future perspectives for theory development in nursing. This analysis is based on the author's experiences and on her study of theory development over the past 15 years.

OVERVIEW OF THEORY DEVELOPMENT

Even though theory development in nursing has progressed a great deal in the past decade, the overall progress has been relatively slow. Actually, there is a dearth of theory in nursing science. The word "theory" as it is used in the titles of some conceptualizations of nursing is really a misnomer. It would be more accurate to consider these works conceptual frameworks or conceptual models. The terminology involved with theory has been used loosely, and sometimes the terms have been used out of context. For instance, in reviewing literature related to theory development, it is found that the terms theory, conceptual framework, theoretical framework, and model are used interchangeably by some individuals. This is confusing to the scholar who has a knowledge of the terms, let alone to the neophyte who is going to be the future nurse-scholar or consumer of the knowledge.

In this paper the terms theory, conceptual framework, and model are used to represent three abstract entities. *Theory* is used to refer to an abstract system of interrelated concepts and propositions that describe, explain, or predict phenomena. The relationship between the concepts is precisely delineated and can be tested empirically. This use of "theory" is similar to Kerlinger's definition. He states that "theory is a set of interrelated constructs (concepts), defini-

tions, and propositions that present a systematic view of phenomena by specifying relations among variables, with the purpose of explaining and predicting the phenomena" (Kerlinger, 1973:9). *Conceptual framework* refers to a group of concepts which may or may not be related to each other, but which are believed to be important in understanding or explaining phenomena. The individual who develops a conceptual framework makes some conjectures as to how the concepts may influence each other. A conceptual framework is more vague and broad than theory and is harder to test empirically (Williams, 1979). *Model* is used to refer to a symbolic representation in logical terms of some phenomena. A model may be used to represent a theory or a conceptual framework.

Approaches to Theory Development

The approaches that can be used to develop theory in any discipline are varied. Theories can be developed through inductive or deductive reasoning. Whereas, in the inductive approach, the theorist moves from specific empirical evidence to make inferences about more general or abstract states, in the deductive approach, the theorist moves from the more general or abstract level to make inferences about more specific states of the phenomena.

Another approach links theory development with inquiry. For instance, in the Baconian approach, research is used to develop theory (Reynolds, 1971). There are laws in nature waiting to be discovered. The theorist makes observations and then develops theory. The opposite approach is to develop the theory and then conduct the research. The theorist imposes his or her description or explanation on the phenomena, then empirically tests the theory. Popper's notion of conjecture and refutations is an example of the theory-then-research approach (1959).

Jacox contends that there are three stages in the process of theory development (1974). The first stage is a period of specifying, defining, and classifying the concepts used to describe the phenomena. A concept is an abstraction of the empirical world. The parameters of each concept must be delineated. The second stage consists of developing statements that propose how two or more concepts are related. The last stage is that of specifying how all of the propositions are related to each other in a systematic way. Each stage in theory development should be tested through research. The theory cannot be tested directly, but only indirectly through testing hypotheses or propositions that are derived from the theory. Research lends support to the theory or assists in the identification of how the theory needs to be modified to agree with the phenomena in the empirical world.

Chinn and Jacobs have constructed a model for theory development in nursing (1978). A theory-development system serves as a guide to a set of operations necessary to evolve theory. In Chinn and Jacobs' system the operations include: (1) concept examination and analysis, (2) formulation and validation of relational statements, (3) actual theory construction, and (4) practical application of the theory. The model can be visualized as a circle, or wheel, that is divided into four quadrants which are further delineated. All aspects of the system influence each other. For instance, concept examination and analysis influences formulation of relational statements. Within the system there are some separate functions and outputs. Whereas analysis of concepts and formulation and validation of relational statements result in descriptive and explanatory knowledge, the theory construction and practical application aspects of the system provide predictive knowledge. The system has boundaries which connote limits regarding the concerns of a particular science. Chinn and Jacobs contend that "to endlessly extend boundaries and encompass the whole of reality, a discipline weakens the power of its scientific endeavors" (1978:8). Chinn and Jacobs's model is useful in understanding the process of theory development, the linkages with research endeavors to test or build theory, and the value of diverse scientific approaches. Chinn and Jacobs do not advocate the development of one kind of theory over another. They stress the importance of developing theory regarding any phenomena that the theorist believes is within the domain of nursing. According to Chinn and Jacobs, theory development is the process through which nursing will establish a defined area of concern.

Another approach to theory development is the derivation of a theory through the use of an existing conceptual model in nursing. Here the theorist uses a conceptual model that is congruent with his or her belief system and knowledge system. After selecting a conceptual model, the theorist delineates which concepts are pertinent to the phenomena to be described, explained, and eventually predicted. The theorist then uses the four levels of theory expounded by Dickoff et al. (1968a) to develop theories regarding the phenomena. These are the factor-isolating, the factor-relating, the situation-relating, and the situation-producing levels. Factor-isolating is the lowest level of theory and focuses on identifying pertinent factors or concepts in a situation. On the factor-relating level relationships between the factors are determined. The situation-relating level predicts what will occur in the situation and assumes that a causal relationship exists between the factors. The situation-producing theory level, which is the highest, is prescriptive in that it tells how to alter aspects of a situation in order to have a specified outcome. It is important to start with lower level theories initially, since they serve as the basis for more sophisticated theories (Kritek, 1978; Menke, 1978). This approach to theory development involves a long commitment on the part of the theorist, but it leads to a refinement of theory that results in cumulative knowledge regarding the phenomena.

HISTORICAL REVIEW OF THEORY DEVELOPMENT

Interest in theory development in nursing can be traced back to the time of Florence Nightingale

(1969; Johnson, 1978). In 1859, in her book *Notes on Nursing*, Nightingale presented the first attempt to theorize about nursing. She included definitions of health, disease, and nursing and emphasized the environmental aspects of nursing care. She advocated systematic observation in order to discover the laws of life and death, which is definitely one approach to theorizing. Nightingale was actually recommending the development of nursing science. There were few other attempts at theorizing from Nightingale's time until the middle of this century. Nursing science was rarely mentioned in the literature until the late 1950s (Carper, 1978). Except for Nightingale and a few other individuals, nursing was in its prescientific era before 1960.

The first scientific conceptualizations about knowledge in nursing appeared in the literature around 1960. Abdellah identified a group of nurse-scholars whom she labeled as the pioneers in identifying nursing theories (1968). The group included Florence Blake, Rita Chow, Lydia Hall, Eileen Hasselmeyer, Madeline Leininger, Ida Orlando, Hildegard Peplau, Reva Rubin, and Ernestine Wiedenbach. Abdellah pointed out that these nurse-scholars were schooled in the field of maternal-child health, psychiatric nursing, or some other defined clinical content area. Other theorists who should be added to the list are Dorothy Johnson, Dorothea Orem, and Martha Rogers. Since the time of these pioneers, other theorists have come forth, for instance, King, Newman, and Roy (King, 1971; Riehl and Roy, 1980). In the 1970s, the state of knowledge in nursing evolved to the place where it could be labeled scientific.

Generally speaking, the majority of theorists have developed conceptual models from which nursing theories can be derived. Some nurse-scholars have worked on refining their conceptual models (Orem, 1980b; Rogers, 1980; Roy, 1980). Others have taken some of the key concepts in the models to test through research. Some new conceptual models have been developed by nurse-scholars and are in the process of being tested. The cadre of nurse-scholars has increased.

There is evidence that these professionals are committing themselves to theorize about and research specific phenomena in more systematic ways. A few scholars have been studying specific phenomena for more than a decade. And nurse-scholars are meeting regionally and nationally to discuss the process of developing, testing, or refining theory relating to specific phenomena. There is a spirit of inquiry among nurses who want to advance the development of nursing knowledge.

STATUS OF THEORY DEVELOPMENT

The number of metatheorists has increased within the past several years. A metatheorist is an individual who analyzes the status of theory development in nursing. The primary metatheorists are faculty members teaching in graduate programs in nursing, doctoral students in nursing, and graduates of doctoral programs in nursing. There have been regional and national efforts to bring these groups of nurse-scholars together to discuss theory development. Several ideas of these metatheorists will be analyzed.

Dickoff, James, and Wiedenbach are metatheorists who stimulated a great deal of controversy regarding theory development. Dickoff and James are philosophers and Wiedenbach is one of the early nurse-scholars. In 1968 they presented a theory of theories paper that was revolutionary in relation to the status of theory development in nursing. This paper discussed the nature of nursing theory and presented an interpretation of the status of theory development in nursing. Dickoff et al. contended that nursing needed to develop situational-producing theory which was prescriptive and which could guide actions in practice to achieve desired goals. They defined situational-producing theory as the highest level of theory and described three other levels of theory—factor-isolating, factor-relating, and situational-relating—as descriptive, explanatory, or predictive in nature (1968a, 1968b).

Dickoff et al. outlines the components of situational-producing theory as:

1) goal-content specified as aim for activity, 2) prescriptions for activity to realize the goal content; and 3) a survey list to serve as a suplement to present prescription and as preparation for future prescription for activity toward the goal-content. (1968a:421)

Dickoff and James advocated that practice theory needs to be more sophisticated conceptually than "pure" theory, or that theory which is concerned with describing, explaining, or predicting phenomena (1968). Each level of theory is a "conceptual invention for some purpose" (Dickoff et al., 1968b:552). Dickoff and James state that

all theory exists finally for the sake of practice (since in a sense every lower level of theory must be theory at the highest level since either the nursing aim is practice or else nursing is no longer a profession as distinct from some mere academic discipline). (1968:199)

When the theory of theories paper was presented, nurse-scholars were quite critical of the notion of advocating the development of prescriptive theory when there were few conceptual frameworks in nursing. However, when the theory of theories paper is analyzed, it appears that Dickoff et al. were making a case for the ideal and were quite futuristic in their thinking. They recognized the need for other levels of theories but believed that the theorist should continue with theory development of a phenomenon until the situational-producing level has been reached. In other words, the theory must ultimately be able to guide action in practice to reach a desired goal.

Dickoff et al. contended that situational-producing theory does not exist in nursing. They believed that embryos of nursing theory existed in the literature and recommended that nurse-scholars develop theories regarding phenomena that have utility for practice. They suggested that these approaches might be different, depending upon the theorist's perception of reality. In essence, they advocated varied approaches to the development of theories regarding phenomena and not of a theory of nursing (1968a).

Beckstrand is a metatheorist who makes a logical argument for not requiring practice theory to be useful to the progress of nursing science (1978a: 1978b; 1980). She states that "the knowledge used to control phenomena in practice is the knowledge of lawlike empirical relationships, and hence it is identical to scientific knowledge" (1978a:132). Beckstrand has taken issue with the notion of Dickoff et al. concerning the need for the development of practice or prescriptive theories for nursing. In actuality, if practice or prescriptive theory is derived from valid deductive arguments, it can be considered one type of scientific theory. One can derive hypotheses which can be empirically tested from a set of propositions regarding specified critical conditions. If the consequences predicted by the hypotheses occur empirically, there is support for the facet of the theory. If the consequences occur repeatedly, one has established the lawlike, empirical relationship of the phenomena and can prescribe when they will occur, which is the aim of prescriptive theory. In that Beckstrand is building a case for the development of predictive theory in nursing, she is supportive of some of the ideas of Dickoff et al. regarding theory.

Similarly, Beckstrand (1980) takes issue with Jacox's (1974) set of rules practice theory. In the set of rules practice theory, a certain group of actions will result in a specific outcome. Beckstrand contends that the locus of prescribing the goal is taken away from the individual practitioner and given to an external authority, the theorist. Beckstrand believes that the nurse using the set of rules practice theory needs to conform not to his or her own belief system in carrying out practice but to a set of rules imposed by an external authority. Beckstrand has taken Jacox's idea of a practice theory out of context. Jacox is advocating theory regarding specific nursing interventions that can result in predictive outcomes. In essence, Jacox is supporting the idea of situation-producing theory put forth by Dickoff et al. The practitioner would use the theory only if it were congruent with his or her belief system. In this it is similar to a counselor deciding which intervention strategy to use to attain a specific client goal. There should be more than one practice theory for each desired outcome but this will occur only when there is acceptance of the idea that there is more than one abstract way to view reality in nursing.

Beckstrand delineates three parameters for quantifying knowledge that is to be useful in practice (1978b). First, practice needs knowledge of change as its goal to improve phenomena, and practice needs knowledge of action to bring about change. Second, the knowledge required is scientific, empirical, ethical, and psychomotor in nature. Third, the practitioner's scientific and ethical knowledge delineates the relevant conditions for change and the desired outcomes. Thus the knowledge used in practice is science, ethics, and logic. Beckstrand's parameters for knowledge useful in practice are congruent with Carper's patterns of knowing in nursing (1978).

Beckstrand contends that nurse-scholars need to develop scientific and philosophical knowledge for the discipline. She supports the notion that conceptual frameworks are useful to developing theory in nursing. For instance,

> When a conceptual framework of nursing entails scientific assumptions explaining the operation of a group of empirical phenomena and how intervention can be accomplished with respect to these, then these assumptions may form a basis for scientific investigation. (Beckstrand 1980:76)

Beckstrand thinks some of the existing conceptual frameworks are ideologies and can be considered practice theories. However, she is not using the term "practice theory" to mean a scientific theory or to mean a theory that has been empirically validated, but only to name a framework that can serve as a reference for guiding one's practice.

Hardy contends that nursing science is at the preparadigm stage in its development (1978). She utilizes Kuhn's (1970) paradigm regarding scientific revolution to analyze the status of theory development in nursing. The preparadigm state is characterized by uncertainty, ambiguity, and divergent schools of thought regarding phenomena in the discipline. Similarly, there is little agreement among the scholars about what entities are important to the development of theory within the discipline. Hardy states that "until there is a prevailing paradigm and exemplar paradigms to give focus to the thinking and work of nurse-scientists, knowledge in nursing will develop slowly and somewhat haphazardly" (1978:39). A paradigm provides the broad parameters for a discipline, and exemplar paradigms are various divisions or ways of viewing the phenomena in the discipline. There are some competing conceptual models in nursing, such as Roy's "adaptation model" or Orem's "self-care model," but none has achieved the status of a scientific paradigm as defined by Kuhn's classification scheme (Carper, 1978). If there were a prevailing paradigm, some of the existing conceptual models might evolve into exemplar paradigms.

Nursing science is primarily at the conceptual framework stage in theory development. Williams (1979) and Fawcett (1978a) concur that nursing has many conceptual frameworks but a dearth of theories. Concentrated efforts by nurse-scholars are necessary if nursing is to advance as a science. Fawcett contends that rapid progress in theory development and theory testing through research is crucial if nursing is to retain and increase its respectability as a science (1978a). It is hoped that more scholars will use existing conceptual frameworks to derive theories that can be validated through research. Some efforts are currently underway based on this approach; examples are seen in Rogers's "unitary man model" and Roy's "adaptation model" (Riehl and Roy, 1980). Likewise, in that there is consensus that the purpose of the discipline is promotion of health and that the focus is man, nursing has the base for a paradigm. Barnard delineates the foci more specifically from her analysis of nurse-philosophers or theorists. She states that "the foci of nursing are the individual in relation to health, the environment, and the change process, whether it be maturation, adaptation, or coping" (1980:208).

Barriers, real or artificial, have impeded the development of nursing theory. One of the primary barriers has been the lack of consensus among nurses that nursing science exists or that it has value for practice (Jacobs and Huether, 1978; Johnson, 1974). There has been no comprehensive body of knowledge or research tradition established in nursing's evolution from an apprenticeship model. Similarly, the linkage between theory and research has not been strong. Only recently has there been more emphasis on research pertaining to theory testing or theory building (Fawcett, 1978a).

Another barrier to the development of nursing theory has been the idea that there needs to be one grand theory of nursing or a unification model of nursing that is accepted by the majority of nurses in the scientific community. This idea has served as an excuse and a rationale for not pursuing theory development. No discipline has a grand theory; all disciplines have many theories pertaining to the phenomena of their particular domain.

A commitment to the development of scientific knowledge is essential for the advance of nursing science. The laissez-faire approach to theory development has hindered progress (Johnson, 1974; Menke, 1978). Each individual in the field has followed his or her own interests and scientific orientation in studying phenomena rather than building upon the ideas of other nurse-scholars. Nursing can no longer afford the laissez-faire direction in theory development. Nurse-scholars need to work together to develop cumulative knowledge about phenomena.

FUTURE PERSPECTIVES FOR THEORY DEVELOPMENT

In this era of nursing science, nurse-scholars have the potential to develop a paradigm and exemplar paradigms for the discipline. If theory development is to become a reality in nursing, it will require more collaboration and colleagueship among scholars, as there must be concentrated, systematic efforts in evolving theory about the phenomena that are important for nursing.

Nurse-scholars need to commit themselves to theory development about specific phenomena for a substantial period of time. The nurse-scholar must develop, test, and refine theory about the phenomena. Initially, the kind of theory developed might be descriptive or explanatory, depending upon what is already known about the phenomena, but the long-range goal would be to develop predictive or prescriptive theory. This approach could result in building systematic, cumulative knowledge about specific phenomena in the discipline.

The academic community is the logical group to assume leadership in advancing theory development, as the majority of nurse-scholars are housed in university settings. Nurse faculty with doctoral preparation need to assume the major responsibility. They need to commit themselves to developing, testing, and refining theory and to serving as mentors for students who will be the future nurse-scholars. Inherent in this plan is the belief that the nurse-scholar is also a nurse-researcher with whom students can work to advance the state of knowledge about specific phenomena.

Some nurse faculty at a university might as a group commit itself to develop theories about specific phenomena. More than one approach to developing theory would probably occur at a university because of the variety of educational backgrounds of the doctorally prepared faculty. As Chinn and Jacobs state, "a sense of mutual respect needs to exist between scientists whose styles may be different" (1978:9). As a result of collaborative endeavors within specific university settings, various universities may become known for their theories regarding some particular phenomena.

There also needs to be collaboration among nurse-scholars from various university settings, nurse-scholars who can share with each other the research they are conducting and who can develop strategies together to build upon one another's theories. State, regional, and national conferences pertaining to specific theory development offer opportunities to facilitate such collaboration. Different scientific camps that serve as the base for the development of exemplar paradigms might develop between and within universities.

The research productivity of nurse-scholars needs to be strengthened. Fawcett advocates the research-theory helix for the development of knowledge (1978a). Research and theory development can be considered as a cyclic process. Research is used to test and build theory, and theory guides research endeavors. Regardless of the theorist's style, research is necessary to validate theory. The same kind of collaborative endeavors as those previously suggested for theory development are needed in conducting research.

Conceptual models that have been developed by some nurse-scholars can be used to derive theories. Here the theorist would delineate which concepts are pertinent to the phenomena for which a theory is to be developed. Another approach would be to test a theory from another discipline to determine if it is valid for phenomena in nursing. There must be a spirit of inquiry in nursing.

Throughout their lifetime, nurse-scholars must continue to be committed to advancing knowledge within the discipline. More effort needs to be spent in postdoctoral study and in continuing educational endeavors related to theory development. Nurse-scholars are responsible for developing strategies to implement tested theory in practice. There must be communication between nurse-scholars and nurses in other settings in order to develop, test, and refine theory necessary for the advancement of the discipline as a science.

EDITOR'S QUESTIONS FOR DISCUSSION

Which scholars of nursing science would agree with Menke that the purpose of nursing is to promote health and that the focus of nursing science is the "phenomenon of man"? Present arguments for and against the statement that there is a dearth of theory in nursing science. Would you agree with Menke that there is little consensus among scholars as to which entities are important to theorize?

What strategies can be suggested to resolve the confusion regarding terminology related to theory development? Compare the basic definition of terms in Santora's chapter (Chap. 8) with Menke's. What similarities and differences exist in theoretical perspectives presented in the chapters by Fawcett (Chap. 14), Newman (Chap. 28), Chinn (Chap. 29), Walker (Chap. 30), Menke (Chap. 31), Hardy (Chap. 32), Meleis (Chap. 33), and Roy (Chap. 34)?

Which scholars of nursing science utilize an inductive and which use a deductive approach to theory development? Provide examples as to how each method can be employed. Which scholars make observations to develop theory and which formulate theory and then test it through research? Is there any relationship between those methods and the inductive and deductive approaches? What is meant by the term scientific inquiry? What is the difference between Dickoff, James, and Wiedenbach's concept of prescriptive theory, Jacox's set of rules practice theory, and Chinn and Jacox's practical application aspect of their model for theory development? Which scholars would agree with the importance of developing theory regarding any phenomena believed to be within the domain of nursing? Which scholars advocate the development of one kind of theory over another? Which scholars have been studying specific phenomena of nursing?

To what extend would you agree with Menke's interpretation and applicability of Dickoff, James, and Wiedenbach's work to the present status of theory development in nursing? Is there an inherent conflict between situation-producing (prescriptive theory) and Beckstrand's notion of practice theory as portrayed by Menke? What is different among theory, law, and principles? What is different among prescriptive theory, policies, and procedures in nursing practice? What strategies can be employed to bridge the hiatus between theoretical concepts and language utilized by scholars of nursing theory and accurate interpretation, meaningfulness, and use by practitioners? How can practice theory be derived from valid deductive arguments to be one type of scientific theory? To what extent do you agree with Menke that Beckstrand has taken Jacox's idea of practice theory out of context? What may be the missing link or focus not addressed in resolving issues regarding the apparent conflict between prescriptive theory and practice theory as portrayed by Menke? What considerations, besides one's belief system, are essential for the practitioner in choosing a framework in practice?

REFERENCES

Abdellah, Faye G.
  1968 "The nature of nursing science." Nursing Research 18:390-393.
Andreoli, Kathleen G. and Carol E. Thompson
  1977 "The nature of science in nursing." Image 9:32-37.
Barnard, Kathyrn E.
  1980 "Knowledge for practice: Directions for the future." Nursing Research 29:208-212.
Beckstrand, Jan.
  1978a "The notion of practice theory and the relationship of science and ethical knowledge to practice." Research in Nursing and Health 1:131-136.
  1978b "The need for a practice theory as indicated by the knowledge used in the conduct of practice." Research in Nursing and Health 1:175-179.
  1980 "A critique of several conceptions of practice theory in nursing." Research in Nursing and Health 3:69-80.
Carper, Barbara A.
  1978 "Fundamental patterns of knowing in nursing." Advances in Nursing Science 1:13-24.
Chinn, Peggy L. and Maeona K. Jacobs
  1978 "A model for theory development in nursing." Advances in Nursing Science 1:1-13.
Dickoff, James and Patricia James
  1968 "Theories of theories." Nursing Research 17:197-206.
Dickoff, James, Patricia James, and Ernestine Wiedenbach
  1968a "Theory in a practice discipline, part 1: Practice oriented theory." Nursing Research 17:215-435.
  1968b "Theory in a practice discipline, part II: Practice oriented theory." Nursing Research 17:545-554.
Donaldson, Sue K. and Dorothy M. Crowley
  1978 "The discipline of nursing." Nursing Outlook 26:113-120.
Downs, Florence S.
  1979 "Clinical and theoretical research." Pp. 67-87 in F. S. Downs and J. W. Fleming (eds.), Issues in Nursing Research. New York: Appleton-Century-Crofts.
Fawcett, Jacqueline
  1978a "The relationship between theory and research: A double helix." Advances in Nursing Science 1:49-62.
  1978b "The 'what' of theory development." Pp. 17-34 in Theory Development: What, Why, How? New York: NLN.
Gortner, Susan R.
  1980 "Nursing science in transition." Nursing Research 29:180-183.

Hardy, Margaret E.
  1978 "Perspectives on nursing theory." Advances in Nursing Science 1:37–48.
Jacobs, Maeona K. and Sue E. Huether
  1978 "Nursing science: The theory-practice linkage." Advances in Nursing Science 1:63–74.
Jacox, Ada
  1974 "Theory construction in nursing." Nursing Research 23:4–13.
Johnson, Dorothy E.
  1974 "Development of theory: A requisite for nursing as a primary health profession." Nursing Research 23:372–377.
  1978 "State of the art of theory development." Pp. 1–10 in Theory Development: What, Why, How? New York: NLN
Kaplan, Abraham
  1964 The Conduct of Inquiry. San Francisco: Chandler.
Kerlinger, Fred N.
  1973 Foundations of Behavioral Research. 2d ed. New York: Holt, Rinehart and Winston.
King, Imogene M.
  1971 Toward a Theory of Nursing. New York: Wiley.
Kritek, Phyllis B.
  1978 "The generation and classification of nursing diagnoses: Toward a theory of nursing." Image 10:33–40.
Kuhn, Thomas
  1970 The Structure of Scientific Revolution. 2d ed. Chicago: University of Chicago Press.
Menke, Edna M.
  1978 "Theory development: A challenge for nursing." Pp. 216–222 in N. L. Chaska (ed.), The Nursing Profession: Views through the Mist. New York: McGraw-Hill.
Newman, Margaret A.
  1979 Theory Development in Nursing. Philadelphia: Davis

Nightingale, Florence
  1969 Notes on Nursing. New York: Dover.
Orem, Dorothea E. (ed.)
  1980a Concept Formalization in Nursing Process and Product. 2d ed. Boston: Little, Brown.
  1980b Nursing: Concepts of Practice. 2d ed. New York: McGraw-Hill.
Popper, Karl R.
  1959 The Logic of Scientific Discovery. New York: Basic Books.
Reynolds, Paul D.
  1971 A Primer in Theory Construction. New York: Bobbs-Merrill.
Riehl, John P. and Sister Callista Roy (eds.)
  1980 Conceptual Models for Nursing Practice. 2d ed. New York: Appleton-Century-Crofts.
Rogers, Martha E.
  1970 An Introduction to the Theoretical Basis of Nursing. Philadelphia: Davis.
  1980 "Nursing: A science of unitary man." Pp. 329–337 in J. P. Riehl and C. Roy (eds.), Conceptual Models for Nursing Practice. 2d ed. New York: Appleton-Century-Crofts.
Roy, Sister Callista
  1976 Introduction to Nursing: An Adaptation Model. Englewood Cliffs: Prentice-Hall.
  1980 "The Roy adaptation model." Pp. 179–188 in J. P. Riehl and C. Roy (eds.), Conceptual Models for Nursing Practice. 2d ed. New York: Appleton-Century-Crofts.
Stevens, Barbara J.
  1979 Nursing Theory. Boston: Little, Brown.
Williams, Carolyn A.
  1979 "The nature and development of conceptual frameworks." Pp. 89–106 in F. S. Downs and J. W. Fleming (eds.), Issues in Nursing Research. New York: Appleton-Century-Crofts.

Chapter 32

Metaparadigms and Theory Development

Margaret Hardy, R.N., Ph.D., F.A.A.N.
Associate Professor
School of Nursing
Boston University
Boston, Massachusetts

INTRODUCTION

In her examination of the current status of nursing knowledge, Margaret Hardy posits a discriminating approach. She clearly argues that nursing knowledge is in the preparadigm stage. According to Hardy, the terms *metaparadigm* and *preparadigm* are essentially different. In general, both terms refer to the nature of scientific knowledge; preparadigm refers to an early developmental stage in the progress of science while metaparadigm refers to a discipline's perspective on reality.

Hardy states that Kuhn never clearly defined the term *paradigm*; she indicates that Masterman's synthesis of Kuhn's 21 meanings of paradigm includes metaparadigms as one of three basic types of a paradigm. The term *metaparadigm,* as used by Masterman, is acknowledged by Kuhn as being similar to his concept of paradigm. According to Hardy, Kuhn refers to paradigms as a set of beliefs, a way of seeing, an organizing principle governing perception—something which determines a large area of reality with a shared commitment among a scientific community. She tends to agree with Kuhn's original view of preparadigms. He characterized preparadigms as divergent schools of thought. Although the same phenomena are addressed, usually they are described and interpreted in different ways.

Hardy makes a clear distinction between metaparadigms and preparadigms. Extracting from Kuhn, she further defines a metaparadigm as a gestalt, global perspective, total world view, or cognitive orientation that is held by the majority of the members of a scientific community. Metaparadigms define the domain of interest, questions to be addressed, and identify appropriate theories, methods, and instruments to be utilized.

Hardy insists that in the preparadigm stage, there are no common set of beliefs, no agreement on theories or concepts that are relevant, nor consensus on methodologies and instruments. The critical point made by Hardy is that nurse-scientists do not act

This chapter is based on a paper presented at the 1979 Rozella M. Schlotfeldt Lectureship, Case Western Reserve University, April 21, 1979. The author thanks W. L. Hardy, Ph.D., for his assistance with this paper.

as a community of scientists with a *common* perspective, set of assumptions and cognitive orientation as to the nature of nursing knowledge. This, she claims, reflects the preparadigm stage of knowledge development and the lack of a metaparadigm. Thus she prefers the term *preparadigm* rather than *metaparadigm* to describe the present stage of nursing science.

Hardy defines and provides a rationale for the term "a community of scientists." She emphasizes the necessity of a scientific community as a prerequisite to metaparadigms and paradigms in order for nursing to be established as a science. There may exist subcommunities or several communities focusing on varying aspects of the same or different paradigms. Hardy advocates that attention be directed to the presence and meaning of a scientific community for nursing.

Hardy views metaparadigms as determining the structure, development, nature of the scientific knowledge, and activities of scientists. A science does not become established until there is consensus on a metaparadigm as a community. Initially the scientific community focuses on solvable problems. Once questions are raised that cannot be addressed through the use of a particular metaparadigm an alternative one may arise. However, consensus regarding the new metaparadigm by the majority of the scientific community needs to occur before knowledge is further advanced as a science. An example of a metaparadigm is biological evolution as proposed by Darwin.

Hardy provides examples of paradigms and discusses particularly the social definition paradigm in sociology. She identifies the agreed upon cognitive orientation of its subject matter, the theories subsumed, and the research tradition in using the paradigm. She offers examples of nurses conducting research based on this paradigm and concludes it may be termed a preparadigm in nursing science.

Hardy concludes her chapter with a specific discussion about the community of nurse-scientists and the practicing professional nurse. She notes that there are several embryonic communities of nurse-scientists. No group has achieved consensus as to a metaparadigm or set of paradigms for nursing. It may be unrealistic to expect a common paradigm to evolve due to the diverse academic disciplines nurse-scientists represent. Hardy is optimistic that the development of multiple paradigms and subcommunities is feasible. She cautions the community of nurse-scientists to heed the profession's societal mandate and the needs of society in evolving paradigms. At the same time she urges tolerance for paradigms which initially may not appear to be of direct value to the practitioner. The community of professional practitioners is viewed as implementing scientific knowledge to guide practice. Hardy offers to both groups the challenge for concerted effort to interact constructively and effectively.

The current status of theories in nursing can only be termed chaotic. It is difficult to identify a core of scientific nursing theories. There is even considerable confusion and dissent in defining "theory," "conceptual framework," and "model"—terms basic to theory development. Nursing theories are hard to identify, if they do in fact exist. Furthermore, both the location of the domain in which scientific knowledge for nursing is to develop and the boundaries of that domain are difficult to determine.

The development of nursing knowledge has been of concern for over 20 years for those nurses who have seen the need for a more rational scientific knowledge base for their profession. Over time the problem has become more pressing; it now requires more systematic thought than it is receiving. Faculty members in the area of theory or teaching courses on theory development are aware that there is a critical need to analyze and solve the problem, especially since the increasing number of doctoral programs and students has resulted in a growing number of graduate level courses in theory development.

Because of these changes in graduate education, there has been a marked increase in the number of nurses who raise significant questions about nursing knowledge. Fortunately, there also has been a noticeable increase in the sophistication of the questions posed.

In nursing we have individual scientists who function independently rather than as members of a community of scientists. Some of these scientific entrepreneurs may identify with a particular nursing theory or theory relevant to nursing, while others claim to be eclectic or atheoretical. This diversity of allegiance to scientific theory probably is related to nursing's unproductive position of having a variety of schools of thought which have very little, if any, empirical base. These schools of thought generate little basic research, and the nursing research which is undertaken is relatively random in focus and often superficial in nature. An outsider attending any of our research meetings or surveying our research journals would have difficulty identifying the focus and the domain of nursing science. He would quickly become aware that nurse-scientists do not function as a community of scientists; they have no common perspective, no common set of assumptions, and no common cognitive orientation as to the nature of nursing knowledge.

Consensus upon a perspective or a cognitive orientation to the domain and nature of a discipline's knowledge is a relatively simplistic interpretation of the term "metaparadigm," a term which will be explored much more fully in the latter part of this paper. The value of a global paradigm is that it channels the work of scientists by structuring their theories and subsequent research. I believe that a fuller understanding of metaparadigms in general and of potential metaparadigms in nursing in particular will advance our understanding of knowledge development in nursing.

PREPARADIGM STAGE OF DEVELOPMENT

My analysis of the current status of nursing knowledge indicates that it is in a preparadigm stage of development. Eventually nursing may develop multiple competing paradigms; it is hoped that when nursing becomes a mature science it will evolve a dominant metaphysical paradigm.

The preparadigm stage of a science—nursing's present location—is, according to Kuhn (1970: 15, 17), characterized by divergent schools of thought which, although addressing the same range of phenomena, usually describe and interpret these phenomena in different ways. There is no common set of beliefs, no agreement on theories, no agreement on methodologies and tools, and no agreement on what facts are relevant. Furthermore, the data are very superficial, being close to common, everyday type of observation, and the tools used to collect the data are unsophisticated. One need only compare how nurses investigate death and dying with how physiologists study the transport of ions across cell membranes to see the difference in the level of scientific development and the marked contrast in precision of terms and methods for obtaining data. This difference is not due to the complexity of the subject matter but to the paradigmatic status of one field versus the other.

Kuhn (1970:19,20), in his discussion of the preparadigm stage in a science, comments on how each scientist doing research during this period must start anew rather than being able to build on preceding work. To build in this sense means to continue on to the next piece of obvious research without need for justification. Scientists working in the preparadigm stage spend inordinate time and effort justifying their approach, their focus, the significance of their research, their methodology, and their interpretations. Furthermore, it is not until a paradigm exists that a community of scientists begins functioning. From Kuhn's perspective (1970:10,11) a paradigm and community of scientists develop concurrently.

COMMUNITY OF SCIENTISTS

My preference for the phrase "community of scientists" over the more common term "discipline" is based on the following. First, the phrase implies the existence of a group of persons who have a common bond and a common social commitment to a unique perspective which directs their scientific activities. Second, the existence of both a community of scientists and a paradigm are prerequisites to normal science.[1]

Third, since "community of scientists" may refer to an entire discipline, to subgroups within a discipline, or even to interdisciplinary groups, it is a less restrictive term than "discipline."

At this point, let me clarify my meaning of the term "community." I use it to refer to a group of persons who are aware of their uniqueness and the separate identity of their group. They have a special coherence which separates them from neighboring groups, and this special bond means they have a shared set of values and a common commitment which operates as they work together to achieve a common goal. Coordination of their activities may include interaction among and coordination of institutions, organizations, groups, and individuals. Such coordinated groups hold a common perspective, common values, and common bonds, and they have common sets of activities and functions which they carry out to achieve a common outcome. Groups with these characteristics form the scientific subcommunities of our society. Such groups work under a common cognitive umbrella or metaparadigm, whether they be biologists, psychologists, or physicists. Depending upon the complexity of the evolvement of a particular discipline, it is possible for there to be a single community of scientists working under a single dominant or metaphysical paradigm, or there may be several subcommunities of scientists working on different aspects of the same paradigm.

[1] It must be noted that the presence of a paradigm and the existence of a community of scientists do not guarantee that normal science will develop. Nor can the development of a community of scientists and a paradigm be artificially hastened, for Kuhn's theory is not prescriptive. In Kuhn's words: "I claim no therapy to assist the transformation of a proto-science to a science nor do I suppose that anything of the sort is to be had . . . . If . . . some scientists take from me the view that they can improve the status of their field by legislating agreement on fundamentals and then turn to puzzle solving, they are badly misconstruing my point." (1970:245)

In less mature disciplines where several paradigms may exist, several communities of scientists may coexist, each believing that its paradigm should be the one adopted by the entire discipline.

Nurse-scientists are not yet at the point of seeing themselves as a community of scientists developing a body of knowledge that is distinct from other groups in the health field. Although there are meetings of nurse-scientists where research papers are presented, these meetings have not yet fostered the characteristics of a community of nurse-scientists with a common cognitive focus.

In this section I have suggested that we should attend to the existence and meaning of scientific communities as we consider the impact of paradigms on structuring knowledge in nursing. In the next section, I will explore Kuhn's meaning of the concept, "paradigm," and Masterman's explication of the metaphysical paradigm. I believe that paradigms and metaparadigms are necessary bases for a science which is progressive and productive.

PARADIGMS AND METAPARADIGMS

The term "paradigm," although never clearly defined by Kuhn (1970), was used frequently and with a wide variety of meanings as he posited the nonrational, noncumulative nature of the development of scientific knowledge. Masterman (1970) synthesized Kuhn's more than 21 meanings of paradigm to three basic types: metaphysical (or metaparadigm), sociological, and construct paradigms. One, the metaparadigm, appears to be the most useful type for understanding the development of knowledge in emerging scientific fields such as nursing.

The term "metaparadigm" covers Kuhn's concept of paradigm as a set of beliefs (1970:4), as a way of seeing (1970:117–120), as an organizing principle governing perception (1970, 121), as something which determines a large area of reality (1970:129), and as "global, embracing all the shared commitments of a scientific group . . ." (1977:460). This metaphysical meaning, which has been termed "metaphysical paradigm" or "metaparadigm" by Masterman (1970:65), has now been acknowledged by Kuhn (1977:400). Drawing upon Kuhn's 1970 postscript (1970: 174–225) and his "Second Thoughts on Paradigms" (1977), one can obtain a reasonable definition of a metaparadigm as a gestalt, a global perspective, a total world view or cognitive orientation which is held by the majority of the members of a discipline or scientific community. The metaparadigm defines the domain of interest, determines the questions to be asked, and identifies the appropriate theories, methods, and instrumentations for answering the scientific questions raised by a community.

Metaparadigms include the cognitive umbrellas under which communities of scientists work. Such paradigms are articulated with reality through the development and testing of theories. Such theories can be termed "paradigm theories" to indicate that they are not isolated entities but are developed in relation to a prevailing metaparadigm.

METAPARADIGMS AND THE STRUCTURE OF KNOWLEDGE

"Normal science" does not become established until there is a consensus on a metaparadigm and a community of scientists exists. To reach this state, one or more past scientific achievements must have occurred, and these achievements must have been acknowledged by a scientific community as providing the foundation for further scientific activity (Kuhn, 1970:10). The commitment of a scientific community to a metaparadigm is a commitment to a set of ideas, a set of rules, and standards for scientific research.

When scientists work in the "normal science" phase of knowledge development, they accumulate knowledge through testing paradigm theories. Some of these theories may be altered or abandoned if the empirical support proves insufficient. Other paradigm theories may be developed more fully, become more precise in their predictions, and increase in their generality. The knowledge

which accrues during this stage is consistent with the metaparadigm. Any theoretical or empirical anomalies are usually unobserved, ignored, or accounted for by examining the theory or research from which they emerged, since metaparadigms are basic beliefs and are not open to change or criticism under normal circumstances.

Metaparadigms, because they determine the cognitive perspective of the scientists and define researchable questions, the appropriate research strategies, and the data admissible, actually determine the *structure, development* and *nature* of the scientific knowledge which will be accumulated. Metaparadigms also circumscribe the *activities* of scientists. These activities include cognition, problem identification, research methods, and standards relative to theories and general scientific practice. Metaparadigms and normal science are closely related and result in a rapid growth of scientific knowledge. When multiple paradigms exist, the knowledge growth is less rapid, but the growth far exceeds any that occurs in the preparadigm stage of knowledge development.

During the stage of normal science few, if any, unanswerable questions are raised; scientists work on solvable problems and are relatively unaware of problematic ideas or data which do not support their guiding framework. It is only when a significant number of anomalies develop and when many scientific problems cannot be accounted for that scientists begin to question the appropriateness of a metaparadigm. It is Kuhn's thesis (1970:66–159) that when a majority of scientists begin to question the adequacy of a metaparadigm and seriously consider adopting an alternative one, a crisis exists. If an alternative metaparadigm arises which is empirically more successful and can account for the anomalies and scientific problems and if it is accepted by the majority of scientists in that field, then a scientific revolution has occurred. With acceptance of a new and superior metaparadigm, scientists are able to resume the work of normal science. For these scientists consensus on the new metaparadigm provides a fresh gestalt or cognitive perspective which redefines the subject matter, domain of interest, researchable questions, research practices, and appropriate theories. Thus the establishment of a metaparadigm profoundly affects the nature of the knowledge developed by a community of scientists.

Biological evolution as proposed by Darwin is an example of a metaparadigm, as are the works of Newton and Einstein. Examples of paradigms which are likely to be familiar to nurses are behaviorism and psychoanalytical thought in psychology; social learning, psychoanalytical thought, the cognitive framework, and the field approach in social psychology; Marxism and capitalism in economics; and social facts, social definition, and social behavior in sociology.

Since 1970 there have been many publications relating to Kuhn's work. Some authors in the social sciences have utilized the notion of paradigm to organize loose bodies of knowledge (Denisoss et al., 1974; Friedrichs, 1970; Gamson and Modigliani, 1974; Ritzer, 1975). Not surprisingly, scientific knowledge has generally been identified as it relates to multiple paradigms rather than to a metaparadigm. These paradigms, however, do enable communities of scientists within social science disciplines to add to a growing body of scientific knowledge. In contrast, in the preparadigm period there is a multiplicity of competing schools; evidence of progress, except within schools, is hard to identify and the efforts of scientists during this period do not add up to science as we know it (Kuhn, 1970:163). Nursing appears to be in the preparadigm stage, for the work of nurse-scientists has not yet resulted in an identifiable body of scientific nursing knowledge.

AN EXAMPLE OF A PARADIGM

Having discussed metaparadigms in the abstract along with a few examples, I will move to a more concrete level by discussing a paradigm used by some scientists in nursing to illustrate some of the basic characteristics of paradigms. I have selected the *social definition paradigm* (Ritzer, 1975: 84-140) because it can be classified as a school

of thought in nursing and also because it is, according to Ritzer, one of three paradigms presently vying for the position of a metaparadigm in sociology.

Publications based on the social definition paradigm are used in nursing education courses and have formed the basis for some nursing research. Many research courses in nursing draw upon *Discovery of Grounded Theory* (Glaser and Strauss, 1967) and *Issues in Participant Observation* (McCall and Simmons, 1969). Clinically related theory courses may use *Awareness of Dying* (Glaser and Strauss, 1965), *Passing On—The Social Organization of Dying* (Sudnow, 1967), and *Becoming a Diabetic: A Study of Emerging Identity* (Quint, 1969). Examples of writings based on the social definition paradigm which may be used in a course on role theory or professional socialization in nursing are "Institutionalized Practices of Information Control" (Quint, 1965), "Initiation into a Woman's Profession: Identity Problems in the Status Transition of Coed Student Nurses" (Davis and Olesen, 1963), and *The Silent Dialogue* (Olesen and Whittaker, 1968). There are many other publications based on research related to the social definition paradigm used in teaching graduate nursing students.

It is clear that some nurses are doing research based on this paradigm, as evidenced by the publication of "Role Supplementation" (Meleis and Swendsen, 1978) and "Alone into the Alone" (Paige, 1980). Dissertations coming out of the doctoral program in nursing at the University of California, San Francisco, have been primarily based on the social definition paradigm.

Having established that the research tradition of the social definition paradigm and research based on theories in that paradigm are taught at the graduate level and that some current nursing research is based on theories related to it, I conclude that the social definition paradigm may be termed a preparadigm in nursing science.

The major perspective of this paradigm is that a person develops a sense of self and of the characteristics associated with human nature through social interaction and subjective interpretation of his or her own behavior and the behavior of others. A scientist who does research from the perspective of the social definition paradigm seeks an objective understanding of how a person evaluates, appraises, uses, creates, and destroys various social relationships. The scientist also seeks to understand how all these activities are influenced by others and the social situation. The scientist sees the person as a decision maker, an active creator of his or her own social reality.

Three theories articulate the social definition paradigm with reality: role theory, symbolic interaction theory, and the phenomenological approach. The social definition paradigm has a recognizable research tradition. Scientists engage in field research to obtain data as objective as possible on subjective interpretations of events and processes. Verbal accounts and writings such as letters, diaries, and interviews are a major source of data. Various forms of scientific observation are used to obtain data on social behavior. From these data, inferences are made about social and subjective processes which may be occurring. Research is reported in the form of biographies, case studies, and descriptive studies supported by anecdotal data to illustrate concepts and processes.

This brief overview of the social definition paradigm identifies the agreed upon cognitive orientation of its subject matter, the theories subsumed under the paradigm, and the research tradition. It has not become a metaparadigm in nursing so far, since it has not resulted in a major scientific nursing achievement and has not gained support from the majority of nurse-scientists. It has not yet been identified as a perspective upon which a significant number of nurse-scientists can base their research.

THE COMMUNITY OF NURSE-SCIENTISTS

Earlier I stated that a community of nurse-scientists does not yet exist in nursing. I suspect, however, that there are several such embryonic communities. One outcome of the nurse-scientist program of the 1960s was the creation of basic scientists with similar academic backgrounds and with commitments to the paradigms of their own academic discipline. These nurses have published research but a common paradigm for nursing has not yet emerged. Some efforts, however, have been exerted by graduates of these different disciplines to create group identities. For example, the nurse-sociologists had a membership of 15 in 1974; by 1978 there were 150. There are similar groups of nurse-scientists in physiology, anthropology, and psychology. None of these groups has yet achieved the status of a community of scientists, nor have members achieved a consensus as to a metaparadigm or set of paradigms that should guide their activities. Groups like the Council of Nurse Researchers and the Western Society for Research in Nursing, although providing an excellent opportunity to communicate nursing research, seem even further from accepting a common paradigm to guide their activities, since these groups draw upon all nurse-scientists regardless of their academic orientation. Can nurse-scientists from different academic disciplines really be expected to develop a common paradigm or even a multiple of paradigms relative to nursing?

No faculty or school yet has conclusive knowledge of what "school of thought" will be most useful to nursing. Programs which are truly of graduate level will present their students with divergent schools of thought, including nursing theories and theories and paradigms relevant to nursing, and will allow students the freedom to determine the focus of their scientific activities. Through critical thought, empirical testing, infinite patience, creativity, and open-mindedness, we may yet see nurse-scientists move beyond the preparadigm stage. This will occur when some schools of thought gain acceptance as they develop stronger empirical support and as other schools of thought are abandoned for lack of usefulness and empirical support. Some schools of thought may merge, and paradigms may be imported from other disciplines. The profession of nursing science will then be in a position to move into the multiple-paradigm stage, with paradigms of a character unimagined today. The diversity of the educated nurse-scientists, the strength of the doctoral programs in nursing, and the commitment in nursing to development of a scientific knowledge base may result in the creation of paradigms and subcommunities of nurse-scientists. From these may then emerge a metaparadigm and a community of nurse-scientists engaged in the normal activities of science.

THE RELATIONSHIP BETWEEN THE COMMUNITIES OF NURSE-SCIENTISTS AND THE PRACTICING PROFESSIONAL NURSE

Should a community of nurse-scientists develop, how will the activities of its members relate to the activities of practicing professional nurses? What should be the link between the two groups is not clear. Currently the activities of the community of practicing professional nurses are determined by societal needs and society's mandate. Both groups of nurses are members of the nursing profession, and therefore both groups need to respond to the profession's societal mandate. There is, however, a strong possibility that the two groups will function independently. If nursing develops a scientific community with specialized journals and meetings, members of that community could alienate the practicing professional community. If the community of nurse-scientists develops the typical division of labor, then communication, perspective, language, and values of the scientific and the practicing communities may diverge, unless a concerted effort is made to overcome barriers. Given the fact that the two groups have some common aims, every effort should be made to have the groups interrelate and affect each other constructively, just as, for example, physicists and engineers now do.

If we accept the premise that the nursing profession draws upon a scientific body of knowledge to guide practice, then it follows that nursing practice would be greatly affected by any para-

digms which might develop in the community of nurse-scientists. Furthermore, it is reasonable to assume that some of these paradigms will have a direct and obvious link to the profession's societal mandate. The paradigms of the community of nurse-scientists must at some point in their evolution take into account such a mandate. Tolerance, however, must exist at the same time for paradigms which do not directly relate to the immediate needs of society; in the long run, knowledge derived under these paradigms may be of greater value to society than paradigms which intially appear to directly reflect society's needs from nursing.

From my perspective, I see the community of nurse-scientists eventually working from multiple paradigms, testing out the theories associated with each. The purpose in theory development and testing will be to explain, predict, and control phenomena which are of concern to the community of practicing professional nurses. Unless members of the latter group are both nurse-scientists and practitioners, their major function will be to implement the knowledge developed by the community of nurse-scientists. The community of practicing professional nurses, however, must also exert direct pressure upon the activities of the scientific community of nurses to solve very pressing, practical, socially relevant problems. This pressure, if concerted, may have a significant impact upon the paradigms which emerge in the scientific community. Nurses in the scientific community should obtain some of their ideas, data, and support from their coprofessionals. They should be informed as to what knowledge is irrelevant and what knowledge needs to be more fully developed. It must be remembered that the "community of nurse-scientists" that develops will ultimately facilitate the nursing profession in meeting its social responsibility.

SUMMARY

I have suggested several ways in which a paradigm may structure the professional science of nursing.

The existence of a metaparadigm makes the activities of normal science a natural course of events. The existence of a visible, active community of nurse-scientists speedily generating knowledge that the community of practicing nurses is able to use should contribute markedly to a renewed cohesiveness within the profession and should raise the profession's morale and the profession's expertise in meeting the needs of society.

It will take time for our profession of nursing to develop a community of nurse-scientists, to develop paradigms, and ultimately to obtain a dominant paradigm, or a metaparadigm. Certainly, progress has been made in the area of nursing science, and some budding communities of nurse-scientists do exist. For today's nurse-scientists there is much work to be done. There is scientific work to be engaged in, and there is a need to share our work and our commitment to a scientific base for nursing with our doctoral students and with other scientists.

The sense of frustration—and, yes, even despair—with the quality, orientation, and value of ongoing research will need to be endured by the growing number of nurse-scientists. However, if some of the concerns about ongoing research are shared, we will be able to focus on improving the quality of our scientific work, and it will become a challenge to be shared with coworkers.

With time, hard work, and a growing community of nurse-scientists, the profession of nursing can move out of the frustrating, ill-focused, preparadigm stage of science to the paradigm and metaphysical-paradigm stages of science. Who of us would not like to carry out the activities of normal science and be part of a committed community of nurse-scientists developing sound, scientific knowledge for the professional science of nursing?

EDITOR'S QUESTIONS FOR DISCUSSION

What is the difference between the terms *preparadigm, metaparadigm,* and *paradigm* as used by Hardy? To what extent does Hardy appear to use the term *metaparadigm* as one type of paradigm according to Masterman, and/or synonymously with the term *paradigm?* If paradigms can be defined as models of reality (Newman, Chap. 28), could "models of reality" be distinctly defined as three stages: preparadigm, metaparadigm, and paradigm? How could a metaparadigm then evolve to a paradigm? What is the difference between a paradigm and a theory? What relationship is there between Hardy's discussion and Santora's (Chap. 8) definition of the terms: *model, framework, theoretical, conceptual?* What is the relationship between Walker's (Chap. 30) description of the metatheoretical movement and Hardy's definition of a metaparadigm? What is the difference between Menke's definition (Chap. 31) of a metatheorist and a metaparadigm?

Provide examples in current development of nursing theory of scientists starting anew and scientists building upon preceding work of their own and/or others. What is meant by the term "normal science"? How is the development of a science a dialectical process? Provide examples of this process in the advancement of knowledge in nursing science.

To what extent would Hardy agree with Fawcett (Chap. 14), Newman (Chap. 28), and Chinn (Chap. 29) as to consensus regarding the major concepts of nursing? Is there a dilemma between the importance of developing theory regarding any phenomenon that is perceived to be within the domain of nursing as discussed by Fawcett (Chap. 14), Newman (Chap. 28), Chinn (Chap. 29), and Menke (Chap. 31), and the need for consensus on a metaparadigm for a community of scientists to exist as proposed by Hardy? How does Hardy indirectly address a possible dilemma and foresee the development of paradigms? On what basis should nurse-scientists from different academic disciplines be expected to contribute to the development of a common paradigm or multiple paradigms relative to nursing? Provide examples as to the specific contributions that might be made by nurse-scientists from different disciplines. What perspective is similar between Fawcett (Chap. 14) and Hardy regarding the type of research relevant for knowledge and practice?

Which group or groups in nursing may be a single community of scientists working under a metaparadigm? Which subcommunities of scientists in nursing are working on different aspects of the same paradigm? Are there subcommunities of scientists co-existing in nursing who believe their paradigm should be the one adopted by the entire discipline? If you perceive this to be true, justify your rationale, proposing arguments for and against the appropriateness of the paradigm(s) for nursing and the adoption of a single paradigm for the discipline.

To what extent would you agree with Hardy that nurse-scientists are not yet at the point of seeing themselves as a community of scientists? What characteristics of a scientific community are present and do not exist in nursing? What strategies can be suggested for directing attention to and developing a scientific community? What are the implications for the profession as a community and society with the development of a community of scientists within nursing? What strategies can be suggested for the community of practicing professional nurses to be both nurse-scientists and practitioners? What link do you perceive should exist between the communities of nurse-scientists and professional practitioners? What strategies can be suggested to prevent alienation and barriers, alluded to by Hardy, between the two groups?

REFERENCES

Davis, F. and V. Olesen
1963 "Initiation into a women's profession: Identity problems in status transition coed to nursing student." Sociometry 26:89-101.

Denisoss, R. S., O. Callahan, and M. H. Levine
1974 Theories and Paradigms in Contemporary Sociology. Itasca, Ill.: F. E. Peacock.

Friedrichs, R. W.
1970 A Sociology of Sociology. New York: Free Press.

Gamson, W. and A. Modigliani
1974 Conceptions of Social Life. Boston: Little, Brown.

Glaser, B. G. and A. L. Strauss
1965 Awareness of Dying. Chicago: Aldine.
1967 The Discovery of Grounded Theory: Strategies for Qualitative Research. Chicago: Aldine.

Kuhn, T. S.
1970 The Structure of Scientific Revolutions. 2d ed. Chicago: University of Chicago Press.
1977 "Second thoughts on paradigms." Pp. 459-482; 500-517 in F. Suppe (ed.), The Structure of Scientific Theory. 2d ed. Urbana: University of Illinois Press.

Olesen, V. and E. Whittaker
1968 The Silent Dialogue. San Francisco: Jossey-Bass.

Masterman, M.
1970 "The nature of a paradigm." Pp. 59-89. in I. Lakatros and A. Musgrave (eds.), Criticisms and the Growth of Knowledge. Cambridge: Cambridge University Press.

McCall, G. J. and J. L. Simmons
1969 Issues in Participant Observation. Reading, Mass.: Addison-Wesley.

Meleis, A. I. and L. A. Swendsen
1978 "Role supplementation: An empirical test of a nursing intervention." Nursing Research 27:11-18.

Paige, S.
    1980   "Alone into the Alone." Unpublished dissertation, Boston University.
Quint, J. C.
    1965   "Institutional practices of information control." Psychiatry 28:119–132.
    1969   "Becoming a diabetic: A study of emerging identity." Unpublished dissertation, University of California, San Francisco.

Ritzer, G.
    1975   Sociology: A Multiple Paradigm Science. Boston: Allyn and Bacon.
Sudnow, D.
    1967   Passing On-The Social Organization of Dying. Englewood Cliffs, N.J.: Prentice-Hall.

Chapter 33

A Model for Theory Description, Analysis, and Critique

Afaf Ibrahim Meleis, R.N., Ph.D., F.A.A.N.
Professor
School of Nursing
Department of Mental Health
and Community Nursing
University of California
San Francisco, California

A unique and exceptionally thorough, relevant model for critique of theories and paradigms in nursing is offered by Afaf Ibrahim Meleis. Although various models have been proposed for theory critique, none appear to be as appropriate for nursing, comprehensively and aptly portrayed as that developed by Meleis. She insists that systematic study of existing theories is essential in order for nursing to become a scientific discipline. She provides four major objectives of theory critique, emphasizing the importance of evaluation, commitment of a group of researchers to a theory, knowledge of the scientific process, and a critical attitude for scholarliness. Meleis cites three objectives of the model proposed. Essentially the model provides a framework for understanding, analyzing, and evaluating theories and conceptual models in nursing. The boundaries clearly defined in her model and discussed are: structural components, functional components, relationship between structure and function, paradigmatic origins, diagramming of theory, and external components. The major portion of the chapter is concerned with the first two aspects of the model.

Meleis considers the structural components of theory in terms of internal structure and dimensions of theory. In her discussion of the former she includes critical definitions of "theory," "assumptions," "concepts," and "propositions." In asserting that propositions manifest a theory's power for explanation, description, or prediction, she differentiates between explanatory, existential, and relational propositions. Meleis carefully explicates nine dimensions of theory. These are: the rationale, system of relations, content, beginnings, scope, goal, phenomenon, abstractness, and method of theory development. Some dimensions are outlined more than others. Regarding theory beginnings, Meleis differentiates between constructive (deductive) and principled (inductive) types. Discussing the scope of theory, she delineates grand, middle-range, and single-domain theories. Considering the goal, descriptive, explanatory, predictive, and prescriptive theory are clearly represented. Meleis believes the ultimate goal of nursing theory development is prescription and change. Addressing the central phenomenon of theory she speaks to theories concerning knowledge of order, disorder, and control. Careful assessment of the method of theory development is urged. Some methods that Meleis speaks to are: the dialectical, the logical, and those organized around nursing problems or methods of intervention.

In Meleis' model, the functional assessment of a theory includes five spheres: goals and consequences; potential for practice, research, education and administration. She focuses upon the first three areas. Seven salient sets of questions are posed to examine the goals and consequences as a theory. The professional practitioner is urged to assess the theory according to its function, meaning, goals, consequences, and potential for practice. Meleis advocates questions related to possible testability as the criterion for a theory's research potential.

In making a critical assessment of the relationship between structure and function of the theory, Meleis illustrates that the method used dictates the critique. Three major questions are suggested to provide answers regarding the paradigmatic origins of the theory. She further points out that visual representation will enhance the clarity of theories and models. The final aspect of Meleis' theory critique model includes analysis of five external criteria: personal values, congruence with values of other professions, congruence with values of societies, the significance of society, and the theory's adoption by others. She cautions that no one theory will completely satisfy all criteria. Meleis has formulated numerous extraordinary, major questions throughout the explication of her model. In addition she offers many examples to demonstrate the utility and value of the model.

Theory in nursing has several important functions. It gives boundaries to the field; it provides a reservoir from which propositions evolve; it provides the basis for formulation of principles and laws; and it is pivotal to the development of an evolving body of knowledge. All these functions are essential in the establishment of the discipline of nursing. The objective of theory is to formulate a minimum set of generalizations that permit the explanation of a maximum number of observable relationships among the variables of a given field of inquiry. Thus far, discoveries and developments in the discipline of nursing have resulted in a number of coexisting conceptual structures that are referred to as models by some and as theories by others. None of these structures has yet achieved the status that Kuhn called a paradigm (Kuhn, 1970). None of them, when competing in proposition formulations or in hypothesis testing, can move unequivocally ahead. Their descriptions and explanations of practice are at the basic and beginning stages of development typical of a premature science. They have been used successfully as frameworks for curricular development; nonetheless, it is not this usage that moves a field to maturity.

Today more than ever before, nursing, the premature science, has a great need for theories to guide its practice and for research to give it a scientific base. It has long been accepted, if not in reality at least in principle, that nurses need to understand and apply nursing theory, that nurse researchers need theoretical frameworks for their research explorations, and that nurse-educators need to build curricula on some theoretical basis. However, after many years the debate continues on what paradigms to use, what theories to implement, and which types of theories are most appropriate for the discipline of nursing.

As more theories develop in nursing and the debate on the usefulness of such theories becomes more objective and profound, and as one or more of the theories receives more research documentation, nursing will come closer to the critical period in its transition from a preparadigmatic to a paradigmatic stage (Kuhn, 1970). As the distance between the two stages grows shorter, it becomes more imperative to focus on understanding, evaluating, critiquing, and extending existing theories. This will help bring about the needed critical period and the scientific revolution for nursing.

Inquiry in science involves an awareness of craft skills associated with all levels of research and theory development as well as a continued search for new ones to master. Therefore, learning the process of theory development is as imperative as learning the logic and procedures of research. Learning such processes involves realizing that styles of theory development differ from one theorist to another, just as styles of inquiry differ from one researcher to another. It is the wisdom gained from understanding the different styles and the epistemology of theories that is essential in utilizing, extending, or developing theories in nursing (Meleis and May, 1981). However, the many issues that have evolved surrounding the discipline of nursing cannot be resolved, nor can any progress be continued, nor can clarification be brought about simply by becoming conversant with different styles by informal means or by intuitive interpretation of theories. A formal and explicit study and critique of existing theories in nursing and of paradigms that are influencing nursing has to be pursued systematically in order for nursing to become a discipline. When critiquing, one critiques against a norm or a set of norms. If a critique is done haphazardly or unsystematically, such evaluation could result in misuse of theory or perhaps even in the discard of a useful theory. Therefore, to critique theories objectively, one has to consider and measure theories in terms of certain norms and criteria. This will promote understanding of the components of the theory, it will direct the reader to ways of using theory, and it will also uncover gaps that require further development.

Different models have been proposed for theory criticism, and many norms have been developed to assess them. Each set of norms has considered and evaluated theories from some specific aspects or angles. All have provided us with significant components and different ways of looking at theories. None is completely congruent with nursing and its theories.

Within the last decade systematic theory examination and criticism have been addressed by a number of writers in nursing. Ellis (1968) took the position that nurses ought to engage in theory development and that there are essential components of significant theories to be incorporated in the development of any theory in nursing. A number of criteria were articulated by Hardy (1974) based on those advocated by sociologists. Significant questions were developed, each considering the evaluation and criticism of a theory from a different perspective (Duffey and Muhlenkamp, 1974). Along the same lines, McFarlane (1980) used criteria that were developed by Dickoff and James (1968). These examples of pioneer work in theory have focused our attention on the significance of theory criticism just as Leininger (1968) had done with research criticism.

Theory criticism in nursing has several objectives:

1 Evaluation is essential in providing the researcher and the practitioner with tools for decision making and utilization of the most congruent model for their purpose.

2 Commitment of a group of researchers to a theory helps in the continuation of the particular research tradition and eventually in the development of a scientific discipline. Such commitment and the selection of a theory to guide the search for scientific generalization can only be profitable if the selection is based on careful consideration of the different paradigms and theories, new and old, in the field. Only then can applicability be carefully judged.

3 Knowledge of the scientific process is essential to help find new ways to organize relationships between old and new theoretical concepts.

4 Skepticism is essential for the development of scholarliness (Meleis, Wilson, and Chater, 1980). Critical examination of theories is an area that has

not been given its due importance, perhaps because a critical attitude usually has a negative connotation in nursing.

It is because of this lack of critical examination that a model for theory criticism in nursing was developed. It is the purpose of this chapter to provide and discuss a model for understanding, analyzing, and evaluating theories and conceptual models in nursing. The model has several objectives:

1 To provide the framework that facilitates and enhances the accurate assessment and evaluation of theories and the reliable description of their components

2 To provide the means by which knowledge and methodologies inherent in theory development are understood

3 To make explicit the rules that govern or ought to govern the acceptance or rejection of theories, which is an important task of the philosophy of science

4 To show how the theories we have might be analyzed and how such an analysis eventually shows whether or not they should be accepted, why they are accepted, and whether or not their acceptance is based on sound principles

5 To utilize the model in theory criticism to delineate gaps and needs for extension and clarification

6 To help the theorist, epistemologist, or researcher to explicate and appraise principles and paradigms influencing theories from both analytical and philosophical perspectives

The model is designed to be used by any student of scholarly endeavors, including established researchers and theoreticians as well as doctoral students in nursing.

The proposed model critique considers each theory in terms of:

I Structural components of theory
II Functional components of theory
  A Goals and consequences as a nursing theory
  B Its potential for practice
  C Its potential for research
  D Its potential for education
  E Its potential for administration
III Relationship between structure and functions of theory
IV Paradigmatic origins of theory
V Diagramming of theory
VI External components

Just as with research evaluation and critique, a critic of a theory should address the boundaries within which the critique is developed. More specifically, the critic should indicate whether or not the critique is based on readings, personal contact with theorists, utilization of theory in teaching, practice, or research, and/or any other involvements of the critique with theory. Biases of the critic, if indeed any exist, as well as mechanisms used to enhance objectivity and deal with such biases, should be indicated.

I STRUCTURAL COMPONENTS OF THEORY

Structure of theory is considered in terms of its internal structure and dimensions of theory (Table 33–1).

A The Internal Structure

To enhance understanding and effectiveness of theories one begins with a definition of a theory. A theory is a coherent articulation of reality as

Table 33-1 Structural Components of Theory

Component	Unit of analysis
1. Internal structure	Assumptions
	Concepts
	Propositions
2. Dimensions of theory	Rationale
	System of relations
	Content
	Beginnings
	Scope
	Goal
	Phenomena
	Obstacles
	Method

perceived by the theorist. It encompasses a set of implicit and explicit assumptions guiding the delineation of distinct concepts and systematic theoretical propositions that are independent of time and space. Every theory begins with a set of givens that have either been empirically tested or are not amenable to empirical proof because of the state of our knowledge. These givens constitute the premises upon which a theory is built and without which a theory cannot be understood or critiqued. Therefore, a student of epistemology and theory development should carefully search for the inherent assumptions, being careful not to overlook the implicit ones. Theories that are more effective to a practice discipline and more amenable to empirical testing are theories in which authors explicitly state the assumptions guiding their thinking.

Other components of theory that should be delineated before any further assessment or evaluation of a theory can be made are its major concepts. Concepts are the building blocks of a theory. A reader considers concepts in terms of clarity, conceptual definitions, observable properties, and whether or not its boundaries are clear. While concepts should have internal properties, the theorist is expected to carefully demonstrate logical interrelationships between them, what is peculiar or special about the phenomenon the theory addresses, and what it shares with a larger class of phenomena. In addition, concepts are analyzed along both primitive-derived (Hague, 1972) and concrete-abstract continua.

A theory's power of explanation, description, or prediction is manifested by its propositions. Propositions are the very reasons theories are developed. In fact, such power is manifested in the ratio between assumptions and propositions. An inverse relationship, with the number of propositions being higher than the number of assumptions, allows more explanatory power.

Propositions with the power of explanation link concepts; therefore, they are expected to have more than two concepts. They are formulated to explain and assert something pertaining to the reality embodied in the theory. *Existence propositions*, however, are constructed around one phenomenon and therefore only describe and assert the existence of this one phenomenon. *Relational propositions*, on the other hand, encompass many kinds, e.g., those that just describe the existence of a relationship and those that describe the direction of such a relationship.

Further analysis of propositions could be done along dimensions specified by Zetterberg (1963: 69–71). Not only does it permit labeling propositions along certain dimensions, such as reversibility, determinism, sequentiality, sufficiency, and substitutability, but such labeling allows appropriate assessment of propositions and their power of explanation and predictability. The clarity and systematization of propositions are also considered when we analyze the selected ordering and sequencing of propositions.

B Dimensions of Theory

Once the internal structure of theory is carefully delineated and analyzed, the student of theory can move to consider the theory descriptively along a number of dimensions. Knowledge of such dimensions has two functions. It enhances the understanding of the internal structure of theory and it helps the critic in delineating gaps. The first dimension to consider is the *rationale* upon which the theory is built. Questions to be considered to describe the theory along this dimension include: Are components of theory united in a chain-link fashion? Is it a theory of the factor type? Is the theory developed around concepts and therefore a concatenated theory? Or, is it based on certain sets of laws that are deduced from a small set of basic principles and therefore hierarchical in nature? The former has fewer explanations that converge on a central point and therefore embodies existence propositions, while the latter embodies an interpretive model and is more likely to contain relational propositions (Kaplan, 1964).

The second dimension to consider is that of the

system of relations. Questions to be asked are: Do relations explain elements or do elements explain relations? A monadic approach in theory construction is that which considers single irreducible units as opposed to a field approach, which considers its unit of analysis in terms of a number of other miniunits. An example of the former is cell theory and an example of the latter is a theory of personality in terms of roles.

Content of theory is a third descriptive dimension (Kaplan, 1964). Content is distinguished by the range of laws and group of individuals to which the theory refers. A theory could be classified as *molar* or *macrotheory* or as *molecular* or *microtheory*. Organizational theories in sociology are macro in content while role theory is micro. Martha Rogers's work (1970) is an example of macrotheory while Dorothea Orem (1979) is a microtheorist.

Where a theorist begins articulating ideas and whether a theorist addresses a theory of extant nursing or one of existing practice specifies another dimension, namely that of theory *beginnings* (Kaplan, 1964). A constructive beginning is hypothetical and intended to build up a picture of more complex phenomena while a principled beginning is more empirically grounded (discovered). The former tends to be more complete, clear, and adaptable and tends to consider relationships hypothetically; the latter is more analytical and addresses the "is" rather than the "ought to be." Others call the former *deductive* because it emphasizes a conceptual structure deduced from another conceptual structure (Duffey and Muhlenkamp, 1974). Its laws are logically interrelated. It is through such deductive logic that theories are derived. It is intended to stimulate and direct empirical research. The major criticism of deductive theories is the lack of empirical support. The inductive beginning, on the other hand, consists essentially of summary statements or empirical relations. An example of the former in nursing is Martha Rogers's (1970) theoretical conceptualization of man in his symphonic harmony with the environment. Her theory evolved

from principles of physics, thermodynamics, and evolution, among others. An example of the latter, that is, principled theory, is a conceptualization of issues surrounding dying evolving from Glaser and Strauss (1965) and Benoliel's (1967) work, even though the latter has not been formally labeled a nursing theory.

Many theorists have addressed the *scope* of theory and its significance in describing the capability of the theory. The basic question that considers a theory's scope is: How many of the basic problems in nursing or one of its specialties could be addressed by the same theory? One of the ways by which we consider and assess the scope of a theory is by comparing and contrasting the number of derived and primitive concepts of the theory. The higher the ratio of derived to primitive concepts, the wider the scope. The significance of scope stems from the notion that, as theories have wider scopes, they tend to be more general and last longer (Kuhn, 1970). In addition, the significance of theory increases as its scope broadens (Ellis, 1968). Therefore, to answer questions related to scope, we also address generality.

Theories with a very wide scope are also called *grand theories*, as opposed to *single domain theories* which could be placed at the other end of a scope continuum. The two major criticisms associated with both ends of the scope continuum (i.e., grand theories and single domain theories) are their attempts to explain everything surrounding a set of phenomena, which is also why they explain nothing [as has been the major criticism of Talcott Parsons' (1949) attempts at a theory of sociology] or address only simple abstract isolated facts and principles. The empiricist and methodologist, Robert Merton (1968), is credited for advocating middle-range theories, thus avoiding those criticisms. Middle-range theories consider a limited number of variables, focus on a limited aspect of relationship, are more susceptible to empirical testing, and could be consolidated into more widely ranging theories. Jacox (1974), following Merton's ideas, urged the development of such theories for only limited aspects within the discipline of nursing, such as pain alleviation or promotion of sleep.

Questions to ask in considering the *goal* of the theory are: Why was the theory developed? What is its aim and intent? Theories are constructed to describe, to explain, to predict, or to prescribe. A descriptive theory gives information related to phenomena under consideration but does not make a claim beyond that, nor does it tell us what to expect in the future. When a beginning linkage and description of relationships between derived concepts are provided, the theory becomes an explanatory theory. Correlative studies to test such theories provide empirical evidence for support of explanatory theories.

Another goal explicated in some theories is that of prediction. A predictive theory encompasses propositions of an "if-then" nature in a consequential manner. The ultimate goal in nursing theories is to prescribe; therefore, prescription is another goal. Theories might have all these goals or only explicate one goal or another. The ultimate goal of development of nursing theories is prescription and change. At this time in the developmental history of nursing theory, all theories representing each of the goals are essential.

The nature of the central *phenomenon* addressed by the theory is yet another dimension for theory evaluation. Johnson (1959) called for the need in nursing for theories addressing knowledge of order, knowledge of disorder, and knowledge of control. The knowledge of order addresses phenomena that are central to objects, events, and interactions in a healthy situation. They describe regularities in such phenomena. They describe the normal state and natural schema of things. They provide baseline data. An example of such knowledge is provided by Auger (1976) in her explication of Johnson (1959) and Riehl and Roy's (1980) normal patterns of a person's behavior within systems of behavior. Knowledge of disorder, on the other hand, recognizes phenomena of those disorders with which nurses deal. An attempt at the development of such knowledge, not yet bound together in a theoretical schema, was

manifested in the conferences on nursing diagnosis (Gebbie, 1976). To prescribe a course action which, when implemented, could change the sequence of events in a desired way is to have knowledge of control. Examples of theories addressing such knowledge are Orem's "self-help" (1979), Meleis' (1975) and Meleis, Swendsen, and Jones' "role supplementation" (1980), among others.

Abstractness, another theory dimension, is evaluated by length of reduction and deduction. A highly abstract theory has an explanatory shell with a small radius (Kaplan, 1964). It is a theory with wide spaces in between its propositions and a conceptual schema that is highly removed from reality but still pertains to it. If abstractness is put on a continuum from high abstractness to low abstractness, Rogers and Johnson would be at the high end and Orem at the low end.

Finally, the *method* of theory development should be carefully assessed. Stevens (1979) proposes that there are four methods utilized in developing theories. One is to be able to assess these methods by considering the reasoning upon which the theory is built, the system of action, and plan for progression. A dialectical method is exemplified by Rogers's work (Stevens, 1979) and is based on Socrates and Hegel. It emphasizes relationship with a whole and, in fact, each whole explains parts and each part is a whole explaining other parts. A dialectical method encompasses contradictions, apposition, and dilemmas, but order evolves out of the interaction among all of them. Erikson's developmental theory (1963) is an example of the resolution of conflict and crisis in the process of moving into the next level of development. A dialectical method defies the Aristotelian logic. The latter is another method of theory development, the logical method. This is a method in which the parts are organized to describe the whole systematically and categorically. A theory of this nature offers description of each part, and the whole is the sum total of all parts. Stevens (1979) considers Johnson and Roy in this category.

The other two methods of theory development are those of problem theories and operational theories. Problem theories (Henderson, 1966; Nursing Theories Conference Group, 1980) are organized around nursing problems, while operational theories (Orem, 1979) are those organized around methods of intervention.

II FUNCTIONAL COMPONENTS OF THEORY

Unlike structural analysis of theories, a functional assessment of a theory carefully considers the raison d'être of the theory and its purpose. Components describe and evaluate theories from a generic perspective and consider whether or not they encompass the elements necessary to any theory. Functional components consider the theory's value to the discipline of nursing and its consequences (Table 33-2). A functional assessment of a theory encompasses five areas:

1 Goals and consequences as a nursing theory
2 Potential for practice
3 Potential for research
4 Potential for education
5 Potential for administration

Only the first three areas will be discussed here.

Table 33-2 Functional Components of Theory

Components	Units of analysis
1. Goals and consequences	Recipient-client
	Definition
	Sources of nursing problems
	Focus of intervention
	Guidelines for intervention
	Action
	Consequences
2. Potential for practice	Direction
	Applicability
	Generalizability
	Cost effectiveness
	Relevance for today
	Central potential
3. Potential for research	Consistency
	Testability
	Predictability

There are several reasons for the omissions and the commissions. Through the commission the author is reaffirming a stand that only when theories are considered adequate to explicate phenomena related to clients and nursing practice can they become frameworks for curricula in nursing and for nursing administration. The omission is because the nursing intelligentsia have supplied the nursing literature with ample guidelines and criteria for evaluating theoretical frameworks for education and administration. Therefore, only the goals and consequences of a nursing theory, its potential for practice, and its potential for research are considered below.

A Goals and Consequences as Nursing Theory

1 "Who is acted upon?" This is the major question that begins to consider the function of theory. Does the theory identify the focus of the theory as the client, family, community, or society or does the theory consider the target as one to the exclusion of others? The target of action here denotes both the target of assessment as well as intervention: The target in nursing should be the client (in the broadest sense) in health or illness.

2 What definitions does the theory offer for nursing, client, health-illness, environment, and nurse-client interactions? Are definitions explicit and clear?

3 Does the theory offer a clear idea of what the sources are of the nursing problem, whether the sources lie within or outside of the individual?

4 Does the theory provide any insights in the forms of intervention for nursing? Are the variables to be manipulated well delineated? Is it clear what are the points of entry for a nursing intervention? Is the focus of intervention within the conceptual area of the theory? Points of entry could vary from manipulating outside stimuli (adaptation theories) and interactions and transactions between client and nurse (King, 1971) to manipulating behaviors within systems (Auger, 1976).

5 Are there guidelines for intervention modalities? Are they specified? And, is there potential for the evolution of such intervention modalities?

6 As a nursing theory, does it provide guidelines for the role of the nurse?

7 Are the consequences of nurses' actions articulated in the theory? Are they intended or unintended, positive or negative, anticipated and delineated? Is there a plan for dealing with such consequences?

B Potential for Practice

A thorough review and assessment of theory has to consider its potential for operationalization and utilization in nursing practice. A practitioner who is considering utilizing a theory in some practice should assess the theory only in terms of its function, meaning, goals, consequences, and potential for practice. Therefore, the theory should be able to respond to these questions or have a framework to help the clinician respond to them.

A critic asks a number of questions in evaluating the theory's potential for practice. These are: Does the theory provide enough direction to affect practice? Does it have a framework for prescriptions? Does the theory include abstract notions that are not applicable to practice? Does the level of abstraction or understandability render it applicable or unapplicable? Does the theory cover all areas of nursing? Should it? Does the theory currently apply to practice? Who pays for utilization of the theory in practice? Is it a timely nursing-practice theory? In other words, does it have relevance for the way nursing is practiced today? Where does the theory fit in terms of nursing process? Is the theory understandable to the practitioner? What is the assessment of practitioners of the theory, its uniqueness, and the esotericism of its language? To what extent can we manipulate its phenomena?

C Potential for Research

The very raison d'être of theories is to guide research and be guided by research; therefore, a critique of a theory should include questions related to assessment of a theory's potential for testability. The concepts and propositions should eventually be related in a consistent manner to a systematic set of observable or testable data. Otherwise, if a theory remains untested its usefulness is in question. Schrag (1967) emphasizes the significance of a theory's potential for research, which he calls "the empirical adequacy" of a theory, and such potential is realized through congruence between "theoretical claims and empirical evidence." He asserts that

. . . credibility refers to the goodness of fit between claims and existing evidence, while predictability estimates how well the claims will hold true in the future. (Schrag, 1967:250.)

Theories are established on current information; it usually remains for the future to provide evidence that corroborates them or demands information from them. While the aim of research is not to establish the absolute truth of the theoretical propositions, it is essential that it begin to indicate a degree of confidence based on empirical evidence. It is noteworthy that any supportive corroboration between theory and data uncovered through research is bound to give support to the entire theory structure, however premature that might be. The reverse, unfortunately, could also be true. Therefore, the type and extent of empirical corroboration should be skeptically considered.

While it is significant to the theory critique to note that theories are tested on a "piecemeal" basis, the critic should still consider finding responses to the following questions: Does the theory build on previous research? Was research done using the theory? What propositions were being tested? How replicable is the research? Can the findings be generalized? What research designs have been used? Why? How appropriate are they? Can prescriptive and predictive studies be designed? Are the research results relevant to other fields? Is the research used appropriately? Did the research fail to provide propositions with potential for generating hypotheses? Do the theories state what research is to be completed to support central theory propositions?

Research potential of a theory should not be critiqued lightly. As Berthold (1968) maintained and stressed, the ultimate criteria for evaluating a theory's usefulness are whether it generates predictions or propositions concerning relevant events and whether it stimulates new observations and insights that could subsequently be corroborated.

III RELATIONSHIP BETWEEN STRUCTURE AND FUNCTION OF THEORY

The critic then continues to make critical assessment and judgment of the relationship between the different components of the theory (Table 33-3). In doing so, the critic cannot judge the logic inherent in the development of a dialectic theory by the same criteria used in judging a logical theory; rather, the method used dictates the critique. A general assessment of tautology, in other words, needless repetitions of an idea in different parts of the theory, is considered. A careful consideration of causes and consequences, which are kept separate to avoid teleology on the part of the theorist, is another dimension in the relationship between structure and function. Therefore, the critic should consider questions such as: Are concepts operationally defined? Do they seem to have content and construct validity? Has there been empirical verification of their properties? How consistent are its propositions with other theories and laws? Is there evidence for corroboration (Schrag, 1967)? And finally, can one detect any spuriousness in the theory's components?

Table 33-3 Relationship between Structure and Function

Operationalizability
Tautology
Teleology
Logic
Corroboration
Spuriousness

IV PARADIGMATIC ORIGINS OF THEORY

Most conceptual models in nursing evolve from a prototype theory or can be traced to theories utilized in other fields. Examples are such theories as Johnson's system paradigm (Riehl and Roy, 1980), Roy's adaptation paradigm (1976), and Paterson and Zderad's existentialist philosophy (1976).

Therefore, for a careful consideration of this component the critic should become conversant with paradigmatic origins of the theory under consideration and address such origins in the critique. Description and critique of theory in relationship to this component provide answers to three major questions:

1 Is the theory derived from and built upon an accepted paradigm?
2 What are the origins of the paradigm?
3 Why was this particular paradigm used?

More specifically: On what prototype theory do the theorists build their conceptual structures? How extensively is the original paradigm or theory used? Is the use of paradigm, obvious to the reader, made explicit or implicit by the writer? Does the theorist present the rationale for his selection of the theory or parts of the theory used? From where do theory inadequacies originate, from prototype theory or nursing theory? Are the problems detected those of borrowed theory or of translation? Does nursing theory improve on prototype theory? How congruent or incongruent is the use of components of prototype theory with nursing theory? How about definitions? Are goals the same? Is justification for variance included? Are the other nursing theories derived from prototype theory? What are they?

V DIAGRAMMING OF THEORY

Clarity of theories and models is enhanced by visual representation of the theory. Major questions to be addressed in relationship to this component are:

1 Was the theory visually and graphically presented?

2 Did graphic representation enhance understanding of different components of the theory?

More specifically: How clear is the visual representation? Is it an accurate representation of the text? Does it include major concepts? Are linkages clear? Are linkage directions indicated? Is representation logical? Are there overlaps? Are there gaps? Is representation a substitute for words and explanation or is it a supplementation? Is the diagram clear and well defined?

VI EXTERNAL COMPONENTS

Finally, the theory should be assessed against several external criteria (Table 33-4). These are: personal values, other professional values, social values, social significance, and circle of contagiousness.

A Personal Values

Ellis (1968) emphasized the importance of recognizing values inherent in theories and in making them explicit. A critical consideration of values should take into account those of the theorist and critic. In the latter the fit between the theorist's and critic's personal and professional values

should be considered. It is through such careful assessment that biases can be delineated.

B Congruence with Other Professional Values

A similar assessment of the values espoused in the theory should be made against values of other professions. Health care professionals will be able to enhance patient care through collaboration and complementarity of value systems. Awareness of such complementarity and/or competition in professional values enhances the potential of the development of a collaborative working schema to close the professional value gaps.

C Congruence with Social Values

Beliefs, values, and expectations of different societies and cultures within societies shape and direct the type of theory that is most useful. While self-help, self-care (at its different levels), and individuality are goals congruent with some cultures' value systems, they are the antithesis of those espoused in others. Therefore, theories with such goals and consequences would be incongruent and inappropriate, and consequently should be avoided. Careful critical assessment of societal values and theory values is an integral part of a thorough theory analysis. Questions such as the following should be addressed: Is the role

Table 33-4 External Components of Theory

Component	Units of analysis
1. Personal values	Theorist implicit-explicit values
	Critic implicit-explicit values
2. Congruence between values of theory and other professions	Complementarity
	Esotericism
	Competition
3. Congruence of theory with social values	Beliefs
	Values
	Customs
4. Social significance	Value to humanity
5. Circle of contagiousness	Geography
	Type of instruction
	Influence of theorist vs. theory

of the nurse within the model congruent with the role of the nurse as perceived by society? And, are actions and outcomes congruent with societal expectations of nursing?

D Social Significance

In our attempt to enhance nursing science and articulate the discipline of nursing, we must not neglect the significance of its practice to humanity and society. The philanthropic Bacon's profound words of the seventeenth century still hold true today:

> Lastly, I would address one general admonition to all; that they consider what are the true ends of knowledge, and that they seek it not either for pleasure of mind, or for contention, or for superiority to others, or for profit, or fame, or power, or for any of these inferior things, but for the benefit and use of life; and that they perfect and govern it in charity. For it was from lust of power that the angels fell, from lust of knowledge that man fell; but of charity there can be no excess, neither did angel or man ever come in danger by it. (Bacon, in Ravetz, 1971:436.)

Therefore, a critic should ask philosophically whether the goals and consequences of theory make a substantial and valued difference in lives of people. (Consider questions from perception of clients and from perception of health professionals.) The critic should also ask whether intended and unintended consequences are carefully considered.

E Circle of Contagiousness

The final test of any theory is whether or not it is adopted by others. The units of analysis here are geographical location and type of institution. It is much easier to consider a theory for adaptation or experimentation when the theory is developed and implemented within the same geographical region. When the theory begins to cross several concentric circles from which it originated, its contagiousness begins to receive supportive corroboration. The critic should research the literature for answers to such questions as: Where has the theory been used or where is it being used both geographically and institutionwise? What is it used for (research, education, administration, clincial practice, etc.)? How influential was the theorist in prompting the implementation of the theory? Where was it first introduced? What happened in the interim? Has the theory been considered and utilized cross-culturally and trans-culturally?

CONCLUSIONS

In spite of the many critics who have been skeptical of Kuhn's attempts at delineating criteria that govern choices of good theory and have labeled them as futile, because "the decision of a scientific group to adopt a new paradigm cannot be based on good reasons of any kind, factual or otherwise" (Shapere, 1966), Kuhn continued to assert that indeed we can do so and that accuracy, consistency, broad scope, simplicity, and fruitfulness in research (Kuhn, 1977:321) are essential as objective criteria in judging competing theories. However, Kuhn also maintained that, "Every individual's choice between competing theories depends on a mixture of objective and subjective factors, or of shared and individual criteria." (Kuhn, 1977:325). The latter is based on idiosyncratic factors and therefore "dependent on individuals'" preferences and personalities. Therefore it does not have a place in our understanding of the philosophy of science. The discussion provided here emphasized the former. It provided norms for theory analysis and criticism in an attempt to decrease the margin of subjectivity and enhance that of objectivity. The model of theory criticism (Fig. 33-1) is designed not only to provide the basis for understanding the internal structure of theory but also the social, intellectual, and structural context that surrounds its development. It delineates a comprehensive framework for all the norms and parameters against which theories ought to be analyzed and critiqued.

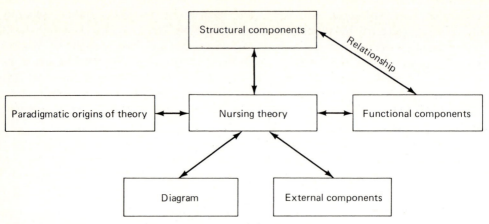

Figure 33-1 Model for description, analysis, and critique of nursing theory.

When using the delineated criteria in critiquing theories, it is important to note that theories may be superior in some points and evolving in other aspects. No one theory will satisfy or be able to address all criteria. Styles of inquiry and personal preferences for theory design affect the configuration and function of theory. Throughout the analysis one should not lose track of the ultimate purpose of theory which is to systematize data and provide its users with unique insight in the matter at hand. Nor should we underestimate the test of time. It is finally the temporal dimension that will determine which theory is adequate and useful and therefore survives and dominates.

EDITOR'S QUESTIONS FOR DISCUSSION

What theories, models, paradigms, and conceptual frameworks in nursing have been critiqued according to any of the criteria offered by Meleis' model? Utilizing Meleis' model, critique each of the current nursing theories, models, preparadigms, paradigms, and conceptual frameworks. Determine the extent to which each of the questions raised for each section of the model can be applied and/or answered. Have other criteria been utilized to critique theories, paradigms, and conceptual frameworks fairly, accurately, and thoroughly? Should the same norms for a critique be applied to all levels in theory development? For example, should conceptual frameworks be critiqued against criteria for a theory? To what extent is there agreement between Hardy (Chap. 32) and Meleis regarding a preparadigmatic stage and the means for transition to a paradigmatic stage in nursing theory? Would the two scholars agree on the importance of commitment of a group of researchers to a theory? What is the relationship between Jacox's set of rules (Menke, Chap. 31) and Meleis' definition and description of a theory? Outline the process of theory development using terminology according to Meleis. What comparisons can be made between the authors in this section as to the steps in theory development? Provide examples of the differences among assumptions, premises, concepts, and propositions.

What discussion by Menke (Chap. 31) and which questions pertaining to inductive and deductive methods posed by the editor are addressed by Meleis? Regarding critique of theory, what previous discussion by Newman (Chap. 32) and editor's questions are addressed by Meleis? What agreement is there between all of the previous authors in this section regarding grand, middle-range, and single-domain theories? What scholars of the previous chapters would agree with Meleis that the ultimate goal of developing nursing theory is prescription and change? What relationship is there between Meleis' questions and presentation considering the goal of theory and Dickoff, James, and Wiedenbach as discussed in Chaps. 30 and 31? What is the relationship between the central phenomenon, suggested by Meleis to be addressed by a theory, and the consensus concerning the phenomenon of nursing as indicated by Fawcett (Chap. 14)? Newman (Chap. 28), Chinn (Chap. 29), Menke (Chap. 31)? How does Meleis' explication of addressing central phenomenon apply to the phenomenon of nursing as discussed in the above chapters? What agreement exists between Meleis, Menke (Chap. 31), and Hardy (Chap. 32) regarding the role of the professional practitioner? Which conceptual models in nursing have evolved from a prototype theory or can be traced to theories utilized in other fields?

REFERENCES

Auger, Jeanine R.
1976 Behavioral Systems and Nursing. Englewood Cliffs, N.J.: Prentice-Hall.

Benoliel, Jeanne Quint
1967 The Nurse and the Dying Patient. New York: Macmillan

Berthold, F. S.
1968 Symposium on theory development in nursing," Nursing Research 17(3):196–197.

Dickoff, James and Patricia James
1968 A theory of theories: A position paper." Nursing Research 17(3):197–203.

Duffey, Margery and Ann F. Muhlenkamp
1974 "A framework for theory analyses." Nursing Outlook 22(9):570–574.

Ellis, Rosemary
1968 "Characteristics of significant theories." Nursing Research 17(3):217–222.

Erikson, Erik
1963 Childhood and Society, 2d ed. New York: W. W. Norton and Co., Inc.

Gebbie, K. (ed.)
1976 Summary of the Second National Conference: Classification of Nursing Diagnosis, St. Louis, March 4–7.

Glaser, B. G. and A. L. Strauss
1965 Awareness of Dying, Chicago: Aldine.

Hague, Jerald
1972 Techniques and Problems of Theory Construction in Sociology. New York: Wiley.

Hardy, Margaret
1974 "Theories: Components, development, evaluation." Nursing Research 23(2): 100–107.

Henderson, V.
1966 The Nature of Nursing. New York: Macmillan.

Jacox, Ada
1974 "Theory construction in nursing: An overview," Nursing Research 23(1):4–13.

Johnson, Dorothy
1959 "The nature of a science of nursing," Nursing Outlook 7(5):291.

Kaplan, Abraham
1964 The Conduct of Inquiry. San Francisco: Chandler Publishing Co.

King, Imogene
1971 Toward a Theory for Nursing. New York: Wiley.

Kuhn, Thomas S.
1970 The Structure of Scientific Revolutions, 2d ed. International Encyclopedia of Unified Science.
1977 The Essential Tension. Chicago: The University of Chicago Press.

Leininger, Madeline
1968 "The research critique: Nature, function and art." Nursing Research 17:444–449.

McFarlane, Elizabeth
1980 "Nursing theory: The comparison of four theoretical proposals." Journal of Advanced Nursing 5:3–19.

Meleis, Afaf I.
1975 "Role insufficiency and role supplemen-

tation: A conceptual framework." Nursing Research 24:264–271.

Meleis, Afaf I. and Kathleen May
1981 "Nursing theory and scholarliness in the doctoral program." Advances in Nursing Science 4(1):31–42.

Meleis, Afaf I., Leslee Swendsen, and Delores Jones
1980 "Preventive role supplementation: A grounded conceptual framework." P. 2 in Current Perspectives in Nursing: Social Issues and Trends. Michael H. Miller and Beverly Flynn (eds.). C. V. Mosby Company.

Meleis, Afaf I., Holly Skodol Wilson, and Shirley Chater
1980 "Toward scholarliness in doctoral dissertations: An analytic model." Research in Nursing & Health 3(3):115–124.

Merton, Robert
1968 Social Theory and Social Structure, revised ed. New York: Freso Press.

Nursing Theories Conference Group
1980 Nursing Theories: The Base for Professional Nursing Practice. Englewood Cliffs, N.J.: Prentice-Hall.

Orem, D. E.
1979 Nursing: Concepts of Practice. New York: McGraw-Hill.

Parsons, Talcott
1949 The Structure of Social Action. New York: The Free Press.

Paterson, J. G. and L. T. Zderad
1976 Humanistic Nursing. New York: Wiley.

Ravetz, Jerome
1971 Scientific Knowledge and its Social Problems. New York: Oxford University Press.

Riehl, Joan and Sister Callista Roy
1980 Conceptual Models for Nursing Practice. New York: Appleton-Century-Crofts.

Rogers, M.
1970 An Introduction to the Theoretical Basis of Nursing, Philadelphia: F. A. Davis Co.

Roy, Sister Callista
1976 Introduction to Nursing: An Adaptational Model. Englewood Cliffs, N.J.: Prentice-Hall.

Schrag, Clarence
1967 "Elements of theoretical analysis in sociology." Pp. 220–253 in Sociological Theory: Inquiries and Paradigms, Llewellyn Gross (ed.). New York: Harper and Row.

Shapere, Dudley
1966 "Meaning and scientific change." Pp. 44–85(3) in Mind and Cosmos: Essays in Contemporary Science and Philosophy, R. G. Colodny (ed.). University of Pittsburg Series in the Philosophy of Science, Pittsburg.

Stevens, Barbara
1979 Nursing Theory: Analysis, Application, Evaluation. Boston: Little Brown.

Zetterberg, Hans
1963 On Theory and Verification in Sociology. Totowa, N.J.: Bedmeister Press.

Chapter 34

Theory Development in Nursing: Proposal for Direction

Sister Callista Roy, R.N., Ph.D., F.A.A.N.
Associate Professor and Chairperson
Department of Nursing
Mount St. Mary's College
Los Angeles, California

After the previous chapters analyzing the past and present stages in the evolution of nursing theory and offering a model for the critique of theory, it is appropriate to conclude this section with a proposal for future direction. Sister Callista Roy deems that theory development and testing are nursing's highest priority. She proposes that the focus be on theories of the human person and of nursing practice.

Roy includes numerous points in her rationale. Some are as follows: nursing needs to take an active stance to be a prominent force in the health care system; the profession cannot expend its limited energy simultaneously in all directions; theory development can respond to the needs of the people and the profession. Regarding the last, she specifically addresses the contribution of theory development.

Roy emphasizes that the common denominator of nursing practice needs to be defined. The commonality is based on shared understandings of the nature of nursing. She views shared understandings being developed theoretically on broad and specific levels. According to Roy, accomplishing this task would enable nursing to meet health care needs. She perceives it is essential for nursing to systematically develop its knowledge base, not only to deal with issues confronting the profession, but also to demonstrate what nurses can do for their clients in various settings in a unique way. Roy cites that a theoretically developed and tested body of knowledge could decrease divisiveness among nurses. She believes the commonality of differing specialty areas could be identified. In so doing parts of nursing could be related to the whole, and nursing science related to other sciences.

Roy, like many of the previous authors, comments on the lack of clarity and conflicts in the use of terms in theory development. She submits specific definitions and meanings for the terms *conceptual model* and *theory*. These are then used as a guide to

Special acknowledgement is given to Dorothy E. Johnson for her writings, teaching, and personal contact with the author, that have so influenced the position presented here.

3

describe the type of theory nursing needs. Roy includes a model indicating the human person and goal of nursing are critical in directing theory development. The profession's theory or theories of the human person can guide the development of nursing practice theories. Roy applies Johnson's three types of knowledge (order, disorder, and control) to theories of the human person and nursing practice.

Roy provides examples of both types of theory development. The first example cited is the effort to develop a theoretical framework for the classification of nursing diagnosis. She outlines the work of the theorists in this area and affirms it contains the rudiments of a theory of the human person. The second example illustrated is Roy's adaptation model, which identifies the person as an adaptive system. The adaptive models are: physiological needs, self concept, role function, and interdependence. Roy briefly demonstrates the role function mode of her model as a piece of theorizing about the person as an adaptive system. She shows how this relates to knowledge of order. In addition, Roy projects how the adaptation model's illustration of the goal of nursing can contribute to knowledge of disorders as well as knowledge of control. Roy concludes that nursing needs a commonly accepted view of the human person and of the goal of nursing. She indicates examples of trends in the direction of some common views. Roy advocates multiple middle-range theories of the human person providing nursing knowledge of order and disorder. She further subscribes to multiple middle-range theories of nursing practice to include knowledge of control, diagnosis, and prescription regarding disorders for nursing intervention.

Numerous strategies are noted to achieve the direction proposed. Some of the suggestions are in progress, such as leadership positions assumed by academic scholars, the involvement of graduate students, and the organization of a community of scholars or "think tank" for theory development. Additional strategies are offered by Roy. These are: monitor and study defining the client and goal of nursing according to a systems model; conduct controlled comparisons as to which descriptions of the client are most useful in assessing, diagnosing, and planning care; dialogue with other health care professionals; reorganize titles and departments within graduate schools of nursing according to phenomenon nursing studies or evolving theories of nursing; chairpersons of departments coordinate the systematic development and testing of the body of nursing knowledge of order, disorder, and control. Finally, Roy offers the challenge to schools utilizing divergent concepts to collaboratively conduct systematic comparative studies.

The nursing profession of the early 1980s has reached a point in time that demands setting priorities for action. The premise of this chapter is that theory development in nursing and testing of the theories developed is nursing's highest priority. After briefly establishing the rationale for this premise, this chapter will explore the kinds of theory development that nursing needs. We will then give examples of these kinds of nursing theory. Finally, based on this view of the need for theoretical progress in nursing, we will propose directions and strategies for further theory development.

RATIONALE FOR THEORY DEVELOPMENT AS HIGHEST PRIORITY

Too often throughout history, the nursing profession has been on the defensive, responding reactively to demands from outside the profession. In World War II, nurses took on increased medical assistant functions and added auxiliary personnel to help with nursing tasks. More recently nurses throughout the many states of this country have been expending needless energy fighting legislation that can have regressive effects on the nursing profession. This legislation is often conceived by men and women who know little about nursing.

There are, however, hopeful signs that nurses are ready and able to turn around that posture, to offensively and aggressively take deliberate action to create a nursing profession for the year 2000 that nurses believe in. In the experience of reacting to poor legislation and in developing new nurse practice acts for some 30 to 40 states, nurses have learned modes of acting in their own behalf. The educational level of nurses is rising, with the number of nurses holding a baccalaureate degree increasing from about 80,000 in 1972 to nearly 250,000 in 1977. Likewise nurses holding master's and doctoral degrees have increased in the same years from about 35,000 to approximately 60,000 (American Nurses' Association, 1977). Some of the most controversial issues in nursing provide unique opportunities for growth as a profession—the credentialing studies, stands on entry into practice, and efforts to unify nursing service and nursing education.

If nursing is to take an active stance in being a *significant* force in the health care system, the profession cannot dissipate its limited energies in all directions at once. The needs of the health care consumers are great—Americans are troubled by economic and security issues, threatened by an unsafe environment, struggling with caring for their elderly family members or for the increasing numbers of persons with chronic illness, and trying diet and exercise fads to ward off such illnesses.

The needs of the nursing profession are great—divisiveness among nursing specialists and organizations splinter needed energies. In 1977 to 1978 the American Nurses' Association spent over $50,000 on a project entitled "The Year of the Nurse" (Kuehn, 1980). Though the campaign may have achieved its minimal goals, including being a vehicle for affirming a positive image for nurses themselves, William L. Kuehn, Director of the American Nurses' Association's communications department, conceded that in the context of a general public audience, it "hardly broke the surface of much stereotyped imaging and thinking" (1980). One year later, in 1979, the American Academy of Nursing conducted a study designed partially to obtain concensus among its members regarding the relative importance of critical issues confronting the profession. The results (Minckley, 1979-80:2) showed that the top two issues perceived as most critical by academy members were:

1 Public image of nursing
2 Reformulation of the role of nurses

Thus because the health care needs of the people of this country (let alone of the world) and nursing's own professional identity demand it, nursing must set priorities for action. Of the many directions such priorities could take, the thesis proposed here is that theory development in nursing and testing of the theories developed constitute nursing's highest priority. How, then, can theory development respond to the needs outlined?

More than 20 years ago, Dorothy E. Johnson (1959) began to sound the warning that nurses must define the nature of their practice. What is the common denominator of what nurses proposed to do for people, whether they be in a rural clinic, or in a metropolitan hospital's intensive care unit, or in a health way station orbiting the earth in outer space? This commonality of nursing is based on shared understandings of the nature of nursing. These shared understandings are to be developed theoretically on the broad level and on more specific levels. Then nursing will be in a position to answer questions related to how it shall meet health care needs of the end of this century and the beginning of the next. The exploration of the nature of our service can give direction to the specific roles to emphasize, for example, hospice care, emergency room triage, nursing home care, or preventive care.

Secondly, both in meeting health care needs, and in dealing with issues facing the profession, nursing must confront the vital question of the systematic development of its knowledge base. Nursing claims to be a profession, that is, a group that uses a well-defined and well-organized body of knowledge to provide a service vital to human and social welfare. We have noted that nursing must clarify the nature of that service, and based on this, can develop its organized body of knowledge. When this body of knowledge demonstrates what nurses can do for their clients in a variety of settings, nursing will be in a position to meet health care needs in its own unique way. This theoretically developed—and research-tested—body of knowledge can also decrease divisiveness among nurses by emphasizing the commonality of what different specialty nurses do and by showing the parts of nursing in relation to the whole and nursing science in relation to other sciences. Nursing practice based on this body of knowledge, then, can demonstrate the social usefulness of nursing as a distinct profession. Perhaps, it is only in this way that nursing can effectively deal with problems of its public image and own divisiveness.

Though discussion of nursing theory and nursing theory development made great strides in the decade of the 1970s, for the sake of those needing nursing care and for the survival and further growth of the nursing profession this chapter maintains that theory development efforts must receive the highest priority for nursing action in the decade of the 1980s.

KINDS OF THEORY DEVELOPMENT NEEDED

One of the major issues crystalized by the discussions of and efforts toward theory development in nursing in the late 1960s and in the 1970s has been the question of the kind of theory development that nursing needs. Does nursing need grand theories or middle-range theories? A unified theory or plurality of theories? Theory *of* nursing? or theory *for* nursing?

The issue about what kind of theory is needed has been clouded by lack of clarity and at times contradictions in the use of the various terms related to the question. For example, one text (The Nursing Theories Conference Group, 1980) considers various conceptualizations of nursing as grand theories. Another text (Riehl and Roy, 1980) unifies the presentation of the work of many of the same authors by discussing them as models for nursing practice. Some feel that the terms *conceptual framework* and *conceptual model* may be used interchangeably (Newman, 1979:5). Another writer (Fawcett, 1978:18–19) calls for a distinction between conceptual and theoretical models.

In defining theory, some authors emphasize the form and function of the system (Roy and Roberts, 1981; and Hardy, 1974). These authors allow for ordering levels of theory by their degree of abstractness from grand theory to abstracted empiricism. In other discussions of theory in nursing, the level of abstraction is used as the distinction between frameworks and theory (Fawcett 1978; Williams 1979).

To pursue the proposal for the kind of theory development needed in nursing, we will submit specific definitions and meanings for the terms *conceptual model* and *theory*. The two concepts will then be related for the purpose of describing the kinds of theory development needed in nursing.

Johnson, as cited by Riehl and Roy, defines a conceptual model for nursing practice as a "systematically constructed, scientifically based, and logically related set of concepts which identify the essential components of nursing practice together with the theoretical bases for these concepts and the values required in their use by the practitioner" (1980:7). Newman (1979) further clarifies the meaning of the term conceptual model by noting that it represents a matrix of concepts which together describe the focus of inquiry. The concepts are linked together by broad generalizations, and the purpose of the model is to provide a focus which directs the questions one asks and the theories one proposes and subsequently tests.

Hardy (1978) introduces Kuhn's notion of a *general paradigm (metaparadigm)* with a meaning related to Johnson and Newman's views of models. She notes that the metaparadigm refers to a total world view or *gestalt*. This sense of an overview providing direction is noted in her list of characteristics of a *prevailing paradigm*, one that: (1) is accepted by most of the members of a discipline, (2) serves as a way of organizing perceptions, (3) defines what entities are of interest, (4) tells scientists where to look to find these entities, (5) tells them what to expect, and (6) reveals how to study them (Hardy, 1978:76).

We are, then, viewing a nursing model as a conceptual scheme of the essential components of nursing which directs the inquiry of the discipline of nursing. Among the essential components of nursing we identify the model's view of the human person and of the goal of nursing as most critical in directing theory development and research.

The definition of theory being used here is that developed by Roy and Roberts: A theory is a system of interrelated propositions used to describe, predict, explain, understand, and control a part of the empirical world (1981:18). The literature (Hardy, 1974; Newman, 1979; Roy and Roberts, 1981) distinguishes among the various types of theoretical statements such as postulates, axioms, and theorems. However, the meaning given to their terms is often different, especially when one is drawing from writings in other fields. For this reason, in our definition of theory, we use the generalized term *proposition* to describe statements that assert relationships between variables. An example of a proposition might be: Decreased levels of stress lead to increased levels of wellness. Furthermore, we note, as does Zetterberg (1954), that propositions themselves are not theory but that to form a theory propositions must be combined into interrelated systems. Burr (1973) provides a clear example of this step in theory building.

The uses of theory listed in the definition are related to the goals of scientific knowledge as discussed by Reynolds (1971). Theories contribute to organizing and categorizing phenomena, to predicting future events, to explaining past events, to understanding what causes events, and to eventual controlling events when appropriate. This definition of theory includes theory developed by induction, deduction, or an axiomatic procedure. Furthermore, it can refer to theory at all levels of abstraction, that is, the scope of a theory can range from all the empirical events of an entire science or discipline to an isolated occurrence in the real world.

Given these specific meanings of the terms models and theory, we can explore the relationships between the concepts and how this view of their relationship can guide us in submitting an answer to the question of the type of theory nursing needs.

Johnson has outlined her view of the relationship between nursing models and nursing theory (Riehl and Roy, 1980:8). In an earlier article, Johnson (1968) described the nature of the knowledge required for practice in nursing. Combining these two explanations, and elaborating on the interrelationships between the various elements, we can create the diagram presented in Fig. 34-1.

We have said that the model's view of the human person and of the goal of nursing are critical in directing theory development. Based on the model's view of the person, nurses will select, or create, basic science theories about how the person functions. For example, if a model views the person as a developmental being, from that perspective the nurse would need a knowledge base of theories about human development.

Many of these theories are available from theorists in other fields, for example, such authors as Erikson (1950), Piaget (1955), and Sullivan (1953). In this instance, the nursing theories might

NURSING MODEL

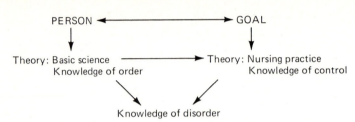

Figure 34-1   Nursing models related to theory development in nursing (*based on Johnson 1968; Riehl and Roy 1980*).

be what are commonly termed "borrowed" theories from the basic sciences. On the other hand, because of the influence of the goal of nursing upon one's view of the person, nursing may be in a position to develop theories of the human person that are unique to nursing. For example, as nurses generate developmental models of the human person, they will also specify more clearly the goal that nurses will have in dealing with their developing clients. Or, stated in the terms used earlier in the chapter, they will clarify the nature of nursing practice. This view of nursing's particular contribution to health care will then sharpen nursing's unique perspective of the human person. This more specific focus can lead to nursing's own development of theories of the human person.

Likewise, the goal of nursing, as influenced by the discipline's theory or theories of the human person, will guide the development of nursing practice theories. Nursing practice theories have been discussed by other authors (Wald and Leonard, 1964; Kline, 1978). In the context of this chapter, nursing practice theories are systems of propositions drawn from nursing models that are related to the diagnosis and treatment of the clients of nursing. When the goal of nursing is clear, we know in general terms the desired state or condition we hope to aid all clients in achieving. As we theorize based on this goal, we begin to describe and classify the occurrence of client problems which are impeding that goal. Thus, we can develop a nursing diag-

nostic classification system. Descriptions of nursing interventions related to these diagnoses can then be outlined.

In our theorizing, as we move beyond the level of describing and classifying, we will develop systems of propositions that relate variables that help us predict, explain, understand, and control how nurses intervene with clients having given diagnoses. Again, we may be borrowing some theories of intervention from other fields, for example, crisis intervention theory. However, if the unique goal of nursing is clearly understood, nursing will be in a position to develop unique theories of nursing practice. Since these theories will need to deal with multiple problems, there will tend to be many theories of at least the "middle-range" level. The plea for development of this level of theory was made some time ago by Jacox (1974). She pointed out the need for developing theories related to specific phenomena, for example, pain.

Below we will be looking at some examples of the two types of theory just described, *theories of the human person* and *nursing practice theory*. In the meantime, we can expand on these concepts by relating them to Johnson's (1968) description of the nature of knowledge required for practice in nursing. Johnson saw her three-part general types of knowledge as perhaps an oversimplification, with some overlapping of boundaries and unclarity of description. At that time, though, she noted that the division seemed reasonable and analytically useful. When reconsidered today in relation to our more recent developments in theory development, they would seem able to help clarify the direction of our theory development.

Johnson's three types of knowledge are: *knowledge of order, knowledge of disorder,* and *knowledge of control.* In considering knowledge of order, Johnson notes that an essential assumption of science is that there is order in nature and that this order can be discovered and understood (1968:206). Nightingale (1859) had long ago viewed the human person as an instrument of nature responding to the same laws whether healthy or sick. As a nursing model describes nursing's view of the human person, and basic science theories are then developed based on that view, we will be describing the patterns of order in the human person (see Fig. 34–1).

Though science looks for basic patterns or laws of order, it is also interested in the deviations from order. Johnson gives examples of phenomena such as wars, riots, earthquakes, disease, and the like. She labels these events *disorder,* though they probably have different laws of order related to them (Johnson, 1968:206). However, she finds the label useful in classifying that knowledge which helps us to understand those events which pose a threat to the well-being or survival of the individual or society.

Nursing can focus on the "normal" patterning of the person, that is, knowledge or order, in the light of the goal of nursing. By identifying threats or deviations from the goal and utilizing the practice theories which describe diagnostic classifications, nursing can discover the concepts, theories, and perhaps some day nursing's laws of disorder.

The final type of knowledge that Johnson discusses is *knowledge of control* (1968:206). Knowledge of control, related to nursing practice theory and based on a clear goal of nursing, prescribes specific actions for nursing intervention. It is nursing's way of changing the sequence of events tending toward disorder into specified outcomes related to nursing's goal.

Using the definitions and meanings given above to the terms *nursing models* and *theory in general* and drawing upon the relationship between these terms outlined in Fig. 34-1, we may return to our question of the kind of theory that nursing needs. According to the position developed here, nursing needs a commonly accepted view of the human person and of the goal of nursing. The theory development that follows will deal with middle-range theories of the human person that provide nursing with its knowledge of order and of disorder. Likewise, nursing needs the development of middle-range theories of nursing practice which include knowledge of control or diagnosis and prescription regarding disorders of the person identified as nursing's specific focus. Thus, though we argue for a common focus on the phenomena of nursing (Johnson, 1978; Hardy, 1978; Donaldson and Crowley, 1977), we are not proposing a grand theory, a unified theory, or a theory *of* nursing. Rather we see, within some commonalities of perspective on the discipline of nursing, the need for development of a plurality of middle-range theories of the human person and theories of nursing practice *for* nursing as an applied science.

EXAMPLES OF THEORIES OF THE PERSON AND OF NURSING PRACTICE

In describing the kind of theory development that nursing needs, we have focused on the need for theories of the person as viewed from nursing's perspective and for theories of nursing practice based on an overall description of the unique goal of nursing. Though a number of theorizing effects currently in progress could be used to illustrate this process, two specific examples best known by the author will be used. The first example is the joint effort of a group of nurse-theorists to develop a theoretical framework for the classification of nursing diagnosis being generated by the National Conference on Nursing Diagnosis. The description of this work and a historical perspective on it is given in detail in the proceedings of the third and fourth national conferences (Kim and Moritz, 1982).

Here, were can simply show how the conceptual scheme being developed is an example of the direction being proposed for theory development. After 4 intensive meetings of about 12 persons nationally known for their work in nursing theory, the group has focused on the phenomenon of the human person called *unitary man—an open system*. In describing this person four basic assumptions were agreed upon, then delineated. First the person is a developmental process that is growing, evolutionary, and negentropic. Second, the human person represents a four-dimensional field with pattern, organization, unity transaction and arbitrary boundaries. The next assumption involves the person's patterning of energy including rhythm, ordering, and mutual simultaneous interaction. Last, the unitary person is seen as goal-seeking.

To move toward the task of the group of providing a framework for the classification of nursing diagnosis, the theorists further described the characteristics of the unitary person according to his major patterns. Nine patterns were grouped under three major factors. Factor 1, *interaction*, included the patterns of exchanging, communicating, and relating. For factor 2, *action*, the patterns of valuing, choosing, and moving were identified. Finally, factor 3, *awareness*, comprises the patterns of waking, feeling, and knowing. The theorist group worked on developing assessment factors and empirical indicators for each pattern.

We noted earlier that theory development in nursing, according to the proposal presented, could profitably focus on theories of the human person and theories of nursing practice. The work of the theorist group described briefly here is still in the early stages of development and has a goal in relation to the Nursing Diagnosis Conference Group, rather than being a theorizing project. Still it contains the rudiments of a theory of the human person. As unitary persons are further described, we can develop systems of

propositions related to their patterns of functioning, or as expressed earlier, we can develop nursing science's knowledge of order about the person.

Originally the group defined the goal of nursing as to promote health. It would seem that, with the later work describing patterns of the unitary person, that goal can be stated more specifically in a way that will be unique to nursing. This then, also gives us the potential for the development and testing of nursing practice theory as described earlier in relation to knowledge of disorder and knowledge of control. The work of this group is used as an example here, not because it exemplifies the total process of theorizing proposed; rather, it can be an example of the beginning stages of this process. More importantly, the project has unusual significance in that it is a joint effort of a number of nurse-theorists and commentators on nursing theory.

The second example of theorizing about the person and about nursing practice will be based on the work developing out of the Roy *adaptation model of nursing* (Roy, 1971; Roy, 1976). The model identifies the person as an adaptive system. In this system, external and internal stimuli, particularly the person's own adaptation level, form the inputs of the system. The internal processes of the system are the *cognator* and the *regulator*. These primary or functional subsystems act as connectives between the *adaptive modes*. The adaptive modes, identified as *physiological needs, self-concept, role function,* and *interdependence,* are the secondary or *effector* subsystems (Roy and Roberts, 1981). The output of the system is adaptive and ineffective responses. Interrelated series of propositions have been developed for the primary and secondary subsystems. These theories draw from other sciences but are integrated into the total view of the person indicated by the Roy model. We will give one illustration of this process of theorizing taken from the work on the role function mode of theorizing.

The role function mode also can be viewed in a systems theory framework. Based on the

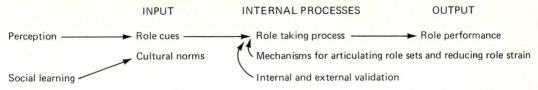

Figure 34-2   The role system.

central processes of the cognator subsystem, the person's functioning in relation to roles can be outlined as in Fig. 34-2.

Perception and social learning provide the basis for role cues and cultural norms which act as input for the role taking process. Mechanisms for articulating role sets and for reducing role strain act as self-regulation while internal and external validation provide feedback. The combination of this input and these internal processes leads to the output of role performance.

The terms of the outline are the concepts of the theory. An exploration of each term is beyond the scope of this paper but is described in Roy and Roberts (1981).

Once the concepts of theory have been specified, the process of theorizing calls for relating the concepts in meaningful propositions. A major proposition that can be postulated from an understanding of the role system can be stated as follows: The amount of clarity of input in the form of role cues and cultural norms positively influences the adequacy of role taking. Going back to the antecedents of role cues and cultural norms, we can have two propositions: (1) Accuracy of perception positively influences the clarity of input in the form of role cues and cultural norms; and (2) Adequacy of social learning positively influences the clarity of input in the form of role cues and cultural norms. A final proposition in the system sequence could be stated thus: The level of role taking positively influences the level of role mastery. The propositions stated here are all interrelated by means of the system diagram. Furthermore, they are a basis for description, explanation, prediction, and control regarding the person as an adaptive

system functioning in relation to the role-function mode.

We have here, then, a small piece of theorizing about the person as an adaptive system. It is basic science theory used to delineate nursing's knowledge about the human person. Specifically, it relates to the order apparent in the functioning of the person. It is, then, theoretical knowledge of order that is developed for nursing. We have noted that, in addition to the knowledge or order stemming from basic and nursing science, nursing also needs knowledge of disorder and knowledge of control. This kind of knowledge will provide us with theory for nursing practice. Through the long process of theorizing, we will eventually come to a prescription of what the nurse in practice can actually do to help his or her patient.

Our brief theorizing with the role function mode has given us some knowledge of the order expected in the role performance of the person. If we add to this knowledge the adaptation model's view of the goal of nursing, we have some knowledge of disorder. The goal of the Roy adaptation model is to promote adaptation in regard to the four modes. Adaptation problems occur when the inputs to the adaptive system are outside the zone of coping as determined by the adaptation level. A proposition related to the knowledge of disorder in regard to role function might thus be stated: Role cues or cultural norms that are above or below the zone for coping set up by the adaptation level will negatively influence the adequacy of role taking. Furthermore, inadequate role taking negatively influences the level of role mastery. This sequence contributes to our knowledge of disorder.

Let us apply this theory to a clinical situation.

A young child is admitted to a pediatric unit. The child has croup and the mother is very frightened. She has never been in a hospital, except for the birth of her child 2 years ago. She can't imagine how she will relate to her child in the strange croupette. She comes out to the nurses' station every 2 to 3 minutes to check on some detail of the child's condition or treatment. When she is at the child's bedside she cries, wrings her hands, and avoids looking at the child. This mother is having difficulty in taking the role of the mother of an ill and hospitalized child.

In terms of our theoretical model concerning role function, we can describe the mother's difficulty in the following way. Her constricted perception and lack of former socialization has led to inadequate role cues for the role-taking process. The role cues are below the minimum amount needed in her present condition for her to make a positive response. The result is inadequate role performance, that is, she fails to carry out a number of appropriate parenting functions in relation to her hospitalized child.

Our process of theorizing now comes to the theory of nursing practice which involves knowledge of control. In other words, what can the nurse do for the distraught parents of a child with croup?

One way of expressing control is to derive a hypothesis from the various propositions of the knowledge of order and knowledge of disorder. Thus, in the series of theorizing we are doing, this hypothesis may be derived: The level of role adequacy will increase more when role cues based on principles of accuracy of perception and adequacy of social learning are specifically introduced than when these cues are not specifically introduced.

In relation to our clinical example, we are prescribing that the nurse introduce role cues in order to increase the parent's role adequacy in relating to the hospitalized child. The type of role cues to be used with parents of hospitalized children have been previously specified in a pilot study and then tested in a clinical re-

search project (Roy, 1967). To provide effective role cues, the nurse first focuses her or his attention on the parents' focus of attention. Secondly, the nurse communicates with the parents concerning the child's general condition, treatment, or activities. Finally, the nurse tells the parents what they might do for their child. The role theory alluded to earlier explains why these simple actions by the nurse can be so helpful to the parents. That is, the cues facilitate role taking by helping the parents focus on the other, recognize the present position of the other, and, finally, identify the response that is expected of them.

Our hypothetical nurse thus enters the child's room and focuses first on the parents' own anxiety. Then he or she explains the child's general condition, the croup tent, and the child's activities, including need for fluids. Last, the nurse explains how the parent may help by observing the child's respirations and by giving the child fluids once each hour. Soon the parent is functioning adequately in the modified parenting role.

In this way, then, the beginning theory relating to the role system, when combined with the model's view of the goal of nursing, is used to describe knowledge of disorder and ultimately knowledge of control. That is, it prescribes nursing actions.

Again, we can say that this example of theorizing for nursing represents beginning efforts. Further elaboration of the theory is needed, especially in relation to seeing the parts of the adaptive system interrelating in holistic behavior. Still the example has perhaps served to further clarify the direction for theory development that is being proposed here.

DIRECTIONS AND STRATEGIES FOR THEORY DEVELOPMENT

In submitting the kind of theory development needed in nursing and in giving examples of efforts representing this type of movement, we have already identified our proposal for direction in theory development in nursing. This direction can be summarized in the following steps:

1 Describe the discipline's common view of the human person and of the goal of nursing
2 Develop theories of the human person providing nursing with its knowledge or order and disorder
3 Develop the multiple middle-range theories of nursing practice that include knowledge of control and knowledge of disorder, that is, the diagnoses and prescriptions relevant to nursing's unique focus or goal

These steps, of course, are not absolutely sequential. Logically, our work of developing the related theories would proceed more orderly and quickly if we could accomplish the first task, that of describing the common view of the discipline of nursing. There are hopeful signs of a trend in the direction of some common views. For example, the analysis made by Donaldson and Crowley (1977:18) noted the following commonalities in the ideas of nursing writers:

1 Concern with principles and laws that govern life processes; well-being; and optimum functioning of human beings, sick or well, for example, Nightingale and Rogers.
2 Concern with the pattern of human behavior in interaction with the environment in critical life situations, for example, Rogers and Johnson.
3 Concern with the processes by which positive changes in health status are effected, for example, Peplau, Kreuter, and Leininger.

Secondly, in the work of the Nurse Theorist Group of the National Conference on Nursing Diagnosis, some of the apparent inconsistencies in philosophical assumptions underlying the concepts of nursing of these authors may be reaching a point of reconciliation.

In spite of this hope, nursing has not yet reached agreement that this task needs to be done, nor can we predict that the task will be completed even in the next 5 years. Thus, it will be important to continue the divergent efforts regarding theorizing indicated in steps 2 and 3. Perhaps we can count on nursing's intuitive sense of what nursing is to provide enough direction to this work that it will find its place in the scheme of the science of nursing that is envisioned when that intuitive sense has been articulated, agreed upon, and theorized and tested.

If this specific direction for theory development has been proposed, then what strategies can be offered to move in this direction? Some of the strategies relative to this proposed direction have been suggested before and have begun to take shape. Johnson (1974) discussed the dissimilar bodies of knowledge that would result from basically different types of models, for example, developmental models and system models. This chapter has expanded on her argument for coming to a common view of the person and nursing's goal. DeBack reports that in a survey of curriculum models in National League for Nursing accredited baccalaureate programs, of the 270 schools responding, 50 percent were categorized as systems models, 19 percent as developmental models, and 6 percent as interaction models, while 24 percent were identified as mixed models (1981:51-66).

Menke (1978) submitted that the academic community should assume a leadership position in the ry development. In recent years, most master's degree programs have introduced courses in which conceptual models and theory development are explicated. There is a sense (in correspondence with theorists and in attendance at theory conferences) that these students are well initiated into the value of nursing models for practice and research. In some schools, the student's thesis research must be drawn from one of the existing conceptual models for nursing. Examining the catalogs of the rapidly developing doctoral programs in nursing, we find a heavy emphasis on nursing theory. In the author's experience of contact with many of these schools, about half the programs have the doctoral students proceed beyond theory analysis to participation in the process of formal theory construction. An example of this work is given by Hill and Roberts in Roy and Roberts (1981:30–39).

Another suggestion made by Menke (1978) was the organization of a community of scholars or "think tank" for theory development and metatheory discussions. The initiation of the Nursing Theory Think Tank group by Pennsylvania State University School of Nursing, coordinated by Margaret Newman, was reported by Chinn (1980).

What can be added to these strategies in progress? First, it is submitted that the apparent natural trend toward defining the client and goal of nursing according to a systems model be monitored and studied. This can be done formally and informally, in nursing education and practice. Controlled comparisons can be made as to whether these descriptions of the client are most useful in assessing, diagnosing, and planning care. At least one such study has been completed (DeBack, 1981:51–66). Dialogue can be established with our clients themselves to see if this view is congruent, or could be made to be congruent, with their perceived needs and expectations. Client support groups such as colostomy clubs could be contacted for this dialogue. Likewise, dialogue with other health care professionals is strongly suggested. Nursing's autonomy is a value to be maintained. Still new insights as well as growth in mutual understanding can result from sharing our developing notions of how we view the client and what we hope to accomplish with him or her with those who also provide care for the same person.

In regard to the role of the academic community, we advocate continuing and intensifying efforts to develop a core group of nurse-scientists who can help us accelerate the pace of progress in all three tasks of theory development. Furthermore, based on current efforts to clarify the nature of our body of knowledge, it may not be too soon to recommend the reorganization of the departments within our graduate schools. If the phenomenon that nursing studies is not the biological person, then we will not have

specialties in cardiovascular nursing or respiratory nursing. What might some of our new specialties look like? Based on the two examples of beginning theories of the human person cited earlier, we might see such titles as: Department of Human Awareness, including the nursing science of waking, feeling, knowing, and perceiving; or Department of Adaptive Cognator Processes focusing on the nursing science of self-concept and role function.

Though the think tank concept has begun, since the interaction of these communities of scholars are on the cutting edge of our progress forward, we urge finding every creative approach possible to intensify these efforts. Too often the constraints of time, money, and energy deter us from such important projects. However, such meetings may become increasingly easier as advancing technology based on other sciences can be used to serve the development of our own science. For example, Rogers claims that a high-speed transit "tubecraft," which can carry persons from New York City to Los Angeles in 21 minutes, is already on the drawing board (1980:334).

However, we cannot wait for the technically easier ways to communicate. The methods available to us now must be utilized. Just as the scholars must interchange ideas, we propose that chairpersons of the departments of our graduate schools coordinate the systematic development and testing of the body of nursing knowledge of order, disorder, and control. Schools using similar concepts of the person could make their work cumulative. Schools using divergent concepts could produce the controlled comparative studies needed. Hopefully, collaboration on design of such studies would eliminate the too often present bias based on regional or personal loyalties to given theorists.

In this chapter we have made a specific proposal for direction in theory development in nursing and urged strategies to be used in moving in that direction since we are convinced that such theory development and testing constitute the highest priority in nursing.

EDITOR'S QUESTIONS FOR DISCUSSION

After reading the seven chapters in this section, and Chaps. 8 and 14, define all the terms used in theory development. Aim for accurate understanding of the definition and meaning of the terms. Cite the degree that there is consensus for definitions and meanings between specific scholars. Are there terms which may legitimately be used synonymously? Which terms appear to be used interchangeably where in fact the meanings are different? What is the essential difference between a proposition in a theory and concepts in a conceptual model?

Discuss pro and con that nursing's highest priority should be the development of theory in nursing. To what extent would you agree with the rationale presented? What other priorities can be offered? Justify the rationale for those priorities.

To what extent is there agreement between Roy and Hardy (Chap. 32) regarding a community of scientists; consensus of a paradigm for nursing; multiple theories; and grand, middle-range, and single-domain theories? What other scholars address these issues? How do the characteristics of a paradigm as indicated by Roy compare with Hardy's description (Chap. 32)? Is there incongruence between a commonality of perspective on the discipline of nursing and plurality in theory as advocated by Roy? What agreements exist between Roy and Meleis (Chap. 33)?

To what extent is Roy in agreement with other scholars as to a nursing diagnostic taxonomy evolving from a nursing conceptual base? Compare Roy's perspective regarding nursing practice theory with those presented by Fawcett (Chap. 14), Walker (Chap. 30), Menke (Chap. 31), Hardy (Chap. 32), and Meleis (Chap. 33). What relationship is there between the types of knowledge needed for nursing as portrayed by Fawcett (Chap. 14) and Johnson's three types of knowledge as applied by Roy? Present arguments for and against Roy's belief that the work of the Nursing Diagnosis Conference Group contains the rudiments of a theory of the human person. What relationship is there between Roy's presentation of the conference group work and Roger's theory? Argue for or against Roy's adaptation model having evolved into a theory? If you perceive the Roy model as a theory, are Roy's and Rogers's formulations competing theories?

REFERENCES

American Nurses' Association
  1977 National Sample Survey of Registered Nurses. Kansas City, Missouri: American Nurses' Association

Burr, Wesley R.
  1973 Theory Construction and the Sociology of the Family. New York: Wiley.

Chinn, Peggy L.
  1980 "From the editor." Advances in Nursing Science 2(4):xiii–xiv.

DeBack, Vivien
  1981 "The relationship between senior nursing students ability to formulate nursing diagnosis and the curriculum model." Advances in Nursing Science 3(3):51–66.

Donaldson, Sue K. and Dorothy Crowley
  1977 "Discipline of nursing: Structure and relationship to practice," Pp. 1–22 in M. Batey (ed.), Communicating Nursing Research, Volume 10. Boulder, Colorado: Western Interstate Commission on Higher Education.

Erikson, Erik
  1950 Childhood and Society. New York: W. W. Norton.

Fawcett, Jacqueline
  1978 "The state of the art of theory development in nursing," Pp. 1–33 in Theory Development: What, Why, How? New York: National League for Nursing.

Hardy, Margaret E.
  1974 "Theories: Components, development,

evaluation." Nursing Research 23:100–107.

1978 "Evaluating nursing theory," Pp. 75–86 in Theory Development: What, Why, How? New York: National League for Nursing.

Hill, Betty J. and Carolyn S. Roberts
1981 "Formal theory construction: An example of the process." Pp. 30–39 in Sister Callista Roy and Sharon Roberts, Theory Contribution in Nursing: An Adaptation Model. Englewood Cliffs, N.J.: Prentice-Hall.

Jacox, Ada
1974 "Theory construction in nursing: An overview." Nursing Research 23:4–13.

Johnson, Dorothy E.
1959 "A philosophy of nursing." Nursing Outlook 7:198–200.
1968 "Theory in nursing: Borrowed and unique." Nursing Research 17:206–209.
1974 "Development of theory: A requisite for nursing as a primary health profession." Nursing Research 23:372–377.
1978 "The state of the art of theory development in nursing," Pp. 1–10 in Theory Development: What, Why, How? New York: National League for Nursing.

Kim, Mi Ja and Derry Moritz
1982 Classification of Nursing Diagnosis: Proceedings of the Third and Fourth National Conferences. New York: McGraw-Hill.

Kline, John
1978 "Theory development in nursing," Pp. 223–231 in N. Chaska (ed.), The Nursing Profession: Views Through The Mist. New York: McGraw-Hill.

Kuehn, William L.
1980 Unpublished personal communication, June 23.

Menke, Edna M.
1978 "Theory development: A challenge for nursing," Pp. 216–222 in N. Chaska (ed.), The Nursing Profession: Views Through The Mist. New York: McGraw-Hill.

Minckley, Barbara B.
1979–80 "Program committee report." News From The American Academy of Nursing 1(2):2. Kansas City, Missouri: American Academy of Nursing.

Newman, Margaret A.
1979 Theory Development in Nursing. Philadelphia: F. A. Davis Co.

Nightingale, Florence
1859 Notes on Nursing: What It Is, and What It Is Not. A facisimile of the first edition with foreword by Annie W. Goodrich. Philadelphia: J. P. Lippincott Co., 1966.

Nursing Theories Conference Group, Julia B. George, Chairperson
1980 Nursing Theories: The Base for Professional Nursing Practice. Englewood Cliffs, N. J.: Prentice-Hall.

Piaget, Jean
1955 The Language and Thought of the Child. New York: World.

Reynolds, Paul Davidson
1971 A Primer of Theory Construction. Indianapolis: Bobbs-Merrill.

Riehl, Joan and Sister Callista Roy
1980 Conceptual Models for Nursing Practice. 2d edition. Englewood Cliffs, N. J.: Prentice-Hall.

Rogers, Martha E.
1980 "Nursing: A science of unitary man." Pp. 329–337 in J. Riehl and Sister Callista Roy, Conceptual Models for Nursing Practice. 2d edition. Englewood Cliffs, N.J.: Prentice-Hall.

Roy, Sister Callista and Sharon Roberts
1981 Theory Contribution in Nursing: An Adaptation Model. Englewood Cliffs, N. J.: Prentice-Hall.

Roy, Sister Callista
1967 "Role cues and mothers of hospitalized children." Nursing Research 16:178–82.
1971 "Adaptation: A basis for nursing practice." Nursing Outlook 19:254–57.
1976 Introduction to Nursing: An Adaptation Model. Englewood Cliffs, N. J.: Prentice-Hall.

Sullivan, Harry Stack
1953 The Independent Theory of Psychiatry. New York: W. W. Norton.

Wald, Florence S. and Robert C. Leonard
1964 "Towards development of nursing practice theory." Nursing Research 13:309–313.
Williams, Carolyn A.
1979 "The nature and development of conceptual frameworks." Pp. 89–96 in F. Downs and J. Fleming (eds.), Issues in Nursing Research. Englewood Cliffs, N.J.: Prentice-Hall.
Zetterberg, Hans
1954 Theory and Verification in Sociology. Totoux, N. J.: Bedminster Press.

Part Five

Nursing Practice

A time for healing; . . .
a time for planting, . . .
a time for mourning,
a time for dancing

Nursing practice does, in fact, include healing, planting, mourning, and dancing. The professional nurse heals the patient/client through the application of nursing knowledge to perform nursing interventions. The quality of the interaction between the nurse and patient is critical in the healing process. The professional nurse also plants the seeds of health maintenance through health education and teaching. Mourning occurs when the goals of nursing interventions are either not achieved or when the interventions were not effective in themselves. It is a time for dancing as the professional nurse and patient/client *together* assess and plan for the patient's nursing needs and evaluate the effectiveness and outcomes of nursing interventions.

Nursing practice is more clearly being defined than in previous decades. The development of a classification system for nursing diagnoses has made distinctions between a nursing and medical intervention possible. Humanistic nursing care for the well and the ill is increasingly advocated. The patient/client as a consumer of care is the central focus. Multiple changes have occurred in modes of providing nursing care, roles in nursing care, the scope of nursing practice, qualifications and accountability for professional practice, and the amount of control over nursing practice. This section portrays nursing practice today as well as evidence of concerns, hopes, and ideals for the future.

Chapter 35

Consumerism and the Nursing Profession

Juanita W. Fleming, R.N., Ph.D., F.A.A.N.
Professor and
Assistant Dean for Graduate Education and
Director of Graduate Studies
College of Nursing
University of Kentucky
Lexington, Kentucky

The reason for the existence of nursing as a profession is for the provision of a unique service to the patient. It is significant that Juanita Fleming's chapter is first in this section. She calls attention to the consumer's role and rights in health care. The role of five federal agencies concerned about the health of consumers is defined. Fleming cites examples of involvement of nongovernmental organizations with consumer concerns, such as the American Nurses' Association, the American Medical Association, and the American Hospital Association.

Fleming focuses predominantly on understanding consumers, their concerns, and their influence in health care. She further identifies nine expectations consumers have of health professionals. In addition to competency, the majority of the expectations pertain to courtesy and personal consideration of the consumer. Some of the concerns of consumers include the cost of drugs, hospitals, and physicians; the shortage of nurses; and the quality of care provided. She indicates that consumers are likely to increase their political power through participation in various health systems agencies, advisory and licensure boards. Fleming perceives that views about health care between providers and consumers are not in harmony.

Fleming offers two major challenges to the profession of nursing in relation to the consumer. The first is to help society clearly understand how the nursing role has changed and communicate what the present role is. The second is to identify how nurses can improve their service and how consumers can help nurses clearly understand their health care needs. Fleming suggests avenues for meeting the challenges, for example, using open and closed circuit television to teach consumers. She views research in the area of humanistic helping and advocacy as being essential.

The health care industry is one of the largest industries serving consumers in the United States. It is a complicated, costly, and constantly changing industry which has several professional disciplines involved in the delivery of services. Often the industry seems to be controlled by vested interests and caught up in power and profit motives. The consumer's role prior to the 1960s was practically nonexistent.

In 1962 the creed and manifesto of the consumer movement as articulated by President John F. Kennedy included:

1 The right to safety—to be protected against the marketing of goods which are hazardous to health or life.
2 The right to be informed—to be protected against fraudulent, deceitful, or grossly misleading information, advertising, labeling, or other practices, and to be given the facts he needs to make an informed choice.
3 The right to choose—to be assured, wherever possible, access to a variety of products and services at competitive prices; and in those industries in which competition is not workable and Government regulation is substituted, an assurance of satisfactory quality and service at fair prices.
4 The right to be heard—to be assured that consumer interests will receive full and sympathetic consideration in the formulation of Government policy, and fair and expeditious treatment in its administrative tribunals. (Kennedy, 1962)

The consumer movement, based on the impact of the 1960s which was labeled the "Decade of the Consumer," has succeeded to some extent in advancing consumer rights in the areas spoken of by President Kennedy. The achievements have come from the combined efforts of consumer groups, business-sponsored initiatives, and government. Consumers are the largest economic group in the country. Two-thirds of all spending in the national economy is by the consumers.

GOVERNMENT AND NONGOVERNMENT ROLES

All levels of the federal government, as well as many nongovernment agencies—associations, manufacturers, and professional groups—have important and unique roles in consumer protection. Whether government's role in protecting the consumer will continue at the level it has in the past is questionable. Some of the agencies may not survive and others may change markedly their methods of surveillance.

The five federal agencies listed below are selected examples of agencies which are concerned with the health care of consumers. Most states also have a consumer affairs office and other agencies which monitor activities in areas which would affect the health of the citizens. The attorney general's office in many states provides support and protection for consumers.

The United States Consumer Product Safety Commission is one of the primary federal agencies. It was activated in May, 1973. Its role in product safety is to protect the public against unreasonable risk of injury; to evaluate the comparative safety of consumer products; to develop uniform safety standards for consumer products and to minimize conflicting state and local regulations; and to investigate cause and prevention of product-related deaths, illnesses, and injuries. This agency has the responsibility for implementing several laws, among them the Flammable Fabrics Act, the Federal Hazardous Substances Act, the Poison Prevention Packaging Act, and the Refrigerator Safety Act.

The Occupational Safety and Health Administration which develops and promulgates occupational safety and health standards and regulations and investigates compliance with these regulations and standards is also concerned with consumer safety.

The Mine Safety and Health Administration also develops and promulgates mandatory safety and health standards. It ensures compliance with standards and cooperates with and provides assistance to states in the development of effective mine safety and health programs. Training programs are designed with the aim of preventing accidents and occupational diseases in the mining industry.

The Center for Disease Control administers national programs for prevention and control of communicable diseases and other preventable conditions, including urban rat control.

The Food and Drug Administration, established in 1907, is one of the oldest agencies. Its activities are directed toward protecting the health of the nation against impure and unsafe goods, drugs, cosmetics, and other potential hazards.

Professional nursing organizations, nationally and statewide, are involved in recommending nurses to serve on advisory committees and boards which consider consumer well-being. For the most part, the input nurses have in federal and state agencies which deal with consumer health is as members of these boards.

The American Medical Association is an example of a nongovernmental organization which has a specific activity in the interest of the consumer. The AMA publishes several pamphlets designed for consumer protection. One of these is entitled *Health Quackery* and another, *Merchants of Menace*.

In 1973 the American Hospital Association published "A Patient's Bill of Rights." These rights were presented with the expectation that their observance would contribute to more effective patient care and greater satisfaction for the patient, the physician, and the hospital organization. Some of these are the right to considerate and respectful care; the right to reasonable information about diagnosis, care, treatment, and alternatives for treatment and care; the right to opportunity to give informed consent; and the right to confidentiality of records.

This document does not, however, speak directly to nursing. The Code for Nursing published by the American Nurses Association clearly delineates how nurses are to function in relationship to the individuals they serve. The code calls for treatment which respects human dignity, safeguards the client's right to privacy, and protects confidential information. The nurses' code specifically indicates that the nurse must maintain competency and assume responsibility and accountability for nursing judgments and actions.

UNDERSTANDING THE CONSUMER

A basic understanding of that aspect of human nature which relates to human needs as a consumer is often overlooked. Yet it may aid nurses in better serving those who enter the health care system. According to Hadley,

Human beings

1 want security both in its physical and psychological meaning to protect gains already made and to insure a beachhead from which further advances may be staged
2 crave for sufficient order and certainty in [their lives] to enable [them] to judge with fair accuracy what will or will not occur if [they do or do not] act in certain ways
3 continuously seek to enlarge the range and to enrich the quality of their satisfactions
4 [are] creature[s] of hope
5 have the capacity to make choices and to exercise this capacity
6 require freedom to exercise choice in those matters in which [they are] capable of making the decision
7 want to experience their own identity and integrity; in other words, want personal dignity
8 want to experience a sense of [their] own worthwhileness. (1971:53–57)

Consumers, of course, behave according to the Gaussian curve, with extremes from "very docile" to "very militant." The more vocal consumers will demand better service and explanations and will pressure the health care industry providers to be more responsible and correct in its dealings with them. Many consumers view the industry providers as perhaps concerned about delivering quality care but acting from its own perspective and without consulting the consumers. In other words, the providers in the health care system are not in tune with the practical realities of consumer opinion.

Nurses, like other health care providers, must assume that consumers will act rationally and that consumers have something of value to contribute to their care. Models of rationality which apply to health care consumers are built on several propositions.

1 Goals and objectives must be known.
2 There must be a set of alternatives from which to choose.
3 The effect of each alternative on achieving the decision maker's goal must be discernible.
4 There is a payoff representing the utility of each alternative to the decision maker.
5 Knowledge about the prevailing state or information as to the consequences of choosing either alternative must be available.

Simon, in discussing a behavioral model of rational choice, notes that the flavor of various rational choices stems primarily from the specific assumptions that are introduced as the givens or contraints within which rational adaptation must take place. Among the constraints are the set of alternatives operational in the choice, the relationships that determine the payoffs, i.e., satisfaction, goal-attainment, and preference orderings among payoffs (Simon, 1955:100).

The consumer needs an explanation as to the goals and objectives of nursing. In fact, ideally the goals and objectives should be developed with the patient, if possible, and the family. The patient may be informed of the goal of the medical care, but how many are informed of the goals of nursing care? The goals are likely to be complementary, but they will not necessarily be the same. The consumer's right to be informed suggests that the right to information about nursing care objectives is critical.

Nurses make care plans based on their assessment of the patient's needs. Alternatives from which the patient can choose should be clearly delineated in the plans nurses make. The importance of developing alternatives cannot be overstated. Consumers have a right to choose; consequently, if the nursing profession offers services, alternatives within the services offered should be available. Each alternative must be clear so that the consumer can understand the effect of selecting one alternative over another.

CONSUMER CONCERNS

Consumers are concerned about the cost of drugs, hospitals, and physicians. The cost of nursing is usually not an issue. This may be because in many hospitals or agencies where nursing care is given nursing costs are not itemized on the bill. Drugs and physician charges are itemized, but nursing is usually buried or not reflected in the item labeled "hospital cost."

Consumers are also concerned about physician and nurse availability. The shortage of nurses and an inability to get the attention of those available was seen as a problem by about 300 of 600 patients surveyed to elicit information regarding how they viewed hospitals and hospital personnel (Watterson, 1971). The quality of nursing care received is identified as a consumer concern (Watterson, 1971; Fleming, 1979); it is interesting to note, however, that in one of the studies the item most highly correlated with consumer satisfaction in quality care was courtesy and consideration shown by nurses. Consumers reported in one study that they had received enough attention from nurses, but they expressed concern about consumer surveys unless there is a willingness to use the information gained (Houston and Pasanen, 1972). Consumer concerns are not limited to those described here; consumer desires are tied very closely to consumer concerns.

CONSUMER INVOLVEMENT IN HEALTH CARE

Consumers have gained political power, and that power is likely to increase. Public Law 93-641, a piece of federal health legislation requiring consumer participation, was impressive evidence of the political clout of consumers. The National Health Planning and Resources Development Act of 1974 creating health systems agencies, the State Health Coordination Councils (S.H.C.C.), the various state health advisory boards, and facilities for certificate of need and licensure boards are all further examples of the influence of consumers in health care.

There seems to be some frustration, however, on the part of consumers as well as on the part of those who provide health care. In the case of nursing, for example, many nurses do not believe consumers understand what nursing care entails. On the other hand, some consumers do not believe nurses can do anything for them without being told to do so by physicians. The lack of understanding on the part of both the nurse and the consumer suggests a need for better communication.

The critical questions seem to be:

1 How can nurses better articulate to consumers the nature and purpose of nursing care?

2 How can nurses better serve consumers who enter the health care system?

3 How can consumers help nurses better understand their health care needs?

Nurses must recognize that the society is, perhaps, moving to an era when emphasis on patient involvement in care necessitates that the consumer have the essential role in his or her own care. The knowledge needed to effectively manage that care must be provided. The assumption that consumers are passive information receivers, at least when it comes to their health care, is a false assumption. Health is important and the consumer is generally motivated to actively seek information if there is an impairment of health. The assumption that the nurse is a better judge of what is happening would place the nurse in an authoritative position. The consumer, to the extent he or she is able, assumes much of the responsibility in his or her own care.

Physicians and nurses are the largest group of health care providers consumers encounter. Consumers seem to want health professionals who

1 Are dedicated and committed, and who care about those to whom they give care; 2 Are competent and have the appropriate knowledge and skills to provide the care needed; 3 Are aware of cultural differences among consumers; 4 Speak and use language the consumer understands; 5 Take time to explain care and problems associated with care; 6 Treat the consumer with dignity and respect; 7 Listen to consumer concerns about problems of care and management; 8 Help the consumer evaluate the significance of certain symptoms; and 9 Demonstrate to the consumer the appropriate self-care techniques.

CHALLENGE TO THE PROFESSION

Two major challenges seem to be evident in terms of the profession and the consumer. The first relates to the profession itself. Though many people are cognizant of what members of the profession do and how they contribute to care, there still seems to be a wide gap in consumer understanding of the role of the nurse.

Aydelotte states that:

Each discipline has its own social goals, its domain (that is, the phenomena with which it deals), its methods of study, and its structure. There is agreement that nursing has practical consequences and a strong service orientation. . . . . Social purpose may also change over time as society changes the junctions it assigns to professions. (1977:47)

Jelinek and Dennis note that nursing must move away from purely technical and clerical tasks, absorb more physician procedures, provide more health maintenance, and gain recognition as having the major responsibility for psychosocial care. Members of the nursing profession are trying to rid themselves of their image as "subservient handmaidens in white" (1976).

Obviously, the role of nursing is changing. Whether the public perception of the role is clear is the question.

The profession might well make a concerted effort to better educate the consumer about nursing. The use of public service announcements on television sponsored by the professional nursing organizations may well be one approach. The messages, of course, would need to be carefully developed, designed to appeal to needs of consumers rather than to promote nursing organizations. There are many other approaches to consumer education, but this chapter is not designed to enumerate them. The challenge to the profession is to help society understand better how the role of nursing has changed and to provide society a clearer indication of what that role presently is.

Though there is some confusion regarding the role of nurses in health teaching, it is clear that health education is important from a nursing perspective and is valuable for consumers, in that it aids them in living lives as healthy as possible. A number of studies regarding nursing and health teaching can be found in the literature.

In planning health care, clear goals must be delineated. The use of open- and closed-circuit television to teach consumers how to care for themselves seems desirable. Closed-circuit television in hospitals and clinics has tremendous potential for educating individual patients and groups of patients and their families. Open-circuit television can be used to teach consumers about preventive health.

Eventually computers are likely to be as common as telephones, and most homes will have them. Giving information on health care to clients via computers which are tied up with hospitals and clinics is another method nurses might use to aid consumers in the future. Computer-assisted instruction has several advantages, the most widely accepted one being that the individual is actively involved in the learning process. Reinforcement is immediate and systematized; consequently, learning is thought to be more effective. The use of technology, not only to enhance consumer understanding of nursing but also to provide the knowledge that will facilitate self-care, is very promising in the future of health education. And nurses have a tremendous stake in improving the health of people in this nation and the world through the teaching of self-care.

The second challenge to nurses is to respond to the critical questions posed earlier. Chapman and Chapman, in citing their belief in humanism, noted:

. . . the essence of humanism is experiences between people in a dynamic interpersonal process and it cannot be politically and financially mandated. To be humanistic is more than talk. It is to hold both an attitude and a set of behaviors that allows one to express visibly the dignity that one perceives in oneself and others. (1975:31)

The nature of helping, the interpersonal process, and advocacy are described well by the Chapmans. However, controlled research is sparse in the areas of humanistic helping and advocacy. How to help consumers of all ages—those who have acute, chronic, and physically disabling conditions; those who are dying; and those who are attempting to prevent ill health—enter the health care system and receive the care they need with dignity is a tremendous challenge. More research in the area of humanistic helping and advocacy is needed.

The future of nursing, as it relates to the consumer, offers substantive challenges.

EDITOR'S QUESTIONS FOR DISCUSSION

Discuss the contributions from consumers that are most desirable in being members of health systems agencies, health advisory and licensure boards. What type of input and representation should be sought from consumers? Identify pros and cons pertaining to the number of consumers represented on health and professional boards. Are there specific qualifications that are desirable to be met by consumers in seeking their representation on government and nongovernment agencies, associations, and professional groups?

What factors contributed to the development of the consumer movement? Is it being sufficiently recognized? Indicate examples in practice as to how "A Patient's Bill of Rights" has contributed to more effective patient care and satisfaction. What mechanism exists for implementing and enforcing "A Patient's Bill of Rights?" How is the "Code for Nursing" enforced in practice? How are the rights of health professionals protected?

Provide examples of disagreement between consumers and providers regarding health care needs and quality care. How can differences in perspectives effectively be dealt with as to the components of high quality care? To what extent should there be a balance between the consumer and provider in identification and evaluation of health care needs and care? What relationship exists between Fleming's list of nine expectations for health professionals and findings in Hardy's study (Chap. 24) regarding patients' evaluation of care?

What similarity exists between Fleming and Chinn (Chap. 29) as to the differences between the role of medicine and nursing? What implications are there for communication with patients if the goals of nursing and medical care may differ at times as suggested by Fleming? What alternatives in providing nursing services might be offered for the consumer? What relationship exists between Flemings' chapter and those by Williams (Chap. 25) and Brown (Chap. 26)?

If the profession of nursing does not have a shared understanding of nursing, as pleaded for by Roy (Chap. 34), how can nursing effectively communicate to society the role of the professional nurse today? Address the three critical questions raised by Fleming regarding understanding and communication. What nursing theorists specifically include involvement of the consumer in his or her own care as components of theory development? How can theoretical language used in the discipline of nursing be translated for meaningfulness to the consumer?

REFERENCES

Aydelotte, Myrtle E.
   1977 "Clinical nursing investigation and structure of knowledge." Pp. 46–52 in Michael Miller and Beverly Flynn (eds.), Current Perspectives in Nursing. St. Louis: Mosby.
Chapman, Jane E. and Harry H. Chapman
   1975 Behavior and Health Care and Humanistic Helping Process. St. Louis: Mosby.
Fleming, Gretchen V.
   1979 "Using consumer evaluations of health care." Hospital Progress 60 (August): 54–60, 68.
Hadley, Cantril
   1971 "The human design." Pp. 53–57 in Edwin P. Hallander and Raymond G. Hunt (eds.), Current Perspectives in Social Psychology. 3rd ed. New York: Oxford Press.
Houston, Charles I. and Wayne E. Pasanen
   1972 "Consumer views: Patients perceptions of hospital care." Hospitals 46(April 16): 70–74.

Jelinek, Richard C. and Lyman C. Dennis
  1976 A Review and Evaluation of Nursing Pro-
        ductivity. U. S. D. H. E. W. Public Health
        Service, Health Resources Adm. Bureau
        of Health Manpower, Division of Nursing.
Kennedy, John F.
  1962 Message from the President of the United
        States Relative to Consumers Protection
        and Interest Program. Document No. 364,
        House of Representatives, 87 Congress,
        2nd session, March 15.

Simon, Herbert A.
  1955 "A behavorial model of rationale choice."
        The Quarterly Journal of Economics 69
        (February): 99–118.
Watterson, Robert
  1971 "Public relations: Determining public
        attitudes." Hospitals 45 (October 16):
        57–59.

Chapter 36

Humanizing Patient Education

Donald A. Bille, R.N., Ph.D.
Associate Professor
Department of Nursing
DePaul University
Chicago, Illinois

Don A. Bille's chapter exemplifies a specific means to meet the challenge posed by Fleming for humanistic helping and advocacy. He explicates an approach to the humanization of patient care–teaching. Bille views humanizing the teaching-learning process as a successful way to increase outcomes for patients and to promote their self-care ability. A paternalistic attitude by either physicians or nurses toward patients is presented as an impediment to learning or applying what has been taught.

The issue of competition in patient education is addressed in relation to who, what, and when teaching may begin. Bille indicates that as long as the Nurse Practice Acts provide for "counsel," the nurse does not need a physician's order to teach. He specifies that when the variables of continuity of care, trust, rapport, and communication are lacking, effective teaching is hindered.

Bille advocates the contractual model of patient care–teaching, whereby the patient agrees to explicit performance levels and the nurse arranges a reward for the achieved levels. He identifies the type of patient care setting condition where the contractual model is appropriate. The goals are: ensure that the patient will experience a sense of success and control over the situation encompassing care–treatment; add to self-esteem and dignity; and promote motivation to learn and humanization of the teaching-learning process. Thus he urges the sharing of care-teaching decisions.

Bille portrays problems that may occur when control in humanized patient education is diverted from the professional to the patient. The occurrence of difficulties is primarily related to a difference between quality of life–health values held by the patient and health professional. Bille cites 10 suggestions based on research as a means for resolution of such disparities, encouragement of learning behaviors, and humanization of the patients' teaching-learning process. These are: identify and teach what the patient wants to learn first, begin to build from the present knowledge base of the patient, assess the physical readiness for learning, maximize the patient's active participation and practice in learning, provide feedback for reinforcement and correction of behavior, adjust the level of material presented for each individual patient, minimize distractions in the learning environment, develop an interpersonal relationship prior to teaching, and aim toward the level of motivation already evident in the patient. Bille concludes that humanizing patient teaching will not only enable the patient to learn more effectively, but also will encourage the development of a more positive view of the hospitalization experience and health care system.

When a person experiences disease or injury, whether or not hospitalization is involved, lifestyle adjustments may become necessary in order to adapt to limitations imposed on the body by that disease or injury. In spite of this, evidence exists that patients have not learned important self-care information. This evidence presents itself in the form of broken clinic appointments, unpaid physician and/or hospital bills, malpractice suits, lack of compliance with prescriptions and medical regimens, and spiraling costs of health care (Green, 1976; Levin, 1978).

Health care providers often feel that they have taught the patient and that the patient either did not learn or chose to ignore what was being taught. A closer examination of *how* patients are being taught may shed light on why patients are not learning or not applying what has been taught. This examination must include a view of physicians and nurses and their approach to the humanization of patient care-teaching Humanizing the patient's teaching-learning process may significantly increase the teaching-learning outcomes and promote the patient's self-care ability.

PHYSICIAN AS CAPTAIN OF THE SHIP

Health care systems have traditionally been arranged according to a hierarchical order, with the physician being the "leader" of the patient's care and treatment. In some cases, however, this leadership position has been transferred to other activities within the health care system. Phillips states that " . . . the physician has been identified as having the greater amount of knowledge and has therefore been placed (or placed himself) at the top of the pecking order" (1979:739). Thus, at the top of the pecking order, physicians may not be subject to the

same amount of control over their activities by others or by society as a whole, since these nonphysicians obviously know less about medicine than the physician does. Consequently, "the physician has been able to demand deference both from other health care providers and from the public" (Phillips, 1979:739).

The physician undoubtedly knows the best methodologies for treatment of disease or injury, at least as far as the "textbook case" is concerned. But what about the individual patient who does not resemble the classical textbook patient? If the physician makes all the necessary decisions about a patient's care and treatment, without actively considering the patient's own values and life-style, the physician is functioning under the paternalistic, "priestly model" of ethics, in which the physician is perceived as "playing God" and may try to convince the patient to undergo a procedure "for his own good" (Aroskar, 1980:18).

The tendency to "parentify" the physician can probably be seen in many health care settings. For instance, "the patient is expected to trust his physician, but the physician need not trust his patient; the patient is expected to submit intimate bodily and personal experiences to the physician, while the physician may withhold vital information from the patient" (Szasz, 1975:131). The patient must have appropriate self-care information in order to regain independence after disease or injury. This information must be presented in a style that is humanistic, not paternalistic.

Hofmann states that "humanistic health care is not paternalistic in its orientation. . . . Personnel who adopt paternalistic attitudes toward patients encourage and reinforce inappropriate dependent relationships that compromise a patient's ability to retain an active, responsible role in his own care" (1979:80). Paternalism also results in a sense of loss of dignity and self-worth. "The patient's loss of dignity often generates a reciprocal loss of respect for him by those around him, especially by his family and physicians. This unfortunate process of degradation is often concealed ... by the imagery and vocabulary of paternalism—family and physician treating the patient as if he were a child (or child-like), and the patient treating them as if they were his parents (or superiors)" (Szasz, 1975:131).

Although the physician may have a great responsibility to teach patients about their diseases or injuries, and the patient needs this information in order to practice self-care, a priestly attitude, a paternalistic view of the patient, and/or a withholding information from the patient will serve to both dehumanize the patient and detract from the benefits of self-care after leaving the physician's surveillance. Dehumanization and lack of dignity will eventually lead to lack of motivation to learn about self-care, resulting in further evidence that patients are not learning or are not applying what has been taught.

NURSE AS ADVOCATE FOR HUMANIZATION

In the traditional health care hierarchy, the nurse has been placed in a position subordinate (if not subservient) to the physician. Because of this, nurses have for too long believed that a physician's order is required before patient teaching can begin. As already noted, knowledge is power, and physicians have typically had greater knowledge (due to advanced educational degrees). As nursing education moves towards higher academic degrees, then, nurses are able to "compete" for power bases. Part of the current competition centers around *who* is in control of the patient's teaching plan, *what* each competitor may teach, and *when* that teaching may begin (i.e., with or without explicit physician's orders).

Nurses already have statutory authority to provide "care and counsel of the ill" as spelled out in the majority of the Nurse Practice Acts.

As long as this counsel (read "teaching") is within the scope of nursing practice, the nurse does not need a physician's order to teach. Therefore, if the nurse can perform the care measure, the nurse can teach about that care measure. Most statutes, however, prevent the nurse from diagnosing disease and prescribing medications. Thus, it may be inferred that the nurse cannot teach about patients' diagnoses or what medications they *should* be taking as a result of their diseases[1] without the physician's explicit permission.

Statutory authority to conduct patient teaching, however, is not enough to humanize the teaching-learning process for optimizing the teaching-learning outcomes. The system for delivering nursing care may actually preclude any effective teaching owing to lack of continuity, lack of trust and rapport, and/or lack of communication.

Lack of Continuity

Many variables exist within the modern health care setting which hinder continuity of care. Nurses who rotate to various shifts, part-time employees, lack of consistency in care assignments, and the recent impediment posed by agency nurses all contribute to less than optimally effective nursing care since the patient may not see the same care provider 2 days in a row. This certainly will do little to humanize the patient's care or to optimize teaching-learning outcomes, since trust and rapport take time to develop.

Lack of Trust and Rapport

The adult patient will learn most effectively from the teacher who develops a base of trust and shows warmth in human interactions. Once the patient comes to trust the nurse for the care provided, a new trust does not have to be

[1] The reader should note that teaching the patient about medications already being administered *is* a function of nursing, since these are already ordered by the physician. Teaching about medications that have *not* been ordered is part of the Medical Practice Act.

developed in order to teach. Trust will be transferred from situation to situation, wherever
the individuals who have set up the trust relationship function.

Lack of Communication

Since many different individuals and many different practitioners come in contact with the
patient on a daily basis, it is obvious that communication channels need to be initiated and
maintained to facilitate not only nursing care,
but also patient teaching. "No man is an island"
is an old saying (quotation from John Donne)
that has significance when it comes to patient
care-teaching. Each practitioner who comes in
contact with the patient must establish a means
of communicating with each of the other practitioners if optimal patient care-teaching is to
occur.

The nurse is closer to the patient's environment for a greater length of time each day than
any other professional. Because of this, the nurse
is in the best position to coordinate activities
centered around humanizing care and teaching.
The nurse must act as an advocate in the care-
teaching plan of the patient. This position, however, must be seen as one which does not control
the patient but rather controls the health care
delivery system. Control of the patient, regardless of whether it is done by the nurse or the
physician, leads to paternalism and its detrimental
effects on the patient's dignity.

Aroskar identifies a model of patient interaction which all nurses should consider using in
their own care-teaching. This is the *contractual
model* whereby "patients are viewed as having
control over the significant decisions affecting
their own lives and bodies. Both patients and
health professionals are considered as ends, not
simply as means to an end (the health of the
patient). The aspects of care related to values
are articulated and the health professional takes
no major action without consulting the patient"
(Aroskar, 1980:18).

The contractual model of patient care-teaching
is certainly not applicable to every patient care
setting. Thus, there may be instances within the
patient care setting in which the nurse must
make all decisions for the patient. The types of
nursing systems described and defined by Orem
(1980:96–97) give the best guidance to the locus
of decision making in patient care-teaching.
Contracting for care-teaching decisions would
be clearly inappropriate when patients are too
ill to make decisions regarding their own physical and/or psychological status, such as when
a patient is critically ill or in a life-threatening
situation ("wholly compensatory"). When the
patient is able to exercise at least partial control
in meeting health requirements and performing
selected activities of daily living ("partially compensatory"), however, decision making must be
shared between the nurse and the patient. When
the patient is in a situation in which the ability
exists to manage health care needs independently
("supportive-educative"), the locus of decision
making is centered within the patient. This patient
requires education for promotion of health,
guidance or support for prevention of disease,
and/or provision of an environment for growth.
All decisions about health care needs at this
point must come from the patient.

The contractual model for patient care-teaching all but guarantees that the patient will experience a sense of success and control over the
situation surrounding care and treatment. This
sense of success and control will add to self-
esteem and dignity, promote motivation to learn,
and further humanize the teaching-learning process (Steckel and Swain, 1977:81).

Any contract contains expectations which
become obligations for both parties entering
into the contract. In the case of contracting
for patient education, the patient agrees to certain performance levels while the nurse arranges
a reward for that performance. Many patients
request (as a reward) extra time with the health
care provider, as well as "assistance in untangling
the bureaucratic red tape necessary in order for
them to obtain benefits, referrals, and consulta-

tions" (Steckel and Swain, 1977:84). The nurse's part of the contracting process, which provides a reward for the patient's learning then may entail helping the patient to "survive" in the modern health care system—the advocacy role. These same advocacy activities further humanize the teaching-learning process.

PATIENT AS CONSUMER OF HEALTH CARE

Adult patients face many dilemmas when they enter the health care system. Until that moment, they have been responsible for making their own decisions and providing for most of their own needs. Healthy adults have a need to make their own decisions and have learned to accept the responsibility for the consequences of a wrong decision. Adults perceive themselves as being able to run their own lives. Adults also "tend to avoid, resist and resent being placed in situations in which they feel they are treated like children —told what to do and what not to do, talked down to, embarrassed, punished, judged" (Knowles, 1967:267).

When the adult is hospitalized, at least some degree of dependence on others becomes necessary. This dependence may range from the need to have medications brought to the bedside to the total dependence of being critically ill (requiring someone else to meet all needs). Since dependence on others may not be a normal part of the adult's self-concept, the adult may also resist learning under conditions that are incongruent with the self-concept of an autonomous individual. Henderson has defined nursing as assisting individuals (sick or well) to perform health activities they would do unaided if they only possessed the strength, will, or knowledge to do so (1964:62). Care-teaching decisions, then, should be shared with the patient to promote a sense of autonomy and motivate patient learning.

In many cases, however, the advocacy role does not exist, and patients are not allowed to participate in the decision-making process. As a result, the patient's self-esteem is lowered, and the patient feels dehumanized. Under these conditions, "patients may in fact prefer depersonalized service, as provided by drugstore sphygmomanometers, dial-a-tapes, and self-administered inhalators. These services offer anonymity and may be considered humanistic, because they enhance patient autonomy, permit individuals to share in the responsibility for their care, and satisfy the special needs of particular patients" (Howard and Derzon, 1979:76).

As one means to aim toward humanization of patient teaching, the American Hospital Association (1974) has drafted "A Patient's Bill of Rights." This document provides a guideline for more effective patient care and spells out many aspects, which include patient teaching (such as informed consent, information about procedures, and information necessary for self-care after discharge from the hospital). Other organizations, such as the enterostomal therapists, mental health associations, etc., have published bills of rights for various groups, including the mentally ill, the ostomy patient, the handicapped, the dying, Jewish patients, children, and pregnant women. These bills of rights are often used against the health care system as patients go to court. "The public is angry with health care providers for what they perceive as indifference to patients as human beings and individuals. Rightly or wrongly, they seek justice through the courts and through legislation" (Hogan, 1978:113).

Complaints of dehumanization are heard as patients demand their rights. These complaints center around health care providers who function with "the perception of people as objects ("things"); the instrumental use and exploitation of people; coldness and indifference in social interaction; the repression and limitation of human freedom (loss of options); and social ostracism and alienation" (Howard and Derzon, 1979:76).

The dehumanized patient does not learn. The teaching-learning process, when conducted in a dehumanizing manner, hinders (if it does not prevent) the patient from learning. What, then, can the nurse or other health care provider do to assure patients' rights and increase the effectiveness of patient teaching?

HUMANIZING PATIENT EDUCATION

Humanized care and teaching constitute an activity which "enhances the dignity and autonomy of patients and health professionals alike" (Howard and Derzon, 1979:76). Although humanization is an end in itself, it also contributes to several other goals within health care, including effective care and optimal teaching-learning outcomes. Humanized care and teaching derive their goals from the *patient's* perceived needs and preferences, regardless of whether or not they conform to the health professional's perceptions of the patient's needs. "It is the learner who determines the desired outcomes in accordance with his decisions as to which risks he chooses to avoid (or not avoid); similarly, content is learner-determined, learner preferences for educational methods are honored, and evaluation is in terms of criteria proposed by the learner" (Levin, 1978:171).

Humanized patient education shifts control from the professional to the patient. Problems may occur when the patient's values differ from those of the health professional, but it must be realized that the patient will make decisions about whether or not prescriptions and teaching material are going to be followed after discharge anyway. These decisions will often reflect a quality of life value in preference to the quality of health values. The patient makes these decisions (right or wrong) because of a value system built up during the years it took to become an adult. By examining the literature on adult education, then, a means for humanizing the patient's teaching-learning process can be developed.

Miller suggests several conditions which encourage learning behaviors in the adult (1964:37 ff.) Since these suggestions were based on research conducted with healthy subjects, adapta-

tion to the health care setting as follows is required because the adult is now a patient.

1 Teach What the Patient Wants to Learn Adults already know a great deal about themselves and their life-styles before their illness. Thus, adults know at least some of the things they must learn in order to take care of themselves. Health care professionals may want a patient to know certain things, such as their own objectives for the patient's learning, and may see these objectives as essential for the patient's adjustment and self-care after hospitalization. If the teaching program starts with these "externally generated" objectives, however, the patient will surely become frustrated and feel dehumanized. The essential starting place in patient education is, therefore, the identification of what the patient wants to learn first—the internally generated objectives. This is not to say that externally generated objectives have no place in patient teaching, but rather that the *starting* point must be the patient's.

The patient whose *own* learning needs are identified and satisfied first will not only learn the material being taught but will also come to trust and respect the health care provider.

2 Build on a Knowledge Base Learning is an activity during which remodeling and remolding of certain intellectual structures occurs and new knowledge and skills are blended into what the learner knows already. The patient's life experiences must be elicited and utilized in the current teaching plan. Once learning needs are identified, the teacher must decide and negotiate with the patient what preliminary knowledge (or base) is necessary in order to reach the identified teaching-learning objectives. The teacher must begin with the patients' present knowledge and then slowly build on that knowledge base until objectives are met.

3 Physical Readiness Is a Prerequisite for Learning The patient who is tired, has been medicated with central nervous system depressants, or has a high fever or an electrolyte imbalance is less than ready to learn. Teaching, if done at all during this time, must be clear, concise, and to the point and for shorter periods of time. The patient's activity schedule must be coordinated to allow for adequate rest periods, as well as adequate periods of time to learn and study.

Unfortunately, there are some situations in which the patient seems too sick to learn. The patient who is comatose, for instance, is not ready to learn about self-care after hospitalization. The care giver should still "teach" this patient what is being done at the moment the activity is being carried out. This not only demonstrates concern for the patient but may help to lower the patient's anxiety or stress levels while it humanizes the care-teaching activities.

4 Participation and Practice Enhance Learning The patient's active participation in the teaching-learning process can be maximized through such methods as verbal interchange, psychomotor activities, and involvement of as many of the body's senses as possible. Thus, while the nurse is providing care measures, the care measure itself is being demonstrated, discussed, and observed. The patient is involved through sight, sound, and touch.

The teaching-learning process must also include practice of self-care behaviors to be performed by the patient after hospitalization. The nurse cannot simply teach principles to the patient and expect the patient to bridge the gap to application but must show the patient what is to be done and then give him or her a chance to do that same task. The patient must also be allowed to make mistakes and learn what was done wrong and why. This trial-and-error behavior increases the ability to learn and increases retention of material already learned.

5 Feedback Guides Learning of Correct Behavior The patient must be given verbal reports on progress toward learning goals. When something has been learned correctly, the patient should be reinforced (rewarded) with verbal praise. This reinforcement of behavior increases the chances for repetition of the behavior at a later point.

Incorrect behavior (mistakes) also needs to be pointed out to the patient and the correct behavior demonstrated again. Negative feedback should be provided in a manner that is not perceived as punishment or reprimand. Humanizing the teaching-learning process requires trust and rapport, which can be easily enhanced through warmth in interpersonal relationships, constructive criticism when deserved, and, most importantly, praise when positive accomplishments are achieved.

6 Material Must Be Adjusted to the Patient's Level Considerable differences in learning ability exist in all people, and the hospitalized adult is certainly no exception. The outcomes of the teaching-learning process are affected by the wide range of these differences. Thus, the level of material presented, as well as the rate of presentation and the length of each teaching-learning interaction, must be adjusted for each individual patient.

The amount of prior education is not a direct indicator of ability to learn about self-care. Thus, the patient educator must listen and observe closely during the teaching-learning interactions. The patient will give clues about the level of understanding verbally or behaviorally. For instance, someone who does not ask questions after a teaching session either may understand everything that was taught or may be so lost as not to know enough information to ask questions. The patient who is restless or begins to look away from the teacher may be trying to politely relay the message that the teaching-learning activities should cease for this session.

7 Distractions Interfere with the Teaching-Learning Process Most clinical units are filled with noisy equipment which interferes not only with communication itself but also with the teaching-learning process. The teaching program which begins amidst the sighing of a respirator or beeping of cardiac monitors may be less effective than the one which occurs in a more relaxed, quiet environment. Physical features of the environment, such as lighting and noise, and other activities unrelated to the teaching-learning interaction must be controlled by the teacher to the extent possible in the setting. If the patient's room is not conducive to the teaching-learning interaction, the patient should be moved to an area more conducive to concentration.

8 A Warm Interpersonal Relationship Enhances Teaching-Learning Outcomes The benefits of trust and rapport in the nurse-patient relationship have already been discussed. The patient will learn best from a person who is trusted. This trust helps to strengthen the credibility of all communications, including the teaching material. Because of this, the best teacher of a patient is the person who also delivers the care. An individual who is unknown to the patient (such as an in-service instructor, patient education coordinator, etc.) will have to take the time to develop trust and rapport before any significant learning will take place.

Even though audiovisual materials have been found to be effective in promoting the teaching-learning process, the extensive use of media may hinder a patient's learning, especially if the patient is working through the emotions of adapting to disease or injury. The warmth of human interaction cannot take place through a television set.

9 Build Self-Esteem to Increase Motivation to Learn Many patient educators have been heard to say, "That patient just isn't motivated to learn!" when in reality they should have said, "That patient isn't motivated to learn what I am motivated to teach." Once again, the learner knows best what learning is needed. Thus, patient teaching must aim toward the level of motiva-

tion already present in the patient. This level of motivation can be increased by striving to improve the patient's self-esteem (Gellerman, 1968). Two very important aspects of increasing the patient's self-esteem are open, two-way communication and granting the patient the power to make decisions about his or her own life.

Two-way communication is enhanced by the feeling that the patient and teacher are equals. Thus, an authoritarian relationship will hinder the patient's desire (if not ability) to learn from someone. Communication makes the patient feel valued, thus adding to feelings of self-worth and self-esteem—it humanizes the teaching-learning process.

The patient has been making decisions about his or her own life for some time now. This activity needs to continue if feelings of usefulness and cooperation are to be maintained. Patients should be included in planning their own patient education programs, that is, allowed to make decisions about what they are to learn. Rosenberg states that the only route to successful patient education programming is one which involves the patient in the decision-making process by planning with and for the patient those educational experiences needed to achieve optimal self-care (1976:94–95). Although the physician, as "captain of the ship," is in control of the patient's treatment plan while the patient is still hospitalized, once discharge from the hospital occurs, "it is the patient's decision to take the medication properly, to adhere to a diet, to maintain a proper exercise regimen. To put it another way, the physician makes the decision regarding therapy. The patient makes decisions regarding adherence, and in order for him to correctly make his decisions, he needs to know not only what and how, but why, what if, what if not, etc." (Rosenberg, 1976:94–95).

SUMMARY

Patients who experience life-altering disease or injury need to learn how to exercise self-care measures. When the patient does not learn or does not apply what has been taught, the fault may lie with how the teaching-learning process was conducted. Humanizing the teaching-learning process requires each health care practitioner to examine his or her own professional activities. Patients who are treated with respect, approached from their own values rather than the health professional's, and allowed to participate in the decision-making process about their care and counsel, will not only learn better but will also come away from the experience of hospitalization with a more positive view of the health care system. Humanizing patient teaching, then, is not only an end in itself but also a means to eliminate other problems within the health care system.

EDITOR'S QUESTIONS FOR DISCUSSION

Bille says that the leadership position of the physician in patient care and treatment has been transferred to other activities within the health care system. What examples illustrate whether or not transference has occurred? What are the implications for the dominant role of the physician in health care and the profession of nursing related to leadership transference by physicians to other activities? Are there situations or circumstances in which the physician should or should not be considered "captain of the ship?"

In addressing paternalistic attitudes of some physicians toward patients, Bille implies some nurses have similar attitudes. What examples can you provide that attitudes exist which reflect control of the patient? Are there any differences between physicians and nurses as to how paternalistic attitudes may be manifested? Are there limitations as to the amount of control a patient should have regarding decisions concerning his or her care? What examples can you provide to illustrate humanization of patient education and care?

Can the competition for power bases between physicians and nurses result in disadvantageous effects for patients? How can accurate, adequate information be provided for patients to ensure their confidence in the health care team? What suggestions can be offered to enhance collaboration and cooperation between health professionals and minimize competition for power bases? To what extent do you agree with Bille that "if the nurse can perform the care measure, the nurse can teach about that care measure?"

As an advocate in the care–teaching plan of the patient, how can the nurse control the health care delivery system without controlling the patient? To what extent can or should the nurse control the health care delivery team? How can optimal communication with other health practitioners be ensured for effective patient care-teaching to occur? Does the term "advocate" used by nurses in relation to patients reflect the nursing profession's effort to delineate the role of nursing? Should the advocate role be considered an unique domain of nursing and/or a shared role with other health professionals?

What are the advantages and disadvantages of the contractual model of patient care-teaching? Under what conditions and settings is it most applicable? What assumptions are inherent in using the contractual model? What other advocacy activities might be suggested, in addition to Bille's suggestions, as rewards for patients' learning? What ethical implications are there in utilizing the contractual model?

How can health professionals effectively assess the readiness of a patient to participate in health care decisions and a teaching-learning process for health behaviors? What methods are most effective for health professionals, on first contact with patients, to evaluate differences between the patients' perceived needs and preferences in health care-teaching and the professional's perceptions of patients' needs? What strategies may be utilized to reconcile value differences between a quality of *life* value in preference to quality of *health* values? When differences occur in values between a patient and a health professional, what are the ethical implications regarding care-teaching?

REFERENCES

American Hospital Association
1974 A Patient's Bill of Rights. Chicago: The American Hospital Association.

Aroskar, Mila Ann
1980 "Ethics of nurse-patient relationships." Nurse Educator March–April, 18–20.

Gellerman, S. W.
1968 Management by motivation. American Management Association, Inc.

Green, Lawrence W.
1976 "The potential of health education includes cost effectiveness." Hospitals 50: 57–61.

Henderson, Virginia
1964 "The nature of nursing." American Journal of Nursing 64:62.

Hofmann, Paul B.
1979 "Can hospitals afford to care less?" Hospitals 53:80–82.

Hogan, Norma Shaw
1978 "Patient's rights: Voluntary or mandatory." Hospitals 52:111–116.

Howard, Jan and Robert A. Derzon
1979 "Prospects for humane care are hopeful." Hospitals 53:76–79.

Knowles, Malcolm
1967 "Program planning for adults as learners." Adult Leadership 16:267.

Levin, Lowell S.
1978 "Patient education and self-care: How do they differ?" Nursing Outlook 26:170–175.

Miller, H. L.
1964 Teaching and Learning in Adult Education. New York: Macmillan.

Orem, Dorothea E.
1980 Nursing: Concepts of Practice (2d ed.) New York: McGraw-Hill.

Phillips, John R.
1979 "Health care provider relationships a matter of reciprocity." Nursing Outlook 27:738–741.

Rosenberg, S. G.
1976 "Patient education: An educator's view," in A. R. Somers (ed.), Promoting Health: Consumer Education and National Policy. Germantown, Maryland: Aspen.

Steckel, Susan and Mary Ann Swain
1977 "Contracting with patients to improve compliance." Hospitals 51:81–84.

Szasz, Thomas S.
1975 "Illness and Indignity." Nursing Digest 1975 Review of Medicine & Surgery. Wakefield, Mass.: Contemporary Publishing, Inc.

Chapter 37

The Nurse as Helper:
Today and Tomorrow

Elaine L. La Monica, R.N., Ed.D., F.A.A.N.
Associate Professor of Nursing Education and
Director, Institute of Research and Service in Nursing Education
Teachers College, Columbia University
New York, New York

It follows that humanistic helping and advocacy cannot be operative if consumers remain in a state of confusion as to the role of nursing. Progressing from the thrust evident in the chapters by Fleming and Bille, Elaine L. La Monica concretely defines the role of nursing as a "helper" to clients in maintaining and optimizing their healthy state. She identifies an identity crisis among nurses related to unclear expectations about themselves, confusion of professional colleagues and patients, uncertainty of positions for services, and preparation of nurses at numerous educational levels. In viewing tomorrow's nurse, La Monica predicts nurses will practice collaboratively with all health care providers, will control and coordinate all health services, and be the primary health care provider. She indicates that the nurse will be interdependent with the physician when cure or rehabilitation is the priority.

La Monica discusses each of the rationales for her projections: need, quality, and cost-effectiveness. Points are made pertaining to health maintenance and prevention of the major diseases to justify the need for a helper role. The focus of her chapter is the rationale for quality care. La Monica addresses the issue by posing answers to two questions: What does nursing do best and what group of health care professionals is best able to meet primary health care needs of consumers? In responding to the first question, La Monica draws particularly from the nursing theoretical perspectives of Roy, Rogers, and Orem. She further indicates that all nurse theorists share a unified approach that can be summarized under the umbrella called "helping" and identifies this as nursing's "domain." She also views the "nursing process" as a recognized and accepted scientific method for delivering services.

La Monica emphasizes the need for investigating the theories of helping. She advocates "helping behavior" as the most important facilitative process for nurses to use

This chapter results from a paper delivered to Teachers College, Columbia University Alumni and friends on 12 April 1980 at the annual "Saturday Symposia." The presentation and chapter are supported by Grant No. NU 00640 from the Division of Nursing, Department of Health and Human Services, DHHS.

and students to learn, perceiving it to be the gestalt of nursing practice. In her description of the helping process, La Monica clearly portrays empathy as a process, rather than an internal state, and an essential ingredient to helper effectiveness. The point is further made that a helper must be at a higher level of functioning than the helpee. The helping process can either help or harm growth, depending on the level of facilitative skills of the helper.

In answering the second question, La Monica identifies the knowledge and skills necessary to meet clients' primary health care needs. She outlines the knowledge components to be: person, health and illness, human behavior in health and illness, and learning theory. Specific skills which build upon knowledge are indicated: client assessment, pedagogy, and helping behavior. La Monica strongly argues that nursing has the requisites to lead the primary health care team, although she admits areas need further development.

Remarks regarding the third rationale—cost—are directed to the expense of health insurance, physicians' fees, depersonalization, and lack of continuity in providing care. La Monica firmly believes nursing can offer a system of primary health care delivery that is cost-effective. The aim would be to decrease the need for patient admissions into hospitals.

La Monica concludes her chapter with a plea for research on helping conditions, including systematic methods of assessing and teaching helping skills. She discusses the foci of her research, the measurement of empathy, and the development of the La Monica Empathy Construct Rating Scale. Currently one of her objectives is to study the relationship of empathy and outcomes of nursing care. La Monica encourages nurses to study the relationship among empathy, educational levels in nursing, and areas of nursing practice. She indicates the need to test various helping models for nursing practice. Finally she foresees that research concerning the process of helping will add to the body of knowledge requisite in basic nursing education.

No other time is more important than today to emphasize the helping aspects of nursing practice. It is well known that health care delivery in the United States and abroad is changing rapidly in both content and process. Not only must nursing practice keep up with such advances, but nurses must become leaders in what nurses do best. Yesterday nurses were recognized clearly and widely as the technical assistants of physicians. Today, with their expanded roles, nurses suffer an identity crisis: (1) nurses themselves are unclear about role expectations; (2) health care colleagues remain confused about the various roles of nursing and what nurses specifically do; (3) health care systems do not have places for our expanded services; (4) nursing educative systems prepare nurses for a variety of roles across four generic educational levels; and (5) consumers remain in the greatest state of confusion and ignorance concerning what they can expect from us, mainly because mass media still portray the nurse as the physician's handmaiden. Given nursing's rapid growth during the past two decades, today's confusion is to be expected, but can be used powerfully to build nursing practice tomorrow. The question that nurses must answer is how to employ today's confusion in a rapid growth cycle for the profession.

Confusion, which is a normal, predictable outcome of change, usually results in a temporary dissipation of personal power in leaders. According to Etzioni (1961), the best situation for leaders is when they have both *personal power* and *position power*. Position power is delegated and personal power is derived from intrinsic sources. Etzioni (1961) asserts further that if leaders cannot have both position and personal power, personal power alone is more important than is position power alone. It is still a well-known fact that the health care system in the United States is controlled by the American Medical Association and its constituents. This situation has been due to the focus on curing disease that has controlled health practices. Contemporary health care, however, emphasizes prevention first and cure second. Such a shift threatens the control of the American Medical Association and places it in a defensive fight for survival.

The profession of nursing poses the greatest threat to the American Medical Association in terms of taking over that top position of control; forces that are driving us include consumers, who are now voicing constant dissatisfaction with health care, and the United States government, which is sympathetic with consumer viewpoints. The American Medical Association may still have position power but its personal power is threatened. Nursing can grasp this personal power to paint tomorrow's portrait of health care in the United States and carve its unique place in that picture. Nursing can capitalize on this confusion by taking leadership from a personally powerful vantage point; it will be the more potent in the absence of both position power and personal power. In order to do this, nursing must move out of a confused state to one of clarity concerning its role and services.

Nursing's confusion has resulted from a process of positive growth due to expansion of technology and advanced opportunities, resulting from higher education. The present stage of nursing's development in providing health care as a profession should include examining nursing practice in terms of quality (what nurses do best) and cost effectiveness (what is best for clientele). Energies must then focus on developing those few roles (which may be only one), preparing students to assume them, and concomitantly educating our professional and lay publics.

Recognizing the current trends, this author believes that tomorrow's professional nurse will be primarily an independent primary health care practitioner—a *helper* to clients as clients seek to maintain and optimize their individual healthy states. These nurses will practice collaboratively with all health care providers, calling in consultants such as the physician, for example, when cure of disease is necessary or the social worker, as another example, when that expertise is warranted. Such a nurse will control and coordinate all health services for the client and be *the* primary health care provider. She or he will be in private practice or will be a leader in a multidisciplinary health care team such as that seen at the present time in health maintenance organizations and clinics. Professional nurses will admit and follow clients in hospitals, planning the comprehensive, individualized nursing care that follows the nursing process together with technical nurses, who will be employed by the hospital, and other health care personnel. When health maintenance is the principal focus for a client, the professional nurse will function independently. When cure or rehabilitation is the priority, the professional nurse will be interdependent with the physician and others. When life sustenance is predominant, the nurse may be independent or interdependent with physicians or psychologists, for example, as needs warrant such additional expertise. Rationale for these projections center on three points: need, quality, and cost effectiveness.

NEED

It is well known that health care in the United States is advancing rapidly toward foci of health maintenance and prevention of disease. The Kaiser Foundation model of the 1950s, John Kennedy's physical fitness programs of the 1960s, and the health maintenance programs of the 1970s are a few examples of this revolution. Further, in the early part of this century, the morbidity and mortality rates of Americans had a high positive relationship with infectious diseases; now those rates have a high positive relationship to chronic disorders caused by our lifestyles (Stachnik, 1980:8). Medicine found cures for infectious disease mainly through antibiotics; now cures for disorders of life-styles are required. This cannot be accomplished through pills, nuclear medicine, or any other technique, for cure involves altering behaviors—unique response patterns of individuals.

Our major killers are heart disease, cerebrovascular disease, respiratory disease, and various cancers. There is abundant evidence that how people live—for example, what and how much they eat and drink, how they exercise, how they handle everyday stress, and whether or not they have a smoking habit—play a part in whether or not Americans develop the killer diseases.

The scope of these problems is vast. Susser (1975:5-8) reports, for example, that of approximately 2 million American deaths in 1969, 40 percent were due to heart disease, 10 percent were due to strokes, and 16 percent were due to various cancers. More appalling is the fact that 178,000 people between the ages of 45 and 64 died of heart disease and 1.2 million people in that same age group were chronically disabled because of heart disease. Obesity is a major predisposing factor to degenerative arthritis of the hips, knees, and ankles, injuries, gastrointestinal cancer, diabetes, strokes, and heart attacks. Yet Stachnik (1980:9) currently reports 16 percent of Americans under the age of 30 are obese and 40 percent of the total population (80 million people) are approximately 20 or more pounds overweight. Stachnik (1980:9) further discusses essential hypertension: (1) it affects 25 to 35 million Americans and half of those are not aware of the problem; (2) of those aware, only about 4 million receive adequate treatment. Hypertension kills 60,000 people a year and is the significant causative factor in about 1.5 million heart attacks and strokes per year in living people. There is valid evidence that a diet high in protein produces high cholesterol levels and saturated fat levels in blood; this hastens the appearance of cardiovascular disease. Upon examining American soldiers killed in the Korean War, 35 percent of them were found to have more than 15 percent

narrowing of their coronary arteries due to abnormal collections of plaque—"their average age was 21" (Stachnik, 1980:9)! Even while sparing the reader further statistics on cigarette smoking, in particular, and a host of other behavioral risk problems, it is safe to conclude that the need for health education of Americans is ubiquitous.

QUALITY

In discussing quality, two questions must be answered: What does nursing do best? Which group of health care professionals is best able to handle the primary health care needs of Americans?

First, what does nursing do best? Riehl and Roy (1980) assert that the ultimate concern of nursing is the total person, with nursing supporting and promoting adaptation of the individual within the context of the person's own health-illness pattern, environmental process, and stimuli available for use. Rogers (1970) maintains that nursing implies a deep respect for the individuality of each person. This reflects study of the relationship between persons and their environments with the goal of facilitating effective nursing care outcomes. In Rogers's (1970) model, disease is low-keyed, with the unified person and human functioning taking priority. The well-being of society, as the suprasystem of persons, must also be a focal point. Orem (1971) focuses on nursing's responsibility as that of moving a person to a state where she or he can maintain care of her/his own health needs. Many other nurse-theorists state nursing's domain similarly. All share a unified, comprehensive, helping approach to the study of humans that includes all that is known about humans in a dynamic, interactive system. Moreover, nursing has a recognized and accepted scientific method for delivering services—the nursing process. Nurses have had more than two decades of concentrated experience in developing these aforementioned goals—their best efforts—they can be summed and called nursing's "domain." All fit under the umbrella called "helping." Nurses know it, can teach it, and have experienced it.

Moving to the second question, what group of health care professionals is best able to handle the primary health care needs of Americans? In order to answer this question, the requisite general skills and knowledge necessary to meet the primary health care needs must be identified. These can be outlined as follows:

Content:

1 Knowledge of humans—biologic, psychologic, and sociologic
2 Knowledge of health and illness
3 Knowledge of human behavior in health and illness
4 Knowledge of learning theory

Process (which builds on knowledge):

1 Client assessment—physiologic and psychologic
2 Pedagogy—the art of instruction
3 Helping behavior operationalized

There is extensive recent medical literature that expounds on the humanistic and holistic expansion of medical practice. Pellegrino (1979) speaks of humanism in medical practice; his thrust is an integration of the humanities into medical practice—physicians should be more humane. Cousins (1979:11-23) speaks of holistic health with medicine recognizing the mind-body relationship. There is now a medical specialty called family medicine. These strides forward should not be negated because medical treatment for too long tended to forget that there was a human being beneath the skin of disease. But, in reality, physicians treat disease; their research is primarily aimed at cure and their long formal education is consumed by study of physiologic humans. The need to treat disease is immortal.

In a recent issue of the *American Psychologist* (Stachnik, 1980), a publication of the American Psychological Association, psychologists state their role in health care delivery. They assert that changing human behavior is their domain. However knowledgeable psychologists may be in human behavior and learning and given that the theory in these areas is rightfully credited to them, knowledge of health and illness and client assessment in both psychologic *and* physiologic domains are not currently part of psychology. Psychologists will most certainly be members of the health care team but they lack the requisites to *lead* the primary health care team.

Nursing has the aforementioned content and process requisites with the benefit of experience in practicing with these requisites. Areas in these requisites, however, need further development and will be discussed after the third area of rationale for nurses to become leaders in primary health care.

COST

The cost of health care continues to skyrocket (Feldstein, 1979:341-391; Raffel, 1980:1-4). Yet, health care is missing in many American lives. Health insurance is often too expensive to purchase and Medicare and Medicaid systems are abused by financially suffering institutions. The United States does not have "socialized medicine" yet we have the symptoms on which a medically socialized state can be predicted. Public hospitals are coming under pressure from government to cut costs; private hospitals suffer great economic burdens. Yet, the hospitals, public or private, profit or nonprofit, are all influenced greatly by the physician. Physicians set the stakes and their fees elevate continuously. They exercise great control over hospital services while maintaining private practices and lobbying, with less effectiveness in recent years, against third-party reimbursement for other health care professionals. What results is that fewer Americans can afford private physicians and a greater number are forced to use clinics. Here, depersonalization peaks, time elapses in blocks, and people no longer can choose to be cared for by a particular person. Is this not socialized medicine?

It is essential to point out that the inability of clients to identify with their care givers may have serious consequences. Hornstein (1976) eloquently asserts that the difference between a person acting toward another as cruel or kind (antisocial or prosocial) involves feelings that others are either like ("we group") or unlike ("they group") that person's self. We-group behavior is generally helpful and they-group behavior is often unhelpful. Numerous research studies done by Hornstein (1976) and his colleagues point out that cooperative social agencies must be grounded on personnel who feel a part of the we group; this involves identifying with another or others. Given these research findings, is it possible or probable, then, that the interaction between health care providers and clients can be optimal when both persons are always meeting for the first time or when continuity of care from one person is not feasible during the majority of visits?

Medicine is under challenge to change; nurses should not stand by waiting for this to happen or not happen. Nursing can offer a system of primary health care delivery that is lower in cost and is effective with the aim of keeping people out of hospitals. There would also be less need for techniques and equipment. It is mandatory that nursing increase the pool of research findings that suggest to the public that nursing's promises of quality health care *and* cost effectiveness have been and will continue to be maintained.

What does professional nursing need in order to achieve the goal of primary health care providers—helpers of people who wish to maintain an optimal healthy state? If one refers back to examine the aforementioned requisites for meeting this goal, it can be noted that knowledge components are at the profession's fingertips—nurses have them and teach them: (1) knowledge of humans—biologic, psychologic, and sociologic; (2) knowledge of health and illness; (3) knowledge of human behavior in health and illness; and (4) knowledge of learning theory. Processes

become focal in further development. It should be underscored that processes imply "doing," not just "knowing about." Experience in doing is mandatory. Complete client assessment such as that found commonly in nurse-practitioner courses needs to become integral in basic nursing education.

Pedagogy, the art of instruction built on the theories of learning, is also essential. The role of the nurse is currently seen as that of a teacher to clients, but emphasis in applying theory in practice is often superficial. Do nurses, for example, diagnose, according to a theoretical model, a client's level of maturity in learning to monitor his or her own diabetes and then build a strategy that has a theoretical base for teaching that person? This author's answer is: Not to the degree that is necessary. Are nurses with basic education cognizant and experienced in the group method of instruction—are they recognized leaders? This author is doubtful.

Perhaps the most important process is *helping behavior* because it is the gestalt and unfortunately is overlooked with frightening frequency. Helping behavior involves teaching and guiding people's journey to help themselves. It is not "doing for," it is "facilitating another." It is not "asking," it is "exploring with." It is not "telling," it is developing alternatives together and letting the client decide knowledgeably. At the present time, helping behavior is acknowledged in basic nursing education but mere acknowledgment is insufficient. From theoretic emphasis, educational systems must move to operational emphasis. Not only must the theories of helping be taught, but educators and other nursing leaders must facilitate a student's experience in *being* an effective helper and must ensure that no one graduates or is permitted to practice unless one has the competencies necessary to fill that role.

The theories of helping on which instruction can be based exist. Numerous studies in psychology have documented that counseling works (Gladstein, 1977). Adams, in a July 1979 issue of *The New York Times*, concluded that no matter what form of counseling is used—behavioral, humanistic, client-centered, or eclectic—counseling works. Nursing educators must investigate what theories of helping are valid for nursing care—what theories, when applied by nurses, result in satisfactory outcomes of client care. Then these results must be consumed by educators of basic nursing programs and transmitted to students.

A helping theory applied to nursing practice that has been the focus of this author's research interest for the past 7 years, as well as that of many colleagues, is Carl Rogers's and Robert Carkhuff's helping model (Carkhuff, 1969b; Rogers, 1961). The basic assumption of their comprehensive helping model is that "all effective interpersonal processes share a common core of conditions conducive to facilitative human experiences" (Carkhuff, 1969b:7). Core conditions receiving impressive backing from research are: empathy, respect, warmth, genuineness, self-disclosure, concreteness, confrontation, and immediacy of relationship or a focus on the here and now (Berenson and Mitchell, 1968; Carkhuff, 1968, 1969a; Collingwood, 1971; Collingwood and Renz, 1969; Mitchell et al., 1970; Muehlberg et al., 1969; Truax, 1970a, 1970b; Truax and Carkhuff, 1967; Truax and Wittmer, 1971; Truax et al., 1971). Empathy has been found to be the key ingredient. Research in psychology suggests that increasing one's level of empathy does increase one's effectiveness in a helping relationship. Most of our past and current research focuses on empathy in nurses and nursing students.

The most recent definition of empathy describes empathy as a process rather than an internal state, operating throughout a helping relationship. Empathy signifies a central focus and feeling *with* and *in* the client's world. The empathic process involves accurate perceptions of the client's world by the helper, communication of this understanding to the client, and the client's perception of the helper's understanding (La Monica, 1980).

Even though the goal of nursing is to provide growth-facilitating support and assistance, there is quantitative and qualitative evidence that the transactions between helpers and clients often do not prove beneficial. Research on helping conditions suggests, in fact, that the helping process can be destructive rather than enhancing to growth, depending on the level of facilitative skills of the helper (Anthony, 1971; Berenson, Mitchell, and Laney, 1968; Berenson, Mitchell, and Morauec, 1968; Carkhuff and Burstein, 1970; Friel et al., 1971). Carkhuff (1969a) underscores that the "helpee's" level of functioning has a strong positive relationship to the helper's effectiveness. Further, if a helper does not possess empathy, the results to the helpee may be detrimental, actually causing more harm than good. There is no neutrality in interactions; they either help or harm. Carkhuff (1969a) further posits that a helper must be at a higher level of functioning than the helpee, otherwise helpee growth will not take place.

Such writings apply to other helper/helpee situations as well: practicing nurses are helpers to clients; nurse leaders are helpers to practitioners; and educators are helpers to students. Effective helping processes of helpers are modeled in each dyad; ineffective helping processes of helpers, unfortunately, follow the same pattern but in the opposite direction. It is therefore critically important that nursing educators and administrators be concerned with their own helping skills as well as with the helping skills of their students and employees. Systematic methods of assessing and teaching helping skills must be developed.

The results of research and other writings in the field led this author to raise three research questions:

1 Does nurse empathy make a difference in nursing care outcome?
2 What are the empathy levels of practicing professional nurses, educators, and students?
3 Can formal educational offerings improve nurses' levels of empathy?

These questions have been the foci of this author's

research and could only be studied if a reliable and valid instrument to measure empathy was available. Empathy measurement research has been the subject of major criticism over the past years because of disagreement on definitions of the concept and the reliability and validity of the instruments used to measure empathy (Conklin and Hunt, 1975).

The Department of Health and Human Services' Division of Nursing funded this author's 2-year investigation (November, 1977, through February, 1980) to study the construct validity of empathy instruments (La Monica, 1980). This investigation resulted in a clearer definition of empathy than had been articulated previously and in an instrument called the *La Monica Empathy Construct Rating Scale* for measuring this clearer construct. Based on a sample of 900, this instrument has high internal consistency (coefficient alpha .96), excellent content validity, discriminant validity that was determined by applying Campbell and Fiske's (1959) multi-trait–multi-method approach, and further construct validity that was determined through factor analysis.

A 3-year renewal grant from the Division of Nursing was funded on March 1, 1980. The primary objectives are: (1) to determine whether nurse empathy can be improved through group instruction and (2) to study experimentally the effects of the level of nurse empathy on selected client outcomes of nursing care. These outcomes are: anxiety, depression, hostility, and satisfaction with care. It is hypothesized that as nurse empathy increases, client's anxiety, depression, and hostility will decrease. Further, as nurse empathy increases, client satisfaction with care will increase. Previous research and literature have suggested that client anxiety, depression, hostility, and dissatisfaction with care are counterproductive to the effective development of coping and adaptive behaviors (Joel and Collins, 1978). Helping the client cope and adapt are our responsibilities.

If the results of the present research suggest that nurse empathy is important, the implications are vast. Change will be indicated in nursing curricula, continuing education programs, hospital and community agencies, and professional disciplines that are involved in health care services. Nurses must also then study the relationship between empathy and (1) educational levels in nursing and (2) areas of nursing practice. The significance of this author's research on helping as well as that of others is evident. However given that, more research is indicated to test different helping models in the nursing environment. Nurses must research how the process of helping, not simply the theory, can be taught and evaluated in the formal educational process.

What may result from research is that the body of knowledge and experience in helping will be an added requisite in basic nursing education. Adding more content to basic professional nursing education is often challenged as impossible within our present 4-year framework. It is agreed that it is not effective only to add to a curriculum. Rationale for addition(s) needs to be clearly defined. The content needs to be consistent with the conceptual framework of the curriculum. Perhaps different models of teaching might be reviewed and recalled. Supervised internship post-baccalaureate education model is one example. Even if a master's degree specializing in primary health care is a minimal, basic educational expectation, though the demand for such specialization has been indicated in a recent position by the National League for Nursing, October, 1979, nursing will have developed a career ladder that does not move the nurse away from the client. Instead it will bring the nurse closer to the client and impute responsibility and accountability for nursing's services. This is exciting, and many colleagues will echo that this is already being done. It is, but it remains imperative as nursing gains greater control over health care in this country, that nursing educators and other leaders prepare students more *fully* to meet the needs of our nation's people.

This is not simply a responsibility, it is a moral and an ethical obligation.

At present nurses fall short on the helping aspects of nursing and it is known that if nurses are not helping, they may be harming. This no longer suffices if nurses are to become leaders in services that are recognized clearly as professionally theirs because nurses are the experts.

EDITOR'S QUESTIONS FOR DISCUSSION

What factors have contributed to an identity crisis for nurses? Discuss whether the identity crisis is of an individual nature or an identity crisis for the profession. What suggestions might be offered for resolution of a crisis?

Do you agree with La Monica that nursing poses the greatest threat to personal power of the American Medical Association? What are the implications for the patient and each of the health care professions if nursing should capitalize on the present confusion in health care as La Monica advocates? What should be the role of the nursing profession if and when any one health professional group is under attack? What relationship exists between La Monica's and Bille's (Chap. 36) statements regarding leadership in the provision of health care? What Questions for Discussion raised in Bille's chapter also apply to La Monica's?

Discuss the circumstances indicated by La Monica for interdependence of nurses with other health professionals in providing care. Is there a need for awareness of interdependence among health care providers to be more emphasized than autonomy? Are there other issues not addressed by La Monica in perceiving tomorrow's nurse primarily as an independent practitioner? How valid are the arguments presented for the nurse to be the primary health care provider? What specific requisites are necessary for a nurse to fulfill that role? What areas in the requisites indicated by La Monica need further development by nurses? What planning, preparation, negotiation, and precautions might be recommended prior to nurses assuming a role as primary health care providers? Is nursing in a position to give specific assurances to the public regarding quality and cost-effectiveness as providers of primary health care? What systematic means of evaluation may be essential in undertaking a role as a primary health care provider?

Which, if any, of the nursing theorists writing Chaps. 28 to 34 might concur with La Monica that nurse theorists share a unified approach and definition of the domain of nursing that could be summarized as "helping"? In reviewing Fawcett's (Chap. 14), Walker's (Chap. 30), Menke's (Chap. 31), and Roy's (Chap. 34) writings, would theories of helping be considered as an example of prescriptive or practice theory? How might a theory of helping be developed to meet criteria for a nursing theory as presented by Meleis (Chap. 33)? What agreement may or may not exist between La Monica's knowledge requisites and Fawcett's (Chap. 14) discussion of the knowledge base for nursing practice?

What relationship exists between Bille's (Chap. 36) and La Monica's discussion of teaching-learning principles and the art of instruction? What relationships and applications are there in La Monica's discourse on teaching-helping skills for Peterson's (Chap. 7) and Clayton's (Chap. 10) presentations on education issues and professional competencies?

What change has occurred regarding empathy research? Discuss qualities of effective helper-helpee interactions. Do you agree with La Monica that "there is no neutrality in interactions; they either help or harm?" What empirical and/or experiential evidence is there to support your point of view? How can the level of facilitative skills of the helper specifically enhance or be destructive to growth of the helpee? What additional research questions might be addressed in empathy research?

REFERENCES

Adams, V.
1979 Consensus is reached: Psychotherapy works. The New York Times: July 10, 1979, C-1.
Anthony, W.
1971 "A methodological investigation of the minimally facilitative level of interpersonal functioning." Journal of Clinical Psychology 27:156-157.
Berenson, B., and K. Mitchell
1968 "Therapeutic conditions after therapist-initiated confrontation." Journal of Clinical Psychology 24:363-364.
Berenson, B., K. Mitchell, and R. Laney
1968 "Level of therapist functioning, types of confrontation and type of patient." Journal of Clinical Psychology 24:111-113.
Berenson, B., K. Mitchell, and J. Moravec
1968 "Level of therapist functioning, patient depth of self-exploration and type of confrontation." Journal of Counseling Psychology 15:136-139.
Campbell, D. and D. Fiske
1959 "Convergent and discriminant validation by the multitrait-multimethod matrix." Psychological Bulletin 56:81-105.
Carkhuff, R.
1968 "The differential functioning of lay and and professional helpers." Journal of Counseling Psychology 15:117-126.
1969a Helping and Human Relations: A Primer for Lay and Professional Helpers (vol. 1). New York: Holt, Rinehart & Winston.
1969b Helping and Human Relations: A Primer for Lay and Professional Helpers (vol. 2). New York: Holt, Rinehart & Winston.
Carkhuff, R., and J. Burstein
1970 "Objective therapist and client ratings of therapist-offered facilitative conditions of moderate to low functioning thera-

pists." Journal of Clinical Psychology 26:394-395.
Collingwood, T.
1971 "Retention and retraining of interpersonal communication skills." Journal of Clinical Psychology 27:294-296.
Collingwood, T., and L. Renz
1969 "The effects of client confrontations upon levels of immediacy offered by high and low functioning counselors." Journal of Clinical Psychology 25:224-226.
Conklin, R., and A. Hunt
1975 "An investigation of the validity of empathy measures." Counselor Education and Supervision 15:119-127.
Cousins, N.
1979 Anatomy of an Illness as Perceived by The Patient. New York: Norton.
Etzioni, A.
1961 A Comparative Analysis of Complex Organizations on Power, Involvement and Their Correlates. New York: The Free Press.
Feldstein, P.
1979 Health Care Economics. New York: Wiley.
Friel, T., B. Berenson, and K. Mitchell
1971 "Factor analysis of therapeutic conditions for high and low functioning therapists." Journal of Clinical Psychology 27:291-293.
Gladstein, G.
1977 "Empathy and counseling outcome: An empirical and conceptual review." The Counseling Psychologist 6:70-79.
Hornstein, H.
1976 Cruelty and Kindness: A New Look at Aggression and Altruism. Englewood Cliffs, N. J.: Prentice-Hall.
Joel, L., and D. Collins
1978 Psychiatric Nursing: Theory and Application. New York: McGraw-Hill.

La Monica, E.
1980 Validity of Empathy Instruments. Progress Report of Dept. of Health and Human Services Grant NU 00640.

Mitchell, K., R. Mitchell, and B. Berenson
1970 "Therapist focus on clients' significant others in psychotherapy." Journal of Clinical Psychology 26:533–536.

Muehlberg, N., R. Pierce, and J. Drasgrow
1969 "A factor analysis of therapeutically facilitative conditions." Journal of Clinical Psychology 25:93–95.

National League for Nursing
1979 Position Statement on the Education of Nurse Practitioners. New York: National League for Nursing, Publication No. 11-1808.

Orem, D.
1971 Nursing: Concepts of Practice. New York: McGraw-Hill.

Pellegrino, E.
1979 Humanism and the Physician. Knoxville: The University of Tennessee Press.

Raffel, M.
1980 The United States Health System: Origins and Functions. New York: Wiley.

Riehl, J., and Sr. C. Roy
1980 Conceptual Models for Nursing Practice. Englewood Cliffs, N.J.: Prentice-Hall.

Rogers, C.
1961 On Becoming a Person. Boston: Houghton Mifflin.

Rogers, M.
1970 An Introduction to the Theoretical Basis of Nursing. Philadelphia: F. A. Davis.

Stachnik, T.
1980 "Priorities for psychology in medical education and health care delivery." American Psychologist 35(1):8–15.

Susser, M.
1975 "Prevention and health maintenance revisited." Bulletin of the New York Academy of Medicine 51:5–8.

Truax, C.
1970a "Length of therapist response, accurate empathy and patient improvement." Journal of Clinical Psychology 26:539–541.
1970b "Therapists' evaluative statements and patient outcome in psychotherapy." Journal of Clinical Psychology, 26:536–538.

Truax, C., and R. Carkhuff
1967 Toward Effective Counseling and Psychotherapy: Training and Practice. Chicago: Aldine Publishing Company.

Truax, C., and J. Wittmer
1971 "The effects of therapist focus on patient anxiety source and the interaction with therapist level of accurate empathy." Journal of Clinical Psychology 27:295–299.

Truax, C., J. Wittmer, and D. Wargo
1971 "Effects of therapeutic conditions of accurate empathy, non-possessive warmth, and genuineness on hospitalized mental patients during group therapy." Journal of Clinical Psychology 27:137–142.

Chapter 38

Collegial Staff Relations and Assertiveness in Nurses: Do They Make Any Difference in Patient Care?

Sharon J. Reeder, R.N., Ph.D., F.A.A.N.
Professor
Center for Health Sciences
School of Nursing
University of California at Los Angeles
Los Angeles, California

After reading about consumer rights, humanizing patient care-education, and the role of the nurse as a health professional, it is timely to focus more specifically on interdisciplinary relationships. Sharon J. Reeder aptly portrays the phenomenon of collaborative effort among nurses and physicians as members of the health team. Furthermore, she discusses assertive behavior in nurses and investigates the relationship between this interpersonal characteristic and collegiality. She attains those objectives by presenting a study in which she examines assertiveness, collegiality, and the relationship to patient care practices judged important for effective hospital infection control.

Reeder characterizes collaborative team effort by a high degree of information exchange, clarity of communication, and mutual respect. She defines collegiality as relationships among individuals of both equal and unequal status. It includes readiness to be mutually helpful and communicate. Collaboration is inherent in order to accomplish goals of the group or organization. Reeder reviews perspectives on collegiality and assertiveness. She indicates that there is a fair degree of consensus that the concept of collegiality includes professional equality, a shared base of knowledge, autonomy, self-directedness, accountability, peer review, and interdependence. It is pointed

The author expresses her appreciation to the Center for Disease Control for making available the data analyzed herein; and to Robert Haley, Howard Freeman, Bertram Raven, David Redfearn, Patricia Yokopenic, and Susan Rakow for comments and suggestions.

out that consensus may exist *within* a single profession but not necessarily *between* professions.

Reeder traces the disparity in colleagueship perspectives between the professions of nursing and medicine. The traditional sex-role socialization of men and women is discussed. Particularly, the early sex-role and professional socialization of women is portrayed as having a diminishing effect on the development of assertive qualities. Other contributing factors suggested by Reeder are: low esteem women have for each other, conditioning of women to "fear" achievement, and the "obedience training" of early nursing education. Lack of equal educational opportunity, blocked mobility to higher occupation levels, and the "doctor-nurse game" are all attributed as significant factors that have prohibited a true "company of equals." In describing the "doctor-nurse game," Reeder perceives it has direct relevance for patient care practices, the development of collegiality, and why assertiveness has become a predominant characteristic for nurses. Negative results in playing the game are cited with the patient ultimately being the innocent victim. Reeder offers as a solution the efforts of the National Joint Practice Commission to define the nature of collegial relations. Four requisites are defined which focus on goal consensus, equality, shared knowledge with complementary expertise, and mutual trust-respect.

In her investigation Reeder obtained a random sample of 7188 staff nurses from 433 hospitals in 48 states. This chapter reports data from a subsample of 5435 nurses in 345 hospitals. Reeder developed a Patient Care Practice Index which describes appropriate patient care relating to the control of nosocomial infections. Two scales of assertiveness were also designed. The first dealt with the nurse's ability to speak to persons who were observed violating infection control procedures, and the second scale was utilized to measure the likelihood of the nurse to report colleague violators to a supervisor. Reeder created two measures of acquiescence: (1) to indicate nurses' willingness to conform to a medical order which prohibited isolation of a patient and (2) to determine nurses' willingness to accede to a physician's continuation of a procedure with contaminated equipment. Finally, a Collegial Relations Scale was developed to determine the type and degree of communication between nurses and physicians.

The findings of Reeder's research show that collegial relations, assertiveness, and the ability to restrain acquiescence under pressure were significantly related to increased rigor in patient care practices. The best single predictor was the measure for conformity to a medical order. She suggests further empirical analyses of issues and data, which reflect collegial communication, as a foundation in providing high-quality patient care.

The provision of high-calibre patient care by both physicians and nurses appears to be becoming increasingly difficult in the modern bureaucratized health milieu. Nowhere is the problem more pointed than in relation to the prevention of hospital-acquired (nosocomial) infections. These infections represent a major health care problem from the standpoint of patient morbidity and mortality. It is estimated that of the 2 million patients who sustain a hospital-acquired infection yearly, 15,000 die. Moreover, the prolongation of the hospital stay and the additional services needed to treat the infection markedly increase the costs of the original hospitalization (Haley et al., 1981).

Authorities in the nosocomial infection field differ in their opinions regarding the efficacy of the various prevention and control practices. There is, however, rather general agreement that the way in which work and working relationships are organized in the hospital does influence the quality of patient care and hence, indirectly, the incidence of hospital-acquired infections (Kass, 1970; Williams, 1970; Schaffner, 1977; Raven, 1978; Raven and Haley, 1980).

In the rhetoric of the nursing profession, two constructs have received considerable attention recently. One construct relates to the character of the role relationships between physicians and nurses; thus we have the plea, even the demand for the "health team," with emphasis on collaborative team effort among the members. The second construct relates more to an assumed intrapersonal characteristic, that of the ability to be assertive. This latter characteristic is seen to be very important for the nurse, who by virtue of sex-role and professional socialization may not be able to be appropriately assertive in patient care situations.

Indeed, a body of expert opinion and research stresses the point that a collaborative team effort leads to high-quality patient care. This team effort is characterized by a high degree of information exchange, clarity of communication by nurses in apprising physicians of their patient's needs and progress, and a mutual respect among the members of the team (Coser, 1958; Friedson and Rhea, 1963; Herman, 1978; Smoyak, 1977; Kramer, 1974; Reeder and Mauksch, 1979).

In this paper, we will delineate an aspect of this team effort. We have termed it "collegiality" and defined it as relationships among individuals of both equal and unequal status within an organization, relationships which allow for readiness to be mutually helpful, as well as readiness to communicate constructively in order to accomplish the goals of the group or organization. Collegiality involves mutual collaboration.

A growing body of literature attests to the fact that assertiveness by nurses in dealing with their peers and physicians is also seen to contribute to a high calibre of patient care. In the complex hospital system of today in which a variety of medical specialists, interns, residents, and technicians may have responsibility for a portion of the care of each patient, the staff nurse becomes a crucial link between the patient and a cadre of care providers. Her continued presence, when accompanied by articulate communication and determined efforts to assure conformity to appropriate patient care practices, may protect patients from incompetent actions and unintended consequences of hospitalization (Herman, 1977, 1978).

This chapter will be primarily a discussion of the phenomenon of collaborative effort (collegiality) among nurses and physicians as members of the health team. In addition, assertive behavior in nurses will be discussed to examine the relationship between this intrapersonal characteristic and collegiality and the relationship to rigorous, appropriate patient care practices deemed important for effective hospital infection control. It is hoped that discussing the above relationships will lend insight into the complex functioning of what has become known as the "health team" and the relevance that this functioning may have for appropiate patient care practices.

The Study on the Efficacy of Nosocomial Infection Control (SENIC Project), sponsored by the Center for Disease Control (CDC), is a national evaluation of programs and activities to prevent hospital-acquired infections (Haley et al., 1980, 1981). It has provided an unusual opportunity to examine various aspects of relationships between health care providers in relation to the quality of patient care. Data in this report is from a preliminary analysis. Subsequent analyses are being prepared and will be reported elsewhere (Reeder and Stevens, forthcoming).

PERSPECTIVES ON COLLEGIALITY AND ASSERTIVENESS

Colleagues as a Company of Equals

When we speak of professional colleagues and collegial relations among the professions, most of us have an intuitive sense of what is meant by the term. Upon closer examination, however, we find some variety in interpretation and definition. An overview of the literature on the topic helps illuminate this diversity. In the late 1950s and 1960s there was increasing attention paid to the dilemma of professionals and scientists working in formal organizations (Wardwell, 1955; Ben-David, 1958; Solomon, 1957; Goss, 1961; Kornhauser, 1962; Freidson and Rhea, 1963). Much of the discussion revolved around the issue of control—and hence, indirectly, the problem of accountability. Debate arose as to whether or not conventional bureaucratic methods are appropriate or practical for controlling the work of scientists and professionals, particularly the physician. A consensus of sorts was reached when it was generally agreed that those workers require a kind of autonomy that is antithetical to Weber's model of rational-legal bureaucracy (Weber, 1947) and, indeed, that the value of their work is substantially reduced when done "by the book" or otherwise subjected to the often detailed and tedious directives of an administrative hierarchy. Over time, it evolved that the proper way for such individuals to work is as members of a self-regulating "company of equals" (Freidson and Rhea, 1963).

But what exactly is a company of equals? Barber provides a descriptive definition when he says:

> [A company of equals is] a social group in which each permanent member . . . is roughly equal in authority, self-directing and self-disciplined, pursuing the goal [of his work] under the guidance of the morality he has learned from his colleagues and which he shares with them. The sources of purpose and authority are in his own conscience, and in his respect for the moral judgments of his peers. If his own conscience is not strong enough, the disapproval of others will control him or will lead to his exclusion from the brotherhood. (Barber, 1962:195)

Barber's definition reflects the then-current state of mind which took for granted the exclusivity of male dominance in the professions. Nevertheless, the notions of professional equality, a shared base of knowledge, autonomy, self-directedness, accountability, peer review, and interdependence have come to be the warp and woof of that which we call collegiality.

A more thoughtful appraisal of the above definition reveals why there may be some problems in the application of the concept among a variety of coworkers. The fact of male dominance in the professions is today still a reality; moreover, some individuals believe that that is an appropriate state of affairs, since men have always been in the forefront of education and general achievement. Thus, given the above definition, when collegial collaboration is defined and discussed among professionals, there may be a fair degree of consensus regarding the definition of the concept *within* a single profession but not necessarily *between* professions. This is especially true if there is a perception that the other profession is "subordinate" in some way; that is, the "majority" sex does not prevail, there is not a requisite knowledge base, control of practice does not exist, and so on.

The Health Team and Collegial Collaboration

Medicine and nursing are the oldest health professions and form the nucleus of what we call the "health team." Their long history of working together is starred by documented instances of outstanding collaborative effort. Unfortunately, it is also marred by other instances of interprofessional and interpersonal conflict. Smoyak (1977) has pointed out that, before there arose the disharmony which is now evident between the two fields, there was a period of little animosity; indeed, "colleagueship" would aptly describe the state of affairs. A century ago, physicians had no antibiotics, no tranquilizers, no operating and delivery suites, no intensive care units. All of the monitoring and transplant technologies were nonexistent. Surgery and anesthesia were just developing. The physician could do little more than nurse the patient. The nurse allowed this, and the two worked closely together; neither was dismayed by territorial invasion. Disparity in economic compensation between the two professions was not a big issue, nor was the disparity in skills so great.

However, traditional sex-role socialization, together with new sciences, new discoveries, and the burgeoning of technologies in this century, encouraged a broadening gulf between the two fields, and hence collegiality suffered. Men were encouraged and, indeed, mandated to learn and study; women were not. Men went to the universities; women stayed home and raised children. Their mandate was to provide a stable environment where their families might thrive and flourish in increasingly hectic times. Subtly, sexual segregation and discrimination became deeply embedded in the world of work. Male-dominated professions, including medicine, developed with leaps and bounds. Nursing and other "women's occupations" faltered, suffering from a debilitating suppression of intellectual activity brought on by sexist ideology and traditional sex-role socialization (Smoyak, 1977; Bullough and Bullough, 1975; Ehrenreich and Deirdre, 1974; Scully and Bart, 1973; Spock, 1971; Reeder, 1978; Levinson, 1976; Feather and Simon, 1973, 1975).

In a cogent analysis of sex discrimination in health care, Bullough and Bullough (1975) point out that the lack of equal educational opportunity is of major importance in explaining sex segregation in the health occupations themselves. The relatively low representation of women in the high-status health professions is mediated through the professional schools, where women students have been more or less systematically excluded except for token representation. Blocked from the higher levels, they have tended to congregate in the health occupations at the middle and lower levels. This is particularly true for nursing, which has come to carry a double image of serving not only the patient but also the physicians. This, of course, mitigates against a true "company of equals" image and reinforces the subordinate, handmaiden aspect so often associated with nursing.

Health care for the patient also suffers, because sex segregation and the concomitant dominant-subordinate posturings have created communication barriers between members of the health team. In an in-depth study of a community hospital, Duff and Hollingshead (1968) concluded that a lack of effective communication between the members of the health team, particularly nurses and physicians, was a significant factor in explaining the poor patient care they found. Other authors have also called attention to maladaptive communication and its relevance for patient care (Stein, 1967; Bullough and Bullough, 1975; Hoekelman, 1978; Reeder and Mauksch, 1979). It is important to note that the communication gap between physicians and nurses is not the normal gap that often occurs in complex organizations with multiple levels of workers, but rather is exaggerated to the point of becoming what one author called the "doctor-nurse game" (Stein, 1967; Bullough and Bullough, 1975).

A brief summary of the "game" is in order, since it has direct bearing on the implementation of collegiality and its relevance for patient care practices.[1] It also gives a perspective on why assertiveness becomes such an important characteristic for nurses. Physicians ordinarily see patients a short time each day and thus must depend on nurses and other health personnel for a good deal of information about their patients. In contrast, nurses have many more opportunities throughout a 24-hour period to observe and listen to patients. These nursing observations and assessments are crucial and, in fact, constitute diagnoses; moreover, they must be acted upon and recommendations made to the physician. However, under the rules of the game, nurses must pretend that they never diagnose nor can they make recommendations directly and honestly to their physician coworkers. This maladaptive interaction has been well documented by Stein (1967). He was fascinated by the way in which nurses did, in fact, make recommendations

---

[1] For a thorough discussion of the pernicious effects of this type of interaction and suggested remedies, see Stein, 1967, and Hoekelman, 1978.

to physicians, the pretense by the physicians that the nurses were *not* making the recommendations, and then the care that successful physicians took *to* follow these recommendations. According to Stein, the game is played to allay the physicians' fears that they make errors of judgment in managing patients (because of lack of observation, among other things). Thus, through the game, nurses are allowed to share in the medical decision making concerning patient care without seeming to and without sharing in the responsibility for those decisions. This allows both sides to develop and maintain the fantasy that the physician is omniscient and omnipotent and that the nurse is really knowledgeable, indispensable to the physician, and to some degree powerful. The single most important rule of the game is that open disagreement between the players must be avoided at all costs. The reward for playing well is ostensible respect and cooperation from the other discipline. The penalites for playing poorly are loss of respect and sabotage. More importantly, and in reality, there are penalites for all concerned for playing the game at all. For nurses, there is the suppression of initiative and intellect and the betrayal of true professionalism; for physicians, there is self-deception, dishonesty, and betrayal of professionalism. For the patient, the innocent victim, there is a diminution in the quality of care that is his or her due. Poor communication causes trouble. Misinterpretation, lack of follow-through, failure to write and read orders and notes, self-serving priority setting, all contribute to mishaps that result in poor patient care practices (Hoekelman, 1978; Smoyak, 1977; Coser, 1958).

Efforts have been made since 1971 to lessen the need for game playing and to enhance teamwork. The interorganizational efforts of the AMA and the ANA resulted in the National Joint Practice Commission (NJPC). This body has been defining the nature of the health care team and the nature of collegial relations. Briefly stated, nurses and physicians work best as colleagues where there is (1) mutual agreement on a goal; (2) equality in

status and personal interactions; (3) a shared base of scientific and professional knowledge with complementary diversity in skills, expertise, and practices; and (4) mutual trust and respect for each other's competence (Smoyak, 1977). If these requisites prevail, there should be improved communication among members of the health team. Nurses should feel free to approach physicians, apprise them of current information regarding their patients (as well as mistakes or problems they see), and make suggestions regarding the total management. Physicians are to encourage this behavior and actively seek collaboration. A true collegial atmosphere, with its heightened communication, results ultimately in improved patient care.

It is expected also that, with continued emphasis on affirmative action, the effort some professions are making to include women and men in their ranks, and the more open opportunities for female advancement, will help mitigate the basic problem of sex segregation; this, in turn, is expected to maximize collegiality between the professions.

Assertive Behavior and the Nurse

We will now turn to a construct that is closely related to collegiality. The point has been made elsewhere that nursing has been inextricably bound to the history of women (Reeder and Mauksch, 1979). The word "nurse" derives from the Latin, *nutrire*, to suckle, and the so-called innate attributes of woman and especially mother, evoke perceptions which still influence the image of nursing and nursing education today. With the absence of formal boundaries to a mother's area of competence and society's demand that she perform the managerial tasks associated with homemaking, the true potential of the nurse's role often becomes blurred in the minds of many, especially those outside of the profession.

As stated previously, since nursing is mainly a woman's field, nurses have been constrained by early sex-role socialization as well as by professional socialization. These types of socialization have tended to blunt, if not erase, any assertive qualities in the aspiring professional.

Women tend to perceive themselves and be viewed by others as stereotypically passive, accommodating, helpless, dependent, submissive, emotional, security-oriented, and expressive (Parsons, 1954; Broverman et al., 1970; Millet, 1970). Nurses, in particular, have described themselves as dependable, methodical, capable, and submissive. Their major expectations for their nursing role have been to be industrious, methodical, and dependable individuals who can sustain subordinate roles while being cooperative, considerate, conventional, adaptable, and ready to "serve" the physician (Reeder and Mauksch, 1979). Early in life women are socialized out of the desire to be decision makers in our society. The health professional literature, particularly, helps continue the myths of innate female inferiority, a specific "role" for a female in our society, and gender-linked emotions rather than culturally learned emotions and desires (Broverman et al., 1970; Marlow, 1973; Cook, 1973; Willson et al., 1975).

It has been demonstrated also that women's general lack of achievement is due, in part, to traditional sex-role socialization which teaches them to make choices which do not result in occupational or educational advancement. A growing body of literature suggests that this socialization contributes to the low esteem that women have for each other and, moreover, that women are conditioned to "fear" achievement, particularly in the male-oriented areas, thus depriving themselves of opportunities for advancement (Levinson, 1976; Feather and Simon, 1973, 1975; Horner, 1972).

Education in nursing, until the last two decades, often occurred in a rigid, regimented, and often theoretically sterile environment which emphasized, essentially, obedience training. Any self-assertion was strongly negatively sanctioned (Reeder and Mauksch, 1979). Socialization messages were contradictory: be an equal member of the health team and be independent in knowledge

and practice, but do not question, assert your knowledge and competence, or disagree with physicians. Although you must practice with sound scientific knowledge, be "professional" by keeping the environment tension-free, remain affectively neutral, ignore conflict, and when all else fails, remain silent (Bullough and Bullough, 1975; Reeder, 1978). All of this served to eradicate any kind of assertive behavior in nurses.

More recently, in the broader society and in nursing as well, there have been concerted efforts by feminist groups and leaders in nursing to raise the consciousness of women. These efforts have helped many women to reassess themselves and to develop practical career goals. Assertion-training workshops for nurses have had surprisingly good results in that the participants were found to be more outspoken and less willing to be noncommittal after such training (Herman, 1977, 1978). While such consciousness raising and training are undoubtedly helpful, it will still take time before the basic early socialization processes change.

DATA AND METHODS

The development of the SENIC Project has been described elsewhere (Haley, 1981; Raven and Haley, 1980). To summarize, a random sample was selected from 433 hospitals, representative of all general medical and surgical hospitals that offer short-term care, are not federal or state-owned, have at least 50 beds, and are located in the contiguous 48 states. Each sampled hospital participated in the Hospital Interview Survey (H.I.S.) phase of the data collection. Three hundred and thirty-eight of them also participated in the second phase, the Medical Records Survey (M.R.S.).

The HIS objective was to measure the characteristics of each hospital's infection control activities practiced in 1976. Thus, a set of personal, structured interviews was administered to hospital staff who play important roles in hospital infection control, including the infection-control nurse, hospital epidemiologist, chairman of the infection-control committee, hospital administrators, and others. Since care by staff nurses is central to controlling hospital-induced infections, a final random sample of 7188 staff nurses were given self-administered questionnaires. This paper reports data from a subsample of 345 hospitals with a nurse population of 5435. The original indices and scales were built on this subsample. Subsequent verification of the measures with the total sample, as well as analyses in progress, indicate that the measures and results tend to replicate.

Measures

The Dependent Variable The dependent measure was the type of care nurses gave their patients. A seven-item proportional summed index, termed the Patient Care Practice Index, was developed. This index described appropriate patient care, care relating particularly to the control of nosocomial infections, but also having relevance for general nursing care. "Correct" practices were defined from current published recommendations (Bennett and Brachman, 1979). The questions dealt with procedures relating to urinary catheter care, proper handling of breathing units or respirators, replacement of intravenous cannulas and administration sets, and whether or not patients had been taught proper breathing techniques before undergoing surgery.

The Independent Variables Perceptions of intrapersonal characteristics of assertiveness and acquiescence and perceptions of collegial relations with physicians served as the independent variables.

The first set of variables dealt with assertiveness and acquiescence. Two scales of assertiveness were developed using factor analytic techniques (principal components analysis with varimax rotation). It is important to note that the assertiveness (and acquiescence) questions were hypothetical situations and not actual ones. Hofling et al.

(1966) found that nurses were more likely to react differently in actual situations than they were to ideological, hypothetical situations.[2]

Assertiveness 1 was composed of items which dealt with the nurses' ability to speak to a variety of individuals who were observed violating different infection-control procedures. A scale ranging from 1 to 19 was developed (mean 13.607; SD 3.752; Cronbach's alpha .80), which indicated good replicability and reliability.

The second assertiveness scale, *Assertiveness 2*, dealt with whether or not the nurse was likely to report to a supervisor those colleagues whom she observed violating various infection-control procedures. The response categories and the nine hypothetical situations used for this scale were identical to those used in the Assertiveness 1 scale; the only difference was that in the first scale the nurse was asked how likely it would be that she would speak to the offender. In the second scale, Assertiveness 2, the nurse was asked how likely it would be that she would report the offender to a superior. This scale was less normally distributed, with more tendency of skewing toward the more assertive end of the scale (mean 13.618; SD 4.898; Cronbach's alpha .90); however, it was reliable.

Two operational measures of acquiescence, *Acquiescence 1 and Acquiescence 2*, were utilized. Acquiescence 1 dealt with the nurses' willingness to acquiesce to a medical order which *prohibited* isolating a child with a purulent wound. Acquiescence 2 dealt with the nurses' willingness to accede

---

[2] Berrelson and Steiner (1964) have pointed out, however, that there is a positive correlation between attitudes and behavior. Others have noted that both attitudes and behavior are affected by the social frame of reference in which they occur (Raab and Lipset, 1959). A recent study of the relationship between attitudes may provide a baseline for decision making about action toward the relevant issue. Against this base line, the individual raises other considerations, such as the views held by the reference group and possible sanctions for acting one way or the other (Acock & DeFleur, 1972).

to a physician's request to continue a urinary catheterization with contaminated equipment.[3]

The second set of independent variables dealt with nurses' perceptions regarding the degree of collegiality or openness of communication between physicians and nurses in their hospital. A Collegial Relations Scale was developed. In order to ascertain the type and degree of communication between nurses and doctors regarding patient care, nurses were asked a series of questions relating to whether or not it was characteristic in their hospital for nurses to approach physicians to report patients' progress, needs, signs, symptoms, errors in treatment and orders, and so on. These situations were utilized as indicators of the type of communication patterns that existed between the two disciplines. A scale ranging from 0 to 14 was developed using factor analytic techniques. Higher scores indicated more collegiality or collaborative communication; lower scores, less collegiality. The scale formed a relatively normal distribution with the majority of cases in the 7–12 range (mean 8.883; SD 2.411; Cronbach's alpha .68). Thus, an acceptable scale was constructed for the collegiality items.

Selected demographic and professional background characteristics were also obtained. These related to age, sex, type of professional education (R.N., L.P.N., etc.), amount of time the nurse had practiced, type of work she usually did (staff, team leader, etc.).

---

[3] Using Pearson product moment correlations, we found the four assertive and acquiescence measures to be correlated with each other. The first assertiveness scale, Assertiveness 1, correlated with the Acquiescence 1 measure at $-.23$, $p = .001$; and the Acquiescence 2 measure at $-.20$, $p = .001$; The Assertiveness 2 scale correlated with Acquiescence 1 measure at $-.14$, $p = .001$ and the Acquiescence 2 measure at $-.12$, $p = .001$. Thus, high assertiveness was associated with low acquiescence. While the associations are not of a great magnitude, they are significant and indicate that a relationship exists. These measures may be measuring the obverse of each other. However, there is the problem of multicollinearity. Subsequent analysis is indicating that Assertiveness 1 is the single best predictor, and hence Assertiveness 2 and the acquiescence items may be dropped without softening the relationships.

Description of the Sample

Our sample was overwhelmingly female. Ninety-eight percent ($N = 5396$) were women and only 2 percent ($N = 39$) were men. With respect to age, 28 percent were over 41 years old; 38 percent were between 27 and 41 years of age; and 34 percent were under 27 years. Thus, our nurses were fairly evenly distributed throughout the three categories. Ninety-two percent of the respondents gave the United States as their country of birth; 8 percent stated other countries, predominantly Canada and England.

The ethnic distribution and the first language of the sample were as follows: the majority were white Anglo (84 percent), with black being the next most prominent category (10 percent). Asian/Oriental constituted about 4 percent of the sample. Ninety-five percent of the nurses claimed English as their first language.

The majority of the sample were registered nurses (68 percent), 32 percent held L.V.N. or L.P.N. licensure and 0.3 percent claimed an "other" type of license. The majority were employed full-time (87 percent). Diploma programs contributed the highest percentage (41 percent) of the nurses. The associate of arts program was represented by approximately 18 percent, and the baccalaureate programs produced about 10 percent of the respondents. These findings are interesting in the light of the pool of registered nurses in general. Given the extremely large number of associate degree graduates and the increasing number of baccalaureate-prepared nurses in the last decade, the fact that over half of the registered nurse sample is diploma-prepared indicates that the diploma programs appear to still be a viable source of nursing personnel.

When asked about the highest academic degree that was achieved, approximately 69 percent listed "none." This is commensurate with the findings regarding type of nursing program completed, since the associate of arts programs and baccalaureate programs constitute about 28 percent of the degrees.

With respect to the professional nursing experiences of our respondents, we found a linear distribution from less than 6 months to 10 years or more. About 52 percent of our nurses had been practicing in the field 5 to 10 years or more. Thirty percent of these had been practicing 10 years or more. Thus, a little more than half of the sample was quite experienced.

When asked the year they completed their nursing program, a little more than half (53 percent) indicated post-1970. The next largest category, with about 25 percent of the respondents, finished in the decade between 1961 and 1970. Thus, three-quarters of those sampled completed programs after 1960. The comparison of the percentages between number of years of practice versus the year the program was completed may reflect the tendency of many nurses to practice their profession intermittently but to continue practice.

A little more than half (53 percent) of our sample were staff nurses. Another 27 percent held administrative positions with some staff duties.

In summary, the great majority of our nurses' sample were white, Anglo, female, English-speaking registered nurses, who were born in the United States. There was a good age spread, and they could be considered well experienced in nursing, with over half of the sample being in practice 5 to 10 years or more.

The Relationship of Collegiality and the Intrapersonal Characteristics to Patient Care Practices

In order to examine the relationship among collegiality, assertiveness, acquiescence, and patient care practices, we first did bivariate correlations between the practices and the other measures. To complete this preliminary analysis we then examined the three-way relationship among the patient care practices and collegiality, controlling or partialing out the effects of the assertiveness and acquiescence measures.[4] We would expect that

[4] Subsequent analysis, using a slightly modified patient care practices index and collegiality scale, tested the effects of the background and demographic characteristics

nurses who were more assertive (and less acquiescent) and who perceived more collegial relations existed in their work milieu would have higher patient care rigor scores.

Bivariate correlations were calculated on the above data (Table 38-1), yielding .12 for collegiality and patient care practices rigor ($p = .001$); when the effects of Assertiveness 1 were partialled out from this association, the correlation decreased to .07 ($p = .001$), indicating that Assertiveness 1 is a viable copredictor of patient care rigor and, in fact, contributes more to the equation than does collegiality.

When the effects of the Assertiveness 2 situation were partialled out, the correlation between collegiality and patient care rigor dropped from .12 to .10 ($p = .001$), indicating that collegiality and Assertiveness 2 together may also better predict rigor than if each measure were considered separately. The Assertiveness 2 measure, however, contributes less to the equation than does Assertiveness 1.

Finally, we explored the relationships between collegiality and patient care rigor controlling for the effects of acquiescence. When the effects of acquiescence were partialled out, the correlations between collegiality and patient rigor rose slightly from -.12 to -.11 for Acquiescence 1 and dropped from -.09 to -.12 for Acquiescence 2. These findings indicate that both acquiescence measures add little to the predictive power of the equation.

A multiple regression further elaborated the partial correlations. When collegiality and the four intrapersonal characteristics were used together to predict patient care practice rigor, the multiple r was .35, indicating that all five variables taken

and selected hospital characteristics and the above measures. Only having an in-service training program, nursing staff ratio and the proportion of R.N.s were significantly related to rigorous patient care practices. An in-service training program was also related to collegiality and assertiveness. Analysis is being undertaken to determine orthogonality between the collegiality and assertiveness measures (Reeder and Stevens, forthcoming).

Table 38-1   Bivariate and Partial Correlations Between Patient Care Practices Rigor,
Collegiality, and Intrapersonal Characteristics*

Relationship of patient care practices rigor with	Bivariate correlations (N = 3515)	
	r	p
Collegiality	.12	.001
Assertiveness 1	.34	.001
Assertiveness 2	.23	.001
Acquiescence 1	−.12	.001
Acquiescence 2	−.09	.001
Relationship of patient care practices rigor with colleg- iality partialing out	Partial correlations (N = 3514)	
	r	p
Assertiveness 1	.07	.001
Assertiveness 2	.10	.001
Acquiescence 1	−.11	.001
Acquiescence 2	−.12	.001

*r = .35 R .12

together were not necessarily better predictors of patient care rigor than Assertiveness 1 (r = .34). The R, however, was .12, indicating that 12 percent of the variance in the above equation was explained by the variables of collegiality and intrapersonal characteristics. While this does not appear large at the outset, given the type of social science data, the amount is creditable.

DISCUSSION AND SUMMARY

To summarize, we found collegial relations and perceived ability to be assertive and not to acquiesce under pressure to be significantly related to increased rigor in patient care practices. The magnitude of the correlations was small, with the exception of Assertiveness 1, and should hence be viewed with caution. Assertiveness 1 appeared to be, of the behavioral measures, the best single predictor of rigorous patient care practices. These results need further research and substantiation, but they do give rise to some interesting speculation.

It may be that assertive behavior may be more important for patient care than the establishment of a true collegial team effort. This sounds somewhat heretical at the outset, since much of the rhetoric of both professions has been stressing collegial activities. Yet we know the pitfalls that become apparent when attempts are made to actually put collegiality into practice. Certainly collegial team effort is much harder to come by; assertiveness training appears to be feasible and workable according to Herman (1978). One also might speculate about the relationship between assertive behavior and a collegial milieu. For instance, one can take the point of view that working in a collegial atmosphere requires (and allows) the nurse to act in an equalitarian way, to share her ideas, and to assertively press her point when necessary. Hence, assertiveness can be viewed as part of a generalized pattern of collegiality. On the other hand, one can maintain that assertive behavior derives from the individual's "social personality makeup" (Borgotta and Cattrell, 1957) and is therefore superordinate and independent of the occupational role or any other role or role sets. In this view, individuals, depending on their overall socialization experiences, will differ in the extent to which they will act to encourage conformity to what they believe right and appropriate. This issue needs to be assessed empirically, since peer relations among the health providers are said to be such a cornerstone of quality patient care.

Future analyses should be completed at the hospital level to test the hypothesis that in hospitals where there is perceived collegial communication between nurses and physicians, there will be more positive, vigorous patient care practices. These an-alyses should include multivariate analyses of the complex relationships among the hospital charac-teristics, the intrapersonal characteristics, and collegiality as they relate to patient care rigor—and eventually to hospital infection rates. An interac-tional model for the joint effects of collegiality and the intrapersonal characteristics holds promise. The collegiality scale should be refined and re-tested. Some actual assertiveness measures need to be developed. More refined sophisticated analyses such as these would allow us to see more clearly the contribution of each variable to the total vari-ance of the completed equation that leads to quality patient care.

EDITOR'S QUESTIONS FOR DISCUSSION

How is self-regulation, professional autonomy antithetical to Weber's model of rational-legal bureaucracy? How does the issue of control and problem of accountabil-ity of a professional manifest itself in a bureaucratic setting? What strategies can effectively be utilized to minimize conflict of a professional employed in a bureau-cratic organization?

What are the issues and problems in the application of the concept professional equality? What factors may influence a difference in consensus between professions and within a single profession regarding a definition of collegial collaboration?

Is there a difference how collegiality manifests itself in professional settings where males are predominantly employed versus where women are the predominant group? Would you agree as suggested by the literature that women have a low esteem for each other? If that is true, what are the implications for the development of collegiality among professional women? How does the phenomenon "fear achievement" display itself among professional women? To what extent is the phenomenon unique among women? What strategies can be suggested for prevention and/or intervention of the phenomenon?

What factors have contributed to an emphasis on collegiality among professionals? Has collegiality been eroded by other dominant concerns and issues? Differentiate by example(s) between assertiveness and aggressiveness in collegial relationships. To what extent do you perceive collegiality as existent within a single profession and between professions, historically and at present? What suggestions can be offered for increasing collegiality among individual professional men and women, between both sexes as members of a single professional group, and among representatives of varying disci-plines on a health team?

Illustrate how patients and students may become victims as the result of differences in definition of collegial collaboration. What contradictory ("double") messages may be given to patients, students, and to a professional where differences in perspectives exist regarding collaboration in providing health care and the education of students? What strategies can be offered to prevent the effects of discrepant definitions and perspectives?

Discuss the validity and reliability of the measures utilized in Reeder's research. What additional data analyses might be suggested? What differences in the findings might one explore in relation to the demographic and professional background characteristics of the subjects? What alternative explanations might be offered for the findings? What explanations of the findings are supported by the data? How likely is it in future research to find that assertive behavior is more important for patient care than the establishment of collegial team efforts? Regarding the speculations presented, what are some implications for design and measurements utilized in future research concerning assertiveness and collegial relationships?

REFERENCES

Acock, A. and M. Defleur
1972 "A configurational approach to contingent consistency in the attitude behavior relationship." The American Sociological Review 37:714–26.

Barber, B.
1962 Science and the Social Order. New York: Collier.

Ben-David, J.
1958 "The professional role of the physician in bureaucratized medium." Human Relations 11:225–274.

Bennett, J. V. and P. S. Brachman
1979 Hospital Infections. New York: Little, Brown.

Berrelson, B. and G. A. Steiner
1964 Human Behavior: An Inventory of Scientific Findings. New York: Harcourt, Brace and World.

Borgotta, E. F. and L. S. Cattrell, Sr.
1957 "Directions for group research in group behavior." American Journal of Sociology 63 (July):42–48.

Broverman, I. D., et al.
1970 "Sex role stereotypes and clinical judgements of mental health." Journal of Consulting and Clinical Psychology 54: 211–13.

Bullough, B. and V. Bullough
1975 "Sex discrimination in health care." Nursing Outlook 23(1):40–45.

Cook, W. R.
1973 Essentials of Gynecology. Philadelphia: Lippincott, 59–60.

Coser, R. L.
1958 "Authority and decision-making in a hospital: A comparative analysis." American Sociological Review 23:56–63.

Duff, R. S. and A. B. Hollingshead
1968 Sickness and Society. New York: Harper & Row.

Ehrenreich, B. and E. Deirdre
1974 Complaints and Disorders: The Sexual Politics of Sickness. Glass Mountain Pamphlet Series. New York: Feminist Press.

Feather, N. and J. Simon
1973 "Fear of success and causal attribution for outcome." Journal of Personality 41:524–541.
1975 "Reactions of male and female success and failure in sex-linked occupations: Impressions of personality, causal attribution, and perceived likelihood of different consequences." Journal of Personality and Social Psychology 31:20–31.

Freidson, E. and B. Rhea
1963 "Process in a company of equals." Social Problems 2(2):119–131.

Goss, M. E.
1961 "Influence and authority among physicians in an outpatient clinic." American Sociological Review 26:39–50.

Haley, R. W., D. R. Schaberg, S. V. Van Allman, and J. E. J. McGowan
1980 "Estimating the extra charges and prolongation of hospitalization due to nosocomial infections: A comparison of methods." Journal of Infectious Disease February.

Haley, R. W., J. V. Bennett, D. Quade, and H. E. Freeman
1981 "Study of the efficacy of nosocomial infection control (SENIC project): Sum-

mary of study design," American Journal of Epidemiology.

Herman, S. J.
1977 "Assertiveness: An answer to job dissatisfaction for nurses." Pp. 14–17 in R. Allurti (ed.), Assertiveness, Innovation, Application, Issues. San Luis Obispo, Calif.: Impact.
1978 Becoming Assertive. New York: Van Nostrand.

Hoekelman, R. A.
1978 "Nurse-physician relationships: Problems and solutions." Pp. 330–35 in N. Chaska (ed.), The Nursing Profession: Views through the Mist. New York: McGraw-Hill

Hofling, C. K. et al.
1966 "An experimental study in nurse-physician relationships." Journal of Nervous and Mental Diseases 143:171-90.

Horner, M. S.
1972 "The motive to avoid success and changing aspirations of college women." In J. M. Bardwick (ed.), Readings in the Psychology of Women. New York: Harper & Row.

Kass, E. H.
1970 "Surveillance as a control system." In Proceedings of the International Conference on Nosocomial Infection Control. Center for Disease Control (August 3-6): 292-293.

Kornhauser, W.
1962 Scientists in Industry: Conflict and Accommodation. Berkeley: University of California Press.

Kramer, M.
1974 Reality Shock: Why Nurses Leave Nursing. St. Louis: Mosby.

Levinson, R.
1976 "Sexism in medicine." American Journal of Nursing 31(March):426–431.

Marlow, D. R.
1973 Textbook of Pediatric Nursing. 4th ed. Philadelphia: Saunders, 61.

Millet K.
1970 Sexual Politics. New York: Doubleday.

Parsons, T.
1954 "An analytical approach to the theories of social stratification." Pp. 69-88 in T.

Parsons (ed.), Essays in Sociological Theory. Glencoe, Ill.: Free Press.

Rach, E., and S. Lipset
1959 Prejudice and Society. New York: The Anti-defamation League of B'Nai B'rith.

Raven, B. H.
1978 "Social power, social influence, and nosocomial infection control." UCLA/S–A9–1, February.

Raven, B. H. and R. W. Haley
1980 "Social influence in a medical context." Pp. 255–278 in L. Buckman (ed.), Applied Social Psychology Annual. 1: Beverly Hills, Calif.: Sage.

Reeder, S.
1978 "The social context of nursing." Pp. 235–245 in N. Chaska (ed.), The Nursing Profession: Views through the Mist. New York: McGraw-Hill.

Reeder, S. and H. Mauksch
1979 "Nursing: Continuing change." Pp. 206–230 in H. Freeman et al. (eds.), The Handbook of Medical Sociology. New York: Prentice-Hall.

Reeder, S. and S. Stevens
(Forthcoming) "Assertive behavior in nurses and collegial staff relations: Implications for patient care practices."

Schaffner, W.
1977 "Humans, the animate reservoir of nosocomial pathogens." Pp. 57–70 in K. R. Cundy and W. Ball (eds.), Infection Control in Health Care Facilities. Baltimore: University Park Press.

Scully, D. and P. Bart
1973 "A funny thing happened on the way to the orifice: Women in gynecological textbooks." American Journal of Sociology 78:1045–1050.

Smoyak, S. A.
1977 "Problems in interprofessional relations." Bulletin of the New York Academy of Medicine 53(Jan.-Feb.):51–59.

Solomon, D.
1957 "Professional persons in bureaucratic organizations." Pp. 253–266 in Symposium on Preventive and Social Psychiatry, Washington, D.C.: Walter Reed Army Institute of Research.

Spock, H.
  1971 Decent and Indecent. New York: Fawcett.
Stein, L. I.
  1967 "The doctor-nurse game." Archives of
         General Psychiatry 16:699–703.
Wardwell, W. I.
  1955 "Social integration, bureaucratization and
         professions." Social Forces 34:356–359.
Weber, M.
  1947 The Theory of Social and Economic
         Organization. New York: University Press.

Williams, R. E. O.
  1970 "Changing perspectives in hospital infec-
         tions." Pp. 1–10 in Proceedings of the
         International Conference on Nosocomial
         Infection Control. Center for Disease
         Control. August.
Willson, J. R., C. T. Bechman, and E. R. Carrington
  1975 Obstetrics and Gynecology. 5th ed. St.
         Louis: Mosby.

Chapter 39

The Cooperation Model for Care in Health and Illness

Patricia MacElveen-Hoehn, R.N., Ph.D.
Research Fellow
Department of Parent and Child Nursing
School of Nursing
University of Washington
Seattle, Washington

As evident in the previous chapters, the importance of cooperation/collaboration among health professionals in providing health and illness care cannot be overstated. It is equally essential that the client be included in collaboration. Patricia MacElveen-Hoehn aptly presents a model for cooperation that is overdue. She examines cooperation as a concept, describes the cooperation model, empirical testing, and indicates implications for nursing practice and education.

In its simplest form, cooperation implies two or more persons acting together to achieve a mutual goal. Five elements of cooperation are vital. For a clearer understanding of the concept, the characteristics of cooperation are contrasted with those of competition. This is done by utilizing nine factors: goals, means, attributes, mutuality, power, conflict, communication, resources, and internal forms (alliances/coalitions). Four stages are identified as being necessary in developing cooperation. These include members having an individual model of what is expected, agreeing on goals, developing mutual trust, and learning each others' working styles.

MacElveen-Hoehn reports research that indicates cooperative groups tend to view themselves as more interdependent. She speaks to the issues of shifting politics in health care, patient power, and incongruent perspectives between the client and care provider. A negotiated level of health between the client and care provider is advocated. The process used to accomplish this is essentially cooperative.

MacElveen-Hoehn explicates the cooperative triad model in health care: the consumer, a person important to the consumer (family), and care provider. She emphasizes that relationships are interdependent, power and status differences are deemphasized,

Development of this model was supported by Grants Nos. 5T32 NU-07004-03 and 5T01-05008 and Grant NU00472, from the Division of Nursing, Bureau of Health Manpower, Health Resources Administration, Department of Health and Human Services.

and the triad feels more satisfied with the management of care. A variety of health and illness situations and settings are discussed for application of the model. Factors which may inhibit development of cooperation are illustrated.

Empirical testing of the model occurred within the home dialysis triad. In Mac Elveen-Hoehn's research four factors, previously identified by Jordan as significant for cooperation, were included. These were shared common goals, consensus on the means to pursue goals, trust, and mutuality of perception. She also included five patient outcome measures of physical, psychological, and social factors: physical status, adherence to the medical regimen, total activity, morale, and positive affect. A combined measure was developed for cooperation. Data were gathered during home interviews from patients, the family member who assisted in the dialysis, and the care provider. Two studies were conducted—the first in Denver with a patient sample of 21 and the second in Seattle that included 36 patients. The findings indicate that common goals and means are related to the patient's total activity. Mutuality of perception and trust are related to physical status, adherence, total activity, and morale. Analysis of the dyads within each triad show that the patient-partner dyad was significantly related to total activity. The patient-doctor dyad was significantly related to physical status and to adherence to the medical regimen. The findings support the general hypothesis that cooperation would be associated with better patient outcomes.

MacElveen-Hoehn transfers the application of the cooperation model to the hospice home care triad, the hypertension management triad, and the prenatal care triad. In so doing, she notes quality of life issues of concern to patients and provides specific examples of negotiating health goals. Application of the cooperation model where children are part of the triad is also considered. She offers the cooperation model for nursing practice stressing the interdependence of all who are involved with a client's care. MacElveen-Hoehn demonstrates application of the model to nursing education, specifically in her discussion of faculty role modeling and the relationship between a teacher and student. She suggests provocative questions for research concerning cooperation in care. Strategies to improve outcomes in adherence behavior are offered for problematic situations. The value in testing the cooperation model in acute care settings and with control groups is recognized.

INTRODUCTION

Cooperation in the delivery of health and illness care is almost an obvious assumption, an unquestionable good. Cooperation implies two or more persons or entities acting jointly for their mutual profit or common benefit. In the delivery of care there is minimally a provider and a consumer. On a larger scale, a group including several disciplines might cooperate in providing health and illness services to an entire community. The major goals for all the above would be achieving the highest level of wellness for the consumers of the care. The care providers experience rewards from those health outcomes as a result of their partici-

pation and activities. Satisfactions for the care providers also accrue from the opportunities for mastering challenges, solving problems, and providing services and from the economic and social benefits of their professional status.

A more formal definition of cooperation derived by Marwell and Schmitt (1975:5-9) from numerous studies suggests the complexity of cooperation and the spectrum of situations in which it may occur. This definition includes five elements. Most writers characterize cooperation first by *efforts toward a desired outcome or goal* and second by the fact that *all the participants are rewarded. Distributed responses*, the third element, refers to whether a division of labor is or is not required for goal achievement. The fourth element, *coordination*, becomes necessary if the responses need to occur in an order or in relation to one another. Finally, if participants synchronize their activities by monitoring cues from each other's behavior, the fifth element, *social coordination*, obtains.

Thus, while many people desire a vaccine or cure for cancer, only a relatively small number of individuals are actively involved in the search. When a vaccine or cure is discovered, large sectors of the population will share in the benefits. In this case, the first two elements apply. In contrast, operation of an intensive care unit would involve all five elements from the identification of shared goals to social coordination. Given that cooperation has advantages for everyone involved, it follows that people should want to cooperate in most situations. What do we know of the occurrence, development, maintenance, or deterioration of cooperation? In health and illness care does cooperation make a difference, or do people working cooperatively simply get along better? A crucial question is: Do we have any evidence that cooperation makes a difference for persons receiving care?

In this chapter, cooperation as a concept will be explored and the cooperation model will be described. Empirical testing of the model will be discussed, and its implications for nursing practice and nursing education will be presented.

HISTORICAL ROOTS OF COOPERATION

A Strategy for Survival

Working together for the good of the group is frequently demonstrated in animal life. In herds the female and the young are often gathered into the center with the males on the perimeter protecting against predators and other dangers. Migrating geese generate enormous aerodynamic efficiency by flying together in V formations. Bees have specialized tasks that are highly coordinated for the maintenance of the hive. There is

little doubt that cooperation among groups of early peoples contributed to their survival.

Human organization from the family to the United Nations is enhanced by cooperative efforts. A concern today is that contemporary civilization has the capacity for total destruction if nations of the world cannot live together cooperatively. How strange it is that something as essential to evolution and the survival of the human race is in jeopardy! When not cooperating, an individual, group, or nation might choose to minimize interaction and remain withdrawn or isolated. Sometimes the interactions are dominated by competition, everyone wanting the prize or power to the exclusion of others. The nature of a particular relationship might include all the above.

From a systems perspective, we can observe members of an athletic team competing with one another for positions on the first team. They also cooperate in practice sessions and especially when they are out to win a game against another team. The teams cooperate to play the scheduled game and to participate in their league activity (their common goals). They do this by agreeing to sets of rules governing play of the game and membership in their league. This type of analysis can be applied to families, small groups, organizations, and international relations.

Development of the Concept of the Cooperative Triad

The study of cooperation in the social sciences emerged with a concomitant interest in competition (Maller, 1929; May and Dobb, 1937; Mead, 1937). Inquiry focused on the differences between these phenomena, on their effects on individuals, groups, societies, and on the relative outcomes of socialistic versus capitalistic forms of economies. In the next decades emphasis shifted to more specific questions about the choice between cooperation and competition and the study of power and conflict within a competitive ethos (Deutsch, 1949a; Mills, 1954; Caplow, 1956, 1959, 1970; Vinacke and Arkoff, 1957; Stryker and Psathas,

1960). This work was influenced by two factors: renewed fascination with Simmel's (1950) triad and the use of game theory in controlled laboratory experiments. [Detailed discussions of these studies can be found in MacElveen, 1971; MacElveen et al., 1975a.]

The high propensity for the three elements of the triad to shift into a 2-against-1 configuration identified by Simmel (1950) fostered the investigation of coalition formation and other strategies for winning. These studies were theoretically productive. Findings, however, were not verified when coalition theory was applied to families in the world outside the laboratory (Strodtbeck, 1954; Caplow, 1959).

Less attention has been addressed to the research of triads not dominated by the instigation of conflict and the acquisition or protection of power. Addition of a third element often strengthens the relationship of an existing dyad by providing a channel for new mutual interests and concerns, as when the birth of a child produces another perhaps indirect bond between parents (Simmel, 1950). An issue raised for this researcher was that maximal benefits available to the child in that triad depends on the measure of harmony and cooperation between the parents. According to Haley (1969) the presence of coalitions in families was an indication of their pathology. In healthy families alliances that do form tend to be transitory and situational. The term *alliance* is used here to mean a strengthened bond between two members directed towards maintaining the triad as beneficial to all members. This is in contrast to the definition of coalition defined as 2 against 1.

Alliance in triads has also been described in relation to cotherapists working with one client or one family (Burgess and Lazure, 1970; Rubenstein and Weiner, 1967). These triads fulfill the characteristics of cooperative triads although the authors do not identify with that concept. The use of triad dynamics as interventions in family therapy has grown out of the seminal work by Haley (1969), Zuk (1971), and Stachowiak (1975).

The significance of cooperative triad dynamics goes beyond the three-person nuclear family as natural triads are everywhere, e.g., parent-student-teacher, labor-management-arbitrator, buyer-seller-real estate agent. Triads have been emphasized here because of their frequent occurrence in health and illness care settings. The basic elements of the care triad involve the relationships among: the consumer of the services; a person important to the consumer, usually a family member, close friend, or partner; and the care provider who might be, e.g., a nurse practitioner, physician, social worker, nutritionist, or counselor.

Before leaving the issues of cooperation and competition, major differences between cooperative and competitive triads will be articulated. This comparison will provide cues which signal whether cooperation is indeed operating, to what degree, or how frequently. Nine factors derived from the literature cited above are used to compare ideal types (extreme cases) of these two kinds of triads: (1) goals, (2) means to achieve the goals, (3) member attributes, (4) mutuality, (5) power, (6) conflict, (7) communications, (8) resources, and (9) internal forms.

Cooperative triads	Competitive triads
1 Goals	
The common goal(s) are shared by each member and available to all or none. Members' other goals are complementary or irrelevant to the common goals. Conflict between personal goals and the common goals must be resolved.	All members strive to attain the same goal(s), which are available only to one to the exclusion of the others. Most goals are oriented to superior positions or power to control others and to monopolize the available advantage.

Cooperative triads	Competitive triads
2 Means	
Activities and strategies towards goal attainment are defined, and members' individual contributions are agreed upon. The division of labor is integrated and coordinated.	Individual and private efforts are used to pursue the goals. No division of labor exists except to the degree necessary to maintain a coalition if it is present.
3 Attributes	
Each member's contributions are essential and may be related to the member's characteristics or resources. Differences are unimportant and in the division of labor they are often complementary.	Only attributes related to power or member's vulnerability are important.
4 Mutuality	
Interdependence and reciprocity are high. Behavior related to the common goals is predictable. Trust is critical to interdependence. Rewards and satisfaction are exchanged en route to the goal. An alliance compensates for temporary inability of one member to perform.	Interdependence is low. Reciprocity is dictated by the relative power positions. Members are in association either because of proximity or because they interact in their contention for the goal. The level of trust is low.
5 Power	
Differences in power are expected and modified by interdependence. A democratic process dominates decision making and other processes. Members' domains of knowledge and skills are recognized. Leadership is a reflection of expertise salient to specific tasks or phases and therefore exercised by different members at different times.	Power differences and rivalry for control or the superior position are the primary focus here. Autocracy prevails; coalitions occur as power strategies. Leadership is tied less to knowledge and skill than to the locus of power and control.
6 Conflict	
Discord can emerge around, e.g., goals, means to goals, or members' contributions. Overt conflict can be a useful impetus toward tension reduction, positive change, creative problem solving, and increased cohesiveness. Covert conflict is short-lived as a function of trust and openness of the communication channels.	The major source of contention is implicit in the struggle for individual power. Conflict is a frequently used strategy to prevent the formulation of coalitions: divide and conquer. While two members are occupied in dispute, the third may gain some advantage. Both covert and overt conflict may persist for long periods.
7 Communication	
The free flow of accurate information expedites all triad interactions and activities. Control of content is minimal. Results of effective communication are: minimal tensions, understanding of goal-related activities, sharing of resources, and mutual	Dissemination of information is limited and selective. Transfer of inaccurate information is a strategy using lies and propaganda. Exchanges are often formal and guarded and may exclude a third member (secrets). This type of communication results in ambiguity, discomfort, fear,

Cooperative triads	Competitive triads
support. Breakdown of good communication is a danger signal and can threaten survival of the cooperative triad.	suspicion, and distrust.

8 Resources

Cooperative triads	Competitive triads
Member assets necessary for goal attainment and for exchanging satisfactions and rewards might include: knowledge, skills, strength, health, status, values, motivations, wealth, emotions, personnel, physical facilities, equipment, and access to assets external to the triad. Resources are shared primarily in relation to the common goal but sometimes also in response to individual members' needs.	Members tend to hoard their assets, which are similar to assets listed for the cooperative triad. Little concern is expressed for other members. Sharing occurs in coalitions only to the extent required for maintenance of that bond. Every advantage is used to gain control over resources of other members.

9 Internal Forms

Cooperative triads	Competitive triads
Temporary alliances of two members may occur in response to attempted withdrawal or inadequate performance of a third member. The alliance strives to prevent isolation of the third member and to preserve the integrity of the triad by increasing inputs of the members in the alliance. Prolonged necessity for an alliance can threaten to exceed the endurance of the two members. In this case, replacement of the nonperforming member may occur, the triad may strain toward dissolution, or the nature of the triad may change from its original purpose.	Formation of coalitions of 2 against 1 is determined by the distribution of power, bargaining positions, and temporal situation of the triad. Coalitions shift the balance of power, e.g., two weak members may use their combined strengths to be stronger than the strongest individual member. Other coalitions are used to ensure the position of the individual with the greatest power. Which members will form coalitions is predictable in specific situations if the initial distribution of power is known. Formation of the coalition occurs with little concern for the fate of the triad itself. Dissolution of the triad may even be to the advantage of those in the coalition.

Agreeing to work together does not always guarantee that cooperation will occur. Jordan et al. (1963) identified four stages necessary to the development of cooperation in a task-oriented group. At first, all members had an *individual model* of what they were supposed to do, the components of the tasks, the nature of the desired outcome, and how to achieve them. In the second stage, through interaction and learning about each other, a *homologous model* evolved, the members reaching agreement on the goals to be pursued and how they would be achieved. The third stage was the manifestation of *trust*. Members perceived that the others had the necessary competencies and were reliable. While trust is essential to cooperation, trust alone is not enough to generate cooperation. The fourth stage involved the lengthy and comprehensive process by which members learned each other's working styles, developed clear communication and the most comfortable and efficient patterns of working together, i.e., *learning to cooperate*. The development of cooperation is a process which takes time and interaction among the people working together. However, in addition to achieving the shared end goals, there are other payoffs which make cooperation rewarding.

In comparing small groups motivated by cooperation or competition, Deutsch (1949b) found vast differences between them. The cooperative groups perceived themselves as more interdependent: allowed more "substitutability" for similarly intended actions and showed more positive affect, less resistance, and more helpfulness to each other than groups motivated by competition. The latter showed less coordination of efforts, less subdivision of activities and diversity of contributions among members, less attentiveness to fellow members and comprehension of communications, less orientation and orderliness, less productivity per time unit, lower quality of product and discussions, less friendliness, and other unfavorable characteristics. The author concluded that greater group or organizational productivity results from cooperative relationships.

Emphasis on the concept of cooperation does not deny that there are many situations where individuals make independent decisions to deal with health problems alone. For example: a woman with stress incontinence chose to manage her symptom by herself with perineal exercises, by not jumping a lot, and by crossing her legs when sneezing. This personal decision continued for many years to avoid the surgery of a vaginal repair, involving neither a care provider nor her family in this matter.

Many people maintain dyadic relationships with care providers who never see the client's family. Adult family members often do not accompany one another to the care provider for routine visits or for minor complaints. A partner may never meet the woman's gynecologist or she may never meet her partner's internist of long association. At other times individuals purposefully maintain an exclusive dyadic relationship with the care provider because they do not want their family involved. Care providers are rarely interested in meeting family members. Not surprisingly, care providers and family members often collide in the emergency room or the coronary care unit as strangers participating in the same crisis. Sometimes, even among patients with long-term health problems and life-threatening illness, a dyadic relationship with the primary care provider is maintained. This may work well unless trouble or a severe illness occurs, when indeed cooperative efforts among the care triad members would be necessary.

The Politics of Care

Inherent in the shifting politics of health care as a right rather than a privilege is the issue of patient power. In the past, patients exchanged their power and control for being taken care of and for a reduction in their role responsibilities (Parsons, 1964:436-447). This was a paternalistic dictatorship model: the wise doctor knew what was best for the patient, who was expected to follow the doctor's orders. This model was congruent with the educational level of the population about health, the position of high-status males, and the concept of health care as a privilege in our society.

Today's population is better educated and more knowledgeable about health. Many people are interested in such self-care programs as stress management, weight control, and exercise. There is a growing willingness to assume conscious responsibility for one's own health. Many people want more information about being healthy, disease processes, treatment alternatives, and drugs they are taking. The advent of birthing centers and living wills points towards greater consumer participation in the planning and decision making of their own care. These and other consumer issues are eloquently described in The Rights of Hospital Patients (Annas, 1975).

The old model is becoming obsolete, and the move to a democratic, cooperation model is evident. The collaboration of clients, their family members, and care providers to maximize the health potential of the client is logically and politically appealing. Goals and means to achieve the goals are germane to cooperation. Compliance to regimens (often an important means to health goals) is rarely perfect and sometimes as such can be life-threatening. This raises cogent questions about agreement of the health goals and how to achieve them.

Treatment goals of patient, therapist, and

family member were compared in an inpatient mental health center in an effort to evaluate treatment outcomes. Only a random relationship was found among these goals. Therapist prediction of how patients would rank-order their own goals was used as a measure of empathy and failed to achieve more than a random relationship. If treatment success is premised on achievement of treatment goals, the failure to identify a common goal or even its emergence over treatment time has gross implications for the establishment of cooperation among those involved in the efforts to get the patient "well" (Polak, 1970).

A Negotiated Level of Health

Most care providers perceive a level of wellness potentially available to an individual if the specified regimen is followed. They also have expectations about the long-term consequences of health-related behaviors. They want the people they care for to have as long and healthy a life as possible.

The client's perspective on the cost-benefit ratio of the regimen differs from that of the care provider. Clients experience costs in such terms as expenses, time, energy, and space. Conflicts may exist between the regimen and the client's lifestyle, values, and self-image. Part or all of the regimen may be congruent with other psychological, social, cultural, or religious factors. Benefits from following the regimen might be relief from discomforting symptoms or their prevention or control. A sense of successful self-management can generate feelings of mastery and competence and relief of pain, itching, burning, nausea, dyspnea, etc., reinforcing the use of the regimen. No experience of impact or negative consequences from adherence to the regimen tends to reduce adherence behavior. A classic situation is the management of the asymptomatic condition of high blood pressure. Following the regimen does not make the client "feel better"; in fact, side effects of the medications may make him or her feel worse. Severe side effects, such as impotence for the rest of a male client's life, may be too

high a cost for the benefit promised. The benefit is a probability (not assurance) that he will not die of stroke, renal failure, or heart disease. If the drugs necessary to maintain his blood pressure at the safe 140 over 90 mmHg level are unacceptable, he may abandon treatment and be completely unprotected.

An alternative to either treatment or no treatment options is what I term a *negotiated level of health*. Client and care provider would collaborate to find the drug which would provide the greatest control of the blood pressure within the tolerance of the client. The negotiated level of health might be control at 200 over 110 mmHg. This is far preferable to no control at all. The basic question is: Do we as care providers believe that the individual has the right to make an informed choice, and are we willing to negotiate the level of health we will agree to work on together? [See Enos and Nilsson (1975) for a detailed description of client goals theory, which addresses this and other goal issues.]

Cooperation in the Nursing Tradition

The medical model has focused on disease and pathological processes and has yielded the care and/or control of many previously fatal diseases. Because of the medical-biotechnologic advances, large segments of the population now have years of extended life within the framework of disability or chronic illness. Such compromised levels of health often include a multitude of challenges for the individuals, their families, and even their communities.

In contrast, from Nightingale in the mid-1800s to the theorists of the last three decades, nursing has focused on the promotion and maintenance of health (The Nursing Theories Conference Group, 1980). This concept addressed the maximal level of wellness available to the individual (group or community) and included physical, psychosocial, cultural, spiritual, and environmental factors. Clients' active participation in goal setting and care plans to achieve the goals (major components of the nursing process) are described by, e.g., Peplau (1952), Orem (1971), Weidenbach (1964), Rogers (1970), Roy (1976), King (1971), Enos and Nilsson (1975), and in ANA (American Nurses' Association) Standards of Care III, IV, and VIII (1973). Emphasis has been on needs of the patient as a total person and as a member of a family (Bowar-Ferres, 1975).

Client goals theory is based on the belief that it is appropriate to involve clients in all phases of the nursing process. This involvement will "enhance the quality of care, facilitate higher levels of health for the client, and change the role of the nurse from 'care giver' to 'care collaborator'" (Enos and Nilsson, 1975:3). The basic concepts of the theory include "(1) client involvement, (2) a holistic approach, (3) negotiated health goals, (4) nurse advocate, (5) increased nurse satisfaction, and (6) increased health care satisfaction" (Enos and Nilsson, 1975:11). The described process by which goals are negotiated and the plan for goal pursuit established are essentially cooperative although there is no emphasis on the triad per se. This theory is used as the basis for nursing practice and nursing education.

In the Veterans' Administration health facilities, increasing emphasis is placed on patients' participation in the efforts for recovery from illness and in self-care responsibilities for promoting and maintaining their health. Hefferin (forthcoming) investigated the effects of an intervention designed to facilitate the collaboration of patients and their nurse in: (1) setting their health goals; (2) setting target dates for achieving the goals; and (3) establishing responsibilities of patients and nurses in pursuit of the identified goals. The experimental design compared 288 experimental subjects with 288 control subjects; 50 nurses participated. In the experimental group, patients and nurses developed the goal statements together; nurses independently defined goals for the control group. Goal attainment scaling was used to measure changes in patients' health status, and questionnaires were developed to measure patient and nurse satisfaction with selected health care ac-

tivities. Hefferin concluded that patients who helped develop their care goals had more positive change in their health status in fewer days than did the control group. Patients from the goals development group were more satisfied than the control group. Nurses themselves experienced greater satisfaction when working collaboratively with patients than they did with the control group. These significant findings suggest that participation of patients in their own care had positive outcomes for them and for the nurses.

DEFINITION OF TERMS

Client, patient, and *consumer* are terms used interchangeably here, although with some special emphasis as follows:

Client implies the existence of an *ongoing relationship* for the purpose of obtaining specific professional services. The client may be, e.g., an individual, couple, family, group, organization, or community.

Patient implies a person *receiving care or treatment for a pathological condition* or a sick person unable to care for him or herself who receives care and assistance.

Consumer implies a *user of goods or services to satisfy a need* (rather than to resell them or produce other goods with them). The phrase "to satisfy" suggests an evaluation of the goods or services and an accountability for their quality.

Care provider designates the entity furnishing health-illness services. The care provider may be an individual, e.g., a pediatric nurse practitioner, a nutritionist, or a nephrologist. The care provider might also refer, for example, to an interdisciplinary team including health and illness professionals and some members of the patient's family.

Family here refers primarily to those most apt to be involved in a person's health-illness care and whose lives are most apt to be affected by the level of that person's well-being. Family is used in the broad sense meaning those people bonded by affection and/or mutual obligation. Thus, family here includes not only kin related by blood or legal ties but also close friends or those persons regarded as important or significant others. Often unrecognized is the homosexual patient's partner, who is usually the primary support person. When such a partner, for example, is excluded from the intensive care unit because of not being "family," the patient is deprived of an important component of his or her therapeutic environment.

Partner is used here with two connotations. First, as a family member sharing the life with another and usually living together, e.g., spouse, homosexual mate, significant other, parent, sibling, son, or daughter. The second connotation is that of being the family member who is most involved with the health or illness regimen.

Collaborate and *cooperate* are used interchangeably and both mean to work or labor together. The term *cooperation* is more commonly associated with a joint effort in which the benefits or profits are shared by all who are involved.

THE HEALTH CARE CONSUMER, SELF-CARE, AND COOPERATION

In order to participate effectively in planning and decision making, health care consumers usually require information, knowledge, and skills. In making these available, the care provider affirms the client since these experiences promote competency and legitimize the right to self-determination. This process empowers the client, whereas the traditional medical approach exchanged power for care. In the cooperative triad model, inclusion of the family allows for its participation and for the formation of an alliance of care provider and family when the client is unable to be actively involved. This model of providing services alters the role of the care provider, as when the client and the family do the dialysis treatment themselves at home. The care provider's role is not diminished by that transfer of care procedure responsibility. Instead, other role behaviors are expanded, e.g., assessing, teaching, supporting, and preparing those involved for changes that may be coming or emergencies that may happen.

The relationships are interdependent, with power and status differences deemphasized and the consumer, the family, and the care provider feeling more satisfied in the management of the situation.

The Actors and Their Roles

Consideration of the cooperation model in a variety of health and illness situations indicates its underlying salience with respect to the functions of relationships in the nursing process. In seeking means to higher levels of health, clients approach the care providers as consultants who are resources for special knowledge, have information about availability of services, options, and strategies, and are often the teachers from whom to learn new skills and knowledge. The occasions for increasing the level of health might include: a visit for help with family planning decisions, classes to understand pregnancy and prepare for childbirth, visits to a well baby clinic, a workshop in holistic health, a clinic program for stress management, a weight reduction program, and a group for women in transition. Contact with the care provider in these instances is often limited, intermittent, and highly specific. In some the individual may approach the care provider alone, and in others we readily see the consumer-family–care provider triad.

In acute care settings patients are often temporarily incapacitated by: pain and other distresses, altered levels of consciousness, effects of pathological process on body integrity, and impact of therapeutic interventions. The care providers may need to act quickly by applying knowledge and skills in an intensely focused manner, as is seen in acute care hospitals, especially in emergency rooms, trauma and burn units, intensive care units, and operating rooms. The presence of family to support the patient and/or to enter into an alliance with the care provider is evident. In other inpatient units, the relationships reflect the critical nature of interdependence, patient and family participation, accountability of the care providers, and the efforts of all to work together effectively. Patient contact with the care providers is frequent, intimate, and continuous. The dynamics of how all members of the care triad participate in efforts toward their common goals are important to optimal outcomes for patients whether they are experiencing, for example, a cerebral vascular accident, herniorrhaphy, leg amputation, extensive burns, a myocardial infarction, chemotherapy for cancer, insulin reaction, or diagnostic tests.

When the health care problem is long-term, it may be comparatively stable (e.g., hemiplegia, diabetes), have remissions and exacerbations (e.g., multiple sclerosis, chronic leukemia) or may be a progressive deterioration (e.g., muscular dystrophy, amyotrophic lateral sclerosis). During the course of these long-term health problems, care may occur in the full range of health facilities: outpatient clinics or doctor's office, acute care hospital, rehabilitation program, limited care facility, nursing home. However, for the majority of these clients the greatest amount of care is at home. Self-care regimens involve monitoring and controlling symptoms and doing treatment procedures. Managing an optimal quality of life within the limitations imposed by the pathology and the regimen itself is a major life challenge.

The interaction of long-term health problems and the client's life-style depends on many factors. The greater the life-style change required, the greater the number of coping skills that are necessary. Change for the clients reverberates in the family system. It is the client and family who must deal on the everyday, year-after-year basis. Role relationships, use of family system resources, and power, goals, and dreams of the future are some of the areas affected by long-term health problems. The family must respond to changes in a member's health status, to the grieving for the inevitable series of losses, and to the shifting nature of its hopes and must provide opportunities for all to meet their needs for healthy growth and development. That in itself would be a demanding agenda if that were the total list. In addition, the system must respond to the many factors in all members' lives and to factors in the external environment.

Sensitivity to the contributions of the family in the cooperative triad as well as those of the client is paramount. Support from the care provider to family members acknowledging the challenges they face, the responses they make, and the right to take care of themselves can influence their continued cooperation in the care triad. In a sense they pool their resources and engage in high interpersonal risk, i.e., they invest much and risk how well their lives will fare under the threat of the long-term health problem. The result of feeling exploited in this situation is likely to be withdrawal of cooperation; reduction of that sense of risk of exploitation could conceivably allow for the reestablishment of cooperation (Marwell and Schmitt, 1975:181–186).

The care providers have limited knowledge and skills to respond to the physical and emotional manifestations of many long-term health problems. It is the successful clients who create the reward in their lives, who are innovative problem solvers, who manage the demands of their health limitations while creating opportunities for high-quality life experiences. It is the special clients whom the care providers see the least who have the most to teach us. They are a tremendous (and, too often, untapped) resource for care providers and other clients facing the same challenges. Many long-term care clients have contact with numerous care providers with various frequencies at various times depending on their health needs. Lack of a consistent care provider who provides continuity over a period of time has implications for the triad dynamics, especially in terms of the accumulated history of experiences together, consistency of approach, and definition of the situation. Clients and family carry the bulk of the responsibility over time, but the intermittent contacts with their care provider are critical and the strength of an established cooperative relationship is a source of great comfort and security even when it is not being actively used.

Other Important Factors

The establishment of cooperation may be confounded by factors that make up the less than perfect real world of clients and families. At any given time individuals have their own particular dynamics, life-style, levels of functioning, developmental tasks, coping resources and patterns, psychological assets, social network resources, life-change events, and other stressors. It is important to recognize that for some people illness, with all its discomforts, inconveniences, and disruption of life, provides an opportunity to meet needs that sometimes cannot be met in more healthy ways. Illness can justify and legitimize time away from a stressful job, a needed rest, or not performing family role obligations. Being sick can elicit caring behaviors from others for people who are unable or unwilling to ask for what they want to meet their dependency needs. Sometimes, if the perception is that no caring person is available, being hospitalized is a way to be taken care of, at least for a brief period. Usually these processes occur unconsciously. In such cases the issue of the need to use illness for secondary gain cannot be ignored because of the difficulty in defining common goals in the care triad.

Families, being ongoing systems, also have dynamics, levels of functioning, developmental tasks, coping resources and patterns, psychological assets, network resources, and stressors. Illness of a family member at times may serve some important function in the maintenance of the family system. This is likely to be out of awareness of the family members, and the illness of that member may be promoted rather than his or her health. Such a problem works against potential treatment goals when the latent motivation of the family is not wellness. Family therapy may be necessary to assist with the movement towards health for all family members.

A client's or a family's priorities may differ from those of the care provider. Addressing their priorities in the plans for care is essential before they can invest in the efforts towards promoting the client's health goals. If the care provider does not hear those other priorities or if the climate of trust is inadequate to allow them to be verbalized, the care provider may be working against conflict-

ing goals or may find that the client and family are not contributing to the efforts toward achievement of the identified goals.

Situations also occur in which the behavior of the care providers inhibits the establishment or maintenance of cooperation. Most often this happens while the care providers have the best interest of the client at heart. They may not acknowledge the expertise that someone with a long-term health problem has about his or her own care and ignore or try to oppose that self-care knowledge. Biases related to sexuality may preclude their recognition or appreciation of the many sexual issues in health and in illness. Personal experience may limit their ability to envision the potentials a disabled person may have for independent living, work, relationships, or parenting. Prejudices about the superiority of the illness care system may render them closed about alternative approaches and less familiar treatment modalities. Stereotyping of people based on age, race, ethnicity, socioeconomic status, or specific group membership reflects ignorance and is unlikely to generate that trust among client, family, and care providers which is essential to cooperation.

These issues are raised here to alert the care provider to some of the subtle factors that may inhibit the development of cooperation or even sabotage the plans and decisions which appear to have been a collaborative enterprise. As can be seen, disruptive influences can be located in any corner of the triad.

EMPIRICAL TESTS OF THE COOPERATION MODEL: THE HOME DIALYSIS TRIAD

The two treatment options in response to end-stage renal disease (ESRD) are transplantation and dialysis. The latter treatment consists of either hemodialysis or peritoneal dialysis, both procedures which can be managed at home or in a dialysis center. Empirical testing of the cooperation model occurred within the context of the home hemodialysis triad. Someone, often a spouse or parent, assists the patient with the dialysis treatment and related tasks. Care providers are exceedingly important during the home training period and during the period of maintenance dialysis which follows.

This highly technological treatment is paired with a demanding regimen of fluid and diet restrictions, medications, blood chemistries, care of the shunt or fistula, and the unending dialysis schedule. The psychosocial impact of dependence on the artificial kidney machine permeates the life space of the patient and of the family (MacElveen, 1977).

The patient must be highly motivated to live in order to deal effectively with the many real and potential losses that may be confronted. These losses relate to life itself, to health, and to physical and mental capacities. The self-image and self-esteem are jeopardized by resulting changes in physical appearance; reduced libido and potency; alterations in family and in occupational and social role performance. Self-sufficiency, independence, and control—important to many people —are under assault. Membership in groups and in community and recreational activities are commonly curtailed. There are the losses of time, energy, freedom, and often future plans and dreams. The monumental challenges, fears, and dysfunctional responses have been recognized as profound obstacles to be overcome in the efforts toward an acceptable quality of life (Abram, 1968; Anger, 1975; Ebra and Tolt, 1972; Fredrich, 1980; Jackle, 1974; Levy, 1974; Pierce, 1975; Hedenberg, 1980).

Dialysis introduces a profound new element into the family system which elicits adaptation to the changes in the patient. The initial adjustments are the beginning of a long series of issues and complications. The differences in the patient's sense of self, interpersonal dynamics, and role performance resonate within the family system. Therefore, spouses, parents, children, and partner experience their own set of real or potential losses and challenges (Hoover et al., 1975). Responses to dialysis reflect the family's psychosocial resources and coping patterns: some families become closer and more competent; some struggle just to survive;

some are overwhelmed; some vacillate among many of these states (Alexander and MacElveen, 1978; Kossoris, 1970). All families, however, have their limits in their ability to transcend trouble that is too great, too frequent, or of too long a duration. Care providers need to be sensitive to the cumulative impact of troubles on families with ongoing major health challenges.

In spite of the formidable demands of life with the artificial kidney machine, many patients and families do manage to integrate it into a satisfying and productive life-style. In addition, home dialysis is far more economical than in-center dialysis. Patients have greater flexibility and control over their treatments and schedules, enjoying greater independence, fewer physical problems, and less hepatitis. Home dialysis patients have been reported to have higher rehabilitation rates than their in-center peers (Blagg, 1972).

My interest in the importance of cooperation in ESRD was generated during several months of nonparticipant observation in a hemodialysis center. The uniqueness of the important contributions of the patients themselves, their families, and the center staff was highly visible in this setting. When everyone was collaborating, the chances of success for the person on dialysis seemed to be remarkably potentiated. The successful achievement of desired outcomes was generally related to uneventful, fairly comfortable dialysis runs; adherence to the regimen; optimal health within the parameters of ESRD; and the ability to fulfill work, family, and social roles and to maintain high morale in spite of the limitations and demands of a life dependent on the artificial kidney machine. Achievement of these goals was fundamental to everyone involved. When goals were being achieved, the quality of the patient's life was enhanced and good feelings of accomplishment were shared by all. When there was conflict about the goals or everyone's efforts were not forthcoming, complications, trouble, illness, frustration, helplessness, anger, sadness, and depression were often observed. When there was unresolved conflict or prolonged inadequate performance of patient or family or the major care provider, success as described above was impossible.

Characteristics of Cooperation Critical to Care

In applying the cooperative triad model to care situations, all the factors used above to contrast the cooperative and competitive triad are salient. From Jordan et al.'s (1963) work on how co-operation develops, four factors emerge as germane. All members must *share common goals* that they understand in the same way. There must be a *consensus on the means* to pursue those goals; members must know their roles and what each one will contribute. Members must be able to *trust* each other, knowing the others can be relied upon to do what is expected of them relative to the goals. Getting to know other members well enough to cooperate involves a lengthy process and eventual predictability of each other's goal-related attitudes and behaviors, i.e., *a mutuality of perception.*

When these factors are operating, the social environment is fertile for good communication, sharing of resources, interdependence, efficient coordination of activities, and other benefits associated with cooperative behavior.

In the Denver study (MacElveen, 1971, 1973), the first two characteristics were combined into *goal and means*. This compromise occurred because the methodological feasibility of generating data to determine a consensus on means to achieve goals was beyond the limits of that work. Co-operation was a combined measure of the following:

1 Triad *goals and means:* a calculation of

$$3 \times \begin{matrix} \text{Common} \\ \text{Goals} \end{matrix} - \begin{matrix} \text{Conflicting} \\ \text{Goals} \end{matrix} + 3 \times \begin{matrix} \text{Means to} \\ \text{Common} \\ \text{Goals} \end{matrix}$$

$$- \begin{matrix} \text{Means in Conflict} \\ \text{with Common Goals} \end{matrix}$$

2 *Trust:* A measure of triad members' perceptions that the others were willing to help, were able to help, and were caring people

3 *Mutuality of perception:* A measure of each triad's members' ability to accurately predict how the two other members would rate themselves and the others on ability, selfishness, honesty, willingness to help, and caring

Cooperation then was the mean of each triad's rank on goals and means, trust, and mutuality of perception.

Outcome Measures

Patient outcomes reflecting a holistic approach included five measures of physical, psychological, and social factors:

1 *Physical status:* An assessment from the patient record by the physician of the presence and seriousness of complications common to dialysis patients.

2 *Adherence to the medical regimen:* An evaluation by the physician of the sodium, protein, and phosphate binder intake, efficiency of dialysis treatments, and fluid intake from dialysis logs and monthly reports of blood chemistries.

3 *Total activity:* Patient report of the mean number of hours per week devoted to paid employment and/or household tasks plus mean hours per week of leisure time that was enjoyed or which felt really good. This eliminated, for example, extended TV watching simply to fill time.

4 *Morale:* An average of scores from two independent observations of verbal and nonverbal behavior by the interviewer and the clinic nurse.

5 *Positive affect:* The inverse of a measure of anxiety, depression, and hostility from a list of adjectives checked by the patient.

Methodology

Data were gathered during home interviews from patients and the family members who were their partners in the dialysis runs. The care provider in each triad was the person from the training center identified by the patient and partner as the staff member most important to them. This was usually the nurse, although the medical director, social worker, and technician were each chosen also.

The second study, conducted in Seattle (Mac-Elveen et al., 1975a), was similar to the first, with minor improvements in the strategies for eliciting goals and for evaluating adherence. In these triads the care provider was the patient's private physician in all cases. Data were collected three times at approximately 3-month intervals.

Findings

Findings in the Denver study suggested that there was a positive relationship between the amount of cooperation in the triad and desired patient outcomes, especially with regard to adherence to the regimen, total activity, and morale (see Table 39-1). In the Seattle study results were similar to those found in the Denver study: adherence, activity, and morale were again associated with cooperation in the care triad (see Table 39-1). Physical status was also found to be related to cooperation. In neither study was positive affect of the patient related to cooperation in the triad. The nonsignificance of this correlation is important because it invites speculation that the importance of the patient's anxiety, depression, or hostility may somehow be modified within the triad dynamics. At the least, it suggests that it is not only those patients with positive affect who manage to have cooperative triads.

Were any parts of cooperation more important to any of the outcomes? When the three subfactors

Table 39-1 Correlation Coefficients (r_s) of Triad Cooperation and Home Dialysis Patient Outcomes in Two Programs*

Patient outcomes	Cooperation	
	Denver (N = 21)	Seattle[‡] (N = approx. 36)
Physical status	.28	.49[§]
Adherence	.40[‡]	.53[§]
Total activity	.45[‡]	.48[§]
Morale	.45[‡]	.37*
Positive affect	.33	.20

*Adapted from MacElveen et al. (1975a:155)
[†]r_s from $\overline{X}$'s of T_1, T_2, T_3 (for 1-yr period)
[‡]$p < .05$
[§]$p < .005$

of cooperation were correlated with the five patient outcomes, the common goals and means factor was related to the patient's total activity (work and leisure) (MacElveen et al., 1975b). Mutuality of perception and trust in the triad were both related to physical status, adherence, total activity, and morale (see Table 39-2). These two subfactors require a history of interactions and point to the importance of continuity of care in that the care provider and the other two members work together over time, usually on an intermittent basis.

Three dyads exist within each triad: patient-doctor, patient-provider, and partner-doctor. Each

Table 39-2 Cooperation Subfactors and Patient Outcome Coefficients (r_s) in Home Dialysis Triads for a 10-Month Period (N = approx. 36)*

Patient outcomes	Cooperation subfactors		
	Common goals and means	Mutuality of perception	Trust
Physical status	.09	.42[†]	.55[‡]
Adherence	.07	.47[‡]	.68[‡]
Total activity	.31*	.52[‡]	.31[†]
Morale	.01	.34[†]	.27[†]
Positive affect	.20	−.20	.12

*From MacElveen et al. (1975b:96)
[†]$p < .05$
[‡]$p < .005$

dyad was correlated with the five patient outcomes (MacElveen et al., 1975b). The patient-doctor dyad was significantly related to total activity ($p < .05$) suggesting that the patients' number of work and leisure time hours was closely tied to the amount of cooperation between them and their partners.

The patient-doctor dyad was significantly related to physical status and to adherence to the medical regimen ($p < .05$). This is particularly interesting for the Seattle sample of patients, of whom 34 percent had been on dialysis from 3 to 10 or more years. Many of these patients managed their treatments and regimen quite independently, seeing their doctor only when something was happening for them. For example, in the 10-month data collection period numerous patients (35 percent) made zero to three visits to their doctor. These data would imply that even though doctor contacts were not as frequent as we might expect, the relationship between doctor and patient was nonetheless important to the patients' physical status and their adherence to the regimen.

The final dyad, partner-doctor, did not yield any relationships between dyad cooperation and any of the five patient outcomes. It is not possible to ascertain if this finding reflects the fact that many of the members of this dyad were not well acquainted with one another.

Limitations of the design of these two studies do not imply causation, i.e., that cooperation in the care triad was responsible for better patient outcomes. The findings did however support the general hypothesis that cooperation would be associated with better patient outcomes. The importance of each triad member is suggested by the findings from the dyadic cooperation analysis: partners are associated with work and leisure time, which contribute greatly to the quality of life; the physician is linked with physical complications and adherence behavior. The implications of the cooperation model for the problem referred to as *noncompliance* are interesting.

The generalizability of the model to other health and illness situations is promising. Obviously

cooperation has been occurring in the past in many situations and among many people. Knowledgeable, systematic efforts to apply the cooperation model is likely to enhance the associated desirable patient-client outcomes.

EXAMPLES OF CLINICAL APPLICATIONS

Cooperation and the Hospice Home Care Triad

The delivery of hospice care for terminally ill patients in this country frequently occurs within a framework respecting patients' rights to determine how they will live out the final stage of their lives. In the hospice concept, patient and family are the unit of care; provision of comfort and control of the patient's distressing symptoms are emphasized; staff is available on a 24-hour-per-day basis; survivors receive bereavement follow-up, and all care providers (lay and professional) receive support. The holistic concern for patient and family needs (physical, emotional, spiritual, social, legal, etc.) requires an interdisciplinary team approach (e.g., nurses, doctors, clergy, social workers, physical therapists). Volunteers are a major component of most hospice programs (Standards of Hospice Care, 1980).

This integrated pattern of family and patient participating with care providers is another example of a natural care triad. Benefits for all those involved are sometimes far-reaching. Patients who die with their pain and distress well controlled and in familiar surroundings with their loved ones have opportunities to satisfy their final goals in life. Family members whose goal was to provide care during this difficult time feel good about being able to respond to the needs of the person who is dying. During bereavement, they seem to suffer less from guilt feelings than is observed generally. They have acquired knowledge and skills they may not have had before, coming out of this experience with new competencies and problem-solving skills. Hospice care providers, both staff and volunteers, report great satisfaction in their work when patients "die well" and families achieve new levels of coping with difficult life situations. An important aspect of hospice care when viewed from a cooperative triad perspective is the availability of support during the process for all members of the triad. This goal and means to achieve it are especially significant if hospice staff are to grow and develop in this work, avoiding the emotional exhaustion often associated with becoming involved and caring about terminally ill patients.

Cooperation and the Hypertension Management Triad

Management of hypertension may extend for decades in the lives of persons with elevated blood pressure. Education about high blood pressure, its symptoms, and treatment strategies is critical. Knowledge and understanding makes it more possible for the client and family to participate in care planning and decision making in an informal way. Control of the blood pressure to maintain levels as close to normal as possible greatly reduces the risk of damage to the heart, kidneys, and brain. The severity of the hypertension dictates the treatment of choice, which usually includes: drugs, diet restrictions, physical exercise, monitoring of blood pressure, and strategies for promoting healthy responses to intense emotions and stressors within family and work relationships.

The fit between the optimal regimen and the clients' life-style may be disparate. Finding the drugs with the least side effects requires collaboration among members of the triad. In the cooperation model proposed here the care provider cannot dictate the level of health at any cost to client and family, an issue which was discussed earlier. Learning to negotiate care goals and collaborating on finding the best means to achieve them is not business as usual for most care providers. The alternatives to not negotiating the health goals may lead to treatment dropouts, who then are totally unprotected. A negotiated level of health may provide maintenance of a less than perfect blood pressure but be better than no protection at all.

When drastic changes in the clients' life-style are considered necessary, the family can provide support for new patterns of work and leisure activities that are health-promoting. Adjusting to diet restrictions and drug therapy may impact the clients' view of self and loss of the sense of normal good health. Following the regimen makes denying the presence of a chronic health problem very difficult. For many people this process of accepting the need for the health regimen takes time and can be enhanced by various kinds of support from the family.

The care provider makes information available and teaches necessary skills such as self-monitoring of blood pressure. Referrals to other health services for diet management, meditation, relaxation techniques, and weight control facilitate efforts to support the common goal of controlled blood pressure. Continuity in the triad relationships enhances adherence behaviors, especially in this situation which requires lifelong monitoring of blood pressure and treatment strategies.

Cooperation and the Prenatal Care Triad

Prior to the arrival of a new baby, the pregnant woman-partner–childbirth education instructor might be a natural triad if the expectant parents are enrolled in a prenatal class. Recently there has been an increase in the participation of partners in the management of the pregnancy, birth, and new baby. In prenatal care, the care provider (e.g., nurse-practitioner or doctor) might identify with the woman and her partner's general goals of a healthy pregnancy and delivery of a healthy baby. Each triad member may have other goals which are more specific subgoals and complementary to the general goals. The woman may want to have her baby naturally, to breast-feed, and to get her figure back as soon after delivery as possible. The partner may want their dyadic relationship not to be changed by the baby's arrival and may also want to share in the labor and delivery process. The care provider goals for both mother and partner might include, e.g., promoting understanding of the physical and emotional changes associated with pregnancy and childbirth; adequate nutrition, daily exercise, and prenatal care for the mother; preparation of the couple for labor and delivery, and realistic expectations of a newborn.

The triad members' goals as described above are individually expressed. None appears to be in conflict and many are interrelated, for example, the mother's desire to have a natural birth, the partner's desire to participate in that process, and the care provider's goals of their gaining an understanding of the pregnancy and birth and being prepared for labor and delivery. Members articulate their goals, objectives, or concerns within the triad interaction. This facilitates awareness of each other's aims and priorities that could influence the strategies for moving toward the shared goals. Sequencing and temporal order influence the establishment of means to the goals. Some couples might request reading materials or classes with other prospective parents or might prefer to work closely with the care provider as the resource for their needed information and skills.

The partner's concern with how the baby might change his or her relationship with the woman is an important question to be addressed. The care provider might facilitate a discussion about their expectations of themselves and of each other following the birth. This might also be a topic in the parental class, where couples might share their feelings and concerns. Information from a care provider could increase their understanding of the postpartum phase and some experiences commonly associated with it.

The care provider who has contact with both parents prior to and following the birth has the opportunity to support a couple in maximizing their growth with this experience. As the physical, emotional, and social health of the parents is promoted, their ability to respond to the baby's needs is enhanced and the care provider's satisfaction is increased.

Cooperation and Children in the Care Triad

Application of the cooperation model in which children are part of the triad is an important

consideration. Too frequently, the abilities of children to be involved in planning and problem solving are grossly underrated by parents and care providers. In some settings 4- and 5-year-olds are taught to give their own insulin injections and to catheterize themselves using clean techniques. Involving a child in his or her own care is more likely to be successful if he or she participates in the planning. Obviously, the degree to which this can occur is relative to the developmental level of the child. The tendency, however, is to discount the ability of the child to contribute to the cooperative approach and to only show him or her what someone wants him or her to do. The older the child is, the greater the involvement and responsibility that can be expected. Children may also be significant as members of the family corner of the triad, not only as offspring but as siblings and as significant others. In some cases, as with adolescents, we may want to promote more personal accountability for health care and to deemphasize the role of parents or family. This can be most effectively done within the cooperation model where the expectation of all those involved can be articulated and mutually agreed upon. For some aspects of health, especially sexual health issues such as contraception, venereal disease, pregnancy, and abortion, the adolescent may insist that there be no family involvement. The adolescent who can be supported by his or her family when dealing with sexual concerns is fortunate. On the other hand, a solely responsible adolescent may be demonstrating developmental progress toward more independent and mature behavior. The presence of an important other person, such as an intimate friend or relative, may be encouraged when the situation is likely to be very stressful. The nurse may want to legitimize sharing when there may be a need for social support, as with pregnancy or abortion.

IMPLICATIONS FOR NURSING

Reeder (1978) describes how the evolving profession of nursing has been influenced by changes in society. Currently we observe consumerism, the self-care movement, the women's movement, and the ever present politics of how to pay for care. The burden of tradition groans on and in many institutions and agencies former means have become ends and clients have become objects rather than subjects in the pattern of interactions. The expensive new technologies tend to generate their own demand for use. Cost effectiveness and bureaucratic efficiency program the parameters of care. Sophisticated tests provide empirical evidence, which often serves primarily to validate clinical judgment. These currents seem to be gathering strength and momentum like streams swollen with the spring runoff. Nurses themselves could be lost in that torrent. It is critical that they resist those forces, as they have the greatest amount of contact with patients, clients, and family members. One of nursing's most crucial responsibilities now and in the future is to assist people to obtain needed services without being dehumanized in the process. The cooperation model is a humanistic approach to care, emphasizing the strengths of client and family and promoting relationships of mutual respect among care providers and the consumers of their services.

The rights of self-determination and understanding are concomitant with the responsibility for informed participation in planning, decision making, and activities related to the promotion of health and reduction of illness.

Nursing Practice

The cooperation model is congruent with the nursing process and stresses the interdependence of all those involved with a client's care. Increasingly, nurses will need to emphasize clinical skills related not only to direct care but to other aspects of nursing as well. Assessment and diagnostic skills sensitive to client and family cues will be reflected in nurses' ability to facilitate the identification and prioritizing of common goals. The nursing approach to the needs of the total person addresses many aspects of well-being and illness, e.g., physical, psychological, social, spiritual, and cultural. Such an approach is likely to generate realistic goals sometimes more crucial to the client and family than to the traditional care provider. Communication and interpersonal skills are required for resolution of goal conflict and attainment of a consensus on the individual contributions towards the identified goals. The process of deciding with client and family the plan for organizing these contributions and for evaluating the movement toward goals role-models a problem-solving and growth-promoting process of people working together which simultaneously acknowledges their individual strengths and interdependence.

One of the greatest resources of nurses is their knowledge of normal growth and development as well as the possible courses of events within a specific acute illness or long-term health problem. Given this base of knowledge they can provide information to clients and families to help prepare them for what may be ahead. Anticipatory guidance contributes to people's ability to respond from a less ambiguous, fearful, or helpless position. Such good nursing reduces the amount of management by crisis and operates more from a preventive, healthy stance in which people experience less distress and more control in their lives.

Other clinical skills of growing importance are: providing opportunities for learning needed knowledge and care skills; collaborating with persons from other disciplines; coordinating the communications and care activities among all those involved with a client; consulting with other professionals and clients; and developing health education strategies for targeted high-risk groups.

Empowerment of clients and families implies their greater control over their own health. However, when interacting with nurses around health and especially around illness events, clients and families often need support and understanding for the challenges they confront, recognition and affirmation for their self-care efforts, and comfort and compassion for their losses and grieving.

The cooperation model for nursing practice can be applied to the variety of settings in which nurses provide services, whether primary, secondary, or tertiary situations.

Whatever model for delivering care is used, it structures consumer-provider interactions and influences the nursing process. Nurses need to identify their personal values and expectations for client and family behavior. They need to be aware of the model of care they use that guides their practice and determines the kind and quality of care they provide.

Nursing Education

Implications of the cooperation model for nursing education relate first to the role modeling by faculty and by nurses in the clinical area. Second, the implications of the model relate to the relationship between the teacher and the student.

When students observe their own teachers applying classroom teaching to their own nurse-client interactions, the learning environment is especially enhanced. This generates congruence between what is received and studied cognitively and what is observed and heard, adding power by the demonstration of the teacher. Awareness of the importance of such role modeling is not new.

To take this assumption another step is to believe that nurse-client interactions recapitulate teacher-student interactions (Parkinson, 1978). Both are helping relationships. Ideally, clients and students are encouraged to grow in their acquisition of health, skills, and knowledge. Their individual uniqueness is recognized and their own goals (related to health and learning, respectively) are elicited and valued. Thus, rather than observing the role modeling, the students experience with their teachers what we hope clients will experience with their nurses. Perhaps much of the degree to which nurses fall short reflects the degree of beneficient dictatorship that guided their education.

In applying the model to nursing courses I have enlisted increasing amounts of student input. The students articulated personal goals within the framework of the course objectives and we negotiated individual and classroom strategies for learning. This is the process of defining common goals and the means to achieve them. Determining

criteria for goal attainment and intermittent evaluation during the term to check our progress were extremely helpful. We shared the learning process in a democratic and mutually responsible manner. This was often done with individual learning contacts, similar to the individualized care plans negotiated for patients and clients. Feedback from students both objectively and subjectively has been very rewarding in these classes. The consistency of the students' educational experience is clearly important in helping them to appreciate and apply the cooperation model in their clinical practice. The rationale for protecting clients from dehumanization in the health care system may also apply to the protection of students from similar experiences in large, impersonal educational systems.

The work of Enos and Nilsson (1975) is very helpful in providing guidelines rich with clinical examples for assisting students to learn and implement a model focusing on the clients' goals. There is a need for more educational materials to integrate the cooperation model into nursing curricula.

Nursing Research

Studies are needed to expand our knowledge and understanding of the relationships between cooperation among those involved with the health and illness issues of others and desirable outcomes, especially for clients. Testing of the model in acute care settings and with control groups would be valuable, e.g., determination of what would happen in application of the cooperation model to those situations in which clients' health is frequently compromised by their choice of not adhering to the regimen. The interrelationships among cooperation in care, the nature of the regimen, and the results of adherence and nonadherence behavior constitute a research thrust that has interesting potential. The importance of the cooperative process is likely to be variable across the range of regimen-adherence behavior. Where following the regimen results in an ongoing reduction of symptoms, as in pain control, adherence is not usually a problem. The resulting experience (comfort) of following the regimen is a positive reinforcement for the adherence behavior. When deviation from the regimen generates a strong and undesirable response, adherence behavior again tends to be reinforced, e.g., if a diabetic person omits the daily insulin injection or omits the food intake when insulin is administered, the negative feedback for nonadherence is fairly rapid and specific. The person with epilepsy who has a seizure during a short period off medications has strong negative reinforcement. This is often a function of the social stigma associated with seizures in public places. If long periods of time that are seizure-free follow discontinuance of medications, then nonadherence is probably reinforced.

In acute illness events such as cystitis, the tendency of many clients is to relate the medications to urgency, pain, and burning. Symptom control often results in premature termination of treatment. Explanation of the necessity for continuing medication for the prescribed period is not always enough. Perhaps greater involvement in the cooperative process might yield better outcomes in adherence behavior.

The most difficult adherence challenges occur when clients experience little or no distress until the prevention or treatment program is initiated. Thus, rather than having a positive relationship between symptom reduction and health regimen, we see a negative relationship in which the health regimen produces discomfort and symptomology. The person whose hypertension regimen causes more problems than no regimen is in a situation of negative reinforcement for adherence behavior (or positive reinforcement for nonadherence). The person on dialysis who must contend with the demanding treatment schedule and fluid and diet restrictions also must deal with the monotonous frequency of large doses of phosphate binders

(e.g., aluminum hydroxide), the result of which makes them feel as if they have just chewed a mouthful of chalk. The fluid restrictions severely limit the natural impulse to "wash it down" with liquids. This problem (for the client) of phosphate binder intake is crucial to the prevention of calcium loss from bones, which promotes susceptibility to pathological fractures and bone pain. Another complication of the calcium-phosphorus imbalance is the deposition of calcium in soft tissues, which may compromise pulmonary status or brain function. However, the persons struggling with trying to swallow their aluminum hydroxide do not have any symptoms of calcium problems until they have deviated for an extended period of time. Again, short-term negative reinforcement for adherence, positive reinforcement for nonadherence. A cooperation strategy might be to shift the feedback system so as to involve the client in appreciating how he or she can influence lab values and exercise control over important physiological processes. In these problematic adherence situations the means to achieve the health goals require creative collaboration of client and care providers.

SUMMARY

The benefits of the cooperation model, especially in the care triad, are appropriate for the numerous situations and settings in which nurses deliver services for those seeking assistance with health and illness. The model is also appropriate to the needs of health care consumers in these times of high cost for health care. Nurses could be the leaders in this system change as well as advocates for patients and clients in the prevailing system. We can facilitate the ability of clients and families to grow and take more responsibility for their own health and own care during illness.

EDITOR'S QUESTIONS FOR DISCUSSION

What are the essential components of the Cooperation Model? How does it differ from other models for care in health and illness? How congruent is it with the various nursing theoretical perspectives offered by nursing theorists? Is there any one nursing theory that may be related to the model more than another? What relationship is there between the model and components of the nursing process? What assumptions are there in utilizing the model? Does the model have limitations? What empirical evidence is there that cooperation makes a difference in outcomes of patient care?

Apply the concept of the cooperative triad to the nursing profession. Using the nine factors to compare cooperative and competitive triads, what example(s) can be indicated for each factor being evident within the nursing profession? How does the choice between cooperation and competition manifest itself within nursing? What are the effects of cooperation and/or competition on nursing practice, education, and research? What strategies can be suggested to elicit cooperation and reduce competition within the profession? Utilizing the previous questions posed for queries within the profession, examine the nursing profession as a cooperative dyad with other professions. How can bonds be strengthened between other professions? How can Jordan's four stages necessary in the development of cooperation be applied to the nursing profession? What is the significance for nursing regarding research findings indicating a relationship between interdependence and cooperative groups?

Are there situations in health and illness care where dyadic cooperative relationships may be more effective for client outcomes than triad? Specify conflicts which may arise in negotiating levels of health. What strategies can be suggested for resolution of conflicts? What relationships exist between MacElveen-Hoehn's focus and Bille (Chap. 36) and La Monica (Chap. 37)? What additional factors to those cited may confound establishment of cooperation? What other cooperation strategies can be suggested to improve adherence behavior? What implications are there of the findings reported by Chaska (Chap. 20) for improving adherence behavior?

What issues may need to be addressed in applying the cooperative triad model in different types of settings, for example, acute care? What other settings may be amenable for implementation of the model? What other type of clinical applications are there for the model than those discussed? In viewing nursing students as clients in the cooperative model, what process is necessary to assist the development and growth of students? In making contracts with students, what type of limitations may be warranted and under what conditions? How does MacElveen-Hoehn's emphasis on humanization of nursing education apply to issues posed by Peterson (Chap. 7), Sargis (Chap. 9), and Dalme (Chap. 11)? What are the relationships between the cooperation model, Bille's (Chap. 36) discussion of the contractual model, and application to nursing education?

Discuss the methodological testing of the cooperation model. What are the strengths and limitations of the studies? How valid and reliable are the measures? Can alternative explanations be offered for the findings? How generalizable are the findings? What methodological suggestions can be made for future testing and application of the model?

REFERENCES

Abram, H. S.
   1968 "The psychiatrist, the treatment of chronic renal failure, and the prolongation of life." American Journal of Psychiatry 124:1351–1358.

Alexander, R. A. and P. M. MacElveen
   1978 "Are we assessing the needs of home dialysis partners?" Self Dialysis Monograph. Chicago: American Association of Nephrology Nurses and Technicians.
American Nurses' Association
   1973 Standards of Nursing Practice. Kansas

City, Mo.: American Nurses' Association.

Anger D.
1975 "The psychological stress of chronic renal failure and long term dialysis." Nursing Clinics of North America 10:449–60.

Annas, George
1975 The Rights of Hospital Patients: An American Civil Liberties Handbook. New York: American Civil Liberties.

Blagg, C. R., T. J. Cole, G. Irvine, T. Marr, T. L. Pollard.
1972 "How much should dialysis cost?" Pp. 54–60 in R. Freeman (ed.), A special publication of transactions of The American Society of Artificial Organs, Washington, D.C.: Georgetown University Press.

Bowar-Ferres, Susan
1975 "Loeb Center and its philosophy of nursing." The American Journal of Nursing 75:810–814.

Burgess, A. and A. Lazure
1970 "Dual therapy by nurse and psychiatrist." American Journal of Nursing 70:1292–1298.

Caplow, Theodore
1956 "Theory of coalitions in the triad." American Sociological Review 21:489–493.
1959 "Further development of a theory of coalition triad." American Journal of Sociology 64:488–493.
1970 Two Against One: Coalitions in Triads. Englewood Cliffs, N. J.: Prentice-Hall.

Deutsch, M.
1949a "A theory of co-operation and competition." Human Relations 2:152–179.
1949b "An experimental study of the effects of cooperation and competition upon group process." Human Relations 2:199–231.

Ebra, G. and J. Tolt
1972 "Chronic hemodialysis—some psychological and rehabilitative considerations." Rehabilitation Literature 33:2–10.

Enos, Marian S. and Beverly Nilsson
1975 A Faculty Manual on Client Goals Theory. Vermillion, S. D.: South Dakota State University.

Fredrich, R. M.
1980 "Patient perception of distress associated with hemodialysis—a state survey." Jour-

nal of the American Association of Nephrology Nurses and Technicians 8: 252–258.

Haley, J.
1969 "Toward a theory of pathological systems," Pp. 11–27 in Gerald H. Zuk and Ivan Boszmormenyi-Nagi (eds.), Family Therapy and Disturbed Families. Palo Alto: Science and Behavior Books.

Hedenberg, A. D.
1980 "Limited care hemodialysis—an appropriate treatment modality for end-style renal disease." Journal of the American Association of Nephrology Nurses and Technicians 8:243–244.

Hefferin, Elizabeth A.
Forth-   "Patient nurse collaboration in health
coming goal setting." Military Medicine.

Hoover, P. M., P. M. MacElveen and R. A. Alexander
1975 "Adjustment of children with parents on haemodialysis." Nursing Times, London, 71:35.

Jackle, M. J.
1974 "Life satisfaction and kidney dialysis." Nursing Forum 4:360–370.

Jordan, N., B. T. Jensen, and S. J. Terebinsky
1963 "The development of cooperation among three-man crews in a simulated man-machine information processing system." Journal of Social Psychology 59:175–184.

King, Imogene M.
1971 Toward a Theory of Nursing: General Concepts of Human Behavior. New York: Wiley.

Kossoris, P.
1970 "Family therapy: An adjunct to home dialysis and transplantation." American Journal of Nursing 70:1730–1733.

Levy, N. B.
1974 Living and Dying: Adaptation to Hemodialysis. Springfield, Ill: Charles C Thomas.

MacElveen, P. M.
1971 "Exploration of the cooperative triad in investigation of home dialysis patient outcomes." Unpublished dissertation, University of Colorado.
1973 "Cooperative triad in home dialysis care and patient outcomes." Pp. 134–147 in M. Batey (ed), Communicating Nursing Research, vol. 5. Boulder, Colorado:

Western Interstate Commission for Higher Education.
1977 "How does home dialysis fit into the family life cycle?" Self Dialysis Monograph, Chicago: American Association of Nephrology Nurses and Technicians.

MacElveen, P. M., P. M. Hoover, and R. A. Alexander
1975a "Patient outcome success related to cooperation among patient, partner and physician." Journal of the American Association of Nephrology Nurses and Technicians 2:148–156.
1975b "Cooperation and successful outcomes in home dialysis." Proceedings: Clinical and Dialysis Transplant Forum V, 93–97. Washington, D. C.: Columbia Planograph.

Maller, J. B.
1929 Cooperation and Competition: An Experimental Study in Motivation. New York: Teachers College, Columbia University Contributions to Education, No. 384.

Marwell, Gerald and David R. Schmitt
1975 Cooperation: An Experimental Analysis. New York: Academic Press.

May, M. A. and L. W. Doob
1937 Competition and Cooperation. New York: Social Science Research Council.

Mead, M.
1937 Cooperation and Competition among Primitive People. New York: McGraw-Hill.

Mills, T. M.
1954 "The coalition pattern in three person groups." American Sociological Review 19:657–666.

Nursing Theories Conference Group, Julia B. George, Chairperson
1980 Nursing Theories: The Base for Professional Nursing Practice. Englewood Cliffs, N.J.: Prentice-Hall.

Orem, Dorothea E.
1971 Nursing: Concepts of Practice. New York: McGraw-Hill.

Parkinson, Margaret H.
1978 "Nurse-Teachers are role models whether they like it or not." New Zealand Nursing Journal 71:14–16.

Parsons, T.
1964 The Social System. New York: Free Press, pp. 436–447.

Peplau, Hildegard E.
1952 Interpersonal Relations in Nursing. New York: McGraw-Hill.

Pierce, P. F.
1975 "Listening with a research ear: Communication with hemodialysis patients." Journal of the American Association of Nephrology Nurses and Technicians 2: 157–170.

Polak, P.
1970 "Patterns of discord: Goals of patients, therapists, and community members." Archives of General Psychiatry 23: 277–283.

Reeder, Sharon J.
1978 "The social context of nursing." Pp. 235–246 in The Nursing Profession: Views through the Mist, Norma L. Chaska (ed.), New York: McGraw-Hill.

Rogers, Martha
1970 The Theoretical Basis for Nursing. Philadelphia: Davis.

Roy, Callista
1976 Introduction to Nursing: An Adaptation Model. Englewood Cliffs, N. J.: Prentice-Hall.

Rubenstein, D. and O. Weiner
1967 "Co-therapy in teamwork relationships in family psychotherapy," Pp. 206–220 in Gerald Zuk and Ivan Boszmormenyi-Nagi (eds.), Family Therapy and Disturbed Families. Palo Alto: Science and Behavior Books.

Simmel, Georg
1950
1980 The Sociology of Georg Simmel. Tr. K. H. Wolff. New York: Glencoe Free Press.

Stachowiak, James
1975 Helping Families to Change. New York: Aronson.

Standards of Hospice Care
1980 Washington, D.C.: National Hospice Organization.

Strodtbeck, F. L.
1954 "The family as a three-person group." American Sociological Review 19:23–29.

Stryker, S. and G. Psathas
1960 "Research coalitions in the triad: Findings, problems, and strategy." Sociometry 23:217–230.

Vinacke, W. E. and A. Arkoff
  1957 "An experimental study of coalitions in the triad." American Sociological Review 22:406–414.

Weidenbach, Ernestine
  1964 Clinical Nursing, A Helping Art. New York: Springer-Verlag.

Zuk, Gerald H.
  1971 Family Therapy: A Triadic-Based Approach. New York: Behavioral.

Chapter 40

Models of Hospice Care

Inge B. Corless, R.N., Ph.D.
Program Director
St. Peter's Hospice
Albany, New York

In the previous chapter the application of the cooperation model was made to the hospice home care triad. It is appropriate that further investigation of hospice care and trends be delineated. The hospice movement may well represent a prime example of humanization in care. Inge B. Corless presents an enlightening chapter concerning the hospice concept, models of care, issues, and directions of programs. Essentially, the concept is one approach aimed toward enabling terminally ill persons to live until they die when other care is no longer considered appropriate. She defines 10 parameters essential to effective hospice care and 10 dimensions along which hospice programs vary. She further describes the multiple models of hospice care that exist. Data are shown to support the discussion and indicate the professional leadership of programs, role of volunteers, and sources of resistance to hospice care programs. Data were secured through mailed questionnaires sent to listings of the National Hospice Organization (N.H.O.) participants at the Third International Seminar on Palliative Care, key informants, visitation of hospice programs, and participant observation at local through national level hospice meetings. The response rate for the 153 N.H.O. groups was 74 percent, while for another 80 non-N.H.O. hospice groups it was 41 percent.

In the United States the emphasis has been on hospice care for the terminally ill cancer patient with an usual time period of six months. There is considerable variation in the organizational type of hospice facilities. The first model in the United States was established in 1974 in Connecticut. The models portrayed include inpatient hospital unit; home care programs; a combination of both inpatient and home care; free-standing hospices operating as pilot projects; a collaborative model arranged between an inpatient unit and a Visiting Nurse Service; one affiliated with a university to provide ambulatory, home, and inpatient care; one formed by a consortium of hospitals. Services also vary with distinctions made between consultations provided, the length of bereavement care, follow-up with clients at home or as an inpatient, and

This is a revision of a paper presented to Sociologists for Health and Consumer Concerns, at the annual meeting of the American Sociological Association, August 29, 1979; the study was made possible by a Research Facilitation Grant from the University of Michigan College of Nursing.

day care programs. Diversity is encouraged to meet the needs in different communities. Although articulation between home and inpatient care is increasing as an important aspect of any hospice program, criteria for acceptance into home care programs frequently exclude persons without family or friends to act as primary care givers. In addition some patients who received hospital team consultation services when initially admitted may not be readmitted for terminal care.

Most hospice programs provide home care either directly through their own nurses or through contractual arrangements with the Visiting Nurse Service. A major issue is where to send clients who require inpatient care. Another issue surrounds the question of physician referral-approval of hospice care. A third question pertains to the composition of the hospice team and the position of volunteers versus paid professionals. The majority of programs currently delivering hospice care have administrators who are professional nurses, followed by a lesser number identified as social workers. Another area of concern in acceptance of hospice care is financial exigency. Leadership as well as resistance in the hospice movement is coming from health professionals. The question of reasonable standards needs to be addressed. Few programs meet all of the criteria established by the N.H.O., nor provide comprehensive care. Committed to the unique service and value of hospice care, Corless raises significant questions to be answered in the future.

The "happy death movement" has emerged in what formerly had been considered a "death-denying" society (Lofland, 1978). The denial of death is manifested in the relegation of the dying to rooms farthest from the nurses' station, in a decrease in the number and time of interactions between medical personnel and the dying, and in a general abandonment of the dying in favor of those for whom "something can be done." The "happy death" movement is characterized by activities organized around the central principle of rescuing the dying from ignominy and restoring the death event to a status befitting a once-in-a-lifetime occurrence. As a concomitant, a dying role has emerged, and with it a number of new organizational approaches embodying a value complex which focuses on the totality of the individual in health and illness. The nomothetic term for these activities is "hospice."

What then *is* hospice? It is variously referred to as a concept of care, a program of care, and a place of care. The *Oxford English Dictionary* describes hospice as "a house of rest and entertainment for pilgrims, travellers or strangers, or a 'home' for the destitute or the sick." And so it was in medieval times. Today the hospice concept is an approach which is directed toward enabling persons to live until they die. Hospice is a concept of health care which involves the availability of interdisciplinary services to clients either in the home or in a specially designated unit or in scattered beds throughout an institution, on a 24-hours-per-day, 7-days-per-week basis. This care is provided to terminally ill persons and their families when treatment aimed at cure or prolongation of life is no longer considered appropriate. Hospice care consists of palliation of pain and symptom control, as well as attention to the psychological, social, spiritual, intellectual, and financial concerns of clients (Saunders, 1967; Woodson, 1976; Lack, 1978).

Lack identifies the following as essential to the delivery of effective hospice care.

1 Coordinated home care-inpatient beds under a central autonomous hospice administration.
2 Skilled symptom control (physical, sociological, psychological and spiritual).
3 Physician directed services.
4 Provision of care by an interdisciplinary team.

5 Services available on a 24 hour a day, 7 day a week on-call basis with emphasis on availability of medical and nursing skills.

6 Patient/family regarded as the unit of care.

7 Bereavement follow-up.

8 Use of volunteers as an integral part of the interdisciplinary team.

9 Structured staff support and communication system.

10 Patients should be accepted to the program on the basis of health needs, not ability to pay. (1978:42)

Support services for the terminally ill person and his or her family and professional and community education are also aspects of the hospice concept of health care. Although, theoretically, comprehensive hospice care incorporates all of these elements, in practice only some of the various aspects of the hospice concept are utilized in the numerous models of hospice care currently available in the United States and Canada. For example, delineation by the Connecticut Hospice (described elsewhere) of the nature of the interdisciplinary team and the professional representation required further specifies this component of the hospice concept of care. It also distinguishes the "haves" in hospice programs from the "have-nots." A Matthew effect ensues, whereby those hospice programs already financially well placed elaborate standards, which, while necessary, serve to enhance their own position relative to newcomers to the hospice movement.

In addition to the basic parameters discussed previously, hospice programs may be described as differing in the following dimensions:

1 The focus of programming

2 The type of hospice services provided

3 The professional leadership of the program

4 The types of professionals involved

5 The use of community agencies

6 The degree of association with an acute care facility

7 The number and type of in-patient beds available

8 The use of volunteers in the program[1]

9 The type and number of clients served[2]

10 The requirements for admission to the program

These dimensions will be noted in the first part of this paper which describes the various models of hospice, or palliative care programs as they are called in Canada.

Emphasis will be given here to the data which describe differing models of hospice care, the professional leadership of hospice programs, the role of volunteers on the hospice team, and sources of resistance to hospice programs of care.

Data were obtained by sending questionnaires to all hospices listed in the *Preliminary Directory of the National Hospice Organization* (1978) and to other hospice organizations not listed but known to the author to be engaged in the delivery of services or to be in one of the planning phases. Questionnaires were also sent to all individuals attending the Third International Seminar on Palliative Care held in Montreal, Canada, in November of 1978. This list of participants expanded our knowledge of groups in the United States and at the same time provided a source of information on developments in Canada. Additional observations were made by visiting a number of ongoing hospice programs and by holding discussions with groups currently planning hospice programs. Participant observation at local, state, regional, and national hospice meetings provided data supplementing and complementing those secured in the survey and in personal interviews.

One of the obstacles to doing research in this area is that hospice planning groups come into existence and dissolve with a rapidity which is breathtaking to chroniclers of the movement.

[1] Although volunteers are considered an essential component by Lack, one finds considerable variation here.

[2] Lack states that need, and not ability to pay, is the key consideration. In fact, the existence of a family member or friend to act as care giver is the proxy for ability to pay in other parts of the health care system and serves to discriminate in much the same way as does lack of financial resources.

Methodologically, this makes it difficult to know the precise size of the population. Using the listings of the National Hospice Organization, the Third International Seminar, and the suggestions of key informants, a total of 472 questionnaires were mailed. One hundred and fifty-three questionnaires were sent to groups listed by the National Hospice Organization, or the N.H.O. The response rate for these was 74 percent or 96 groups. The remainder of the questionnaires were mailed to groups located through the other sources mentioned, with the goal of obtaining responses from groups not listed by the National Hospice Organization and from committees at the early stages of hospice formation. Responses from another 80 non-N.H.O. hospice groups were obtained in this way, for a response rate of 41 percent and an overall response rate of 54 percent. It had been anticipated that the overall response rate might be low, as far more questionnaires were mailed in the hope of capturing all of the groups in the United States and Canada who were in any manner involved in the delivery of hospice services or who were preparing to do so. The response rate of 74 percent for N.H.O. listed groups is not as high as might be desired, and the results must be interpreted with this in mind. The response rate does include questionnaires returned from the international leaders in hospice care as well as from many lesser-known groups.

In the United States, hospice programs have emphasized the care of the terminally ill cancer patient. This is in part a by-product of the fact that the funding agency for a number of pilot projects has been the National Cancer Institute. In other instances, the focus on the cancer patient is a result of the decision that hospice care be provided to those persons and their families whose remaining lifetime can be measured in days, weeks, or months, rather than years. The usual time frame is 6 months. Needless to say, not all disease processes lend themselves to such prognostication.

Another element which differentiates various hospice programs is the degree of association with an acute care facility. One type of hospice is that which is a unit in an acute care hospital.

Such a model of care is provided by the Palliative Care Service of the Royal Victoria Hospital in Montreal, Canada. Their inpatient unit consists of 12 beds and provides services to those individuals who are (1) "difficult to manage in other departments because of poorly controlled physical symptoms or difficult psychosocial situations" and (2) patients in home care who require admission (Mount, 1976:63). In addition to an inpatient unit, the Palliative Care Service provides consultations throughout the rest of the hospital. Their four home care nurses provide care to 25 to 35 patients, and more at times. A strong component of this program and most others is bereavement care for the family of the terminally ill person. Bereavement care is usually continued for a period of 1 year after the death of the family member. In some programs, especially where children are involved, bereavement care is provided for 2 years. While hospice services at the Royal Victoria Hospital encompass inpatient, home care, consultation, and bereavement services, some programs in the United States provide only home care or only inpatient components. The Palliative Care Service is also distinctive in that it has its own staff of home care nurses. In most hospice programs in the United States, services are contracted from such community groups as the Visiting Nurse Service. Examples of hospice models of this sort will be given shortly.

While the Palliative Care Service is located in an acute care hospital, Rogers Memorial Hospice in Oconomowoc, Wisconsin, has a 10-bed unit in a wing of a mental hospital, and rather than an urban setting, Rogers Memorial Hospice is located in a rural area 20 miles from Milwaukee. This hospice has the interesting feature of an enclosed sun porch, in the corner of which is a self-service bar for patients and their friends. On one occasion, a patient and her husband gave an anniversary party for themselves and their relatives on that porch; they truly entered into the spirit(s) of living until they died.

The first and one of the most well-known hospice programs in the United States began in

March 1974. Hospice, Inc., of New Haven, Connecticut, now renamed the Connecticut Hospice, calls itself "the first American hospice" (Lack and Buckingham, 1978). The Connecticut Hospice has a home care program which serves an average of 40 to 50 patients. At times, they have a waiting list of from 20 to 30 persons. The Connecticut Hospice has built an inpatient facility with a 44-bed capacity which was designed with explicit consideration for the needs of the terminally ill and their families.

Inpatient units vary in size from 4 beds to a 62-bed facility at the Hospice of Rockland in Pomona, New York.[3] Units of 10 to 12 beds are more typical of current inpatient units. Some professionals suggest that, with an emphasis on home care, inpatient units of four to six beds are more appropriate.[4] The Hospice of Marin in California, which is currently a home care program caring for 30 to 40 patient/families per week, also seems to be veering toward an inpatient unit as a backup for clients who, for one reason or another, can no longer be cared for at home. At the moment, individuals who require institutional care are admitted to the hospital with which their own physician is affiliated. The Marin Hospice team then does follow-up with their client in the chosen hospital. Affiliation with any one hospital would alienate the professional community associated with other institutions. As a result, they are considering a six-bed, freestanding unit as their inpatient facility. The politics of health care make a detached unit desirable in this community.

Many of the new hospice programs are starting with home care programs. This may be a consequence of the nature of the sponsoring group. Community groups are likely to start with home

care, whereas institutional groups usually start with inpatient units. The major decisions for most groups are whether an inpatient unit should be a component of the program and whether that unit should be part of an existing facility or a separate entity. The articulation between home care and inpatient unit is getting increased attention as an important feature of any hospice program. Although previously elaborated by Lack as an essential ingredient of hospice, the concern for articulation has been given a new impetus by the Health Care Financing Administration (HCFA) demonstration program.

Another model of hospice care is provided by the St. Luke's Hospice team in New York, which is hospital-based and was begun in April, 1975. St. Luke's Hospice is located in St. Luke's–Roosevelt Hospital Center and is composed of a team which provides a consultation service for patients located throughout the St. Luke's hospital and for others who have chosen to go home. As of this writing, there is no separate hospice inpatient unit.

The home care program for hospice patients at St. Luke's is managed through the hospital's home care program. A hospice family nurse practitioner conducts a physical and psychosocial assessment of patients for hospice home care. Follow-up is provided by the hospital's own home care nurses. Most of their patients live in multiproblem families where terminal illness is just one of numerous issues. Some of their patients live alone and are cared for at home until it is no longer safe for them to be there. At that time additional help must be mobilized by enlisting family, friends, and volunteers so that the patient is able to remain at home, or admission to an extended care facility must be arranged. The hospice patient is *not* readmitted to St. Luke's for terminal care on an inpatient basis other than for the aforementioned consultation prior to discharge.

In contrast to these models of hospice care, three freestanding hospices are operating as pilot projects as part of a grant from the National Cancer Institute. These are the Riverside Hospice in New Jersey, Hillhaven Hospice in Arizona,

---

[3] Based on collation of information presented in the Preliminary Directory of the National Hospice Organization, (New Haven, Conn.: The National Hospice Organization, 1978).

[4] I am indebted to Dr. Gary Jacobsen of the Oregon Comprehensive Cancer Program for his insights into this question.

and the Kaiser Permanente Hospice in California. Riverside Hospice in Boontown, New Jersey, located in the home of a former corporation president, is replete with a number of amenities, including a bomb shelter. The inpatient unit has 16 beds arranged in 2- and 3-bedded rooms. Riverside has a pool and patio beyond which is a good-sized pond, playing fields used by the local community, and woods in which to walk. The living room, which opens onto the patio, has a fireplace. The library with leather chairs provides a quiet sanctuary. Riverside Hospice is physically and aesthetically one of the most beautiful hospices in the United States.

The home care program at Riverside provides care for 50 patients. This program has been most innovative in helping those who live alone to remain at home to die; neighbors are brought together to organize care for the dying person. The Hospice of Marin has also gathered neighbors together to help terminally ill persons who live alone to die at home.

In many hospices, persons without family or friends to act as primary care givers are not accepted into home care programs. Thus, although ability to pay, i.e., financial status, does not bar an individual from hospice care, absence of a primary care giver, i.e., familial status, is used as a discriminating factor for admission to hospice programs. Other criteria for acceptance include a prognosis of limited life. A diagnosis of cancer is specified in many instances, as is physician approval. The approval by the primary physician of the patient's hospice involvement has been incorporated as an essential ingredient so that, for one thing, hospice physicians will not be accused of "stealing" patients. A more benign interpretation and a more beneficial outcome is the desire on the part of most hospice programs for the continuation of the primary physician's involvement in the care of the terminally ill person. Physician referral, although desirable, is not always necessary. Referrals from other professionals, family, and friends are also accepted by most hospice programs. The question of physician referral-approval is one of the

key elements to hospice development and will be discussed shortly.

Another freestanding hospice, which has an inpatient capacity of 39 beds and offers home care services through their own hospice nurses, is located in Tucson, Arizona. Initially, Hillhaven Hospice utilized the Visiting Nurse Service, supplemented by hospice nurses during the evening and on weekends. Hillhaven Hospice, which began offering services on April 17, 1977, was unique in that it offered day care services for patients who spent part of the day at the hospice. In this way, persons who might otherwise have needed to be institutionalized were able to reside in their own homes. A day care program for hospice clients also made it possible for those who were employed to participate in the care of a terminally ill family member, while continuing their work. Due to financial exigencies, Hillhaven Hospice was not able to continue offering day care to clients.

Respite care, either on a day care basis or for short periods of time, such as a weekend or for a week to 10 days, provides the terminally ill person with care while allowing family members to have an opportunity for some rest and recreation. Short periods of respite care away from their loved ones make it possible for some families to continue to provide home care to members who are dying.

Another model of hospice services is given by the Toledo Hospital and the Toledo Visiting Nurse Service. A collaborative service has been arranged between the 17-bed inpatient oncology unit of the Toledo Hospital and the Visiting Nurse Service. Toledo Hospital hospice patients are discharged to the home care of the V.N.S. Hospice home care patients experiencing problems call the Visiting Nurse Service directly during the day. However, during the hours from 4:30 P.M. to 8:00 A.M., home care clients call the oncology ward. If the nurse on duty thinks a home visit is required, she utilizes the hospital's long-range beeper system to contact the visiting nurse on call.

By way of contrast, the hospice program of the Visiting Nurse Service in Hartford, Connecticut, offers 24-hour-per-day, 7-days-per-week care for its terminally ill patients without a direct linkage to an inpatient unit. This program, namely the Hartford Visiting Nurse Service Hospice program, is nurse-directed, as are some others. For example, in Dayton, Ohio, a nurse-directed hospice program, not associated with the Visiting Nurse Service, provides home care services. This has been accomplished because local hospitals each contribute one nurse to the community hospice program.

The Veterans Administration is now investigating hospice care. A 15-bed inpatient unit has been established at the Wadsworth V.A. hospital in Los Angeles. One of those beds is reserved for patients who require care but have no family member or friend to serve as primary care giver in the home. The V.A. Hospice is investigating various facets of hospice care in its research program. Program evaluation is also emphasized, and these efforts are supported by a unique relationship with academicians at UCLA.

Another hospice group which is affiliated with a university is located in Springfield, Illinois. The University of Southern Illinois and St. John's Hospital have coordinated their efforts in starting a Continuum of Health Care Program. They plan to provide ambulatory and home care as well as a 20-bed inpatient facility. What is most interesting about this program is that it will be placed in physical proximity to a day care program for the elderly. A home care program for the elderly is also available. This mutlifocal programming is characteristic of St. Christopher's Hospice in London, England, but is not found in most programs in the United States. For example, St. Christopher's Hospice has a Draper Wing for housing the nonsick elderly. St. Christopher's also has a day care program for staff children. St. John's Hospice plans to accept patients with nonmalignant processes such as multiple sclerosis and motor-neuron disease, as well as those with cancer. This, too, distinguishes the program as St. John's, for the overwhelming majority of hospice programs, as mentioned previously, give care only to those with cancer.

Another model of hospice care is that represented by the Southeastern Michigan Hospice, Inc. This hospice, which will have a 40-bed inpatient unit as well as a home care program, has been formed by a consortium of hospitals in the Detroit area. The unit, which will be a floor of an extended care facility, will be independent and separate from the parent hospitals and yet have the advantage of an affiliation with the acute care institutions in the region. Theoretically, at least, this tie-in would seem to reduce the possibility of a lack of referrals to their facility which, according to both personal interviews and our mailed questionnaire, is a problem for many of our respondents.

Most hospices do not currently provide comprehensive care programs. An example of a limited program, which nonetheless is an innovative attempt to meet the needs in their community, is found in the Lake Orion, Michigan, Hospice Group, which is a committee of Oxford-Orion Fish (Friends in Service Here). Their emphasis is on the training of volunteers who engage in various family support activities rather than in the provision of direct physical care to the patient. The Lake Orion group has also organized a series of lectures as part of their focus on community education.

It can be seen from this account that there are numerous models of hospice programs currently in operation. Undoubtedly even greater diversity exists. This diversity has been encouraged as a means of meeting the needs of the people in various communities. It also has been encouraged as a means of investigating the utility of various models of hospice care. In an effort to forestall premature closure on this issue, leaders of the hospice movement in Oregon have temporarily delayed the setting of standards and hospice accreditation (Jacobsen, 1979). The emphasis has been one of encouraging innovation without, at the same time, abandoning a concern for the danger of exploitation.

To put the first part of this chapter in some perspective, data from the mailed questionnaire will be utilized to supplement the findings. To obtain this data, the following questions were asked:

- At what stage of development would you say your group is?
  - A. Informal discussion
  - B. Formally organized process for examining issues and information
  - C. Development of plans for hospice care—beginning implementation
  - D. Delivery of services

Depending on the stage of development, respondents were directed to the appropriate part of the questionnaire. For example, those actively engaged in the delivery of services were asked:

- Do you currently provide home care?
- Do you have your own inpatient unit?
- Is your inpatient unit:
  - A. Freestanding
  - B. Part of an acute care hospital
  - C. Part of a nursing home
  - D. Other

Of the 50 respondents who said they were actively engaged in the delivery of services, 30 (or 60 percent) provide only home care, 18 (or 36 percent) engage in both inpatient care and home care, and 2 programs are doing neither.[5] Most hospice programs provide home care either directly through their own home care nurses or, more typically, through contractual arrangements with the Visiting Nurse Service or some other home health agency. Hospice groups providing home care are far less likely to have a direct inpatient linkage than the reverse. In fact, one of the major problems confronting hospice home care groups is where to send their clients who require inpatient care.

The argument as to the benefits of a freestanding versus attached hospice is one of the minor strains in the hospice movement. Those who favor a detached, or freestanding, unit speak to the hominess of their facilities and to the fact that hospice programs are attempting to get away from the "traditional model of medical care." It is argued that one needs to get out of the system so as to be able to transcend the medical model. Proponents of hospice units in acute care facilities note that other medical services are readily available in these facilities and so may be utilized as needed for rendering high quality care to the terminally ill. Furthermore, it is argued that, by setting up a caring system in close proximity to curative activities, one is in the best position to influence other aspects of the medical care system. Lastly, it is suggested, detached units separate and isolate the terminally ill from the rest of the health care system, and for that matter, society.

Whatever the merits of either position, our data indicate that for those groups indicating they have inpatient units, 62 percent are part of an acute care facility while only 11 percent are housed in a detached, or freestanding, unit. Part of the explanation for this may be found in the cost of constructing new units as well as in the over-beddedness of some geographical areas.

In response to a question on the professional identification of the administrator-director of the hospice program, it was found that in those programs currently delivering services 40 percent of the directors were nurses, while 14 percent of the directors identified themselves as social workers. The programs currently delivering hospice care are predominantly headed by women (76 percent). It will be interesting to see if these ratios, that is, women and nurses as directors, are maintained in those programs which are now in the formative stages. As hospice becomes an accepted program of care, one would expect to see a shifting, if not a reversal, of these ratios. It seems likely that many current programs have nurse-directors who perform the role of coordinator of care. This position, with the expansion of hospice programs, may be superseded by the position of a nonnurse administrator. Unless nurses assert themselves, future

---

[5] These two programs are providing psychological and social support services to patients and families.

surveys may not show the same percentage of nursing leadership. Furthermore, the role of the physician in hospice programs is emphasized both in written materials and in public meetings (Lack, 1978). Although there are political reasons for such an approach, the result is to emphasize the status quo, with medicine as the dominant profession in the interdisciplinary team. This shift in the collegial roles of hospice team members is not the only change which is occurring.

As hospice home care programs are becoming more well known, the composition of the hospice team appears to be changing. And by composition I am referring here only to the position of the volunteer versus the paid professional. According to our survey data, in established hospice home care programs, a smaller proportion of the programs are staffed by volunteers ($N = 8$) than are staffed by a combination of paid professionals and volunteers ($N = 23$).

For those programs at the beginning implementation stage, slightly more are staffed by volunteers ($N = 22$) than are staffed by paid professionals ($N = 21$). One would expect that volunteers will be incorporated into these programs in a different manner once the delivery of services commences. The volunteers in these newer programs will more likely fill a role which supplements the efforts of the paid professionals. By way of contrast, in the first few programs in the United States, volunteer professionals were devoting time not only to planning but also to the ongoing delivery of services. Interviews with hospice leaders suggest that the difficulty of maintaining what are essentially two full-time jobs (one for which one is paid, and the other on a volunteer basis) combined with the nature of the work has contributed to the transition from all-volunteer groups to those staffed by paid professionals combined with part-time volunteers. Although there is some debate as to the precise mix, there is a consensus that it is desirable for volunteers to be part-time. The English advocate that even the paid professionals work part-time, but, that is another issue and is related to staff stress.

Several sources of resistance to the hospice movement were mentioned by groups currently delivering hospice care. According to questionnaire responses, physicians were the greatest source of resistance (50 percent of all sources mentioned); social workers and health system agencies (12½ percent each) made up the next largest groups. In marked contrast, hospice groups still at the beginning implementation stage mentioned visiting nurse services and public health nurses as their major source of resistance 30 percent of the time, followed by home health agencies and physicians (15 percent each). However, other questions in the survey, as well as observations made by participants, suggest an overwhelming concern with potential physician resistance, since such resistance could mean a lack of referrals. At the beginning implementation stage, this concern is verbalized as a need for the education of the medical community. The increasing opposition of visiting nurse services and home health agencies may be explained by the fact that these groups claim to be doing hospice care already. Some home health agency respondents to our survey said, in effect, "I don't know what all the fuss is about—we've been caring for the terminally ill at home for a long time now." And indeed these home health agencies have rendered such care. The crucial question is whether there are any meaningful differences between this care and that provided by hospice programs.

In summary, our survey data are consonant with the results from data derived from interviews and participant observation. These results indicate that multiple models of hospice care currently exist, particularly in the United States. Exceedingly few of these programs meet all of the criteria for a full-service hospice program as elaborated by the National Hospice Organization. For example, even those groups which provide both inpatient and home care may not employ the services of a pharmacist, a professional considered an essential member of the interdisciplinary team. The counterposition to those advocating standards and criteria is that the movement needs flexibility at this time to experiment with various hospice models.

Strict regulation, it is argued, is premature and would inhibit exploration of the various options. Those who favor regulation at this time are concerned with the need to maintain standards so as to avoid the "nursing home scandal." This debate is a source of strain within the hospice movement.

Another cause for concern within the hospice movement is that, although the leadership in hospice is coming from professionals traditionally concerned with health care, so is the resistance. The emphasis on professional education is, therefore, an important aspect of most hospice programs. Ultimately the acceptance of hospice care into the health care system may not be a question of professional prerogative or ownership of the patient, but one of financial exigency. Can hospice care be delivered in a financially feasible manner and without any erosion in standards? The next several years should provide the answer.

EDITOR'S QUESTIONS FOR DISCUSSION

In reviewing the differences in models of hospice care, how can the cooperation model (Chap. 39) be applied as a triad in the provision of care? Can it be used to resolve issues of concern to patients, health professionals, and organization facilities for care? How effective might it be to develop strong dyad prior to triad relationships in prevention and/or resolution of problematic situations? What variables exist which influence attitudes toward dying and death?

What factors contributed to the different models of hospice care in the United States and Canada? What social, economic, professional, and organizational issues are involved in implementation of hospice care? What are the "driving" and "restraining" forces for and against progression of the hospice movement? What factors have contributed to the effectiveness of the Connecticut Hospice? How has the politics of health care affected the development of hospice models? To what extent are services provided in hospice care determined by availability, interest of health professionals, and other personnel resources, rather than need to provide more comprehensive services? What strategies and avenues might be explored to provide more comprehensive services? What are the advantages and disadvantages of day care programs for the client, care provider, and facility? Are there dangers of exploitation in hospice care? How can standards be enforced without strict regulation?

What factors involve criteria for admission of clients to inpatient, home, or a combination of both models of hospice care? How justifiable are current criteria for most models of care? What alternatives might be explored for admission of persons into home care programs who do not have someone to act as a primary care giver? What issues would need to be addressed in developing models of hospice care for patients who have long-term incurable illnesses? Is there evidence of equal concern and care for patients with incurable illnesses as exists for those who have terminal cancer? What strategies can be offered to resolve the issues of physician referral-approval for hospice care and readmission of clients to hospital facilities?

What is the role of professional nurses in hospice care? What implications exist for the nursing profession in the high proportion of administrator-directors of hospice programs being nurses? How might staff stress-burnout be prevented or managed? Is there evidence of a need to educationally prepare nurses for hospice care that may differ from roles in visiting nurse services or home health agencies?

How might empirical evaluation of hospice care be conducted? What essential research questions need to be addressed? How might resistances to the hospice movement by health professionals be studied? Discuss the reliability and validity of the data base secured to describe differing models of hospice care. What strategies might be suggested to effectively deal with the methodological obstacles in conducting hospice research?

REFERENCES

Jacobsen, Gary
  1979 Personal communication. Oregon Comprehensive Cancer Program.
Lack, Sylvia A.
  1978 "New Haven (1974): Characteristics of a hospice program of care." Pp. 41–52 in Glenn Davidson (ed.), The Hospice Development in Administration. Washington, D.C.: Hemisphere.
Lack, Sylvia A. and Robert W. Buckingham III
  1978 First American Hospice. New Haven, Conn.: Hospice, Inc.
Lofland, Lyn H.
  1978 The Craft of Dying: The Modern Face of Death. Beverly Hills, Calif.: Sage.

Mount, B. M.
  1976 Report of Pilot Project, January 1975–January 1977. Montreal: Palliative Care Service, Royal Victoria Hospital.
Preliminary Directory of The National Hospice Organization
  1978 New Haven, Conn.: NHO.
Saunders, Cicely
  1967 The Management of Terminal Illness. London: Hosp. Med. Publ.
Woodson, Robert
  1976 "The concept of hospice care in terminal disease." Frontiers of Radiation Therapy Oncology, vol. xi, 161–179. Basel, Switzerland: S. Kargen A. G.

Chapter 41

Conceptual Issues in Nursing Diagnosis

Marjory Gordon, R.N., Ph.D., F.A.A.N.
Professor
School of Nursing
Boston College
Chestnut Hill, Massachusetts

One cannot have a comprehensive view of consumer care without specifically considering the diagnosis for treatment. Treatment follows from diagnosis. The nursing profession has long been involved in formulating a means in nursing practice to describe and implement standards for what nurses do. Inherent in this process is the differentiation between a nursing and medical diagnosis. Legal, professional, and social responsibilities require that distinctions be made. Marjory Gordon focuses on underlying conceptual issues in nomenclature development. Diagnostic terms are needed for nurses to summarize the nursing process data of assessing, planning, implementing, and evaluating nursing care.

Gordon offers a structural definition of a nursing diagnosis. It has three components: the health problem, the probable cause, and defining signs and symptoms. She contrasts potential health problems with actual problems. The latter requires specification of etiological factor(s), which is critical to nursing intervention. She asserts that signs and symptoms exist as clusters of critical defining characteristics for each diagnostic category. The high probability of signs and symptoms being present for a specific category leads to accuracy and differentiation in diagnosis. Legal certainty is not possible due to behavioral data being included in diagnostic judgment. Conceptual definitions are also presented which pertain to dysfunctional health reaction patterns and responses amenable for nursing intervention. Concepts used by various nursing theorists serve as the bases for the definitions. Although little agreement exists among theorists on conceptualization of a nursing diagnosis, there is consensus for the "working" definition, "a phrase or term which is a synthesis of a cluster of empirical indicators describing characteristics of a unitary man."

An issue that is considerably discussed pertains to the condition a diagnosis describes. It is recognized that nurses are confronted not only with actual and potential problems but also with conditions that are not a health state. Gordon believes that developing a nomenclature and classification system should accommodate all of these areas. She illustrates by numerous examples the dissimilarities between a medical and nursing diagnosis. Gordon notes patient conditions where the use of a pathophysiological concept is actually a rewording of a medical diagnosis. She maintains that if nurses assert they treat a state, they are viewing health problems as being treated under protocols or have not defined the problem from a nursing perspective. It is emphasized that a nursing diagnosis does not require a medical referral.

The work of the National Conference Group for Classification of Nursing Diagnoses is outlined. The group has established guidelines for submission and review of diagnoses. Once a diagnostic category is accepted it is considered ready for clinical testing. Validation is essential of the existence, incidence, and utilization of the diagnostic category in determining nursing therapy. Different approaches, methods, and projects are described for nomenclature identification and classification into categories. Although there is concern that many systems will be developed, the ultimate criterion of acceptability will be clinical usefulness. The objective is to create a standardized language for describing client problems.

Gordon speaks to controversies regarding the implementation of nursing diagnosis. The nurse's professional role concept is cited as a critical factor in her readiness to use diagnosis. The frequent changing of perspectives in the overall focus of clinical practice is another factor. She concludes progress will increase in resolving all the issues due to the commitment of nurses.

"Nursing process" is a term widely used in North America and other parts of the world to describe what nurses do. Standards for this component of practice have been written (ANA, 1973), but in actuality these standards cannot be fully implemented until nursing diagnoses (Standard II) are developed and integrated into clinicians' practice. Two deterrents exist. One is diagnostic skills; many nurses have not had opportunities to learn and develop expertise in this area. The second, closely related factor, is the profession's need to develop diagnostic terms and concepts for summarizing assessment data and for planning, implementing, and evaluating nursing care. These two factors are interdependent. For the present discussion, skills will be ignored in order to focus on the underlying conceptual issues in nomenclature development and utilization.

CONCEPTUAL FOCUS

The development of nursing diagnosis requires that the practitioner, educator, researcher, or theorist answer, not abstractly and not superficially, the question: What is nursing? To use diagnosis in clinical practice, a reasonably concrete idea of the focus of nursing is needed. Discriminations have to be made between clinical problems which are, or are not, within the scope of nursing practice; that is, boundaries must be drawn to delineate the aspect of practice that requires judgments independent of another profession's orders or protocols.

For consumer protection there are legal and professional boundaries in diagnosis and treatment. Also to be considered in diagnosis are a profession's social responsibilities. These considerations bring the abstract question of what is the focus of nursing and its domain of diagnosis and treatment to the practical level (i.e., the concrete reality of practice) and require that nursing theoreticians and nursing practitioners seek answers together.

Since nursing diagnosis was first described by McManus (1950), many authors have offered their own definitions. Gebbie and Lavin (1975) define it as a product of nursing assessment. Campbell (1978), in her study of students' diagnoses, views it as a human response and resource limitation, and Gordon (1976:1298) sees it as concise terms describing an actual or potential health problem, or the state of the client. In McLane's (1981) survey of educators the latter is a commonly used definition.

Structural Definition

A structural definition of a nursing diagnosis permits a greater grasp of the idea. Such a definition addresses structural components necessary for recognition and utilization. The three components are (1) the health problem amenable to nursing intervention (P), (2) the probable cause or etiological factors (E), and (3) defining signs and symptoms(S). This has been described as the PES structural format for a diagnosis (Gordon, 1976).

Potential health problems requiring preventive intervention do not require etiological specification. The risk factors or defining signs and symptoms are also the cause of the high-risk state. For example, bed rest, incontinence, inadequate nutrition, and decreased perceptual awareness produce a high risk for potential skin breakdown. These signs define the state and also the etiology, or cause, of the state.

In contrast, *actual problems* require specification of etiological factor(s). This is critical for planning nursing intervention. For example, McCourt and her colleagues (1981) have delineated a set of etiological factors involved in a total self-care deficit (bathing, dressing, toileting, feeding, and grooming). The treatment of this problem is entirely different when it is related to hyperactivity in a psychiatric patient than when it is related to an uncompensated sensory-perceptual deficit following a cerebrovascular accident. In both instances, the treatment may involve basic assistance in self-care, a technical intervention; yet, a professional intervention would also include bringing the patient to an optimal functional level of self-care. The probable cause of a health problem is a critical factor for planning nursing intervention.

Each diagnostic category has a cluster of critical defining characteristics. These are the signs and symptoms that *must* be present for the diagnostic label to be used correctly. From an assessment perspective, defining characteristics are the signs and symptoms manifested by a client.

The critical defining characteristics for diagnostic labels are probabilistic criteria. They are the best predictors for judging the presence or absence of a health problem. This implies two things. One, a number of signs and symptoms may be present, but the ones that lead to high accuracy in diagnostic judgment are those that have a high probability of being present when a particular state of the client is actually present. In addition, critical defining criteria permit differential diagnosis. This means they differentiate one category from another.

The second implication of probabilistic diagnostic criteria is that logical certainty usually cannot be attained. Nursing diagnosis, medical diagnosis, and social casework diagnosis involve uncertainty-based judgments. This results from the variability of the human behavioral data used in judgment. Diagnosticians have to learn how to deal with uncertainty-based judgments, a situation not always stressed in nursing education.

Conceptual Definition

Development, classification, and standardization of nursing diagnoses require agreement on the focus of nursing. Various types of word labels to describe this focus can be generated, argued for, and accepted. *Systematic* development of scientific concepts requires a more formal process of factor isolating and naming. Dickoff et al. (1968:415–435) and Diers (1979) have emphasized this particular point and discussed the process. The focus of nursing has been conceptualized as patterns of unitary man (Rogers, 1970), self-care deficits (Orem, 1980), adaptation (Roy, 1976), and behavioral systems (Johnson, 1980). Out of the popular "patient needs" framework have come conceptualizations such as "need deprivation or alteration in meeting human needs" (Yura and Walsh, 1978:114–115) and "conflict in needs" (Soares, 1978:275). "Needs" here are constructs inferred by clients' responses.

Others have conceptualized the response itself. Little and Carnevali (1976:46) view a diagnosis as a "concise, precise, neutral statement of client response to a stressor or potential stressor in the health area." A "patient's response which is actually or potentially unhealthful" is the conceptual focus used by Mundinger and Jauron (1975:97). Gordon (1982), Shoemaker (1980:60), Durand and Prince (1966:52), and Jones (1979:67) use the term "pattern," such as "dysfunctional pattern" or "reaction pattern." At the level of abstraction represented by any of these conceptualizations, agreement as to the focus of nursing could probably be reached.

At a more concrete level, though, one may ask, What types of unhealthful human responses, reactions, or functions do nurses diagnose and treat? This question will bring diverse viewpoints to the fore. For example, Aspinall includes in her concept of nursing diagnosis the impaired functioning of a body system (1976:434). She states that this construct contrasts with medical diagnoses which focus on the underlying cause or include the etiology of the body system disturbance. Aspinall's view represents a perspective that would be consistent with certain currently identified nursing diagnoses: alterations in cardiac output, impaired gas exchange, fluid volume deficit, or alteration in tissue perfusion (Kim and Moritz, 1981). But these states are not amenable to nursing intervention as that intervention is discussed in nursing textbooks. They are a rewording of medical diagnoses using a pathophysiological concept. In this author's opinion, when a person manifests signs and symptoms of these states, a medical referral is indicated for the protection of both nurse and consumer. A nursing diagnosis does not require referral. When a biological organ or system focus is used, it leads logically to medical diagnosis or diagnoses such as those above. It must be noted that criticism of this conceptual focus and the aforementioned diagnoses is made from a particular viewpoint. Criticism is warranted only if nursing diagnosis is defined as a condition amenable to nursing therapy.

When nurses argue that they treat a state such as alteration in cardiac output, their line of reasoning reveals two things: they either view health problems treated under protocols as within the

concept or definition of nursing diagnosis, or they have not defined the patient's problem from a nursing perspective. Questioning usually elicits treatments for alteration in cardiac output that are appropriate therapy for various nursing diagnoses. These include decreased activity tolerance, ineffective coping pattern, knowledge deficits, decreased home maintenance management, or independence-dependence conflict.

An alternative conceptualization of problems treated by nurses is dysfunctional health patterns (Gordon, 1982). These patterns are defined as composite client-situations that are nonproductive; this concept of nursing diagnosis does not lead so readily to physiological alterations usually treated by a physician.

Actual dysfunctional health patterns can result from pathology or can, over time, produce disease. Potentially dysfunctional patterns describe risk states and are the basis for preventive nursing care. Table 41-1 provides a brief summary of a typology. Within each area problematic patterns can exist which have traditionally been assessed and treated by nurses. Many are currently described in diagnostic terms (Kim and Moritz, 1981). Applicability to clinical specialty areas and varied clients (persons, families, and communities) has led to suggestion that the areas provide the format for a standardized basic data base for nursing (Gordon, 1982).[1]

The National Conference Group for Classification of Nursing Diagnoses has viewed nursing diagnosis as a judgment or conclusion based on a nursing assessment (Gebbie and Lavin, 1975). No explicit conceptual focus has been accepted by this group because of the diversity of views in nursing and because diagnostic categories have been generated inductively from nurses' clinical experience.

In conjunction with this national body, a group of the major nursing theorists in the United States

---

[1] The publications of Faye McCain and Dorothy Smith especially contributed to concept and typology development.

Table 41-1 Functional Health Patterns Typology

I. *Health perception-health management pattern.* Describes client's perceived pattern of health well-being and how health is managed.

II. *Nutritional-metabolic pattern.* Describes patterns of food and fluid consumption relative to metabolic need and pattern indicators of local nutrient supply.

III. *Elimination pattern.* Describes patterns of excretory function (bowel, bladder, skin).

IV. *Activity-exercise pattern.* Describes pattern of exercise, activity, and leisure-recreation.

V. *Cognitive-perceptual pattern.* Describes sensory-perceptual pattern and functional cognitive patterns.

VI. *Sleep-rest pattern.* Describes patterns of sleep, rest, and relaxation.

VII. *Self-perception–self-concept pattern.* Describes self-concept pattern and perceptions of self (e.g., body comfort, body image).

VIII. *Role-relationship pattern.* Describes role-engagement and relationships pattern.

IX. *Sexuality-reproductive pattern.* Describes client's patterns of satisfaction-dissatisfaction with sexuality pattern. Also describes reproductive patterns.

X. *Coping-stress tolerance pattern.* Describes general coping pattern and effectiveness of the pattern in terms of stress tolerance.

XI. *Value-belief pattern.* Describes patterns of values, beliefs (including spiritual), or goals that guide choices or decisions.

Source: M. Gordon: Nursing Diagnosis: Process and Application, McGraw-Hill Book Company, New York, 1982:81.

is developing a conceptual framework for identification and classification. At the Fourth National Conference the group's working definition of nursing diagnosis was "a phrase or term which is a synthesis of a cluster of empirical indicators describing characteristics of unitary man" (Kim and Moritz, 1981). At present, the characteristics are being identified. "Relating" and "choosing" are two examples of the type of unitary characteristics that have been proposed as classification system categories. It will be interesting to watch the progress of this work in regard to diagnostic classification system development. It will also be interesting to note its potential influence on theory development in nursing.

Implicit or explicit in many discussions is the issue of what condition a diagnosis describes. Do nurses diagnose and treat health states, health problems, or both? Agreement exists that actual and potential problems are included in the concept, but discussions have occurred at national conferences regarding health states that are not problems, potential problems, or risk states. (A condition requiring anticipatory guidance is a potential

problem, not a health state.) Examples of health states are seen instead in situations in which a person, family, or community desires to reach a higher level of health functioning (Gottlieb, 1981). McKeehan (1978) has suggested the example of prospective parents desiring to attain self-growth through the experience of parenting. The couple has no knowledge, skill deficits, nor anticipated deficits; according to current expectations, values, and standards, no problems or potential problems exist in this situation, Jacob's proposal (1981) of the diagnosis, "family coping, potential for growth," was accepted by the National Conference Group for Classification of Nursing Diagnoses. This is seen as a health state in which there is a desire to "optimize wellness" and "readiness for enhanced health and growth" (Kim and Moritz, 1981).

Nurses are confronted with a myriad of health problems in clinical practice. Perhaps at times, promotion of higher levels of growth through health counseling is overlooked. Granted, current nursing resources in this country are not sufficient to treat the population's actual and potential health problems; yet, there are those who desire the type of health care described above and those who wish to practice it. The developing nomenclature and classification system will have to accommodate these diagnoses whether or not, in a practical sense, insurers provide reimbursement for personal growth counseling.

IDENTIFICATION, STANDARDIZATION, AND CLASSIFICATION ISSUES

In 1973 when participants in the First National Conference for Classification of Nursing Diagnoses initiated the process of classification, diagnosis was a vague entity to most nurses. Today, a large number of articles and one book have been published, three other books are in progress, and four national conferences have been held. Regional, state and local conferences have provided opportunities for nurses to become involved in identification of diagnostic nomenclature. The sustained effort and enthusiasm of nurses leads one to believe this is not a "passing fad" in nursing.

Identification and Standardization Issues

A number of projects for identification of diagnostic nomenclature are currently in progress. The National Conference Group for Classification of Nursing Diagnoses is the most representative group. It includes nurses from all areas and levels of practice, education, and research, as well as experts in nursing theory and its construction. All clinical specialties are represented, as well as areas of the United States and some provinces of Canada.

The Conference Group is loosely organized but closely held together by interest, enthusiasm, and commitment. It has received no outside funding for its task force, meetings, or research. Structural and funding problems have actually been assets to open, participatory development in the early years of this project.

Diagnostic concepts that describe actual or potential health problems amenable to nursing

therapy can be identified inductively from practice or deductively from a conceptual model. The National Conference Group has used the inductive approach. Nurses have labeled problems they have observed and treated in their clinical practice. Although every nurse participating undoubtedly has a set of beliefs about what nursing is, no explicit conceptual framework has been adopted for the project. Guidelines for submission and review of diagnoses are mainly structural.

The National Conference Group publishes a list of accepted diagnoses and the defining characteristics (signs and symptoms) presently identified (Kim and Moritz, 1981). Acceptance of a diagnostic category by this group means the particular category meets the guidelines and is sufficiently developed for clinical testing. Although majority agreement has been reached at each conference, most participants recognize that the list of accepted diagnoses contains terms at various levels (Kim and Moritz, 1981). For example, fear and rape-trauma syndrome are different levels of abstraction. As another example, alterations in parenting is a broad category, no doubt encompassing more specific and useful diagnoses.

Because of these ambiguities, some have suggested that a more scientific approach to identification and naming is required (Taxonomy Consultant Group, 1979). The Conference Group recognizes that clinical testing of diagnostic categories is a necessary step in validation. Testing would provide data on whether a diagnostic entity exists, its incidence, and its utilization in determining nursing therapy (Gordon and Sweeney, 1979). It has also been recognized that translation of the conference list of diagnoses would permit clinical testing in other countries and cultures, an eventual necessity for development of an international classification system. Thus far, notification of translation has been received only from Japan (Kondo, 1979).

A second project related to nomenclature identification was completed in 1980 (Simmons). The Community Health Nursing Field Project was done under contract to the Omaha Visiting Nurses Association. Although not labeled as diagnoses, many of the "nursing problems" identified were consistent with the National Conference list. In this project, problems were identified from visiting nurse records and then field-tested in various community agencies of other states. Jones (1979) also developed a list of nursing diagnoses during an exploratory research project in Canada; the second and current phase of the project is designed to test and refine the nursing diagnosis. Jones's list includes the diagnoses accepted by the National Conference.

Campbell, in a study of undergraduate students' care plans, identified a large number of nursing diagnoses (1978). This work was in progress before the First National Conference, and overlap is minimal. Under the auspices of a children and youth project, another classification system of nursing problems was developed (Minnesota Systems Research, 1976), but many of the categories are at a very concrete (symptom) level.

Some concern exists among those who envision a proliferation of nomenclature systems, which could present a situation similar to that described in the biblical story of the Tower of Babel. The objective of developing diagnostic labels is primarily the creation of a standardized language for describing client problems. The language would be a means of coding and communicating observations. The development of different word-symbols or labels for the same phenomenon certainly would deter communication, and, theoretically, the concern expressed is a legitimate one. But in actuality, attempts are continuously made by the National Conference Group to bring together individuals and groups working on classification projects. National meetings provide a forum where differences are discussed and debated. As McKay (1977:223) points out, "classification systems are of value only when they are adopted by the majority of practitioners." Thus, the ultimate criterion of acceptability will be clinical usefulness, a criterion of the so-called market place.

A number of clinical studies of nurses' utilization of the diagnosis list accepted by the National Conference are reported to be underway. These are being carried out in psychiatric, obstetrical-gynecological, and medical-surgical settings. Some preliminary reports indicate, as expected, that the accepted list is incomplete (Gordon et al, 1980; Leslie, 1981; Sweeney and Gordon, 1982). These studies provide some indication of utilization but do not take into account the reliability of the nurses using the diagnostic nomenclature. Lacking further analysis, the findings rest on the assumption that nurse subjects are not in actuality overdiagnosing or underdiagnosing (Gordon and Sweeney, 1979).

As implied above, further development and research is required before standardization of diagnostic labels is contemplated. One issue relevant to eventual standardization, as well as to current usage, is the present lack of critical defining characteristics for each accepted diagnostic category. These are the signs and symptoms that must be present for the diagnostic label to be applied. Although listings of characteristics are provided for the accepted diagnoses (Kim and Moritz, 1981), they require further study and review.

Two rather simple steps are required to identify defining characteristics. The first is a review of literature to determine the description of a category, as, for example, independence-dependence conflict. The second step is to utilize the diagnosis clinically. Each time the diagnosis is made, data should be collected on the presenting signs and symptoms and etiological factor(s). As cases accumulate, probability of each sign and symptom can be determined. The result is the identification of client characteristics highly correlated with the presence of the health problem—the critical defining characteristics. Further study could identify variations that may exist in various client populations.

When terminology is finally standardized, all nurses will have to use the existing nomenclature. Policies will be established for adding, deleting, and revising diagnostic categories at periodic intervals. The eventual standardization of terminology has implications for the present. One is that nurses wishing to influence diagnostic nomenclature development should be involved *now*. The second implication is that theoretical and clinical studies need to be done *now*.

Classification Issues

Ordering or arranging diagnostic categories into groups or sets is the process of classification. Its purposes can be multiple. For example, diagnoses can be classified into certain categories that will facilitate the process of using assessment data. Another alternative is to develop groupings of diagnoses on the basis of complexity or nursing care time quantifications, this may assist in utilization of diagnostic-related groupings for the planning of unit staffing (Halloran, 1980). Present efforts of the National Conference Group are directed toward establishing a system of conceptual organization that could provide a basis for other more sophisticated uses of the classification system.

IMPLEMENTATION ISSUES

Resolution of issues and work in progress could be facilitated if every professional nurse identified the problems used as a basis for intervention, shared insights, and reported difficulties encountered.[2] Yet in reality, a number of factors tend to militate against this.

The "Controversial" Issue

Some clinicians consider diagnosis to be outside nursing's role. One basis for this is lack of understanding that nursing diagnosis is not a usurpation of the physician's role in medical diagnosis—unless, of course, Florence Nightingale usurped the role of the army surgeons in diagnosing nutritional deficits in Crimean hospitals.

Other reasons that nursing diagnosis is a controversial issue are also related to an erroneous

[2] Reports could be disseminated by publication in nursing journals or by the Task Force of the National Conference Group. (Write to Dr. Marjory Gordon, Boston College, School of Nursing, Chestnut Hill, MA 02167.)

concept of the nurse's role. If nursing is seen exclusively as assisting the physician in disease treatment, then nursing diagnosis is an inappropriate role. A related reason is, as one staff nurse said, "nursing administration doesn't enforce it." Underlying this is the dominant "employee" orientation of the nursing role. Yet another version of this refrain is "the doctors may react." This too is an indication of whom the nurse views as significant and what type of atmosphere should be maintained in colleague relationships. Seemingly, nursing supervisors or administrators, unlike doctors, do not "react," or, if they do, it is not a situation to be avoided.

These are not isolated comments or conceptions. Neither are they related only to nursing diagnosis; they are signs of a deeper, more comprehensive problem. Implementation of nursing diagnosis in some practice settings must begin with a consideration of the nurses' self-conception as professionals. Ignoring this basic issue is a violation of the principle of readiness. In order to use diagnosis, nurses have to perceive autonomy and accountability as their professional characteristics.

The "Consistency" Issue

How difficult it is for human beings to shift perspectives! Changing one's global approach from task to task produces cognitive strain. Yet this is what is expected when there is a lack of consistency in the overall focus of clinical practice.

Consider an example of inconsistency. Nursing diagnosis is part of nursing process, and this is the accepted approach to patient care. Evaluation, whether for purposes of salary or position change, is based on such things as neatness, interpersonal relations, and assuming responsibility. Staffing is based on patient's need for medically delegated treatments or bathing. Documentation is provided by the traditional nurse's note, emphasizing the presence or absence of disease signs and symptoms. To everyone's satisfaction, "appears to be bleeding" has virtually disappeared. Rounds or shift reports focus on tests, treatments, and other observations.

In-service education is up to date on new procedures, (usually medical), new developments in treatment of disease, and current changes in organization methods. Orientation for new staff includes nursing process, its use, importance, and the nursing philosophy in regard to this. Quality assurance programs focus on populations with certain diseases, disease complications, or therapeutic objectives of nursing. Clearly, depending on the activity, the nurse's perspective is constantly shifting from one framework to another.

This rather extended and extreme example does have value. How much easier it would be if clinical activities were consistently organized in terms of the clinical problems of clients. Care, reports, quality assurance, and in-service education (to some extent) could be based on nursing diagnoses, and evaluation of nurses could emphasize competency in nursing process. This would provide consistency in thinking about practice, and it would facilitate implementation of nursing process and its component, nursing diagnosis.

SUMMARY

A number of issues need to be resolved in the current efforts toward identification, classification, and implementation of nursing diagnoses. Some issues relate to the development of nursing's clinical science, others to the clinicians' concept of their role. The current classification system of nursing diagnoses consists of a set of defined, and some ill-defined, conditions nurses say they treat in their practice. The system is a momentous step, taken in less than 10 years, toward describing the domain of nursing practice from a clinical perspective. The next 10 years should show even greater progress because of the commitment of nurses to solving the conceptual issues, implementing nursing diagnosis in educational settings, and studying its clinical usefulness.

EDITOR'S QUESTIONS FOR DISCUSSION

Why cannot standards for nursing practice be fully implemented until nursing diagnoses are integrated into clinician's practice? How does nursing diagnosis enable the question, "What is nursing?" to be answered? What means can be suggested for integration into practice? What evidence is there of commitment by nurses in practice to use nursing diagnoses? Are mechanisms available to enforce the implementation and use of nursing diagnoses? In Gordon's discussion of nursing diagnosis as a controversial issue, what implications are there for nursing education, nursing administration, and nursing practice? What strategies can be suggested to resolve the issue?

Would you agree with the difficulties Gordon cites in shifting perspectives from task to task in nursing practice? Could cognitive strain in the implementation of nursing diagnoses also occur due to a need for a change from a task to task perspective to a global approach and focus of clinical practice? How might possible strain and difficulty be prevented in planning for change and implementation of nursing diagnoses? To what extent do you agree with Gordon's solution for providing consistency in viewing nursing practice? Indicate by examples how nursing care, reports, quality assurance, in-service education, and performance evaluation could be based on nursing diagnoses.

What is meant by probabilistic criteria for diagnostic labels? Contrast medical diagnoses with nursing diagnoses. What is the focus in a nursing diagnosis? How possible is certainty in a nursing diagnosis when compared with certainty in a medical diagnosis? Do you agree with Gordon that the rewording of a medical diagnosis by using pathophysiological concepts to describe a patient state is not a nursing diagnosis? Would you agree that such identification in rewording patient's conditions require a medical referral? Would you agree that when nurses treat a state under protocols that they are not utilizing a nursing perspective or diagnosis? What implications are there in the findings of Monnig's survey (Chap. 3) for nursing diagnoses? What relationship exists among the competency findings of Clayton's study (Chap. 10), the development of diagnostic skills by nurses, and nursing diagnoses?

Would you agree that potential problems, risk states, prevention of illness, health maintenance, and optimizing wellness are areas of nursing practice which require a different nomenclature and classification system than for actual problems? How might nomenclature be developed to include these states? What examples can you provide of the inductive approach being used to identify diagnostic concepts? What deductive examples can be cited from conceptual models of nursing theorists? What are the relationships among the development of diagnostic nomenclature, a classification system, and nursing theory? What are the implications for nursing theory development in the work by the National Conference Group for Classification of Nursing Diagnoses?

Review Sweeney's and Gordon's Chap. 23 as a clinical study of nurses' utilization of the diagnostic list accepted by the National Conference Group. What implications are there from Gordon's discussion of conceptual, classification issues and findings showed in Chap. 23 for future utilization studies?

What are the advantages and disadvantages of standardization of diagnostic labels? How can the current lack of critical defining characteristics be developed for each diagnostic category? In the formulation of groupings of diagnoses, should the professional level of health personnel available to provide care be considered? What policies might be established for adding, deleting, and revising diagnostic categories at periodic intervals? What progress would you predict in resolving conceptual issues, identification, classification, implementation, and utilization of nursing diagnoses in the next 10 years?

REFERENCES

American Nurses Association
1973 Standards for Nursing Practice. Kansas City, Mo.: ANA.

Aspinall, Mary Jo
1976 "Nursing diagnosis—the weak link." Nursing Outlook 24:433–437.

Campbell, Claire
1978 Nursing Diagnosis and Intervention in Nursing Practice. New York: Wiley.

Dickoff, James, Patricia James, and Ernestine Weidenbach
1968 "Theory in a practice discipline: Part I. Practice-oriented theory." Nursing Research 17:415–435.

Diers, Donna
1979 Research in Nursing Practice. Philadelphia: Lippincott.

Durand, M. and P. Prince
1966 "Nursing diagnosis: Process and decisions." Nursing Forum 5:50–64.

Gebbie, K. and M. A. Lavin
1975 Classification of Nursing Diagnoses. Proceedings of the 1st National Conference. St. Louis, Mo., October, 1973. St. Louis: Mosby.

Gordon, Marjory
1976 "Nursing diagnosis and the diagnostic process." American Journal of Nursing 76:1298–1300.

Gordon, Marjory
1982 Nursing Diagnosis: Process and Application. New York: McGraw-Hill.

Gordon, Marjory and Mary Ann Sweeney
1979 "Methodological problems and issues in identifying and standardizing nursing diagnosis." Advances in Nursing Science 2:1–15.

Gordon, Marjory, Mary Ann Sweeney, and Kathleen McKeehan
1980 "Clinical utilization of nursing diagnoses." American Journal of Nursing 80:672–674.

Gottlieb, Laurie
 1981 "Small steps toward the development of a health classification system for nursing." Pp. 203–213 in M. J. Kim and D. A. Moritz (eds.), Classification of Nursing Diagnosis. Proceedings of the 3rd and 4th National Conference. St. Louis, Mo., April, 1978, and 1980. New York: McGraw-Hill.

Halloran, Edward
 1980 "Analysis of variation in nursing workload by patient and nursing condition." Unpublished doctoral dissertation, 8106567, University of Illinois. The Medical Center, Chicago.

Jacob, Dorothea
 1981 "Diagnoses submitted to Fourth National Conference." Pp. 287–290 in M. J. Kim and D. A. Moritz (eds.), Classification of Nursing Diagnosis. Proceedings of the 3rd and 4th National Conference. St. Louis, Mo., April, 1978, and 1980. New York: McGraw-Hill.

Johnson, Dorothy E.
 1980 "The behavioral system model for nursing." Pp. 207–216 in J. P. Riehl and Sister Callista Roy (eds.), Conceptual Models for Nursing Practice. 2nd ed. New York: Appleton-Century-Crofts.

Jones, Phyllis E.
 1979 "Terminology for nursing diagnoses." Advances in Nursing Science 2:65–72.

Kim, Mi Ja and Derry Ann Moritz, (eds.)
 1981 Classification of Nursing Diagnoses. Proceedings of the 3rd and 4th National Conference. St. Louis, Mo., April, 1978, and 1980. New York: McGraw-Hill.

Kondo, Yunko
 1979 Director, Continuing Education, St. Luke's College, Tokyo, Japan. Personal communication.

Leslie, F. M.
 1981 "Nursing Diagnosis: Use in long-term care." American Journal of Nursing 81:1012–1014.

Little, Delores and Doris Carnevali
 1976 "Diagnostic statement: Problem defined." Pp. 45–64 in J. B. Walter, G. P. Pardee, and D. M. Molbo (eds.), Dynamics of Problem-Oriented Approaches: Patient Care and Documentation. Philadelphia: Lippincott.

McCourt, Ann
 1981 "Measurement of functional deficits in quality assurance." Pp. 1–5 in American Nurses Association (eds.), Quality Assurance Update. 5:1–5. Kansas City, Mo.: American Nurses Association.

McKay, Rose
 1977 "Research Q and A." Nursing Research 26:222–224.

McKeehan, Kathleen
 1978 Doctoral student, Case Western Reserve, Cleveland, Ohio. Personal communication.

McLane, Audrey
 1981 "Nursing diagnosis in baccalaureate and graduate education." Pp. 105–119 in M. J. Kim and D. A. Moritz (eds.), Classification of Nursing Diagnoses. Proceedings of the 3rd and 4th National Conference. St. Louis, Mo., April, 1978, and 1980. New York: McGraw-Hill.

McManus, Louise
 1950 "Assumptions of functions of nursing." Pp. 54–55 in Regional Planning for Nursing and Nursing Education. New York: Bureau of Publications, Teachers College, Columbia University.

Minnesota Systems Research, Inc.
 1976 Nursing Problem Classification for Children and Youth. Rockville, Md.: Public Health Service.

Mundinger, Mary O'Neil and Grace Dotterer Jauron
 1975 "Developing a nursing diagnosis." Nursing Outlook 23:94–98.

Orem, Dorothea E.
 1980 Nursing Concepts of Practice. New York: McGraw-Hill.

Rogers, Martha
 1970 Introduction to the Theoretical Basis for Nursing. New York: Davis.

Roy, Sister Callista
 1976 Introduction to Nursing: An Adaptation Model. Englewood Cliffs, N.J.: Prentice-Hall.

Shoemaker, Joyce
 1980 "How nursing diagnosis helps focus your care." RN 42:56–61.

Simmons, D. A.
  1980 Classification Scheme for Client Problems
        in Community Health Nursing. D.H.H.S.
        Publication #HRA 80–16. Department of
        Health and Human Services. Washington,
        D.C.: U.S. Government Printing Office.
Soares, Carol A.
  1978 "Nursing and medical diagnoses: Com-
        parison of variant and essential features."
        Pp. 269–278 in Norma Chaska (ed.), The
        Nursing Profession: Views through the
        Mist. New York: McGraw-Hill.
Sweeney, Mary Ann and Marjory Gordon
  1982 "Nursing diagnosis: Implementation and

incidence in an obstetrical and gynecological population." Pp. in Norma Chaska,
(ed.), The Nursing Profession: A Time to
Speak, New York: McGraw-Hill.
Taxonomy Consultant Group
  1979 American Nurses' Foundation Taxonomy
        Project (P. Brimmer, Director). Kansas
        City, Mo.: American Nurses' Foundation.
Yura, Helen and Mary Walsh
  1978 Human Needs and the Nursing Process.
        New York: Appleton-Century-Crofts.

Chapter 42

The Role and Function of the Clinical Nurse Specialist

Grayce M. Sills, R.N., Ph.D., F.A.A.N.
Professor, Director
Advanced Psychiatric/Mental Health Nursing
School of Nursing
The Ohio State University
Columbus, Ohio

Following the essay on nursing diagnoses, it is timely to focus on a professional role, which could be the prime avenue for successful implementation of diagnoses in nursing practice. Furthermore, it is essential in this era of specialization for health professionals to be knowledgeable as to the evolvement and present status of specialized roles in nursing. Grayce M. Sills uniquely examines the specific role of the clinical nurse specialist (C.N.S). She delineates the historical and societal forces which created a need for the profession to respond. In 1980 over 75 graduate programs existed to prepare nurses for the role. Dimensions of the role, concerns related to positions and setting of employment, and educational preparation are portrayed.

Early history indicates a number of factors contributed to the development of specialization in nursing. A shift from a model of private duty nursing to hospital-based nursing was one factor. Other factors were the hierarchical nature of hospitals with bureaucratic requisites of standardization and governing notions regarding women in a bureaucracy. The result was an emphasis for expertise in the areas of teaching, administration, and supervision. Sills remarks about the early trends to award certificates upon completion of programs, which varied in length, in a specialized area. She notes that the varying type of programs present today to prepare nurse practitioners may be a resurrection of historical trends. The first graduate level program to prepare clinical specialists was developed in psychiatric nursing in 1954 by Hildegard E. Peplau at Rutgers. Titles for the advanced practitioner have always been an issue. The 1980 American Nurses' Association's (ANA) social policy statement officially clarified the situation. Even so, there exist about 20 organizations outside the ANA which represent various types of "specialized" practice.

Admitting that there is a low level of consensus, Sills conceptualizes the dimensions of the clinical specialist position. These are addressed under the categories of clinical competence, organizational responsibility, and the practice component. She identifies the philosophical matrix for practice, maintains that the specialist must come to the practice setting with an in-depth theoretical base relevant to the area of specialization, test practice against the available standards for care, and demonstrate expertise in implementing the functions of a specialist. Sills presents the debate as to the appropriate position for the specialist within the organization: staff versus line authority and responsibility. She indicates the type of settings and arrangements by and in which clinical specialists are employed. These include hospitals, individual or groups of physicians, outpatient settings as Health Maintenance Organizations (HMOs), and solo practitioners or in joint practice with other nurse specialists and/or physicians. She cites the ANA's Social Policy Statement which urges the development of negotiated positions without standardization.

Two aspects of the practitioner dimension are explored. In the direct practice component, Sills maintains that advanced educational preparation at the master's or doctoral level is essential for the continuous development of a theoretical knowledge base. Experience is also emphasized, preferably through a network of support as a mentor/coach, or at least with peers. The indirect practice roles explored are educator, consultant, supervisor, and researcher. Sills views the specialist as a provider of formal or informal teaching-learning experiences for nursing staff and the consumer. Knowledge of teaching-learning theories is deemed as a requisite. She provides guidelines for functioning as a consultant and cites instances where the specialist may need to be a consultee. It is indicated that the specialist may be expected to be not only a skilled clinical but also a managerial supervisor. The research role requires the C.N.S. to be an intelligent consumer of research findings, generate research questions from practice and collaborate in the research process, and report case studies connected from a conceptual framework to describe, analyze, and evaluate nursing care. Sills perceives that inherent in all the roles is a requisite knowledge base regarding change: types, processes, theories, and strategies.

Numerous concerns are delineated. A major issue is the need for the C.N.S. to be able to assess the setting where she plans to be employed. This includes inquiry regarding philosophical stance, type and structure, and geographical and power location of nursing within the organization. Sills makes a strong distinction between autonomous and independent practice. The former connotes power and control over one's area of expertise allowing for interdependence to thrive. The latter implies individual practice, results in accountability dilemmas, and is not viable in the evolving health care system. Sills argues for autonomous contextual settings. She proposes nurse-corporations as an alternative rational solution to the problems that exist for specialists in bureaucratic settings. The professional nurse would not be an employee of the hospital or agency, but a member of a professional corporation that provides nursing services on a fee-for-service basis. Sills foresees her proposal as a means for clearer accountability, direct reimbursement for services, and a solution to problems of the collective bargaining program. Clinical nurse specialists would have the option to incorporate in group practice models and contract with agencies and organizations. It is suggested corporations could be developed locally and nationally, the latter as the American Nurses' Corporation.

Sills urges C.N.S. to be influential in health affairs and policy groups at the local through national levels. She exhorts participation in the ANA, national advanced practice groups, the women's movement, and development of certification for areas of specialty competence. In conclusion, Sills focuses specifically on the preparation and education of the C.N.S. A master's degree, if not a Doctor of Nursing Science degree, is advocated as the minimal educational preparation, to be followed by 2 to 3 years of clinical experience. She emphasizes the need for commitment to life-long learning, common and in-depth content for practice, role modeling, and familiarity with the ANA standards for practice in the area of specialty. Sills predicts that the role will be the entry level for the profession in 50 years.

HISTORICAL DEVELOPMENT OF THE CLINICAL NURSE SPECIALIST POSITION

Before beginning a discussion of the position of clinical nurse specialist (C.N.S.), it will be useful to highlight the historical developments which presaged the emergence of this relatively young idea in the overall development of the profession of nursing.

Smoyak (1976) attributes a very early beginning to specialization and cites an article in the first issue of the *American Journal of Nursing* in October, 1900, by Katherine DeWitt titled "Specialities in Nursing." Several authors support the idea that specialization in nursing occurred quite early in the profession's development. The private duty nurse, who became skillful in certain types of nursing care, developed an idiosyncratic base for practice. This practice, based on experience, was likely a prototype of what was to emerge in a somewhat different form after World War II (Peplau, 1965; Norris, 1977; Burd, 1966). Peplau (1965) delineates societal forces that have led the development of specialization in any field as (1) an increase in knowledge germane to the field, (2) the development of new technology, and (3) the response to a hitherto little-known public need and public interest.

Norris (1977) reviews some of the historical elements which combined to create graduate education in nursing. She suggests the present trend began during World War II, when nurses had great authority and responsibility in patient care, especially in different situations and field hospitals. When they returned home, these nurses had the G.I. Bill, which afforded the opportunity to pursue bachelor's and then master's degrees. The National Mental Health Act of 1946 greatly abetted graduate education for psychiatric nurses, and in 1964 the Nurse Training Act facilitated educational opportunities for nurses in other areas of clinical practice. Graduate education in nursing began in the 1950s. Norris notes that it was 1952 before there was a subject heading in the *American Journal of Nursing* index for graduate education and only as recently as 1960 did the NLN publish a list of accredited programs. These graduate education programs began through the work of faculty and students to develop intellectual competence to test out the conceptual skills needed for expert practice. Norris's paper has 68 citations, with only a few authors cited more than once, all representing the crucial work in concept and theory development that has facilitated the development of the C.N.S. position.

As graduate education in nursing developed, many of its early leaders were prepared at Teachers College, Columbia University. As has been noted by others, this artifact of nursing's history contributed greatly to the early conceptions of specialization in nursing. Specialization was thought to be the development of functional expertise in the areas of teaching, administration, and supervision. However, this is a singular view and requires understanding of the post-World War II increase in demands for hospital care and treatment and nursing's subsequent shift from a model of private duty nursing to almost exclusively hospital-based nursing. In the latter instance, the bureaucratic and hierarchial nature of the organization, the hospital, was to shape the profession in ways that are as yet not fully understood. Further, the fact that nursing was, and is still, largely a woman's profession, with all the attendant issues and problems of women in the work force of organizations largely dominated by men, created situations which were inimical to the growth of clinical practice in nursing (Ashley, 1976; Sills, 1976). Out of this ambience the notion emerged that nurses were something less than full-fledged professionals; they had to be managed, guided, and directed. Further, the demands of the bureaucratic organization were for standardization of the parts.[1]

Likely as a product of this bureaucratic model, there has been and continues to be a pervasive force in nursing for a coercive homogeneity of the field. This has led nursing educators to think that what was needed in advanced preparation was not more theory in nursing, but more theory in teaching and management. Although as early as 1949 the idea of specialization had been introduced at a conference of directors of graduate programs in nursing convened at the University of Minnesota, the earlier trend consisted of many postgraduate programs; a postgraduate program could mean anything from postdiploma to postbaccalaureate. These programs typically ranged in length from 3 months to a year and sometimes 2. Such programs awarded certificates which had little or no value in academia, but they did provide for the development of a cadre of nurses who had better-than-average preparation in some specialized area of nursing. The program for preparation in nurse midwifery began in this way, and some of the programs still continue outside the mainstream of conventional graduate preparation within the university. One is tempted to include here the recent spate of programs to prepare nurse practitioners in short-term, nonuniversity- or university-based programs. These can be seen as a resurrection of the trend to minimize nursing's claim to legitimacy in specialized areas of nursing practice and to once more yield to the organization's demand for certain kinds of skills to perform certain kinds of tasks.

In any kind of social change, there are driving forces and restraining forces. The major driving force for the preparation of clinical specialists at the graduate (master's) level was the work of Peplau at Rutgers, The State University of New Jersey. In 1954, Peplau developed the first program that focused exclusively on the development of an advanced practitioner in psychiatric nursing. The extensive contributions of this remarkable nurse to the development of clinical specialization at the graduate level are legion (Smoyak, 1976; Sills, 1978). In 1963, the Surgeon General's Consultant Group on Nursing recommended that the Professional Nurse Traineeship Program be expanded to permit the training of clinical specialists. Hence, with the impetus from federal monies, the clinical specialist movement began to allow for increased numbers of students in more graduate programs in nursing.

However, several restraining forces continued to operate within the movement. The issue of titles was hotly debated in the nursing literature. Nurse clinician, advanced clinical nurse, nurse practitioner—all such titles had different meanings, differing descriptions of the preparation needed and of the performance expected. Recently, the social policy statement of the American Nurses Association made clear the professional organization's official position on this issue.

> The specialist in nursing practice is a nurse who, through study and supervised practice at the graduate level (master's or doctorate), has become expert in a defined area of knowledge and practice in a selected clinical area of nursing. Specialists in nursing practice are also generalists, in that they hold a baccalaureate in nursing, and therefore are able to provide the full range of nursing care. In addition, upon completion of a graduate degree in a university graduate program with an emphasis on clinical specialization, the specialist in nursing practice should meet the criteria for specialty certification through nursing's professional society. (ANA, 1980:23)

One would be remiss not to point out that there exist outside the framework of the ANA 20 or so specialty organizations representing

---

[1] Dorothy Smith, former dean of the College of Nursing at the University of Florida at Gainesville, once referred to this as the syndrome of "nurses as interchangeable parts" after the assembly-line industrial model.

various types of "specialized" practice in nursing. In many instances these groups have acted as restraining forces in the effort to develop clinical expertise at the graduate level; in other instances they have spurred the development of graduate education. From this view, then, these specialty organizations are a mixed blessing. It is this author's hope that by the year 2000 there will have been developments permitting a unification of all these specialty efforts into a coherent whole that serves the nurse, nursing, and the public well.

The past two decades have seen remarkable growth in the preparation for specialization in graduate programs. In 1980, there were over 75 such programs in colleges and universities around the country.

It is clear, then, that the societal forces Peplau referred to did create the need for specialization, the profession responded, and nursing is now faced with the challenges provided by this established trend.

DIMENSIONS OF THE POSITION OF THE C.N.S.

Some of the challenges set forth by the trend toward increased clinical specialization in nursing are reflected by the voluminous literature extant in the field (Lewis, 1970; Riehl and McVay, 1973; Rotkovitch, 1976). This discussion of the dimensions of the position of clinical nurse specialist assumes that there is, at the present time, a low level of consensus about what should be the normative dimensions of the position. This presentation is a contribution toward an effort at clarity and toward an emerging consensus, at least at the 51 percent level. It is based on understandings gleaned from the literature, from the experience of more than a decade in the educational preparation of clinical specialists, and from observations of the subsequent performances of these nurses. Much of the literature speaks to the role or roles of the C.N.S. This discussion will focus on what is more broadly conceptualized as dimensions of the position of the C.N.S.

Clinical Competence and Responsibility

First and foremost, the C.N.S. must have a personal philosophy of care. In this philosophical matrix are located the essences of the practice—the rationale for the practice, the belief in the theoretical and conceptual frameworks which guide the practice, the commitment to inquiry which governs the practice, the ethical and moral values which metagovern the practice, the value for the ongoing development of the profession of nursing, and the value for the ongoing explication of the humanistic and scientific bases for the discipline of nursing.

Second, the C.N.S., through advanced preparation and training developed through graduate study, comes to the practice setting with an in-depth theoretical base relevant to the particular area of specialization. The competencies to be developed

> . . . include ability to observe, conceptualize, diagnose, and analyze complex clinical or non-clinical problems related to health, ability to consider a wide range of theory relevant to understanding those problems, and ability to select and justify application of theory deemed to be most useful in understanding the problems and in determining the range of possible treatment options. Ability to foresee and discuss short- and long-range possible consequences is also to be demonstrated. While this is not an exhaustive list, the foregoing intellectual competencies are of the utmost importance in specialization. (ANA, 1980:23)

Third, the C.N.S. must constantly test the practice against the available standards for care. Where the standards are absent or wanting, the C.N.S. is responsible for reporting this to the profession and for working for the establishment of more adequate standards. Martin and Finneran (1980) report a teaching model for the use of standards of practice as a basis for peer review. They deem the experience a useful one and hypothesize that the practitioners using this model will be both more effective and more efficient.

Fourth, the ability of the C.N.S. to demonstrate expertise can best be demonstrated by the characteristic ways in which functions are implemented in the practice itself. "Expert competence is an abstraction—the difference between a generalist and a specialist cannot be seen until it has been made concrete through practice, over time" (ANA, 1980:25).

However, the call for theory-based practice by the C.N.S. requires that the C.N.S. must be aware of the extent of support for the theory based on an entire body of relevant studies. Hardy cogently frames this issue thusly:

> If nurses are taught 'theories' that have little or no empirical support, the nursing care interventions based on such 'theories' may have deleterious effects on clients who believe in the nurse's skill, expertise and competence. . . . For example, even if a conceptual framework for crisis intervention makes intuitive sense to a nurse, using it as a basis of action when it does not have sound empirical support is a serious error in judgment and one that has considerable ethical implications. There is a need to develop and use empirically sound scientific knowledge if nursing is to retain its reputation as a profession. (1978:47)

Hardy's caveat is timely. Moreover, it poses serious ethical questions which every C.N.S. must carefully consider.

Organizational Responsibility of the C.N.S.

Perhaps no single issue has been as widely discussed in the literature about the C.N.S. as that of the appropriate position of the C.N.S. within the organization. The debate centers around staff vs. line authority and responsibility. To the best of this author's understanding, there have been no evaluative studies which might shed some light on the issue, but considerable heat has been generated from one polemic position or another. Stevens (1976) speaks to the administrative view-point and suggests that contracting for accountability is one way of reducing the mismatch of the C.N.S. with the bureaucratic organization. Blake (1977) suggests that for the C.N.S. to function as a consultant, she or he should be in a staff rather than a line position. Crabtree (1979) reviews the advantages and disadvantages of the functioning of the C.N.S. in staff, line, and matrix type organizations. Her conclusions are in favor of the C.N.S. as a clinical nursing supervisor with responsibility for nursing care and nursing personnel.

The ANA's social policy statement is very opened ended on this issue:

> When nurse specialists are employed in health care settings, descriptions of their position and functions ought not be standardized. The work rules for the specialist must be jointly determined and negotiated by the applicant and the employing institution. The emphasis should be on developing negotiated positions and organizational arrangements that are most likely to result in freedom and responsibility for maximum use of the abilities of the particular specialist in the particular health care setting. In joint practices and partnerships, in which nurse specialists practice on a private basis with other nurses or other professionals, joint determination of working arrangements and shared responsibility also apply. (ANA, 1980:26–27)

Clearly, the C.N.S. needs to have some set of organizational concepts and theories to determine if a given setting for practice will enable the fullest utilization of the potential inherent in the C.N.S. position.

Typically, the C.N.S., when employed by an organization, is in either a staff or line position. Recently, some C.N.S.s have been employed by a physician or group of physicians. In this position, the C.N.S. is responsible to both patients and physicians. The relationship with organized nursing service is typically less than clear-cut. Often, it seems, the C.N.S. opts for this type of organizational arrangement because it seems to offer more flexibility than a position within a nursing department. C.N.S.s who are working in Health Maintenance Organizations (H.M.O.s) or other outpatient settings are also often not formally attached to any organized nursing service department. Some C.N.S.s are engaged in joint practice arrangements with physicians (National Joint Practice Commission, 1977). Some C.N.S.s practice their specialty as solo practitioners or in joint practice with other C.N.S.s or other health care professionals. It can be seen, then, that a variety of organizational arrangements exist for the position of C.N.S. The issues and concerns related to these sets of arrangements are discussed in another section of this paper.

The Practitioner Dimension

For purposes of this discussion, it is assumed that there are two aspects of the dimension of practitioner. The first is direct practice, which involves the delivering of expert nursing to an individual, family, group, or community. The second is indirect practice, which involves the delivery of expert nursing to other health care professionals, potential consumers of nursing services, indeed, almost anyone and everyone.

The Direct Practice Component In the first instance, the C.N.S. must possess and continually develop a body of knowledge, organized in theoretical and conceptual modes, to guide and direct the work. This demands advanced preparation, either at the master's or the doctoral level, and represents the profession's efforts to provide the most exquisite and highly skilled nursing to those in need of such service. The ability to successfully perform in this dimension of the C.N.S. position is greatly enhanced by experience, wherein the thoughtful considerations of the intellect are constantly brought to bear in a continuous evaluation of the performance.

Obviously, ability to give such a high quality of care does not emerge full-bloom from a master's program, but requires nourishment to grow and flourish. Such nourishment often comes from a mentor who helps to guide, support, model, and, most of all, critique the clinical work of the novice. All of this might be subsumed under the genre of coaching, and the lucky C.N.S. will have the experience of working with a seasoned coach. In the absence of a mentor/coach, peers can be used to aid the ongoing growth of the C.N.S. Peers can and must effectively support one another with what Stevenson calls "tough love" (1980:75).

C.N.S.s must be able to effectively network to each other in order to provide a continuous cutting edge for the development of new knowledge and the testing of what is already known. Without such networking of support, the C.N.S. is easily and effectively coopted into a system and often loses sight of the original vision of the position.

The potential theory base from which the C.N.S. derives the pertinent prescriptions for practice spans the scope of human knowledge. It is graduate education that functions to narrow that scope to the specialty area of concern. Thus, study in philosophy, physiology, biochemistry, sociology, and other fields together with the study of contemporary nursing theories, allows the C.N.S. to pursue direct practice with competence and with an open, inquiring mind.

The Indirect Practice Component The most commonly cited roles of the C.N.S. in indirect practice are the roles of educator, consultant, supervisor, and researcher.

The educator role, as well as all roles within the position of C.N.S., implies an "other" as necessary complementary, i.e., educator-educatee or teacher-student. In this conception, then, almost anyone can be a target for the efforts of the C.N.S. to provide formal or informal teaching-learning experiences based on some assessment of need. The permutations of this role are numerous. The C.N.S. in this role provides leadership for nursing staff development activities. Intradisciplinary conferences among nursing staff from differing services is a component of this role. Educational efforts with client groups are an important element of this role. Notable examples of client groups include the various types of planned parenthood groups such as Lamaze and special groups organized around shared life experience, e.g., bereavement groups. Formal teaching may be done with nursing, medical, and other students as is appropriate. Clearly, a requisite for these learning activities is that the C.N.S. be cognizant of teaching-learning theories and is able to tailor the educational efforts to the situational requirements.

In many ways, this teaching function of the C.N.S. is a vital one for the profession of nursing and its growth and development. It seems likely that, as nursing moves forward in its efforts to strengthen the discipline base of the profession, the C.N.S. is strategically located at the interface of theory and practice and is ideally situated to bring a focus to theory testing in the empirical setting.

The consultant role of the C.N.S. seems likely to have inherent in its function many of the aspects of what is meant when "professionalism" is invoked in discussions about nursing. The C.N.S. who is a "professional" does not require management or supervision in the traditional sense. What is required is that the C.N.S. know how to function as a consultant and a consultee. As a consultant, the C.N.S. is requested by an individual, group, family, organization, or community to facilitate some kind of resolution to a perceived problematic situation. There are many excellent models in the literature for the practice of consultation. Therefore, a model will not be discussed here, but some thoughts are presented for the general consideration of the C.N.S. who is involved in this function.

- Be sure you are asked directly by the person or group requesting the consultation. Often someone in a power position decides that a person or group needs your intervention. Such a coercive consultation mode has low probability of success.
- Define, as early as possible, the model and time frame to be used for the consultation. Some

will expect the C.N.S. to be an instant expert; the tendency here is to solve a problem prematurely or for the consultant to take on ownership of the problem and solve it for the client. Further, consultation always ends!

- Identify clearly that the concern is one which you have the skill and knowledge to handle effectively and one that needs to be resolved. Many organizational problems are one-time-only phenomena and may not, in fact, require resolution. Here a solution may create more problems than it solves, an oft-recurring phenomenon in organizations.
- Time is money, so be prepared. Do your homework. Become as familiar with the situation as possible before the process begins.
- Consider the cost involved in the time expended in consultation and use that information to fix charges for consultation or to negotiate for appropriate trade-offs.
- There are inherent dangers in consultation within one's own hierarchial organization. Be aware of these and suggest consultants from outside the organization when appropriate. Remember that "a prophet is often without honor in his own country."
- When both consultant and consultee are viewed as having expertise and strengths, albeit different ones, the result is likely growth and learning.

While the above list is not exhaustive, it does contain some pragmatic considerations for the C.N.S. in the consultant role.

The C.N.S. also functions in the reciprocal role of consultee. It is useful to consider that, no matter what the level of expertise, the C.N.S. is likely to require assistance in areas that may be beyond his or her scope or that may require an additional perspective. The C.N.S. should expect that such services will be available and accessible in any clinical setting for practice. The availability of such assistance should be a consideration included in the negotiation for the position of C.N.S.

The role of supervisor may also fall to the C.N.S. In some organizational contexts, supervision of the clinical work of others is expected;

in other organizational settings, the expected supervisory function may be more managerial and related to nonnursing policies, procedures, and tasks. The clinical review of nursing actions, outcomes, and problems is clearly within the purview of the C.N.S. Indeed, part of the often-cited function of role modeling includes the ability to function as a skilled clinical supervisor. Less attention has been paid to this aspect of the C.N.S. position than perhaps is its due. The best of teaching-learning is often accomplished through the skillful processing of the clinical work in the supervisory relationship. It is understood that this function is similar to, yet different from, peer review. Peer review involves coequals; supervisory review requires one with more skill experience than the other, but each with valuable information. Both peer review and supervisory review are a part of the C.N.S.'s function.

The research role is conceptually closer to a function than a role in the social-psychological sense and is clearly within the purview of the C.N.S.'s position. Research to date has focused on the C.N.S. as person and the roles and utilization of the C.N.S., specifically, the characteristics of the C.N.S., the roles of the C.N.S., descriptions of the work of the C.N.S. Less research has focused on the clinical practice issues and on measures of outcome differences based on the C.N.S.'s application of theory. Padilla (1973) provides an excellent review of five early studies related to the C.N.S. In her summary of these studies, she reports that four of them strongly point to the effectiveness of the C.N.S. in improving nursing behavior under certain conditions. However, much more work needs to be done. First, the C.N.S. needs to be an intelligent consumer of research findings. Second, the C.N.S. needs to generate research questions emerging from practice and to inform the researchers and collaborate with them in the research process. Third, the C.N.S. can report case studies. Case studies, when they are carefully documented and connected to a clear diagnostic nomenclature and a conceptual or theoretical framework, can be used to describe, analyze,

and evaluate nursing care. The case study can then be replicated by other C.N.S.s, and thus the body of nursing knowledge is expanded.

This somewhat brief discussion of the major roles of the C.N.S. is not complete without some discussion of the pervasive feature of all of the roles. Indeed, central to the position of the C.N.S. is a set of ideas about change. Inherent in all that the C.N.S. does is the fundamental notion of attempting to alter or change the course of some human experience in a negentropic rather than entropic direction. Thus, the C.N.S. must have a working knowledge of types of change, processes of change, and theories of change, as well as of experiential strategies and tactics for dealing with change. Learning about change and testing ideas about change bring a verve and excitement to the work of the C.N.S. In this respect, more is needed to be known about the failures of C.N.S.s, for what is sinful is not to have tried and failed, but to have tried and not to have learned from the experience and not to be willing to share the knowledge gained from the failure. For too long, nursing has generally attributed success and failure to personality variables. Such an approach has some utility, but it also prevents the appropriate study and documentation of processes and their structures from which beginning conceptual frameworks and theoretical hunches can be developed. Nursing could use a "National Center for the Study of Change in the Nursing Care System." Such a think tank could begin with smaller units also, and C.N.S.s could provide the leadership for such an effort.

ISSUES AND CONCERNS FOR THE C.N.S.

Contextual Set

Wherever the C.N.S. position is enacted, it is always embedded in some set of contextual variables. The C.N.S. needs to be able to do a contextual assessment of the system in which he or she plans to enact the position. Some of the more important of these variables to be considered are (1) the philosophic stance of the social organization; (2) the type of structure of the social organization; and (3) the location of the social organization.

In considering the philosophic stance of the organization certain questions arise. What does the organization purport to believe about its mission in the society? What are its values? The C.N.S. will profit by getting answers to these questions and determining if there is a match or mismatch with the C.N.S.'s philosophic position. It is preferable to do this type of comparative analysis before committing to employment in an organization. Too often the C.N.S. belatedly discovers that there is a profound mismatch between the two philosophic sets.

The type and structure of the organization are also to be considered. Is the organization bureaucratic in its rules and policies and to what extent and degree? Is the organization organized hierarchially? If so, is the hierarchy steep or rather flat? What is the history of the organization? Is it relatively new or very old? Is there great tradition and relative inflexibility in the norms that govern the social relationships in the organization, or is the organization fairly open vis-a-vis the norms and the role relationships? Are these flexible and negotiable? What are the actual power modes in the organization? Who has power? Who has input into decision making? How are conflict and controversy viewed and resolved? What are the power styles of the extant leadership in the organization?

When the C.N.S. collects data to answer these questions, an assessment can be made with respect to the "goodness of fit" between what the C.N.S. values and is comfortable with and the characteristics of the social organization. Such an assessment will go a long way to militate against failure of the C.N.S. to thrive and survive in an organization (Donnelly et al., 1980).

Consideration of the location of the social organization concerns both the geographical location and the location of power and influence in the organization. Is the facility in a rural, urban, or suburban area? If it is in an urban area, is it lower-, middle-, or upper-class oriented in its service delivery? Is the organization well integrated into the community, or is it somewhat apart from its community in the sense of geographic location? Further, where in the organization are the power and influence positions and networks? The questions at issue in this instance are: Where is nursing in relationship to hospital administration and other disciplines with respect to who makes decisions? How are decisions made about the mission and goals of the organization? How are decisions made at operational levels about implementation of the goals?

When the above considerations are taken into account, the C.N.S. gains a clear view of the contextual set in which the functions of the position will be enacted and is then in a position to make an informed choice about whether or not a match exists between the contextual set and the preferred contextual set of the C.N.S. When a match does not exist and the C.N.S. enters the position, a rather low probability exists for a successful outcome. The size of the mismatch may only become apparent over time. If this is the case, then in the usual course of events, the C.N.S. will show symptoms of burnout, there will be organizational uproar and unbridled conflict, and the C.N.S. may quit or be fired. Often then the next step for the C.N.S. is to undertake the search for another setting—a setting free from what is perceived as onerous constraints on professional practice. The search for such a setting has led in part to the movement toward independent practice (Jacox and Norris, 1977).

Autonomous Nursing Practice

In this discussion preference is given to the use of the term "autonomous" nursing practice rather than "independent." "Autonomous" is selected for its connotation of power and control over one's area of expertise. Such power and control allow for interdependence in the delivery of health care services, while preserving the autonomy of one's own practice base. Further, the term "independent" sometimes seems to connote a solo or individual practice, and this model seems fraught with some dilemmas, especially in regard to 24-hour responsibility and other dimensions of accountability. Whitaker, who functioned in this mode, reflects on the experience thusly:

> I do not advocate solo-provider health care delivery. Health team linkage is a must. Health care cannot be provided by one individual alone. Primary health care is and should be a 24-hour per day, 7-day per week service. This requires a multidiscipline team of people in addition to a well developed referral system. (1977:262)

In a similar manner, Ford offers the following opinion:

> Independent practice, for nurses as well as for all health professionals, is passe, a myth; it is 50 years too late and is not viable in today's evolving health care systems. (1977:152)

C.N.S.s who become disillusioned, disappointed, or frustrated in organizational settings opt for the emotional and psychic appeal of independent practice, only to find that that model too has its pitfalls, especially if it is conceived of as solo practice. What is argued for here is for the C.N.S.s to find or create contextual settings in which autonomy can flourish and interdependence can thrive to the ultimate benefit of the recipient of services. To this end, many C.N.S.s leave hospital-type settings for community-based settings in the hope that the latter will offer fewer constraints and greater flexibility. However, the area of expertise of some C.N.S.s does not allow this option. And there are some C.N.S.s who choose to stay in the organizational setting and work for change.

Several years ago, I attempted to reframe this organizational dilemma in an effort to generate thinking about possible alternative futures for C.N.S.s in bureaucratic settings. A proposal for nurse-corporations has evolved from this effort.

The conceptual key to the corporation proposal is that it changes the fundamental nature of the social contract. The professional nurse would no longer be an employee of the hospital or agency, but rather a member of a professional corporation which provides nursing services to patients and clients on a fee-for-service basis. The dimension of accountability becomes much clearer when nursing services are not computed in with the costs for housekeeping, overhead, etc. Such a change in the nature of the social contract is, it seems to me, fundamentally necessary for the survival of nursing as a profession rather than an occupational group of workers employed by other organizations.

Our history is clear—that we began practice in this way. We did private duty in hospitals and were directly reimbursed by the client. In present day society, that mechanism would be too simplistic, but the corporation of nurses could be the agent in present day society.

The corporation at the national level might be called the American Nurses' Corporation. Then local corporations could develop their own names, but the structural patterns, etc., would come from the American Nurses' Corporation.

Such a proposal is no pie-in-the-sky, but represents, I think, a rational solution to a serious problem which besets the collective bargaining program. It provides for allowing nursing to become whole again, both in nursing service delivery and in the professional association. Such wholeness would be both desirable and possible and needed, I believe, for the health of our profession. (Sills, 1979)

Thus one option would be for C.N.S.s to incorporate in group practice models and to contract with agencies and organizations. Clients would then be billed specifically for X units of Y level of nursing service. This dimension of the corporate practice would need careful working out, but it can be done. Clearly, the name of the game at the organizational level in health care is economics. Money equals power. To deny or ignore this reality is to live periously close to the brink of disaster. Thus, the central thesis here is that for the C.N.S. to practice autonomously, an organizational pattern different from what presently exists must emerge. There are some reports that some small steps in the direction just discussed are being taken in various regions of the country. It is hoped that the conceptual frame presented here will contribute to the ongoing development of such efforts.

THE C.N.S. AND THE LARGER COMMUNITY

The C.N.S., as an articulate, able, competent person, must seek, find, and use positions of influence in communities. The process may begin with the health committee in a local church, with consultations for a local school, or with the health policy group of a political organization. For in the networking that takes place between and among local communities—counties, regions, states, and federal government—are the opportunities to make your presence a vital force in the policy decisions about health affairs. It will seldom happen that the president of the United States will reach out and pluck you from obscurity to serve on a presidential panel; it is more reasonable to expect that your link to community is through consumer groups and health advocacy groups (e.g., P.T.A.s, Action for Newborns). You should actively seek positions on boards—little ones, then bigger ones. For if the C.N.S. is to become institutionalized into the system of health care, the process must also occur at the organizational level and the societal level; the process cannot be achieved without pervasive presence of the C.N.S. at all levels of the health care system.

The C.N.S. and the Community of Nursing

To exhort the C.N.S.s to membership in ANA is perhaps superfluous. Rather, what seems needed is to exhort them to activity in the professional organization. This activity must go on at all levels —local, state, and national. Each C.N.S. should have, or, if not, should create, an advanced practice group at the national level. These groups have the potential of becoming a powerful leadership cadre for the next era of ANA's history. But this will not just happen. C.N.S.s must work to make it happen.

There are two other areas of special interest to the C.N.S. and they are interrelated: certification and third-party payment. The development of certification for areas of specialty competence has had a rough trajectory. Nevertheless, such certification remains the best likely avenue for claiming the right to third-party payment. Third-party payments have become a reality for some of us; but though some have already achieved this goal, more work is needed. C.N.S.s need to know each other, use each other, and network in effective ways. Those who have been or are undergoing certification must share the process and help others; they must act in ways that bespeak concern for each other and the profession, in ways that are collaborative rather than competitive. There is often bickering about who came from the "best" graduate program. There is often the complaint that C.N.S.s are too different from one another; yet, I think there need not and should not be a move toward homogeneity too soon. We need to find ways to reward excellence of practice. Such recognition should be given at all levels of C.N.S. practice. Some district and state nurses' associations have begun this process, but not all. What prevents this? Competition? Envy? Insecurity? The values of the C.N.S. would seem to lie with cooperation, collaboration, and sharing. One trusts this will continue to be so and that the spirit will grow and be useful to nursing and those we serve.

The C.N.S. and the Community of Women

Some of the concerns already discussed are concerns that are related to our status as women. Several comments are in order here. First, nurses are *not* in the forefront of the women's movement. In a recent book (Reverby, 1976) a nonnurse wrote a five-page article titled, "Health is

Women's Work." The analysis, I think, is flawed, but, be that as it may, the unpleasant fact remains that most often, even in the literature of the women's movement, nursing is woefully underrepresented, and where it is represented, it is represented by others. To illustrate further, a recent National Conference on Research on Women and Health Care had but one paper by a nurse, Jeanne Quint Benoleil. What does this suggest? Among other things, it tells us that more nurses must get credentials equal with those held by other health care workers—credentials such as the master's degree, the doctor of nursing science degree, or the doctor of philosophy degree. Armed with these credentials, we must write and speak in ways which will assure the coming generations in our discipline that we have created a climate in which they can grow and work in an ambience of health.

Preparation and Education of the C.N.S.

Clearly, the C.N.S.'s educational preparation is at least at the master's level. Recently initiated programs leading to the doctor of nursing science degree augur well for the future of advanced preparation for clinical specialization in nursing.

The principle of equifinality is useful when thinking about the variety of extant programs of preparation for clinical specialization. Each program has its unique elements as well as elements that are similar to other programs. Programs vary in the amount of time required for completion; the range seems to be from 9 months to 24 or 28 months. The likely argument here is that the educational program plus 2 or 3 years of clinical work are required to finely hone the skills and knowledge of the C.N.S.

A review of the literature about the nature of the types of graduate programs yields no clearcut consensus about what ought to be normative. This is as it should be, and additional time is required before any such consensus can be expected. However, there are some concepts and theories that I believe are salient in the preparation of the C.N.S. First and foremost, if the student does not already know how to learn, then learning how to learn, together with the concomitant commitment to life-long learning, is the aim of graduate study.

The need for knowledge of and experience with theories of change has already been discussed. Further, teaching-learning theory and methods have great utility for the C.N.S, irrespective of clinical area of specialization. C.N.S.s will be well served if they develop a framework for understanding inquiry in nursing and methodological approaches to research. In addition, a valuing of theory and of critical ability to develop and examine theoretical concepts and constructs will both enhance practice and add to the knowledge base for practice.

The above has focused on ideas that are thought to be essential content for the education of the C.N.S. However, there is more involved in graduate education. First and most obvious is the need to couple common content with the more restricted but in-depth content that provides the focus for the practice. This, of course, varies widely from one specialty area to another. Second, the C.N.S. needs to be exposed to learning contexts where experts are at work. For the neophyte this modeling of roles done by the seasoned C.N.S. cannot be underestimated in terms of its value for learning. However, such opportunities do not always exist; the C.N.S. may find that pioneering, while more difficult, can yield useful experiences. However, what is needed in both instances is the ability to engage in the systematic practice of evaluating one's own performance and changing and learning in that process.

Every C.N.S., early on, should be familiar with the ANA standards for practice in the area of specialty. If none exist, then the C.N.S. must take the opportunity to create them—first for himself or herself, then to share them with a peer group, and later to move them to the state or national level as and when appropriate. Certification for C.N.S.s in psychiatric nursing began in just this way in New Jersey, and that movement eventually helped to create the momentum for certification in this field.

The mix suggested, then, for the creation and development of the C.N.S. is a blend of values, theories, and concepts as content, specialized areas of knowledge, and experiential learning. The philosophical underpinnings for all of this are to be remembered. Whitehouse has stated:

> Philosophy is the seed from which the practice germinates and finds expression. Philosophy is the persistently haunting spirit which continues to motivate the mind. One cannot develop an

effective practice with the necessary insight and flexibility without a clear concept of philosophy. Practice is, in turn , the test of the quality of a philosophy (1962:9).

The future for the C.N.S. is unlimited in its potential. The prediction offered here is that this will become the entry level for the profession 50 years hence. The health of persons in families, communities, and nations will be the better if this significant direction for the nursing profession achieves its promise. The belief here expressed is that it will!

EDITOR'S QUESTIONS FOR DISCUSSION

What particular relationships and implications are there regarding issues and trends in nursing education among Conway (Chap. 2), Monnig (Chap. 3), Williamson (Chap. 5), Peterson (Chap. 7), Santora (Chap. 8), Sargis (Chap. 9), Clayton (Chap. 10), Dalme (Chap. 11), Grace (Chap. 12), O'Connor (Chap. 13), and Sills' contribution? What Questions for Discussion posed from those chapters are addressed by Sills?

What pendulum and trends have existed in the history of graduate nursing education? What forces have contributed to the changes in focus of graduate education? How have rationales for changes/trends been established? What is the basis for legitimacy of the rationale? How likely are present foci in graduate nursing education to continue? What restraining and driving forces may influence the present foci? Apply the previous queries to the history of undergraduate nursing education. Are there significant differences regarding trends, change, foci between undergraduate and graduate education? Should there be differences? Indicate specific rationale for your viewpoint. What has been the impact of trend changes in nursing education on patient care, nursing practice, education, research, theory development, the profession of nursing, other health professions, the health care system, and society at large? What strategies might be utilized to assess, plan, implement, and evaluate change in nursing education for undergraduate and graduate nursing education?

What are the implications for the ANA and the profession with numerous organizations representing various types of "specialized" practice in nursing existing outside of the ANA? How have these groups acted as restraining and/or driving forces toward efforts for the development of clinical expertise at the graduate level?

Debate the appropriate position for a C.N.S. within an organization vis-à-vis staff versus line authority and responsibility. What criteria might be suggested in contracting for accountability with a bureaucratic organization? Is there a trend toward the C.N.S. fulfilling the role as a clinical nursing supervisor with responsibility for nursing care and nursing personnel? What factors may contribute to the dual responsibility? To what extent should core management content be included in the educational preparation of the C.N.S. for dual roles?

How can a C.N.S. effectively evaluate an organizational setting for appropriateness to practice? How can a C.N.S. determine whether the "right" questions have been asked in assessing a setting? How can the power and influence of nursing in relation to other disciplines be assessed during the interview process? What strategies can be offered to change an organizational situation and/or prevent conflict if a mismatch is detected after employment between the C.N.S. and the organization? To what extent and under what conditions should strategies be used to resolve differences between a C.N.S. and the setting of employment?

What economic issues influence the type of position and setting a C.N.S. chooses in which to practice? Does a C.N.S. employed in HMOs, solo or joint practice settings function differently from a nurse practitioner? What are the advantages and disadvantages for the C.N.S. not to be formally attached to an organized nursing service department? Does a mentor/coach relationship exist in most settings for the new C.N.S. graduate? How economically feasible is a mentor system? To what extent does "reality shock" exist for the newly employed C.N.S.? How might this be prevented? What alternative networks for support can be suggested?

Why does Sills prefer to use the term "autonomous" rather than "independent" nursing practice? From the previous chapters, which contributors would agree with Sills' rationale and choice of terms? What are the "pitfalls" of independent practice?

Discuss Sills' proposal for nurse corporations. What are the advantages of nurse corporations? How is certification for areas of specialty competence related to third party payment? Are there disadvantages not addressed by Sills? How similar is the concept to that utilized by some physicians? Are there factors inherent in the nursing profession which would hinder the development of nurse corporations? What implications would nurse corporations have for the ANA, nursing practice and nursing education, and the profession of nursing? What impact might nurse corporations have on collective bargaining programs? What assessment and planning would be essential before implementation of nurse corporations? How do you account for the underrepresentation of nursing in community/national health organizations and activities as well as in the women's movement? Are there alternatives other than nurse corporations to the issues raised by Sills?

Debate the differences in perspective regarding graduate education as presented by Williamson (Chap. 5) and Sills. Would you agree with Sills that the C.N.S. will become the entry level for the profession in 50 years? How should the clinical specialist be prepared educationally and experientially? What should be the "common content" for nurses in a graduate program that has clinical specialist as the major area of concentration? What should be the in-depth content? If the major content of a graduate program is that identified for a clinical specialist in direct practice what should be the content for preparation for the indirect practice roles of educator, consultant, supervisor, and researcher? Does Sills imply postmaster's educational preparation for indirect practice roles? Should the clinical specialist program be a functional role option with the major area of concentration being the "generalist" content of master's programs with such titles as *Adult Nursing* or *Medical-Surgical Nursing?* If a graduate program is a "generalist" program with options to choose a secondary area (minor/functional role) as a clinical specialist, educator, or administrator, what content should be provided in a major "generalist" program and for each of the role options? How should the content of a doctoral program in nursing science differentiate from content of a masters program?

Discuss Sills' considerations for the C.N.S. role as consultant. Can the C.N.S. be an effective consultant without an educational knowledge base of management and organizations? What inherent dangers exist in consultation for bureaucratic organizations? In Sills' discussion of the role of supervisor, is it implied that experience skill development is the "best" teacher? How does Mayer (Chap. 17) address the specific needs in the research role of the clinical specialist as cited by Sills? What are the implications of Hardy's findings (Chap. 24) for the clinical specialist role?

Would you agree that knowledge of change theory is inherent in all of the roles of the C.N.S.? Is change theory of more importance to the C.N.S. than knowledge of other theories? What nursing theoretical knowledge base should the C.N.S. possess? What applications from Fawcett (Chap. 14), Hardy (Chap. 32), Meleis (Chap. 33), and Roy (Chap. 34) should be considered in the development of nursing theoretical content for C.N.S. graduate programs? Which theoretical and conceptual nursing frameworks are evident as guides in the practice of the C.N.S.? To what extent does Hardy's advice in 1978, as quoted by Sills, apply today? In reviewing Hardy's chapter 32, does the same perspective exist? Is there evidence of the use of conceptual frameworks or nursing care interventions completed with little or no empirical support? What ethical considerations need to be considered in utilizing frameworks or interventions without empirical support? What research methodology would you propose to evaluate the role and functions of the C.N.S.?

REFERENCES

American Nurses Association
  1980 "Nursing: A social policy statement." Kansas City, Mo.: ANA.

Ashley, Jo Ann
  1976 Hospitals, Paternalism, and the Role of the Nurse. New York: Teachers College Press.

Blake, P.
  1977 "The clinical nurse specialist as nurse consultant." Journal of Nursing Administration 7(10):33–36.

Burd, S.
  1966 "The clinical specialization trend in psychiatric nursing." Unpublished doctoral dissertation, Rutgers, The State University of New Jersey.

Crabtree, M.
  1979 "Effective utilization of clinical specialists within the organizational structure of hospital nursing service." Nursing Administration Quarterly 4:1–11.

Donnelly, G. F., A. Mengel, and D. C. Sutterly
  1980 The Nursing System: Issues, Ethics, and Politics. New York: Wiley.

Ford, L. C.
  1977 "Perspectives on professional practice." Pp. 151–168 in A. Jacox and C. Norris (eds.), Organizing for Independent Nursing Practice. New York: Appleton-Century-Crofts.

Hardy, Margaret E.
  1978 "Perspectives on nursing theory." Advances in Nursing Science 1:37–48.

Jacox, A. and C. Norris (eds.)
  1977 Organizing for Independent Nursing Practice. New York: Appleton-Century-Crofts.

Lewis, E. (ed.)
  1970 The Clinical Nurse Specialist. New York: American Journal of Nursing.

Martin, E. and M. Finneran
  1980 "A teaching design: Standards of practice as a basis for peer review." Perspectives in Psychiatric Care 18:242–248.

National Joint Practice Commission
  1977 Together: A Casebook of Joint Practice in Primary Care. Chicago: National Joint Practice Commission.

Norris, C. M.
  1977 "One perspective on the nurse practitioner movement." Pp. 21–33 in A. Jacox and C. Norris (eds.), Organizing for Independent Nursing Practice. New York: Appleton-Century-Crofts.

Padilla, G. V.
  1973 "Clinical specialist research: Evaluation and recommendations, conclusions and implications." Pp. 283–334 in J. Riehl and J. McVay (eds.), The Clinical Nurse

Specialist: Interpretations. New York: Appleton-Century-Crofts.

Peplau, H. E.
1965 "Specialization in professional nursing." Nursing Service 3:268–287.

Reverby, S.
1976 "Health is women's work." Pp. 346–350 in R. Baxandrall; L. Gordon, and S. Reverby (eds.), America's Working Women: A Documentary History—1600 to the Present. New York: Vintage.

Riehl, J. and J. McVay (eds.)
1973 The Clinical Nurse Specialist. Interpretations. New York: Appleton-Century-Crofts.

Rotkovitch, R. (ed.)
1976 Quality of Patient Care and the Role of the Clinical Nursing Specialist. New York: Wiley.

Sills, G. M.
1976 "Nursing, medicine, and hospital administration." American Journal of Nursing 9:1432–1434.
1978 "Hildegard E. Peplau: Leader, practitioner, academician, scholar, and therorist." Perspectives in Psychiatric Care 16:122–128.

1979 Letter to the ANA Board of Directors. Unpublished, March 26.

Smoyak, S.
1976 "Specialization in nursing: From then to now." Nursing Outlook 14:676–681.

Stevens, B.
1976 "Accountability of the clinical specialist: The administrator's viewpoint." Journal of Nursing Administration 6(2):30–32.

Stevenson, J. S.
1980 "Developing staff research potential: Overcoming nurse resistance to research." Pp. 73–78 in Lorraine Machon (ed.), The Practitioner/Teacher Role: Practice What You Teach. Wakefield, Conn.: Nursing Resources.

Whitaker, C.
1977 "A family nurse clinician in a rural setting." Pp. 257–262 in A. Jacox and C. Norris (eds.), Organizing for Independent Nursing Practice. New York: Appleton-Century-Crofts.

Whitehouse, F. A.
1962 "The Rationale of Nursing." Rehabilitation Record 3(4) (July-August):9–12.

Chapter 43

Problems with Implementing Primary Nursing

John F. Klein, R.N., Ph.D.
Associate Professor
Department of Sociology
John Carroll University
Cleveland, Ohio
and
Staff Nurse
Department of Psychiatry
St. Luke's Hospital
Cleveland, Ohio

At approximately the same time as the emergence of a defined role for the clinical nurse specialist (C.N.S.) the mode of providing nursing care called *primary nursing* has evolved. Relationships between high quality care for the client and implications for the profession exist with the occurrence of those phenomena. The nursing profession is concerned that high quality care be provided to the consumer through the most effective means. It can happen that consideration is not sufficiently given to relevant factors before a mode of providing health care is implemented. John F. Klein aptly provides a service in identifying specific problems associated with the implementation of primary nursing. He focuses primarily on the Manthey/Minnesota Model which requires 24-hour accountability on the part of the primary nurse.

Primary nursing is defined and the components are outlined to include: assignment of each patient to a specific primary registered nurse who personally assesses, plans and provides the care and is responsible for the plan on a 24-hour basis; close communication and coordination among and between all care givers; patient and family involvement from the initial history through discharge planning; and a head nurse who fulfills the role of staff leader, clinician, validator, and facilitator. Nurses who assume on-site responsibility when the primary nurse is absent are called *associate nurses*. Accountability to the level of the registered nurse at the bedside is the central feature in primary nursing. It is perceived that improvements in patient care emerge due to the increase in continuity, comprehensiveness, coordination, and patient centeredness of care as well as increase in patient, nurse, and physician satisfaction with the provision of primary care. Evidence is reported that staff turnover is decreased and staff development has occurred on units where primary nursing is utilized.

Klein notes that primary nursing contributes the advancement of professional nursing and legitimacy as a profession. He emphasizes the criteria of consultative rather than hierarchical relationships, self-supervision, and collaboration with the patient and family. Behavioral expectations like accountability, responsibility, collegial relationships, and communication linkages unique to primary nursing are explored. These are perceived as increasing the degree of professionalism.

Explication of major problematic areas are presented. The main issue discussed in implementation is change itself, which requires alteration in the role and functions of the professional nurse with corresponding changes in colleagues. The primary nurse is seen as the pivotal planner of nursing care and coordinator of all care activities. Specific changes are necessary, such as, the head nurse being defined as the clinical expert, attitudinal orientation toward roles and relationships, communication patterns, and reorientation of the consumer, and family. Innovative role changes take time for incumbents to accept, interaction to occur, and to be accepted by others.

Items are identified that have the potential to create major difficulties. The necessity for up-to-date, comprehensive care plans, changes in the nature and use of the Kardex, patient records, and insightful content in charting are deemed essential. Additional factors are described as contributing to problems and questions in need of resolution. A major factor is the nurse-patient assignment process; another is staffing, including the use of part-time and ancillary personnel. Evaluation and cost-effectiveness of primary nursing are addressed. Problems like time and effort to find and consult with the primary nurse and her "gatekeeping" function are cited as sources for potential conflict.

No simple answers are provided. In determining the appropriate number of patients for one primary nurse, consideration needs to be given to the professional level of functioning of the nurse in terms of knowledge, expertise, experience, and complexity/severity of the patient's condition. Associate nurse assignments, intra- and extraunit patient transfers, and staffing for three different shifts of service create difficulties in providing for continuity of care. Part-time nurses might assume a primary or associate nurse role for short-term patients. It is maintained that the licensed practical nurse is not prepared nor legally supported to be a primary nurse. There is evidence that nursing attendant positions are being eliminated, for reasons of cost-effectiveness and to enable the primary nurse to have total contact and care for the patient. Behavioral performance and cost-effectiveness are advocated as the central foci in evaluation of primary nursing. Some limitations of experimental research are presented.

Klein insists that two major kinds of preparation are essential for planning and implementing primary nursing: in-service/administrative support for nursing staff and a reexamination of basic nursing education. Serious discrepancies exist between research pilot programs reported in the literature and the reality evident in settings as to the actual time frame needed for implementation. He maintains that the typical, present education programs for nursing practice still remain below university standards when compared with programs for other health professionals. Furthermore, it is stated that present programs do not prepare the nurse to assume the role expected in primary nursing. Many in-service education programs are viewed as enabling little more than the nurse to be informed of technical/mechanical unique differences among hospitals.

Klein urges careful examination of the settings from which research findings are reported as well as a realistic assessment and understanding of the hospital setting for nursing practice before primary nursing is implemented. He perceives that the typical general hospital setting is crisis oriented and lacks the resources to implement luxurious modes of providing patient care. Klein insists the quality of patient care depends on the individual nurse, regardless of the nursing care framework utilized. He maintains that primary nursing may only ensure a heightened visibility of care in the total health care model but cannot ensure provision of the highest level of nursing care.

In conclusion, Klein indicates such exposure should demonstrate what nursing *is* and *can* potentially do for patients. In essence, he views primary nursing as the opportunity for nurses to recapture their "roots"—the patient's bedside.

Credit for the development of primary nursing is given by Robinson to the University of Minnesota Hospitals in 1958, although the operational plan emerged as a nursing modality in the middle of the 1960s with small-scale experiments (1974:31). Logsdon has defined primary nursing as "the nursing care provided to the patient by one nurse who plans with the patient the care that the patient and the nurse decide is needed—care that results from coordination with other disciplines and collaboration with the primary physician" (1973:284). Wolff has further summarized the details of primary nursing, based upon the Nursing Services Department at the University of Minnesota Hospitals:

> 1 Assignment of each patient to a specific primary nurse (RN) who makes major assessment, from which she derives the plan of care. She is responsible for the plan on a 24-hour basis. When on duty, this nurse personally provides care for "her" patients.
> 2 Close communication among care givers, between nurses and across disciplines, including coordination of medical and nursing plans of care.
> 3 Patient and family involvement from the initial history through discharge planning, necessarily entailing a close primary nurse/patient relationship.
> 4 Head nurse serving as staff leader, clinician, validator of clinical experience and communication facilitator. (1977:25)

Other nurses assume on-site responsibility for the patients of an absent primary nurse. The nurse in this role is called the associate nurse.

At any given time a nurse may be acting as primary nurse for one set of patients and as associate nurse for another set. Elpern points out that "The associate nurse is responsible to the primary nurse for contributing to and implementing the primary nurse's plan of care, and for evaluating and reporting the patient's status and response to therapy" (1977:208).

Two models of primary nursing exist, their difference being denoted by the degree of accountability. The Loeb Center model (Alfano, 1969), initiated by Lydia Hall in 1963, requires only 8-hour accountability on the part of the primary nurse, while the Manthey model (Manthey et al., 1970), developed at the University of Minnesota, requires 24-hour accountability. Since a good deal of the literature either directly or indirectly addresses primary nursing through the Manthey/Minnesota model, this article will focus primarily upon the 24-hour accountability model.

There has been some discussion to the effect that primary nursing is not really a new concept of nursing care, but rather a revision and further extension of the case method which is still used for clinical exposition in nursing education (Logsdon, 1973).

SOME RESULTS FROM PRIMARY NURSING

Ciske indicates that the accountability feature in primary nursing is the very essence of this modality of nursing care, entailing numerous responsibilities of a technical and decision-making nature (1979). This in turn gives visible criteria for assessment and evaluation of the nursing care given to patients. Furthermore, such criteria provide a basis upon which a nursing unit may be judged. Smith indicates that, besides accountability, the substantive factors of primary nursing that emerge are improvements in patient care because of an increase in continuity, comprehensiveness, coordination, patient-centeredness, and better staff development (1977).

Some evidence has been provided that the professional nursing staff not only accepts the implementation of primary nursing, but also believes it is providing better patient care (Manthey, 1973; Bakke, 1974). Physicians' comments have been favorable where primary nursing has been instituted (Manthey, 1973), and it has been reported that patients perceive that they are receiving better nursing care (Daeffler, 1975). There is also some evidence that staff turnover is decreased on units with primary nursing (Page, 1974) and that staff development has taken place more readily on those units (Ciske, 1974).

Caution has been noted by Ciske in regard to some misconceptions that have emerged about primary nursing (1979:892). It is not an exclusive, possessive relationship between nurse and patient, nor is it an overdependence of the patient on the nurse. It is not the sacrifice of private, away-from-the-job time of the primary nurse, and it is certainly not misplaced idealism. These features, to the primary nursing modality of care, are obvious dangers that should be guarded against by the nursing staff.

One of the major implications of primary nursing is the advancement it contributes for nursing in general toward the quest for professional standing. Criteria for professionalism generally include some elements of collegial relationships in the practice of service, of independence of the practitioner, and of a mandate from the public in addition to licensure (Bixler and Bixler, 1945). The previously mentioned features of responsibility and accountability on the part of the nurse may be defined as a major contribution to increased independence for the practicing nurse. When staff nurses re-

late to one another on a consultative, rather than on a parallel or even a competitive basis, and when the head nurse and other nursing supervisors are defined as clinical experts, the long-standing, rigid hierarchial conflict in nursing administration between "rank and file" is curbed. Christman indicates that this form of self-supervision is professionally exciting for nursing (1975). The involvement of the patient and family by the nurse in planning comprehensive nursing care may be defined as an impetus to heightened awareness on the part of the public that health care is not the exclusive responsibility of medicine and nursing and that high quality health care can only be achieved through individual and family collaboration with health care professionals.

The preceding review provides a base line to proceed to the purpose of this paper, which is to define some of the major problem areas in the successful implementation and continuation of primary nursing in the typical general hospital setting. The comparison of primary nursing with other modalities of nursing care will not be discussed, since this subject is extensively addressed in the literature (Marram et al., 1974).

THE PROBLEM OF CHANGE

While it has been suggested that primary nursing is not a new concept for patient care, it does represent a change from the more familiar themes of team nursing and functional nursing which permeated nursing care shortly after World War II. The introduction of a major alternative in nursing care delivery denotes the introduction of a major change within the organizational confines of the hospital. Such an introduction of change has rippling effects within the organization on an individual, unit, and interdepartmental level. The nature of change that is demanded by primary nursing includes an alteration in the mode of operation of the professional nurse and a corresponding change in other professional workers who have contact with the patient. The primary nurse is pivotal as the key planner of nursing care and the major coordinator of *all* care activities that are directed to the patient. The primary nurse is responsible and accountable for this planning and coordination. This position of centrality for the primary nurse demands a change in the traditional thinking of most health care personnel. No longer can a fragmented every-person-for-self approach be tolerated in the delivery of service to the patient.

A consequence of such major change within the organizational setting has frequently been denoted as an uncomfortableness felt especially at the individual level. But such feelings are generally identified with the movement away from what is an old and familiar way of doing things to what is new and unfamiliar. The unfamiliar can create uncertainties and doubts which decrease efficiency of operation because of hesitation and vacillation between the old and the new.

The innovative features associated with the introduction of primary nursing represent the new and relatively unfamiliar. These features have the potential for creating a climate of personal and group uncomfortableness in the face of change. Change items that possess the potential to create major problems in the successful implementation of primary nursing are identified and discussed below.

Care Plans, Kardex, and Charting

Comprehensive and up-to-date care plans become an absolute necessity to guide not only the primary nurse, but all other personnel who have contact with the patient. This is especially so in the absence of the primary nurse. The nature and use of the Kardex must usually undergo some kind of change to reflect either a capsulized version of the care plan or an expansion of the patient's total treatment regime involving all services (Bakke, 1974; Manthey, 1973).

The nature of patient charting must also usually undergo some kind of change. The use of problem-oriented charting frequently becomes a necessity in order to reflect the comprehensive thrust of the nursing care plan and the components of the plan specifically related to patient response. Not only must the form of charting be modified but the content must become more insightful. No longer can standard phrases such as "up and about" or "tolerating . . . well" satisfy the in-depth nursing care approach that is entailed in primary nursing. While more informed charting and up-to-date Kardex and care plans have been a desirable mode of operation for some time, they are crucial to the operation of primary nursing. Prendergast provides a detailed account of the role of problem-oriented records in a primary nursing system and the extensive planning involved in the transition (1977:235). In a rather conservative and modest estimate, she labeled such an implementation a "challenging endeavor." However, she indicated that this endeavor could move primary nursing from a stagnated plateau to a level of providing even better patient care. Despite the importance of such accurate record keeping, Spoth (1977) reports this area remained an unresolved problem in the setting she described.

Patient Assignment Process

The nurse-patient assignment process becomes more problematic under the primary nursing framework. No simple answer can be given to the question of how many primary patients are appropriate to any one primary nurse. Daeffler's (1975) ratio of between one and four patients for each nurse is representative of the literature. Page (1974) proposes that one function of the head nurse is to assign nurses to patients, keeping in mind a variety of factors known about individual patients and nurses that should ensure a successful nursing care outcome. Consideration must be given to the level of functioning of the nurse in terms of knowledge, expertise, and experience and to the complexity and severity of each patient's illness. Further complicating the assignment process is the choice of the associate nurse assigned to the case in the absence of the primary nurse. If continuity of patient care is to be maintained, associate nurses should be assigned and the schedules of primary nurse and associate nurse should be coordinated so that at least one is present each day.

Intraunit and extraunit transfers of patients further complicate the nurse assignment process. This is demonstrated by the movement of patients through the hospital such as is observed in obstetrical care. The nurse assigned when the patient is admitted to the labor area should, theoretically, follow the patient through to the delivery and the postpartum area. This assignment should also include the newborn in the nursery in order to maintain total family involvement. It has been proposed that the assigned primary nurse begin responsibility prior to the admission of the patient and continue care through to discharge from the hospital. Such ideal continuity of care by the primary nurse presents not only assignment problems but also staffing problems as the nurse moves from unit to unit with the patient. This state of affairs could hardly be tolerated by those in the central nursing office who mechanically attempt to staff hospital units.

Staffing Problems

A hint of staffing problems emerges here. If primary nurses follow their patients through the hospital, staffing individual units becomes dependent upon patient transfers into, through, and out of the hospital. The involvement of primary nurses prior to admission and after discharge reduces nursing time within the organizational setting. These two features alone drain already critically low numbers of nursing professionals for unit assignment.

Serious problems arise when there is a significant difference in numbers of nursing personnel among the three shifts of the day. Sustaining primary nursing through the evening shift may require either increasing the number of nurses or creating a nurse-patient ratio that is inconsistent

with the nature of primary nursing. Elpern indicates that primary nursing for the night shift has not been successful (1977:209). The reasons for this lack of success are obvious. Sleep patterns of hospitalized patients, important yet unpredictable, are sufficiently erratic to undermine primary nursing.

An additional staffing problem that complicates primary nursing is the use of part-time help. Elpern's report of a trial in primary nursing indicated that part-time staff were kept at a minimum because such staff cannot give the needed amount of time to patients and families on a consistent basis (1977:211). However, Ciske admits that a part-time nurse, working at least 2 consecutive days consistently, might assume a primary or associate nurse role for short-term patients (1977:63). Many hospitals, though, depend extensively upon the use of part-time nurses. In such settings any large-scale attempt to have part-time nurses as primary nurses may well reverse the role of the primary nurse and the associate. Since the part-time nurse is in contact with the patient for such a short period during hospitalization, the continuity of care might be completely short-circuited.

Another problem that has arisen in the area of staffing is the use of ancillary personnel. Ciske observes that the licensed practical nurse (L.P.N.) is not prepared or legally supported to be a primary nurse (1977:63). However, Elpern's report showed L.P.N.s were being used as primary nurses after they passed a refresher course in drug administration (1977:209). As a cautionary note, Manthey et al. admit that "an LPN is not assigned a patient whose care required technical skills or nursing interaction skills beyond her ability" (1970:71). The implication is that the L.P.N.s were given technological surgery to transform them into some kind of an "approximate" R.N. This kind of manipulation can produce professional Frankensteins, who can then in turn threaten their creators. If there is any credibility in defining a difference between L.P.N.s and R.N.s, it is simply in that the former cannot do the same kind of service as the latter. Nor can the former be "tinkered with" in order to mimic R.N.s. Such kind of occupational intervention threatens not only the survival and image of L.P.N.s as a group, but also casts doubt on the status of professional nursing.

If the question of survival for practical nurses is raised, the future existence of nursing attendants becomes even more open to question. There is ample evidence that established primary nursing units are alive and well where the position of nursing attendant has been gradually eliminated. Ciske's report indicates that nursing aides were not involved in direct care on some shifts and that they acted mainly as messengers (1974). Dahlen (1978) reports that her organization has eliminated nursing aides altogether. Examples profiling a primary nursing system typically indicate a phasing out of the nursing attendant position, either directly or by attrition.

The elimination of nursing attendants allows the primary nurse total contact with the patient for all nursing needs. Such contact provides a social situational context that enhances communication between the nurse and the patient, laying the groundwork for information flow and for the establishment of a trusting relationship. Thus, the simple tasks that nursing once passed to ancillary personnel, tasks which medicine had passed to nursing long before, are recaptured by primary nursing for the purpose of sustained contact with the patient. The question of efficacious use of relatively limited numbers of R.N.s to sustain this close contact cannot be ignored. There are many hospitals, sorely dependent on ancillary personnel, that would find it impossible to implement primary nursing on this basis alone.

Evaluation Problems

Where primary nursing exists, nursing administration is faced with an evaluation problem. For the nursing profession that may be a *felix culpa*. The classical approach for evaluating staff nurses on the basis of task efficiency, personal appearance, and respect for authority has little association with the basic concepts underlying primary

nursing. While personal neatness, on-time punch-in, deference to administrators, and speed of technical task performance may have merit in oiling the wheels of the assembly line, these traits seem secondary in importance to patient planning, coordinating professional services, and accountability to others. The length of patient care plans and the quality and the individualized nature of such plans need assessment. Under the primary nursing model it is the actual practice of nursing in its behavioral performance for the benefit of the patient that must be the central focus in evaluation. Thus, there is need to move beyond the obvious level of the traditional concrete externals used for nurse evaluation to the more intricate, subtle, and professional dimensions demanded by primary nursing.

Cost-Effectiveness

While many advantages may be evident in the primary nursing care model, administrators are quick to ask, "At what cost?" There is evidence to indicate that primary nursing, even in models that eliminate ancillary personnel and staff units with an all-R.N. work force, may still cost less than other models of nursing care (Marram et al., 1976; Osinski and Powals, 1980). It has been noted that the "down time" of ancillary personnel, highlighted by increasing militant unionism that presses for further narrowing of job description, has increased the overall costs of units that include such positions. The advantage, then, is that an all-R.N. staff is kept in near-perpetual motion, involved with a wide array of tasks ranging from the most complex to those bordering on menial. To carry the notion of the favorable cost-effectiveness aspect of primary nursing to an extreme, it might also be considered that since cleanliness of the physical environment plays some role in the safety of the patient, it is not inconceivable that nurses could be scrubbing the walls and floors of the patient's rooms. This activity could promote further situational contact between the nurse and the patient, while eliminating the costs of environmental services. Thus, the outcome of further reduced costs through primary nursing care is even more evident!

Typical research models employed to determine the cost-effectiveness of primary nursing retain the problems of the "experimental effect." This effect pertains to the isolation of one unit, or even a few units, within a major medical setting, units staffed by nurses hand-picked from a large pool or by a motivated set of "volunteers." It also pertains to the "thrill effect" of participating in a new and experimental nursing program, and it undoubtedly influences performance outcome, not only in the quality of nursing care but also in the ability of nurses to maintain technical-task accomplishment in the absence of ancillary personnel. Maintaining this exhilaration over a period of time in a typical hospital setting throughout an institution may be a completely different kind of challenge, one bringing quite different results.

Role Changes

What appears to be at the core of primary nursing is a set of role changes necessitated by the increased degree of professionalism. Elpern noted that the project for patient care reorganization at Rush demanded "extensive role changes. These role changes left no categories of nursing staff untouched" (1977:210). The fact that the concept of role is associated with that of status (position) is indicative of the shared expectations that self and others have of behavior performance in a given status (Shaw and Costanzo, 1970:327–344). The new behavioral expectations associated with primary nursing—such as accountability, responsibility, collegial relationships, and communication linkages—are extensions of behavioral expectations for nursing. Manthey et al. have pointed out that a common failing with other modalities of nursing care is that the "buck" could always be passed to someone or, at least, passed back and forth (1970:66). But the location of where the "buck" stops in primary nursing is very clear. It is the primary nurse who is responsible for quality of patient care and who is accountable to all.

A major problem with such innovative role changes is the need for sufficient time, not only for role incumbents to familarize themselves with the new behaviors expected so as to become comfortable with a different kind of performance, but also for others with whom the role incumbents interact to accept such new kinds of behavior. Thus, role change is actually a two-way street which interacting parties must carefully navigate, accepting and respecting the newly demarcated lanes of traffic. Elpern's previously noted remark on the necessary role changes demanded in primary nursing can well be extended far beyond the nursing personnel level. Besides the adjustment to new kinds of responsibilities on the part of the staff nurse, head nurses and nursing administrators are forced to revise their mode of management. No longer can the head nurse be expected to function as the all-powerful central force of the nursing unit. Rather, the head nurse is more appropriately defined as the clinical expert, the immediate resource person for consultation and resource access for the staff nurse (Elpern, 1977:213; Ciske, 1977:62). Additionally, the head nurse refers matters of patient inquiry from other services to the primary nurse for concise information and status reporting. The basic change from hierarchy to lateral collegial relationship between head nurse and staff nurse necessitates a change of attitudinal orientation which can differ markedly from more traditional socialization patterns for head nurses.

Other health care professionals cannot escape necessary role changes that are brought about by primary nursing. Since the primary nurse is the central figure in the patient care schema, physicians, social workers, dietitians, and others need to have increased contact with the primary nurse for information and coordination of efforts. For many such personnel this demands increased time and closer dealings with more nursing personnel; no longer can they expect all communication flow to be with the head nurse. The notorious problems of nurse-physician communication are well known, but a recently reported incident by Shubin emphasizes the gravity of the problem (1979:90). A patient who had had a tracheotomy and who was attached to a ventilator was reintroduced to solid foods by the nursing staff. Four months after the task was initiated, an order was written by the attending physician to introduce the patient to solid foods! Not only does this represent a failure of verbal communication, it also makes written communication in the Nursing Notes a worthless aid in determining patient progress.

Other professionals are frequently irritated by the time and effort it takes to seek out and consult with staff nurses about patient concerns and progress in specific areas. The typical phone call or momentary visit, usually directed to the head nurse, is a demand for instant information about any number of patients. Spoth reports that

> Support services had difficulty responding in an appropriate manner to the increased demands and expectations being placed upon them. The resultant friction and conflict required a great amount of time and energy in order to restore communication and facilitate a cooperative relationship. Total resolution of these recurring conflicts has yet to be achieved. (1977:226)

Spoth identifies this "gatekeeping" function of the primary nurse as an important source of conflict with other departments. She points out that extensive and continuing socialization is required for those so involved.

Lest the most important person involved in primary nursing—the patient—be forgotten, attention must be directed to the necessary role change demanded of the consumer. One of the objectives of primary nursing is to actively involve the patient and family in the planning and implementation of a plan of care that will most benefit the patient and hasten return to the highest possible health level. Characteristically, this demands a reorientation on the part of the patient. The literature on the person's response to illness documents a passive role at best, and frequently a mystified one (Denton, 1978:130-149). The

startling advances in chemotherapy and surgical-mechanical techniques have frequently created an aura of the miraculous and the mysterious. The history of silence on the part of the patient resulted in a large number of patients who are quite willing to let the health care industry do their "magic" and pay the price. Thus, not only do patients pay in dollars but they also pay in forfeiting a knowledgeable and active participation in their own well-being. Perhaps a notable fallacy of primary nursing is the assumption that patients are able to participate in their own health care. It might be more reasonable to assume a need to sensitize and socialize both patient and family to recognize their responsibility to communicate as a necessary antecedent to participation. Such socialization may well transcend any one hospitalization period and demand more intensive and extensive follow-up work on the part of health professionals in general.

THE PREPARATION FOR CHANGE

The planning and implementing of primary nursing within the organizational confines of the hospital require at least two major kinds of preparation: in-service administrative support for the nursing staff and a reexamination of basic nursing education. The literature cautions against change by administrative edict (Manthey, 1978). Indeed, many of the reports on primary nursing discuss specific case examples showing the amount of energy and the length of time that was directed to preparing for primary nursing on selected units. Wolff (1977:27) states that 1 year was devoted to building the organizational structure for primary nursing, while Corn et al. (1977:19) indicate 6 months as the time period necessary for implementation. However, Olsen states that "We have been in the process of implementing primary nursing on our unit for three years" (1977:54). The discrepancies that so frequently exist between the experimental research pilot programs reported in the literature and what happens in the everyday work place are startling. A recent inquiry by the author to a member of the nursing administration at a moderate size hospital (600 beds) in a large metropolitan area revealed uncertainty by the administrator as to the number of units in the hospital that were using primary nursing. This administrator then produced a folder which contained a partial bibliography on primary nursing and several pages of rationale and operating procedures from two of the units in the hospital that were utilizing primary nursing. This folder constituted the extent of involvement of the central nursing office with primary nursing in that hospital. The author discovered through interviewing the staff on two of the units using primary nursing that the entire implementing process had been a self-taught program on the part of the staff. Apparently, the central nursing office of this hospital knew only that, at some unspecified time, primary nursing was implemented on unit X. This posture on the part of nursing administration demonstrates both apathy and a lack of sensitivity to the needs and concerns of nursing personnel and patients. The example also indicates the courage and tenacity of a group of nurses who were sufficiently motivated to implement a change in nursing care style in the face of complete detachment on the part of nursing administration.

Such an example can easily be passed over as an isolated incident of inconsequential proportions. However, more often than not, nursing administration is concerned with multidimensional problems and relegates fundamental nursing care to a lower priority than it deserves. Curtin (1980) reports on one New England hospital where the vice-president for nursing affairs is a laboratory technician with only an associate degree. While the literature cites nicely controlled studies showing the classic stages of planned change, such accounts should not be taken as the standard by which all hospitals and their administrative departments operate. The aloof, noninvolved role of nursing administration in any kind of change other than what is required for more cost-efficient technical operation is a very evident and pervasive

mode of operation. Contemplating the precarious pathway which major nursing care changes may have to follow gives rise to a distinct feeling of discouragement.

The second kind of preparation necessary for extensive change in nursing is the basic education process that prepares practitioners for service to the client. The early twentieth century tradition of nursing education was based upon the principle that nursing was subordinate to just about everything and everyone in the health care system. Early nursing education in the hospital diploma school enhanced this perspective as nurses were educated in seclusion from other disciplines and relied on physicians for a portion of their knowledge. The percentage of diploma schools has declined in the last 10 to 15 years, giving way to the increase in associate degree nursing programs. But this latter form of education remains in limbo as to its professional standing, both in nursing and in comparison with other service delivery occupations. A minority of nurses holds educational credentials at the baccalaureate level and above.

Thus, the typical educational basis for nursing practice is of highly questionable standards when compared with that of other professions, especially in the health field. Furthermore, subject matter that promotes conceptual thinking and independent decision making based upon presenting clinical data within the health field is not extensively offered. An examination of the content of nursing education reveals a "smattering" approach, one composed of "a little of this and a touch of that." With this kind of background, how is a young graduate to assume responsibility for planning and implementing the total realm of care for the patient, be accountable to all concerned, and, theoretically, be competent in all nursing clinical specialities at the basic level? In effect, the young graduate is expected to be a person prepared in everything for everyone. It is little wonder that dissatisfaction is rampant and turnover in staff is high as nurses begin an early search for some kind of organizational sanity—a search that is more often than not in vain. Yet, the concept of any kind of apprenticeship or internship has never really captured the fancy of nursing.

It is suggested that the typical educational program for nursing practice still remains below the university level and ill-prepares the typical young nurse to assume the role that is expected in primary nursing. Furthermore, the typical orientation program and in-service education programs of many hospitals do little more than assist the nurse in keeping informed of technical and mechanical uniqueness that exists from one hospital to another.

THE PROMISE—IDEAL VERSUS REAL

For the past several years the literature addressing primary nursing has cast a rosy hue. Many hospital personnel who encounter primary nursing are at least as satisfied with this modality of nursing care as with other forms, if not ecstatic about it. The nurses involved feel more professional and like the greater patient contact. Patient satisfaction increases because of a sense of "my nurse" and a sense of greater personal attention. Physicians consider this form of nursing care as good as, if not slightly better than, other models. Of course, we have not heard from ancillary workers whose positions are either eliminated or greatly endangered, but their sacrifice might be a necessity and worthwhile if patient care is truly as good as, or better than, before, with no increase in cost. The move toward primary nursing can help nurses recapture their "roots" in the work place—the patient's bedside.

The promise of utopia, however, is tempered by a careful examination of the settings from which results are obtained and a realistic understanding of the typical hospital setting in which nursing care is practiced. Most of the reports detailing primary nursing implementation come from large hospital medical centers in major metropolitan areas. These settings are able to draw from among the best personnel in all health care

professions and are usually the "trend setters" in all areas of health care. The personnel are the best educated and experienced that the professions, including nursing, can muster. The administration of such health care settings is usually sufficiently enlightened to both permit and foster elements of change within the organization.

The promise of primary nursing is lofty, for the patient, for nursing, and for the organization. However, the stark reality is that the typical hospital—faced with personnel turnover for numerous reasons, increasing union militancy of ancillary workers, competition for patients and professional staff, the daily crunch of meeting staffing needs, and a precarious monetary basis in the face of rising consumer activism for both greater fiscal responsibility and lowered costs—is hard pressed to deal with esoteric models of patient care. The typical general hospital setting is still one that is crisis-oriented in its organizational functioning and in its orientation to the patient's situation of life or death in discrete terms.

Unfortunately, many nurses continue to be concerned with those features of nursing care that deal only with avoiding death and maintaining life, they give only passing consideration to the more abstract features that contribute to the quality of the life that is saved or maintained. One nurse was recently heard to say that "we don't want to make it too comfortable for the patient, after all this is not his home." The tempering of such stark realism must be taken into account in the expanded framework of nursing care.

Daeffler states that the quality of patient care depends on the individual nurse, regardless of what nursing care framework is used (1975:22). The continuing problem for all professions is how to ensure that the individual practitioner will indeed deliver quality service. Neither primary nursing nor any other model of nursing care can ensure that nurses will deliver the highest level of nursing care. What primary nursing can ensure is heightened visibility of care in the total health care model. Such exposure should demonstrate what nursing *is* doing for patients and what it *can* do for patients.

Primary nursing is still in its infancy. In order to acquire greater maturity this mode of nursing care needs continued refining and pruning. Advancement must take place at both the conceptual level and especially at the concrete operational level. As health care personnel become more familiar with primary nursing, the misunderstandings and uncomfortableness will give way to increased acceptance, no matter how retarded the pace. Other problems, however, are more resistant to solution. Until such time as adequate numbers of truly professionally educated nurses are available, primary nursing will continue to be a luxury that only a few units of selected hospitals will be able to enjoy.

EDITOR'S QUESTIONS FOR DISCUSSION

Define primary nursing. What are the purpose, goal, and objectives of primary nursing? What are the basic concepts underlying primary nursing? What are the innovative features of primary nursing? What factors have contributed to the emergence of primary nursing? How is 24-hour accountability demonstrated in primary nursing? How is a change from hierarchical to lateral collegial relationships demonstrated in primary nursing? How does primary nursing increase professionalism? How is decentralized decision making evident in primary nursing? How does alteration in the professional role of the nurse through primary nursing effect a corresponding change in roles of other health professionals? What misconceptions have emerged about primary nursing?

How similar are the concepts underlying primary nursing and private duty nursing? What are the differences between primary, modular, team, and functional modes of providing nursing care? In other modes of providing nursing care, where is the responsibility and accountability for the quality of patient care? How is modular nursing an appropriate initial stage towards primary nursing? What structural environmental factors are most conducive to modular nursing? What conditions concerning organizational setting, geographic location, personnel, patients, and attitudes are essential for successful implementation of primary nursing? Are there considerations and/or circumstances in which any one of the other modes of care may be more appropriate to utilize? How does one assess a setting for the most appropriate and effective mode of providing nursing care?

What level of preparation educationally and experientially is essential to be a primary nurse? Present the rationale for your position. How essential is it to have an all R.N. staff to effectively use primary nursing? Is it possible to compromise and still have the essence of primary nursing? In utilizing an all R.N. staff, to what extent is the professional nurse expected also to accomplish technical and environmental tasks? If that expectation is there, how might that be contradictory to the appropriate role for a professional nurse?

Would the role of the C.N.S. differ in settings of primary nursing where there is an all R.N. staff? Would Sills (Chap. 42) agree with Klein regarding the head nurse and other nursing supervisors being defined as clinical experts where primary nursing exists? How does the primary nurse role differ from the role of the C.N.S.? How does the role of the head nurse differ from the role of a primary nurse? Do interfaces exist between the roles of the primary nurse and clinical specialist?

How can isolation of the primary nurse be prevented? How might staff resource systems be developed for continuity of care in primary nursing? What alternative activities and functions can be considered for nurses to maintain primary nursing throughout night shifts? How can "burnout" be prevented in primary nursing? How can primary nursing groups organize to promote development and support for primary nurses? What relationship is there between clinical ladders and primary nursing? How can clinical ladders be developed to interface with primary nursing? What should be the levels and components of clinical ladders?

What has been the impact of primary nursing for the licensed practical nurse (L.P.N.) and nursing attendants? What is the future of the licensed practical nurse? Are there conditions under which the L.P.N. may be a primary or associate primary nurse? What is the future for nursing attendants? What empirical evidence is there that it is cost-effective to phase out the utilization of nursing attendants, not only where primary nursing is the predominant mode of care, but also in settings where other modes of care are used?

In geographical areas where the number of professional nurses is limited, what alternatives are there to provide and ensure high quality nursing care? Discuss the issues raised by Klein regarding the need of many hospitals to depend on ancillary personnel. How do trends in providing nursing care that are initiated in large hospital/medical centers in major metropolitan areas influence typical hospital settings in other geographic areas where health personnel resources are more limited? To what extent do "bandwagon" effects occur with innovative modes of providing care? What avenues can be used by hospitals to change from a crisis orientation to multiple problems as turnover, union militancy, competition for staff and patients, and fiscal urgencies to an orientation of prevention, planning and innovation? What communication should occur between the large hospital/medical centers in major metropolitan areas and smaller community, suburban, rural hospitals to share the realities of providing patient care? Are there differences in perspectives and problems between the two types of settings similar to the "reality gap" that has existed between nursing education and nursing practice? How can the two types of settings collaborate?

What factors need to be considered in determining the appropriate ratio of patients for one primary nurse? Review Dorothy Walker's chapter 4 regarding the legal responsibilities of the nurse. What implications may exist, particularly regarding contracts and the professional level of the nurse assigned as a primary nurse? What implications exist regarding reimbursement for nursing service by third party payers in the assignments of a primary nurse? What applications are there from Bille (Chap. 36) and La Monica (Chap. 37) for the role of the primary nurse? What implications are there for the development and testing of nursing theory in primary nursing?

What is the basis for needed changes in the nature of patient charting and utilization of care plans, Kardex and patient records in primary nursing? Is the nursing history used differently in primary nursing than with other modes of nursing care? What strategies can be suggested to provide continuity of nursing care in primary nursing? What proposals can be offered to resolve the issues presented concerning three different shifts of service? How can part-time personnel most effectively be utilized in primary nursing?

What potential conflicts may evolve in primary nursing? How can the effort and time required to seek out and consult with the primary nurse be minimized? How does the "gate-keeping" function as identified by Klein necessitate interfaces and negotiations with the head nurse, clinical specialists, other health professionals, and departments? Is a "gate-keeping" function essential to the role of a primary nurse?

What are the key issues concerning change in modes of providing nursing care?

What nursing theory framework(s) or model(s) might be applicable in implementation of primary nursing? What data need to be available and assessment completed in planning for a change to primary nursing? Propose stages in planning and identify all the components of implementation and evaluation. Who should be involved in the earliest stages of planning and to what extent? What strategies are most effective in obtaining administrative support and commitment by nursing staff? What changes in attitudes and by whom are essential for implementation of primary nursing? How can the transition and uncomfortableness associated with change be effectively minimized? What strategies can be posed to promote role change as needed in primary nursing? How is nursing staff more readily developed through primary nursing as suggested by Klein?

What are the implications for in-service education based on Klein's perception of "typical" hospital programs? Would major graduate programs for the preparation of leaders and teachers in continuing education and staff development be offered in schools of nursing? Are there philosophical differences between graduate nursing education programs and continuing education and staff development programs? If so, how can these differences be resolved? What alternatives might be suggested for location of major graduate programs in continuing education? How appropriate would it be for major programs in continuing education to have as an additional mission to develop strategies and programs for the purpose of resolving the nursing shortage? What considerations and issues would need to be addressed to undertake such a mission? What approaches are available to resolve the nursing shortage without compromising professional standards?

To what extent do you agree with Klein's perception of "typical" basic nursing education? How true is it that content that promotes conceptual thinking and independent decision making are lacking in basic nursing education? Why has not the concept of an apprenticeship/internship period for the young graduate never really been accepted by the profession? How are the diverging views on internship related to a discrepancy in educators' conceptualization of education, behavioral expectations in outcomes of programs, professionalism, and employers of new graduates expectations for performance? How can the differences in expectations for practice be reconciled between educators and prospective employers of new graduates? Should internships/preceptorships be required after graduation for the new graduate? If so, who should bear the cost for such programs, to what extent, and for what frame? Should the new graduate be expected to practice as a primary nurse? Would Williamson's suggestions (Chap. 5) regarding the professional entry degree be an acceptable solution to the questions raised by Klein? Review Peterson's (Chap. 7), Santora's (Chap. 8), and Clayton's (Chap. 10) ideas. If Klein's view of undergraduate nursing education is accurate, should primary nurses be prepared at the graduate level? Would an acceptable, realistic solution be to resolve the issues in undergraduate education rather than to expect a higher level of professional education for the primary nurse?

What empirical evidence exists that the quality of patient care provided in primary nursing is higher than other modes of providing care? What empirical evidence exists that primary nursing increases nurse satisfaction/professionalism, decreases staff turnover, and increases physician satisfaction? What empirical evidence is there regarding cost-effectiveness of primary nursing? What research designs can you propose to cope with the problems noted with previous experimental studies? What independent and dependent variables are essential to include? What structure and process variables need to be considered to evaluate outcomes of primary nursing? How can behavioral performance be most effectively evaluated? What is the importance of nursing audits in measuring quality of care?

Would you agree with Klein that the quality of patient care depends on the individual nurse, regardless of what nursing framework is used? Regardless of the setting, what might be the unifying force to resolve probems and differences in modes of care? Should the prime goal be to seek methods and solutions to *ensure* that the individual practitioner will deliver high quality service? If so, *how* and to what degree can ensurance be provided and accountability by the profession be fulfilled?

Would you agree with Klein that neither primary nursing nor any other mode can ensure the provision of the highest level of nursing care? Is the main achievement of primary nursing the exposure of nursing and demonstration of what nursing *is* and *can* potentially do for patients? Will primary nursing continue to be a luxury only selected hospitals can enjoy? What future do you foresee for primary nursing and/or other alternative modes for providing nursing care?

REFERENCES

Alfano, Genrose J.
  1969 "The Loeb Center for nursing and reha-
        bilitation." Nursing Clinics of North
        America 4:487–493.
Bakke, Kathy
  1974 "Primary nursing: Perceptions of a staff
        nurse." American Journal of Nursing
        74:1432–1434.
Bixler, Roy and Genevieve Bixler
  1945 "The professional status of nursing."
        American Journal of Nursing 45:731–
        735.
Christman, Luther
  1975 "Primary nursing care." Paper presented
        at meeting of Sigma Theta Tau, Case
        Western Reserve University, December 4.
Ciske, Karen L.
  1974 "Primary nursing: An organization that
        promotes professional practice." Journal
        of Nursing Administration 4,1:28–31.
  1977 "Misconceptions about staffing and
        patient assignment in primary nursing."
        Nursing Administration Quarterly 1,2:61–
        68.
  1979 "Accountability—The essence of primary
        nursing." American Journal of Nursing."
        79:890–894.
Corn, Florence, Margot Hahn, and Kathleen Lepper
  1977 "Salvaging primary nursing." Supervisor
        Nurse 8,5:29–26.

Curtin, Leah L.
  1980 "My cup boileth over." Supervisor Nurse
        11,1:7.
Daeffler, Reidun Juvkam
  1975 "Patients' perception of care under team
        and primary nursing." Journal of Nursing
        Administration 5,2:20–26.
Dahlen, Alice L.
  1978 "With primary nursing we have it all
        together." American Journal of Nursing
        78:426–428.
Denton, John A.
  1978 Medical Sociology. Boston: Houghton
        Mifflin.
Elpern, Ellen Heid
  1977 "Structural and organizational supports
        for primary nursing." Nursing Clinics of
        North America 12:205–219.
Logsdon, Audrey
  1973 "Why primary nursing?" Nursing Clinics
        of North America 8:283–291.
Manthey, Marie
  1973 "Primary nursing is alive and well in the
        hospital." American Journal of Nursing
        73:83–87.
  1978 "If you are instituting primary nursing."
        American Journal of Nursing 78:426.
Manthey, Marie, Karen Ciske, Patricia Robertson,
    and Isabel Harris
  1970 "Primary nursing: A return to the con-
        cept of 'my nurse' and 'my patient.'"
        Nursing Forum 9:65–83.

Marram, Gwen, Kathleen Flynn, Wendy Abaravich, and Sheila Carey
1976   Cost-Effectiveness of Primary and Team Nursing. Wakefield, Mass.: Contemporary.

Marram, Gwen D., Margaret W. Schlegel, and Em O. Bevis
1974   Primary Nursing: A Model for Individualized Care. St. Louis: Mosby.

Olsen, Anna
1977   "Change takes time." Nursing Administration Quarterly 1:51–59.

Osinski, Elsie G. and Jill G. Powals
1980   "The cost of all R.N. staffed primary nursing." Supervisor Nurse 11,1:16–21.

Page, Marjorie
1974   "Perceptions of a head nurse." American Journal of Nursing 74:1435–1436.

Prendergast, Judith A.
1977   "Implementing problem-oriented records in a primary nursing system." Nursing Clinics of North America 12:235–246.

Robinson, Alice M.
1974   "Primary-care nursing at two teaching hospitals." RN 37,4:31–35.

Shaw, Marvin E. and Philip R. Costanzo
1970   Theories of Social Psychology. New York: McGraw-Hill.

Shubin, Seymour
1979   "Communicating (or, make that *non* communicating) with doctors." Nursing 79 9,2:90–94.

Smith, Constance C.
1977   "Primary nursing care—substantive nursing care delivery system." Nursing Administration Quarterly 1,1:1–8.

Spoth, Juliann
1977   "Primary nursing: The agony and the ecstasy." Nursing Clinics of North America 12:221–234.

Wolff, Kathleen G.
1977   "Change: Implementation of primary nursing through ad hocracy." Journal of Nursing Administration 7,10:24–27.

Chapter 44

Reimbursement for Nursing Practice

Virginia S. Cleland, R.N., Ph.D., F.A.A.N.
Professor
College of Nursing
Wayne State University
Detroit, Michigan

Following treatises on roles and modes in providing nursing care, it is timely to focus on payment for nursing services. Direct acknowledgment through reimbursement for the services provided by nurses in practice has long been supported by the nursing profession. The incorporation of nursing services into the per diem hospital charge has been a source of lamentation for departments of nursing and confusion to the consumer. Accountability for the cost or effectiveness of nursing care is neither possible nor can the consumer know or control what is purchased through insurance without direct reimbursement. Virginia S. Cleland identifies some of the existing problems in health economics, strongly advocates the need for changes, and provides an enlightening description of the perplexing issues associated with reimbursement for nursing care. She notes how the cost of nursing service is subsumed in a patient's billing statement and illustrates cost-effective services nurses frequently perform which are not the role of the professional nurse.

Cleland cites economic inequities in health care, for example, the variation in practitioners of medical service for the different socioeconomic classes of patients. She explains the reimbursement mechanism used for physicians on the basis of his or her actual charge, his or her customary charge, or the area's prevailing charge. Inequities of the billing system for physicians and other health professional services are indicated. Cleland maintains many institutions offer duplicative services that add to unnecessary health service costs. She speaks to the economic dissimilarities between nonprofit and profit institutions. The argument is presented that a strong health industry alliance exists between health agency administrators and physicians. It is perceived that spiraling costs of health services cannot be controlled without legal restrictions implicating the practice of medicine. Four reasons are provided as to why the health system economy does not respond as a normal market: the consumers' lack of information about services, control of demand by providers, third-party payment of medical hospital bills, and the rewards for nonprofit hospitals for being large and providing multiple services rather than being well managed and efficient. Cleland predicts that changes in reimbursement procedures will be made by the state and federal government for more

596

rational dispersement policies, reliable cost accounting techniques, and valid documentation of costs and effectiveness.

In the discussion concerning reimbursement for organized nursing services, Cleland emphasizes that nursing can become an income-producing hospital service when the profession is ready to demand it, defend the patient's right to know what nursing care costs, and be prepared for scrutiny when the patient makes a comparison between what was paid for and received. She proclaims patients cannot and should not be charged for care that was not available. The reasons provided as to why nursing services have not been converted to a revenue-producing department are lack of nursing power and control by hospital administrators over nursing. Cleland offers the suggestion for nursing leaders to develop the case for identifiable reimbursement with the Health Care Financing Administration of the Department of Health and Human Resources. She warns that the practice of "substitutability," where nurses prepared for one level of practice are projected to a higher level without the appropriate experience or education, should not be permitted.

Strategies are suggested for reimbursement. The levels of nursing care and requisite academic and experiential qualifications of nurses need to be defined, clarified, and interpreted for the public. Research is needed to examine the relationship between levels of nursing practice and nursing care provided, patients' needs, and costs of care per the defined levels. Examples of potential and actual abuses are cited regarding the use of nursing personnel for specified levels of care. Two approaches are indicated for research: classification of patients into three to five levels of care depending upon their nursing needs and the development of Diagnosis Related Groups.

Cleland predicts reimbursement for ambulatory care by group master's-prepared nurse practitioners of health promotion and disease prevention is the greatest arena. She advocates autonomy to practice nursing not delegated medicine, with separate provider numbers for nurse practitioners, which permits evaluation for quality and costs of services to occur. Three economic models for autonomy of practice are offered, those utilized by dentists, clinical psychologists, and one in use at the University Health Center in Detroit based upon a fee-for-visit concept. Cleland concludes with six specific strategies for reimbursement in ambulatory care. These are: define the group of nurses who qualify as those with a master's degree in nursing who have earned ANA advanced certification; compute charges from a predetermined formula; advocate inclusion of health promotion and illness prevention services in all health plans; promote specific nursing services for definable populations; foster demonstration projects to help third-party payers obtain data; and promote the concept of freedom of choice in selecting a primary care provider. Political processes and unity are indicated as being essential to make changes a reality.

Reimbursement for practice in a direct and publicly identifiable manner will become a major professional issue for nursing in the 1980s.[1] As the

[1] Portions of this paper were used originally by the author in the keynote paper honoring Jessie Scott upon her retirement as Director, Division of Nursing, Department of Health and Human Resources, May 25, 1979. "Old Dreams, New Visions," *Prospectives for Nursing: Symposium.* Nurse Planning Series #15. Health Resources Administration, 1980, pp. 1–9.

educational framework defining levels of nursing practice is constructed by the profession, it will become possible to pursue the issue of reimbursement with determination. Direct reimbursement has not been an appropriate or productive undertaking while the philosophy "an R.N. is an R.N. is an R.N." has been operational within the health care system.

The cost of nursing care in service institutions

is reimbursed today. However, the costs are not identified in a patient's billing statement and instead are obscured along with food service, housekeeping service, laundry, etc., in the so-called routine services which make up an institution's per diem charge. In ambulatory care, the nurse-practitioner's services are commonly subsumed under a physician's fee-for-service.

It is unlikely that there can be substantial or widespread improvement of nursing care without research to devise techniques to relate patient needs, services, costs, and charges in a manner which leaves nurses answerable to their clients for the quality and costs of services rendered. Nor is improvement likely without an organized effort among a significant number of nurses.

Nursing is a human service profession. The services offered must be *effective* or the profession can be charged with quackery. The service must be *cost-effective* or society will find a substitute. Nurses have certainly been cost-effective. They are cost-effective when substituting for hospital administration on the evening and night shift. They are cost-effective when substituting for medical house officers and attending physicians when those persons are not available. Nurses substitute for social workers, pharmacists, physical therapists, and inhalation therapists. Nurses keep records of charges for the business office and act as secretaries to remind physicians to complete their charting. Nurses have been in high demand to do chart audits for utilization review and quality assurance programs. They have been hired in large numbers to assist insurance companies in processing claims appropriately.

There was a 23 percent increase between 1972 and 1977 in the number of registered nurses; yet simultaneously there is a great national unmet demand for nurses (U.S. Department of Health and Human Resources, 1978:18,128). Yes, the employment of the nurse has been cost-effective.

The public pays for nursing care, but individual consumers have had little knowledge and less control over what they have purchased through insurance, what they actually needed, what they received, or what they must pay out-of-pocket because it was not included in their insurance.

The nursing profession can not be held accountable for the cost or effectiveness of nursing care until nurses have more control over the appropriate utilization of nursing resources. Only with appropriate use of nurses by level of education and experience can nursing have a significant impact on the availability, continuity, quality, and cost of health services. Health system goals cannot be achieved without active participation by nurses in the documentation and quantification of their contributions.

ECONOMIC IMPLICATIONS OF HEALTH CARE

This paper does not attempt a broad overview of the economics of the health care system. A useful introductory text that presumes no prior reader background in economics is that by Philip Jacobs, *The Economics of Health and Medical Care* (1980). Because many nurses are so trusting and accepting of the economic practices of their own employing hospital or of the physicians with whom they work, certain economic inequities will be mentioned here.

Certain economic rules and regulations of health care are quite predictive of who gets what medical service from which practitioner in what facility. For example:

Welfare class: Cared for by interns and residents in public hospitals

Working class: Cared for by general and family practitioners in private community hospitals

Upper middle class: Cared for by board-certified specialists in private teaching hospitals

It is no accident that medical students and house officers learn their skills on welfare patients. These relationships are economically determined and have little correlation with "service" attitudes and "caring" philosophies of individual practitioners.

Many private, nonprofit hospitals maintain

outpatient departments to recruit low-income patients who are fully covered by Medicare or Medicaid. These patients become "clinical material" for the training of house officers. Attending physicians are provided with the assistance of house officers but at the same time can protect their private patients from being used by residents in training. The residents have clinic patients on whom to develop skills in the use of intrusive procedures; the attending physicians have their off-time protected while the hospital gets the prestige and status of being a "teaching hospital," and the costs are passed back to state and federal governments.

Medicine, the occupation which meets all the sociologists' criteria for a "profession," practices great subtlety economically. Physicians, through the Political Action Committee of the American Medical Association, are repeatedly the largest contributors to the election campaigns of members of Congress—$1.6 million to candidates for Congress in 1978 (Demkovich, 1979:2021). In return for this continuing largesse, Congress has been very sensitive to the wishes of physicians. To illustrate, Congress instructed the Social Security Administration to designate physician fees under Medicare-Medicaid legislation to be the "prevailing and customary" charges currently being paid. With this vague authorization language, Congress removed itself from any influence over physicians' fees. Rules and regulations were developed during Social Security Administration hearings mainly attended by physicians and administrators.

The physician is reimbursed on the basis of the lowest of (a) his actual charge, (b) his customary charge, or (c) the area's prevailing charge. The actual charge is self-explanatory. The customary charge is the physician's median billed charge for that service during the previous calendar year. The prevailing charge may be the 75th percentile of the distribution of all customary charges by "similar" physicians within a geographic market area. Under Blue Cross, the prevailing charge is set at the 90th percentile and commercial insurers, because of higher billing costs,

pay at the 92d percentile of the prevailing charges (Gabel and Redisch, 1979).

Thus, under the rubric of "customary and usual" fees, the physician can charge any fee he wishes and then actually collect a fee set at 90 percent of those customary in that locality. The difference between the actual and the customary can be billed directly to the patient. In the case of the retired and the elderly on fixed incomes, the uncovered portion not paid by Medicare can be troublesome. Even if the excess charge is *never* collected, it goes into next year's computations of that physician's "customary" charges and that community's "usual" fee for that particular service.

Anesthesiologists may send professional service bills to patients whose anesthetic was given by a nurse-anesthetist. Thus, the patient, or his or her insuring party, may pay twice for the same procedure—first as a part of the hospital bill because the nurse-anesthetist receives a hospital-based salary and second in a professional service bill from the anesthesiologist. While it is appropriate for the anesthesiologist to be paid a salary for administrative and supervisory functions, a professional fee for service per patient cannot be justified.

Radiologists and pathologists negotiate percentages of those departments' gross or net receipts. Are patients paying for professional services as "piecework," or should these be called "commissions" on sales?

Hospital administrators and their employees stand behind their institutions' nonprofit status and view their institutions as valuable community resources. In truth, many of these institutions are offering duplicative services which add unnecessarily to health service costs in their area. The nature of hospital payments by third-party payers is such that duplicative services do not produce competitive pricing.

Many hospitals in this nation have board members who are in direct conflict of interest because of economic relationships with their institutions. An attorney may sit on a hospital board while his partner handles an institution's business and labor contracts. The president of the local bank may sit on a board while the hospital keeps its accounts in that bank or the bank lends the hospital money for a new facility. Nonprofit hospital board members should be required to sign annual statements that they have no personal or family economic interest in the financial affairs of the institution. Hospitals which derive significant portions of income from governmental funds should be required to provide a list of board members upon request and to hold open board meetings.

Nonprofit status in most states sets no limits on administrators' salaries but rather only restricts the disbursement of net receipts to avoid showing a profit. All over the country, hospitals have expanded their physical plants, added new services, and built medical office facilities for physicians who agree to bring their patients for hospitalization to that institution. Because these medical office buildings are built by the hospital, usually with tax-exempt bonds, rents do not reflect the usual property taxes and return on investment costs. The decreased rents are a legally acceptable reward to the physician for bringing patients to that hospital.

Hospitals, like physicians, have been treated very generously in Medicare-Medicaid legislation. Claiborne, author of *The Great Health Care Rip-off*, has reported:

> . . . Social Security Administration allowed hospitals to depreciate the full cost of buildings that had already been partly, or even wholly depreciated. They could depreciate buildings constructed with federal grants—meaning that the government was paying twice for the same building. They could write off the cost of the equipment well before its useful term of life. And so on.
>
> Perhaps most important, hospitals were not required to "fund" their depreciation allowances, to actually set them aside for use only in replacing obsolete plants. Instead, they could (and did) use the funds for additional buildings and equipment—whose "reasonable costs" then became a ground for demanding still higher government payments. (1978:16)

Hospitals which are frankly incorporated as "for-profit" institutions tend to be more honest in their goals. Stocks in these for-profit chains can be purchased on the stock exchanges. The for-profit hospitals seek out hospital admissions which are short-term and highly predictable and for which bills will be fully paid and then send the complex, long-term, inadequately financed patients to tax-supported institutions. With inflation and tax limitations due to referenda, many public institutions, particularly city and county hospitals, are closing. These institutions have limited income and very high costs because they are left with patients other hospitals do not choose to admit.

The hospital-medical industry is the third largest employer in the United States, exceeded only by government (local, state, and federal) and the wholesale-retail industry. It is a very complex, very expensive interrelated nonsystem. How does such a nonsystem hang together enough to be commonly referred to as "the health system?" There is one common rule that explains a great deal about the economics of hospital and medical care. This rule is that hospital administrators, singly or as a group, never take a public position which places them between physicians and their ability to make money. The first corollary of the rule is that physicians never place themselves between a hospital administrator and that institution's ability to make money. Thus, it becomes very difficult for health planners and economists to get all the information needed for decisions compatible with the public welfare.

The spiraling costs of health services cannot be controlled without legal restrictions involving the practice of medicine. Physicians initiate nearly all health service charges. At one time it was thought physicians were like other economic commodities, i.e., if society increased the number of physicians, some would establish their practices in rural areas and in urban centers and thus correct the problems of maldistribution. More recent studies indicate that this is not a valid assumption. The health system economy does not respond as a normal market for several reasons: (a) consumer ignorance—consumers do not have requisite information on which to make informed judgments about the services to be purchased; (b) control of demand by providers—the patient generally makes only one decision, that is, to seek medical care; (c) third-party payment of medical hospital bills—70 percent of all services are paid by a third party, the patient is not personally concerned about the size of the bill, and the physician is assured reimbursement; (d) cost-based retrospective reimbursement—nonprofit hospitals have been rewarded both in prestige and financially for being large and having a wide range of services rather than for being well managed and efficient (Wicks, 1979).

The total cost of health service in this nation has continued to grow without control mainly because hospitals have been reimbursed for their costs and physicians on the basis of their customary and usual charges. Recent data of actual and projected expenditures are shown below (Freeland et al., 1980:2).

Despite such evidence that health costs are out of control, congressional lobbying efforts of the American Hospital Association, Federation of American Hospitals (proprietary institutions), and the American Medical Association succeeded in defeating the Carter administration's hospital cost containment bill in the House of Representatives in November, 1979, and passed in its stead a mild "voluntary" program (News, 1980:12).

The majority of labor unions are unconcerned with health care costs as long as an employer is paying the total insurance premium as a fringe benefit and service is reasonably good. Insurance companies are more concerned about their relations with health service institutions and physicians than about holding the costs down. These companies simply add their administrative costs to the service costs and assess the new charges.

However, some new sources of economic pressures on the delivery of health services are developing. City and county governments are rapidly getting out of the business of institutional medical care. State and federal categorical health service programs will have to absorb the cost of care for patients formerly cared for in city and county facilities. The state and federal governments are much further from the site of care delivery and as direct providers of the monies can exert pressures for more rational disbursement policies, more reliable cost accounting techniques, and more valid documentation of costs and effectiveness.

Corporations and institutions with large payrolls are becoming involved in health planning and are studying ways to control health insurance costs or services. Companies which in the past merely passed their health care costs through to the consumers of company products are finding increasing difficulty in remaining competitive against foreign corporations.

It is likely that significant changes will be made in the reimbursement procedures of existing health programs by state and federal executive branch

National health expenditures (in billions)	Proportion of G.N.P. (%)
Historical period	
1965 . . . .$ 43.0	6.2
1970 . . . . 74.7	7.6
1975 . . . . 131.5	8.6
1978 . . . . 192.4	9.1
Projections	
1980 . . . . 244.6	9.5
1985 . . . . 438.2	10.5
1990 . . . . 757.9	11.5

departments (not Congress). There is considerable agreement that past policies have resulted in over-emphasis on medical diagnosis and treatment of pathology and underemphasis on health promotion and disease prevention. With a rapidly increasing population over the age of 65, the cost of continuing these past practices is astronomical, with little benefit economically to be gained from increased production of goods or services from these retired workers.

From this preceding, albeit brief, view of some of the existing problems in health economics and the need for changes to be made, more specific problems relating to reimbursement for nursing care will be introduced.

REIMBURSEMENT FOR ORGANIZED NURSING SERVICES

It is a common practice of hospitals not to charge directly for the services of nutritionists, social workers, and nurses. By incorporating these services into the per diem charge, hospital administrators retain considerable freedom to adjust and modify the budget and the accounts. On the other hand, the hospital does bill separately for radiology, laboratory services, pharmacy, and physical therapy. The reader should not fail to notice the sexism involved. Service departments traditionally headed by men are viewed as "income-producing" and those headed by women as "routine costs."

Nursing can become an income-producing hospital service when the profession is ready to demand it and is prepared to defend the patient's right to know what his or her nursing care costs. Nursing must be prepared to stand the intensity of reaction when patient and family compare what they have paid for and what they have received. When the patient is directly charged for the service, the old explanation of "not enough nurses" becomes difficult to defend. The patient cannot and should not be charged for care that was not available.

Today the typical hospital's accounts cover six distinct areas: (1) outpatient accounts; (2) non-patient care-related overhead accounts; (3) patient care-related overhead accounts; (4) room, board, and other routine (hotel) accounts; (5) ancillary accounts (radiology, laboratory, etc.); and (6) nursing accounts. It is at the last stage of the accounting process that nursing costs become folded into the hotellike costs of a hospital to form the basis for the per diem charge. These nursing costs could as easily be billed separately and then nursing would become revenue-producing like pharmacy, the laboratories, etc.

If converting nursing to a revenue-producing department could be accomplished this easily, why has it not been done? The answer is *power*! Nursing costs generally represent 40 to 60 percent of an institution's budget, depending upon the institution's size and complexity. Hospitals are willing to bill separately for countless items costing less than $5.00 but will not bill for nursing care. If nursing were acknowledged as producing 40 to 60 percent of the institution's income, nursing would gain a very powerful position in the administrative structure. Instead, nursing administrators are kept humble by being constantly reminded of the high payroll costs of the nursing department.

Hospital administrators will not voluntarily give up that control over nursing; however, nursing can force resolution of the issue. Nursing leaders can build a case for identifiable reimbursement for nursing care with the Health Care Financing Administration of the Department of Health and Human Resources. Because such a change in procedure would provide agency officials with better data for improved assessment of costs, they would likely view such a change as supportive of their goals. Whatever is required for Medicaid and Medicare accounting quickly becomes the standard for the industry.

However, nursing should not seek such changes without concurrently demanding professional control of the practice of nursing within the institution. Federal support for research into better methods to relate nursing care and costs of services would immediately follow, as has been the case with physician and hospital reimbursement.

The public assumes an unreasonable burden when employers place nurses prepared for one level of practice at a higher level without the appropriate experience or education. *Substitutability* has meant that a hospital can collect reimbursement for a coronary care unit when, in fact, the nurses have not been prepared to carry out the specialized procedures of cornary care. Substitutability has meant that a hospital can put an L.P.N. in charge of a nursing unit on the night shift and provide "supervision" from a distant nursing office. Substitutability destroys job satisfaction and promotes instability in nursing staffs. High turnover creates waste in the use of human resources through increased costs of recruitment, hiring, orientation, and termination procedures.

STRATEGIES FOR REIMBURSEMENT FOR ORGANIZED NURSING SERVICES

Nursing has begun to accept its responsibility to define, clarify, and interpret for the public the levels of nursing care and the requisite academic and experiential qualifications of nurses to provide this care. There is need for further research on the relationship between levels of nursing practice, levels of nursing care provided, patient needs, and costs of care by defined levels. Faculty members in graduate programs in nursing must devote more attention to this area of research.

There are at least two fundamentally different approaches such research might take. One method is based upon the classification of patients into three to five levels of care depending upon their nursing needs. Then, nursing staff can be categorized into competency levels such as LPNs, RN1, RN2, RN3, and RN4 (Colvecchio et al., 1974). Education and experience define the categories and management determines the level at which a nurse is actually practicing.

If 20 percent of the patients on a particular clinical service have level III needs, then the staff hours (excluding head nurses) provided for these patients should be at the RN3 or RN4 level. If levels of care are defined for groups of patients, it becomes possible to relate nursing staffing costs to nursing charges. Departments of nursing can become more publicly accountable. When an institution either cannot or will not employ appropriate nursing personnel for a specified level of care, then that level of care is not available and the public must not be charged for undocumented service. For example, when institutions fail more than 10 percent of the time to provide a standard level of personnel, it would be appropriate for the third-party payer to reimburse at the rate of the next lower level of care, i.e., if not intensive care then moderate care, if not moderate care then extended care. Currently there are no penalites for downgrading staff, and for too many institutions the incentive is to staff only at a level which avoids successful lawsuits. Similarly, there have been serious abuses by institutions keeping intensive care units constantly filled and failing to move patients to moderate care levels until another patient is available to use the intensive care bed. This practice tends to maximize institutional income and also patient charges.

A fundamentally different method of determining staffing and costs has recently appeared in the literature. This research pertains to the development of Diagnosis Related Groups and may become increasingly significant in the reimbursement of care (Horn and Schumaker, 1979). A total of 383 Diagnostic Related Groups have been defined. For the first time it would be possible to subject an institution's service load to external audit and enable accountants and planners to compare patient mix and costs across institutions.

While there are objections to the concept of the Diagnostic Related Groups (DRGs), it is being used now by Maryland, New Jersey, New York, and Georgia for reimbursement purposes. There has been some research correlating 25 nursing activities and the number of minutes of nursing time involved with a per-diem nursing weight established for each Diagnostic Related Group. In the past, nursing has been ill-served by these operations research methodologies. Nurse researchers must become more involved in such studies so that the questions nursing wants answered will be asked.

REIMBURSEMENT FOR MASTER'S-PREPARED NURSE PRACTITIONERS IN AMBULATORY CARE

Reimbursement for ambulatory care is quite different from reimbursement for institutional practice. This is the arena of greatest opportunity for practice relating to health promotion and disease prevention. It is also the arena of greatest direct conflict with medical practitioners in relation to reimbursement.

There will be few self-employed solo nurse practitioners in ambulatory care, for they will be economically dependent upon private pay patients. Third-party payers do not wish to expand practice opportunities for solo practitioners. Rather, multiple incentives are being created to encourage physicians to move into group practice arrangements where there are better managerial and evaluative services.

It is likely that the profession's standards for the qualifications of nurse practitioners for autonomous nursing practice will be the master's degree with a major in nursing and advanced certification by the American Nurses Association. Such qualifications would afford the public maximum protection and provide third-party payers with criteria easy to administer. The variability of practitioner skills of nurses with lesser credentials is too great for the profession to attest to their competencies for autonomous practice. However baccalaureate-prepared nurse practitioners could be employed in ambulatory practice under the clinical supervision of advanced nurse practitioners as part of a nursing practice group.

Nurse practitioners should strive for complete autonomy of nursing practice within organized practice groups. *Practice autonomy* means the right to practice nursing rather than delegated medicine, to admit and discharge clients, determine frequency of visits, negotiate charges, and collect reimbursement as practitioners of nursing rather than as physician associates. This means that nurse practitioners must have separate provider numbers, which then makes the output of that practice subject to evaluation for both quality and cost of services. Being a part of a group practice setting also means that physician consultation and referral is available.

An economic model for autonomy of practice can be that of dentists engaged in practice in a hospital or medical clinic. The dentists have their own practice organization but coordinate their activities with those of other practice groups in the agency.

Another model, though less desirable, is that of clinical psychologists practicing with medically trained psychiatrists. In some states, these umbrella arrangements are necessary for reimbursement purposes, but the clinical psychologists select their own clients, manage treatment, and negotiate their fees, although insurance claims are submitted in the name of the psychiatrist. These practice arrangements will exist until there is sufficient public support of the service for practitioners to be able to practice in the name of their own profession.

A nurse practitioner appropriately can accept associate status in a medical staff organization during a preliminary period with the understanding that full professional status and a prorated share in the group's profits would be made available after a year of service. In negotiating economic worth, nurse practitioners should be cognizant not only of the value of their own services but also of the value of the physician's released time, which enables him or her to see additional patients.

Still another model, which has been used at the University Health Center in Detroit, is a Medicaid contract with the State of Michigan based upon the concept of a fee-for-visit rather than the more common fee-for-service. The former is a prenegotiated annual fee-for-visit that covers professional services from any primary care health professional plus x-rays and laboratory services ordered at the time of the visit. Clients are seen by physicians, social workers, nutritionists, clinical psychologists, or nurse-practitioners according to the client's needs and choice. Each professional discipline is independently organized and individuals are paid salaries appropriate for the market value of their services. Practitioners can share in group profits deriving from high productivity and effective management.

STRATEGIES FOR REIMBURSEMENT IN AMBULATORY CARE

Strategies for gaining reimbursement for nurses practicing in ambulatory care can be based upon several tactics such as the following:

1 Define the group of nurses who would qualify—registered nurses with master's degree in nursing and who earned ANA advanced certification in their area of practice. Some third-party payers are willing to test a reimbursement model if the profession will define who is qualified to provide the services.

2 Compute charges from a predetermined formula.

$$\frac{\text{Yearly compensation}}{2080 \text{ hours} - (\text{fringe benefit days} \times 8 \text{ hours})}$$

$$= \text{Hourly rate} + \text{overhead assessment}$$

$$= \text{hourly fee}$$

The hourly fee as a basis for charges can be defended. Overhead includes cost of space, equipment, utilities, and support staff. The mode of payment of physicians (fee for service) is directly responsible for producing overspecialization, geographic maldistribution of services, excessively brief office visits, overhospitalization, excess surgery, and skyrocketing costs.

3 Advocate, through political processes, the inclusion of health promotion and illness prevention services in all third-party payment programs and in state and Health Systems Agencies' health plans. Few physicians are academically prepared for health promotion services and fewer yet have

such a career interest. This is nursing's natural arena of practice.

4 Promote specific nursing services for definable populations. For example, physical examinations and health histories for employment, life insurance, and school purposes should be nursing's responsibility. Health assessments for presumed healthy persons are too important as health promotional opportunities to be lost to hurried physicians.

The priority preventive services, i.e., family planning, pregnancy and infant care, immunizations, sexually transmitted disease services, hypertension case finding and control, and cancer screening activities should become nursing's primary care responsibilities. Symptomatic treatment of upper respiratory infections, constipation, insomnia, vaginitis, nonrecurrent urinary tract infections, and life-stress anxieties and depression are other problems more relevant to health promotion and disease prevention than illness treatment.

Health services for the elderly are costly because their problems too often are conceptualized as treatment rather than maintenance. The fact that pathology is present does not mean that it is the primary problem. The client is most often in need of health education, maintenance, and psychological support which can be provided by nurse practitioners in higher quality and at lower costs than by physicians.

5 Foster the development of demonstration projects to assist third-party payers to obtain utilization data upon which large prepayment endeavors can be based.

6 Promote the concept of *freedom of choice* in selecting a primary care provider. This technique has been effectively used by osteopathic physicians and clinical psychologists in demanding inclusion in insurance offerings. Nursing can work with other nonphysician providers to encourage action by the Federal Trade Commission (FTC) to break up the economic monopoly of medicine. It is of interest to note that the medical establishment is sufficiently worried about future activities of the FTC that in February 1980 there was a move by the Senate to completely close off the medical, dental, and other health professions to FTC scrutiny. This was defeated by only two votes (Washington Report, 1980).

CONCLUSION

There is much at stake in nursing strategies for nursing care reimbursement in institutions or in ambulatory care. Timing is the most important consideration. Nursing is not as ready as one might hope, but the steps to be taken are reasonably clear. It is better to move now than to wait another decade when more research is in place. Reimbursement mechanisms can be refined and adjusted after the basic structure is in place. State health plans are being developed which will support the movement of monies from the support of high-technology treatment of infrequent diseases to health promotion and disease prevention.

The effect of loss of foreign medical graduates is being felt by service agencies. While the Graduate Medical Education National Advisory Committee (GMENAC) in its report to Congress in September, 1980, has predicted a surplus of physicians by 1990, these supply predictions in relation to primary care practitioners are quite likely overstated. The predictions are based upon an assumption that continued capitation funding for American medical schools will be available. The data also assume that all osteopathic physicians (of which 45.1 percent are specialists), psychiatrists, obstetrician-gynecologists, and some general surgeons function as primary care providers (Division of Medicine, 1978).

The health industry alliance between health agency administrators and physicians is so entrenched that nursing can expect little from either group. Occasionally there is assistance from individual members, but group support cannot be anticipated. Rather, ploys must be devised which neither group can attack as not being in the public's interest. Then, with full use of the concepts of *freedom of choice of practitioner* and *reduced costs*, the changes must be pushed through politically. Individual nurses and the professional organizations must use political processes with sufficient strength and unity to make needed changes a reality. The decade of the 1980s is the time for action.

EDITOR'S QUESTIONS FOR DISCUSSION

Are there other examples where nurses have been cost-effective for services that are not considered functions of the professional role? How likely is it that nurses will discontinue performing the functions indicated by Cleland? What strategies can be offered to change the situation?

In illustrating the inequities in health care, to what extent can the examples provided also apply to the provision of nursing services? What ethical issues are inherent in variations of type of practitioner for different socioeconomic classes of patients? How can the inequities and abuses cited regarding reimbursement of physicians' services be prevented as well as in implementing reimbursement for nursing services? To what extent is there evidence or data to support the portrayal of duplicative services, conflicts of interest due to economic relationships, differences between nonprofit and profit institutions, and alliances between health agency administrators and physicians? What are the implications for the health professions and consumer of the state and federal governments becoming more directly involved in controlling health insurance roots or services?

How can nursing costs be billed separately? Why has not nursing been converted to a revenue-producing department? What are the predominant issues in need of resolution for nursing costs to be directly reimbursed? How can "substitutability" of nurses be prevented? What implications are there for reimbursement of nursing services in geographic areas where health personnel are more limited? What alternative strategies can be offered for seeking reimbursement in such areas?

Review Dorothy Walker's chapter 4 and discuss what are the legal ramifications of reimbursement for nursing. Do you agree that many institutions are staffed only at a level to avoid lawsuits? How can the relationship between levels of nursing practice and nursing care provided, patient needs and costs of care by defined levels most appropriately be established? Should patient classification systems be standardized? What competencies should be expected if nursing staff were categorized by education and experience? Are there any possibilities for categories suggested in the findings of Clayton's study (Chap. 10)? Should competencies also be expected in application of a nursing conceptual/theoretical base for nursing interventions? How can linkage be established and accepted between nursing theoretical bases and skill competencies in practice? Which of the nursing theorists contributing in Section 4 offer suggestions toward dual competencies? How can management determine the level at which a nurse is actually practicing? Review Chap. 23 by Sweeney and Gordon and Chap. 41 by Gordon. What relationship is there between classifying patients into levels of care according to their nursing needs and the work of the National Conference Group for Classification of Nursing Diagnoses? How does the work of the National Conference Group compare with the work of Diagnosis Related Groups referred to by Cleland? What evidence exists that nursing is prepared to have reimbursement implemented? What steps does nursing yet need to take to prepare for reimbursement? What research questions should be asked and studied for reimbursement purposes?

What implications are there for primary nursing and reimbursement? What possibilities exist for Sills' proposal (Chap. 42) for nurse corporations and reimbursement? What relationship exists between Brown's chapter 26 and Cleland's discussion of reimbursement for nurse practitioners? Compare the viewpoints regarding educational preparation of entry into practice by Williamson (Chap. 5) and Klein (Chap. 43). From those writings what problems evidently would need to be resolved regarding academic qualifications and levels of nursing practice and care provided? What are the suggestions for reimbursement of the clinical nurse specialist (C.N.S.) in Sills' chapter 42? Compare Sills' view (Chap. 42) of practice settings and autonomy for the C.N.S. with Cleland's prediction of group nurse practitioners in ambulatory care settings and definition of "practice autonomy." Is there a relationship between Sills' nurse-corporation proposal and any of the three economic models for autonomy of practice offered by Cleland? What quality of care issues may enter into a fee-for-visit model rather than the more common fee-for-service? How much agreement is evident between Williamson (Chap. 5) and Cleland's proposal for qualifications of nurses for reimbursement who practice in ambulatory care? What implications are there for Fleming's (Chap. 35), Bille's (Chap. 36), and La Monica's (Chap. 47) writings concerning health education, preventive services, and Cleland's discussion of reimbursement for definable services and populations? What impact might the present economic state have on the future direct reimbursement of nursing services?

REFERENCES

Claiborne, Robert
  1978 "The great health care rip-off." Saturday Review (January 7) 10–16, 150.
Colvecchio, R., B. Tescher, and C. Scalzi
  1974 "A clinical ladder for nursing practice." Journal of Nursing Administration (September-October) 4:54–58.
Demkovich, Linda A.
  1979 "The AMA-Reports of its death have been greatly exaggerated." National Journal 11:2017–22.

Division of Medicine, Bureau of Health Manpower
   1978 GMENAC Staff Papers: Supply and Distribution of Physicians and Physician Extenders. Health Resources Administration pp. 25 and 66.

Freeland, M., G. Calat, and C. Schedler
   1980 "Projection of national health expenditures, 1980, 1985, and 1990." Health Care Financing Review 1(3-Winter):1–27.

Gabel, J. R. and M. A. Redisch
   1979 "Alternative physician payment methods: Incentives, efficiency and national health insurance." Milbank Memorial Fund Quarterly 57:38–59.

Horn, S. and D. Schumacher
   1979 "An analysis of case mix complexity using information theory and diagnostic related grouping." Medical Care 17(4 April):383–89.

Jacobs, Philip
   1980 The Economics of Health and Medical Care. Baltimore: University Park Press.

News
   1980 "House rejects cost containment legislation." American Journal of Nursing (January) 80:12.

Washingtion Report
   1980 "Capital comment." Washington Report on Health Legislation 6(12-March 19):1

U.S. Department of Health, Education and Welfare
   1978 First Report to the Congress, Nurse Training Act of 1975. Division of Nursing, Health Resources Administration, Pp. 18 and 128.

Wicks, E. E.
   1979 "Planning, Regulation and the Economics of Health Care" in Health Planning Proceedings, Michigan Health Planning Conference, May 3.

Chapter 45

The Relationship of Nurse Practice Acts to the Professionalization of Nursing

Bonnie Bullough, R.N., Ph.D., F.A.A.N.
Dean and Professor
School of Nursing
State University of New York at Buffalo
Buffalo, New York

The extensive attention paid to numerous aspects of nursing practice in the previous chapters of this section is not complete without an examination of Nurse Practice Acts. The law is fundamentally related to defining nursing, the scope of practice and essential to the professionalization of nursing. Bonnie Bullough offers a distinct perspective on the evolution of professionalism in medicine, the history of the American Nurse Practice Acts, and implications for the professionalization of nursing.

She reviews the varying definitions for defining professions. Definitions are formulated according to attributes possessed, such as possession of specialized techniques for giving service; characteristics such as the five formulated by Greenwood and four by Barber; and elements as the six developed as a scale by Moore. Professions have also been classified by an ethical stance, distinctions made between the professional and amateur, and as an ideal type. More recently the crucial attribute indicated is the power an occupation has to control the terms, conditions, and content of its work. The key attribute for focus is autonomy.

Bullough traces the genesis of professionalism in medicine not only to illustrate the process but also to understand the impact medical licensure has for other health occupations. The key variables cited are the emergence of the university and the sponsorship of the throne which allowed the university practitioners to assert primacy. The basic attributes of medicine as a profession, according to Bullough, are autonomy, institutionalization within the university, organization, and the use of government as an instrument of power. Medicine established the legal precedent for occupational licensure. Licenses for other health occupations became amendments to the medical practice acts.

Bullough divides the history of nursing practice laws into three phases. The first phase is from 1903 to 1938. The nursing organizations, the National League for Nursing (NLN) and the American Nurses' Association (ANA), wanted to upgrade the educational standards for nurses and did the lobbying to facilitate the passing of a registration act in the first state, North Carolina, in 1903. By 1923 all states had a nurse registration act. The term "registration" is appropriate since no state outlined a scope of practice.

The second phase of nursing licensure started in 1938 with the passing of the first mandatory practice act in New York. The scope of nursing functions was established for two levels of nurses, registered and practical. In 1955 the ANA adopted a model definition of professional practice, which facilitated the process of defining nursing and passing mandatory practice acts. By 1967, 15 states had incorporated the language of this model into their state laws, while six others slightly modified the model. It is noted that the 1955 model act included a disclaimer clearly stating that nursing did not include any acts of diagnosis or the prescription of therapeutic measures.

The third phase, 1971 to the present, is the era of expanding functions of the nursing role. Bullough analyzes some of the factors influencing the changes. A major driving force is the dramatic improvement of the nursing educational system. By 1972 the combination of nurses (58%) who graduated from baccalaureate and associate degree programs totaled more than the graduates from diploma schools (42%). Although the number who have graduated from the lower division college level associate degree programs has continued to increase in percent more than graduates from baccalaureate programs, by 1978 a great decrease occurred in the percentage of diploma graduates. The New York State Nurses' Association resolution that the baccalaureate degree be the entry into professional practice by 1985 has served as an impetus toward collegiate education. Similar resolutions have been passed to this date with considerable debate related to the current number of registered nurses who do not hold a baccalaureate degree. The number of nurses completing career ladder baccalaureate and master's degree programs is rapidly increasing. A second driving force for role expansion is related to the increased specialization in medicine and decreased numbers of generalists to provide primary care. The utilization of physician assistants (P.A.s) to fill the need encouraged nurses to rethink their role and functions. Health care technology in specialized nursing units like coronary care and an increase of the aging population also have contributed to the expansion of the nursing role. Nurse practitioners and clinical specialists are being prepared at the master's level for expanded roles. Bullough discusses a number of restraining forces to the expanded role. The resistance of medicine is one factor. The inclination to relinquish procedures to nurses but retain control over formal decision-making processes is noted. The subordination of women, precedents set by Florence Nightingale, and psychological restraining forces related to feminity are other factors outlined. The law also was a factor which limited the expansion of the role.

Bullough addresses the interrelationships between the law and social change. She summarizes the steps taken to legalize an expanded role in 50 states and four other jurisdictions with nurse practice acts. Thirty-seven states used the approach of rules and regulations drawn up by boards of nursing, medicine, or combined boards. In addition a legislative mandate was given to most boards, with the result being state certification as the dominant trend in legal implementation of the expanded role. Twenty-two states require or recognize some sort of national certification for state certification. Since 1977, states have started recognizing certification of nurse practitioners by the ANA. The second major approach has been to expand the definition of a registered nurse to include diagnosis and treatment. In 1972 New York invoked the concept of a nursing diagnosis and a nursing regime, while California in 1974 broadly described the nursing decision-making responsibility. Two other mechanisms utilized for expansion of the law are protocols, or standardized procedures, and practice acts which allow physicians to delegate the right to diagnose and treat. As a result of P.A.s being developed, most states provide exemptions in their medical practice acts for other workers when they act under physician supervision.

Bullough perceives two trends have occurred which impact on the professionalization of nursing. The first is that the role of the registered nurse is being broadly redefined with a disappearance of restrictions on diagnosis and treatment. She supports this trend by citing case law precedents involving registered nurses. The second trend is that of granting a state credential for specialized nurses such as nurse practitioners, midwives, anesthetists, and clinical specialists. The credentialing process is called "certification," although "licensure" is viewed to be the more accurate term. Speciality certification in the professionalization process has previously been reserved to the private professional organization. Bullough concludes her remarks on professionalization by describing the potential impact and conflict in the implementation of the recommendations of the Credentialing Study commissioned by the ANA. She views differences within the profession, the consumer movement, and the federal government's responsibility for occupational licensure as complicating the implementation of the credentialing study. Bullough predicts a compromise position that will include: both basic licensure and speciality certification by the states; acceptance of certification by professional organizations by states as one criterion for state certification; and certain competencies for third-party reimbursement requested by federal regulations. Nursing is perceived as developing an unique limited model of professionalization which shares power with other health professionals and consumers.

In order to give perspective to this discussion of the law as a variable in the professionalization process, some discussion of the definition of the term "professional" is in order. The focus of the many definitions of this term varies. The pioneer sociological work on professions was done by A. M. Carr-Saunders and P. A. Wilson. Their study, published in 1933, compared law and medicine with other occupations, including some they classified as near-professions. The authors concluded that the key attribute of a profession is the possession of specialized techniques for giving service to clients. These techniques are acquired through a substantial program of intellectual study. In addition, members of professions tend to band together in some type of organization or occupational community to enforce standards and control access to the occupation. Often this process of control is carried out in cooperation with the state by the use of licensure laws. These authors distinguished professional workers from business-

men by the fact that professionals are paid salaries or fees, while those engaged in business enterprises seek their income through profit. They noted, however, that within the business community a professional salaried managerial class was developing.

Using a circle to illustrate their definition, Carr-Saunders and Wilson placed medicine and law near the center since these professions have specialized techniques based upon a significant body of knowledge for serving the public. Workers in these professions are paid fees and salaries rather than making profits from the service they give to clients; they are organized to uphold the standards of their profession; they have managed to involve the state in their efforts to secure a monopoly through licensure laws. On the other hand, nursing and midwifery were placed near the periphery of the circle, primarily because their educational system was said to be focused on the techniques of care rather than on a scientific body of knowledge basic to these techniques. Other workers also considered by Carr-Saunders and Wilson to have somewhat of a peripheral professional status include merchant seamen, mine managers, opticians, pharmacists, secretaries, bankers, and journalists (1933).

Since that time, other sociologists have put forth different definitions of what constitutes a profession. Greenwood (1957) published a list of five characteristics of a profession: (1) systematic theory, (2) authority, (3) prestige, (4) a code of ethics, and (5) a professional culture. Barber (1963) reduced this list to four, arguing that such attributes as authority and prestige are not essential to a profession, but are instead derived from the more basic elements of knowledge, commitment, an ethical code, and a focus on achievement rather than on extrinsic rewards. For Barber the essence of professionalism is an ethical stance that separates professional workers from members of all other occupations. Moore (1970) developed a scale containing six elements. In addition to Greenwood's five, Moore argued that a distinction must be made between the professional and the amateur. Therefore Moore added the stipulation that the occupation should be a major source of income to the worker (1970:3-22). He felt such a distinction important in tracing the professionalization process that was taking place in political campaigns, voluntary organizations, and other areas of society where there was a growing trend to turn to experts rather than to leave the task to volunteers. Vollmer and Mills see the term "professional" only as an ideal type, regarding it as valuable for describing a dynamic process but not for describing the realities of any one occupation (1966:7-8).

Recently a somewhat more skeptical outlook on professions has developed among a small group of sociologists. Probably the intellectual leader of this group is Eliot Freidson (1970, 1977), who has studied the professions, especially medicine, extensively. He argues that the crucial attribute of a highly professionalized occupation is its power to control the terms, conditions, and content of its work. In a similar vein, Stewart and Cantor have focused on autonomy as the key attribute of a profession, explaining that the other elements often included in the definitions are either means for achieving autonomy or benefits which flow from having autonomy (1974:1-6). Possibly the most radical member of this school of thought is Daniels (1971) who suggests that the often-cited service orientation of the high status professions is, in fact, the result of a well-carried-out public relations campaign, rather than of any extraordinary commitment to public welfare.

EVOLUTION OF PROFESSIONALISM IN MEDICINE

Overlooked in these definitions is how an occupation becomes a profession, and here the historian can shed some light. Historically, the most important variable in the development of a profession seems to be occupational control of an educational institution, since such control allows the occupation to limit access to the profession, to provide specialized knowledge, and to demarcate the professional from other workers in the field. This can easily be demonstrated in the emergence of medicine as a profession during the later medieval period. One key element here was the emergence of the university, since before that time training had been primarily through apprenticeship, with the secrets of the trade being passed on from father to son or master to pupil. As the universities developed in the twelfth century, either through associations of masters or of students, medicine became institutionalized. The medical universities not only standardized the educational system but acted as barriers to would-be practitioners who lacked university education. At the same time, institutionalization facilitated research by establishing a community of scholars who were interested in each other's findings and who gave each other encouragement and support.

A second key element, in the emergence of the profession was the sponsorship of the crown which allowed the university-trained practitioners to assert primacy over rival groups. For example, in the fourteenth century the Parisian physicians obtained a royal decree allowing them to control and limit the practice of the apprentice-trained barbers, surgeons, and pharmacists (apothecaries). Similarly, in England in the fifteenth century, the king decreed that the practice of medicine should be limited to university graduates, although the surgeons trained on the job were allowed to continue practicing in a subordinate status (V. Bullough, 1961, 1974). This data showing the evolution of medicine as a prototype profession supports the more radical definition of the professionalization process. The basic attributes of medicine as a profession seem to be its autonomy, its institutionalization within the university, its organization, and the use of government as an instrument of power.

In the United States, government is usually represented by legislative bodies and court systems, since the federal structure allocates regulatory power to the states rather than to the central government. Again, medicine established the legal precedent for occupational licensure. The lobbying for licensure was carried out by the American Medical Association (AMA) which was established in 1847. Organizational objectives included raising the level of competence of physicians, lessening competition from other healers, and increasing the power and status of the profession—in short, professionalization. In the beginning, government was almost all important because the AMA lacked control of the teaching institutions. This control came later. In 1873 the association succeeded in getting its first licensure act through the Texas legislature (V. Bullough, 1980). In 1881 a similar statute passed in West Virginia was challenged in court by its opponents. Finally, in 1888 the Supreme Court ruled that occupational licensure was a valid exercise of the political powers of the states (U.S., 1888). After that date medical licensure spread rapidly throughout all of the states.

The fact that medical licensure came first

had implications for other health occupations; their subsequent licenses became, in effect, amendments to the medical practice acts. Nurses also used the medical acts as models, but the nursing laws were necessarily limited in scope.

THE NURSE PRACTICE ACTS

The history of American nursing practice laws can be divided into three phases: (1) 1903 to 1938—the early nurse registration acts, (2) 1938 to 1971—the era in which the scope of nursing function was defined, and (3) 1971 to the present—the era of expanding functions for registered nurses. The first phase was instituted in a manner similar to the early medical practice law; nursing moved first to organize and then to use the organization to further professionalize the occupation.

The organization which was to become the National League for Nursing (NLN) was established in 1894, and a precursor to the American Nurses Association (ANA) was set up in 1896. The collective goals of these two groups were similar to the goals of the AMA. In basic terms, the groups sought recognition for the trained nurse in order to cut out competition from untrained nurses. To do this they wanted to upgrade the educational standards for nurses and to increase the power and prestige of nursing.

To facilitate the registration campaign, the nursing organizations set up constituent state groups to do the necessary lobbying in the legislature. This was not an easy task in an era when women did not have the vote, but by force of enthusiasm and numbers they were able to convince various legislatures. North Carolina, in 1903, became the first state to pass a registration act, followed almost immediately by New York and New Jersey in the same year. One by one, other states followed suit until, by 1923, all of the states then in the union had a nurse registration act. These first phase acts are properly called registration acts rather than practice acts because none of them included a statement outlining a scope of practice. The term "registered nurse" was defined as someone of good character who had completed an acceptable nursing program and passed a board examination (B. Bullough, 1980).

The second phase in the development of nursing licensure started in 1938 when the first mandatory practice act was passed in New York. This law established two levels of nurses, registered and practical, restricting nursing functions to members of these two groups (American Journal of Nursing, 1939; Jacobson, 1940). This event marked the beginning of a new thrust in the efforts of nurse activists whose primary goal now became the achievement of mandatory licensure.

While mandatory licensure can be thought of as a long-range aspiration, dating from the beginning of the century when abortive attempts were made to restrict the use of the title "nurse," the goal did not seem a realistic one until the New York nurses broke the barrier. Their efforts, and those of nurses in several states which followed their precedent, were facilitated by the development of licensure for practical nurses. Employment patterns for nurses were changing in this period from private duty to hospital nursing, and hospital administrators argued with some justification that all nursing functions did not require the standard 3-year training period which was by then the norm. The development of the practical nurse as the basic bedside practitioner allowed registered nurses to argue more successfully for licensure for all practitioners.

Besides being linked with the stratification of the nursing role, mandatory licensure included another interesting implication. In order to pass a mandatory act of any kind, it was necessary to spell out the scope of practice of the occupation which was being protected against encroachment. The older nursing laws merely made it illegal for an unauthorized person to use the title "registered nurse," but it was not illegal for such a person to practice nursing. If the new mandatory laws were to make it illegal for an unauthorized person to practice nursing, a definition of the scope of practice had to be written into the law in order that

violations of the mandatory provisions could be identified. Eventually the definition even came to be thought of as a goal in and of itself, with the result that nurses and legal advisors of the day advocated that the scope of practice be defined in nurse practice acts (Lesnick and Anderson, 1947: 47).

The process of defining nursing and of passing mandatory nurse practice acts was facilitated in 1955 when the Board of Directors of the American Nurses Association (ANA) adopted a model definition of nursing. Professional practice was defined as:

> . . . the performance, for compensation, of any acts in the observation, care and counsel of the ill, injured or infirm or in the maintenance of health or prevention of illness of others, or in the supervision and teaching of other personnel or the administration of medications and treatments as prescribed by a licensed physician or a licensed dentist; requiring substantial specialized judgment and skill and based on knowledge and application of principles of biological, physical and social science. The foregoing shall not be deemed to include any acts of diagnosis or prescription of therapeutic or corrective measures. ("ANA Board Approves," 1955)

This definition became the new model for changing nurse practice acts, so that, by 1967, 15 states had incorporated the language of this model into their state laws; another 6 states had used the model with only slight modifications (Fogotson et al., 1967b). A notable aspect of this model act, as well as the other similar definitions of practice, is the disclaimer which clearly spells out the fact that nursing did not include any acts of diagnosis or the prescription of therapeutic measures. Before the era of mandatory licensure, nurse registration acts did not define nursing, with the result that they did not include any such disclaimer. Moreover, some of the definitions passed before the ANA model act was formulated used other language which did not forbid diagnosis and treatment.

Actually, by 1955, when the model act was issued by the ANA, nurses were a fairly well-educated group of workers. They were observing patients, collecting data about their conditions, and acting on those data to deliver nursing care. They were, in fact, making diagnostic decisions and treating people on the basis of those decisions. The disclaimers in the scope-of-practice statements were out of date at the time they were written.

The behavior on the part of nurses seems like a manifestation of a minority group withdrawal. It is a type of alienation or anticipatory self-discrimination. Rather than risk a rebuff or a possible boundary dispute with medicine, nurses almost unconsciously decided to deny their role in the patient care decision-making process. Similar patterns of anticipatory self-discrimination are fairly common phenomena among other minority groups; the ghetto walls are often as well policed from the inside as the outside. Feelings of powerlessness and fear prevent people from challenging discriminatory practices (B. Bullough, 1967).

THE THIRD PHASE IN NURSING LICENSURE

The third phase in the history of nursing licensure can be dated from 1971 to the present. It is marked by an expansion of the nursing role. Before describing the changes in the law during this phase, some analysis of the factors influencing the changes in the nursing role seems appropriate.

If the social change framework associated with Kurt Lewin is utilized, the variables behind role expansion can be categorized as driving forces and restraining forces (Lewin, 1958; Benne and Birnbaum, 1969). Probably the major long-range driving force for this current change in functions is the slow but dramatic improvement of the nursing educational system. Although nursing education in this country is more than a century old, throughout most of this period it was purely apprenticeship training. Finally in 1972 a watershed mark was reached. For the first time there were more nurses graduated from collegiate than diploma schools; 21 percent of the new graduates

were awarded baccalaureate degrees; 37 percent earned associate of arts degrees, and 42 percent were from diploma programs. This movement toward collegiate education, albeit primarily at the lower-division level, has continued (ANA 1974: 73). In 1978, 23 percent of the new graduates were from baccalaureate schools, 47 percent from community college associate degree programs, and only 23 percent from diploma schools (Vaughn and Johnson, 1979). The movement for the first time gave nurses control of their own education, free from interference by hospital administrators and staff physicians.

Though hospital schools remained, the competition from the college-based schools and the rising expectations of student nurses forced the existing hospital schools to upgrade their programs by hiring more and better-prepared instructors and avoiding the exploitation of their students. In the process nurses gained more control. Although these costly improvements are a major factor in the continued closing of hospital programs, they have also substantially improved the quality of education in the diploma schools. These changes in education are crucial elements in the professionalization process.

The fact that the recent rapid move toward collegiate education was primarily at the associate-of-arts rather than the baccalaureate level is distressing to many educators who believe that a stronger knowlege base is needed. A resolution, originating in New York, expressed this concern by calling for legislation to make the baccalaureate level the entry point into professional nursing by 1985 (N.Y.S.N.A., 1974). This resolution quickly became the focus of national discussion, and in 1976 the Council of Baccalaureate and Higher Degrees of the National League for Nursing passed a similar resolution. The idea gained ground when a package of three entry-into-practice resolutions was passed by the American Nurses Association in 1978 ("ANA Convention," 1978). Various other nursing organizations have debated the issue, and some, including most notably the American Association of Operating Room Nurses, have supported the movement. Although there are differences of opinion as to what they mean, whether or not they should be implemented, and what their implementation would do for the profession, the resolutions are emerging as one of the major issues facing the profession today. The major deterrent to implementation seems to be the problem of what to do about the current registered-nurse work force, 80 percent of whom do not hold baccalaureate degrees.

Though legislation requiring the minimum of a baccalaureate degree has not yet been enacted, the demand for higher standards for entry into practice has had effects on the professionalization of nursing. There is a danger that in the long run the consequences may be negative because internal fighting might decrease nursing's political clout in state houses across the country. But in the short term the resolutions have motivated nurses to seek more education, clearly a positive force for professionalization. This educational upgrading is most apparent in the registered-nurse continuation programs for diploma and associate degree graduates. While there were 3003 registered nurses graduating from baccalaureate programs in 1974, this number had doubled by 1978 when it reached 6146 (Vaughn and Johnson, 1979). The number of nurses attaining master's degree programs is also increasing rapidly; in 1970, 1988 master's degrees were awarded while the figure in 1978 was 4271 (ANA, 1979:114, Vaughn and Johnson, 1979). Since both the career ladder baccalaureate and the master's degree programs emphasize advanced clinical specialties, including critical care and practitioner specialties, these developments are a significant factor in the recent more rapid expansion of the roles of registered nurses.

A second driving force for role expansion comes from outside nursing. Throughout the last century the science and technology of medicine expanded at a rapid rate. As medicine became more complex it became more specialized. In 1910 most of the doctors were general practitioners; now specialists outnumber generalists by nearly four to one

(U.S.D.H.E.W., 1976). Thus, the major gap in services developed at the primary care level, resulting in a shortage of providers who could treat the common episodic and chronic illnesses at a price that ordinary people and government third-party payers could afford.

Nurse practitioners are not the only group which responded to this need. Within medicine the specialty of family medicine developed; residencies in that area opened up in 1969. Physicians' assistants (P.A.s) also moved in to fill the breach, and as a new concept they were highly newsworthy. They demonstrated publicly that the delegation of a significant number of medical tasks was possible. Once this became apparent, some physicians remembered that nurses existed and thought about them as perhaps better-prepared assistants, probably more tractable, and certainly more plentiful than ex-independent-duty corpsmen who were the first candidates for P.A. training (Bergman, 1971). The physician's assistant movement also gave courage to nurses to rethink their own traditional avoidance of overt expansion of their functions onto the medical turf of diagnosis and treatment.

Inside the hospital the expanding health care technology furnished the major impetus for the development of specialized nursing units. New monitoring devices and life-saving techniques require on-the-spot experts who can make diagnostic decisions and treat patients appropriately without waiting to consult a physician.

Coronary care units, the model for many of these nursing awards, evolved during the 1960s when it was realized that most post-myocardial-infarction deaths were due to cardiac arrhythmias and that a significant number of lives could be saved if the aberrant rhythms could be converted back to normal rhythms. Staffing coronary care units with full-time physicians was briefly considered, since diagnosing and treating an arrhythmia is clearly a complex medical function, but it was simply not economically feasible. Instead, nurses were given advanced preparation and they now staff all of the units (Berwind, 1975). The success of the specialized coronary care units in cutting the death rate due to heart attacks has encouraged other special nursing wards for patients suffering from trauma, renal, and respiratory problems.

The sociological importance of these units for the expansion of the nursing role should not be overlooked. Because these units are increasing at such a rapid pace, the nurse-clinicians who staff them are probably more important than the ambulatory nurse practitioners in bringing about change in the scope of function, power, and income of nurses. The functions of the specialized intensive care nurses are complex, their knowledge base is intensive, and their level of autonomy is greater the that of most other nurses. They represent a significant incursion into what was formerly considered medical territory.

Demography also enters the picture as a variable in the expansion of nursing functions. The nation's population is aging, and many elderly people live for long periods of time with either chronic illness or the infirmities of old age. These patients need the concerned attention of a practitioner who is prepared in the social as well as the medical sciences, who wants to spend time, and whose time is not so expensive as to be unaffordable for the agency or third-party provider. Consequently, nurse practitioners and clinical specialists are moving into the geriatric field.

These, then, are the major driving forces which caused the role of the nurse to expand slowly during the first 90 years and then more rapidly during the last decade. The fact that the progress was so slow and that the role is still restricted is partly explained by the restraining forces—the most important of which is medicine. Medicine, which was the impetus for change, is also the most significant factor in restricting the expansion of the nursing role. Although physicians in the past were willing to turn procedures such as temperature taking, blood pressure reading, and patient observation over to nurses, they tried to retain control over the formal decision-making process relative to patient care. Because they could not be present

at all times, it became impossible for them to actually make all of the decisions about patient care, and elaborate games were developed to pretend that physicians made all of the diagnostic and treatment decisions.

Physicians, however, could never have achieved this expansive definition of their prerogatives if nurses had not allowed it. The reason nurses seemed to allow it was because most of them were women, and nursing, probably more than any occupation except housewifery and prostitution, reflects the stereotyped role of women. The norms and values of nursing are feminine, and the relationships between nurses and physicians have reflected the extreme subordination of women, with all of the male-female game playing which tends to go along with that subordination. Moreover, the educational system has, at least in the past, tended to reinforce this feminine and subordinate picture of the role of the nurse, so that new generations of students have been taught to be ladylike, subservient, and manipulative.

Florence Nightingale set a precedent for this behavior pattern, although she was undoubtedly merely accepting the norms of her day. In Scutari, although she came with significant power delegated to her by the secretary of war, she refused to allow the nurses under her command to give any care to the suffering men until the surgeons "ordered" them to do so (Woodham-Smith, 1951:98–110).

After the war she retired from public view, gradually secluding herself more and more until she finally simply took to her bed where she stayed for the last 50 years of her life. Sitting in her bed she wrote letters, collected data, and wrote lengthy, well-documented position papers aimed at reforming the army and the health care delivery system, but she never appeared in public to defend these positions. Instead she convinced her various male friends and admirers, including Sidney Herbert who had been secretary of war, that they should wage the public fight for reform. She claimed that she was a weak, feeble woman and that the work of public struggles had to be handled by great strong men. While this modus operandi was probably the key to her effectiveness, the precedent which she set for women and nurses has not been without negative consequences (Woodham-Smith, 1951).

In fact the games played by Nightingale helped set the stage for the nurse-doctor game which was noted in the decade of the sixties. As described by Leonard Stein (1967), this game was marked by circular communication patterns in which nurses pretended to avoid making recommendations about patient care and physicians pretended they were gathering all of the data and doing all of the decision making. Yet nurses actually made recommendations and successful physicians actually followed these recommendations. Stein called the pattern a transactional neurosis.

These tortured communication patterns and feminine withdrawal from open admission of decision making acted as deterrents to the development of new nursing roles. The force which has been most helpful in overcoming these psychological barriers to role expansion has been the women's movement. At first this movement had difficulty gaining a foothold in nursing. Some feminists looked upon nurses as the worst possible examples of subordinate women and decided to avoid them. Now, however, nurses themselves have joined the movement. Assertiveness training has become a popular offering in continuing education programs throughout the country. As nurses become more assertive some are willing to try new roles. They are assisted in this quest by the increased numbers of men entering nursing. The psychological restraining forces related to femininity are still present, but they are lessening.

For a time the law also served as a major restraining force limiting the expansion of the nursing role. Sociologists and political scientists have long been interested in the complex interrelationships between the law and social change (Ross et al., 1970; Friedmann, 1964; Nagel, 1969; Becker, 1973). In some cases it is possible to trace changes in the law to changes that have already occurred in the society (Dienes, 1970);

in other cases, the opposite causal sequence can be traced, with new laws creating significant changes in the society (Lewis, 1969). Here, both processes can be observed. Before 1971 the nurse practice acts, which forbade nurses the right to overtly participate in diagnosis and treatment, were a deterrent to role expansion. Employers worried about malpractice suits and the legitimacy of billing patients for nurses' services; nurses worried about the morality and safety of violating existing laws. The laws were a significant barrier to role change. As the laws were revised, this barrier was removed or lessened.

PHASE III REVISIONS OF THE NURSE PRACTICE ACTS

Table 45-1 summarizes the steps that have been taken through nurse practice acts to legalize an expanded nursing role in the 50 states and the 4 other jurisdictions. Only Rhode Island, Ohio, Oklahoma, and the four nonstate jurisdictions (Washington, D.C., Guam, the Virgin Islands, and Puerto Rico) have not revised their practice acts in some way since 1971.

As shown in Table 45-1 the major mechanism for accomplishing this goal has been through rules and regulations drawn up by the state boards of nursing, medicine, or some combination of boards. Thirty-seven states have adopted this approach. In most of these states a legislative mandate was given to the boards to devise a mechanism for dealing with the expanding functions of nursing. However, in Wisconsin, Delaware, and Tennessee the boards of nursing were able to take on this responsibility without new statutory law. As the board rules shape up, state certification seems to be the dominant trend in implementation. To date this certification has focused on midwives, nurse practitioners, and nurse anesthetists, but in a few states clinical specialists of various types are included. As can be noted, 28 jurisdictions are now certifying nurse midwives, 29 certify nurse practitioners, 22 certify nurse anesthetists, and 6 states certify a generalized nursing specialist or one or more specific type of clinical nurse specialists.

Since the American College of Nurse Midwives and the American Association of Nurse Anesthetists are the oldest accrediting bodies, states started by recognizing national certification by these groups as a criterion for state certification. However, more recently (since 1977), states have started recognizing certification of nurse practitioners by the American Nurses Association (ANA), the National Board of Pediatric Nurse Practitioners and Associates (NAPNAP), or the National Association of the American College of Obstetricians and Gynecologists (NAACOG). As can be noted, 22 states require or recognize some sort of national certification for state certification.

The second major approach used by states to broaden the scope of practice has been to expand the definition of functions of a registered nurse to include diagnosis and treatment. In 1972 New York and in 1974 California adopted this mechanism. California merely described the nursing decision-making responsibility in broad terms; the New York act is more problematic because it invoked the concept of a nursing diagnosis and a nursing regime. That state defines a nursing diagnosis in the following way:

> Diagnosing in the context of nursing practice means that identification of and discrimination between physical and psychosocial signs and symptoms are essential to the effective execution and management of a nursing regime. Such diagnostic privilege is distinct from a medical diagnosis. (N.Y.S.L., 1972)

This language suggests that the act of diagnosis is somehow different when performed by a nurse rather than by a phsyician, but the law lacks clarity in actually operationalizing that difference. Members of a nursing in-group who are familiar with the argument that the nursing diagnosis should be psychosocial rather than physical might well understand the language, but to the uninitiated the wording suggests that when nurses examine patients they place the signs and symptoms in two piles—one physical and one psychosocial; physicians presumably are allowed to be cognizant of the essential interplay between the psyche and the soma. This seems a peculiar way to distinguish a nursing from a medical diagnosis, particularly in light of the fact that the nursing educational system has for many years stressed the importance of the interplay between the biologic and psychosocial factors in illness. In spite of this apparent lack of clarity, 13 states have used this definition of diagnosis, and several others mention a nursing diagnosis or a nursing regime.

Probably the only operational definition of a nursing diagnosis and therapeutic plan that would hold up over time and empirical study would be a definition which differentiates a diagnosis and therapeutic plan done by a nurse from one carried out by a physician.

This was, in fact, the approach used by some nurse practitioners for a time. They claimed that the work role of the practitioner fell under the general rubric of the terms "nursing diagnosis" and "nursing regime." However, more recently a backlash movement led by at least one conservative member of the New Jersey Board of Medicine has pointed up the problematic aspect of this conceptualization of the scope of nursing function. The New Jersey board member has claimed that the nurse practitioner role is illegal (AJN, 1978; "Regional Review," 1978).

In addition to these two major approaches—board rules with or without certification and expanded definitions for all registered nurses—there are two other mechanisms for expansion of the law that have been utilized in some states. Protocols or standardized procedures were called for in the early Idaho and Tennessee regulations, as well as in the California law. More states now mention protocols; 13 such citations appear in Table 45–1. Although protocols have been criticized as a "cookbook approach," they probably have value in this transition period in that they assure physicians and the public that nurse practitioners are caring for their patients in an orderly fashion.

Table 45-1 Phase III Revisions of the Nurse Practice Acts

Western states	Year expanded role recognized	Board regs.	Expanded definition of R.N.	Protocols	NP or blanket specialty certification	State certification specific mention		Nat. cert. recognized	Prescription drugs	Remarks
						Midwives	Anesthetists			
Alaska	1974	Nurs & Med			Advanced NP; adv. NP in remote location			Required*	Yes-Class I and II	Interim preceptorship permits issued until nationally certified*
Arizona	1973	Nurs & Med	Yes		PNA; FNP; ANP; OB-GYN NP	Yes		Yes	Prepackaged in rural areas	Exam required nat. exam can be used
California	1974	Nurs	Yes	Yes	Including ANP; PNP; OB-GYN NP; FNP	Yes		Yes	Experimental projects only	
Colorado	1974		Yes		Advanced practice of nursing	Yes		Yes		
Hawaii	1979	Nurs			Expanded role*	Yes	Yes	Yes		ANA standards for clinical specialists and NPS used*
Idaho	1971	Nurs & Med	Yes	Yes	NP	Yes*	Yes		with protocol	Midwives considered NP specialty*
Montana	1976					Yes				
Nevada	1973	Nurs	Yes	Yes	NP			Yes	Protocol*	Controlled substances only with Board of Med. approval*
New Mexico	1975	Nurs	Yes		NP	Yes	Yes	Yes	Yes	

State	Year	Authority		Title				Comments
Oregon	1973	Nurs	Yes	NP including FNP; PNP; ANP; GNP; Psych/Mental Health NP; Women's Health NP; School Health NP; College Health NP		Yes*		As NP*
Texas	1979	Nurs		Advanced NP				Regs. being challenged by Med. & Hosp. Association
Utah	1975	Nurs	Yes			Yes		
Washington	1975	Nurs & Med	Yes	Certified RN		Yes	Required; CRN with 30 h pharm.	Advanced RN & specialized RN discontinued 1980
Wyoming	1975	Nurs & Med	Yes	Yes				Midwives, anest. and NP included in common regs.
Midwestern								
Illinois	1975	Board of Opinions on prof. nursing	Yes					
Indiana	1974	Nurs & Med	Yes					
Iowa	1976		Yes	ARNP-including FNP; School NP; PNP; Mental Health NP	Yes*	Yes*		Types of ARNP*
Kansas	1978	Nurs	Yes	ARNP				
Michigan	1978	Nurs	Yes	NP		Yes	Required	

continued

Table 45-1 Continued

Midwestern states	Year expanded role recognized	Board regs.	Expanded definition of R.N.	Protocols	NP or blanket specialty certification	State certification specific mention		Nat. cert. recognized	Prescription drugs	Remarks
						Midwives	Anesthetists			
Minnesota	1974		Yes							
Missouri	1976		Yes							
Nebraska	1974	Nurs & Med	Yes							Board of Nursing blocked from promulgating rules by Attorney General
North Dakota	1977	Nurs	Yes							
Ohio										
Oklahoma							Yes	Required*		For anesthetists*
South Dakota	1972	Nurs & Med	Yes		NP	Yes	Yes	Required*	Yes	Practice agreement required; national cert. for anesthetists*
Wisconsin										Board memo indicates NP congruent with law
Northeastern										
Connecticut	1975	Nurs	Yes							
Delaware	1978	Nurs			ARNP			Yes		Statement by Board of Nursing; no law or regulations yet

State	Year	Board		Title / Certification			As agent of MD	Remarks
Maine	1974	Nurs	Yes	Nurse Associate or NP		Yes	As agent of MD	
Massachusetts	1975		Yes	NP Psych/Mental Health Clinical Spec.	Yes	Yes		
New Hampshire	1974	Nurs & Med	Yes	ARNP (PNA; FNP; OB-GYN NP; Pediatric Nurse Clinician, Community Health; Psych/Mental Health)	Yes*	Yes*	Emergency; Required†	Midwife one type of ARNP*; national cert. required for nurse anesthetists & midwives†
New Jersey	1974	Nurse*	Yes			Yes		Guidelines
New York	1972	Nurse	Yes*		Yes	Yes		Guidelines for NP programs;* special provisions for School NP† counsel to state education dept. has ruled diagnosis and treatment illegal
Pennsylvania	1973	Nurs & Med	Yes	Cert. reg. NP	Yes*	Yes	Required for anes.	Medical Board exam given*
Rhode Island	Not yet*							No prohibition against diagnosis and treatment*
Vermont	1974		Yes					
Southern								
Alabama	1975	Nurs	Yes		Yes	Yes	Required*	Can practice while waiting results of first writing of exam in anes.*

continued

Table 45-1 Continued

Southern states	Year expanded role recognized	Board regs.	Expanded definition of R.N.	Protocols	NP or blanket specialty certification	State certification specific mention		Nat. cert. recognized	Prescription drugs	Remarks
						Midwives	Anesthetists			
Arkansas	1979	Nurs			Reg. NP		Yes	Yes for anest.		
Florida	1975	Nurs & Med	Yes	Yes	ARNP (FNP; Fam. Plan. NP PNP; Geriatric NP, Adult Primary Care NP)	Yes*	Yes*			Categories of ARNP*
Georgia	1979	Nurs		Yes	NP*	Yes	Yes	Required		Rules in draft form; master's degree by 1990*
Louisiana	1976	Nurs	Yes		Advanced Prac. of Nurs. (primary nurse associates; clinical specialists)	Yes	Yes	Yes		
Kentucky	1978	Nurs	Yes		ARNP	Yes		Required		
Maryland	1974	Nurs	Yes							
Mississippi	1976	Nurs & Health		Yes	PNP or PNA; ANP; Family Planning NP; FNP; Primary Care NP; OB-GYN NP	Yes	Yes	Required*		Graduates of NP, anest. & Midwifery programs can practice up to 18 months while they attain nat. certification*

State	Year	Board			Recognized titles	Yes*		Required*	Special formulary	Statutory power
North Carolina	1973	Med & Nurs			FNP; Family Planning NP, PNP	Yes*				Statutory power is Med. Board; nursing only recommends**; midwives a type of NP*; national certification for midwives*
South Carolina	1975	Nurs	Yes	Yes		Yes		Required		For Nurse Midwives and Anest. Board Statements for Acute care NP; additional acts for LPN; Psych/Mental health clin. spec. Comm. health clin. Spec.; FNP; Family Planning NP; Occupa. Health NP; PNP; School NP.
Tennessee	1972	Nurs		Yes						
Virginia	1975	Med & Nurs*		Yes	NP (FNP & PNP programs approved)	Yes	Yes		Yes	Statutory coverage of NP in Med. Practice Act*
West Virginia	*	Nurs			ARNP*	Yes	Yes		Yes	Draft not adopted yet*

continued

Table 45-1 Continued

Other Jurisdictions	Year expanded role recognized	Board regs.	Expanded definition of R.N.	Protocols	NP or blanket specialty certification	State certification specific mention		Nat. cert. recognized	Prescription drugs	Remarks
						Midwives	Anesthetists			
Guam										
Puerto Rico										
Virgin Islands						Yes				
Washington, D.C.						Yes				

* The remarks column with * or † are explanatory statements for * or † in the table.

† Abbreviations:
ANP – Adult Nurse Practitioner
ARNP – Advanced Registered Nurse Practitioner
FNP – Family Nurse Practitioner
GNP – Geriatric Nurse Practitioner
NP – Nurse Practitioner
OB-GYN NP – Obstetrical-Gynecological Nurse Practitioner
PNA – Pediatric Nurse Associate
PNP – Pediatric Nurse Practitioner
RN – Registered Nurse

An approach to role expansion not covered in Table 45–1 is exemplified by Maine's Practice Act, which allows individual physicians to delegate the right to diagnose and treat. It indicates that professional nursing includes

> . . . diagnosis or prescription of therapeutic or corrective measures when such services are delegated by a physician to a registered nurse who has completed the necessary additional education programs. . . . (Maine Rev. Statutes)

Even before the current phase in nursing licensure there were state medical practice acts, including those of Arizona, Colorado, Florida, Kansas, and Oklahoma, which gave physicians broad powers to delegate medical acts to other workers (Fogotson et al., 1967a; Fish, 1974). As a consequence of the development of the concept of physicians' assistants, most other states now provide exemptions in their medical practice acts for other workers acting under physician supervision. This mechanism is, in fact, a major source of legal sanction for physicians' assistants, who had no basic license of their own, although a quasi license-certification mechanism has developed in some states. The delegatory statutes are a less satisfactory mechanism for nurses, who do have a basic license and who carry independent functions as well as physician-delegated functions.

IMPLICATIONS FOR PROFESSIONALIZATION

What are the implications of these changes for the professionalization of nursing? Changes in the law are clearly intertwined with the professionalization process. Throughout the first 70 years of this century, legal sanction for nursing slowly expanded as nurses became more professionalized. In the past 10 years this process has escalated. The movement has not occurred without barriers and backlash, but it has nevertheless occurred. There are two concomitant trends. First, the basic role of the registered nurse is being redefined in broader terms,

and the restrictions on diagnosis and treatment by registered nurses are disappearing.

This trend in statutory law is supported by some significant changes in case-law precedents involving registered nurses. The landmark decision was made in the 1965 Darling case. The plaintiff, who broke his leg while playing football, was taken to a local hospital where he was treated with traction and a plaster cast. The cast was apparently too tight since his toes became swollen, painful, and dark. His physician notched his cast, but soon after that blood and then a foul-smelling drainage were noted by the nursing staff. Eventually, he was taken to another hospital where his leg was amputated.

The case was vigorously defended by both the physician and the hospital. The hospital argued that it was not responsible for what happened to the patient, since it merely housed and supported him while doctors made all of the diagnostic and treatment decisions. This line of reasoning failed to impress the court. The hospital and its nurses were held negligent, primarily because the nurses did not test the circulation in the patient's foot frequently enough, did not realize that the developing symptoms were dangerous, and did not call hospital authorities when the attending physician failed to act (Ill. St. Supreme Court, 1964, 1965; "Darling Case," 1968:1875).

A recent West Virginia case reiterates these findings. In this case the patient entered the hospital suffering from a comminuted fracture of his wrist. During his hospital stay an infection developed; his arm became swollen and black, with a foul-smelling drainage. He became feverish, was unable to retain oral antibiotics, and finally became delirious. While he survived, his arm had to be amputated. The nursing staff reported these symptoms to the treating physician, but he failed to act. The jury found, and the appellate court upheld, the fact that the hospital was negligent because the nurses did not report the failure of the attending physician to his department chairman. The nursing procedure manual called for this further reporting, so simply accepting the patient's deteriorating condition was considered negligent (Va. Code Sec. 54–275).

These cases suggest that more judgment is being called for by nurses. They are not only being held accountable for their own actions but are also being held responsible for monitoring the care given by other health professionals. This clearly places nurses in a more powerful position; it demands more of the profession; it necessitates a stronger educational system; it will, in the long run, bring to nursing more of the rewards of a higher status occupation. This is a move towards professionalization.

The second trend which is reflected in licensure is the development of a smaller cadre of specialized nurses: nurse practitioners, midwives, anesthetists, and clinical specialists. There is evidence of a clear trend toward granting these specialists a state credential. Although the states are calling this credentialing process "certification," "licensure" may actually be a more accurate term, since previous usage has reserved the term "certification" for a credential granted by a professional body rather than by the state. There seems to be a second level of licensure for registered nurses developing. The implications of this development for the professionalization process are somewhat complex, since a pure professional model, or at least the medical model of professionalization, has reserved specialty certification to the private professional organization (the American Medical Association) rather than to the state. Nursing has in recent years moved to develop such a thrust, and a major credentialing study has been completed —a study commissioned by the resolution of the 1974 House of Delegates of the American Nurses Association (ANA, 1979). The resolution led to the formation of a study committee and to a major research project at the University of Wisconsin. After assessing the current status of all of the governmental and professional credentialing mechanisms in operation, the study group decided that the current system was much in need of reform, fragmented as it was and marked by both gaps and overlaps. The study group recommended that one single credentialing body, directed by a coalition of nursing organizations, be set up. (ANA, 1979;

Committee for Credentialing, 1979; "Positions," 1979). This body could accredit nursing programs run by schools of nursing or other institutions, license nurses, and certify all of the advanced specialties that are now handled by a variety of large and small nursing organizations, as well as by state governments (ANA, 1979).

This is also a move in support of professionalization, but it is in the opposite direction from the states' efforts to take on the certification of nursing specialists. The situation may well create conflict, at least within the ranks of the profession. Unfortunately, nursing is seeking more professional autonomy at a point later in time than most other professions. Law, medicine, education, and social work have already achieved professional status, and in the process they often gave the concept a bad name, stretching their span of control a bit too far and robbing consumers of legitimate decision-making power. Thus, nursing is in the position of making its move for greater control at the height of the consumer movement, and as a result, implementation of the credentialing study will be difficult.

The federal government may also move to complicate this picture. Although, as indicated earlier in this paper, occupational licensure is clearly a responsibility of the state governments, the federal government has developed an interest in the field because of the implications for cost and quality of health care. In 1970 Congress instructed the Department of Health, Education, and Welfare to study the problems associated with the credentialing of health personnel. Two reports were issued outlining some significant problems in the proliferation of licensed categories as well as in the artificial barriers to upward mobility within the system (U.S.D.H.E.W., 1971; Cohen and Miike, 1973). As a consequence, a 2-year moratorium on licensing of new categories of workers was called for in 1971. In 1973 this moratorium was extended to 1975; in the meantime, some attempts were made to think through the whole issue of health licensure in order to make it more functional for consumers.

Unfortunately, one of the first approaches tried was the establishment of two experimental projects using institutional licensure as an alternative. For a variety of reasons these efforts failed; institutionalized licensure did not seem to protect the patient or facilitate career mobility any better than did the old system (Kelly, 1980). Because this failure did not solve the underlying problems, it seems reasonable to expect that the Department of Health and Human Services will try again to intervene in the problem. If this does happen, the mechanism for federal entry into the licensing system will probably be through the reimbursement aspects of Medicare and Medicaid, rather than through any direct challenge to the states power of licensure.

CONCLUSION

Although nursing is clearly more professionalized than it was 70 years ago, with improvements in both its educational system and its power position, it seems unlikely that it will ever achieve the level of control of the older medical model. With all of the various currents and crosscurrents related to credentialing, the best that can be hoped for is a compromise position. That compromise will probably include both basic licensure and specialty certification for nursing by the states. The states do, however, seem ready to accept certification by the professional organizations as one criterion for their certification. Federal regulations will probably call for certain competencies for third-party reimbursement. Thus, nursing is clearly developing its own unique limited model of professionalization. It is a model which shares power with other health professionals and with consumers, but the compromise may be a reasonable model for this time and place in our history.

EDITOR'S QUESTIONS FOR DISCUSSION

What relationships are there among Conway's prescription for professionalization (Chap. 2), the law as a variable in the professionalization process as portrayed by Dorothy Walker (Chap. 4), and Bullough's perspective on the evolution of professionalism in nursing? How might nursing theorists respond to the conclusion by authors that the "key attribute of a profession was its possession of specialized techniques for giving service?" Would La Monica (Chap. 37) agree to that conclusion? Compare D. Walker's chapter 4 with Bullough's in regard to how standards are enforced and the process of control in a profession is carried out in cooperation with the state. In reviewing Conway's chapter 2, what effect does the establishment of a community of scholars have on control in a profession? Would Cleland (Chap. 44) agree with Carr-Saunders and Wilson's view of medicine and law as professions? What "ethical stance" separates professionals from members of other occupations? Present arguments for and against Freidson's belief that the crucial attribute of a profession is its power to control the terms, conditions, and content of its work. Is there a difference between that attribute and autonomy? In the evolution of nursing as a profession, are these attributes the predominant forces more than the development of a nursing knowledge base? Would you agree with Daniels that the cited service orientation of the high status professions is more the result of an effective public relations campaign rather than extraordinary commitment to public welfare?

Compare the professionalization process and four basic attributes of medicine as a profession as perceived by Bullough with the professionalization process of nursing and attributes present to this date. Is the process different? If so, what are the contributing factors? Has nursing had advantages in achieving professional status which have not been available to other professional groups?

What impact have the medical practice acts had on the nursing laws? What is the difference between registration acts and practice acts? How and why did two levels of nurses in practice become established? What stratifications in nursing roles exist today? Argue for and against different levels of mandatory licensure for all practitioners.

What different interpretations exist today of the ANA's 1955 model definition of nursing? What difficulties have occurred in making distinctions between a nursing diagnosis and a medical diagnosis that may be related to the 1955 model? Would you agree with Bullough regarding patterns of anticipatory self-discrimination by nurses in denying their role in the patient care decision-making process?

What impact has the development of associate of arts degree programs had on programs for practical nurses and diploma programs? How similar in content and expected performance outcomes are programs to prepare licensed practical nurses (L.P.N.), associate of arts degree (A.A.) nurses, and diploma nurses? Should programs for practical nurses be phased out? What is the role of an L.P.N.? Are there similarities in content and expected performance outcomes between diploma and associate degree programs? What factors have influenced the phasing out of diploma programs? To what extent do educational career ladders exist in nursing programs at the undergraduate level? What empirical evidence exists in professional performance between graduates of practical nurse, diploma, associate degree, and baccalaureate degree programs?

Present arguments for an against different types of licensure for nursing practice. How should the levels of nursing practice be defined? Should differences in practice be defined by categories such as technical or professional? What criteria might be utilized in defining the levels of practice? Should each level of nursing practice require a different licensure examination and license? Should some levels of nursing practice be combined for an identical examination and license? What suggestions for solutions to these questions may be found by Williamson (Chap. 5), Sargis (Chap. 9), Clayton (Chap. 10), Grace (Chap. 12), Brown (Chap. 26), Sills (Chap. 42), and Klein (Chap. 43)?

What differences of opinion exist today as to the meaning of the New York State resolution in 1974 for legislation to make the baccalaureate level the entry point into professional nursing by 1985? Should this and similar emerging resolutions be implemented? What impact would their implementation have on practice and the profession? What strategies have been proposed to resolve the problem of the large number of current registered nurses who do not hold a baccalaureate degree? What alternatives does Sargis (Chap. 9) propose? How has the demand for higher standards for entry into practice affected the professionalization of nursing? What factors have influenced the demand for higher standards for entry into practice? How should questions be resolved regarding the quantity and quality of nurses prepared for practice?

What is the sociological importance of the expanded nursing role? How congruent are the chapters by Williams (Chap 25) and Brown (Chap. 26) with Bullough's description of the development of physicians' assistants and nurse practitioners? Would Williamson (Chap. 5) and Sills (Chap. 42) perceive clinical nurse specialists being the predominant nurses to be employed in technologically complex, specialized nursing units as coronary care? Would Williamson, Sills, Williams (Chap. 25), and Brown (Chap. 26) agree with Bullough that nurse clinicians who staff specialized units are more important than ambulatory nurse practitioners in changing the scope of function, power, and income of nurses? Present arguments and rationale for and against Bullough's suggestion. Provide examples of physicians relinquishing procedures to nurses yet retaining control over the formal decision-making process relative to patient care. What guidelines are available in negotiating for performance and control?

Would Palmer (Chap. 1) agree with Bullough's portrayal of Florence Nightingale and the precedent she perceives Nightingale set for women's behavior? To what extent might such a precedent account for Sills' (Chap. 42) note regarding the sparse involvement of nurses in the women's movement? What effect has assertiveness training had on women individually, within the nursing profession, between other professions and society? What findings of Reeder's study (Chap. 38) indicate a change in norms for professional behavior? To what extent have males, who are members of the nursing profession, been subject to the same or different psychological and role restraining forces cited by Bullough? What suggestions can be offered to constructively counteract these forces?

Provide examples of the interrelationships between the law and social change in the professions. What applications can be made from Dorothy Walker's chapter 4 to the approaches used to legalize the expanding functions of nursing? Debate the professional appropriateness of the four different approaches toward legislation for expanded definitions of the role and functions of a registered nurse. Compare the definition of a nursing diagnosis as provided in Gordon's chapter 41 with the New York definition. How can these discrepancies best be clarified? Would you agree with Bullough regarding the operational definition of a nursing diagnosis that would withstand the test of time and empirical study? What implications are there for the work of the National Conference Group for Classification of Nursing Diagnoses and the development of a theoretical knowledge base for the profession in the legislative trend toward disappearing restrictions on diagnosis and treatment by registered nurses? What evidence indicates how, what, and for whom nurses are being held accountable? What implications in the legislative events and trends exist for Cleland's discussion (Chap. 44) on direct reimbursement for nursing practice? How can the nursing profession most effectively plan to meet the needs Bullough suggests are associated with professionalization?

Debate the issues concerned with the establishment of a national nursing credentialing center. What is the difference between certification and licensure? Is a second level of licensure for registered nurses occurring with states granting certification? What is the implication for the professionalization process with specialty certification being granted also by the state rather than being reserved to the private professional organization? What is the present status in implementation of the recommendations of the Credentialing Study? Have the potential conflicts suggested by Bullough occurred? To what extent has the compromise position forseen by Bullough related to credentialing been realized? What future changes can be predicted in legislation, licensure, and credentialing for nurses?

REFERENCES

American Journal of Nursing

1939   "All those who nurse for hire!" AJN 39: 275–277.

1978   "News: Nurse practitioners fight moves to restrict their practice." AJN 78(August):1285, 1308, 1310.

American Nurses Association

1974   Facts About Nursing: 1972–3. Kansas City, Mo.: ANA.

1979   The Study of Credentialing in Nursing:
A New Approach. Kansas City, Mo.:
ANA.

"A.N.A. board approves a definition of nursing
practice."
1955   American Journal of Nursing 55(August):
1474.

"A.N.A. convention: 1978."
1978   Nursing Outlook 26:500–507.

Barber, Bernard
1963   "Some problems in the sociology of
professions.' Daedalus, 92(Fall):669–688.

Becker, Theodore Lewis
1973   The Impact of Supreme Court Decisions:
Empirical Studies. 2nd ed. New York:
Oxford University Press.

Benne, Kenneth D. and Max Birnbaum
1969   "Principles of changing." Pp. 328–334 in
G. Bennis, D. Benne and R. Chin (eds.),
The Planning of Change. 2nd ed. New
York: Holt.

Bergman, A.
1971   "Physician's assistants belong in the nursing profession." American Journal of
Nursing 71(May):975–977.

Berwind, A.
1975   "The nurse in the coronary care unit."
Pp. 82–94 in B. Bullough (ed.), The Law
and the Expanding Nursing Role. 1st ed.
New York: Appleton-Century-Crofts.

Bullough, Bonnie
1967   "Alienation in the ghetto." American
Journal of Sociology 72(March):469–
478.
1980   The Law and the Expanding Nursing Role.
2nd ed. New York: Appleton-Century-
Crofts.

Bullough, Vern L.
1961   "Status and medieval medicine." Journal
of Health and Human Behavior 2(Fall):
204–210.
1974   The Development of Medicine as a Profession. New York: Neale Watson Science
History.
1980   "Licensure and the medical monopoly."
Pp. 14–22 in B. Bullough (ed.), The
Law and the Expanding Nursing Role.
2nd ed. New York: Appleton-Century-
Crofts.

Carr-Saunders, A. M. and P. A. Wilson
1933   The Professions. Oxford: Clarendon Press.

Cohen, Harris S. and Lawrence H. Miike
1973   Developments in Health Manpower Licen-
sure: A Follow-up to the 1971 Report on
Licensure and Related Health Personnel
Credentialling. U.S. Department of Health,
Education and Welfare Publication No.
(HRA) 74–3101. Washington, D.C.: U.S.
Government Printing Office.

Committee for the Study of Credentialing in
Nursing
1979   "Credentialing in nursing: A new approach." Report of the Committee. American Journal of Nursing 79(April):674–
683.

Daniels, A. K.
1971   "How free should the profession be?"
Pp. 39–57 in E. Freidson (ed.), The
Professions and Their Prospects. Beverly
Hills: Sage.

Derbyshier, Robert C.
1969   United States Reports: Cases Adjudged
in the Supreme Courts. Dent vs. West
Virginia, 129:114–128. Medical Licensure
and Discipline in the United States.
Baltimore: The Johns Hopkins Press.

Dienes, C. T.
1970   "Judges, legislators and social change."
American Behavioral Scientist 13(March–
April):511–521.

Fish, M. S.
1974   "Nursing vis-a-vis medicine: A proposal
for legislation." Pp. 14–22 in Licensure
and Credentialing: Proceedings of the
ANA Conference for Members and Professional Employees of State Boards of
Nursing and the ANA Advisory Council
1972. Detroit: ANA.

Fogotson, E. H., Ruth Roemer, R. W. Newman,
and J. L. Cook
1967a "Licensure of physicians." Report of the
National Advisory Commission on Health
Manpower.   2:294.   Washington,   D.C.:
U.S. Government Printing Office.
1967b "Licensure of other medical personnel."
Report of the National Advisory Commission on Health Manpower 2:407–
492. Washington, D.C.: U.S. Government
Printing Office.

Freidson, E.
1970   Professional Dominance: The Social Structure of Medical Care. New York: Atherton.

1977 "The future of professionalization." Pp. 14–38 in M. Stacey (ed.), Health and the Division of Labor, 1977. New York: Prodist.

Friedmann, W. G.
1964 Law in a Changing Society. New York: Columbia University Press.

Greenwood, Ernest
1957 "Attributes of a profession." Social Work 2:45–55.

Illinois State Supreme Court
1964 Darling vs. Charleston Community Hosp-
1965 ital. 200 NE 2d 145, 211 NE 2d 253.

"The Darling Case."
1968 Journal American Medical Association 206:1875.

Jacobson, M.
1940 "Nursing laws and what every nurse should know about them." American Journal of Nursing 40:1221–1226.

Kelly, Lucie Young
1980 "Institutional licensure: Panic or panacea?" Pp. 109–124 in B. Bullough (ed.), The Law and the Expanding Nursing Role. 2nd ed. New York: Appleton-Century-Crofts.

Lesnick, M. J. and B. E. Anderson
1947 Legal Aspects of Nursing. Philadelphia: Lippincott.

Lewin, Kurt
1958 "Group Decision and Social Change." Pp. 197–211 in E. Maccoby, M. Newcomb, and L. Hartley (eds.), Readings in Social Psychology. New York: Holt.

Lewis, T.
1969 The Impact of Supreme Court Decisions: Empirical Studies. New York: Oxford University Press.

Maine
1974 Revised Statutes. Title 32, Chapter 31, Section 2102.

Moore, Wilbert E.
1970 The Professions: Roles and Rules. Gerald W. Rosenblum, collab. New York: Russell Sage Foundation.

Nagel, S.
1969 The Legal Process From a Behavioral Perspective. Homewood, Ill.: Dorsey.

New York State Legislature
1972 Education Law. Op Title 8, Article 130, Section 6901.

New York State Nurses Association
1974 Resolution on Entry Into Professional Practice. Albany: N.Y.S.N.A.

North Carolina State Legislature
General Statutes. Section 90-1814.

"Positions, conclusions and recommendations from the study of credentialing in nursing: A new approach."
1979 Nursing Outlook 27(April):263–271.

"Regional review."
1978 Nurse Practitioner 3(May–June):6.

Ross, H. L., D. Campbell, and G. Glass
1970 "Determination of a legal reform." American Behavioral Scientist 13(March–April): 494–509.

Stein, Leonard
1967 "The doctor-nurse game." Archives of General Psychiatry 16:699–703.

Stewart, P. L. and M. G. Cantor
1974 Varieties of Work Experience: The Social Control of Occupational Groups and Roles. New York: Wiley.

"The Darling Case"
1968 Journal of the American Medical Association 206(November 18):1875.

U.S. Department of Health, Education, and Welfare
1971 Report on Licensure and Related Health Personnel Credentialing. Publication No. (HSM) 72-11. Washington, D.C.: U.S. Government Printing Office.
1976 Health Resources Statistics: Health Manpower and Health Facilities. National Center for Health Statistics. Washington, D.C.: U.S. Government Printing Office.

Vaughn, John C. and Walter L. Johnson
1979 "Educational preparation for nursing—1978." Nursing Outlook 27(September): 608–614.

Virginia Code. Section 54–275.

Vollmer, Howard M. and Donald L. Mills (eds.)
1966 Professionalization. Englewood Cliffs, N.J.: Prentice-Hall.

Woodham-Smith, C.
1951 Florence Nightingale: 1820–1910. New York: McGraw-Hill.

Part Six

Administration: Nursing Service and Education

A time for searching, . . .
a time for throwing away. . . .
a time for speaking. . . .
a time for serving

Nursing administration for providing the delivery of nursing care and nursing education utilizes the management processes of planning, organizing, directing, controlling, and evaluating. As they plan, nurse administrators are required to search for data, resources, and mechanisms to achieve goals. In organizing, the search continues for the most effective means for goal attainment. Through evaluation, they may throw away goals that are unattainable, or ineffective mechanisms for achieving goals. As nurse administrators, direction is essential in their role. Consequently, they speak for and of authority, responsibility, and accountability in the name of nursing staff and faculty who they represent and serve. In fulfilling the management role of controlling, nurse administrators sew to secure the organization or institution in the direction which was planned and organized to achieve specific goals. They sew through continual evaluation of the means and outcome in attaining goals. Particularly, the institution is sewn/ secured through the active participation of nursing staff and faculty in the planning, decision making, and evaluation of and for goals.

Nursing administration is a complex, rewarding challenge for the professional nurse. The complexities are within the multiple, simultaneous issues and demands, with which the administrator is confronted, in being ultimately accountable for providing the delivery of high-quality nursing care and education. The rewards are in working with and for persons who are professionals. The challenges are in the numerous perplexing problems, which require resolution in order for nursing organizations and institutions to fulfill their mission. The chapters that follow represent the great diversity of complex issues, challenges, and rewards that are evident today in nursing administration. Effective leadership in nursing administration is critical for the profession to fulfill its mission.

Chapter 46

Collaboration/Unification Models for Nursing Education and Nursing Service

Jannetta MacPhail, R.N., Ph.D., F.A.A.N.
Dean and Professor of Nursing
Frances Payne Bolton School of Nursing
Case Western Reserve University
Cleveland, Ohio

With the emphasis on the unification of nursing education and nursing practice it is particularly relevant that Jannetta MacPhail's chapter be the first in this section, titled "Administration: Nursing Service and Education." Administration is a key factor in the success of collaboration/unification models. MacPhail succinctly delineates the influences and rationale for collaboration/unification models, describes the three predominant models that have been developed, and cites examples which indicate increasing interest in collaboration/unification between nursing education and nursing service.

MacPhail traces the history and problems inherent in educating students of nursing in hospital schools of nursing. Essentially, service needs took priority over the learning needs of students. Due to the differences between the primary mission of nursing service and nursing education in university schools, the answer to the dilemma was to separate nursing education and nursing service. However, MacPhail indicates the dire consequences and adverse effects this had on both the quality of nursing care and the quality of nursing education. Nursing faculty abdicated responsibility for the quality of nursing care provided, divested themselves of authority to create an exemplary learning environment, and lost motivation to seek opportunities to maintain and increase their clinical expertise. MacPhail further comments on the development of negative attitudes and a dichotomy between nursing staff and faculty. Action was taken by a few nursing education and service leaders to overcome the barriers by developing and testing models to unify education and services.

MacPhail explains the five major reasons for the need to promote and facilitate collaboration/unification between nursing education and nursing service. They are: to work together to provide the best possible quality of nursing care; to provide an exemplary learning climate for nursing students and staff; to develop nursing research; to help resolve problems of nurse supply and demand; to promote the interdependence of a school of nursing and organized nursing services used for students' practice and research. In providing the rationale MacPhail presents legitimate criticisms of nursing education and service. For example, nursing curricula developed by faculty who are not in touch with the realities of current practice are less likely to sufficiently prepare students for practice today. On the other hand, students need an exemplary learning environment, where a high quality of nursing care can be observed and clinical inquiry is supported.

The three collaboration/unification models developed over the past 15 years are: the Case Western Reserve University/University Hospitals of Cleveland model, University of Rochester model, and Rush University model. MacPhail portrays the basic components of each. The first model is an interinstitutional organization and agreement between two private independent institutions implemented in 1966. The organization of nursing service is decentralized with a head of nursing in each institution. Interfaces between nursing education and nursing care occur at the clinical department level. There are three types of joint appointments described. The shared appointment is one where the incumbent has specific responsibilities in both organizations, which involve sharing of cost and time on a proportional basis, selecting one organization to receive salary and fringe benefits, and holding a regular faculty appointment in terms of rank and eligibility for tenure. The faculty-associate appointment is one held by regular faculty, who have full rank, eligibility for tenure in the School of Nursing with an Associate in Nursing appointment in the University Hospitals of Cleveland; they are paid fully by the University with primary responsibilities to the school and no sharing of costs, but have practice and research privileges in the University Hospitals. The third type of joint appointment is the clinical appointment. Clinical appointees are nurses in leadership positions in the University Hospitals and other health care agencies where students practice. They are paid fully by the primary institution where they have responsibility, appointed according to the same criteria as for regular faculty, may participate in teaching, and serve as preceptors, but are not eligible for tenure.

The last two models are in academic health centers in which the university and hospital are under one board of trustees, administration, and budget. The University of Rochester model was initiated in 1972. The head of nursing serves as both Dean of the School of Nursing and Director of Nursing Services in Strong Memorial Hospital, with the School of Nursing having overall responsibility for the delivery and quality of nursing care. Associate deans for practice and education and clinical chiefs collaborate with the dean/director of nursing in providing academic and practice leadership in the University of Rochester Medical Center. The Rush University model is similar in that the head of nursing serves as both Dean of the College of Nursing and Vice President for Nursing Affairs at the Rush–Presbyterian–St. Luke's Medical Center. Associate deans and chairpersons assist in providing leadership for integration of nursing care, education, members and research. Faculty members serve in the role of practitioner/teacher. All three models have the same goals as outlined through MacPhail's rationale.

MacPhail notes numerous examples which indicate increasing interest in the concept of unification of nursing service and education. Some are: a Robert Wood Johnson Foundation sponsored meeting in 1979 with the outcome of a major publication calling for a commitment to unification models as an essential means for nursing to achieve its fullest potential in the delivery of care; the annual meeting of the American Academy of Nursing in 1979, at which the resolution was endorsed for the cementing of relationships between service and education through several mechanisms and papers presented which were published as a book. Other major national meetings identified deterrents to faculty practice, as well as illustrated how faculty involvement could be facilitated, and demonstrated the success of models. Furthermore an organization, the Midwest Alliance in Nursing (MAIN) was established to promote collaboration efforts in 13 midwestern states. MacPhail predicts that in the 1980s new models will be developed and tested, and mechanisms implemented to remove deterrents. She foresees that the interdependence of practice and education will prove to enhance the quality of nursing care and education, and the advancement of nursing knowledge.

INTRODUCTION

The need for collaboration between nursing education and nursing service has been identified as a concern of increasing importance in the past few years. The impetus for the trend emanates from a number of sources. The potential outcomes of a movement to unify nurse educators and nursing service leaders in a common endeavor have far-reaching implications for the quality of nursing care and nursing education and for the advancement of nursing knowledge.

HISTORICAL INFLUENCES

Although collaboration between those who educate practitioners to provide nursing care and those directly responsible for the provision of nursing care seems like a logical assumption, this is not the situation that prevails in nursing education in America (United States and Canada) today. It is generally agreed that faculties have responsibility for selecting learning opportunities for students and for providing an academic environment which holds promise of stimulating their continuous learning. As a result of historic circumstances, however, nursing faculties in general have divested themselves of responsibility for the quality of nursing care provided in hospitals and other health care agencies used for student learning (Schlotfeldt and MacPhail, 1969).

In the early years of the twentieth century hospital schools of nursing were the only institutions responsible for educating students of nursing. Each training school, as such institutions were then termed, was owned and operated by the hospital, which usually was the only clinical setting used for practice. Students staffed the hospital and the only graduate nurses on staff were the matron or superintendent, supervisors, and perhaps some head nurses. Under such circumstances service needs took precedence over the learning needs of students. With the advent of university schools of nursing, which began in 1909 with the establishment of the University of Minnesota School of Nursing, leaders in nursing education faced a dilemma in evolving relationships between a school of nursing owned and operated by a university, whose primary missions were education, research, and service to the community, and a nursing service which was an integral part of a health care agency whose primary mission was providing care, with education and research as secondary goals. In some instances, the university and hospital were owned and operated by one board and one administration; in other instances, the school of nursing and university of which it was a part and the hospital were two private, independent institutions.

The answer to this dilemma was to separate nursing education and nursing service so that educators assumed no responsibility for the quality of nursing care provided in the health care agencies used for students' practice. Indeed, this circumstance eventually prevailed in hospital schools of nursing because of continued exploitation of nursing students to provide care regardless of their learning needs. In choosing this course of action, nursing faculty members also divested themselves of authority to create an exemplary learning environment. Although the clinical settings used for students' practice and graduate students' research are called "laboratories," nursing faculty members responsible for guiding students' learning and research have had little or no control over the nursing care given and little or no influence over the practitioner role models students observe or over nursing research being done (Schlotfeldt and MacPhail, 1969).

Faculty members in most nursing schools today are, essentially "guests" in the hospitals and other health care agencies in which nursing students have opportunities to apply theory about nursing practice and research learned in nursing schools. The role of "guest," unfortunately, has not encouraged them to seek opportunities to maintain and enhance their own clinical expertise or to test hypotheses with a view toward advancing nursing knowledge and improving practice. Indeed, faculty members are often alleged to be not competent to practice and have not earned the respect of nursing staff which would help to engender productive working relationships. Faculty members, in turn, frequently lament the poor quality of nursing care provided and the negative attitudes of nursing staff in the clinical settings in which their students are having clinical experiences.

Within the past 20 years, a few leaders in nursing education and nursing service, concerned about the adverse effects of these circumstances on both the quality of nursing care and the quality of nursing education, took action to develop and test models designed to overcome the barrier and unify nursing education and nursing service in a common endeavor. Their purposes were: (1) to provide optimal standards of nursing care which would benefit both the recipients of care and the learners, i.e., the nursing students and staff, who need exemplary role models to observe and emulate and (2) to have faculty assume appropriate responsibility as professionals for the quality of nursing practice observed by students as well as for the learning opportunities provided them.

RATIONALE FOR COLLABORATION/ UNIFICATION MODELS

At least five reasons exist for nurse-educators and their colleagues in nursing service to attend to the need to promote and facilitate collaboration/ unification between nursing education and nursing service.

A major reason, which should be a major concern to all nurses, is to work together to provide the best possible quality of nursing care. In most schools of nursing faculty members with the benefit of advanced education fail to apply it in patient care because they have no legitimate or effective mechanism for influencing standards of nursing practice in the settings used for students' practice (MacPhail, 1972). Johnson (1980) points out that "faculty may complain to other faculty about the inadequacies of care on a nursing unit, but they seldom share these concerns with the head nurse; even less frequently do they intervene directly to improve the quality of care delivered by the nursing staff." Such an attitude tends to create a dichotomy of "we" and "they" and the problems in nursing care may not be addressed. It is ironic that the majority of nurses who have the most advanced education in nursing are faculty in schools of nursing who do not involve themselves in addressing problems in nursing care. Christman (1979) identified this situation as a major problem and took action to create a unification model at Rush University that has all faculty members assume responsibility for nursing care in their roles as teacher-practitioners.

Some of the critics of faculty members' failure to be involved in practice have focused on finding ways for faculty to do so and thus maintain and enhance their clinical competence and be respected by both students and nursing staff as role models. It is possible that faculty can have such involvement in practice but exert very limited influence on standards of nursing care within the health care agencies used for students' practice. This point was emphasized by representatives from both Case Western Reserve University and the University of Rochester in their presentations at the American Association of Colleges of Nursing "Workshop on Faculty Clinical Practice: A Strategy for Reconciliation," held in Dallas, Texas, in December 1979. Hence, employing such an approach does not really address the problem of the lack of collaboration/

unification between nursing education and nursing services.

A second reason for promoting and facilitating collaboration/unification models is to provide an exemplary learning climate for nursing students and staff. Although one can learn negatively from poor role models, it is a very expensive way of learning and is not supported by learning theorists. If faculty has responsibility for providing an academic environment that holds promise of stimulating students' continuous learning, the students should have opportunity to observe the quality of nursing care they are expected to emulate. They need a learning environment that supports questioning, inquiry, flexibility, and independence of thought and action, rather than an environment that engenders rigidity, conformity, dependence on rules, regulations, and superiors, and adherence to long-standing patterns which lack established scientific bases. The latter is the type of climate found to varying degrees in some of the clinical settings used for students' practice. Moreover, the attitude of nurse administrators and staff in such settings is often not helpful to learners because of their lack of understanding of the goals held for students and the rationale underlying changes in nursing education.

"Closely related to the need for faculty to exercise proper control over the learning environment is the commitment that nursing must become a learned profession in which academic leaders seek new and improved ways to provide exemplary nursing care to all who need it" (Schlotfeldt and MacPhail, 1969:1020). The development of nursing research is the third major reason for promoting collaboration/unification models between nursing education and nursing service. Faculty members need to serve as role models in promoting a spirit of inquiry, identifying researchable problems, conducting sound investigations, and applying research findings. Nursing is handicapped by having far too few nurse investigators and theorists engaged in advancing nursing knowledge. If nursing faculties in university schools of nursing regard themselves as full-fledged members of the academic community, they have responsibility for giving leadership to the profession in advancing nursing knowledge and in closing the gap between available knowledge and its application in the resolution of vexing problems relevant to nursing.

A fourth reason for supporting and facilitating collaboration/unification models between nursing education and nursing service is the need to help resolve problems of nurse supply and demand. Although nurse-educators have produced more nurses to help address the problem of a shortage of nurses to give care and to serve as teachers, administrators, and investigators, there continues to be much criticism by nursing service of the adequacy of the graduates to meet complex needs prevalent in nursing services. Some of the criticism is well founded when one examines nursing curricula which provide very limited opportunities for practice and include nursing courses taught by faculty who are not in touch with current practice. A nursing faculty which is involved in practice and aware of current problems faced by nursing service personnel is more likely to shape a curriculum that provides the type of learning opportunities needed by students to be prepared for practice today and in the future. Faculty and nursing service leaders in a collaboration/unification model view themselves as colleagues in resolving problems rather than in criticizing each other, as occurs in settings that engender strict separation of education and service.

Based on the outcomes achieved by the three recognized collaboration/unification models (Case Western Reserve University/University Hospitals of Cleveland; Rush University; University of Rochester), there is reason to believe that the utilization of nursing personnel can be greatly improved by having well-qualified leaders in nursing service who are a vital component of all the collaboration/unification models. Similarly, they have addressed problems of nurse dissatisfaction and turnover and found that the opportunity to practice as taught is an important influence on retention and job satisfaction. This observation is supported by Kramer's findings (1974) in her extensive study of new graduates and their socialization into the profession.

A fifth reason for promoting the concept of academic leadership for nursing and the development of collaboration/unification models is the interdependence of a school of nursing and organized nursing services utiltized for students' practice and research. Quality nursing care and clinical inquiry are essential to providing an exemplary learning environment for students. Similarly, opportunities for continued learning and clinical inquiry are necessary to develop high standards of nursing practice and a stimulating learning environment for nursing staff.

Expert practitioners of nursing need and want intellectual stimulation from colleagues in an academic environment. Competent investigators are attracted to settings in which they will have access to pursue research interests and opportunity to interact with nurse-clinicians, scientists, and other professionals. If faculty members are to have the opportunity to maintain and enhance their clinical competence, they must have identity and involvement in a setting in which they have practice and research privileges (Schlotfeldt and MacPhail, 1969).

COLLABORATION/UNIFICATION MODELS

The first collaboration/unification model in a university setting was that designed at the University of Florida by Dorothy Smith when she accepted the deanship in 1959. She believed it imperative to unify nursing services and nursing education and implemented this belief by engaging in the practice of nursing herself and expecting her faculty to do the same. Thus, faculty members who taught didactic content and were principally responsible for the students' socialization into the profession also served as their role models in practice (Mauksch, 1980). In her presentation at the October 1979 workshop for four representatives from 10 academic health centers which was sponsored by the Robert Wood Johnson Foundation, Smith identified factors that she believes contributed to the demise of that unification/collaboration model. A major one was failure to apply role theory and theories of planned change in the process of development.

The three collaboration/unification models that have been developed over the past 15 years and which are recognized as models nationally and internationally are the interinstitutional model between Case Western Reserve University and the University Hospitals of Cleveland and the models at Rush University and the University of Rochester. The latter two models are in academic health centers in which the university and the hospital are under one board of trustees, one administration, and one budget. In contrast, the first model is a unique interinstitutional organization and agreement worked out between two private, independent institutions, each with its own board of trustees, administration, and budget. Basic components of the three models will be described.

CASE WESTERN RESERVE UNIVERSITY— UNIVERSITY HOSPITALS OF CLEVELAND

The model at Case Western Reserve University and the University Hospitals of Cleveland is based on the concept of academic leadership for nursing. A pilot project was undertaken in psychiatric nursing and rehabilitation nursing in the early 1960s to test an interinstitutional relationship designed to attain specific objectives:

1 Improve the quality of nursing care
2 Enhance the learning climate for nursing students and staff
3 Promote a spirit of inquiry and the development of research in nursing
4 Promote interprofessional collaboration, particularly between nurses and physicians
5 Improve the utilization of nurses' time and talents

The pilot project provided sufficient evidence that the objectives could be attained to persuade the W. K. Kellogg Foundation in 1966 to support a 5-year demonstration project designed to implement the concept of academic leadership for nursing throughout all clinical services.

The project was designed to change the organization of nursing service to a decentralized pattern similar to the organizational structure in the school of nursing, with a head of nursing for each institution rather than an overall head as in the Rush University and University of Rochester models. The interface of nursing education and nursing care is conceived to occur at the clinical department level. Because the model involved two institutions, several types of joint appointments were designed to promote the concept of a joint endeavor with privileges and responsibilities:

1 The *shared* appointment is designed for an incumbent who has specific responsibilities in both organizations which involves sharing of cost and time commitment. The sharing may be on a 50-50, 75-25, or other proportional basis, depending on the needs of the two organizations as decided collaboratively by the heads of nursing in the two organizations. Examples of the shared appointment are the chairperson-director of each clinical specialty and the faculty-nurse clinician appointee. All hold a regular faculty appointment in terms of rank and eligibility for tenure. Salary and fringe benefits are shared between the two organizations. The incumbent must select one organization from which to receive salary and fringe benefits and that organization cross-charges the other institution for its share of the cost.

2 The *faculty-associate* appointment is held by regular faculty who have full rank and are eligible for tenure in the school of nursing with an associate in nursing appointment in the University Hospitals of Cleveland. They are paid fully by the university with no sharing of costs. Their primary responsibilities are to the school, with the associate in nursing appointment providing practice and research privileges. It entails responsibility for influencing the quality of nursing care to provide the caliber desired for students to observe and emulate. Faculty may influence practice in a variety of ways, such as providing consultation, participating in staff development, serving as a role model for staff, sharing in problem solving in relation to nursing practice or nursing leadership, identifying problems for investigation, and conducting research. The dean holds an appointment as administrative associate in nursing in the hospital, which involves a variety of responsibilities for determining policy pertaining to nursing practice and administration of nursing services.

3 The *clinical* appointment is the third type of joint appointment for nurses in leadership positions in the University Hospitals of Cleveland and other health care agencies used for students' practice. Clinical appointees are paid fully by the hospital or another health care agency in which they have primary responsibility. They are appointed according to the same criteria used for regular faculty but are not eligible for tenure. They are held accountable for the quality of care provided in the clinical setting and make a major contribution if they can ensure that it is of the quality students are taught. In addition, they may participate in teaching, serve as preceptors for students, provide consultation to students and faculty, and participate in curriculum development and committee work in the school of nursing. The school has the opportunity and responsibility to nominate persons who meet the appointment criteria for mutually agreed upon leadership positions in the University Hospitals. To date, the positions have included clinical directors, assistant directors, nurse-clinicians, and selected staff development positions. If the hospital did not approve the nominee, another would have to be found; however, this situation has not been encountered to date. The school does not have the authority to nominate for leadership positions in other health care agencies; however, such agencies frequently seek the school's help in recruiting persons who will qualify for a clinical appointment.

All joint appointees are held accountable for fulfilling role expectations in both organizations through regular ongoing evaluation and by an annual evaluation in writing, which is reviewed by the school's Committee on Appointment, Reappointment, Promotion, and Tenure. Performance in a leadership position in a health care agency is reviewed through the evaluation system of that organization.

On the basis of the 5-year demonstration project, which concluded in 1971, it was determined that the objectives had been attained sufficiently to continue with the joint endeavor. A more detailed interpretation of outcomes may be found in the final report of the demonstration project (MacPhail, 1980). There is no longer a sense of "we" and "they" but rather "us." Regular faculty members have a sense of responsibility for the quality of nursing practice and for maintaining their own competence rather than concern for only education and research, as in most nursing schools. The leadership persons in the University Hospitals and other health care agencies who hold clinical appointments have concern for the quality of education and opportunities for involvement to influence the educational and research programs. They also have access to academic colleagues with whom to discuss ideas and from whom they can seek support and consultation in developing practice and research in the clinical settings.

In the 9 years since the demonstration project, efforts have continued to improve the collaboration/unification model and to test out new ideas that will continue to achieve the goals of quality nursing practice, quality nursing education and research, nurse-physician collaboration, and wise use of nurses' time and talents. The model has been proved to be a viable one which can be adapted to other settings in which a school of nursing and hospital or other health care agency are committed to promoting and facilitating collaboration/unification between nursing education and nursing service for the betterment of patients and students.

UNIVERSITY OF ROCHESTER MODEL

The unification model at the University of Rochester was initiated in 1972 at a propitious time, when a new school of nursing was organized with the help of a grant from the W. K. Kellogg Foundation. The head of nursing serves as both dean of the school of nursing and director of nursing services in Strong Memorial Hospital, which is a component of the University of Rochester Medical Center. The school of nursing has overall respon-

sibility for the delivery and quality of nursing care to hospitalized and ambulatory patients at the hospital. The head of nursing is responsible for providing academic leadership, assuming administrative responsibilities in both the university and the medical center, and formulating top-level policies for programs of education, practice, and research (Ford, 1980).

Collaborating with the dean-director of nursing in providing leadership in the planning and implementation of programs of both practice and education are the associate deans for practice and for education and several clinical chiefs. They also support faculty members in their research, facilitate scholarly efforts, and engage in the generation of new knowledge themselves. These administrative leaders, who hold appointments in both the school and the hospital, maintain their clinical competence and educational skills through practice and teaching. Nursing faculty members who hold clinician II appointments in the hospital teach in the educational programs; maintain their competence through clinical practice and/or service; and use their practice to generate new hypotheses for research, improve the quality of patient care, serve as role models for students and staff, and develop colleague and team relationships with other health care professionals, particularly physicians (Ford, 1980).

"In addition to responsibility for nursing service at Strong Memorial Hospital, the school reaches into the community and region through its educational, clinical, and research activities in community health agencies, schools, industry, health maintenance organizations, and gerontological and rehabilitation nursing services" (Ford, 1980:245).

Ford points out that "through its responsibility for all three components, the school of nursing provides a continuous loop of practice, research, and education. The practice component contributes to education and the education component to practice, and research draws from each and contributes to the advancement of both" (1980:247).

RUSH UNIVERSITY MODEL

The Rush University unification model is similar to the University of Rochester Model in that the head of nursing serves as both dean of the college of nursing and vice president for nursing affairs at the medical center. Assisting the head of nursing in providing administrative leadership are associate deans and the chairpersons of seven clinical departments. Each chairperson is responsible for integrating nursing care, nursing education, and research so that the goals of the department and the medical center are achieved (Nayer, 1980).

All other faculty serve in the role of practitioner-teacher, not only as classroom and clinical teachers of students but also as consultants to nursing staff and as role models for patient care, research, and interdisciplinary collaboration. Christman states that the basic premise underlying the role is that expert clinicians teach and, conversely, teachers should also practice. The practitioner-teacher may serve as unit leader or as part of the nursing staff on a unit with responsibility for a group of primary patients. In addition to having responsibility for direct care of patients and the education of nursing students, the practitioner-teacher is expected to support ongoing research, focus on the continuing education of nursing staff, and work with others in achieving the goals of the department (Rush Presbyterian–St. Luke's Medical Center, 1979).

Although the organizational structures, titles, and mechanisms for promoting collaboration/unification differ in these three models, their goals are the same. All are designed to promote optimal quality of nursing practice and an exemplary learning environment for nursing students and staff. All recognize the interdependence of these two goals and view the outcomes as beneficial to both the recipients of care and the consumers of education. All are designed to promote a spirit of inquiry and facilitate the advancement of nursing knowledge. All value the talents and contributions of the nurse and provide support systems that promote wise use of nurses' time and talents. The role expectations and the status and incentive systems in the three models promote and reward professional commitment and nursing practice of a truly professional nature. All three models recognize the vital importance of interprofessional relationships to the quality of care and education and have demonstrated enhancement of nurse-physician relationships.

RECENT INTEREST AND SUPPORT

A number of recent events and developments reflect a notable increase of interest in collaboration/unification between nursing education and nursing service.

In January 1979 the Robert Wood Johnson Foundation sponsored a meeting of 13 selected leaders in nursing education and nursing service. One outcome of this event was the publication of a "statement of belief regarding faculty practice" (Christman et al., 1979). The statement calls for commitment to the concept of unification of nursing service and education and the development of unification models for nursing faculty as an essential means for nursing achieving its fullest potential in the delivery of health care. Another outcome was a conference held in October, 1979, for selected representatives from 10 academic health centers which was sponsored by the foundation. The conference brought together deans of nursing and medicine, nursing service leaders, and hospital administrators to address issues pertaining to nurse-physician relationships and nursing education–nursing service collaboration/unification. The papers presented are to be published in the near future.

The program of the annual meeting of the American Academy of Nursing held in September 1979 included a section on "The Interface between Nursing Practice and Nursing Education." Six papers were presented which are now available with the publication of a book, *Health Policy and Nursing Practice* (Aiken, 1980). The outcomes of the collaboration/unification models developed at Case Western Reserve University and the University of Rochester are described. At this meeting academy members approved a resolution which was approved unanimously by the American Nurses Association House of Delegates in June, 1980. The resolution "endorsed the idea of cementing the relationship between service and education through such devices as faculty practice, joint appointments, shared salaries, clinical faculty appointments, and collaborative research" (Nayer, 1980: 1114). The resolution also supported the development and testing of new collaboration/unification models.

In December, 1979, the American Association of Colleges of Nursing presented a workshop on "Faculty Clinical Practice: A Strategy for Reconciliation," which addressed the problem of nursing faculty not being involved in practice. The papers presented and the discussion groups that followed not only identified deterrents to faculty practice but also demonstrated the success of collaboration/unification models in promoting and facilitating faculty practice. Moreover, the workshop participants were from both nursing education and nursing service.

In March, 1980, the program meeting of the Council of Baccalaureate and Higher Degree Programs of the National League for Nursing was entitled "Cognitive Dissonance: Interpreting and Implementing Faculty Practice Roles in Nursing Education" (National League for Nursing, 1980). Collaboration/unification models between nursing education and nursing service once again illustrated how faculty involvement in practice could be promoted and facilitated. In her discussion of restructuring of faculty role to include practice, Spero states that "the inclusion of clinical practice in order to maintain familiarity with basic skills and/or to gain stature among our service colleagues is, in and of itself, insufficient reason to restructure our role" (1980:24). She points out that it is justified if involvement in practice is reflected in faculty research, in educators serving as role models for students and staff, and in

reflection upon and analysis of the practice framework.

At the 1980 Biennial Convention of the American Nurses Association, a program was presented on the three collaboration/unification models described above. The program was a joint endeavor by the Commissions on Nursing Education and Nursing Services undertaken as a consequence of a joint meeting to consider possible means of promoting more collaborative efforts.

When the Midwest Alliance in Nursing (MAIN) came into being in April, 1979, one of its major purposes was identified as promoting collaboration between nursing education and nursing service in the 13 midwestern states. Membership in the organization was open to both nursing education institutions and nursing service agencies. To date, the membership is equally divided between the two types of organizations. The topic of MAIN's first program meeting in September, 1980, was "Collaboration Between Nursing Education and Nursing Service." Papers were presented to share the development of new interinstitutional models at the University of Illinois and at Marquette University which have provided added stimulus to the movement.

Nayer (1980) describes several other collaboration efforts, such as the use of selected joint appointments between the University of Arizona College of Nursing and the Veterans Administration Hospitals. She refers to the joint appointments existing at Yale University, the University of Wisconsin-Madison, and several other university schools of nursing. None are developed in the sense of a single administration like the Rochester and Rush models. Nor do any include the comprehensive model of a school of nursing which assumes responsibility for quality controls for a total nursing service, as does the Case Western Reserve University–University Hospitals of Cleveland model.

PREDICTIONS FOR THE FUTURE

The ferment in relation to collaboration/unification between nursing education and service augurs well for the future of nursing practice, education, and research. It is predicted that new collaboration/unification models will be developed and tested in the 1980s. In addition, in settings where a comprehensive model is not feasible, there will be more efforts to implement some mechanisms to remove or reconcile differences between education and service that serve as deterrents to enhancing the quality of nursing care and nursing education.

All these joint endeavors will recognize the interdependence of practice and education and will prove to be beneficial to the recipients of nursing care, to the consumers of nursing education, and to the advancement of nursing knowledge.

EDITOR'S QUESTIONS FOR DISCUSSION

What factors are critical to the success of collaboration/unification models? What incentives can be utilized to promote collaboration? What empirical evidence exists as to the impact of unification models on the quality of nursing care, nursing education, and the advancement of nursing knowledge? What methodological approaches can be suggested to evaluate the development, implementation, and outcomes of collaboration/unification models? Suggest alternative types of models in organizational design, roles, responsibility, and accountability? What are the most effective approaches to initiate collaboration and who should be responsible for them? Suggest strategies for achieving collaboration before organizational models are developed. What are the critical steps, variables, and considerations that are essential in the long-range planning of collaboration/unification models? How can collaboration efforts between nursing practice and education be promoted, particularly in geographic areas where financial and professional personnel resources are scarce? To what extent has the cost-effectiveness of collaboration/unification models been demonstrated? What are the advantages and disadvantages of models developed under a single board of trustees, administration, and budget versus those formulated between two independent institutions? What are the implications of collaboration/unification models for implementation of primary nursing in relation to the discussion and editor's questions posed in Klein's chapter (43)? What effects and relationships might there be among collaboration/unification models, reimbursement of nursing services as advocated by Cleland (Chap. 44), and nurse corporations as proposed by Sills (Chap. 42)?

To what extent do you agree with MacPhail's portrayal of the effects of separating nursing service and education on the quality of nursing care and nursing education? Could those effects have been foreseen and prevented? What other factors may have influenced a dichotomy between nursing practices and education? What differences between the characteristics of a professional and bureaucratic model of practice may have been inherent in the eventual separation of nursing service and nursing education? How are these differences resolved in collaboration/unification models?

Are there other legitimate reasons that may be offered for faculty withdrawing from the practice arena? What alternatives may be available to faculty members to enhance their clinical competency? What negotiation process is essential for those who are involved in practice to influence the standards of nursing care within a health care institution or agency? What strategies can be offered for the prevention and/or resolution of possible role conflict in settings where collaboration/unification models exist? Should there be a difference in the "exemplary learning climate" for nursing students from that for nursing staff? What strategies can be utilized to enhance the type of learning climate in some clinical settings for nursing staff and students? What congruence and implications are there in MacPhail's view of the results of some nursing curricula and the chapters by Williamson (5), Peterson (7), Santora (8), Dalme (11), Fawcett (14), Roy (34), and Sills (42)? The failure to apply role theory and theories of planned change has been identified by Smith as one of the major factors in the demise of the first unification/collaboration model designed in 1959. How was this factor accounted for in the process of development of the present models? Are there other issues that need to be considered which have not been addressed in developing collaboration/unification models? What factors may influence the future of collaboration/unification models?

In models where there are shared appointments, should there be different criteria for faculty appointment, promotion, and tenure (FAPT)? To what extent might the proportion of time allocated to the university be a factor in consideration of criteria? Should FAPT criteria be developed to provide for a two-track system, such as a clinical track and academic track? Who might more appropriately qualify for a clinical track rather than academic? What criteria might be suggested for such a system? How might a two-track system be planned and implemented? Should incumbents have a choice as to which system they might choose? What are the implications for academic and clinical settings if two-track systems are available? What potential conflicting issues are inherent in shared, faculty-associate, and clinical appointments? How might these be prevented? Would the development of two-track systems provide more equity in rewards, responsibility, contributions, and commitment? If so, provide examples of how that result might occur. Would two-track systems potentially raise other issues than are known to occur with the varying type of appointments between and within institutions? How can those potential problems be prevented?

Should tenure be abolished in academic institutions? What are the advantages and disadvantages of tenure for the individual and institution? What alternative mechanisms can be suggested to achieve the purpose of tenure and at the same time prevent adverse effects which may be related to tenure? Discuss whether a nonproductive long-term service employee and/or tenured faculty member should be retained. What ethical considerations for decision making are implicit in such situations? What strategies can be suggested to prevent the evolution of a nonproductive employee and/or faculty member as well as reverse a process of nonproductivity?

REFERENCES

Aiken, L. H. (ed.)
  1980 Health Policy and Nursing Practice. New York: McGraw-Hill.
Christman, L.
  1979 "The practitioner-teacher." Nurse Educator 4,2:8–11.
Christman, L., D. Diers, C. Fagin, E. Fahy, L. Fischer, L. Ford, H. Grace, J. MacPhail, I. Mauksch, M. Murphy, G. Smith, M. Styles, and R. Wilson
  1979 "Statement of belief regarding faculty practice." Nursing Outlook 27,3:158.

Ford, L. C.
  1980 "Creating a center of excellence in nursing." Pp. 242–55 in L. H. Aiken (ed.), Health Policy and Nursing Practice. New York: McGraw-Hill.
Johnson, J. A.
  1980 "The education/service split: Who loses?" Nursing Outlook 28,7:412–15.
Kramer, M.
  1974 Reality Shock: Why Nurses Leave Nursing. St. Louis: Mosby.
MacPhail, J.
  1972 An Experiment in Nursing: Planning, Implementing and Assessing Planned

Change. Cleveland, Ohio: Case Western Reserve University, Frances Payne Bolton School of Nursing.

1980 "Implementation and evaluation of the Case Western Reserve University Unification Model." Pp. 229–41 in L. H. Aiken (ed.), Health Policy and Nursing Practice. New York: McGraw-Hill.

Mauksch, Ingeborg G.
1980 "A rationale for the reunification of nursing services and nursing education," Pp. 211–17 in L. H. Aiken (ed.), Health Policy and Nursing Practice. New York: McGraw-Hill.

National League for Nursing
1980 Proceedings of Semi-annual Meeting of the Council of Higher Degree Programs. Cognitive Dissonance: Interpreting and Implementing Faculty Practice Roles in Nursing Education. NLN Publication #15–1831. March.

Nayer, D. D.
1980 "Unification: Bringing nursing service and nursing education together." American Journal of Nursing 80,6:1110–1114.

Rush Presbyterian–St. Luke's Medical Center
1979 Proceedings: The Dedication of the John H. and Helen Kellogg National Center for Excellence in Nursing, October 30–31.

Schlotfeldt, R. M.
1980 "The development of a model for unifying nursing practice and nursing education." Pp. 218-28 in L. H. Aiken (ed.), Health Policy and Nursing Practice. New York: McGraw-Hill.

Schlotfeldt, R., and J. MacPhail
1969 "An experiment in nursing: Rationale and characteristics." American Journal of Nursing 69,5:1018–1023.

Spero, J.
1980 "Nursing: A professional practice discipline in academia." Nursing and Health Care 1,1:22–25.

Chapter 47

Ethics and Nursing Administration

Anne J. Davis, R.N., Ph.D., F.A.A.N.
Professor
School of Nursing
University of California
San Francisco, California

It can be ethically argued that nursing administrators in service and education need to incorporate the body of knowledge of bioethics into their repertoire of expertise. Nursing administrators in leadership positions need a solid grasp of ethical principles and theories as role models and in fostering a climate for dialogue in resolving specific ethical dilemmas. Although Anne J. Davis uses the service setting to demonstrate salient points, the scholarly presentation also has applicability for administrators and leaders in education settings.

Anne J. Davis specifically addresses bioethics and the role of nursing administration in the nurses' attempt to practice according to the American Nurses Association (ANA) Code for Nurses. As a basis for this discussion, she focuses upon four ethical principles and the process of reasoning. Relevant examples are illustrated and challenging questions are raised throughout her provocative chapter. The sociology of ethical decision making is emphasized due to the unique social position nurses have in their role with patients, families, physicians, and administrators.

In bioethics the underlying question is: What is the ethical thing to do or what ought to be done in a given situation? The areas addressed usually are: clinical problems, human subjects in research, allocation of resources, and health policy issues. Davis identifies major strains which create dissonance for hospital nurses when confronted by ethical issues. One tension is related to what should nurses do with information obtained by virtue of having the most contact with patients who often pose numerous questions. Another strain is due to the multiple loyalties and obligations nurses experience to patients, families, the hospital, physicians, other staff nurses, and their own professional standards and ethics. In addition nurses are accountable to both medical and nursing authorities.

One of the most basic ethical principles in bioethics is autonomy, which means the person has the liberty to deliberate, choose, and then act on a plan of action. Nonmaleficence is another principle which addresses both intentional and the risk of harm. The principle of beneficence requires that one acts to contribute to the well-being of others. The principle of distributive justice has particular application for nursing administrators since it involves criteria on which both risks and benefits are fairly distributed among persons. Other ethical principles are the duty to tell the truth and confidentiality.

Davis explicates two predominant normative ethical systems—utilitarianism and ethical formalism. Normative ethics attempts to justify one form of behavior over another, based on an ordered set of moral standards. The basic concept of utilitarianism is that an act is right if doing it either brings about good consequences, or if it is of such a kind that if everyone did it, it would have good consequences. Davis explains the difference between the standards of intrinsic and instrumental value. Intrinsic value means something as an end in itself has value, not as a means to an end. Utilitarians can know whether an act is morally right only by finding out the consequences of the act and then determine the intrinsic goodness or badness of those consequences. Ethical formalism is based on a theory that holds an action is right only if it accords with a moral role and a principle of duty. In essence it is the kind of action which makes it right or wrong, not the goodness or badness of consequences, and the basis of what is known as the moral rule of conduct. Davis explores a third view of conduct referred to as ethical pluralism. Essentially ethical pluralists argue that both the consequences and rule of obligation can apply to one and the same action; there is no single principle to determine the rightness or wrongness of every action. Both the means and ends of ethical actions are considered in weighing the comparative importance of reasons for or against a given action.

Davis perceives nurses using ethical theories, which can result in dilemmas when conflicting moral claims occur. She advocates that nursing administrators provide opportunities in a formal arena for ongoing dialogue of ethical issues. Understanding one's individual ethical stance is encouraged. Davis maintains there is an ethical obligation inherent in the administrative-leadership role to actively attempt to deal with the ethics of any given situation.

INTRODUCTION

Bioethics usually addresses several interrelated areas: (1) clinical problems, (2) human subjects in research, (3) allocation of resources, (4) health policy issues. The underlying questions raise issues as to what is the ethical thing to do or what we ought to do in a given situation. The literature in the field tends to focus on either ethical problems such as euthanasia, abortion, mental retardation, and behavior control (E. L. Bandman and B. Bandman, 1978; Beauchamp and Walters, 1978; Davis and Aroskar, 1978) or, much less often, on the ethical principles which apply in bioethics (Beauchamp and Childress, 1979). Most of this ever-increasing literature is written predominantly for physicians since they are the ones with special legal and ethical obligations towards patients and their families as well as towards society as a whole. These writings rarely develop the idea that many bioethical issues arise within the context of health care facilities such as hospitals which are complex organizations where numerous individuals have a part in patient care (Davis and Aroskar, 1978; Murphy, 1978). Although mention may be made of the fact that ethical principles are the same for all health care professionals, the sociology of ethical decision making rarely receives any in-depth attention.

Of all the individuals caring for patients in these complex institutions, nurses seem to have a special social position both vis-à-vis the patient and vis-à-vis the physician owing to the nursing role and the nature of nurses' relationships with patients and their families. Historically, as well as in the contemporary scene, nurses can find themselves in a middle position between the system and the patient or between the physician and the patient when ethical questions arise. The nurses are asked questions by patients and their families about care, medical decisions, informed consent, and competency of others which affect the patient's well-being.

Traditionally, nurses have been expected to act with moral passivity to ethical dilemmas or have been expected to join forces and close ranks with other health professionals in the name of loyalty to the institution and/or to the physician. As recently as 1977, a bioethicist discussing truth telling said that health personnel other than physicians should not get involved with ethical problems of truth telling since to do so might cause them to lose their jobs. This statement seems to assume at least two things: (1) the patient and physician exist in some sort of two-person relationship divorced from all other social interaction, and (2) all other health personnel such as nurses are some type of amoral robots who simply have an obligation to carry out orders and do their jobs more or less unquestioningly or to react with moral passivity when ethical conflict occurs. To people with firsthand experience of the sociology of bioethics in health care facilities the above statement not only does not reflect reality in many instances but it also raises some serious questions about the sociology of ethical decision making in these institutions.

Several major strains can be identified which create dissonance for hospital nurses when they confront ethical issues. First, it is staff nurses who often have the most contact with patients and who find themselves being questioned by these patients. Staff nurses also gather a great deal of information as to how patients view and experience a given situation. Do these nurses have an obligation to do something with the data collected, especially when they indicate that patients have questions about their care, do not fully understand what they have consented to, or have some doubts about the medical procedures being performed? What if patients suspect that the physician is withholding information about their diagnosis and/or prognosis? What should

the nurse do? By the very nature of the nurse-patient relationship in which patients give nurses information or raise questions and doubts, nurses are involved. To say that they should not get involved denies the reality of the situation. By their presence and their relationship with patients they are involved.

In the hospital bureaucracy, sociologically speaking, staff nurses are subordinate in the hierarchy of care givers. They are answerable to both medical and nursing authorities for their actions or lack of them. What if the nurse indicates to the physician that a patient is asking many questions about his or her illness (especially when information has been withheld from the patient) or that the patient has not given *informed consent*, and the physician does nothing to deal with the situation? Does the nurse have an obligation to do more? How far does one's obligation extend?

Another strain can develop when a staff nurse questions the ethics of nursing care performed by another nurse. If such a concern is brought out into the open, will the concerned nurse be seen as one who has "squealed" on a colleague and be shunned by the nursing staff? Will this nurse be labeled a troublemaker by the nursing administrator who has the power of the evaluation conference and report detailing the nurse's performance?

In short, what is the nature of the sociology of morals in a hospital? How can and should nurses deal with the possible strain between their professional ethical obligations and their employee status? How can they cope with the fact that they experience multiple loyalties or obligations to patients and their families, to the hospital, to the physician, and to their own professional standards and ethics? The Code for Nurses developed by the American Nurses Association (ANA) (1976) makes it clear that the nursing profession expects its members to have as their primary obligation the patient's well-being. How can and should nurses meet this expectation in light of their multiple loyalties and their own social position in the bureaucracy of the health care facility? Importantly, what is the role of the nursing administration in the nurse's attempt to practice according to the code? This last question, along with selected ethical principles and theories, provides the focus for this chapter. Before developing the focus on nursing administration, it might be fruitful to discuss selected ethical principles and the process of ethical reasoning. Such a discussion will indicate how individuals can think through an ethical problem in a more rational manner and move away from an emotional response or a righteous indignation stance which in the short run may be functional but in the long run may be counterproductive.

SELECTED ETHICAL PRINCIPLES

Autonomy is one of the most basic ethical principles in bioethics. It refers to personal liberty in which the individual has the right to determine his or her course of action in accordance with a plan chosen by himself or herself (Beauchamp and Childress, 1979:56). The autonomous individual deliberates on and chooses a plan of action and then acts on that plan. A truly autonomous person has the ability to act in an independent, self-reliant, and self-contained fashion to make his or her own decisions. In a broad sense, this means being one's own person. There are some situations which can act to diminish autonomy for a person. For example, institutionalized individuals such as prisoners or the mentally ill and retarded often experience a loss of autonomy.

The Patient's Bill of Rights developed by the American Hospital Association (1974) speaks to the autonomy of the patient in stating that the patient has the right to information, the right to give informed consent, and the right to refuse treatment to the extent permitted by law and to be informed of the medical consequences of this refusal. It makes the point that in order for patients to make decisions regarding medical care they must be informed. Without such data patients cannot act autonomously.

It has been common practice for those in the health care professions to violate the patient's autonomy in the name of his or her own good.

This action, called *paternalism*, has been the source of many problems including the lack of trust in relationships with patients. The English philosopher John Stuart Mill wrote on the issue of paternalism in general when he said in *Liberty* (1859) the sole end for which mankind is warranted, individually or collectively, in interfering with the liberty of action of any of their number is self-protection. Mill takes the very strong stance that an individual cannot rightfully be compelled to do or forebear because it will be better for him to do so, because it will make him happier, or because, in the opinion of others, to do so would be wise or even right. This means that the evil involved in advancing the individual's interest by compulsion outweighs the good done. Paternalism in which the use of coercion achieves a good that is not recognized as such by those persons for whom the good is intended obviously acts to diminish their autonomy.

Nonmaleficence, duty to do no harm, encompasses both intentional harm and the risk of harm (Beauchamp and Childress, 1979). Under this duty, intentional harm is prohibited except under special conditions such as self-defense. Risk of harm is allowed under many conditions provided the goals of the actions are sufficiently important to justify such behaviors. When situations of risk of harm arise, both ethical principles and the law recognize a standard of due care. What constitutes due care varies from time to time and place to place. The ANA code addresses the ethical principle of nonmaleficence in at least three ways. First, by stating that nurses should act to safeguard the client and the public when health care and safety are affected by the incompetent, unethical, or illegal practices of any person, it indicates that nurses have the duty to protect patients and others from possible harm. A second way that nurses guard patients from harm is to maintain competence in nursing, while a third way is to seek consultation.

Our ethical duty not only requires that we treat individuals as autonomous persons and not harm them but it also requires that we act to contribute to their well-being. This is the principle of *benefi-cence*. In everyday activities it is sometimes difficult to distinguish between noninfliction of harm and the production of benefits. As has been noted, "the duty to confer benefits and actively to prevent and remove harm is important in biomedical and behavioral contexts, and of equal importance is the duty to balance the good it is possible to produce against the harms that might result from doing or not doing the good" (Beauchamp and Childress, 1979: 136).

Another important ethical principle in bioethics is distributive justice, which comes into play when there is competition for resources or benefits. Essentially, distributive justice has to do with the distribution of both risks and benefits in a society. An underlying issue has to do with the criteria on which resources are fairly distributed among persons. The usual list of criteria includes: (1) to each an equal share, (2) to each according to individual need, (3) to each according to individual effort, (4) to each according to societal contribution, (5) to each according to merit. Some theories of justice accept all five of these principles, depending on what is being distributed.

Other ethical principles detailed in the bioethics literature are veracity or the duty to tell the truth and not to lie or deceive others and the rule of confidentiality. Both veracity and confidentiality are built into professional codes of ethics, including the Code for Nurses.

ETHICAL REASONING

A *normative ethical system* is an ordered set of moral standards and rules of conduct by reference to which, with additional factual knowledge of an event, one can determine in any situation of choice what a person ought or ought not do. Normative ethics attempts to justify one form of behavior over another and to determine the right-making characteristics of action for purposes of carrying out duties and obligations.

Two normative ethical systems are widely discussed and defended in contemporary moral philosophy. The first, *utilitarianism*, is a teleological system which holds that an action is morally right either if a person's doing it brings about good consequences or if the action is of a kind which, if everyone did it, would have good consequences. The basic concept is utility, that is, an act is right if it is useful. But one needs to ask the question, useful for what end? Unless we know the end to which something is to be judged as a means, we do not know how to decide whether it is useful or not. Utilitarianism provides the answer by saying that an act is right when it is useful in bringing about a desirable or good end for the most people, an end that has intrinsic value. By *intrinsic value* is meant the value that something has as an end in itself and not as a means to some further end. There are certain things that we value because of their consequences, such as going to the dentist (instrumental value), but which we do not value in themselves. On the other hand, there are certain experiences or conditions of life that we want to have and to enjoy for their own sake, such as friendship. Such experiences or conditions of life we judge to be intrinsically good. For us they have intrinsic value. The basic principle of utilitarian ethics is that the right depends on the good. In short, we can know whether an act is morally right only by finding out what its consequences are and then determining the intrinsic goodness or badness of those consequences. The moral rightness of an act is itself an intrinsic value. On the contrary, an act is right only when it is instrumentally good and its rightness consists in its instrumental goodness. The standard of intrinsic value by which utilitarians judge the goodness of the consequences of a right act is whether it brings about pleasure or happiness or prevents the bringing about of pain or unhappiness. No act is morally wrong in itself, but rather its wrongness depends entirely on its consequences.

The second normative ethical system is *ethical formalism*, which is a deontological system. Deontological theory holds that an action is right if it accords with a moral rule, wrong if it violates such a rule. Moral rules are based on an ultimate principle of duty. Deontologists hold that it is not the goodness or badness of the consequences of an action that makes it right or wrong but the kind of action it is. An action is right in this view if it is of a kind that all moral agents have an obligation to perform; it is wrong if it is one that all moral agents have an obligation to avoid. This is known as the *moral rule of conduct*, and deontologists believe that the ground of such obligation lies in the fact that the moral rule in question satisfies the requirements of an ultimate norm or supreme principle of duty. It is not a necessary or sufficient condition of a right action that it brings about good consequences.

Some moral philosophers hold that the grounds of right conduct are both teleological and deontological and that there is no single supreme principle from which, ultimately, the moral rightness or wrongness of every action can be derived. According to this view, referred to as *ethical pluralism*, the moral reasons for or against some action lie in the consequences of those actions, while the moral reasons governing other actions arise from their being of a kind required or prohibited by a rule of duty or obligation. Ethical pluralists argue that both sorts of reasons, in fact, can apply to one and the same action. Ethical pluralists weigh the comparative importance of these various reasons to see which reasons outweigh or override any other applicable to the given action. Sometimes the consequences of an action will be so bad that it ought not be done, despite an obligation to do it. At other times, the obligation will be sufficiently stringent to outweigh the badness of the consequences. Ethical pluralism recognized that we as individuals are concerned with both the means and ends of our ethical actions.

Nurses, like other health professionals, use ethical reasoning in determining their actions and often they do this with limited knowledge, if any, of formal ethical theories. This means that it becomes more difficult for them to articulate their ethical stance in ways that can be taken seriously by others. Rather, what often happens is that nurses have ethical concerns regarding a given situation but share it in an emotional manner which can be easily dismissed as not having grounding in knowledge and understanding of the situation.

Ethical dilemmas are situations in which conflicting moral claims occur. This can take various forms, such as a conflict between one's professional obligation and the rights of the patient or one's professional obligation and the limits imposed by one's employee status in which one is expected to follow orders. When a staff nurse confronts an ethical dilemma, what, if anything, should be done about the situation? And importantly, who should be involved in any ethical reasoning which might occur? Does nursing administration have a role grounded in ethical obligations?

THE ROLE OF NURSING ADMINISTRATION

It can be argued that nursing administration, ranging from the head nurse of a unit to the director of nursing, should assume an active role in the ethical issues which arise in a health care institution. Generally speaking, this leadership group should provide a climate in which ethical issues can be discussed in a formal arena. Such an activity has the potential to lessen the burnout problems of nurses who confront these ethical issues (Davis, 1979). Often ethical dilemmas by their very nature do not have easy answers. It is the continuing dialogue around these issues which can assist individuals to systematically view the profound and complex aspects of these situations and to come to realize that others experience similar conflicts as to what is the right thing to do from an ethical base.

Because of the power structure in health care institutions, in some instances individuals from nursing administration will need to take an active role in a given ethical dilemma. If a staff nurse approaches the head nurse, for example, with what she or he considers to be an ethical issue involving a patient and another health professional and over which this nurse believes her- or himself to have little input or control, then the head nurse has the ethical obligation inherent in the administrative-leadership role to collect data about the situation and to assist toward a solution. A solution may be something as simple as having the parties involved discuss their ethical justification for their decision. Not only is it counter-productive to blame another for what seem to be unethical actions, but without a full understanding of the other's ethical stance one could question the ethics of this blaming.

If certain patterns of actions develop which seem to be ethically questionable or which place nurses in what they perceive to be an unethical position vis-à-vis patients and their families, then again nursing administration has an ethical obligation to attend to this. This attention to a situation may entail suggesting to the nurses that they themselves deal directly with the situation but with the knowledge that they have support from the nursing leadership group. Nurses need to know that if they raise legitimate ethical questions about situations, they will not be viewed as "trouble-makers" and "nitpickers" but rather as concerned professionals who have an ethical obligation inherent in their role to be concerned about and to

actively attempt to deal with the ethics of any given situation.

All the above discussion assumes that nursing leadership has a grasp of ethical principles and theories to the extent that it can assume a leader-ship position in creating a climate which fosters dialogue on ethical issues and in dealing with specific ethical dilemmas. Since ethical issues arise in many of the daily activities of health professionals, and on the assumption these issues will continue to grow and become even more complex and exert a profound effect on nursing practitioners, it can be ethically argued that nursing administrators need to incorporate this body of knowledge into their repertoire of ex-pertise. Historically, books on nursing ethics were little more than concerns about etiquette and some aspects of the legal issues. More recently bioethics and nursing ethics have brought into focus the myriad ethical dilemmas, along with the ethical principles and theories to guide our actions. Nursing administrators have an important role in this most basic and human concern in-creasingly found in the health care arena.

EDITOR'S QUESTIONS FOR DISCUSSION

Discuss the extent to which nurses act with moral passivity to ethical dilemmas. What evidence is there from Reeder's study (Chap. 38) that might indicate nurses' tradi-tional patterns to act with moral passivity is changing? How true is the assumption that getting involved with ethical problems of truth-telling may cause a nurse to lose her job? What evidence is there for the two assumptions made by Davis regarding the statement of a bioethicist that nurses should not get involved with ethical problems of truth-telling? What factors may influence the degree to which nurses are assertive in resolving ethical issues? To what extent do nurses have an obligation to do some-thing with the information they collect from patients? How can nurses ethically cope with the multiple loyalties and obligations they experience? Provide examples of how nurses in service and education follow the ethical principles of veracity and con-fidentiality. Discuss whether or not there can ethically be exceptions to following those principles.

Provide examples as to how the ethical principle of autonomy is demonstrated in nursing service and education. What application and congruence is there between Davis's discussion of autonomy and the chapters by Bille (36) and La Monica (37)? Provide examples of where the patient's autonomy has been violated in the name of his or her own good. How can that type of paternalistic attitude and action be changed?

Are there situations where paternalistic attitudes and actions may be appropriate? How does one determine the risk of harm in providing care? What criteria are used to determine what constitutes due care? Provide examples as to how nurses carry out the ethical principle of nonmaleficence as addressed by the ANA Code for Nurses. What other ways and to what extent do nurses follow the principle of nonmaleficence? Discuss examples as to how the principle of beneficence should be applied with patients, students, peers, colleagues, and other health professionals. What criteria can be used to distinguish between noninfliction of harm and the production of benefits? Determine whether and/or how the good done can be balanced against harms that might result. Provide examples as to how nursing administrators in service and education actually do and/or should apply the five criteria of distributive justice. How do and should nursing staff and faculty apply the criteria in relationships with patients, students, peers, colleagues, and other health professionals?

What applications are there from Ketefian's chapter (19) to Davis's discussion of ethical reasoning? How are ethical stances formulated? What variables influence the development of any one normative ethical system? Discuss the impact of theology on the development of one's normative ethical system. Is there a relationship between a person's theological stance and the development of a normative ethical system? Provide examples where dissonance may or may not occur if there is a difference between a person's development theologically and his or her normative ethical system. How can conflicts be resolved should they occur? Debate whether or not as a norm it is possible to be value-free. To what extent does a person tend to be consistent in the application of any one normative ethical system?

Debate the principles between each of the normative ethical systems presented: utilitarianism, ethical formalism, and ethical pluralism. To what extent do you agree with the tenets of any one ethical system? Provide examples of each ethical system in nursing practice, education, and administration. Does a useful end for most persons always justify the means? Can the intrinsic and instrumental value be in conflict? Debate principles of alternative normative ethical systems.

What legal implications are there for nurses and other health professionals in each of the normative ethical systems? Provide specific examples in nursing practice, education, and research where application of any one of the normative ethical systems may result in potential conflict with the law. Determine in Walker's chapter (4) the examples of litigation and Bullough's chapter (45) where specific normative ethical systems may be evident.

What is the role of nursing administration in service and education concerning ethical obligations? What applications can be made between Davis's discussion and Ezell's chapter (6)? How can an administrative leader provide a climate for dialogue of ethical issues? What ethical implications are there for the administrator in the development of a particular ethical stance by nursing staff and faculty? Is it possible to separate one's own ethical stance from a given situation? To what extent should the ethical stance of an individual be respected? How can ethical conflicts between individuals be resolved? To what extent and under what conditions should the nursing administrator take an active role in a given ethical dilemma? Given a conflict between the ethical stance of two or more individuals in a situation brought to an administrator's attention, what criteria might be applicable as to whose ethical perspective should reign? Provide examples of ethical dilemmas in administration, how they were resolved, and the effectiveness of the resolutions.

REFERENCES

American Hospital Association
  1974 Statement on a Patient's Bill of Rights. Chicago: American Hospital Association.
American Nurses Association
  1976 Code for Nurses With Interpretative Statements. Kansas City, Mo.: American Nurses Association.
Bandman, E. L. and B. Bandman
  1978 Bioethics and Human Rights. Boston: Little, Brown.
Beauchamp, T. L. and L. Walters
  1978 Contemporary Issues in Bioethics. Encino, Calif.: Dickenson.
Beauchamp, T. L. and T. F. Childress
  1979 Principles of Biomedical Ethics. New York: Oxford University Press.

Davis, A. J.
  1977 "Ethical dilemmas and nursing practice." The Linacre Quarterly, 44:302–311.
  1979 "Ethics rounds with intensive care nurses." The Nursing Clinics of North America 14:45–56.
Davis, A. J. and M. A. Aroskar
  1978 Ethical Dilemmas and Nursing Practice. Englewood Cliffs, N.J.: Prentice-Hall.
Mill, J. S.
  1974 On Liberty. New York: Penguin (first published 1859).
Murphy, C. P.
  1978 "The moral situation in nursing," Pp. 313–20 in E. L. Bandman and B. Bandman (eds.), Bioethics and Human Rights. Boston: Little, Brown.

Chapter 48

Developing the Head Nurse Role—A Key to Survival in Nursing Service Administration

Maryann F. Fralic, R.N., Dr. P.H.
Assistant Professor
Department of Nursing Administration
School of Nursing
University of Pittsburgh
Pittsburgh, Pennsylvania

Following Davis's entreaty that the nursing administrator has a role in ethical issues, it is relevant to concentrate on the first-line nursing manager—the head nurse, who is the key person representing the organization to the staff. Maryann F. Fralic focuses on the development and maximization of the head nurse role. She argues that the past role and scope of the head nurse position is inadequate for today's needs and that traditional hierarchical structures weaken the authority and accountability, and defines the head nurse as a manager who has an integrator role. Fralic suggests the avenue by which clinical nurses may make the transition to professional management is primarily through the auspices of a staff development department.

Rationales provided for enlarging the range of the head nurse role are: the changing nature of the work and work force, the professionalization process in nursing, diminishing resources for professional nurses, declining applications in professional nurse programs, incongruity between educational and practice settings, and increasing complexities of health-care organizations. Problems such as recruitment and retention of nurses and the variation in the degree of professionalism of nurses and conflicts in managing professionals in an organization are cited. Fralic perceives the need to meet the problems/issues through explicit decision making, accountability, responsibility, and authority at the head nurse level. Specifically, she advocates flat organizational designs to fulfill today's needs. She asserts the head nurse should report directly to the level immediately below the chief nurse executive. Fralic maintains that the traditional supervisor nurse role should be supplanted with relevant staff support such as clinical experts.

Fralic reviews a research project which indicates head nurses are managers through performance in seven major areas of management. She discusses the difficulties of the role, which requires competency in human relations skills, clinical and technical skills, knowledge, and processes of management. The head nurse role is portrayed as a mediator of the environment, staff facilitator, and coordinator of the interdependencies in nursing service. Fralic outlines six transitions that must be made as a new head nurse. She urges the selection of head nurses through behaviors that appear to be predictive of management success.

Specific planning for management education as well as time to acquire the skills are advised. According to Fralic, the length, structure, and format for the program should be individualized to meet the needs of prospective head nurses and the resources of the organization. Elements deemed essential for a program include practicum-type experiences, preceptor-type relationships, and advanced continuing educational support to enhance knowledge and skills. Fralic views expanding the scope of the head nurse role as critical to the long-term organizational viability in nursing administration.

The focus of this paper is the preparation and utilization of the head nurse role—a rethinking of power and structure, a redefinition of roles, and a very necessary realignment of authority.

Nursing administrators have always been required to develop an effective construct for planning and delivering an appropriate level of nursing care in an organized setting. So what's new about that?

What's new is that it now must be done optimally! The margin for error is gone. Let's look at why this is true.

The nature and complexity of nursing service administration in hospitals is of intense interest today. The message is clear that performance must be continually improved despite diminishing resources. The realities of the cost-containment environment and the most serious issue of limited professional nurse supply are presented as clear examples of the imperative to "do more with less."

Yesterday's methods will not permit us to meet the new challenges; a harder look at our strengths and resources is required. Peter Drucker (1964) reminds us that effective business focuses on opportunities rather than problems. The opportunity, and indeed the requirement, exists to maximize the role of the head nurse. This role is particularly chosen since the first-line nursing manager, operating with appropriate responsibility and authority, is the key to the achievement of the organization's goals.

Enlarging the scope of the head nurse role is necessitated by the changing nature of the work force, the professionalization process in nursing, and the urgent need to maintain the attractiveness of hospitals as major employers of professional nurses. These few examples are illustrative of the acute need to develop head nurses as effective contemporary managers and key variables in the performance of the nursing service department. The obligation exists to capitalize on the individual and collective potential of the head nurse, providing a systematic program for deliberate management development. The complexities of health care organizations are increasing geometrically and have created a need for head nurses who are competent in deploying organizational resources, both human and material, and who share real accountability for organizational performance.

Nursing directors, behaving not unlike other managers, have tended to allocate time, effort, and resources to those problems which appear most pressing. Thus, we have structured differently in different settings to meet varying major objectives. Our past typical organizational structures frequently reveal an emphasis on a heavy supervisory layer and multiple levels performing various coordinative functions—with the head nurse role subordinate to them. Since such structures do not permit significant authority and responsibility, with so many administrative layers overhead, we created a "quasi manager" position as the functional role of the head nurse. This model has become unworkable today.

FORCES MANDATING CHANGE

Skillful administrators do not itemize organizational problems without some real thought to planning for their resolution. Key problems that come quickly to mind today—and likely will extend into the future—are nurse supply and retention, incongruence between the educational and practice settings with resultant reality shock, dwindling resources, and the changing nature of the work and the work force. Each of these factors has created alarming concern, causing us to scurry about seeking remedies. And if we take a long look ahead, we know that the scurrying will become even more intense!

Look, for example, at a major force impinging on nursing management today—diminishing resources. Let us look particularly at the scarcity of registered nurses. This situation is presently alarming, and predictions indicate that decreasing supply and increasing demand for registered nurses will intensify this situation. How will nursing service administration cope with this ominous reality? And it is ominous indeed, recognizing the escalating utilization of registered nurses in our acute care settings as patient care becomes increasingly more complex and intensified. And yet, a realistic look at declining applications, enrollment, and graduation from professional nurse programs foretells even greater future problems with nurse supply.

Happily, efforts are underway nationally to stimulate greater interest in nursing as a profession, and major recruitment efforts have begun. But a clear hard look at the future reveals fewer R.N.s generally, and in hospitals specifically—at least in the short run. Hospitals will get less than their traditional share of R.N.s as other settings actively compete for them. What a terrible thought—even fewer nurses or, at best, no more than we have today! The reality of that potential is sobering indeed.

The foresightful nursing administrator will be preparing the nursing organization for this eventuality. Obviously, a look at external forces is first and foremost: What is the source of our supply? Is it reliable? How can it be augmented? What will make us more attractive as an employer? What new relationships must be built with external sources? etc., etc. All those questions and many more must be raised and answered when scanning the external environment and its realities.

Of crucial importance, however, is the extremely critical and methodical analysis of the internal environment that must be undertaken. A basic approach in times of scarcity is to maximize all existing resources. As administrative eyes search the organizational structure, seeking key resources to be developed, they should come to rest upon the head nurse, that key first-line manager.

The potency of the head nurse role should be obvious but, unfortunately, it generally suffers from a "disuse atrophy." The perceptive nurse executive knows that the head nurse represents the organization to the staff. The head nurse in effect is the organization as perceived by the employee. The professional staff nurse, that very limited resource, relates directly to a head nurse who may largely affect the nurse's success or failure in the organization. We tend to forget this critical relationship as we spend huge sums on professional nurse recruitment efforts, always seeming to find expensive new gimmicks with which to entice the prospective employee. We forget, however, that those recruitment dollars may be wasted if the nurse entering the organization encounters an ineffective, inflexible, or nonsupportive first-line manager. And, conversely, the highly proficient head nurse can prove to be the key retention factor! Researchers are just beginning to explore this relationship, and it promises to be a fertile area for study. It seems entirely probable that the quality of direct supervision would prove to be the major independent variable in such studies.

EXPECTATIONS AND NEEDS OF TODAY'S PROFESSIONAL NURSE

The keen competition for professional nurses is illustrative of the alarming problems facing today's health care organizations. Effectively using the head nurse to ameliorate this situation is postulated as a basic and necessary approach to this problem.

When demand outstripped supply, we lost the luxury of complacency in our approach to management. Focus shifted from tolerating the vagaries and idiosyncracies of the manager to concentrating on the needs and expectations of the worker. The recalcitrant manager cannot be condoned—we must "sharpen up" all systems. The head nurse who precipitates or contributes to employee turnover generally, and professional nurse turnover particularly, will no longer be tolerated—certainly not in an era when most hospitals are identifying problems associated with attracting and maintaining excellence in nursing as their top priority. In such an environment, it is incumbent upon the first-line supervisor especially to adapt to the needs of the contemporary nurse-employee.

It is recognized that today's worker is different from the employee of yesterday. The contemporary worker expects good wages and working conditions—those are taken for granted. Other rewards such as quality of work life are sought from the work place today. This is generally true of all workers in all fields and certainly not restricted to health care workers. If you now overlay the additional expectations of the professional worker with higher levels of education and inner-directedness, things become quite complex (Raskin, 1979).

The head nurse is in a unique position to ma-

nipulate the variables in the work environment to accommodate the needs of the employees. Obviously, no intimation is made that the presence of patients merely accommodates staff—rather, how to prioritize the needs of patients while meeting needs of the staff is the real challenge to the head nurse.

A major challenge does arise when managing professionals. Inevitable sources of conflict exist between the professional and the organization, and these sources must be reconciled. For example:

- The organization seeks its own goals, and the professional seeks professional and personal goals.
- The organization must operate bureaucratically, with rules and regulations—the professional seeks autonomy.
- The organization has allegiance to its own standards while professionals come to the organization with allegiance to their profession's standards and their own skills.
- The organization sees the professional as a resource to be utilized—the professional sees the organization as a resource to be used while accomplishing professional and personal goals.

Illustrative of this entire phenomenon is a comment in a recent *New York Times* article. The headline of the article concerning newly graduated M.B.A.s makes the point very well— "Company Loyalty, They Feel, Is an Amusing Anachronism" (Campbell, 1980).

Watchwords of the nursing professional seem to be opportunities for creative flexibility, expanded participation in patient care decisions, and expanded recognition of professionalism and personal worth. The rigid, insensitive manager is anathema to these nurses. The resultant conflict may manifest itself in increased absenteeism, turnover, decreased productivity and morale, and other signs of worker alienation.

Now let's add a final complicating factor to this already difficult situation—the difference among nursing practitioners. Even though all nurses seek to call themselves professional, the degree of their professionalism varies. And this variation is not necessarily related to their respective generic educational programs. The point is that nurses will vary in the degree of professionalism that they bring to a work situation; some wish to be mainly autonomous and exhibit high degrees of self-direction while others perform work in a manner that is routinized and heavily task-oriented, not process-oriented. Thus, we further compound the management dilemma of the head nurse if even within the nursing group there are different degrees of professionals, each with differing expectations. For example, the nurse with a high professional orientation would eagerly respond to a joint practice or primary nursing environment, while the task-oriented nurse would prefer the security of a team or functional nursing care delivery system.

Such a detailing of worker expectations in managing such "mixed breeds" is both overwhelming and intimidating. However, it is "part of the territory" for today's head nurse. Actually, managers in all work settings are facing similar challenges and are responding to them—and so must we.

Only a few short years ago, measures which sought to accommodate the employee so pointedly would have seemed extraordinary indeed; today we must consider these approaches to be ordinary and necessary if we are to assure the long-term viability of our organizations. Development of the head nurse role must include a sensitivity to these issues and assistance in developing realistic management approaches to meeting worker expectations.

A CASE FOR FLATTENING THE HIERARCHICAL STRUCTURE

Departments of nursing traditionally have been depicted as tall hierarchical organizations. It cannot be denied that there is a certain efficiency to such structure. However, the head nurse role consequently is far removed from the locus of control. Functioning as a bona fide manager in this structure can be problematic for the head nurse—real decision making becomes diluted with so many layers of managers understandably seeking to justify their positional power. For example, the head nurse may be required to consult the supervisor, who consults a coordinator, who must discuss the issue with an assistant director, who talks to the associate director, who may finally discuss the matter with the director of nursing. This presents obvious problems with efficiency and timeliness as information and decisions travel up and down the chain of command. More importantly, the system fosters head-nurse dependence rather than self-direction. The danger exists that the nursing staff may view its own manager as a "message carrier," one who only relays the decisions of others, not one who makes decisions.

There is increasing dissatisfaction with old conventional hierarchies. Successful experimentation with flatter organizational structures is occurring with more frequency. The basic good sense that mandates the strengthening of the responsibility and authority of the head nurse dictates that traditional structures are unworkable. The increasing decentralization and dispersion of authority requires that appropriate power and responsibility be vested in the first-level manager. As a result, the role of the nursing supervisor has become increasingly unclear and ill-defined.

The need to strengthen the head nurse role presents a case against perpetuating and proliferating traditional nursing supervisors. Even though supervisors were essentially designed to support the head nurse administratively, they often serve as sources of frustration and ambiguity; this effect, however, is not necessarily a fault of the supervisor but rather an inevitable by-product of structure. It seems much more valid to keep management decision-making at the lowest possible level in the organization, i.e., with each head nurse insofar as is possible. Should we perhaps supplant supervisory line support with relevant staff support for the head nurse? For example, increasing the availability of clinical experts could provide an invaluable and highly appropriate dimension of support for head nurses, who must concentrate on developing management acumen and expertise. These comments are not intended to demean the traditional supervisor; rather, the point is made that traditional structures have made that job most difficult.

A more effective organizational design would have the head nurse reporting directly to an upper division nursing manager at the assistant-associate director level or the level below the chief nurse-executive. This provides for a more direct and unencumbered line of responsibility and authority; it also strongly encourages the maximum amount of decision making at the unit level.

It is clearly recognized that overall coordinative or integrative administrative functions are necessary in every organization. These positions should be developed deliberately within the nursing division without diluting the head nurse role and responsibility.

Certainly, no one structure is suggested for the department of nursing, since each organization must carefully scrutinize its own requirements and resources. The case is made, however, for enlarging the scope of the head nurse position and for eliminating unnecessary and often dysfunctional traditional supervisory levels.

ONE MORE TIME—IS THE HEAD NURSE REALLY A MANAGER

The very fact that this question is raised periodically and repeatedly is indicative of the problem. It is generally acknowledged that the head nurse does indeed manage patient care—but is he or she really a manager in the customary sense? We have generally been quick to defend the management title but reluctant to provide the structure and confer the authority and power needed to really manage.

The management of the overall level of nursing practice within a patient unit is indeed the responsibility of the head nurse (this is as distinguished from the responsibility of the staff nurse to manage the efforts of a nursing team). Inherent

in accepting accountability for overall patient care levels is the acknowledgment that legitimate management, in the fullest sense, must occur. The head nurse must be viewed, and must view him- or herself, as a bona fide manager within the institution.

The fact that the head nurse actually is a manager was established in a research project (Sherman, 1975) which studied nurses in supervisory positions to see if they actually were performing the work of management. The study utilized the seven major functional areas of management that theorists generally agree upon, namely:

Planning
Organizing
Staffing
Leading
Communicating
Decision making
Controlling

Within the seven functional areas 101 tasks (specific activities) were identified. The assumption was that if a nurse does the tasks of management across all seven functional areas and with some regular frequency, then indeed she or he is a manager (a manager being defined as one who performs the tasks of management).

The head nurses in this study provided hard evidence that they are true managers as defined by the tasks which they perform. The study revealed that 77.2 percent of the "core tasks" of management were performed regularly by head nurses. The researcher concluded that the head nurse clearly performed the management function and was unquestioningly as much a manager as those in any other field.

WHY IS THE JOB SO DIFFICULT— AND SO IMPORTANT!

Sasser and Leonard capsulize the inherent difficulties of the first-level manager as follows:

Performing well as a first-level supervisor is like walking the circus high wire. In both positions, the ability to maintain one's balance when shifting forces pull in opposite directions is a measure of one's success. First-level supervisors must be able to harmonize the demands of management, the demands of the collective work force (often represented by unions), and the demands of workers with the requirements for doing the tasks at hand. These needs are more often than not conflicting and even at times mutually exclusive. First-level supervisors usually have mixed emotions about their situation and often lose their sense of identity as they try to perform this precarious balancing act. Today these supervisors are part of management, but chances are they were once among the employees they are now trying to supervise. Although first-level supervisors have the responsibility for implementing the goals of upper management, their organizational authority to carry out the necessary actions is frequently unclear and often insufficient. By allowing these lowest-level managers to use the levers of influence inherent in their position, higher-level managers will be improving the performance of the whole organization (1980:113).

The authors further proceed with the following observation:

Being a first-level supervisor is one of the most difficult, demanding, and challenging jobs in any organization. Buried in an organizational web, this person must be adroit at administering a unit and at perceiving which, among all the daily tasks delegated downward, are the most important to accomplish. Through such administrative competence, he or she must be able to link the unit's accomplishments to the functioning of other organizational subunits (1980:113).

Many factors combine to make the job a difficult one. The societal changes reflected in the nature of the work force are illustrative of these forces. For example, in the past, a safe assumption would be that the worker was dedicated to the job, the department, and the employer. Today, attitudes and values of a multiple-generation worker base complicate the management role. Additionally, the educational level of the work force continues to rise—the manager often will not maintain an educational advantage over the worker.

Human relations skills are increasingly important for the first-level supervisor. The work force is no longer made up of conformists who support management's rules and regulations without question. Indeed, they are more likely to ask "How will you fit into my goals?" rather than ask, as formerly, "How can I fit into this organization's goals?". Seeking congruence between the goals of the organization and the worker's personal and professional goals is a new responsibility for managers (Fralic, 1980).

Technical competence is another imperative for the head nurse who must be able to perform specific tasks in the clinical area and also must understand the processes and technologies being managed. Appropriate technical skills are also necessary to deal with the many specialists needed to accomplish the unit's objectives and to appropriately train subordinates in their tasks (Sasser and Leonard, 1980).

As the head nurse "sits" in a very pivotal position structurally—between the upper management level and the work force—a key function is managing the conflict between the two groups. This is more complicated as traditional authority has decreased and dependency on others to get the job done has increased. Also, some customary operating levers have been lost or have been eroded over time. Formerly, for example, the head nurse would be instrumental in picking and choosing staff nurses—the scarcity of nurses has severely limited this prerogative. Also, in some settings, there are more constraints on the management freedom of job assignments and disciplinary procedures.

A major and frequently underestimated difficulty for the head nurse is the role as mediator of the environment, i.e. housekeeping, dietary, medical staff, laundry services—the list seems endless! The significance of this role is critical since these areas are outside of the head nurse's direct authority, yet they are vital to the effective and efficient delivery of nursing services. The interdependencies are obvious, and their coordination is key to managerial success. It is never pleasant to be responsible for factors over which we have little or no control.

Aside from the various interdepartmental mediating functions, there also are intradepartmental coordinative functions. Various staff support systems, i.e., nursing audit, patient education, and staff development, require mediation efforts since they, too, are seeking to establish a power base, influence the job, and protect their areas of expertise. These "specialists" are responsible for "parts of" the head nurse's job.

These situations are illustrative of the integrator role that has emerged as a new management function—the challenge of high differentiation and simultaneously high integration. The integrator must achieve the unity of effort among the major functional specialists in the environment. The integrator must handle the nonroutine and unprogrammed problems that arise among the various groups and also resolve interdepartmental conflicts and facilitate decisions of various magnitude. Questions then follow regarding what authority the integrators should have and how they get it (Lawrence and Lorsch, 1967). These are relatively new problems for nursing service administrators to consider.

This point is further illustrated by Miles's maxim which states, "The responsibility of every manager exceeds his authority, and if he tries to increase his authority to equal his responsibility, he is likely to diminish both" (Miles, 1979:5). He amplifies by stating that each manager is responsible for effective, economical, and expeditious results; however, no managers should demand or expect to have all the necessary organizational resources and full authority over policies and personnel under their personal command and

control. The head nurse role provides ample illustration of this reality.

Let us consider again, for emphasis, a central variable affecting the performance of the head nurse—the changing nature of the work force. People view their jobs and their employers differently today (Campbell, 1979). This is a highly significant observation since the successful manager knows that human resources comprise the most valuable resource in any organization. And the head nurse manages human resources of "mixed breeds," assuming responsibility for various groups of professional and nonprofessional workers. All of them, however, are challenging the traditional rigidities of the work place and work itself has lost its former primacy in their scale of values. The general trend of workers is to demand more participation in decisions involving their work, more variety in their tasks, and more challenging growth opportunities.

Professional workers' expectations are even more complex. They seek meaningfulness and achievement from their work and they define these very individualistically. They also seek responsibility, knowledge of results, and a real voice in the structure of their work. Formerly, the head nurse could unilaterally and autocratically determine the care delivery system to be employed on the nursing unit. Today she or he wisely assumes a facilitator role with the staff. The astute manager knows that not all change occurs in a "top down" manner; some change is highly legitimate if it issues from the opposite direction. For example, if the professional staff expresses interest in a nursing care delivery system that is new but within the resources and standards of the organization, the astute head nurse would ask, "How can I help you?". Such flexibility has become necessary with a finite and professional staff.

The picture emerges of a head nurse role that is complex, changing, and extremely challenging. With such pivotal functions and responsibilities, it becomes clear that more attention must be focused on the importance of appropriately developing this role. Head nurses will continue to be essential. Even with primary nursing systems, the unit-based manager remains necessary. Some would argue that the professional nurse is quite capable of pursuing patient care goals independently; this is unquestionably true. However, only the manager pursues the organization's goals and coordinates organizational effort.

When considering the importance of competent head nurses to an organization, they should be viewed as a most valuable nonrenewable resource (Rosow, 1979). That is, they are commonly a combination of institutional experience, institutional loyalty, sound clinical judgment, and managerial ability.

HOW CAN WE DEVELOP THE MANAGEMENT CAPABILITY OF HEAD NURSES?

Common practice has been to promote the best clinical nurse to the role of head nurse. We are quickly realizing the fallacy of this approach. Even with the best candidate, role transition problems are inevitable and must be ameliorated. Silber and Sherman (1974) describe this dilemma of leaving the technical (staff nurse) culture and entering the management (head nurse) culture. They indicate the following transitions that must be made as the new head nurse "crosses over" the bridge from technician to professional manager:

- The movement is from a technical (clinical nursing) specialty to a management specialty
- The movement is made from the subordinate culture to management culture (no longer one of the work group, but now its leader)
- Where the technician could "follow the book," the manager must write new charters
- The movement from a proscribed job as a technician, to the freedom and ambiguity of the manager role
- Where you were formerly paid for hours worked, you are now paid for results
- There is relative safety in the technician world and risk and exposure in the world of the

professional manager—instead of receiving expert answers in crisis situations, you will now be expected to provide those answers

It is fairly obvious that the transition to head nurse, under the best circumstances, will be difficult and requires much deliberate effort and planning.

A logical starting point is with good selection procedures. Sherman lists the following behaviors as predictive of management success: an orientation towards achievement and results, interpersonal skills, the ability to derive satisfaction from the development of others, and a healthy desire to exercise appropriate power (1975:18). The literature does not report any association between type of basic nursing preparation and prediction of success in management; rather, those predictors already mentioned appear more reliable. I would add to those the qualities of maturity (not necessarily age-related), a sense of humor, and an ability to adapt to new and ever-changing job demands.

Following the selection process and appointment to the management role, a plan must be developed to provide core content in management in combination with addressing individually personalized developmental needs. (Actually, experienced head nurses require similar education if none was provided for them initially.)

Dinsmore (1975) refers to the Four R's—results, resources, requisites, and responsibilities—as fundamentals of managerial performance.

Results are defined as what happened or what was achieved. The very important point is made that subordinates must be informed of the results that the manager is seeking—then both can move in the same direction, augmenting each other's efforts.

The improvement and enlargement of resources, particularly those directly related to responsibilities and results, are also central to the manager's role.

Requisites are described as the fundamental factors which can be measured and controlled and appear to have the most significant influence on achievement levels. Examples are hiring, firing, and retaining.

Responsibilities in this context relate to minimizing the possibility of conflict between individual responsibilities and those of the organization.

Specific planning for management education is required if head nurses are to have the necessary tools with which to manage. This first requires broad and general management information, planned by persons with management expertise. Sufficient time must be devoted to the acquisition of management skills. It is extremely unfair to criticize a head nurse's deficient performance as a manager when she or he has never been appropriately prepared to be one! The length, structure, and format of the course should be individualized and tailored to the participant's needs and the organization's resources.

Once the basic information has been taught, ongoing educational support must be planned. The level of programming should become increasingly sophisticated so that there can be continued advancement of knowledge and skills. Regularly scheduled, appropriately spaced, and carefully planned educational sessions are certainly more desirable than the random and haphazard approach commonly employed.

It seems particularly essential to provide a practicum-type experience for the new head nurse. We must abandon the practice of expecting people to function effectively as head nurses after only a brief and perfunctory orientation period. As we look at other major industries, we see a very long, deliberate, and programmed preparation for the management role, sometimes involving a series of preparatory jobs. We obviously cannot afford that luxury; however, a substantial preceptor-type relationship with an experienced and capable head nurse seems essential. The practicum should be formalized and accomplished under the auspices of the staff development department. This time period should be considered to be an inviolable developmental period for the beginning management practitioner.

The perceptive nurse administrator will provide a comprehensive program to develop the management skills of new and existing head nurses. This assumes that they deserve trust and support as key managers and that their authority will be expanded appropriately as responsibilities increase. Care also must be taken that suitable rewards accompany this increased responsibility.

Too often the head nurse role is viewed as punitive, not rewarding. For example, head nurses may complain that salaries of some staff nurses may surpass their own; they also report instances of having to work additional shifts if staff members are unwilling to do so. This blurring of manager-subordinate roles precludes the development of a real sense of affiliation with management and commitment to that role by the head nurse. The responsibilities of the job are much more willingly accepted if there is a discernible reward structure. New types of reward systems are emerging. For example, a future benefit is projected to be employer-financed sabbaticals for purposes of mid-career self-inquiry. We must begin to consider such nontraditional approaches if we are to continually enrich the manager's role.

The nursing director is the key element in providing the impetus and developing an effective structure for preparing and maintaining effective unit-level managers.

RESULTS OF THE FOCUS ON HEAD NURSE DEVELOPMENT

As power is decentralized in an organization, individual managers must exercise more independent decision making. In a supportive environment, this results in management growth and an increase in confidence and self-esteem. Managers learn to trust their own judgment, becoming more decisive and garnering genuine staff support.

Competent head nurses also have highly positive effects on upper management in nursing and the organization as a whole. As they become more autonomous, they require less supervision. They can make their own decisions in many areas that would require several levels of intervention in a tall, rigid hierarchical structure. The benefit to the organization is that it gains their trust, their support, and their effectiveness. This, in turn, facilitates overall staff effectiveness, staff satisfaction, and the achievement of departmental and organizational goals.

Expanding the scope of the head nurse role is crucial if we are to assure our long-term organizational viability in nursing service administration. This new breed manager is urgently needed in our contemporary and future health care organization.

EDITOR'S QUESTIONS FOR DISCUSSION

How much congruence might there be regarding the expanded scope and preparation for the head nurse role as presented by Fralic and views expressed by Sills (Chap. 42) and Klein (Chap. 43)? Would Sills consider "clinical experts" as "relevant staff support" for the head nurse as suggested by Fralic? To what extent is there agreement between Klein and Fralic regarding the potential of "typical" hospital staff development programs? How much consensus does there appear to be between Williamson (Chap. 5) and Fralic regarding the basic education of clinical staff nurses? Comparing the discussion and editor's questions posed in Sills' (42) and Klein's (43) chapters, and Fralic's presentation, what distinctions or potential conflict are apparent among the roles of the clinical nurse specialist, primary nurse, and head nurse?

What is the relationship between the professionalization process in nursing and Fralic's perceived need to enlarge the scope of the head nurse role? What positive and negative outcomes may be predicted in expanding the scope of the head nurse role? What considerations are essential in planning for the potential maximation of existing resources? How can an expanded role of the head nurse cope with reality shock of staff nurses, which Fralic suggests is related to the incongruence between educational and practice settings? What empirical evidence exists as to variation in the degree of professionalism among nurse practitioners? What are the implications for the profession, as suggested by Fralic, if the variation is not necessarily related to the respective generic educational programs of the practitioner? What empirical investigation might be proposed? How can the nurse executive appropriately assess the professional qualifications, ability and potential of the staff for managerial positions? How can the head nurse appropriately assess the professional ability and potential of his/her nursing staff? What suggestions can be offered to accommodate for the different degrees of professionalism, expectations, and needs in an organization? To what extent should this be done for professional staff and personnel?

What is the effect of hierarchical structure of an organization and administrative efficiency? What criteria can be suggested for measuring the effectiveness of organizational designs in achieving primary goals? How might reliable and valid criteria for measurement best be established? Debate the pros and cons of decentralized organizations where significant management decision making is made by the first-level manager. How is communication of decisions most effectively made and conveyed to higher levels of management and to nursing staff?

What other factors than indicated by Fralic influenced the "traditional" role of the head nurse to become dysfunctional? How has the nature of the work, personnel resources, and environment changed in practice settings? What impact has the change had on the quality of patient care, nursing and hospital administration and other health care professionals? What impact has the unit manager had on the traditional role of the head nurse? What empirical evidence exists for the effectiveness and role of the head nurse? What empirical evidence exists as to the head nurse being a significant variable in the retention of staff nurses? What are the most effective means for recruitment and retention of professional nursing staff?

How different is the expanded role of the head nurse in specific qualifications and functions as proposed by Fralic from the traditional role? How might the head nurse be in a unique position to reconcile the four sources of conflict, indicated by Fralic, that exist between the professional and the organization? To what degree does the scope and method of performing the seven management functions vary from the first-line level manager through to the chief nurse executive?

What implications are there in Fralic's description of the needed transitions by a new head nurse as a "technician to professional manager"? How significant is the use of the term "technical (clinical nursing) specialty" for professional clinical practice and management today? What assumptions appear to exist concerning the essential preparation of the professional nurse manager?

Discuss Fralic's essential elements for a program to develop head nurses? How might head nurses be best prepared for the "integrator" role? What additional content and preparation should be included? Discuss Davis's chapter (47) and provide examples of the unique position the head nurse had regarding ethical issues. Respond to Davis's and the editor's questions raised for discussion that specifically apply to the role of the head nurse. What application may be made from the chapters by Williamson (5), Santora (8), O'Connor (13), Fawcett (14), Newman (28), and Roy (34) for professional preparation of the head nurse? What other previous chapters have specific implications for the development of the head nurse? What empirical evidence exists regarding reliable and valid predictors of management success? What other issues should be considered in developing the head nurse role?

REFERENCES

Campbell, Earnest G.
1979 "Are you hiring obsolete managers?" S.A.M. Advanced Management Journal Autumn: 33–38.
1980 "Company loyalty, they feel, is an amusing anachronism." The New York Times.

Dinsmore, Francis W.
1975 Developing Tomorrow's Managers Today. New York: AMACOM (a Division of the American Management Association).

Drucker, Peter F.
1964 Managing for Results. New York: Harper & Row.

Fralic, Maryann F.
1980 "Nursing shortage: Coping today and planning for tomorrow." Hospitals 54, 9:65–67.

Lawrence, Paul R. and J. W. Lorsch
1967 "New management jobs: The integrator." Harvard Business Review 12:142–51.

Miles, Tufus, E., Jr.
1979 "Miles's Six Other Maxims of Management." AMA Management Digest 11,6: 4–8.

Raskin, A. H.
1979 "Management challenges in the 21st century." S.A.M. Advanced Management Journal Autumn:25–32.

Rosow, Jerome M.
1979 "The coming management population explosion." S.A.M. Advanced Management Journal Autumn:4–16.

Sasser, W. Earl, Jr. and Frank S. Leonard
1980 "Let first-level supervisors do their job." Harvard Business Review 58,2:113–121.

Sherman, V. Clayton
1975 Nursing and the Management Function. Unpublished Dissertation. Western Michigan University, Kalamazoo, Michigan.

Silber, Mark and V. Clayton Sherman
1974 Managerial Performance and Promotability: The Making of an Executive. New York: AMACOM (a Division of the American Management Association).

Chapter 49

The Nursing Administrator: Advocate or Adversary

Sue T. Hegyvary, R.N., Ph.D., F.A.A.N.
Associate Dean/Assistant Vice President
Rush Presbyterian-St. Luke's Medical Center
Chicago, Illinois

Following Fralic's discussion of the first-line manager, the head nurse, it is essential to call attention to the roles of nursing administrators at the higher levels of management. The first-line managers cannot fulfill their role nor achieve the goals of the institution without the support and structure of upper-level management. Sue T. Hegyvary portrays the nursing administrator as one who does make a difference in nursing care. The concepts, principles, and examples illustrated can also be applied in administration of nursing education.

Hegyvary clarifies concepts and reviews the historical stages of administration. She discusses trends that have influenced changes in the roles of nursing administrators, professional nursing practice, and views of leadership. Considerable attention is paid to the Rush-Medicus studies of quality of nursing care and primary nursing. Hegyvary asserts that current perceptions of administration tend more toward controlling than serving, but successful administrators balance the needs for flexibility in clinical practice and predictability in organizational management through their style of leadership.

In describing the evolution of administration she points out that bureaucracies are necessary, although the problems of clinical practitioners in a bureaucratic setting are cited. Hegyvary indicates the influence of the scientific management school: its emphasis on productivity, standards, task analysis, nursing, and patient care. In essence, she views the human relations movement as a completion of a current triad in management: structure, process, and outcome. The bureaucracy defined structures, scientific management focused on outcomes, and human relations emphasized behavioral processes. Hegyvary maintains a countertrend had to occur in which no one element of the management triad was emphasized more than another. Thus, the rationalistic, open systems model evolved, in which all types of interrelated variables within an organization are considered in relation to its environment. She believes it is essential for nursing administrators to integrate methods of management, the clinical practice base, and their leadership style conducive for high quality professional nursing practice.

Significant trends in the genesis of management roles and perspectives are the development of nursing administrators as a colleague in nursing practice, the issue of quality assurance, and the evolution of primary nursing. Evaluation of the quality of nursing care has focused on either structure, outcomes, or processes, but rarely combining all three variables. One of a series of the Rush-Medicus studies of quality of nursing care focused on an operational definition of the nursing process. Six categories containing 33 variables were selected for study on 104 clients in 19 hospitals. Hegyvary reports that the quality of the nursing process was significantly related to all six categories: hospital characteristics, unit organizational structure, perceptions of unit and supervisory staff, leadership style, and nursing education. The greatest impact was unit organizational structure. Other findings showed that the highest quality units had: a more open, flexible leadership style; a higher level of clinical orientation by the staff; and higher staff satisfaction. Hegyvary suggests implications of the findings for the nursing administrator. Essentially, nursing performance requries a clear not global definition. There is no one specific approach or set of variables that can best be used to address the issue of quality of care. The variables that correlate with the quality of care cover the scope of administrative responsibility. Hegyvary compares and relates the structure, outcome, and process variables included in the study with each of the stages of management development. She suggests that the rational, open-systems approach to quality of care studies is the most comprehensive for inclusion of all the major variables.

Hegyvary portrays primary nursing as the epitome of professional practice. It requires accountability, autonomy, a decentralized structure for decision making, and responsibility for patients over time. As a result a new style of leadership is required by administrators for the primary nurse to have authority to fulfill the responsibilities. She views the primary nurse as the prime decision maker, with the head nurse being a resource person or a colleague who also has primary patients. Supervisors are not necessary, but the role of director changes in a number of major ways. The director needs to provide the structure and support to permit professional practice, interpret, and promote changes related to primary nursing to the medical staff, establish alliances based on patient care, and ensure adequate patient support services. Hegyvary reports studies of clinical management and leadership style. Structuring expectations is reported as a central factor in leadership. Findings from the Rush-Medicus study revealed that the highest-quality units were characterized by leaders described as high in tolerance, sensitivity, and role assumption, and low in the degree of structure. Hegyvary concludes that the norms set, accepted, or condoned by nurses are the key to professional practice. The professionalization of nursing demands leaders who are colleagues and advocates.

The old days of the "snoopy supervisor" are over. Or are they? How do care-giving nurses react to the presence of a supervisor or director of nursing on their units? Are they colleagues on the same team, or is it "we against they"? The answers to those questions vary across institutions and even within the same institution or unit. The real question is whether the administrator makes any difference.

This chapter discusses the nursing adminis-

trator as one who can, should, and usually does make a difference in nursing care. The difference can be all variations of positive or negative. The central theme of this discussion is that nursing administration can enhance or inhibit professional nursing practice. The focus is on upper level management, i.e., directors and assistants, though many concepts, principles, and examples apply to middle and front-line management as well. While the discussion and examples refer to administrators in nursing practice, usually hospitals, the same considerations could likely be applied in nursing education.

To begin the discussion, we first will clarify some basic concepts of administration and the nursing administrator. The next section is a review of the focus and style of leadership, including a brief historical review. Some observations specific to the nurse as administrator will be reviewed as a basis for looking toward the future.

THE CONCEPT OF ADMINISTRATION

The root of the word administer is a Latin word meaning "to serve." To administer means to "have charge of as chief agent in managing, as public affairs; conduct, direct" (McKechnie, 1977:25). Current perceptions of administration frequently tend more toward controlling than serving. Can one control and direct but at the same time serve? Some studies of leadership would suggest that it is not only possible but essential for stability and effectiveness. How often it happens is another issue.

Nursing administration presents an interesting composite of demands. The nursing administrator is responsible for the work of a group of clinical practitioners in a bureaucratic setting. That situation already denotes potential sources of conflict comparable to the professional-bureaucratic dilemma described in other areas of work, such as that of scientists in industry.

The hospital is a highly bureaucratic organization. Even with changes in industry toward human relations and a more open-systems approach, hospitals retain rather rigid structures and resist change (Georgopoulos, 1972:16–22). At the same time, nurses talk a great deal about client or patient-centered care, implying flexibility in routines and exercise of professional judgment. The greater the demand for flexibility and judgment by the nurse, the greater the potential conflict with the rules and regulations that characterize the bureaucratic focus.

The degree of conflict and the nature of the resolution depend on the people involved, the consistency of their philosophy and goals, and their views on nursing actions and patients' rights. Thus, the nursing administrator continuously juggles two parts: the need for flexibility in clinical practice and the need for predictability in organizational management. The former is essential for humane care; the latter is necessary to avoid chaos.

Successful performance of this juggling act requires not only considerable knowledge and skill but also the element of style. Part of one's leadership style is a function of personality; part of it can be learned through education and experience. The successful nursing administrator clearly lives in the eternal triangle of clinical practice, organizational management, and leadership style. Each of these concepts will be discussed in greater detail in later sections, with particular attention to studies of leadership and management.

EVOLUTION OF NURSING ADMINISTRATION

The nature of activities and priorities of nursing administrators cannot be separated from the work place itself—the hospital or other agency that provides patient care. A review of some stages of development of health care institutions gives a view of the concurrent evolution of nursing administration.

The military and religious origins of health care institutions are well known and in fact still are obvious in many countries. The rigidly structured, hierarchical, dogmatic style that plagues many institutions today often is attributed to or blamed on those traditions. While some of that argument is true, using it as an excuse for current stagnation is like the adult delinquent blaming his childhood for all his criminal actions!

Further, one can cite some hospitals operated by the military or by the church that are far more flexible, humane, and progressive than many other public or private hospitals. Clearly, the problem is not with the military or the church per se. Problems arise whenever rigid attitudes, dogmatic authority, and the priority on rules and regulations are so ingrained that the form, the bureaucracy itself, takes precedence over the substance of professional values.

Current styles of organizational management have evolved from numerous forces. The evolution of nursing administration can be linked to many general organizational forces as well as to characteristics of nursing as an occupational group. Let us review our roots, starting with a definition of bureaucracy, to attempt to see what that means for the present and future.

Focus on the Institution

The bureaucracy has a bad reputation in the modern world. In fact, we now refer to such creatures as "complex organizations" instead, perhaps hoping to alleviate some of the negative taste. But bureaucracies are a necessary fact of life in the industrialized world. How could we manage huge enterprises, such as industries, universities, or medical centers, without: (1) some delineation of lines of authority and communication; (2) some kind of division of labor, with people trained for various special skills; (3) an administrative staff to maintain order and keep up with all the rules and regulations of other bureaucracies; (4) a norm of impartiality and fairness in decisions; (5) the ever-present file system? Those characteristics of a bureaucracy were defined more than 100 years ago by Max Weber, a German economist (Newman et al., 1972:8). Weber's work is a classic in the development of organizational theory. He was a man far ahead of his time—seeing and thinking what others had not yet had the insight to define.

His ideas caught on fast, particularly as the industrial revolution gained full momentum. Businesses and industries grew and along with them "the bureaucracy," with strong emphasis on "the institution." By the early part of this century, Weberian ideas and definitions were applied with great zeal.

Unfortunately, they were applied a bit too zealously. Merton (1969:47–58) described the result as the dysfunctions of bureaucracy. In essence, the means—that is, the structure and lines of communication, became the ends in themselves. The purpose of the organization became lost in the red tape as petty bureaucrats placed more emphasis on position and procedure than on purpose. Does this sound familiar? It still persists today in many organizations, though another stage evolved in the first decade of the twentieth century.

The Productivity Stage

The excessive focus on institutional structure clearly was out of place in booming industries that needed to churn out products and profits. So then came "scientific management," with the focus on productivity. A major theorist in this school, Frederick W. Taylor, and his colleagues had a major impact on industrial development by introducing methods of critical analysis and careful evaluation of problems and processes.

They set up standards and specifications for machines, raw materials and procedures. They made quality control checks. They emphasized preventive maintenance of equipment. They carefully selected and trained workers for specifically designed jobs. They introduced assignments to workers, production schedules, and methods for dispatching and transporting materials and products. Then they used time studies to set standards for a day's work (Newman et al., 1972:7).

Their work revolutionized every business or industry it touched. Task analysis became the order of the day. Every activity was analyzed and defined step by step to ensure a standard procedure and a standard product. Workers then were trained to perform the tasks step by step without variation.

Before moving on to the next stage, let us stop and consider the situation at that time in hospitals and nursing. It was far behind that of industry. Many hospitals were still centers of charity, and techniques of patient care were still very limited.

Physicians directed most hospitals; the lay hospital administrator was almost unknown.

Much of nursing care was provided in patients' homes until hospitals grew in such prolific numbers. Then it was necessary to provide nurses around the clock and to organize the work of nursing. With nursing at a low educational and occupational level, with the military and religious orders being quite rigid and beyond questioning, and with the gradual influence of task analysis and concepts of productivity, the response of nurses was natural and predictable.

They organized the work in keeping both with tradition and with the current trends. Schedules were set up for routine activities; tasks were defined in step-by-step detail; training programs were based on these orderly procedures and tasks. More than half a century later, this approach still prevails in many hospitals and even in some schools of nursing.

The Discovery of Human Relations

It would seem that hospitals should have had a more humanistic approach than industries simply because of the nature of their services and clientele. But the human relations movement came straight out of industry. A study that began as another analysis of productivity in the school of scientific management resulted in a landmark report on motivation of workers (Newman et al., 1972). This and subsequent studies, combined with social and economic conditions in the era of the great depression, led to increasing attention to the people involved in organizations.

The human relations era was characterized by its emphasis on behavioral concepts, as opposed to the institutional focus of the bureaucratic era and the stress on productivity in scientific management. Are these concepts in opposition to each other? If we examine them closely, they in fact are another version of a current trichotomy—structure, process, and outcome. The bureaucracy defined structures; scientific management focused on outcomes and how to produce them; human relations emphasized behavioral processes.

Each focus was a response to conditions and forces in effect at the time. As the pendulum went too far in one direction and social or economic conditions changed at the same time, a countertrend had to occur. Each stage made an important contribution to the current view of organizations and their management.

What was happening in nursing during the human relations era? Some nursing took place in the community but increasing emphasis was placed on hospital care. And hospitals seemed to be stuck back at the bureaucratic stage, with a bit of lagging influence of task analysis. Meanwhile, nurses became interested in higher education, and the "educators" split off from the "service people." Barely a dent has yet been made in that tradition!

Nursing administrators were the "directors of nurses," generally functioning in the structured, centralized manner of hospitals. Although words such as patient-centered or family-centered care, even comprehensive care, would have been consistent with the human relations movement, they did not appear until much later. Nor did the emphasis on working conditions, job satisfaction, and staff morale become widespread until very recent years.

Clearly, in a rational and complex system one cannot look exclusively at psychosocial processes any more than one can restrict the view to structures or outcomes. That realization led to a new concept in modern organizational management.

The Rationalistic, Open Systems Model

The concept of the *open system* evolved as a way of looking at all types of interrelated variables within an organization as well as the relationship between an organization and its environment. Typical of this approach is definition of a model to depict factors in the organization and how they relate to each other. Of course, the model can be restricted to one particular part of the organization, such as a problem on a patient care unit or a problem of traffic flow through x-ray.

Many of the techniques used in analyzing such problems grew out of scientific management, i.e., the detailed analysis of tasks or problems. Studies of nursing activities conducted from the perspective of operations research often proceed in this direction. While such studies may be very useful to the nursing administrator, they also may be technically sophisticated approaches that require considerable time and money and still miss the point.

For example, studies of staffing for patient care units in hospitals have been a favorite topic for years. Computer models have been generated so that shift-to-shift changes in staffing can be made from unit to unit. The central idea in that approach is to quantify the workload by shift and allocate staff accordingly. The sensible nursing administrator (and likely the sensible operations researcher) will see immediately that there are more questions raised by this approach. What happens to continuity and coordination of care if nurses are pulled from unit to unit frequently? What about the rate of absenteeism and turnover if nurses go to work not knowing even what unit they will be working on that day? Don't group morale and cohesion decline if stable work groups cannot be formed? Is not the day-to-day workload and staffing numbers game the antithesis of professional nursing practice?

It is not the definition or intent of the open systems model to present such a restricted view. In fact the example given above is more consistent with the 1920s approach in scientific management and does not reflect the concern for interacting variables as defined in the open systems model. Modern-day nursing administrators are faced with the necessity of understanding these approaches to organizational management *in the context of clinical practice.* Systems engineers and operations researchers can help tremendously in providing an extensive data base about hospital operations. But the nursing administrator must distinguish the "sell job" from the helpful colleague, put assorted data together, and make the

appropriate decisions on the basis of both clinical and organizational data.

To what extent do nursing administrators currently put all the parts together—the methods of organizational management, the clinical practice base, and a leadership style conducive to a high quality of professional nursing practice? Though no quantified answer can be given, it would seem to depend on whether the nursing administrator performs as a bureaucrat or a colleague, an adversary or an advocate. To attempt to see whether it makes any difference, let us turn now to some studies of clinical management and leadership style.

MANAGEMENT OF NURSING PRACTICE

In recent years nursing administration has begun to take a broader view of the world than just the bureaucratic model of operations. Trends in education likely had an influence in this regard. It used to be that when one studied "nursing administration," one actually studied neither nursing nor administration. Both were considerably watered down and often were taught by neither practitioners nor administrators.

The nursing administrator did not have legitimacy with nurses as a colleague in nursing practice. At the same time, hospital administration tended to treat the nursing director as a lesser breed to whom important administrative decisions were not entrusted. The chief nurse often learned about decisions for the nursing budget or operational decisions that would greatly affect nurses only after the decisions were final.

Such situations are complex ones, and the causes for them certainly are not limited to academic credentials or preparation. The paternalistic, bureaucratic manner so frequent in hospital administration, the limited level of professionalization of nursing, and the lack of alliance with physicians as professional colleagues undoubtedly affect the performance of the nursing administrator.

Two recent trends within nursing have contributed to changes in the roles and perspectives of nursing administrators: the issue of quality assurance and the evolution of primary nursing as an institutional model of professional nursing practice. These two developments, both emphasizing excellence in clinical practice, are reviewed here in relation to nursing administration.

Quality of Nursing Care

In the evolution of concepts of organizational management, the major stages of development can be characterized by their emphasis on either structures, outcomes, or processes. After a century of development, these discrete parts finally merged, at least in the minds of theorists. While they may be analyzed separately, few modern theorists fail to view them as interrelated variables that must be considered in combination to gain an accurate and full picture of an institution.

Similarly, in the field of quality of nursing care, the very early studies centered on structural measures—the organization chart, the committees, the policies and procedures. We should be proud and relieved that it has not taken a century to move from structural definitions to a more comprehensive view of nursing within a patient care system! As measures of various parts of the system became more accurate, the view emerged of nursing practice within an organization as a set of processes directed toward a range of outcomes and affected at every turn by various structural measures and organizational processes.

One study that attempted to analyze influences on the quality of the nursing process was a part of a series of Rush-Medicus studies of quality of nursing care (Haussman et al., 1976; Hegyvary and Haussmann, 1976:22). The central focus of the dependent variable was an operational definition of the nursing process. The field test of the instrument has shown a high level of reliability and validity (Haussmann and Hegyvary, 1976: 324).

To determine what variables are related to quality of the nursing process, 6 categories containing 33 variables were selected for study on 104 units in 19 hospitals. The categories of variables were: (1) hospital characteristics, (2) unit organizational structure, (3) perceptions of unit staff, (4) perceptions of supervisory staff, (5) leadership style, and (6) nursing education.

The essence of the findings was that the quality of the nursing process was significantly related to every category of variable and to 31 of the 33 individual variables. Further, the nursing process varied according to the adequancy of support services, such as housekeeping, clerical, pharmacy, transport, and other auxiliary and administrative services. No single variable stood out as the key to quality of care. But there were some categories of greater significance than others.

The category of greatest overall impact was unit organizational structure. Compared with the units with lowest scores, the highest-quality units had this combination of characteristics: (1) they were better coordinated across services; (2) they were smaller; (3) they were staffed with more registered nurses, fewer practical nurses, and fewer aides; and (4) they tended toward primary nursing rather than task assignments.

Three other differences were found between highest and lowest scoring units. The highest-quality units showed a more open and flexible leadership style; the unit staffers had a higher level of clinical orientation in their current roles; and staff satisfaction was higher. It is true that many of these independent variables are correlated with each other so that no one variable may be singled out as the causative factor in quality of care.

The picture presented by these findings is one of a highly complex and vulnerable situation in nursing care. What does that mean for the nursing administrator? First, it requires a careful look at the definition of nursing performance, defined in this study as the nursing process.[1] Many nursing administrators in the study had a global definition of nursing and concentrated more on other parts

---

[1] A subsequent study to relate nursing process and patient outcomes showed a diffuse relationship that varied greatly according to patient population. Additional research is required to give a clearer view of the structure-process-outcome association.

of the hospital than they did on nursing practice. Many did not question whether support services were adequate and gave implicit consent that nursing staffers fill in any gaps in poorly performed support services. Defining the expectations for nursing performance led to greater clarity, visibility, accountability, and quality in nursing care.

Second, the variables that correlated with the quality of care covered the scope of administrative responsibility. Structure was highly important, but so was style of leadership and staff attitudes and perceptions. Nursing education explained less variance but also tended to show some effect. Is there a particular set of variables or approach that the administrator can use to tackle the issue of quality of care? No. Every category must be taken into account.

Thinking back to the evolution of nursing administration, let us compare these findings with stages of organizational development. The bureaucratic or institutional approach would look at structure—staffing, division of labor, and so on. Structural variables showed a significant influence on quality of care in this study, so there is some support for a bureaucratic approach.

Scientific management would emphasize the product and the efficiency of the organization. Coordination of services certainly is an aspect of efficiency and was shown to be related to quality of nursing care. Allocation of staff in relation to patient care needs, with systematic calculation of workload, also reflects the approach of scientific management. In this respect, there was some support for this focus. At the same time, though, one could argue that the task specialization found in functional nursing is characteristic of the approach of scientific management. Task specialization in nursing, i.e., the functional method, was not supported.

What about human relations? A major concern in this approach, employee job satisfaction, was shown to be highly related to the quality of nursing care. The finding that a more sensitive, more tolerant, and less structured style of leadership had a positive correlation with quality of care also reflects the importance of human relations.

That brings us to the rational, open systems approach. It requires consideration of inputs, processes, products, and environment—in short, every aspect of operation. The results of this study suggest that anything less than a comprehensive approach by the nursing administrator would be incomplete. While no study can conclude explicitly how to manage in every situation, the variables outlined above indicate some major considerations for the management of nursing services.

The Change toward Professional Nursing Practice

Most people now call it *primary nursing* and regard it as new and unique to nursing. In fact, it is a philosophy of care and an organizational arrangement that brings nursing closer than it has ever been to professional practice—in the true sense of the word. Professional practice of any type requires a specific knowledge base, definition of professional standards and ethics, autonomy to make decisions, individual accountability, a specific and unique service to a specific client over time (Greenwood, 1966:10). A task-centered, shift mentality falls dreadfully short of that definition.

Primary nursing requires the accountability, the autonomy, the decentralized structure for making decisions, the responsibility for clients over time. It is real back-to-the-bedside nursing. It is more difficult to organize and implement than other professional practices, such as medical, dental, or legal services, because of the need for professional staff to be present and providing the service 24 hours a day. Simply being on call is not enough.

As primary nursing has evolved, it has changed not only nursing practice but also the role of nursing administration. Reports from many projects to change from task or team-task assignments to primary nursing tell the story of the new style of leadership required in primary nursing.

The single greatest role change in primary nursing is that of the registered nurse as primary nurse. This person has responsibility and accountability for the nursing care of a small group of patients— this is comparable with the responsibility and accountability of the attending physician for the medical care of those patients. The primary nurse must have authority to carry out those responsibilities.

From where does the authority come? The requirement of decentralized authority means that some other roles must change, such as that of the head nurse. Several authors have reported that, prior to primary nursing, the head nurse made all major decisions, did all the care planning and discharge teaching, conferred with patients and families, made rounds and other contacts with physicians, and filtered relevant information to staff (Medaglia, 1978:32; Bartels et al., 1977: 26). Pity the poor head nurse who was very conscientious in trying to do all that!

In primary nursing, either the head nurse changes or the primary nurse cannot fulfill the role. Decisions about nursing care are made by the primary nurse. When that happens, the head nurse may be a resource. Most reports indicate that, as primary nursing becomes fully implemented, the head nurse is not just the nursing chief of the unit but basically is a professional colleague with personal primary patients (Medaglia, 1978:32; Elpern, 1977:205).

Roles of other supervisory staffers are similarly affected. For example, consider the evening and night supervisors. They are no longer called from unit to unit to make decisions *for* staff. Staffers make their own decisions, short of a hospital emergency. More and more hospitals are finding the old style supervisory roles superfluous and inconsistent with primary nursing. Some have discontinued these positions entirely. Others have changed the responsibilities to unit-based patient care assignments, e.g., as primary or associate nurse, with the additional responsibility of being on call for a shift in case of departmental or hospital emergency.

And what about the director of nursing and top administration? More changes, but they still relate to primary nurses. Because of the decentralization of authority through middle and front-line management, relationships of the director with other managerial staffers change. Perhaps the most significant challenge to the director is to provide the structure and support necessary for professional nursing practice. Three problem areas illustrate this point.

First, as suggested above, the primary nurse needs the structure and support that permit professional nursing practice. The content of practice is up to the nurse; providing the structure and support is the responsibility of several people, particularly the nursing director. Will the director support or resent a very decentralized structure for making decisions? As the primary nurse attempts to coordinate a patient's care, will the director provide the increasing educational opportunities for the nurse to learn more about system coordination? What rewards are there for high-quality professional performance?

Second, the director is in a key position to interpret and promote changes related to primary nursing to the medical staff. Alliances among clinical practitioners have been shown to be very logical, powerful, and effective. Many nurses have shied away from real alliances with physicians, perhaps because of fear of medical domination. Is it better to run track all over the hospital under the control of the hospital administrator?

There is another alternative, and making it happen depends largely on the nursing director— an alliance based on patient care. Those can be just so many pretty words, and probably most directors would insist that they have an excellent professional alliance. But the nature of nursing practice and the structure for making decisions that affect nurses usually speak to the contrary. Do the medical and nursing directors share information regularly, other than the crisis type, about patient care operations? Do they consult each other about new programs in the planning stages, rather than after the fact? Do they work as colleagues?

It is essential that this mutual exchange be a two-way street. The street usually is one way and consists of physicians complaining to the nursing director about nursing care, or perhaps occasionally stopping by to say the "girls" are doing a good job. The alliance handles complaints from both sides, but far more than that it sets the norm and provides stability for the entire organization in the direction of patient care. Establishing the alliance requires changes in the behavior of many nurses and physicians. Those changes have evolved in many settings as nurses have moved closer to true professional practice. They have occurred not as a result of confrontation and clenched fists but from collaboration and open minds.

Similarly, the nursing director has a major responsibility in supporting primary nursing through ensuring adequate patient support services. One of the most frequent complaints of nursing staff and one of the greatest blocks to professional nursing practice is inadequate support services. Study has shown that every part of the nursing process, including routine physical care, suffers when nurses perform the tasks of other services, such as clerical, housekeeping, pharmacy, supply, and transport services (Haussmann et al., 1976:30).

Reports from primary nursing projects have indicated that primary nursing, because of the patient-centered role of the nurse, places a strain on other resources (Hegyvary, 1977:187; Elpern, 1977:205). The more the nurses have filled in the gaps, the greater the strain will be when they insist on being nurses—not messengers, delivery people, and general track runners throughout the hospital. That is where the backing of the nursing director is crucial.

The nurse on the unit lives the headaches but has little power or position to resolve institutional problems. Such strains are top management problems that involve attitudes, territories, job descriptions, union contracts, staffing, and budgets—and administrative accountability. The nursing director who supports professional nursing practice will not assume or ask other nurses to assume responsibility or accountability for a host of nonclinical services. Whether nursing will hold itself accountable for nursing care and other services accountable to do their jobs so nurses can give care is a fundamental dilemma that could make or break the future of professional nursing practice.

Primary nursing, then, places some definite requirements on the nursing director. As nurses move toward a true professional model, the director's role as a colleague and advocate is essential. At the same time, the director must develop all alliances as a colleague with medical and administrative leaders. This type of openness and responsibility requires a change from old patterns of control to a modern style of leadership.

VIEWS OF LEADERSHIP

The above discussion presents a picture of the nursing administrator as a leader rather than a bureaucrat. Of course, some maintenance of the bureaucracy is necessary—files, reports, policies, channels of communication, etc.—but that is not the central focus of a leader. What characterizes a leader? Are there particular traits or behaviors that are desirable for the nursing administrator?

A while back, the usual view of leadership style was one of three choices: autocratic, democratic, or laissez-faire. While we still use the terms in a general way, studies of leadership measure specific traits or behaviors. Some of the most comprehensive studies of leadership have been reported by Stogdill (1974).

In a summary of several studies, Stogdill (1974: 93) reported that the most frequently occurring factors used to characterize the skills of the leader were: (1) social and interpersonal skills, (2) technical skills, (3) administrative skills, (4) intellectual skills, (5) effectiveness and achievement, (6) social nearness, friendliness, (7) supportiveness of group tasks, and (8) task motivation and application.

In a study of two sets of behaviors and their effects on group productivity, cohesion, and satisfaction, Stogdill (1974:418) defined the two sets as person-oriented and work-oriented behaviors. Person-oriented behaviors were described as democratic, permissive, follower-oriented, participative, and considerate. The work-oriented style was autocratic, restrictive, task-oriented, socially distant, directive, and structured. He reported that no one set of behaviors is best at all times. A very important behavior was structuring expectations, which he regards as "perhaps the central factor in leadership."

It is no surprise that the measure of leadership used by Hegyvary and Haussmann (1976:22) in their study of correlates of quality of nursing care reflects some of these dimensions. That tool, developed by Kruse and Stogdill (1973), measured four sets of behaviors: tolerance, sensitivity, role assumption, and structure.

The results from 104 medical, surgical, and pediatric units in 19 American hospitals indicated that the degree of structure was inversely related to the other three sets of behaviors. Persons who maintained a tight and rigid structure were low in tolerance and sensitivity and did not behave as group leader and promoter. More important, the latter three types of behavior were associated with higher quality of nursing care. The highest-quality units were characterized by leaders described as high in tolerance, sensitivity, and role assumption and low in the degree of structure.

Other findings from the Rush-Medicus study of correlates of quality of nursing care, as previously described, further support the view of nursing administration as a complex set of demands for system management. No one behavior or aspect of leadership and management can be applied in isolation.

Stogdill (1974:81) summarized the complexity of the problem of leadership style:

> A leader is characterized by a strong drive for responsibility and task completion, vigor and persistence in pursuit of goals, venturesomeness and originality in problem solving, drive to exercise initiative in social situations, self-confidence and sense of personal identity, willingness to accept consequences of decision and action, readiness to absorb interpersonal stress, willingness to tolerate frustration and delay, ability to influence other persons' behavior, and capacity to structure social interaction systems to the purpose at hand.

Probably few people in any field would score high consistently on every behavior. But production of a few more nursing administrators of this type surely would be the single greatest boost to professional nursing practice.

THE KEY IN A LOCKED DOOR

This chapter has presented some views and reports of studies that indicate the need for continued and rapid evolution in nursing administration. The dogmatic, domineering, snoopy, hard-line bureaucratic style clearly is inconsistent with the modern way of life and work. Changes toward professionalization of nursing increasingly cry for leaders who are colleagues and advocates.

Nursing education and research have promoted many changes in the nursing profession. But the shock of the practice setting to the ideals and goals of the new graduate or even to the conscientious, seasoned nurse are all too obvious. Most of our institutions basically have a locked door on professional nursing practice, which is not due primarily to malicious administrators or frenetic physicians. Our own studies and observations show that the norms set, accepted, or condoned by *nurses* are the key to the locked door of professional practice.

The nursing administrator—the one who leads and serves—can enhance or inhibit professional nursing practice. To the nursing administrators standing guard over the very essence of the profession, we can only say, "Lead, follow, or get out of the way."

EDITOR'S QUESTIONS FOR DISCUSSION

How can Hegyvary's discussion about administrators in nursing practice be applied to administrators in nursing education? What comparisons can be made between Fralic's chapter (48) and Hegyvary's reflections about professional practitioners in a humanistic setting? Provide examples of situations where flexibility and judgment required by the nurse poses conflict with the characteristics of a bureaucracy. What processes may be suggested to resolve such conflicts? What strategies can be suggested for nursing administrators in service or education to simultaneously maintain flexibility and predictability in organizational management? Provide examples of cases in which bureaucratic values take precedence over professional values and vice versa in administration. What organizational and professional variables are present in either case where one set of values take precedence over the other? Provide examples of bureaucratic structures being functional and dysfunctional. What type of strategies might an administrator utilize to effectively use the advantages of bureaucratic structure and prevent or curb the disadvantages? What are the characteristics of a professional administrator?

Discuss the impact of scientific management on nursing practice, modes of providing care, nursing education, administration, and professionalism. What factors in nursing may have contributed to the influence of scientific management? How generalizable and of what value are studies from the perspective of "operations research"? What strategies and methods can be suggested to improve the generalizability and relevancy of data, such as in studies of staffing. Provide examples of the utilization of each management approach presented in administration of nursing practice and education. How can the concepts of a bureaucracy, scientific management, and human relations be integrated by an administrator for effective management? Provide examples of the utilization of a rationalistic, open systems model in the resolution of administrative issues.

How has the issue of quality assurance and evolution of primary nursing contributed to changes in the roles and perspectives of nursing administrators? Provide examples of structure, process, outcome variables that have independently been used and combined in studies of quality of nursing care. What structure, process, outcome measures can be suggested for future studies? What criteria may be utilized for the selection of variables to integrate all three measures in quality-of-care studies? What ethical issues are inherent in conducting quality-of-care research? To what extent should the providers of care be given specific feedback as to the results of quality-of-care research? What alternative explanations might be offered for the findings of the one study presented from the series of Rush-Medicus studies? What factors may influence nursing administrators to have a global definition of nursing? Provide examples of differences between global and comprehensive definitions of nursing? What are the implications for nursing education and the preparation of nursing administrators regarding the type of definition of nursing held by administrators? Discuss whether it is or is not possible to have high quality of care provided in an organization or agency without academic preparation and practice experience in management and leadership. What variables need to be considered in responding to the above question? Why might you expect that the variables that correlated with the quality of care in the Rush-Medicus study cover the scope of administrative responsibility?

Compare the congruence between Fralic's (Chap. 48) and Hegyvary's view regarding decision making by the head nurse and primary nursing. To what extent do they agree regarding the role of supervisors? What discussion by Klein (Chap. 43) and questions posed by the editor apply to Hegyvary's presentation? Provide examples of the new style of leadership which Hegyvary states is required in primary nursing. What issues addressed and questions raised for discussion in the chapters by Williamson (5),

O'Connor (13), and Sills (42) may relate to Hegyvary's views on professional practice, leadership and management? Respond to the editor's questions raised for discussion (Chap. 42) concerning the application of nursing theory to the role of the primary nurse.

How and to what degree should the director of nursing provide the structure and support for professional nursing practice? What type should the director provide? Provide examples of how the director of nursing may most effectively interpret and promote changes related to primary nursing to medical staff. To what extent should someone at the unit level be responsible and accountable for resolution of management problems and strains, such as those related to union contracts and territories? Suggest strategies for resolving issues related to inadequate support services for professional practice. Provide examples as to potential contradictions or conflicts when clinical decision making is decentralized and administrative decision making is centralized. How might these be resolved? What strategies for developing effective alliances for nursing in administration of nursing service and education can be suggested?

Compare and provide examples of the person-oriented and work-oriented styles of behavior. How might administrators as leaders most effectively structure realistic expectations for staff and faculty? Discuss leadership styles of administrators and their relationship to effective professional performance of staff and faculty. What variables may influence the effectiveness of one style more than another? To what extent do environment, organizational structure, and climate influence the style of a leader? How can leaders assess the extent to which they may need to adapt their most consistent style of leadership to an organization's methods and style? How can leaders assess the extent to which they may be able to influence adaptation of an organization's modus operandi to their leadership and administrative style? What ethical implications are there from Davis's chapter (47) for leadership and administrative style? What questions for discussion from Chap. 47 also apply to Hegyvary's presentation?

REFERENCES

Bartels, Diane, Vivian Good, and Susan Lampe
1977 "The role of the head nurse in primary nursing," Canadian Nurse March: 26–29.

Elpern, Ellen Heid
1977 "Structural and Organizational Supports for primary nursing," Nursing Clinics of North America 12(2):205–220.

Georgopoulos, Basil S. (ed.)
1972 Organization Research on Health Institutions. Ann Arbor: University of Michigan.

Greenwood, Ernest
1966 "The elements of professionalization," Pp. 9–19 in Howard M. Vollmer and Donald L. Mills (eds.), Professionalization. Englewood Cliffs, N.J.: Prentice-Hall.

Haussmann, R. K. Dieter, Sue T. Hegyvary, and John F. Newman
1976 Monitoring Quality of Nursing Care, Part 2: Assessment and Study of Correlates. Dept. Health Human Services Publ. No. 76-7.

Haussmann, R. K. Dieter and Sue T. Hegyvary
1976 "Field testing the nursing quality monitoring methodology." Nursing Research 25(5):324–331.

Hegyvary, Sue T.
1977 "Foundations of primary nursing." Nursing Clinics of North America 12(2): 187–196.

Hegyvary, Sue T. and R. K. Dieter Haussmann
1976 "Correlates of nursing care quality," Journal of Nursing Administration 6(9): 22–27.

Kruse, Lorane C. and Ralph M. Stogdill
  1973 The Leadership Role of the Nurse.
        Columbus: Ohio State University Re-
        search Foundation.
McKechnie, Jean L.
  1977 Webster's New Twentieth Century Dic-
        tionary of the English Language (2d ed.).
        Collins-World Publishing Company.
Medaglia, Marlene
  1978 "A coronary care unit implements pri-
        mary nursing." Canadian Nurse May:
        32–34.

Merton, Robert K.
  1969 "Bureaucratic structure and personality,"
        Pp. 47–58 in Amitai Etzioni, A Sociologi-
        cal Reader in Complex Organizations.
        New York: Holt, Rinehart and Winston.
Newman, William H., Charles E. Summer, and
    Kirby E. Warren
  1972 The Process of Management (3d ed.).
        Englewood Cliffs, N. J.: Prentice-Hall.
Stogdill, Ralph M.
  1974 Handbook of Leadership: A Survey of
        Theory and Research. New York: Free
        Press.

Chapter 50

The Development of a
Practice Setting

Lois C. Malkemes, R.N., Ph.D.
Patient Care Administrator
University Hospital and
Professor, College of Nursing
University of Arkansas Medical Sciences Campus
Little Rock, Arkansas

The primary nursing mode for providing care has been equated to the most appropriate form of professional practice. Following Hegyvary's portrayal of the nursing administrator's role for professional practice, it is of great value to be more knowledgeable as to how professional practice settings can be developed. Lois C. Malkemes provides an enlightening description of a program to change a service setting into a setting for professional practice. Clear distinctions are made between the two types of settings. Schein's framework for planned change is utilized. The experience of the change is candidly discussed and analyzed.

Malkemes believes the term "nursing service" implies an organizationally subordinate relationship of nursing in serving an organization. The organization of nursing service refers to those persons employed in occupations, not a setting where professionals practice. Professional nursing practice is characterized by authority, accountability, independent decision making, collaboration, advocacy, and facilitation. The organizational structure for professional practice is essentially decentralized and different from a service setting. The formal organizational structure facilitates, not creates, a professional practice mode. A system of governance is utilized as a mechanism of organizing nursing departments. A by-laws structure provides nursing staff, as members of a department, decision-making rights, and responsibilities. Malkemes uses clinical specialists' responsibilities to demonstrate how formal and governance structures are congruent. For example, clinical specialists are not only responsible for standards of care for their patients but also for monitoring procedures, establishing standards for performance, evaluation, and practice privileges germane to their specialty area. Recruitment philosophy and activities determine the character of a professional practice setting. A philosophy of self-direction and evaluation is essential in staff development.

Malkemes emphasizes the need for a framework of planned change in implementing professional practice settings. This includes collecting data to identify problems, identifying variables which need to be manipulated, and initiating the process of change. She points out that in using Schein's process—unfreezing, redefinition, and refreezing—all three phases in reality occur together. Malkemes's responsibility to change a service setting to a practice setting was for a 3- to 5-year time frame. Motivation for change was strong from the department, hospital, and medical staff. It took about 6 months to gather the data from which 11 problem areas emerged. These were reduced to one—the modality of care—which was viewed as central to the other problems. Primary nursing was the mode established, projecting that this mode of care would have positive effects for the identified problem areas.

Some of the occurrences in Malkemes's experience were: the magnitude of resistance to change by some nurses for direct responsibility and accountability for care; a gap between acceptance of change by professional staff who stayed and new nurses who wanted more change; changes in internal policies to commit the department to recruit nurses who wanted professional practice; the establishment of close ties among all affiliating educational units; and medical staff participating in nursing's decisions only through patient care committees. It took 8 months to develop an effective decision making governance structure. The process of unfreezing took about 12 to 15 months. There were periods of retrogression before progress was made. A core professional staff stabilized upon which to build. A patient classification system was developed in the "redefinition" phase to improve staffing and justify increased resources. After 3 years the professional nursing staff doubled, turnover decreased by one-half, and levels of satisfaction increased.

In the analysis of the change, Malkemes notes that it is critical to identify all of the potential problems before implementation toward professional practice. Role redefinition is difficult and provokes crises. One cannot assume staff will rush to participate in a governance system. There is a difference between saying accountability is desired and being accountable. Decisions generally were made on the basis of patient care concerns. Respect, trust, and confidence in administration must be earned. Malkemes cites the problem oriented system of documentation and the establishment of responsibility for a defined group of patients as highlights of her experience. She concludes that self-direction must be imbued early in educational programs with on-going communication between educational units and nursing practice administrators. A developing profession needs not only education for practice but also the opportunity to engage in professional practice in formulated practice settings.

Increasingly, the nursing literature and indeed the profession subscribes to the concept of *nursing practice* without a clear delineation of the characteristics of practice and the total milieu that supports the professional who is practicing. The following is one attempt to describe a practice setting, delineate the characteristics of professional practice, describe an experience in change, and suggest implications for the nursing profession.

A PRACTICE SETTING

Some recent literature addresses, in part, the concept of a practice setting, but most specifically suggests the delivery of care through the primary nursing modality (Manthey, 1980:12-13; Sample, 1979:13-15). However, to understand the nature and character of practice settings, it has become evident that there is a necessity to understand first the nature of practice and this is the departure.

We are very familiar with the concept of *nursing service* and for the most part use it interchangeably with nursing practice. But, is it the same? According to *Webster's New Collegiate Dictionary*, service refers to "an occupation or function of serving, employment as a servant" 1977:1059). Nursing service, then, implies an organizationally subordinate relationship of nursing with the function of serving the organization.

The organization of nursing service refers to those who function in the department of nursing service, i.e., to those people employed in occupations, not to a setting where professionals practice. This philosophy perpetuates an organizational structure and delivery of care by persons who are controlled and directed and who control and direct.

Practice, on the other hand, has a very different meaning and is associated with the professions. Practice refers to the performance of an indentifiable action, becoming "proficient" at it, and being engaged in it professionally (Webster, 1977: 902). Practice, then, is associated with independent decision making, self-direction, openness, inquiry, accountability, and delivery. The organizational structure, by definition and necessity, will be different from that of a service setting so that it facilitates professional practice.

Having made the above distinction and assertion, it is reasonable to also suggest that nursing administrators choose to develop a nursing service or a professional nursing practice setting. In delineating the two, there is an assumption that nursing practice can be professionally described. The following is a description of a practice setting and the basis for change from a service setting to a practice setting.

The initial question that must be addressed, philosophically and conceptually, is: What type of care will be provided in the particular setting? The mode of delivery, by whatever name, must provide the opportunity for registered nurses to have a defined case load, assume 24-hour accountability, be involved in inquiry, collaborate in practice, continue their education and development, and most especially, have authority for nursing care.

Professional nursing practice is a process in which the nurse is involved with a client and through which the client's health problems are identified and brought to resolution. As such, professional nursing practice incorporates the following characteristics:

Authority	Influencing the process of care through the professional role
Accountability	Responsibility to client, self, profession and to make decisions regarding care
Independent decision making	Making judgments within each phase of the nursing process as client problems are resolved
Collaboration	Sharing relationships with multidisciplines in order to assess the client's problems and help the client solve them
Advocacy	Intervention on behalf of the client to solve problems and interface with the system at large
Facilitation	Maximizing the potential of the organization and client-family system in care

It is reasonable to suggest that this type of nursing practice cannot be implemented in a traditional structure of nursing service, where accountability is to the setting, little or no authority for care is established, independent decisions are frowned upon, and advocacy is the exception rather than the rule. A true facilitator the nurse is not! A setting truly must nurture professional practice.

Manthey suggests that the appropriate structure for nursing practice is the decentralization of the formal organizational structure (1980:12). She further states,

> The elements of decentralized decision making —clear allocation and acceptance of responsibility and accountability—form the foundation for a cohesive administrative structure. . . . (1980:12)

For efficient organizational functioning and for lessening the possibility of role conflict, responsibility at each level must be clearly delineated. The professional nurse, then, is aware of and accepts authority for the day-to-day responsibility of a case load; the coordinating role incumbent assumes responsibility for standards of care to groups of like clients; and administrative incumbents are responsible for facilitating the quality of care and are accountable for the product.

The formal organizational structure will not create a professional practice mode in and of itself, but it will begin to facilitate its development when other conditions are present. It is important that the expectation of self-direction be pervasive in all matters of practice and consequently that administration support the authority and self-direction of the nurse. A system of governance is a mechanism of organizing nursing departments, so that matters important to everyday practice can be decided on through a grass-roots representation and decision-making process.

Questions relating to practice privileges, the nature of practice, the scope of practice, and relevant policies and procedures can be handled by nursing staff through a by-laws structure that gives members of the department decision-making rights and responsibilities. It helps to create a setting where grass-roots participants can feel a sense of responsibility for their own destiny and allows for creative solutions to grass-roots problems.

This discussion so far does not mean to imply that the formal and governance structures are not congruent with each other. On the contrary, they must be congruent philosophically both with each other and with the goals and objectives to which the department subscribes. For instance, within the formal structure clinical specialists are responsible for standards of care of clients within their specialty case load. In addition, they have responsibility for monitoring procedures relevant to their areas of specialty interest and for the establishment of performance standards, evaluation, and practice privileges. For the clinical specialist group then, the governance system provides a mechanism for communication as well as for the establishment of standards for their own practice with a review procedure and reporting line. In relation to professional practice, the clinical specialists have the authority and responsibility to establish and implement standards of care but are accountable for their own

practice and have a defined mechanism for facilitating better care and improvement.

Comment should be made about other programs supportive to a professional practice setting which thus enhance a professional practice. Recruitment activities within health care settings are themselves big businesses. Recruitment philosophy dictates that programs must be based upon retention. The best recruitment sets forth, in a public relations format, the character of a professional practice setting. Coordinated efforts that reflect feedback mechanisms to programs enhance the recruitment efforts. The recruitment effort must not exist in isolation but rather must be a part of and be participated in by the nurses in the practice setting.

In addition, staff development philosophy and strategies must change to reflect the expectation of self-direction in professional practice. Whether it be in orientation, which is individualized, or in staff development programs, the expectations that the registered nurse participate and evaluate her- or himself must be established and sanctioned. This type of program places the responsibility for direction and development squarely on the individual nurse.

A practice setting, in summary, is one that supports and facilitates professional nursing practice and the growth of the individual professionally and that is distinctive from nursing service settings. Authority must be vested in nursing and the responsibility defined at all levels. In addition, self-direction and accountability for that practice is vested in the professional nurse.

A FRAMEWORK FOR CHANGE

It seems fair to assume that ideal practice settings for professional nurses do not exist. Therefore, it is likely that planned change becomes the order of the day. Although Manthey *states* that edicts do not bring about a move toward the development of professional practice settings (1980:13), the risk involved in the declaration and the path it charts are important in establishing the overall goals to be achieved in setting the stage for change.

The framework of planned change (Schein, 1969:99) suggests that having established a workable data base from which to identify problems, strengths, and weaknesses and a goal, the process of change can begin. The process suggests a mechanism of change as follows: unfreezing, i.e., creating an openness; redefinition, i.e., changing the cognitive definition; and refreezing, i.e., reinforcement. Schein's process suggests that the data can be grouped into or can suggest strategies that when prioritized delineate problems to be addressed through planned change strategies.

Establishing the goal of professional practice indicates data that must be collected relative to what has been established as the specifics of professional practice, i.e., numbers of professional nurses, mode of delivery, staffing patterns, experience with professional nurses, competency level, self-direction, skills of collaboration, and the degree to which nurses accept responsibility for their own practice. Specific indicators might be a reflection of a care plan for 24 hours; an assessment and professional identification with 24 hours of accountability; communication regarding progress of the patient; and a responsibility for care givers.

Once the problems within an organization and the variables to be manipulated in change have been identified, the mechanisms of change indicated by Schein (1969:99–107) can be initiated. It must be pointed out that the three phases of change are only analytically separate, but in reality redefinition is going on during unfreezing and reinforcement is occurring during the other phases. The three phases represent emphasis.

AN EXPERIENCE IN CHANGE

The process of change outlined by Schein (1969) was the guide for a broad-based program necessary to change a nursing service setting into a nursing practice setting. A problem-riddled department

of nursing in a steady state of crisis was a positive point from which to initiate any process of change. The motivation for change was strong from within the department, hospital, and medical staff, even though the precise nature of those changes and their effect on others was not readily understood. Having accepted the responsibility for directing this department, the author accepted the responsibility for changes from a service setting to a professional practice setting within a 3- to 5-year time frame. One crisis after another instigated the need for implementing the data-gathering phase of the process, which took approximately 6 months. From that data, the following problem list emerged very quickly:

1 Lack of nursing administration support
2 High turnover
3 Functional care supported by inadequate staffing
4 Inadequate staff development
5 Poor communication patterns
6 Unclear roles
7 Recruitment efforts not associated with programs
8 Unrealistic budget
9 Dominance of the medical staff
10 Negative attitude toward nursing
11 Crisis-oriented problem solving

The problems were reduced to one that was viewed to be central to the solution of the other problems, and that was the modality of care. The previous modality of care was the functional type, characterized by the organization of care by tasks. This modality, which was an outgrowth from industry, emphasized efficiency and reduced patient care to tasks requiring specific individualized skills. If institutionally there was a commitment to solving the "nursing problem," then there would have to be, by necessity, a commitment to changes necessary to changing the modality of care, and such was the case. The target, then, was the establishment of the practice modality that would ultimately effect changes in:

1 Attitude toward administration

2 Turnover and satisfaction
3 Staffing
4 Staff development
5 Communication
6 Clarifying roles
7 Retention and recruitment efforts
8 Budget
9 Attitudes of medical staff
10 Relationships with other departments
11 Orientation toward problem solving

The modality of care projected to be established was primary nursing, the conceptualization of which required, central to its core, the registered nurse to assume the direct responsibility for the care of clients. This included the accountability, authority, and autonomy necessary for nursing care to be delivered to a defined case load of clients. Although modifications of the primary nursing modality were accepted initially, the factor of accountability was not negotiable.

The underlying assumption, as change was contemplated, was that the registered nurse staff wanted to create a professional practice setting and would wholeheartedly support it for themselves and others. With that in mind and with a formal organizational structure already decentralized, the first directive was issued: registered nurses were to assume direct responsibility for care of the clients.

The initial reaction was, "We can't do that on our bare bones staffing." Needless to say, the responsibility for direction and support was placed on the administrative staff and staff development. Over a very short period of time, the staff began to view ways in which modifications could be established, and movement towards the defined goal was observed.

A somewhat unexpected occurrence, at least in the magnitude of the effect experienced, was that some registered nurses did not want to change the mode of operation and indeed were quite content to continue in their old ways. These nurses were quickly identified and pressure, through sanctions, was applied. The end

result was that those who could not make the transition left, leaving a more critical void in staffing, while others were enticed to try primary nursing.

The expectation of caring for clients never waivered, even as staffing seemed to reach a critical low. On the horizon was a group of new graduates, who had been lured to the setting because of the commitment to professional practice. Those who were left were willing to hold the setting together until freshness and relief came through.

The state of the organization certainly required some unpopular decisions. No longer was the medical staff encouraged to participate in decisions by the nursing organization except through patient care committees. Previously, medical direction had dominated decision making at all levels of the organization. In addition, close ties were established between all educational units affiliated with the hospital. Another high-risk decision, which had far-reaching implications, was made to close beds owing to inadequate numbers of professional nurses for providing safe care. With this action nursing symbolically established itself as having authority for nursing care, even though this change in position was not readily evident.

The recruitment program during this period was very important. In the past, we had recruited nurses without regard for their expertise, commitment, or risk-taking behaviors. Now, we wanted creative, thinking, action-oriented nurses who wanted to practice nursing as we had defined it and who were willing to "buy into" an ever-changing environment. It was clear that our internal policies had to change for us to symbolically commit ourselves to these nurses who wanted to practice.

The staff development personnel worked with the nursing administrators and the recruitment coordinator to develop programs that addressed the transition of student to graduate through specialized training and individualized orientation programs that were developed by staff development personnel and offered in schools of nursing statewide, as well as implemented within the department of nursing. All attempts were made to suggest to the recruits that they were special, their needs were unique, and the department would work to support their development.

The governance structure took shape early, too. Nurses suggested that there was little or no participation in the governance of the department, and members of the existing structural committees were interviewed to ascertain what was good about the system and what needed to be changed. After approximately 8 months, a governance structure was developed that reflected grass-roots participation in decision making.

Initially, there was much concentration on matters tangential to practice, but there were many programs and ideas that were supportive of practice at the same time. There was a perceived need to develop a different system of thinking and documentation of nursing practice. An ad hoc committee developed the problem-oriented system and responded to helping personnel on the units learn the system. In addition, no one was expected to do more than he or she could possibly achieve.

There seemed to be a period of going backwards before progress was made, and that was a very frustrating time for everyone. People began to question whether what was being considered would ever work. However, introduction of a new direction was motivating, and a little glimmer of hope continued. The staff did deteriorate until a core was stabilized, and that core was what the staff built upon. There were many suggestions for how staffing could be enhanced such as foreign recruitment and contract services, but all were rejected because they would have: (1) symbolized no progress; (2) been too difficult to accomplish in a short period of time; and (3) been very expensive. Each and every one was encouraged daily to stay on, and any ray of hope was quickly passed on to the staff.

The process of unfreezing took approximately 12 to 15 months before changes became visible.

It was a period of ups and downs, but each time nursing had a solid goal, which emerged unwavering and which guided all aspects of decison making and care. Eventually, nursing established itself as the authority for decisions regarding care, and as each new question arose, the solution was negotiated. Each day, each client, each decision brought a redefinition of what nursing practice was and what it was to become in this setting.

The redefinition did not take place without some resistance as nurses continuously talked of how sick their patients were and how the expectations were too great. This spurred the development of a patient classification system, which was justified to the staff as a mechanism to verify acuity and thus additional resources. They accepted its use, especially when they found it effective.

Just as closing beds was symbolic, so was reopening those beds and then opening new beds. With each passing month, nursing was able to honor its commitment to provide professional care to clients. The medical staff came to appreciate nursing's positive contribution to care and to know what professional nursing care was, and yet, there was a continuing need to demonstrate both the nature and scope of professional practice as each year came to an end.

Now is the time to reflect and reinforce. Over a 3-year time span, the professional nursing staff has doubled, the turnover has been cut in half, and the satisfaction level has increased. Nurses are caring for patients and are involved in self-governance, quality assurance, inquiry, and staff development. What then should be the concern?

AN ANALYSIS OF THE CHANGE

In the process of rapid and massive organizational change, gaining stability must be an intermediate goal, along with the development of what has been initiated so far. The department has reached a point at which stability in redefinition must be achieved. There are many outside system changes, decisions, and pressures which keenly affect the progress and directions of change in an organization. Gaining stability has been a challenge with the threat of losing what has developed and of going backward always present. With all the progress achieved, there need not be complacency. There is much yet to develop and much yet to accomplish.

What is necessary to look out for when initiating a change toward professional practice? A process of planned change must be established and must be implemented as a process, with all the potential problems and pitfalls being identified by the change from the outset. For instance, well-meaning colleagues in other disciplines may have many good suggestions, but many of these may not fit the timing in the process of change. There is a strong force pulling in a multitude of directions. Staying on the course is tough.

The role change that occurs in developing a professional nursing practice setting affects all concerned, but those involved in the nursing care arena are the most affected because clarificatiion of roles is so important. Role redefinition is both essential and frustrating. The difficulty for the nurse providing direct care to a case load has been discussed, but others—administrators, head nurses, and support personnel—also have and will experience role crises in an effort to clarify roles. The hope is that not all experiences hit at once and that positive resolutions can occur. Some of these tasks remain in the development stage.

Just as it was assumed that all registered nurses wanted to be involved in direct care of clients, it was assumed that given a structure they would work like bees to implement the governance. Although this structure was differentially subscribed to, there was not an overwhelming rush to participate. Little by little, nurses are seeing that participation makes a difference for their well-being, practice, and environment. This is, however, still developing.

The programs that have been most effective have been those closest to the care of clients. The problem-oriented system of documentation and the responsibility for a defined case load or for primary nursing seem to be the highlights of their accomplishments. Special project development has consumed a great deal of energy, and a great participation in the overall department affairs is evident.

What of the progress with other identifiable problems? Respect, trust, and confidence in administration must be earned, and this is no easy task. Some days are more positive than others, but this is an area that needs continuous attention and nurturing. Concerns for budgetary matters are closely associated with attitudes toward administration. Commitments to improve nursing practice have brought an increased commitment for resources. It is a time of cost containment, and hard decisions must be made regarding the allocation of resources. Sometimes this is unpopular with staff, and sometimes with administration, but decisions generally are made on the basis of patient care concerns, a guiding force in this practice setting. In addition, the use of a patient classification system will increasingly help to justify increased resources for improved staffing and associated programs.

Nursing has achieved a position as a positive force in the environment. It makes a difference on both the patient care level and administration level. Planning is future-oriented rather than crisis-oriented and continues on the move towards "developing a professional practice setting."

A new group of nurses now enjoy practice privileges within the department. They are energetic, creative, and wanting change now. They have not seen the changes that have occurred. They want more changes toward improved practice. Although this is hard for the core troops to understand without being defensive, they are trying to muster the energy to move ahead. Moving ahead is essential to keeping those innovative, creative, self-directed nurses, who require much time and effort to recruit.

It is with some trepidation that this account is communicated. It is now the beginning of the fourth year of a 5-year commitment. Continuous nurturing will be the key to future development.

IMPLICATIONS FOR THE NURSING PROFESSION

Mundinger presents the question very well (1980: 63): Where are the risk takers in nursing? Nursing practice settings cannot and will not be developed except by those who know or think they know what professional practice is and how to get there. There is no doubt that many risk takers have been burned out in the past; this is something that is unacceptable for the future. The future of nursing education and practice may very well reside in the present and future development of practice settings. Such development needs support from nursing.

Although registered nurses are being held responsible for the care of patients, there is not a keen sense of commitment on their part to their accountability for all plans and actions. Although nurses speak of wanting such accountability and wanting to include the necessary behavior in their practice, there is a resistance to wanting to have all plans and actions reviewed. Being accountable and saying we are accountable are two different reference points. Helping nurses accept their accountability is no easy task but is a necessary goal.

What do we do with the nurse who wants authority and autonomy while not accepting professional responsibility? There is more to professional practice than care of the individual client. Professional development and education must be pursued with self-direction. It will take time for a direction-oriented department to change the expectation from the department providing for the needs of its staff to the nurses seeking to provide for themselves. This approach must be inculcated early and more deliberately in educational programs.

Nursing practice administrators must earn the respect of their nursing colleagues. Authority by position does not ensure that leadership prevails. Being concerned and offering help in the solving of nitty-gritty practice problems is essential to the credibility of nursing administrators. Communication with educational units and understanding of their products is also essential to providing a setting for nurses to practice.

Where is nursing research in the model? It is very much an integral part of that which is being nourished but is slow to take hold. Its importance in verifying practice and developing a knowledge base for the future is essential to the developing setting. Well-prepared nurses who foster questioning and the formal research process within clinical settings are a necessity. The validation of practice, whether we do make a difference, and the validation of roles and educational preparation for those roles will be important research contributions of a professional practice setting. Indeed, this must be a joint education and practice endeavor.

Education for practice is only part of the process of a developing profession. Having the opportunity to engage in professional practice is a crucial next step. There is indeed a need to develop practice settings if we view nursing as a professional endeavor. The choice is ours. The implications are far-reaching.

EDITOR'S QUESTIONS FOR DISCUSSION

What are the relationships between Hegyvary's portrayal of professional practice (Chap. 49) and Malkemes's discussion of practice settings? Provide examples for distinguishing between service and practice settings. What are the relationships among organization structure, service settings, and professional practice? How is accountability demonstrated to the setting in a traditional structure of nursing service?

What criteria can be suggested for determining the mode of care that most effectively can be provided in a particular setting? What administrative functions are most appropriate to be decentralized for professional practice? What variables influence how and to what degree they should be decentralized?

What relationships are there between Sills' proposal for nursing governance (Chap. 42) and Malkemes's discussion of a system of governance? How much congruence is there between the two authors regarding the responsibility of clinical specialists and support systems for that group? How might a by-laws structure most effectively be implemented in a nursing organization? How can an administrator facilitate congruence between formal organization and governance structures? What mechanisms can be suggested to resolve potential conflicts?

What are the most effective recruitment methods for professional practice and education settings? Refer to discussions by D. Walker (Chap. 4), Bullough (Chap. 45), and Davis (Chap. 47) for implications regarding recruitment. What ethical and legal obligations and responsibilities does the administrator have for recruitment purposes, interviewing of candidates, the conveying and obtaining of information to and from applicants and other sources?

Compare Klein's (Chap. 43) discussion concerning problems and issues in implementing primary nursing with Malkemes's experience. How much agreement is there regarding the need for planned change and the identification of potential problems? How typical is Malkemes's experience in implementation of professional practice with others? What differences in strategies, methods, and outcomes can be cited? What suggestions can be offered in planning for the future?

What are the most effective methods to collect valid and reliable data prior to implementation of primary nursing? How might an administrator effectively assess the potential risk-taking behaviors that may be required? How typical are the 11 problem areas identified by Malkemes in service settings? How does primary nursing specifically address each of the 11 areas? What other variables may need to be considered before choosing primary nursing as a mode of care in the 11 problem areas and generalizable to other settings? What questions for discussion in Chap. 43 apply to or are addressed by Malkemes?

How can an administrator most effectively create a "climate" conducive to accepting change? What are the most effective strategies for encouraging internalization of a commitment for change? What comparisons can be made regarding the difficulties in role redefinition between Malkemes's description and evidence from Fralic's chapter (48)? What criteria might be suggested for prioritizing crises should numerous ones appear simultaneously? What alternative explanations can be provided for a discrepancy between desiring autonomy, responsibility, and accountability and actually being accountable? What strategies can be offered to develop and/or change staff and faculty who want authority and autonomy, but are not willing to accept professional responsibility? How can burnout be prevented for high risk takers in implementing change? What criteria can be suggested to assess and evaluate the pace of change? What other implications for the profession, nursing education, and research in implementing professional practice are addressed in the chapters by Conway (2), Williamson (5), Santora (8), Clayton (10), Fawcett (14), Mayer (17), Hardy (24), Newman (28), Chinn (29), Hardy (32), Meleis (33), Roy (34), MacElveen-Hoehn (39), Gordon (41), and MacPhail (46)?

How can an administrator empirically evaluate change? Suggest methodologies for longitudinal studies and critical variables that should be included. How might research concerning organizational change most effectively be accomplished through collaboration and an interdisciplinary team? What criteria need to be established for roles on an interdisciplinary team prior to the research? Refer to the chapter by Disbrow (18).

REFERENCES

Manthey, Marie
   1980   "A theoretical framework for primary nursing." Journal of Nursing Administration 10:11–15.
Mundinger, Mary O'Neil
   1980   Autonomy in Nursing. Germantown, Maryland. Aspen Systems Corp.
Sample, Sally A.
   1979   "Harborview's contribution to nursing practice." Nursing Administration Quarterly 4:13–15.
Schein, Edgar H.
   1969   "The mechanisms of change," Pp. 98–107 in Warren B. Bennis, Kenneth D. Benne, Robert Chin (eds.), The Planning of Change. New York: Holt, Rinehart & Winston.
Webster's New Collegiate Dictionary
   1977   8th ed. Springfield, Mass.: G. C. Merriam Co.

Chapter 51

A Study of Nurses' Perceptions of Participative Management

Lucille T. Mercadante, R.N., Ed.D.
Assistant Administrator
International Hospital
Miami, Florida

Recruitment and retention of staff nurses has been cited as a most perplexing issue. It is not only a critical problem for service settings that have not or are not able to implement primary nursing, but remains an issue (though lesser) in practice settings where professional practice–primary nursing has been established. One way of addressing the problem has been to develop settings and a mode of care for professional practice where committed professional nurses will want to practice. Lucille T. Mercadante suggests another means: to develop organizational structures which allow for professional nurses to share in the control of nursing practice. Control of nursing practice has been cited as the underlying issue of the profession. Control and accountability for professional practice as previously addressed are one alternative. Mercadante views models of participative management through a committee structure as another means for control of practice and as an approach to recruit and retain professional nurses. Mercadante presents the results of a survey conducted at a southeastern medical center to measure how nurses serving on committees perceived committee structure as a model of participative management and shared governance. The five committees created for the purpose of involving nursing personnel in decision making focused on: nursing practice, performance appraisal and promotion, position description, nursing policy and procedure, and nursing audit.

In reviewing the literature, Mercadante notes the escalation of union activity and unionization of professional nurses. Some of the issues raised include the right to bargain about assignments, position descriptions, evaluations, and number of staff and their responsibilities. Dissatisfaction with the work itself is indicated as a possible underlying factor in turnover of nurses. She documents from surveys the need for nurses to be involved in decision making affecting control of their practice for job satisfaction. Mercadante discusses Herzberg's two types of motivators, "job content" and "job context (hygiene factors)." The latter, which includes fringe benefits, salary, and company policy, does not increase productivity or decrease turnover, although when present, it may prevent dissatisfaction. The former as an intrinsic motivator includes opportunities for professional advancement, recognition, achievement, and personal growth, and is associated with job satisfaction. A shared-authority model of

696

governance is also recognized as a motivator. Mercadante concludes that effective communication is the essence of all relationships. To be held legally accountable for the nature and quality of their practice through state nurse practice acts, practitioners need some form of shared governance. Thus, she views participative management as a form of shared governance.

The instrument used for Mercadante's survey was an adaptation of Likert's "Profile of Organizational Characteristics." It consists of 20 questions associated with four patterns of management: exploitive authoritative, benevolent authoritative, consultative, and participative. Seven areas of concern are included in the questions: leadership, motivation, communication, interaction, decision making, goal setting, and feedback control. Forty questionnaires were distributed to and returned by the 40 members of the five committees. Twenty-two (55 percent) of the respondents held positions considered part of nursing management, while eighteen (45 percent) were in non-nursing management positions. Length of service on committees ranged from 3 months to 2 years. Length of employment ranged from 8 months to 14 years. Results of the survey were tabulated by frequency of response and converted to percentages for comparisons. Numerical values from one through four were assigned respectively to the four patterns of management to compute the mean score.

The major finding was that respondents perceived the nursing department's participative management model as falling between the consultative and participative patterns of management. The mean response was 3.29. Four areas of concern had scores above the mean. The questions concerning interaction, communication, decision making, and feedback control in order respectively ranked highest. Mercadante views the results within the section of decision making as indicating respondents see themselves involved in the decision-making process, but final decisions were made by top management. The two sections with the lowest mean scores were motivation and goal setting.

Mercadante concludes that although structuring committees provide a mechanism in decision making and control of practice, respondents view themselves more as consultants than full participants. She proposes a four-step plan of action to alter the system of management to a total participative model. The plan includes: increase involvement of committee members by eliciting goals; pursue potential members who want to be involved in decision making; seek ideas and suggestions from members with assurance for prompt feedback; and establish joint problem-solving sessions between nurse managers and nonadministrative nurses.

Recruitment and retention of professional nurses are the most critical problems confronting administrators of health care institutions, primarily hospitals. Brief concludes that "dissatisfaction with the work itself may be the root causal factor underlying the high rate of turnover exhibited by nurses" (1976:56-57). Other studies of why nurses change jobs so frequently, and even leave nursing, have concluded that many nurses are dissatisfied with their work environment because they have no voice in decisions affecting their practice (Brief, 1976; Godfrey, 1978a, 1978b; Werther, 1978).

A major challenge for nurse administrators is to meet the needs of their professional nurses. Job satisfaction has been identified as the key to meeting these needs. Werther (1978) defines job satisfiers as "those aspects of the job or job setting that appeal to the employee's ego." Rehmus notes that professionals, perhaps more than any other employee group, want important elements of job control (1970). They want significant inputs into their working environment and a major voice in the way their day-to-day work is conducted. Professionals want to be involved in establishing the standards of work performance and to influence levels of compensation paid for their work. Cleland points out that "The resolution of the issue of who will control nursing practice is probably the primary problem facing the profession today" (1978:40). She advises nursing service administrators to develop organizational structures which allow professional nurses and administrators of nursing services to share in the control of nursing practice.

Several years ago, the nursing administration of a large southeastern medical center developed a model of participative management through a committee structure. This structure consisted of a group of committees created for the purpose of involving nursing personnel in the decision-making process. The Nursing Practice Committee was composed of a cross-representation of registered nurses recognized by peers and supervisors for their clinical knowledge and expertise. The committee effectively handled issues relating to quality of practice and performance, and their work resulted in new or revised policies and practices. The Performance Appraisal and Promotion Committee consisted of a representative group of all nursing personnel; they reviewed qualifications and recommended candidates for promotion. The majority of the members were nonadministrative nurses. The Position Description Committee, also made up of a cross-representation of all nursing personnel, was most effective in reviewing job functions and maintaining updated descriptions of expectations and limitations of each job within the nursing department. These committees were recommending bodies to the nursing administrator and played a significant role in maintaining openness of communication, with information flowing upward and laterally, as well as downward.

REVIEW OF LITERATURE

The escalation of union activity in the health care industry has evoked serious concern among boards of trustees, administrators, and consumers. Increased unionization of professional nurses has prompted nursing service administrators to sharply scrutinize factors contributing to collective action. Poor communication between management and its professional staff and the latter's lack of involvement in the decision-making process, particularly as it relates to patient care management, have been well documented in the literature as causative factors leading to unionization (Rehmus, 1970; Conta, 1972; Reece, 1977).

Most of the issues raised by nurses fall within the boundaries of mandatory bargaining (Cleland, 1969). These issues include the right to bargain about assignments, job duties, job descriptions, evaluations, number of staff and their responsibilities, and all conditions related to the work environment. In a survey reported by Godfrey (1978a, 1978b), 70 percent of the respondents indicated they were usually left out of the decision-making process. Sixty-six percent felt that nursing administration was generally unresponsive to their suggestions and complaints. The surveyor reported no correlation between job satisfaction and the actual salary earned by nurses.

The authority to do one's job the way it should be done also correlates positively to job satisfaction (Godfrey, 1978a). The need for nurse involvement in the decisions affecting his or her practice is supported further by Bentley who points out:

> . . . nurse professionals, working in what Etzioni describes as a normative organization rather than an economic one, receive their rewards from the intrinsic values of the job itself, along with the esteem of their peers and the public. As their professional tasks and environment are increasingly controlled from the outside, satisfaction goes down and frustrations multiply. Moreover,

membership and status are important factors to those in all levels of nursing. (1977:3)

Herzberg (1966, 1968) identified two types of motivators, which he labeled "job content" and "job context." The job context motivators, referred to as "hygiene factors," included fringe benefits, salary, and company policy. Herzberg asserted that administrators who manipulate hygiene factors can prevent dissatisfaction, but their efforts will not increase productivity nor decrease absenteeism and turnover. The motivators that have been associated with nurses' accounts of job satisfaction are opportunities for professional advancement, recognition, achievement, and personal growth (Herzberg, 1968; Werther, 1978). Also recognizing the importance of motivation in the shared-authority model of governance, Richardson and Bender (1974) point out that the ability to motivate people to function at higher levels of commitment, promote values, and provide flexibility in dealing with the need for change are vital to the strength and success of the model. It is obvious that if professional nurses have an opportunity to interact with nursing administration, then nursing administration will have more of an opportunity to know what they (the nurses) need and want.

The very essence of all relationships is communication. Establishing and maintaining open channels of communication is another significant factor affecting job satisfaction. Godfrey's survey (1978b) reported that 61 percent of the respondents rated communication with nursing administrators as fair or worse. Truly effective communication requires multiple channels for output of information and input of feedback and suggestions. It requires a mechanism through which employees can be heard and a climate in which they have a sense of freedom and worth and in which they feel secure about communicating openly (Peterfreund, 1976).

Aside from the theories of humanistic behavioral scientists, changes in state nurse prac-

tice acts, which hold nurses legally accountable for their nursing practice, have increased this awareness of and need for more involvement in decisions affecting their practice. To be held truly accountable for the nature and quality of one's practice within an institution, the practitioner must have a voice and must be involved in establishing the standards of practice through some form of shared governance (Cleland, 1978). Increased interest in participative management techniques is viewed as an attempt to interject more humanism into the management of a nursing department and to gain long-range improvements in productivity and labor relations (Christman, 1976; Likert, 1967).

The motivation for collective bargaining can be redirected by encouraging and allowing nurses to share in decision making and by fostering responsibility among them for the improvement of nursing care services (Cleland, 1978). Maintaining openness of communication with information flowing upward and laterally, as well as downward, can be achieved through a committee structure.

PURPOSE OF STUDY

Participative management is a form of shared governance. Commenting on this form of governance, Cleland (1978) emphasizes the need to clearly differentiate which positions and committees have advisory functions and which have decision-making authority. The present study was therefore devised to measure how nurses serving on nursing committees at a southeastern medical center perceived this committee structure as a model of participative management.

PROCEDURE AND METHODOLOGY

A survey was conducted to measure how participants serving on nursing committees perceived the participative management model of the nursing department of a southeastern medical center. The instrument used for the survey was an adaptation of Likert's "Profile of Organizational Characteristics" (see Table 51-1), which appear in his book *The Human Organization*. The Likert scale has been widely tested for validity and reliability (Likert, 1967:13–46). The questionnaire consisted of 20 questions, each having 4 possible responses associated with the exploitive authoritative, benevolent authoritative, consultative, and participative patterns of management. The questions were divided into seven areas of concern: leadership, motivation, communication, interaction, decision making, goal setting, and feedback control.

Questionnaires were distributed to professional nurse members of the Nursing Practice, Performance Appraisal and Promotion, and Position Description Committees. Also included

in the survey were nurse members of the Nursing Audit and Nursing Policy and Procedure Committees. The latter two committees were added to the sample to enlarge the population surveyed. Total number of respondents was 40. A brief profile regarding length of employment at the medical center, position title, and length of membership on present committees was solicited.

Results of the survey were tabulated by frequency of response and were converted to percentages to facilitate comparisons (Table 51-2). The exploitive authoritative, benevolent authoritative, consultative, and participative patterns (systems 1, 2, 3, and 4) were assigned numerical values of 1, 2, 3, and 4, respectively. An arithmetic mean was calculated for each of the 20 questions, each of the 7 areas of concern, and

Table 51-1 Profile of Organized Characteristics (After Likert, 1967:197–211.)

Leadership

1. How much confidence is shown in subordinates?

| None | Condescending | Substantial | Complete |

2. How free do subordinates feel to talk to their superiors about their jobs?

| Not at all | Not very | Rather free | Fully free |

3. Are subordinates' ideas sought and used if worthy?

| Seldom | Sometimes | Usually | Always |

Motivation

4. To what extent do superiors use (a) fear, (b) threats, (c) punishment, (d) rewards, (e) involvement as motivation?

| A, B, C, & occasionally D | D and some C | D and some C & E | D and C based on group-set goals |

5. Do subordinates feel responsibility for achieving organizational goals?

| No, all top level | Little, most at top and midlevel | Fairly general | Yes, all levels |

Communication

6. What is the direction of information flow?

| Downward | Mostly downward | Down and up | Down, up, and lateral |

7. How is downward communication accepted?

| With suspicion | Some with suspicion | With caution | With open mind |

8. How accurate is upward communication?

| Often wrong | Censored for boss | Limited accuracy | Accurate |

9. How well do superiors know and understand problems faced by subordinates?

| Not at all | Some | Quite well | Very well |

Interaction

10. How do superiors and subordinates interact?

| Little, always with fear and distrust | Little, usually with some condescension | Moderate, with fair amt. of confidence and trust | Extensive, high degree of confidence and trust |

11. How much cooperative teamwork is present?

| None | Relatively little | Moderate amount | Very substantial amount |

Table 51-1   Continued

Decision Making

12. At what level are decisions being made?

Mostly at top	Policy at top, some delegation	Broad policy at top, more delegation	Throughout, but well integrated

13. How is technical and professional knowledge used in decision making?

At higher levels only	At higher & middle levels	To certain extent all levels	To a great extent all levels

14. Are subordinates involved in decisions related to their work?

Not at all	Occasionally consulted	Usually consulted	Fully involved

15. Does involvement in decision-making process contribute to motivation?

No, often weakens motivation	Relatively little contribution	Some contribution	Substantial contribution

Goal Setting

16. How are organizational goals established?

Orders used	Orders issued and opportunity for comment	Orders issued after discussion w/subordinates	Group action (except crisis)

17. How much covert resistance to goals is present?

Strong resistance	Moderate resistance	Some resistance all times	Little or no resistance

Feedback Control

18. How concentrated are review and control function?

Highly at top	Relatively high at top	Moderate delegation to lower levels	Quite widely shared

19. Is there an informal organization resisting the formal one?

Yes	Partially resistant	Occasionally resistant	No, same goals as formal organization

20. What are cost, productivity, and other control data used for?

Policing, punishment	Reward and punishment	Reward some self-guidance	Self-guidance problem solving

the total of all responses (Table 51-3). Results of the study were shared with participants, nursing administrative staff, and members of the hospital's executive administrative group.

Assumptions

1 It was assumed that respondents did not feel threatened by the survey and that responses reflected their honest views.

2 It was assumed that respondents understood the meaning of participative management.

Limitations

1 No attempt was made to determine respondents' prior perceptions of nursing management, and findings are limited to their perceptions of the medical center's nursing management model.

2 Respondents' scores were not differentiated between those holding nurse manager positions and those in nonnurse manager positions.

3 Generalizations were limited due to the size and specifications of the group sampled.

Delimitations

1 The population included only registered professional nurses who were members of nursing committees of the medical center's nursing department.

2 Only current members of the committees were surveyed.

Definition of Terms

1 Nurse managers—Head nurses, assistant head nurses and patient care coordinators who were registered professional nurses occupying middle-

management positions in the medical center's nursing department.

2 Participative management—A management system which emphasizes openness of communication, with information flowing upward, laterally, and downward, and which fosters group decisions through cooperative relationships between management and employees.

RESULTS AND DISCUSSION

Questionnaires, which were an adaptation of Likert's "Profile of Organizational Characteristics," were distributed to professional nurse members of committees dealing with nursing practice, performance appraisal and promotion, position description, nursing policy and procedure, and nursing audit. Forty questionnaires were distributed and returned.

Respondents were asked to identify themselves by position title, length of service on committee, and length of employment at the medical center. Names were not solicited. Twenty-two, or 55 percent, of the respondents held positions of assistant head nurse, head nurse, or patient care coordinator. These positions were considered part of nursing management. Eighteen, or 45 percent, of the respondents were nurses in nonnursing management positions. Length of service on committees ranged from 3 months to 2 years, and length of employment at the medical center ranged from 8 months to 14 years.

Results of the survey were tabulated and are shown on Tables 51-2 and 51-3. Table 51-2 contains percentage tabulations for each response to each question on the questionnaire. Questions not answered were counted in the tabulation, and the sum of responses for each question totals 100 percent.

Systems 1, 2, 3, and 4 (the exploitive authoritative, benevolent authoritative, consultative, and participative patterns) were assigned numerical values of 1, 2, 3, and 4, respectively, and these values were used to compute the arithmetic mean. The first column of Table 51-3 contains the arithmetic mean for each of the 20 questions

listed. The second column contains the arithmetic mean for each of the seven areas of concern.

The arithmetic mean for all responses was 3.29. Fifty percent of the questions had answers which yielded scores above the arithmetic mean. Although the arithmetic mean of 3.29 for all responses placed the nursing department's participative management model, as perceived by respondents, between the consultative and participative patterns of management, the survey revealed several significant findings.

There were four areas of concern registering above-average scores. The section dealing with interaction had the highest arithmetic mean, 3.43. Questions 10 and 11, regarding teamwork and degree of confidence and trust between superiors and subordinates, ranked well above the average mean, with scores of 3.35 and 3.50, respectively. Ranking second highest was the communication section, with an arithmetic mean of 3.42. Questions 6, 7, and 8, dealing with flow and accuracy of information, also ranked well above the average mean, with question 7, regarding downward flow of communication, registering the highest score (3.65) of the 20 questions. This was probably due to the fact that many of the respondents were nurse managers who were responsible for some of the downward communication and who perceived it as being accepted with an open mind. Also within this section, however, question 9, concerning how well superiors know and understand problems faced by subordinates, ranked second lowest of those below the arithmetic mean, with a 3.08. This would seem to indicate that, regardless of position, nurses surveyed doubted that superiors really know or understand the problems encountered in the work environment.

The section concerned with decision making scored third highest, with an arithmetic mean of 3.32. Because of the investigator's expectation that the participative management model utilized by the medical center's nursing administration would provide for significant involvement of professional nurses in decision-making proc-

Table 51-2   Patterns of Management as Revealed by Responses to Seven Areas of Concern

	Percentages for each management pattern				
	Exploitive authoritative (System 1)	Benevolent authoritative (System 2)	Consultative (System 3)	Participative (System 4)	No answer
Leadership					
1 How much confidence is shown in subordinates?	0	0	72.5	27.5	
2 How free do subordinates feel to talk about their jobs?	0	2.5	57.5	40.0	
3 Are subordinates ideas sought and used if worthy?	0	12.5	62.5	25.0	
Motivation					
4 To what extent do superiors use (a) fear, (b) threats, (c) punishment, (d) rewards, (e) involvement as motivation?	2.5	5.0	42.5	45.0	5.0
5 Do subordinates feel responsibility for achieving organizational goals?	7.5	20.0	40.0	32.5	
Communication					
6 What is the direction of information flow?	0	7.5	30.0	62.5	
7 How is downward communication accepted?	0	5.0	30.0	65.0	
8 How accurate is upward communication?	0	7.5	30.0	60.0	2.5
9 How well do superiors know and understand problems faced by subordinates?	0	25.0	42.5	32.5	
Interaction					
10 How do superiors and subordinates interact?	0	5.0	55.0	40.0	
11 How much cooperative teamwork is present?	0	0	50.0	50.0	
Decision Making					
12 At what level are decisions being made?	7.5	15.0	50.0	27.5	
13 How is technical and professional knowledge used in decision making?	0	15.0	35.0	50.0	
14 Are subordinates involved in decisions related to their work?	0	10.0	50.0	40.0	
15 Does involvement in decision-making process contribute to motivation?	0	0	37.5	62.5	
Goal Setting					
16 How are organization goals established?	2.5	10.0	50.0	37.5	
17 How much covert resistance to goals is present?	5.0	17.5	37.5	40.0	
Feedback Control					
18 How concentrated are review and control function?	2.5	20.0	35.0	42.5	
19 Is there an informal organization resisting the formal one?	2.5	7.5	50.0	40.0	
20 What are cost, productivity, and other control data used for?	2.5	7.5	25.0	62.5	2.5

Table 51-3 Response for Each Item and Each Area of Concern by Mean Score

	Arithmetic mean*	
	For this question	For this area of concern
Leadership		
1 How much confidence is shown in subordinates?	3.28	
2 How free do subordinates feel to talk about their jobs?	3.38	3.26
3 Are subordinates' ideas sought and used if worthy?	3.13	
Motivation		
4 To what extent do superiors use (a) fear, (b) threats, (c) punishment, (d) rewards, (e) involvement as motivation?	3.20	3.09
5 Do subordinates feel responsibility for achieving organizational goals?	2.98	
Communication		
6 What is the direction of information flow?	3.55	
7 How is downward communication accepted?	3.65	3.42
8 How accurate is upward communication?	3.45	
9 How well do superiors know and understand problems faced by subordinates?	3.08	
Interaction		
10 How do superiors and subordinates interact?	3.55	
11 How much cooperative teamwork is present?	3.50	3.43
Decision Making		
12 At what level are decisions being made?	2.98	
13 How is technical and professional knowledge used in decision making?	3.35	3.32
14 Are subordinates involved in decisions related to their work?	3.30	
15 Does involvement in decision-making process contribute to motivation?	3.63	
Goal Setting		
16 How are organizational goals established?	3.23	
17 How much covert resistance to goals is present?	3.13	3.18
Feedback Control		
18 How concentrated are review and control function?	3.18	
19 Is there an informal organization resisting the formal one?	3.28	3.30
20 What are cost, productivity, and other control data used for?	3.43	

*The arithmetic mean for all responses was 3.29.

esses, each of the questions within this section, and their mean scores, were reviewed in detail. Two questions in the survey had the lowest arithmetic mean, 2.98; one of these was question 12, which dealt with the level at which decisions are made. Conversely, question 15, on use of decision making as a motivational tool, scored well above average and had the second highest mean, 3.63. Questions concerning use of technical and professional knowledge and subordinates' involvement in decisions related to their work also scored above average. Results of this section of the survey seem to indicate that, while respondents perceived themselves as being involved in the decision-making process, they also perceived that final decisions were made by top management.

Scoring slightly above average was the section on feedback control, with an arithmetic mean of 3.30. The question on use of productivity data scored well above average, while the question relating to review and control function was well below average. Question 19 scored slightly below average, indicating occasional resistance from the informal organization toward the formal one.

The arithmetic mean of the leadership section was 3.26, slightly below average. Scores on the first two questions were average and slightly above average, indicating that respondents believed a substantial amount of confidence was shown in subordinates and that they felt free to talk to superiors about their jobs. However, question 3, on use of subordinates' ideas, scored well below average, with a 3.13.

The two sections with the lowest arithmetic mean were motivation, 3.09, and goal setting, 3.18. Question 4, on methods of motivation, scored slightly below average, while question 5, regarding respondents' perceptions of responsibility for achieving organizational goals, had the lowest arithmetic mean, 2.98. Of the two questions concerning goal setting, number 17, regarding presence of covert resistance to goals, had one of the lowest scores, 3.13.

The two questions with the lowest mean score of 2.98 indicate that respondents perceived decisions as being made by top-level management and did not feel responsibility for achieving organizational goals. Additionally, concentration of review and control functions was perceived to be at a relatively high level of management. Apparently, respondents did not consider themselves sufficiently involved in decision making to feel they were participating in goal setting, program planning, and evaluation. Perhaps that is why they also perceived strong to moderate covert resistance (3.13) to nursing department goals.

To paraphrase Richardson and Bender (1974), when goals and objectives are not developed jointly, commitment to their achievement by all members within the organization will be lacking. The other questions with below-average scores indicate that respondents felt that their superiors did not understand their problems and that their ideas were not sought and used.

IMPLICATIONS AND RECOMMENDATIONS

Research relating to business, industry, and the social sciences has demonstrated that in order to effectively reach organizational goals, participation in the establishment of those goals must occur (Cleland, 1978; Herzberg, 1968; Likert, 1967; Richardson, 1974). A model of participative management through a committee structure was developed by the nursing department of a southeastern medical center for the primary purpose of involving nurses in decisions affecting their practice and work environment. Although the structure provided a mechanism for nurses to have a voice and a vote on major issues of concern to them, they perceived themselves more as consultants than as full participants. Results of the study placed the committee structure of this southeastern medical center's nursing department between the consultative and participative patterns of management. And, although the findings were not entirely negative, they fell short of the investigator's expectations.

To help shift the system of management to a total participative model, a plan of action was proposed which incorporated the following goals:

1 To increase involvement of committee members' establishing and achieving goals for the nursing department. (One approach would be to elicit from members the goals they consider important for the nursing department.)

2 To aggressively pursue committee members who want to be involved in decision making.

3 To be more aggressive in seeking ideas and suggestions from committee members and to assure that prompt feedback regarding use of these ideas and suggestions is provided.

4 To establish joint problem-solving sessions so that nurse managers and nonnurse managers can share and better understand each other's problems.

EDITOR'S QUESTIONS FOR DISCUSSION

To what extent is participative management inherent in primary nursing and professional practice? What is the difference between administration and management? Compare a system of governance through committee structure with Sills's discussion of nursing governance (Chap. 42) and Malkemes's views (Chap. 50). Are there implications for shared governance evident in Bullough's discussion on state nurse practice acts (Chap. 45)? What alternative or additional forms are there of participative management? What is the relationship between management by objectives (MBO) and participative management? What factors are essential for participative management to be effective? Provide examples of situations or conditions where participative management may not be appropriate? For those situations and/or conditions what type of management would be effective? To what extent should an organization be flexible as to various modes of management? What implications are there for participative management from Malkemes's experience (Chap. 50) regarding nurses who say they wish to be accountable but are not and the findings of Mercadante's survey? What applications to participative management can be made from Bille's (36) and La Monica's (37) chapters? What nursing theoretical conceptual framework or model may be most applicable to participative management?

Compare the findings of Braito's and Caston's study on job satisfaction (Chap. 27) with Mercadante's review of the literature. What factors most influence job satisfaction? To what extent does the mode of providing care contribute to the control of nursing practice? What alternative models of participative management can be suggested? To what extent is there unionization of professional nurses in settings where primary nursing has been established?

Discuss the methodology utilized by Mercadante. How valid and reliable is Likert's instrument? What criteria should be considered in establishing committees in an organizational structure? How was committee membership established? What criteria might be suggested for membership? What impact may including both nurse-managers and clinical staff nurses on committees have on the findings of participative management surveys? What questions are essential to include in surveys when both management and nursing staff are concerned with decision making? What type of sampling method was utilized? What other limitations are there of the survey? What elements of bias are inherent and accounted for in the findings? What alternative explanations can be offered for the findings? What additional statistical data analyses might have been completed?

Discuss the proposed plan to alter the system of management to a total participative model. What additional data should be obtained before the plan is implemented? What considerations need to be made regarding committee membership? Should joint problem-solving sessions occur within the committee structure? How cost-effective are committees for achieving goals? What on-going evaluation and methodologies can be suggested for assessing the effectiveness of committees as a form of participative management? What alternative methodologies and other critical variables for inclusion can be suggested for future research concerning participative management?

REFERENCES

Bentley, Peter
  1977 Health Care Agencies and Professionals: A Changing Relationship. Publication No. 14-1669. New York: NLN.

Brief, Arthur P.
  1976 "Turnover among hospital nurses: A suggested model." Journal of Nursing Administration 6,8:55-58.

Christman, Luther
  1976 "Nurses seek to influence care." Hospitals 50(April):97-100.

Cleland, Virginia S.
  1969 "Collective bargaining: What is negotiable?" American Journal of Nursing 69,9:1892-1895.
  1978 "Shared governance in a professional model of collective bargaining." Journal of Nursing Administration 8,5:39-43.

Conta, A. Lionne
  1972 "Bargaining by professionals." American Journal of Nursing 72,2:309-312.

Godfrey, Marjorie A.
  1978a "Job satisfaction: Part I." Nursing/78, 4(April)89-102.
  1978b "Job satisfaction: Part II." Nursing/78, 5(May):105-120.

Herzberg, Frederick
  1966 Work and the Nature of Man. New York: World.
  1968 "One more time: How do you motivate employees?" Harvard Business Review 46(February):53-57.

Likert, Rensis
  1967 The Human Organization. New York: McGraw-Hill.

Peterfreund, Stanley
  1976 "Employees must have a sense of freedom, worth." Hospitals, 50(August): 60-62.

Reece, David A.
  1977 "Union decertification and the salaried approach: A workable alternative." Journal of Nursing Administration 7,6:20-24.

Rehmus, C. M.
  1970 "Professional employees and the right to representation." Professional Engineer (American) 70(February)48-51.

Richardson, Richard C., Jr.
  1974 "Governance theory: A comparison of approaches." The Journal of Higher Education 74(May):344-354.

Richardson, Richard C. and Louis W. Bender
  1974 College Governance, 2d ed. Fort Lauderdale: Nova University.

Werther, William B., Jr.
  1978 Unions Do Not Happen, They Are Caused. Publication No. 20-1725. New York: NLN.

Chapter 52

Applying Nursing Theory in Nursing Administration

Barbara J. Stevens, R.N., Ph.D., F.A.A.N.
Director, Division of Health Services,
Sciences and Education
Chairman, Department of Nursing Education
and
Isabel Maitland Stewart Professor
Teachers College, Columbia University
New York, New York

With the requirement that all nursing acts demand a theoretical basis confirmed by research for professional practice and status as a profession, tradition is no longer an accepted rationale for a nursing act, intervention, or decision. The nurse executive faces the challenge of managing nursing in the complex state of transition toward complete professionalization. Barbara J. Stevens examines the new demand for the nurse executive to implement a theory of nursing within the delivery system of the nursing department. She identifies multiple and shifting variables pertaining to the patient, environment, and the nurse which characterize nursing judgments. Nursing has few absolutes, but those also alter with changes in both nursing and medical technology and delivery of nursing care.

Stevens sets the stage for application of nursing theory in nursing administration by first defining a theory of nursing as a description of nursing that identifies those elements that are seen as comprising the critical factors of nursing. She illustrates the contrasting themes and elements of nursing theories through differences between Levine's and Orem's conceptualizations. Stevens asserts there may be theories that are more effective for a given setting than another. She then clarifies the relationship between nursing theory and research. Research questions are formulated from a theoretical base. Researchers differ in theoretical positions. Therefore they may formulate the research question differently though they address the same research problem as other investigators. They may ask different questions concerning the same data, as well as analyze, explain, and offer different conclusions from the same data. Stevens maintains there is no shared "body of knowledge" for all nursing since there is no absolute conclusion from research applicable in all theories. Stevens perceives nursing as "practical action" that must take place "now," but is hoped that what is done is based on some theory of what ought to be done.

Stevens addresses the issues of who decides on the theory to be applied in the administrative setting. Some executives and theorists believe that practitioners should be permitted to apply the theory under which they were educated. Stevens notes that freedom in selection of a theory may result in substitute primary nursing having to apply three or four different theories to different patients; it dictates diverse coexisting formats for Kardex, nursing orders, and charting which would require cost justification; the impact on care may differ as nursing theories are developed and refined. Stevens suggests three options: an organization might select a single theory, implement it institution-wide, and make all policies, practices, and records conform to the theory; allow each department or unit to select a theory for implementation in its own setting; or the nurse executive may choose to ignore theory as a function of management. She offers advantages and disadvantages in choosing any one of the three options.

Stevens emphasizes that few persons use or describe total theories; most use theory elements. A total theory constitutes content, process, and context. She examines the content (subject matter) and process (acts and/or thoughts) formulated by Levine, Peplau, Orlando, Orem, Roy, Rogers, Hall, and Johnson. Stevens comments on the significant differences among all eight theorists. She does not discuss the context for theory application, assuming that nurse executives would automatically eliminate theories incompatible with their setting. However, she suggests that a nursing department may amplify, supplement, or adapt a given or incompletely developed theory. In so doing it is essential that selected elements are compatible.

Stevens advocates a logistic process be utilized in adjusting or adapting theory. She contrasts the different reasoning approaches to utilizing process in nursing. Nursing process is a logistic approach. Problem solving is another popular approach but does not follow a precise formula. The most common form of problematic process in nursing administration is problem-oriented charting. Assessment is not routine but initiated by a perceived problem. Stevens maintains that it is essential for the content and process component to be compatible in instituting a partial theory. Furthermore, she urges that only one process component be used in a given theory. Two other approaches cited are the operational and dialectic processes.

Stevens suggests that the best formula for a nurse executive or management team to apply a selected theory—or components—in an organization is the protocol developed by Coleman. The managerial components of planning, organizing, staffing, directing, and controlling are related to implementation of theory. Examples of the need for congruence between the theory being implemented and each management phase are provided. Stevens concludes that administrative structures need to be modified so as to reinforce use of a theoretical model.

Today's nurse executive faces the challenge of managing nursing when it is in transition toward full status as a profession and an academic discipline. This adds another dimension to an already complex managerial task. The nature of what is being managed is shifting rapidly. Yesterday's nursing acts were relatively well known and easily prescribed. Even the independent nursing component was programmed on the basis of past traditions. Today that is no longer the case. Tradition is no longer an accepted rationale for a nursing act or decision; all nursing acts require confirmation by research, preferably research with a basis in a specified theoretical conception of the nursing field.

Much of nursing substance has yet to be subjected to this process. Hence today's nursing executive manages care delivered by a discipline in which most questions have yet to be raised, let alone answered. Yet it is a profession that cannot put off its services until its acts are confirmed. Today's patient cannot wait for tomorrow's research findings. And today's practicing nurse must make decisions and act, knowing that his or her choices may prove wrong. Today's nurses do not have the security of tradition to assure them of good choices, as did the nurses of the past.

Neither nurses nor nurse executives can ignore the fact that they work in the action domain, where intellectual pursuit alone does not suffice. Both dwell in a domain where choices must be based on partial, inadequate, and incomplete knowledge. Further, nursing is a discipline with few absolutes anyway. What is best for one patient may not be best for another with a similar physiological health status. Nursing is characterized by judgments concerning multiple and shifting variables:

     1 Patient variables: physiological, sociological, economical, intellectual, motivational, psychological
     2 Environmental variables: as illustration, nursing acts under situations of cardiac monitoring might differ from acts for the same patient in a nonmonitored situation
     3 Nurse variables: two nurses may require two different approaches to a similar patient because of differences in their own ages, experiences, or philosophies

Nursing-care absolutes also change with changes in both nursing and medical technology. For example, changes in techniques for laminectomy radically changed the requisite nursing care that such patients require. The same may be said for innumerable situations in nursing care delivery. Other technologies also impact on nursing care delivery. For example, when the domain of drug-dependent learning was explored in the discipline of education, the findings required changes in patient teaching by nurses.

Most nurse executives and their staffs are comfortable today with the impact of nursing research in and on their departments. They understand and use simple action research, such as subjecting two groups of patients to different nursing treatments for the same health need and later comparing patient outcomes. Indeed, nursing quality control systems that measure the patient health status (physiological or behavioral) provide essential research in that they point out instances in which the normal procedures of care are ineffective and new procedures must be proposed and tested. More sophisticated nursing departments are initiating more advanced measures of nursing research at this time, and nurse executives usually are quite capable of evaluating a research proposal submitted for their consideration.

Nurse executives are confronted now with a new demand: that they implement a selected theory of nursing in their department's delivery system. Certainly it is time that this missing link in the theory-research-practice cycle be put in place. Indeed, the profession of nursing is unique in that it substantially incorporated research into its career behaviors before identifying and exploring those implicit theories that were (or were not) confirmed by the research.

WHAT IS THEORY?

What is the theory of nursing? How does it relate to nursing research? What does it *do* to nursing practice? A theory of nursing is a description of nursing that identifies those elements that are seen as comprising the critical factors of nursing. Just as a road map indicates essentials for the driver-roads and their markings (not mountains or valleys or beautiful scenic stops)—so a theory isolates the essentials of nursing from that total environment in which nursing takes place. Analogously, freudian psychology defines essential concepts such as id, ego, superego, consciousness, repression, and suppression. Other essential elements are those that indicate how these major concepts interrelate. Developmental psychology, in contrast, has different essentials—such as developmental tasks and developmental needs—but the process of highlighting and interrelating elements is identical.

Nursing theories similarly have contrasting themes and elements. For example, according to Levine (1967) nursing constitutes *conservation* of that which represents successful adaptation on the part of the patient. Conservation elements consist of: energy conservation, structural conservation, maintenance of personal integrity, and maintenance of social integrity. In contrast, Orem (1971) describes nursing as the provision of *self-care* that patients would provide for themselves were they able. (Self-care is further differentiated as the theory is elaborated.)

Nursing has at least 10 or more different theories in early stages of development. Some will prove fruitful as they develop; others will die out as research shows them to be minimally productive. It is not likely that nursing will ever have only one theory. Nevertheless, there may be theories that are more effective for a given setting than for another. A well-baby clinic may profit from a different theory from that used in an acute care setting, or psychiatric nursing may benefit from a model different from that used in public health nursing.

NURSING THEORY AND NURSING RESEARCH

How, then, does nursing theory relate to nursing research? Every instance of nursing research comes from some theory position, whether or not the researcher recognizes the fact. Qualified researchers know their theory basis; they can elaborate that theory (or conceptual framework) which underlies the given research. The theory determines what questions the researcher asks and how the researcher analyzes and interprets the data collected. To illustrate: the Freudian and the developmental psychologist look at the same data—the patient and his or her actions, beliefs, and values. But they ask different questions concerning those data, formulate different explanations for the data, and prescribe different therapies. Their research results

in different conclusions from the same data. Similarly, in nursing there is no absolute conclusion from research applicable in all theories. There is no shared body of knowledge that is the same for all nursing. Each nursing theory will build its own body of knowledge, even though diverse theories may examine the same raw data.

What is the state of understanding concerning this relationship between theory and research in nursing? Researchers from different theoretical positions (recognized or not) all purport to add to the same body of knowledge. The result is that no single theory (or conceptual framework) is well developed. No single theory has been the inspiration for a group of related research studies. Had this happened, the results of such research would have led to further refinement and development of that initial theory base. Research confirms or disconfirms theory; as knowledge accumulates, the theory is altered to better reflect the reality. Indeed, the chief purpose of research is to discover theories about the world (in this case, the world of nursing) and how it works.

Now, since nursing is *practical action* that must take place *now*, what is done is based on some theory of what ought to be done. Hopefully, the basis for decisions concerning nursing acts will be a theory that has—so far—stood the test of time, even if there is little research yet to confirm it. Clearly, nursing will have more import if it rests on a known, rather than an intuited, theory.

THEORY IN THE ADMINISTRATIVE SETTING

The nurse executive, reflecting on the application of theory to practice, must consider who decides on the theory to be applied: the nursing organization or the individual practitioner. In the typical case of today, both have some decision-making authority. The nursing organization reflects some theory elements in its selected assignment systems, report systems, and charting predilections. For example, a Kardex system that requires the use of a nursing process imposes one theory element, while problem-oriented charting imposes an alternative one. Practitioners also utilize theory when they write specific nursing orders for given patients.

Some hold that nurses themselves are the proper loci of theory decisions. Theorists or nurse executives who hold this position believe that nurses should be allowed to apply the theory under which they were educated. Unfortunately theory choice is not this simple. Choice is constrained by the procedures, policies, and practices of the nursing department as well as by the need for continuity of care for each patient across shifts. Even in primary nursing, there is a problem if each primary nurse selects her or his own theory preference. In this case a relief nurse who substitutes for several primary nurses may have to apply three or four different theories to different patients. Clearly, that level of practice is too complex to expect of the average nurse. Even if the average nurse were capable of shifting the frame of reference with each patient, good administration would dictate a simpler plan for care delivery.

Note that such freedom in selection of a theory would indicate diverse coexisting formats for Kardex, nursing orders, charting. Even if nurses could cope with this complexity, it would present insurmountable difficulties for supportive personnel such as aides, practical nurses, and secretaries. The nurse executive also would have to justify the high cost of having so many different coexisting chart forms and systems of care coordination.

At present these problems of delivery may not appear at a superficial review. Indeed, few nurses understand theory enough to actually apply it to what happens in the organizational setting. In addition, theories in the infantile developmental state do not direct care to a great degree, so they all look alike. But that will change with time. Today, if one asks three nurses practicing under three different theories to take care of the same comatose patient, they generally give the same care (even though from different premises). Tomorrow, the care given by these three may radically differ. This is to be expected as nursing theories develop and are refined; their impact on care will not always be such as to produce identical nursing acts.

Since most of nursing is a coordinated effort among many nurses rather than an independent practice, it is logical that the organizing body select the theories to be utilized. (Even primary nurses are not in independent practice. After all, they are present only 40 hours out of the 168 in a week on the average.) How, then, does a nursing organization apply nursing theory to care delivery? There are several possible answers to this question. First, an organization might select a single theory and implement it on an institutionwide basis, making all policies, practices, and records conform to the theory. The advantages of this scheme are those of consistency, economy of scale, simplicity for nonprofessional staff (improving their flexibility and mobility within the system), and ability to conduct related nursing research (under the aegis of a single theory). The disadvantage is that any theory selected will not give an ideal fit with all units within the average nursing organization. (This disadvantage will be less applicable in a singlepurpose institution, e.g., a maternity center, a psychiatric care center, or a home for mentally retarded.)

Another option open to the nurse executive is to let each department or unit select a theory for implementation in its own setting. The advantages of this plan are that a theory may be selected for its "fit" with the work of the unit, and nurses educated under one theory may be clustered in units where that theory is applied. Further, in this system some comparative data may be collected as to diverse theories' productivity and effectiveness. The disadvantages of the system are loss of flexibility of staff, loss of economies of scale, and confusion for interdigitating professions that must deal with units under diverse care delivery systems.

The third option for the nurse executive is to ignore theory as a function of management. The advantages of this choice are those of allowing freedom of action among staff and providing for easier affiliation with diverse schools of nursing.

The disadvantage is that one cannot really avoid theory by failing to identify it. There will be elements of "hidden theory" as revealed in choices of practices and policies. Further, it always is better to function in knowledge than in ignorance, and to ignore theory elements is to opt for ignorance. Additionally, if theory elements are unexamined, there may be conflicting messages. For example, problem-oriented charting and the Kardex version of the nursing process may be used simultaneously, causing nurses to have to think in two diverse thought patterns at the same time.

STRUCTURES IN A THEORY

The nurse executive will be cognizant of the fact that few people (even nurse-theorists) use or describe total theories; most use theory elements. Indeed, some people insist that such an incomplete theory be called a *conceptual framework* rather than a theory as indication of this incompleteness. (This chapter will not address this minor semantic debate.) What would constitute a total theory? A well-elaborated and interdigitated theory would include:

1 Content—subject matter, i.e., that to which nursing is applied
2 Process—acts and/or thoughts which are applied to the subject matter
3 Context—where and/or under what circumstance that process is applied to that content

Most present theories of nursing are weak in one or more of these aspects.

Theories Analyzed by Content and Process

For nurse executives the context for theory application is that supplied by the nature of their institution. For many nurse executives this will mean the acute care setting or a specialty setting. For simplicity the element of context will be omitted in this comparison, assuming that nurse executives would automatically eliminate theories incompatible with their context. Further, in most nursing theories, the element of context is little elaborated, minimally explored, and often merely assumed by the theory author. An examination of content and process alone will reveal important differences among theories.

Theorist	Content	Process	Comments
Levine (1967)	Conservation Energic Structural Personal Social Adaptation	Reading "messages" sent by the patient Appears to be problematic, though Levine does not say this	Content is clear; process is minimally addressed
Peplau (1962)	Anxiety	Encourage patient to: 1 Recognize anxiety exists 2 Recognize relief-giving patterns 3 Provide data regarding situations that precede anxiety 4 Identify situational causes for increased anxiety	Strong focus on process; content limited and minimally explored
Orlando (1961)	Nurse-patient relationship Patient behavior	Nurse should: 1 Observe behavior 2 Reflect it back without interpretation 3 Encourage the patient to interpret it	Content is limited; process (as in Peplau) is highly specified

Theorist	Content	Process	Comments
Roy (1974)	Modes of adaptation 1 Physiologic needs 2 Self-concept 3 Role function 4 Interdependence	Stimulus-response interference with: 1 Focal stimuli 2 Residual stimuli 3 Contextual stimuli	Both content and process developed but their fit with each other is questionable (Can a biological process interact with a conceptual content?)

Orem (1971)	Self-care
	1 Universal
	  a Air-food-water
	  b Excrements
	  c Rest-activity
	  d Social interaction-solitude
	  e Hazards of life-well-being
	  f Being normal
	2 Health deviation
	  a Change in structure
	  b Change in function
	  c Change in behavior
		Deliberation action:
		1 Adjust ways of meeting universal requirements
		2 Establish new techniques of self-care
		3 Modify self-image
		4 Revise routines of daily living
		5 Develop new lifestyle
		6 Cope with effects of health deviation or its treatment
		Actions specific to nursing:
		1 Acting for another
		2 Guiding
		3 Supporting
		4 Providing an appropriate environment
		5 Teaching
			Both content and process are elaborated, but they may be overlong for easy memorization and retention

Rogers (1970)	Principles 1 Resonancy 2 Reciprocity 3 Synchrony 4 Helicy	Not yet described, but one can assume a dialectic process will emerge	Until the process is further elaborated, it is difficult to say how nursing actions can be directed by this theory
Hall (1966)	Self-mastery	Rogerian techniques	A limited subject matter for nursing, a question of whether a borrowed technique is appropriate as the major impetus for nursing action
Johnson (1968)	Behavioral systems 1 Affiliation 2 Aggression 3 Dependence 4 Achievement 5 Ingestion 6 Elimination 7 Sex	Modes of intervention: 1 Impose external controls and regulatory mechanisms 2 Supply conditions and resources for fulfilling subsystem functional requirements	Fails to identify how subsystems interact at this stage of development, but does have content and process

Even when using an incompletely developed theory, nursing service is forced to have a broad scope of content and a defined process directing thought and action. To achieve this, a nursing department may amplify, supplement, or adapt a given theory. In making such changes in (or additions to) a given model, it is important that the selected pieces be compatible with each other. For example, a systems model (with focus on the separate parts and their interrelationships) is a natural fit with Johnson's model. In this case the process (logistic addition of component parts) fits Johnson's component parts, which are themselves pieces of content in a larger whole (the human behavioral system).

The nursing process is a logistic process that presently is in favor. The elements are sequential (invariant sequence), with each element dependent on the preceding one (nature of interrelationship). In the nursing process, a person is initially assessed simply because he or she is labeled (usually through being admitted) as a patient. There is no other stimulus to start the nursing process. The process has as many steps as the particular user envisions, but the common ones are: assessment, diagnosis, prognosis, goal setting, care planning, care implementation, and evaluation of both the patient outcome and the plan itself. Many forms of the so-called nursing process eliminate one or more of these steps, but the steps, whatever they may be, are envisioned as building upon each other in a cumulative pattern. This process is goal-oriented, with the goal determined before care patterns are planned. Success is measured in terms of achievement of the predetermined goal.

The logistic or systems approach is highly structured and works well when the content components of a given nursing theory (such as Johnson's) are clearly specified and concretely differentiated from one another. Stimulus-response theories typify this approach (such as Roy's), in which a specified goal is brought about in a systematic plan.

The other popular approach to process in nursing is that of problem solving. In the problematic method, nursing action does not follow a highly precise formula; instead the process is brought into being when the nurse detects an obstacle, impediment, or puzzlement, however indefinitely perceived. The nurse then sets about clarifying that puzzle by search of the relevant environment. Obviously, the "environment" will be different for every problem. Indeed, the environment may shift as the nurse further clarifies the problem. Problem solving, then, is a relatively disorderly fluctuation between the problem and its context. When the problem reaches its final state, it will be quite different from the initial fuzzy determination that something was amiss. In problem solving, the focus is upon the delimitation and conception of the problem rather than on its solution. Indeed, the way the problem is cast will determine the potential solutions to be tried. The only "goal" in this system is the successful removal of the problem. There is no single answer (the goal-setting stage of nursing process); the "right" answer is any answer that effectively and efficiently removes the problem.

The most common form of problematic process found in nursing administration is that of problem-oriented charting. Note that while this purports simply to be a charting form, it forces nurses to approach their work (and their patients) in a way that looks for the problematic, the troublesome. In such a system, assessment is not routine but is initiated by a perceived problem, and the assessment is not generalized but is related to that problem.

Here again, it is important that the nursing service instituting a theory or partial theory look at compatibility of process and content. As illustration, a problematic approach would be inconsistent with Johnson's theory; her components (behavior systems) cannot easily be conceived as problems. In contrast, Levine's components, e.g., conserving personal integrity or conserving energy, can be perceived as problems to be resolved.

It is important not only that the content

component and the process component be compatible but that only one process component be used in a given theory. It is inconsistent and confusing, for example, to expect nurses to establish logistic goals on a care plan while requiring that they chart in a problematic mode in relation to the same patient. Tactics such as this will ensure that a nurse has confused processes and will think and act with indecision.

While problematic and logistic thought predominate in nursing, they are not the only possible processes that may be used in theory construction. The operational process operates by discrimination and differentiation. This is the preferred method in medicine, and it is surprising that nursing has so overlooked this option. Operational thought (and action) is dominated by the principle of choice: either one path or another. In medical practice it is typified in differential diagnosis. Orem is the only well-known theorist who appears to instinctively use an operational approach (Stevens, 1979). The dialectic process is similarly overlooked in nursing, with Rogers the only well-known theorist to demonstrate this approach to theory.

THE PRAGMATICS OF APPLYING THEORY IN THE PRACTICE SETTING

What, then, are the mechanisms by which a nurse executive or a management team sets about the process of applying a selected theory, or theory components, in the institutional setting? Coleman (1977) has the best formula for this task; she looks at the managerial components of planning, organizing, staffing, directing, and controlling as they relate to theory implementation in the nursing department. The process is a complex one, but her directives are extremely useful, though they cannot be summarized in a short chapter such as this one. Some recommendations from each managerial component will be highlighted here, but the reader is referred to Coleman for a comprehensive view of the implementation task.

In the *planning* phase, it is important that the

theory be evident in the statements of philosophy and purpose; the objectives of the department should be to deliver care in the manner conceived in the theory. In the *organization* phase, the organization chart and the committee structure should be planned with the theory in mind. Even the types of personnel used may vary, depending upon the theory selected. One historical example of nursing organization that would have major impact on theory is that of progressive patient care. Some nurses may never have heard of this system; others will recall the system as one in which patients are assigned to care units, not on the basis of their medical-surgical, physician-dominated classifications but according to type or level of nursing care required. Indeed, the original intensive care unit arose in conjunction with the progressive care system. Progressive care, as an illustration, is an organizational statement of theory; it perceives nursing as located in what the nurse does, not in what the patient is. Such a system would be compatible with a task-oriented or nurse-oriented theory.

Additional organizing elements would include the Kardex forms and charting requirements. Do the forms reflect the major components of the accepted theory or do they conflict in their demands? Do the unit conferences (if this tactic is used) conform to and reinforce the theory?

The *staffing* phase of administration also may be affected by a selected theory. Does the theory allow diverse staff to be "interchangeable" with professional nurses? Must only professional staffing be used? Or is some component of nursing—such as determining the nursing orders—reserved exclusively for professionals? The *directing* phase also must reflect the theory to be implemented. Is education to the theory provided in orientation and ongoing in-service education? Is the theory reinforced in all documents and reports? Do the assignment systems allow for the kind of practice dictated by the theory? Are the rewards and punishments of the system related to the theory in the *controlling* phase? Are the formats for performance appraisal, quality control, and evaluation of the nursing organization itself done in such a way as to require use of the theory?

Since the Coleman protocol is thorough, there will be no attempt to duplicate it here, but this chapter should serve to make the reader cognizant of the amount of work involved in the actual implementation of theory into a system of nursing care delivery. It is not enough to say that one will use a particular theory, relying upon individuals to follow that format. It is not enough to place educational responsibility with an in-service education department. Even if that department is successful in educating every nurse in the insti-

tution to a given theory, the job is incomplete if the administrative structures are not modified so as to reinforce (or require) use of that theoretical model. Theory implementation begins with the nurse executive; it must be influential on every administrative and nursing process if it is to have an impact on patient care. Theory application is a structural job of reordering a nursing division to express a given theoretical position. Education is an adjunct, but only an adjunct to the structural administrative revision of departmental form and function.

EDITOR'S QUESTIONS FOR DISCUSSION

Compare Stevens's conceptualization of nursing and approach to theory construction with the presentations in the previous chapters by Santora (8), Fawcett (14), Newman (28), Chinn (29), Walker (30), Menke (31), Hardy (32), Meleis (33), and Roy (34). What commonalities and differences exist? To what extent is there agreement among Stevens, Hardy, and Roy regarding a shared body of knowledge in nursing? How congruent is the model for critique of theories and paradigms in nursing developed by Meleis with the form for analysis offered by Stevens? Apply both Stevens' method and Meleis' model to each of the eight theoretical formulations examined by Stevens as a basis for deciding the appropriateness of each for use specifically by nursing administrators in administration of nursing education and nursing service.

Provide examples of the multiple judgment variables by which Stevens characterizes nursing. What additional variables may be suggested? What other factors may influence change in nursing care "absolutes"? Provide examples of nursing care absolutes. What empirical evidence exists concerning the management effectiveness of quality-control systems? Provide specific examples of nursing departments utilizing sophisticated measures in nursing research. Provide examples of nursing theory determining the questions the researcher asks. How are differences in theoretical positions of researchers shown in the analysis and interpretation of data? What obligations are inherent in reporting research findings and interpretation of data? What are the advantages and disadvantages for patient care, nursing administration, and the profession in different theoretical perspectives underlying the basis for addressing the same research problem? What suggestions can be offered for nursing in building its body of knowledge through diverse theoretical formulations?

How much agreement might there be concerning application of theory and the practicing community between Chinn (Chap. 29), Roy (Chap. 34), and Stevens? Provide arguments, rationale, and examples for and against a belief that nursing is "practical action." How would you characterize nursing? To what extent are decisions concerning nursing acts based on theories that have stood the "test of time"? Discuss whether a theory can stand the "test of time," without confirmation by research, and be a legitimate theory. What examples can you provide of a "theory" standing the test of time? What are criteria for a theory? Provide examples of elements of theory in a nursing organization.

Discuss who should decide on the nursing theory to be applied in a nursing organization. What specific factors influence the choice of a theory? What are the implications for patient care, the practitioner, nursing organization, and the profession if only one theory is permitted for implementation in an organization? Should a normative expectation for professional practice be that a nurse be able to proficiently apply different theories to different patients? How much agreement is there between Klein's (Chap. 43) observations of the level of practice of the typical nurse and Stevens's comments? By what criteria can a nurse be able to resolve potential conflicts when more than one theory is being utilized in a setting? Provide examples of three different theories being applied to the care of a single patient and the impact on patient care. To what extent is it necessary for nursing acts to be identical in providing care? How important is the process (how, manner) of providing care versus the nursing act in the application of nursing theory?

Discuss the advantages and disadvantages of the three options Stevens offers in implementing nursing theory for the provision of care in an organization. What rationale can you provide for the option you would choose? What alternative options may be suggested? Besides management and nursing functions and tasks, what behavioral and other variables are critical for the nurse executive to consider in choosing and implementing nursing theory? What application and suggestions may be found or made from Malkemes's (Chap. 50) and Mercadante's (Chap. 51) discussions to the implementation of nursing theory? What implications might be suggested in Stevens's presentation for the experiences offered by Malkemes and Mercadante? How is theory a function of management?

What criteria can a nurse executive utilize to assess the compatibility of a nursing theory for application within an organizational setting? For each of the eight formulations of theory Stevens examines according to content and process, provide examples of the context for application. What organizational characteristics and settings would be most critical for appropriate implementation of each theory? Provide examples as to how a nursing department may amplify, supplement, or adapt an incompletely developed or a given specific theory. Provide specific examples of each of the process approaches used in nursing as described by Stevens in the management role and functions of nursing administration. What is the difference between the approaches to process presented by Stevens and the use and components of process in her examination of theories? To what extent do you agree with Stevens that only one process component should be used in instituting a given or partial theory? How can potential difficulties be resolved if differences between content, process, and context components appear in implementation of a theory? How can the operational and dialectic processes be used in theory construction for an organization? Provide other examples of the relationship between each of the five managerial components described by Stevens and theory implementation in a nursing department. To what extent should an organization adapt to a given theory or a given or partial theory be adapted to the organization? Must the theory be evident in each of the management components prior to implementation or does nursing administration need to plan to reflect the theory into each component of management? To what extent should the nurse executive have a choice as to which theoretical components of a theory will be implemented? What other criteria may be suggested for decision making concerning instituting a theory in a department of nursing?

REFERENCES

Coleman, Leatrice J.
1977 Development of an Administrative Protocol: The Relationship Among Nursing Theory, Practice, and Administrative Theory. Unpublished thesis, University of Illinois, Chicago.

Hall, Lydia E.
1966 "Another view of nursing care and quality." Pp. 47–66 in K. M. Straub and K. S. Parker (eds.), Continuity of Patient Care: The Role of Nursing. Washington, D.C.: Catholic University Press.

Johnson, Dorothy E.
1968 "One conceptual model of nursing." Unpublished paper presented at Vanderbilt University, Nashville, April 25, 1968.

Levine, Myra E.
1967 "The four conservation principles of nursing." Nursing Forum 1:47–53.

Orem, Dorothea E.
1971 Nursing: Concepts of Practice. New York: McGraw-Hill.

Orlando, Ida Jean
1961 The Dynamic Nurse-Patient Relationship. New York: Putnam's.

Peplau, Hildegard E.
1962 "Interpersonal techniques: The crux of psychiatric nursing." American Journal of Nursing 6:50–54.

Rogers, Martha E.
1970 An Introduction to the Theoretical Basis of Nursing. Philadelphia: F. A. Davis.

Roy, Callista
1974 "The Roy adaptation model." Pp. 135–144 in J. P. Riehl and C. Roy (eds.), Conceptual Models for Nursing Practice. Englewood Cliffs, N.J.: Prentice-Hall.

Stevens, Barbara J.
1979 Nursing Theory: Analysis, Application, Evaluation. Boston: Little, Brown.

Chapter 53

Theories of Nursing and Organizations: Generating Integrated Models for Administrative Practice

Norma L. Chaska, R.N., Ph.D., F.A.A.N.
Associate Professor
Chairperson, Nursing Administration
Coordinator, Nursing Research
School of Nursing
Medical College of Georgia
Augusta, Georgia

Stevens has provided the mandate for the application and implementation of nursing theory into departments of nursing for *nursing* practice. Her focus was on the selection of a theory by the nurse executive or management team and contrasting the content and process of theoretical formulations by nurse-theorists. In emphasizing the context, the organizational or institutional setting where nursing theory may be applied, Norma L. Chaska advocates the construction of integrated models for nursing *administrative* practice in health care and academic settings. Her basic premise is that the senior nurse administrator of nursing practice and nursing education must have an underlying scientific knowledge base besides factual knowledge for their practice. Nursing administration is viewed as an unique synthesis of the two disciplines nursing and management and their related theories. It is paramount, then, to develop a scientific knowledge base for nursing administration utilizing concepts from both disciplines, which can be integrated into a conceptual model. A definition is offered for integrated nursing administration conceptual models. The model should be congruent with the goals and objectives of the institution, administratively reflected and implemented in the department of nursing, and congruent with models and theory selected by clinicians for patient care.

Chaska provides additional rationale for integrated conceptual models. These include: the key leadership role of administrators in health care and academic settings to represent and translate nursing at the highest level of administration and to the community; the accurate assessment of appropriate nursing theory or conceptual models for implementation for patient care and education of nursing students given the characteristics of the organization or institution and the conceptual model for nursing administration; the adaptive mode of management desired when the majority of employees in a setting are professionals.

Suggestions are made as to how integrated conceptual models may be formulated, and examples are indicated. It is necessary to first identify the essential elements and concepts of management thought, administrative and organizational theory, nursing concepts, nursing theory, and/or nursing conceptual models that might be most critical to the management role of a nurse administrator. The author does not examine the various methods in theory construction. However, broad guidelines are established for linkage of concepts into a model. Examples of concepts from nursing and management are shown. The necessity for congruence of concepts with organization structure and design is emphasized. Examples are provided for the genesis of integrated conceptual models. One includes the linkage of a portion of the concepts used in Roy's adaptation model, organizational concepts that emphasize the individual, concepts of management processes applied at a micro level, and the concepts of an open system. Another example utilizes the broad concepts of nursing knowledge (man, health, nursing, and environment), with concepts from management, administrative theory, and organizational behavior (interaction, systems, adaptation, development).

Considerations are proposed for validation and implementation of integrated models. Research is essential to validate the relationships between and among the concepts and effectiveness of the integrated model for prescriptions applied to administrative issues. In implementation of the integrated model, critical variables are discussed, including congruence of the model with the environment, readiness of staff and faculty, and the political role of the administrator. In conclusion, Chaska offers the challenge to create integrated models for a scientific knowledge base in nursing administration, as an avenue to ensure accountability of the nurse administrator and enhance unity between the professional practice and education settings.

BACKGROUND AND PURPOSE

Time is overdue for the construction of integrated conceptual models for the practice of nursing administration in providing for the delivery of nursing care and in nursing education.[1] A primary role of an administrator is to facilitate the achievement of organizational and individual goals and objectives. A professional administrator executes the role through the management functions of planning, organizing, directing, controlling, and evaluating. More frequently than not, management experience rather than specific academic preparation for management and leadership has been one of the predominant qualifications for an administrator. With the increasing complexities in providing health care and meeting academic obligations and responsibilities, the potential administrator in this decade is more aware of the need for an educational preparation and a scientific knowledge base for their practice. The most effective administrator may be one who is able to synthesize both the knowledge (intellectual) and action domain for realistic application in practice. The environment with and in which administrators interact most often is complex. It would seem that the more eclectic conceptual approach a potential administrator can develop, the more successful administrators may be in adapting the management role to the organization and individuals they serve—health care professionals and/or faculty. There are essentially three purposes of this chapter: to advocate and provide rationale for the construction of integrated models for administrative practice; to suggest how integrated models may be generated;

---

[1] This chapter has benefited from a careful critique by Cathryn L. Glanville, Associate Professor, School of Nursing, Medical College of Georgia.

and to provide some considerations for validation and implementation of integrated models. The author will not attempt to delve into current debate regarding terminology and semantic differences of theoreticians and approaches to theory construction. Rather, the overall purpose is to offer an essay concerning a challenge to create integrated nursing administration conceptual models for provision of nursing care delivery and for nursing education settings.

DEFINITION OF TERMS

Although the author acknowledges that some of the following definitions are not commonly used by theoreticians, the major terms as applied for this chapter are defined as follows:

Concepts: abstract ideas or thoughts that are based on perceptions about general classes of an object

Propositions: descriptive statements that assert relationships between concepts and/or among variables

Hypothesis: a statement in measurable terms of relationships, between concepts which can be systematically tested

Theory: a system of empirically validated interrelated propositions used to describe, explain, understand, predict, prescribe for, or control a part of reality

Conceptual mode: a set of concepts logically linked by broad generalizations, which are not sufficiently empirically established, but provide a focus for inquiry and testing

Conceptual framework: a structural device for enclosing and supporting abstract, multidimensional concepts, which may or may not be related themselves, for a cohesive whole

Integrated nursing administration conceptual models: a set of concepts, which are linked by broad generalizations, drawn from schools of management, administrative and organizational theory, and nursing theory to identify essential components of nursing administration, which have value connotations and provide a focus for inquiry, testing, and prescription.

ADVOCACY AND RATIONALE FOR INTEGRATED CONCEPTUAL MODELS

It is questionable whether nurse-scientists have a common perspective as to the nature of nursing knowledge. However, there appears to be some consensus that the key concepts are nursing, man (person), health and environment (society). At the same time, one might argue that it is to the benefit of the profession for numerous perspectives to be utilized in the development of nursing knowledge. This may be particularly true for practitioners in nursing administration.

Nursing administration is an unique synthesis of two disciplines, nursing and management, and their related theories. Those persons who argue whether or not administration *is* nursing might refer in this volume to Chap. 1, "From Whence We Came," by Irene Palmer (1983:16). The quotations cited from the original writings of Florence Nightingale may well be the foundation for the discipline of nursing administration in health care and academic settings. Given the essential two disciplines that form the skeleton conceptual base upon which to build a body of knowledge, scholars and practitioners of nursing administration have an opportune challenge. Being in leadership positions, nurse administrators need to utilize a scientific base in practice. There is also a considerable amount of factual knowledge required in the practice arena of administration, such as how to obtain and allocate financial and human resources to operationalize high quality care and professional education programs. The integration of knowledge from nursing, management, and organization is essential for their effectiveness as leaders. Nurse administrators are the significant representatives and translators of nursing at the highest level of administration in an organization. As leaders and managers, they speak for staff and patients' needs as well as those of faculty and students. Nurse administrators in a setting for nursing care delivery and/or education of professional practitioners require a conceptual base of both nursing and management.

As an administrator providing for patient care, the chief nurse (however titled in various settings) must be able to assess, analyze, and evaluate the appropriateness of a partial or complete nursing theory or conceptual model for utilization by clinicians given the organizational setting, characteristics, and mode of care provided. The model applied in patient care and intervention should essentially be based on the client's needs and compatible with the philosophy, goals, and objectives of the department of nursing and the organization. The unique role for clinicians of patient care and education (that is, nursing staff and faculty) is to translate the nursing theory or model into action and outcomes that can be evaluated. The unique role for nurse administrators in patient, health-care, and academic settings is to translate the needs of professional personnel—i.e., nursing staff and faculty—and outcomes to higher levels of administration in settings that can legitimately be evaluated. The conceptual model between and operationalized by clinicians of patient care (clinical nurse specialists), clinicians of management (chief nurse administrators), and the organization need to be congruent. For example, conflicts may arise if the conceptual model of the clinical nurse specialist is based essentially on concepts of self-care, that of the chief nurse administrator and the department of nursing is based on group process, and the context of employment is a highly bureaucratic structure. The bureaucratic structure may emphasize efficiency, to the disappointment of the administrator who advocates group process, and conformity, which may frustrate the clinical nurse specialist who desires autonomy as a professional and for the patient.

As administrators of nursing education, deans of professional programs also need to assess, analyze, and evaluate the appropriateness of a nursing theory or conceptual model given the philosophy and objectives of a particular school, college, or university. Curriculum design begins with the development of a philosophy and selected objectives for a program. It is the nursing theory or conceptual model which makes possible the articulation of both the objectives and philosophy. Curricula offered by an educational institution should reflect the conceptual model chosen by faculty. As it is true for departments of nursing, chief nurse administrators, and clinical nurse specialists, congruence is required among the conceptual model activated by schools, deans, and faculty.

Nurse administrators in professional education, nursing care, and health care institutions or organizations have the additional complexity of adapting their management role for meeting the needs of employees when the majority are professionals. The conflicts of professionals being employed in bureaucratic organizations and institutions are well known. Issues concerning autonomy, authority, responsibility, and accountability are a major challenge for the professional nurse administrator to negotiate. Successful resolution calls for an adaptive management style. Adaptive management is fluid and dynamic. It requires an exciting demand to carry out on-going evaluation of management actions within the settings of nursing practice and education and apply the appropriate theories to effectively cope with emerging trends, changes, and issues in conjunction with the goals of the institution or organization. Nurse administrators must be knowledgeable as to the wide range of factors which influence change, such as the needs of society; the role of the health professions including the profession of nursing; technology, the economics and politics of health care and education; and the role of the federal government.

Professional nurse administrators in health care and academia are looking for a solid base for practice and prescriptions in addressing the many issues with which they are confronted. They want defined the set of circumstances, conditions, or behaviors that result in a given definable outcome, such as high quality of care provided for patients and professional competency in practice for graduates of professional nursing programs. The nurse administrator is faced with the dilemma of how to fuse the elements of management and nursing as their unique knowledge base for administrative practice. One possible solution may be to formulate and test models for nursing administration, which this author has previously defined as integrated conceptual models.

GENERATING INTEGRATED MODELS

In developing integrated models for nursing administration, it is necessary to first identify the essential elements and concepts of management thought; administrative; and organization theory; nursing concepts; nursing theory; and/or nursing conceptual models that might be most critical to the management role of a nurse administrator. It is suggested that an initial phase be to encourage scholars and practitioners of nursing administration to choose specific concepts perceived to be relevant in their practice. This implies that the designated concepts may have value connotations. The value signification may be associated with a specific philosophical stance regarding nursing and management, for example, nursing administration being perceived as a humanistic service. Thus, rationale for choosing the concepts should be indicated. In linking the concepts into propositional statements the basis for asserting relationships between the concepts and the underlying assumptions need to be specified. Finally, hypotheses can be formulated for testing and validation. Examples concerning the choice of concepts are indicated. Note that the various methods for construction of a conceptual model are not examined. The author provides only broad guidelines for consideration. There are numerous texts one can refer to concerning theory construction (Hardy and Conway, 1978; Riehl and Roy, 1980; Roy and Roberts, 1981; Turner, 1978; Zeitlin, 1973; Zeitlin, 1981).

Some scholars and practitioners may view as relevant the concepts of role, decision making, interaction, communication, change, adaptation, motivation, self-actualization, conflict, intervention, power, and leadership. The majority of these concepts are referred to as behavioral processes. They are evident in some of the conceptual/

theoretical formulations in management, sociology, and nursing.

In addition, the management processes of planning, organizing, controlling, directing, and evaluating can be examined as concepts. The concepts from specific schools of management, and administrative and organizational theory, can also be drawn from to develop integrated theory. Management and organizational theory has been classified in numerous ways (Gibson et al., 1982; Hall, 1982; Katz and Kahn, 1978; Mintzberg, 1979). The categorization of traditional and contemporary organizational theories includes structural, group, individual, technological, economic, and contingency theorists (Hall, 1982:309-314). Concepts concerning the structure of an organization, i.e., centralization, size, complexity, and formalization, and designs such as matrix or tall or flat (narrow or wide spans of control) hierarchies should be considered. Concepts from systems of managerial leadership, such as management by objectives (Odiorne, 1979) or participative management through committee structure are recommended to be included.

Nursing theoreticians have focused predominantly on developmental, systems, and interaction models (Riehl and Roy, 1980). Without explicating specific formulations, some of the concepts mentioned are more complex than others. For example, Roy's adaptation model has essentially four modes: physiologic needs, self-concept, role function, and interdependence (Roy, 1980:182). Betty Neuman's health care systems model, which is derived from the theories of gestalt, field, systems, and Selye's stress adaptation, has seven major model units, and is quite complex (Craddock and Stanhope, 1980:160-161).

As has been suggested any one concept, categories of concepts from nursing, management, administrative, and organizational theory might be employed to construct an integrated model. However, it would be essential to be logically consistent in using the concepts to ensure compatibility with the organization structure and design where the model may be tested and implemented. Perhaps the simplest way to demonstrate this point is to utilize open systems theory as a point of reference, since it is a predominant theory in organizations, nursing, and sociology (Katz and Kahn, 1978; Riehl and Roy, 1980:101–106). In an open systems approach interaction with the environment is an essential element. The concept also implies system properties, stable patterns of relationships, and behavior within boundaries (Katz and Kahn, 1978:31). An example of a systems frame of reference being used for a nursing administration model is that developed by Arndt and Huckabay (1980:19–47). However, the model does not include concepts from nursing theory.

To integrate nursing theory with management and administrative and organizational theory, one specific example might be to combine Roy's concepts of role function, interdependence, and self-concept; Neuman's concept of stress; the organizational concepts of decentralization individual perspectives, and motivation with concepts of the management processes (planning, organizing, controlling, directing, and evaluating) as a total open system. The management processes can be focused and applied at a micro level (for the individual) as well as macro level (for groups or the total organization). All of these concepts portrayed are essentially compatible with an organizational structure that emphasizes the individual, decentralized decision making, that is, one which is small in size, not complex, and has few rules and procedures. On the other hand, one might argue that an open systems perspective may also be an appropriate base for incorporating complex and numerous concepts from nursing and management into an integrated model for administration.

What does not appear appropriate is to combine a total nursing model, such as all four modes of Roy's adaptation model, to be integrated with numerous management and organizational concepts for a complex organization. A nursing model that has few categories for analysis may not be adequate for complex organizations. The elements of complex organizations are defined by Hall as horizontal differentiation, vertical differentiation,

and spatial dispersion (1982:78–83). These include multiple subdivision of tasks, job titles, hierarchical levels, and the separation of power or task centers by space. It would seem wise to integrate multiple nursing concepts or partial theories for compatibility with multiple management concepts employed in complex organizations.

A final example is provided for the genesis of an integrated administrative model by using the key concepts—for which there is some consensus among nurse-scientists—concerning the nature of nursing knowledge: man (person), health, nursing, environment (society). These can be integrated with concepts from management, administrative theory, and organizational behavior. This illustration is adapted from portions of the conceptual framework (structural device) developed by the author for the graduate program in nursing administration in the School of Nursing, Medical College of Georgia, Augusta, and applied as the genesis of an integrated conceptual model for administrative practice in providing for the delivery of nursing care and in nursing education.[2] In integrating the two disciplines of nursing and management, concepts of human and organizational behavior, interaction, systems, adaptation, and development can be explored in relation to the role of the nurse administrator. The four major concepts man, health, nursing, and environment are addressed as follows:

Persons (man) in organizations are dynamic bio-psycho-social beings with potential for growth, development, maturity, and adaptation. A person's behavior within an organization is a reflection of the interrelationships of internal and external variables. As persons interact within the organization they seek to meet their professional and personal needs and the needs and goals of the organization. An organization's steady state, or relative wholeness, is reflected in its repeated suc-

---

[2] The author acknowledges Barbara Ponder, Assistant Professor, School of Nursing, Medical College of Georgia, for her contribution and critique of the original conceptual framework developed for the graduate program in nursing administration.

cessful adaptations to stressors. These arise from its internal environments, subsystem needs and goals, and its external environment, such as societal expectations, demands, and resources. Negotiation is a major adaptive mechanism of organizations.

Health within an organization is a dynamic process which exists on a continuum ranging from states of wellness to states of illness. The health of an organization is perceived as the ability of persons to maintain an adaptive range of behaviors cognizant of respect and dignity for others with whom they interact to achieve the goals of persons and the organization. Integrity of persons is essential for health of the organization.

Nursing (health care professional nurse administrators in providing for the delivery of nursing care and for nursing education in academia) seeks to manage the *environment* of health care and professional education for practitioners. They provide a climate and resources conducive to assist professional nursing staff to deliver high-quality care for the client and faculty to provide high-quality educational programs, effective teaching methods, and students prepared for professional competency and accountability. The systems of prevention, assessment, intervention, evaluation and maintenance are utilized.

Nurse administrators perform a humanistic service that assists persons to adapt and develop in order to achieve their highest potential as a professional in providing for the highest quality of care for the client and education for the student. The strengths and resources of health care and academic professionals are developed to respond to stressors threatening the adaptive capacities of persons within the organization in providing health care and professional education.

Professional nurse administrators provide the *nursing leadership* and hold the ultimate *accountability* for nursing care provided to the client and academic programs offered for the student. The quality of nursing leadership is a major determinant of the effectiveness of health care organizations and professional academic institutions. The process of *cooperation, collaboration, negotiation,* and *advocacy* is essential to all health-care professionals in an organization and professional institution. Nurse administrators work with and through all health professionals to achieve the goals of the

organization and institution, and the ultimate goal of providing quality care for the client and quality professional education for the student.

The *environment* (society) expects the health professions to serve the public good and to monitor the performance of the profession's practitioners. Nursing administration holds the accountability for nursing practice and quality of care provided in a health care organization and quality of education offered in professional programs. Nursing administration as a subdiscipline within the profession of nursing provides the leadership for standards and performance in the provision of client care and education of students. Nursing administration serves as a pivotal point at which clients and personnel needs of the organization and needs of students and faculty interface with all other health care professionals. In that role the nurse administrator is responsible and accountable for effectively translating and communicating the needs for client care, of personnel, faculty, and students; to the executive management of health care organizations, educational institutions; and to society at large. Responsibility for meeting the goals of the health care system is shared by individuals and by groups composed of the providers, the clients, and the community as a whole. Nursing administration as a subsystem of the profession of nursing, through its quality leadership and management in the provision of health services and professional education for practitioners, continuously influences the total health care system.

CONSIDERATIONS FOR VALIDATION AND IMPLEMENTATION OF INTEGRATED MODELS

There are multiple settings and conditions under which nursing administration is practiced. No single nursing, management, or integrated conceptual model may be applicable for all settings. At the same time one model may be more appropriate than another for a given setting or set of conditions. Organizations constantly change, although the pace and elements of change vary. Integrated nursing administration conceptual models should not be static but rather contain sufficient elements to allow for change to meet the needs and demands of the situation.

Research and validation of proposed integrated models are essential prior to implementation. The linkage of the concepts must be validated, and effectiveness for administrative prescriptions must be evaluated. One alternative may be to evaluate the relationship of the concepts and the integrated model for effectiveness by focusing on administrative issues, such as recruitment, mode of providing care, or curriculum design. This may be followed by successive testing of the model for numerous administrative problems and situations. Multiple interacting variables, conditions, and settings should be utilized in validating the relationships among the concepts and the effectiveness of the model. Prescriptions for successfully meeting administrative issues may result.

In implementation of an integrated model, what has previously been recommended should be noted, that is, compatibility of the model with the administrative and organizational characteristics of an institution. The critical variables are the personality and administrative style of the nurse administrator, the setting and environment itself, the mode of care provided, the professional level of the nursing staff, the needs of the consumer (client); or the type of curricula offered, the professional level of faculty, and the needs of faculty and students. Readiness of staff and faculty to be involved with the genesis of an integrated model, including the suggestion for specific concepts, needs to be assessed by the nurse administrator. In addition, planning by staff and faculty for implementation and evaluation of the model at each phase is essential. Political decision making is inherent in each phase of implementation. Powerful political forces may emerge if staff, faculty, or both perceive implications for their role that is deemed undesirable. Negotiation is a key process and role of the nurse administrator in resolving obstacles in implementation.

In conclusion, the nurse administrator in health care and/or academia is accountable for either the delivery of nursing care or quality of education programs or both. Nurse administrators must be prepared to be leaders in organized settings for nursing care and education with the requisite knowledge and competencies to ensure both the quality and effectiveness of care and teaching. As executives within a given organization, nurse administrators are accountable to clients, students, the organization, and the community at large. Integrated models for administrative practice in providing for the delivery of nursing care and in nursing education may be the means to establish a scientific knowledge base, an avenue to ensure accountability, and also enhance cohesiveness between the professional practice and educational setting.

EDITOR'S QUESTIONS FOR DISCUSSION

To what extent do you agree that integrated conceptual models are needed for administrative practice? Provide additional rationale for the development of integrated conceptual models for administrative practice in providing for the delivery of nursing care and in nursing education. What concepts from other disciplines not referred to in this chapter might be suggested for integrated models? Why should administrators have a scientific knowledge base for practice? What factual knowledge do administrators in health care and academic settings need to acquire? What is the most effective means to obtain that type of knowledge? Should factual knowledge be incorporated in an integrated conceptual model? If so, how might it be incorporated? How might the role of the nurse administrator be included in an integrated model? Should "tasks," such as completing reports, writing memos, or "skills" as needed in time management be incorporated in models? To what extent should the above or other similar examples be included as technology in an integrated model? Present arguments and rationale for and against developing principles of technology rather than focusing on tasks and skills in themselves. How can principles be used in the development of integrated conceptual models for administration?

Provide examples of adaptive management styles of administrators, given specifically different organizational and institutional settings and personnel. How can an administrator develop political astuteness in a particular setting? What factors influence the ability to be astute to the political climate of the external environment, the organization, and personnel? How might adaptive management be related to contingency theory? What implications does contingency theory have for increasing certainty in organizations and institutions?

Provide examples of prescriptions administrators desire in their practice. What type of scientific base is required for valid and reliable prescriptions for the examples provided? How might the scientific base for prescriptions be formulated through the genesis of integrated conceptual models?

What elements and concepts from management thought, administrative and organization theory, nursing theory, conceptual models, and conceptual frameworks do you perceive essential to include in an integrated conceptual model for administration in providing for the delivery of nursing care and in nursing education? Provide rationale for the concepts you have indicated. How might learning concepts and theories be relevant in an integrated model? Form propositional statements from the concepts you have indicated, indicate the underlying assumptions in your model, and formulate hypotheses. How might you validate your model? Using the concepts of nurse-theoreticians presented in Stevens' chapter (52), and management and organization concepts, formulate an integrated conceptual model for nursing administration.

Given the concepts presented in Chaska's chapter, how might an integrated conceptual model be developed? What concepts of human behavior, organizational structure, and organization processes are indicated? Concerning the concept of organization design, how might the factors of division of labor, departmentalization, span of control, and authority be included in an integrated model? Given the concept of organizational or institutional effectiveness, how might the factors of production, efficiency, satisfaction, adaptiveness, development, and survival be incorporated in an integrated model? What are the elements of an open system?

Diagram the specific example provided of concepts that may be combined for an integrated conceptual model. What are the elements of role function, self-concept, and interdependence that should be indicated in the diagram under each of Roy's concepts? What elements of Neuman's concept of stress should be shown? How can the elements of decentralization be designated? What factors in individual perceptions would be salient to illustrate? What elements of motivation would you show? How can you portray the concepts of the five management processes cited? How can you indicate the elements of an open system? Finally, how would you illustrate the relationships and interaction between and among all of the concepts provided as an integrated conceptual model for administrative practice? Illustrate how this integrated model can be addressed to an administrative issue. How is the example using the concepts: man, health, nursing, environment, as a genesis for an integrated conceptual *model,* in reality a conceptual *framework?*

Discuss theoretical construction for integrated models. Present arguments for support or negation of the definition of terms as applied by the author. Why might prescription and control be salient elements of a definition for theory in administration?

What alternative definition can you provide for an integrated nursing administration conceptual model? How much agreement might there be between Chaska's definition of terms and those utilized by nurse-theoreticians? What initial approach and reasoning process in theory construction appears to be used by Chaska? What level of knowledge in theory development is being addressed? How congruent is Chaska's proposal for integrated conceptual models with the perspectives and theoretical approaches used by nurse-scholars?

How does Fawcett's (Chapter 14) discussion of prescriptive theory relate to Chaska's concept of integrated conceptual models? How can integrated models be goal-directed for application? Can constructing integrated models be an effecitve means to develop scientific prescriptive theory? Why might nursing administration, as a subdiscipline of nursing, be a more fruitful arena for the genesis of prescriptive theory? How might research be designed to validate concepts used in integrated models and to generate prescriptive theory? How does the knowledge base of practice theory as discussed by Fawcett (Chapter 14), Walker (Chapter 30) and Manke (Chapter 31) differ from the knowledge base proposed to evolve from integrated conceptual models? What editor's questions for discussion in those chapters apply or are addressed by Chaska in this chapter? How does Walker's (Chapter 30) critique for theory synthesis apply to Chaska's proposal for integrated models? How congruent is Chaska's approach to theory construction with Steven's (Chapter 52)? What relationship is there between Menke's (chapter 31) discussion of Dickhoff, James, and Wiedenbach's stance in theory construction and Chaska's? How can integrated conceptual models be created from an operational or dialectic reasoning process? Apply Meleis' (Chapter 33) model for description, analysis, and critique of nursing theory to the construction of integrated conceptual models. What applications might there be in integrated conceptual models for the administrative issues portrayed by Malkemes (Chapter 50) and Mercadante (Chapter 51)?

Suggest alternative methodologies for the construction of integrated conceptual models. What research methods may be most effective in establishing the reliability and validity of an integrated model? What additional recommendations can be made regarding the construction, validation, implementation, and evaluation of integrated conceptual models for administration in providing for the delivery of nursing care and in nursing education?

REFERENCES

Arndt, Clara and Loucine M. Daderian Huckabay
　1980　Nursing Administration: Theory for Practice with a Systems Approach. St. Louis: The C. V. Mosby Company.
Craddock, Ruth B., and Marcia K. Stanhope
　1980　"The Neuman health-care systems model: Recommended adaptation." Pp. 159–169 in Joan P. Riehl and Sister Callista Roy (eds), 2nd ed., Conceptual Models for the Nursing Practice. New York: Appleton-Century-Crofts.

Gibson, James L., John M. Ivancevich, and James H. Donnelly, Jr.
　1982　Organizations: Behavior—Structure—Processes. 4th edition. Plano, Tex.: Business Publications, Inc.
Hall, Richard H.
　1982　Organizations: Structure and Process. 3rd edition. Englewood Cliffs, N.J.: Prentice-Hall, Inc.
Hardy, Margaret E., and Mary E. Conway
　1978　Role Theory: Perspectives for Health Professionals. New York: Appleton-Century-Crofts.

Katz, Daniel and Robert L. Kahn.
1978 The Social Psychology of Organizations, 2nd ed., New York: John Wiley & Sons.

Mintzberg, Henry
1979 The Structuring of Organizations. Englewood Cliffs, N.J.: Prentice-Hall, Inc.

Odiorne, George S.
1979 MBO II: A System of Managerial Leadership for the 80s. Belmont, Calif.: Fearon Pitman Publishers, Inc.

Palmer, Irene S.
1982 "From whence we came," Pp. 3–28. in N. L. Chaska (ed.), The Nursing Profession: A Time to Speak. New York: McGraw-Hill.

Riehl, Joan P., and Sister Callista Roy
1980 Conceptual Models for Nursing Practice. 2d edition. New York: Appleton-Century-Crofts.

Roy, Sister Callista and Shara L. Roberts
1981 Theory Construction in Nursing: An Adaptation Model. Englewood Cliffs, N.J.: Prentice-Hall, Inc.

Roy, Sister Callista
1980 "The Roy adaptation model." Pp. 179–188 in Joan P. Riehl and Sister Callista Roy (eds.). Conceptual Models for Nursing Practice, 2nd ed. New York: Appleton-Century-Crofts.

Turner, Jonathan H.
1978 The Structure of Sociological Theory, revised edition. Homewood, Ill.: The Dorsey Press.

Zeitlin, Irving M.
1981 Ideology and the Development of Sociological Theory, 2nd ed. Englewood Cliffs, N.J.: Prentice-Hall, Inc.
1973 Rethinking Sociology: A Critique of Contemporary Theory. New York: Appleton-Century-Crofts.

Chapter 54

Marketing Strategies
Applied to Nursing

Doris J. Froebe, R.N., Ph.D., F.A.A.N.
Professor
Chairperson, Nursing Administration
School of Nursing
Indiana University
Indianapolis, Indiana

One method has been suggested by Chaska for validating integrated nursing administration conceptual models. Confirmation is needed for integrated models as a scientific knowledge base for practice and effectiveness for prescriptions in transacting nursing administrative issues. One problem that has been frequently mentioned and cited for potential attention in scientific testing of integrated conceptual models is recruitment and retention of professional nursing staff and faculty. Doris Froebe addresses the recruitment issue by focusing on marketing strategies. Although she pays particular attention to the service aspects in providing delivery of health services, issues regarding the successful attraction of sufficient professional personnel are also described. In general, marketing is the analysis, planning, implementation, and control of programs designed to bring about voluntary exchanges of values with target markets to achieve organizational objectives.

Froebe emphasizes the exchange relationship that is central to the concept of marketing and ethical implications involved, particularly for the health field. It is essential to take into account the client's needs and concerns *before* developing the service to be marketed; thus, client solicitation cannot occur. In making that point, Froebe discusses a number of issues. These include cost containment, a voluntary exchange process in which consumers help determine the services they need and will use, privacy while delivering health care services, and manipulation of a market.

She identifies four distinct types of constituencies in the organizations of health services: external, which includes regulators, such as licensing and accreditation bodies, and suppliers who provide time or money; internal, which includes boards of trustees, health professionals and employees, and volunteers; client, which includes patients who use the health services; colleague, which includes those persons who work in and for the health organization and other organizations providing similar services. Marketing in the nonprofit sector includes identification of the service and location for accessible delivery of the service to be provided, assessment of the total cost to the consumer, and creating an awareness and promotion of the service.

In developing a marketing program to recruit and retain professional nurses, a number of factors are deemed essential. These include: location of the facility; costs, which should include placement and orientation of the nurse; child care facilities and flexible work scheduling; and advertising.

Administrative control and evaluation of the marketing process is viewed as being critical to the success of a program. Control is geared to monitoring transactions, utilization of services, and adjusting marketing activities to meet planned goals. Utilization of services implies a need for adequate professional nurse staffing, progressive scheduling modes, and participative nurse management. Evaluation includes measuring efforts, outcomes, and public recognition, which should be reflected in the health status of the community. Froebe implies that it is essential for nurse administrators to have a knowledge of marketing concepts to comprehend fully the applicability and limits to marketing in the health field.

Industry must function efficiently and effectively to survive in the 1980s. The health care industry is no exception, although it falls within the realm of nonprofit services. Appropriate goal setting and the direction of resources to the achievement of goals provides the key to efficient and effective operation. The success and even the survival of an organization depend upon the attraction of sufficient personnel and material resources, conversion of resources into goods and services for delivery of health-related services, and the distribution of services to appropriate publics. To achieve these ends, an exchange relationship becomes a central concept. Likewise, exchange is a central concept of marketing.

Marketing processes are not new to industry, but their application within the industries labeled as being nonprofit is new. Thus, before discussing any pros or cons relating to marketing, it is necessary to provide a general definition of marketing. Kotler (1975:5) offers the following definition of marketing:

> Marketing is the analysis, planning, implementation, and control of carefully formulated programs designed to bring about voluntary exchanges of values with target markets for the purpose of achieving organizational objectives. It relies heavily on designing the organization's offering in terms of the target market's needs and desires, and on using effective pricing,

communication, and distribution to inform, motivate, and service the market.

The above definition identifies marketing as an applied science and directs its focus to managing exchanges. Management functions in the form of planning, decision making, implementation, and control are contained within the definition. The definition relating exchange to need and/or desire draws upon motivation and probability theories. Systems theory provides an organizing framework for the marketing activity. It must be emphasized that although marketing concepts have long been a part of the profit sector, there is nothing in the nature of the marketing definition to preclude its application within the nonprofit sector.

Exchange takes the form of services, goods, or money since each can reflect a value for the market exchange. The values ascribed to each exchange must be considered tentative and ever-changing in the health service marketplace. Population and economic, and political factors are major variables influencing these exchanges.

People indoctrinated in the delivery of health services express concern with the movement toward marketing of health services. Their concerns are not too difficult to comprehend and deserve attention.

Marketing is concerned with the expansion of sales or a product. In the health field this could imply the solicitation of clients for existing services or expanding services. Client solicitation has been deemed an unworthy activity within the health services. Expansion of service has gone forward unchecked during the health service industry's illustrious past. If the view is taken that marketing is an exchange rather than selling, the ethical implications of selling a service, whether needed by the client or not, or expansion of service are not problematic issues. Marketing implies taking the client's needs and concerns into the organization's focus before developing the service to be marketed. Whether or not to open additional beds could well depend upon the nurses available in the marketplace. Consumer oriented research and inquiry prior to finalizing decisions is a marketing approach. If a voluntary exchange mechanism is employed, the need for pressing services upon an unwilling market or expanding a service when resources are not available cannot occur.

In the 1960s consumer rights surfaced with Nader, health service agencies, and the legislation of Professional Standards Review Organization (PSROs). The age of consumerism had been introduced. A second concern embraced the issues of cost containment. Two questions arise. Will the addition of marketing activity in the field result in increased cost scrutiny by the government, client publics, and charitable giving? Can we expend money to market a service without increasing a service cost? Proponents of the use of marketing do not become overly concerned with these questions (Cooper, 1979: 243). They maintain that the essence of marketing, the exchange process, offers the secret to cost containment. If consumers help to determine the services which they will be utilizing, the industry will never need hard-sell techniques to stay cost-effective.

A third concern rests with the necessity to maintain privacy while delivering health care services. It is argued that marketing success stems from marketing research. Research seeks a notion of peoples' likes and dislikes. Marketing research used in the health services industry will require

maintaining a sensitivity to the public's feelings where privileged information is a concern.

A fourth and last concern to be considered rests with the manipulation of a market. Is it ethical to create demand where none logically exists in the name of providing a public good? Market proponents (MacStravic, 1977: 13) believe that the involvement of clients in broader decision-making endeavors will provide just the opposite effect. They believe that the fourth concern, market manipulation, exists today because services are developed and then must be sold to the public.

Since exchange has been identified as a key concept within the definition of nursing, it is logical to identify the groups with whom exchanges can occur in the health care industry. An individual is a constituent of an organization who has an important connection with that organization for one reason or another. Constituent groups are distinguished from other groups by likeness between members of the group and the members' differences from members of other constituent groups of the organization. Organizations in the health services category can identify four distinct types of constituencies.

MacStravic (1977: 20) enumerates constituent categories of the typical health organization as follows:

> . . . external constituencies who support, regulate, or otherwise impact on the organization from outside; internal constituencies or those people who work in and for the organization and make it function; client constituencies or people who use or otherwise benefit from the organization's services; and colleague constituencies or those organizations which provide similar or related services and are potential competitors or collaborators.

External constituencies for the health sector include a number of sources. Among these sources are regulators. Regulating bodies take the form of licensing bodies and accreditation commissions. Suppliers and organizations or people who give time or money to the organization are external to the organization. The National League for Nursing, state boards, and advisory committees are examples of external constituencies of nursing. In general, the broad-based community is an external public which does not participate in an ongoing exchange relationship with the organization, but may, at some point in time, be either a client or external support constituency.

Internal constituencies take the form of boards of trustees, internal audit committees, employees who provide services to the organization, and volunteers working within the organization. Physicians are usually included within this grouping. The department of nursing and all its members fall within this category.

Persons benefiting from the services of an organization become a client constituency of the organization. Patient groups utilize the direct health services either as inpatients or outpatients. Clients may be those using blood bank services, laboratory facilities, or other services that are not representative of broader direct care service. The public who benefit indirectly, such as parents of sick children and others who derive health education, also fall into this group. For example, spouses who go to diabetic classes or learn about postoperative cardiac care through preoperative films are included as a public benefiting from the organization's service.

Colleague constituents of an organization include people and organizations providing like services. This group includes other hospitals, private laboratories, proprietary nursing groups, and other free-standing clinics. These groups may be viewed as either competitors or colleagues.

Although constituencies can be separated for illustration or analysis, they are not mutually exclusive. Organizations seek balance and satisfactions from within and between groups. Relationships between the constituency and the organization occur because an exchange occurs. The identification of the organization's constituencies is the first phase of the marketing process.

The term *market identification* is generally used to categorize the constituencies or publics thus far described. By using the marketing process however, it is possible to break these constituencies into smaller components for the purposes of developing a marketing strategy.

A further breakdown of any constituency is termed *market segmentation*. A market segment is a distinct group of constituents that may become a target for the organization to achieve one of its goals. The segmentation is based upon the similarities within the group and the differences among groups. For example, although both physicians and nurses fall within the internal constituent groups of a health industry, they are also segmented from each other by client expectation, education, and relationship to the organization. Similar segmentation can be noted in client groups, donors, colleagues, volunteers, suppliers, regulators, and accreditors. The most useful segmenting attributes are the location, demographics, behaviors, and potential size of a segmented group.

Identification of constituents, further segmentation of constituents, and identification of the broad purposes of the organization are keys to the successful implementation of the marketing process. More specifically, however, marketing in the nonprofit sector must follow the analysis of four factors. First, the service to be delivered must become identified and known; second, a location for delivery that provides access to the service must be determined; third, the cost of the service must be assessed in terms of the total cost to the consumer; and fourth, a mechanism for creating awareness of the service or promotion of the service is needed.

Techniques relating to the preceding factors have been used and refined in the profit sector, and although the nonprofit sector and profit sector are significantly different, the purposes and functions of marketing can be employed by both sectors.

Most health organizations use professional judgment to derive standards of client behavior. Concomitant to this service concept is the health system's orientation, which assumes that the consumer will react favorably to good service and facilities and that very little marketing effort is required. If this attitude is not accepted by the constituents, organizational efforts may become dysfunctional. Within the profit sector, the railroads have suffered impressively from adopting this attitude. It has now become evident that the health community is not immune from constituent opinion, nor is it guaranteed survival by the fact of its existence. The task of comprehending needs, desires, and attitudes of constituents is the basis of marketing.

With constituent input, the product or service aspect of the system is planned. For example, if the internal constituent is nursing, the following concerns might be addressed:

1 Is there sufficient nursing staff available for maintaining and/or increasing the capacity of the organization?
2 Is recruitment for the organization equal to or greater than that which occurs in comparable organizations?
3 Are professional nurse retention statistics available for analysis and planning?

The factor of location for a successful marketing program is especially relevant for the system of nursing. The location of the facility is a factor in nurse recruitment and retention. There is no precise formula for measuring the impact of time or distance on the organization's recruitment and retention practices. Nonetheless, transportation and safety in parking locations are valued by nurses in general, and in particular by recruiters. Inner city institutions vie with surburban ones for the nurses available in the market.

The costs related to marketing nurse positions depends upon the institution's willingness to include everything that can be attributed to the recruitment, placement, and orientation of the nurse. A wider definition of price should make the organization more sensitive to the factors which can influence retention. In the marketing program for nurses, the calculation of price has seldom been related to revenue, aside from the

cost of closing beds as a result of insufficient personnel. Specific alterations in an organization's marketing program may be in order. For example, child care facilities and flexible work scheduling may be included to enhance the recruitment of nurses.

The factor of cost would be significantly different if we were considering the client constituency. In this area, the specific charge is by no means the most important consideration. Many charges are met entirely by third-party payers. Nonetheless, client constituents now tend to consider everything that goes into forming a relationship with the agency. Child care during the visit, transportation, and specific policies of the agency with which the constituent must comply are considered by client publics.

Advertising is the most common mechanism for creating awareness of the marketable product or service. Looking to the internal constituency, we find a dichotomy between the use of advertising for physicians and nurses. The former may occur in strategic ads in professional journals; the latter is a matter of widespread publicity and advertising. The purpose of both methods is to move target markets through a hierarchy of effects from unawareness to awareness, to interest, and finally to a decision to join a particular constituency.

The client constituency sees promotion from a different point of view. In fact, some clients will consider any form of promotion to be unethical. On the other hand, the client must have information about the location, timing, and price of service to effectively utilize the service. When new services are added, promotional efforts will need to be expanded and prolonged.

The colleague constituency will view promotion from still another perspective. The promotion of service in one agency may be seen as competitive by others in another area. In general, areawide planning for service expansion has been developed as one mechanism to allay competitive behaviors. The impact of the marketing process should not promote colleague competition but should be a mechanism to effect the most efficient and effective utilization of services.

Product, place, price, and promotion must be separately addressed each time a marketing strategy is planned. At the same time, it must be remembered that each factor impacts on all the others and the interactions between factors must be recognized.

Planning a marketing program in nursing and the administration of such a program are correlates. Plans need to be flexible enough to cover unforeseen occurrences. For example, it is clearly apparent that the need to market an agency's programs to attract needed nursing personnel requires that the following factors be taken into consideration:

• Nurses are a scarce resource within many communities.
• New opportunities in which nurses may seek employment will add to recruitment planning difficulties.
• Organizing structures in a centralized or decentralized nursing department may add to personnel turnover.
• Environmental changes surrounding the agency's location may add to or subtract from recruiting effectiveness.

Implementation of a program does not mean that marketing strategies cease. Marketing is an ongoing activity. During any stage of implementation, feedback may require service adjustment. For example, population changes, wage disputes, or changing client needs may vary the initial strategy.

Control of the marketing process is an important administrative mechanism. Control is a process for monitoring program activities' outcomes and adjusting activities from time to time to meet planned goals. Management by exception, direct

supervision, and management by objectives fall within the controls implied. Marketing control is geared to monitoring transactions and utilization of services.

There are many different factors to be addressed in attempting to achieve control in marketing. Common control factors relate to overall utilization, the organization's share of a market, the degree of effort implied to achieve a desired level of utilization, and public recognition of an organization's output.

Agency utilization implies the need for adequate nurse staffing, progressive mechanisms for scheduling, and participative nurse management. A patient dissatisfied with nursing care may return to a facility simply because there is no choice but will not recommend the agency to friends. Moreover, if a choice becomes available in the future, that patient may quickly defect to a different agency.

Evaluation as a process parallels control. Its goals embrace long-range and multiple levels of organizational activity. Control assumes that a program will be continued and simply addresses effectiveness and efficiency. Evaluation assumes only that the organization may continue. It covers a broader informational analysis.

Outcomes of the agency and of the nursing division in particular should be reflected in the health status of the community. Measuring such an impact is very difficult. Nonetheless, it must be attempted through audits, committee participation, and organizational structuring.

The application of marketing strategy to the nonprofit sector, and to nursing in particular, has been developed to demonstrate that a knowledge of marketing concepts is essential to fully comprehend both the applicability of and limits to marketing in the health field.

EDITOR'S QUESTIONS FOR DISCUSSION

Review the chapters by D. Walker (4), Sills (42), Cleland (44), Bullough (45), David (47), Malkemes (50), Mercadante (51), Stevens (52), and Chaska (53), and Editor's Questions for Discussion for each. What legal, ethical, reimbursement, and administrative issues can be related to marketing strategies and programs? What specific application and enlightment does Froebe's chapter provide for the role of the nurse administrator in settings for providing the delivery of health care and/or the professional education of students? How is marketing a management function of the nurse administrator? How are motivation, probability, and systems theories applied to marketing? What implications are there for these concepts in the development of integrated conceptual models for nursing administrative practice as presented by Chaska (Chap. 53)?

In nursing administration, in providing for health care and professional education, how is exchange a central concept? What form does exchange take in terms of marketing? What professional implications are there in marketing of health services and for professional personnel? How does the supply and demand for professional nursing care affect the profession of nursing? To what extent does nursing education take into account the needs of society, region, and community before developing professional education programs? Should services in providing nursing care or providing professional education be expanded when resources do not appear to be readily accessible? How can nurse administrators resolve the dilemma between identified needs for nursing care and professional education, and insufficient resources to implement or expand services and programs?

What relationships and implications are there between Fleming's (Chap. 35), Bille's (Chap. 36), and La Monica's (Chap. 37) contributions and Froebe's discussion concerning the consumer of services? How do Froebe's four concerns regarding marketing apply to nurse administrators in health care and education settings? What are the implications for using marketing strategies for determining compatibility between potential personnel and an organization?

What exchange occurs between and among the four constituent groups, described by Froebe, and the profession of nursing? What strategies can be suggested for enhancing the exchange relationships of these groups? What process can an organization use to identify its constituencies? How can organizations maintain and enhance collegial relationships with other potential competing organizations in marketing for professional personnel? Provide examples as to the relationship between segmentation of constituents, identification of broad purposes of the organization, and success of the marketing process. Discuss ethical implications and differences between techniques used in marketing for the nonprofit and profit sectors. How can an organization assess an appropriate balance between providing for consumer needs that have been identified and actual capability to delivery quality care and/or provide professional education? What other factors in addition to those indicated by Froebe should be considered in a marketing program relevant to recruitment and retention of professional nursing staff, faculty, and the profession of nursing? What data are available regarding the total costs of marketing programs in nursing? What data should nurse administrators have in health care and education settings in planning a marketing program? Discuss the ethical implications of advertising and other forms of promotion. What impact have "agencies" for supplementing nursing staff in institutions had on marketing strategies used by and for nursing and the profession of nursing?

How can transactions in marketing be effectively monitored? Discuss the possible relationship between a participative management style of nurse administrators and utilization of health care services and professional nurse education, adequate professional nurse staffing, faculty, and scheduling of services and courses provided. What empirical evidence is available concerning leadership style of administrators and the utilization of services by consumers?

Provide methodological suggestions for the evaluation of marketing programs in nursing. What are the significant researchable questions? How might cost effectiveness be assessed? What measurable structure, process, and outcome variables should be included?

REFERENCES

Cooper, Phillip D. (Editor)
  1979 Health Care Marketing: Issues and Trends. Germantown, Md.: Aspen Systems Corporation.

Kotler, Phillip
  1975 Marketing for Non-Profit Organizations. Englewood Cliffs, N.J.: Prentice-Hall.
MacStravic, Robin E.
  1977 Marketing Health Care. Germantown, Md.: Aspen Systems Corporation.

Chapter 55

The Academic Deanship in Nursing: Challenge or Capitulation

Juanita F. Murphy, R.N., Ph.D., F.A.A.N.
Dean and Professor
College of Nursing
Arizona State University
Tempe, Arizona

Marketing as an applied science outlined by Froebe may well be relevant to the selection and procurement of qualified professionals to assume the numerous vacant deanship positions in academic settings. Juanita F. Murphy aptly examines the crisis state of the academic deanship in nursing. Identified sources of difficulty include competency, conflicting role expectations of the dean by various interconnected constituencies, and increasing external and internal pressures impacting academic governance. Murphy advocates the acquisition of Katz's defined three skills—technical, human, and conceptual—to enhance the efficiency of existing and aspiring deans to assure excellence in academic nursing administration. She portrays the similarities between the three critical skills and Armiger's discussion of deans of the past, present, and future. Murphy maintains that though competence in each of the three skills is essential, the balance of need among the three for a nurse administrator is determined by the situation or condition of the organization.

Murphy explicates the complex issues of the nursing dean's role in academe. There is virtually little consensus as to how to "play" the role. In demonstrating salient points, she cites situations from the literature which academic nurse administrators could easily confirm. For example, though everybody wants a strong dean, nobody wants one *now* unless it is for some other school; strong deans must have their own policies and at the same time must agree with the policies of each constituent. Differing administrative skills are needed for the divergent expectations of various persons with whom a dean interacts.

Some of the external pressures that impinge on the dean's role include increased state and federal regulation and litigation, centralization of power and authority in the university governance board, demand for public accountability, escalation of costs, budget cuts, and retrenchment. The dean is also bombarded by internal pressures from faculty demanding shared governance and students insisting on flexible curriculum. Murphy quotes Dumke and indicates that the concept of university governance via participatory democracy neither exists on a campus nor does it provide for the accountability demanded by the public or students. She credits the annual continuing education seminars offered to deans by the American Association of Colleges of Nursing (AACN) and the National League for Nursing (NLN) Department of Baccalaureate and Higher Degree Programs as a means to resolve the deanship crisis and a source for enrichment.

Murphy focuses on the need to assist and develop future deans to be more effective. Katz's three skills are viewed as essential for nurse administrators. The degree to which the administrator must have the skills will vary according to their managerial level. Technical skill pertains to methods, processes, procedures, or techniques. Human skill comprises ability to be an effective group member and to build cooperative team effort. This skill includes intergroup relationships and leadership. Conceptual skill involves thinking in terms of priorities, probabilities, and patterns among elements. The three skills are needed to accomplish the particular responsibility, understand and motivate individuals and groups, and coordinate and integrate all the activities of an organization toward its mission and goals. At lower levels of administrative responsibility technical and human skills are of the greatest importance, while the need for conceptual skill increases with each level. Murphy views conceptual skill as an absolute requirement for the high-level administrator like the academic dean.

According to Armiger, deans of the past needed technical skill to define nursing as an academic discipline and be a role model for teaching nursing content in academe. Human skill was used to assist insufficiently prepared faculty to change from a hospital-school orientation to assume the rights and responsibilities of an academic faculty. Present deans have surrendered much of their technical skill to associate and assistant deans and to administrative assistants. They use human skill to provide leadership to well qualified clinical and research academic faculty. Conceptual skill is predominantly exercised through the dean's political and professional involvement at the local, state, and national level. Future deans are predicted to have research-based conceptual skills. Human skills will shift toward moving faculty to the discovery and dissemination of nursing science.

In linking Armiger's description of the changing role of nursing deans in academe with Katz's skills, it is indicated that changing conditions or organizational growth in size and complexity determine the differing balance among personal skills. For example, Katz is quoted as associating a specific administrative role with each of the three skills. A remedial role—saving an organization that is in difficulty—calls for drastic human action requiring exceptional conceptual and technical skills. A maintainance role—sustaining an organization in its present state—emphasizes human skills and modest technical skill. An innovative role—developing and expanding an organization—demands high competence in both conceptual and human skills with technical needs provided by subordinates.

Murphy urges incumbent deans to use Katz's role categories to assess the status of their college or school and examine their repertory of skills accordingly. If one or more of the three skills is limited she advises that the dean face reality and look for solutions. She further prescribes an essential preparation and continuing socialization for the deanship role that is well planned and organized. Previous experience, background, professional education, practice, and time are needed for the maturation of essential skills. Murphy discusses examples for acquiring each of the skills, although conceptual skill appears to be viewed as an innate ability. She maintains that attention should be directed toward identifying and nurturing aspiring deans who demonstrate conceptual skill. Murphy believes remedial and maintenance roles have taken precedence over the innovative role, primarily due to less reliance or concern for conceptual skill. Murphy insists a greater balance of conceptual skill is a requisite of all aspiring and incumbent deans to effectively meet the challenges inherent in the role.

There is considerable speculation that the traditional role of the academic dean[1] in institutions of higher and postsecondary education is in jeopardy. The identified sources of trouble are varied but include competing and conflicting role expectations of the dean by numerous interrelated constituencies and increasing external and internal pressures that directly impact the governance of the educational unit.

Among the numerous constituencies that have implicit and explicit role expectations for the academic dean are the students, faculty, associate and assistant deans, administrative assistants, secretaries, academic vice presidents, affirmative action officers, the university governing board, and the general and professional public (particularly in the case of professional colleges) and academic dean colleagues. Consensus on how to play the academic dean's role is almost nil. Marshall, a long-time faculty member, suggests: "It is high time that someone told deans how to play their roles. Except the deans themselves, everyone knows how to be a dean but nobody is sufficiently forthright to say so in public . . ." (1956:636). He further proposes that everybody wants a strong dean ". . . next year; nobody wants one now unless it is for some other school" (1956:639). The desire for a strong dean by faculty could indicate that they believe the present one is weak, ". . . which means that he does not pursue their pet causes relentlessly. Investigation discloses the further nature of this paradigm. The policies of this strong dean must be his own else he is not strong, but they must also agree with the policies of each speaker" (1956:638). Among the numerous constituencies of the academic dean, there are similar

conflicting and competing expectations on how the job should be performed.

While increasing external and internal pressures are a related source of adversity for the academic dean, they are of a different magnitude from the divergent expectations of constituencies on how the role should be performed. Because of these different magnitudes, differing administrative skills are needed to ferret out the relative impact of each in relation to doing what is expected. Among the various external pressures that have increasingly impinged upon the dean's role during the past one or two decades are: (1) increased state and federal regulation and litigation; (2) centralization of power and authority in the governing board; (3) demand for accountability from the general public; and (4) escalating costs, inflation, recession, budget cuts, and retrenchment. It is felt generally that the direct impact of these external pressures is buffered and diffused by the larger institution and thus individual schools or colleges are affected only indirectly. This is far from true, for that which affects the whole also affects the component parts.

The plethora of daily, weekly, and annual accountability reports and documents submitted by deans to the myriad of information seekers has grown geometrically. Along with differing views by constituencies as to how the dean should play the role and increasing regulations imposed by external sources, the academic deanship is bombarded from within by faculty demands for shared governance and by students' demands for increased flexibility in curriculum development. What pattern of university governance is appropriate for the next decade when the university governance board has taken drastic steps to centralize the power and authority of the university system, when faculties have a deep distrust of this concentrated power and want to seize it for themselves, and when students demand programs and

[1] The term *academic dean* is used to designate the chief administrative official of a school or college within an institution of higher education.

curricula that are individually tailored to their own needs? The chancellor of a large university captured the contemporary scenario aptly:

> Higher education during the past several years has been experiencing a tremendous drive on the part of many of its faculties to model educational institutions after the political state, with an approach to the separation of powers concept. . . . Under this concept, faculties would decide on the mission of the institution and the curriculum to carry it out and they would, in effect, elect their administrators and recall them when unsatisfactory, and all this would be accomplished with the cumbersome machinery of participatory democracy and the one-man one-vote principle, with large and complex committees assigned most of the decisions (Dumke, 1973).

He concludes that such a political system does not exist on the campus; the campus does not exist for the purpose of carrying out the will of the faculty constituency; and, above all, this concept of university governance does not provide for accountability demanded by the public or by the students.

With regard to students' demands for more flexibility in curriculum development, an aura of suspicion was created by students in the late sixties as they clamored, demonstrated, and revolted for more relevancy in the curriculum. Although the watchword changed from "relevancy" during the sixties to "flexibility" in the seventies, the unrest and discontent are still apparent, while the strategies developed by students vis-à-vis faculty and deans for input are different.

The following strategies for students' demands proposed by deTornyay are meritorious:

> Our responses must be prompt and reasonable and based on the merit of the demand, not of the politeness or propriety of the demanding students' behavior of the moment. We are required to have statesmanship and although we may not approve of the behavior, we will discuss the complaints because if they are valid,

we are willing to do something about them. The compensation for such patient forebearance is that an attitude of objectivity and fairness will prevent a malcontent from gaining majority support (deTornyay, 1976).

It is rather phenomenal that, since most nursing students are exposed to content in assertiveness training, we do not know how to respond to them when they attempt to implement what they have been taught.

Indeed, the academic deanship is in trouble! Or, at least, incumbent deans are troubled by the multitude of audiences and pressures with which they are expected to deal on a daily basis. While this inventory and exposition of sources of adversity is not exhaustive, it is apparent that the role of the academic dean is being compressed and contracted from all sides as well as from the top and bottom. It is easy to understand why the tenure of the dean is rather short, why there are numerous vacancies annually, and why there is increasing reluctance on the part of qualified individuals to assume a deanship.

During the last decade, the number of deanship vacancies each year created tremendous anxiety within academic nursing. The number of prepared individuals willing to assume deanship responsibilities was far less than the demand.

In an attempt to resolve the deanship crisis there was a decided shift away from identifying available individuals who would assume the position of academic nursing deanship toward identification of educational mechanisms which would enhance the efficiency of existing and aspiring deans and which would assure excellence in academic nursing administration. This shift was based on an increasing recognition that governance and administration had become more complex and difficult in all institutions of our society, including institutions of higher education as well as schools and colleges within the university. It was perceived by many who were concerned with the deanship crisis that more effective skills in administration, management, and leadership were needed as a result of the changing internal and external environments of the university.

But what are these needed skills? If they can be identified, when and how does one develop or accrue them? If procurement mechanisms are available or can be made available, will there be enough "seekers" to mount an educational and socialization enterprise which would result in more academic nursing deans with additional skills? Armiger has presented a thorough description of the actions and processes undertaken by representatives of the American Association of Colleges of Nursing (AACN) and the National League for Nursing (NLN) Department of Baccalaureate and Higher Degree Programs in regard to these questions (Armiger, 1976). Particularly pertinent is Armiger's explication of the needed continuing education for excellence in academic administration in nursing as proposed by incumbent deans.

> Among those listed . . . are budget preparation and management, legislative activity, affirmative action, grievance procedures, student participation in faculty appointments, due process litigation, and other aspects of the wide spectrum of administrative responsibilities" (1976:167).

Unquestionably, the annual continuing education seminars offered by AACN and NLN to deans during the past 5 years have enriched their administrative effectiveness. New steps are needed now to deal with changing conditions and emerging environments which will have impact upon the role and responsibilities of future deanships. What administrative skills will assist the future deans to be more effective?

Katz, in a classic article written some 25 years ago, identifies three basic skills that every effective administrator must have in varying degrees, according to the level of managerial operation. These three basic skills—technical, human, and conceptual —can be developed and can be demonstrated. Katz has defined technical skill as "an understanding of, and proficiency in, a specified kind of activity, particularly one involving methods, processes, procedures, or techniques" (1974:91). Working with "things," which includes processes or physical objects, is of primary importance in developing and demonstrating technical skill. Human skill is defined as "the executive's ability to work effectively as a group member and to build cooperative effort within the team he leads" (1974:91). This skill obviously is needed in working with people toward creating an environment within which the goals and objectives of the enterprise can be planned, developed, and implemented. In a retrospective commentary some 20 years after the original article, Katz indicated that human skills might usefully be subdivided into leadership ability and skill in intergroup relationships. Conceptual skill is defined as:

> The ability to see the enterprise as a whole; it includes recognizing how the various functions of the organization depend on one another, and how changes in one part affect all the others; and it extends to visualizing the relationship of the individual business to the industry, the community, and the political, social, and economic forces of the nation as a whole (1974:93).

In his later elaboration of conceptual skill, Katz indicated that it "involves always thinking in terms of the following: relative emphases and priorities among conflicting objectives and criteria; relative tendencies and probabilities (rather than certainties); rough correlations and patterns among elements (rather than clear-cut cause-and-effect relationships)" (1974:101).

Thus, for the effective administrator technical skill is needed to accomplish the particular responsibility; human skill is needed to understand and motivate individuals and groups; and conceptual skill is needed to coordinate and integrate all the activities and interests of the enterprise toward its common mission and goals. These three skills are interrelated and are needed by administrators at all levels. However, their relative importance varies with the level of administrative responsibility. Technical and human skill have greatest importance, while conceptual skill has lesser importance, at the lower levels of administrative responsibility. At higher levels, technical skills become relatively less important, human skill shifts from intragroup to intergroup concerns, and the need for conceptual skill increases rapidly. In short, for the effective, successful high-level administrator, such as the academic dean, conceptual skill is an absolute essential.

There are obvious descriptive similarities between this trilogy of basic skills and Armiger's erudite exposition of academic nursing deans of the past, present, and future (1976). "Deans of the past exerted leadership in curriculum development, maintained scholarly interests, taught at least one course, and enjoyed considerable autonomy in the direction of the school" (1976:164). In essence, the technical skill of nursing deans of the past was needed primarily to refine and define nursing as an academic discipline and to serve as a role model for teaching nursing content in that context. They used human skill in assisting meagerly prepared faculty to move from a hospital-school orientation toward assumption of the rights and responsibilities of an academic faculty. Armiger's portrayal of the deans of the present indicates that they have relinquished much technical skill to a support cadre of associate and assistant deans and administrative assistants while exercising conceptual skill in state and national political involvement and serving on boards and commissions at the local, state, and national levels. Their time is divided among innumerable competing demands within and outside of the university. Human skill is used by deans of the present to provide leadership to an increasingly well-qualified academic faculty, whose technical skills are sharp in the clinical and research levels (1976:165).

Armiger predicts optimistically that nursing deans of the future will be involved in newly negotiated cooperative arrangements involving interdisciplinary sharing of core courses and clinical learning experiences for students. They will encourage and be the innovators of interdependent relations between the university's programs and the community it serves. Their increasing conceptual skill will be research-based as they seek to identify future directions and to translate research into action. Their human skill will shift toward urging faculty to become involved in the discovery and dissemination of nursing science. Most importantly, nursing deans of the future will keep abreast of changes within the internal and external environment of their colleges and will be able to select and incorporate meritorious changes in various parts of the collegiate enterprise with full appreciation and understanding of the ramifications of such changes on the various parts as well as on the total college and university (1976:166).

Armiger captured adroitly the recent historical development and changing functions and responsibilities of academic nursing deans in a multilinear fashion. Katz, on the other hand, maintains that changing conditions or organizational growth in in size and complexity determine the differing balance among personal skills. For example, "The *remedial* role (saving the organization when it is in great difficulty) calls for drastic human action and emphasizes conceptual and technical skills. The *maintaining* role (sustaining the organization in its present posture) emphasizes human skills and requires only modest technical or strategic changes. But the *innovative* role (developing and expanding the organization) demands high competence in both conceptual and intergroup skills, with the technical contribution provided primarily by subordinates" (Katz, 1974:102).

Thus, all levels of administrators require competence in each of the three skills, but the balance of need among the three is determined by the situation or condition of the organization.

Incumbent deans might well use these role categories to assess the status of their college or school; after determining which category most appropriately characterizes their college status, a self-examination of their repertoire of skills—technical, human, conceptual—could follow. If the repertoire does not contain one or more of the three skills or if one or more of the three skills need to be sharpened, face the reality and look for solutions.

Armiger poignantly concluded that the deanship crisis exists because the present system of preparation is inadequate to meet the needs for deans of the future (1976:166). While remedial programs are being offered by various organizations (including nursing associations) the deanship crisis will not be alleviated until there is recognition that preparatory and continuing socialization must be well planned and organized. If, in fact, there is an intent to develop administrative skills for academic administration in nursing, there must be opportunity for the development of skills through practice and through relating one's own personal experience and background to what is being taught. Administrative development programs may not achieve satisfactory results because of the inability to nurture the maturation of essential skills.

Professional nurses are well grounded in the principles and processes of nursing and, as a part of their socialization process, have considerable practice and experience under the supervision of a master mentor. Thus, the development of technical skills can be procured in institutions of higher education which offer a professional nursing degree.

The knowledge base for the development of human skill is rooted in the behavioral sciences and can be acquired in various departments of most universities. There are various approaches to the development of human skill. For example, Harvard's Institute for Educational Management is well known for the case study approach. Other such organizations use the role-playing approach. While the content and teaching approach may be varied for the development of human skill, the essential outcome is to be able to work effectively with others in both intra- and intergroup situations.

The development of conceptual skill is another matter. Successful approaches and strategies for teaching and learning this skill are not well documented. Mentorships, advisorships, and presentation of complex situations for analysis and problem solving are among the strategies most used in the development of conceptual skill. After many years of dealing with how this skill could be developed, Katz concluded that:

> Unless a person has learned to think this way early in life, it is unrealistic to expect a major change on reaching executive status. Job rotation, special interdepartmental assignments, and working with case problems certainly provide opportunities for a person to enhance previously developed conceptual abilities. But I question how easily this way of thinking can be inculcated after a person passes adolescence. In this sense, then, conceptual skill should perhaps be viewed as an innate ability (1974:101).

This analysis has serious implications as movement is directed toward the procurement of academic nursing deans for the future.

As steps are taken to remedy and alleviate the crisis of adequately prepared academic nursing deans, attention should be directed toward identifying and nurturing aspiring deans who manifest conceptual skill. Aspirants, then, should be encouraged to take advantage of the numerous routes whereby human skill can be developed. Incumbent deans should self-assess their skills. If human skill is lacking or needs to be sharpened, again, various alternatives are available, probably in their own university. If conceptual skill is limited or lacking, every effort should be made to get someone with a gestalt, visionary perspective appointed to the college or school on a full-time basis, for example, as an associate dean, or on a part-time basis, for example as a consultant. Such prescribed action is mandatory if new imperatives of university and college change are to be confronted as challenges rather than met with capitulation.

In summary, the traditional role of the academic dean in institutions of higher education is in peril. Divergent demands and role expectations of the dean have contributed to this perilous situation. There has not been adequate and appropriate preparation of aspiring and incumbent deans to deal with the increasing number of competing and conflicting demands and pressures. Remedial and maintenance roles have taken precedence over the innovative role because of greater reliance on technical and human skill, with lesser reliance on and concern for conceptual skill. This has led to capitulation as the pressures have increased.

For the future academic dean three essential skills are needed for effective administration: technical, human, and conceptual. In order to cope with present and future challenges, a greater shift to conceptual skill is required of all aspiring and incumbent deans.

EDITOR'S QUESTIONS FOR DISCUSSION

Provide additional examples of the type of conflicting role expectations that exist for a dean. What strategies can be suggested for resolution of such conflicts? Identify the competencies a dean is expected to have. What factors influence the lack of consensus as to how to "play" the dean's role? To what extent and under what conditions should deans seek advice from the numerous constituencies with whom they interact? What are the ethical and role implications for the dean in seeking advice from constituents and for constituents who are sought for advice by the dean? What responsibilities and obligations does the dean have in seeking and/or following the advice of constituents? What responsibilities and obligations do constituents have who were sought for or provided advice to the dean? Compare the crisis in academic deanships with that of chief nurse administrators in health and nursing care settings. To what extent do chief nurse administrators have the same difficulties regarding competency, conflicting role expectations, and increasing external and internal pressures? What crisis differences exist between the two roles? Are different strategies required in resolving the chief nurse administrator crisis? If so, suggest alternatives for resolution of the crisis.

How can one account for the statement that everybody wants a strong dean next year, but nobody wants one now unless it is for some other school? What are the implications for nurse administrators in academe as well as in health and nursing care settings if the statement is true? What elements, conditions, or factors do deans and/or chief nurse administrators need to accept as *inherent* in the position? Which ones are negotiable with constituents and which ones would it be recommended not to negotiate, but to have a clear understanding and acceptance of prior to assuming a position of dean and/or chief nurse administrator? How might differences in understanding role expectations which may appear after assuming the highest-level nurse administrator position be resolved? What factors influence the degree to which information is withheld or provided between the prospective dean or chief nurse administrator and the highest level of administration during the interview and assessment phase for the position? How can either party be assured that the "right" questions are being asked and candid responses provided? What suggestions can be offered for achieving that goal? What applications can be made from Froebe's chapter (54) to Murphy's discussion concerning obtaining qualified deans? What ethical implications are there in the assessment phase of procuring a qualified dean or chief nurse administrator which may or may not also apply in procuring other professional employees? Review the editor's questions for discussion in chapters by Davis (47) and Malkemes (50). How can the balance of Katz's three skills be accurately assessed in a prospective high-level administrator to match the needs of the organization according to Katz's role categories?

Provide suggestions/strategies for effectively meeting the external and internal pressures indicated by Murphy. What additional pressures exist for a dean and/or chief nurse administrator? How can the contradiction between a centralized university governance board and demands for shared governance by faculty be resolved? Provide examples of the effects of such differences in governance. Are there situations or conditions where divergent forms of governance are appropriate? If so, indicate and discuss the examples. Present arguments and rationale for and against the conclusion that participatory democracy neither exists on university campuses nor does it provide for accountability demanded by the public or students. What alternative modes of governance can you suggest that are effective? What relationships can be made and which questions are addressed concerning mechanisms of governance between Murphy's chapter and those by Sills (42), Malkemes (50), and Mercandante (51)? How do strategies developed by students, faculty, and deans for input differ? Identify the domains for input and feedback each would want. How might a dean or chief nurse administrator most effectively develop a support base in dealing with all of the external and internal pressures of the role?

Discuss the effectiveness of continuing education seminars and programs offered for administrative effectiveness. What are the prime benefits of such programs? How much of the content provided can realistically be transferred to the immediate administrative setting in academia or nursing care? What additional content do you perceive as vital through continuing education programs?

How might aspiring deans or chief nurse administrators of nursing care best prepare themselves for their role? What is the most effective career route? What factors influence a person to choose a deanship or a chief nurse administrator position? What are the various *meanings* imputed to the position by aspiring and incumbent deans? Provide examples of Katz's three skills which are essential in the role of dean or chief nurse administrator. Review the chapters by Sills (42), Klein (43), Frolic (48), Hegyvary (49), Malkemes (50), Mercandante (51), and Stevens (52). What level and degree of Katz's three skills may be applied as requisites in the management roles indicated in those chapters? Provide specific examples of the varying degree and levels of management where Katz's three skills are essential. What additional skills may be suggested as requisites for high-level nursing administrative positions? How do the skills deemed essential by Murphy relate to those indicated by O'Connor (Chap. 13)? How can Katz's role categories and skills be included in Chaska's suggestion (Chap. 53) for developing integrated conceptual models for nursing administration practice? How do Katz's role categories relate to mediated roles as discussed by O'Connor (Chap. 13)?

To what extent do you agree with Armiger's description of the historical role development of academic nursing deans and Katz's matching of role categories with skill needs? Are there other role categories that might be suggested? Using Katz's role categories assess the status of your college or school and examine your own repertoire of skills—technical, human, conceptual—appropriate for the level and degree of your administrative responsibility. What suggestions can you make for increasing any one or more of the skills in which you may be limited? What additional means can be suggested for developing any one of the three skills?

Discuss the knowledge base for the development of technical, human, and conceptual skills as suggested by Murphy. What additional alternatives may an aspiring dean or chief nurse administrator of nursing care utilize to develop the essential skills? If conceptual ability is an innate ability, to what extent and how can the ability be enhanced? How might administrative residencies in academic and nursing care settings be an effective means in developing all three skills? Discuss the advantages and disadvantages of residency programs developed based on academic preparation for a high-level nurse administrative position in academe and/or nursing care settings. Why has there been more reliance on technical and human skills than conceptual? What strategies and means can be suggested to counteract those tendencies and associated role performance? Provide examples of the balance of need among the three skills which may be determined by the situation or condition of the organization? Provide examples as to how conceptual ability may be demonstrated in identifying potential high-level nurse administrators? How can one accurately assess conceptual ability? What are the implications and consequences for organizations, institutions, and the profession of nursing if conceptual skills are not required for all aspiring and incumbent deans and chief nurse administrators in nursing care settings? What are the implications and relationships between conceptual ability of the high-level nurse administrator and the implementation of nursing theory into nursing practice and professional programs for nursing education, generation of integrated conceptual models for nursing administration practice, and the further development of a scientific knowledge base for the profession of nursing?

REFERENCES

Armiger, B.
   1976   "The educational crisis in the preparation of deans." Nursing Outlook, 24,3:164–168.
deTornyay, R.
   1976   "Changing student relationships: Roles and Responsibilities in institutions of integrity." Paper presented at the Deans Seminar, cosponsored by the American Association of Colleges of Nursing and the Council of Baccalaureate and Higher Degree Programs of the National League for Nursing, Durango, Colorado, July.

Dumke, G. S.
   1973   "Accountability and action." Paper presented at the 13th Annual Meeting of the American Association of State Colleges and Universities, San Diego, November.
Katz, R. L.
   1974   "Skills of an effective administrator." Harvard Business Review, 5:90–102.
Marshall, M. S.
   1956   "How to be a dean." American Association of University Professors Bulletin 42, Winter:636–643.

Chapter 56

Building a Network of Support In Order to Strengthen the Position of the Dean

Claire M. Fagin, R.N., Ph.D., F.A.A.N.
Dean and Professor
School of Nursing
University of Pennsylvania
Philadelphia, Pennsylvania
and
Diane O. McGivern, R.N., Ph.D., F.A.A.N.
Associate Dean
School of Nursing
University of Pennsylvania
Philadelphia, Pennsylvania

After Murphy's enlightening portrayal of the academic deanship in nursing and the multiple difficulties and complexities inherent in the role, even given that the incumbent possesses the identified essential skills, one might ask how the academic dean can not only survive, but succeed in the role. Claire M. Fagin and Diane O. McGivern provide a forceful response to that question by advocating the building of support networks. They explain the dean's leadership role, provide a rationale as to why support networks are crucial to success, delineate the make-up of the network, designate the skills the dean must have to develop and participate in a support network, define obstacles to development of a network, and indicate how the network of support or lack of it may result in resignation.

Fagin and McGivern follow through on Murphy's discussion of strains and exaggerated expectations in leadership. In their view these are related to rapid change, multiple and unsettled goals in the profession of nursing, and unrest in the academic scene. They note the increasing print media visibility of the profession and mortality rate for deans of nursing. A 1979 AACN (American Association of Colleges of Nursing) survey of the academic life expectancy of nursing deans revealed that 121 of 170 respondents (71 percent of the total population) had held their position five years or less. Of the 170, 85 (50 percent) of the respondents were in their positions three years or fewer. They conclude that regardless of the dean's functioning or timeliness of their end, one or more threads in the dean's support network were missing.

Concerning leadership, Fagin and McGivern assume that the dean as an effective leader must understand power, have the capacity to use power for goal achievement, and is viewed as a planner, energizer, initiator, risk-taker who is accountable. They view leadership from the perspective of the quality of one's role within a particular social system and interaction of groups, but not as an enduring role unless the organization was developed in a way that enables the person to retain the leadership role after the contextual purposes of the role are met. Six major responsibilities of the dean are outlined. These include: defining the majoring direction of the school; verifying that instruction and research advances to fulfill objectives; maintaining an up-to-dateness of the practice and education components with the profession; maintaining a plan of internal governance based on collegiality; ensuring the up-to-dateness of faculty; and ensuring the overall quality control of the school or college. Fagin and McGivern conclude that the leadership "fit" may achieve a different degree of success in fulfilling the first three functions from the degree of success achieved in fulfilling the others. Demands of their role require that deans make decisions based on knowledge and facts; that they rehearse scenarios with trusted and knowledgeable critics; that they achieve goals through motivation and guidance of groups at several levels; and that they renew physical and emotional energy which is constantly drained.

A network of support is defined as a matrix of groups and individuals who provide the dean with information, critical review and feedback, completion of work that contributes to goals, and personal and professional support. Fagin and McGivern provide four reasons that support network functions are important. In general, support networks: assist the dean to enjoy the leadership position, develop personally and professionally; are important to the profession via the compatibility of nursing deans' goals with the growth of the nursing profession; contribute to the profession's collective understanding; and compensate for the lack of earlier support groups and mentors. Fagin and McGivern outline three levels of interaction within the network of support.

The first level includes individuals and groups who are peers. These include deans and administrators within one's institution; other professionals, such as lawyers and corporation and political figures; and deans of nursing and organizations of deans and colleagues in the profession. Fagin and McGivern emphasize the reciprocal nature of a support network and the need for deans to assess correctly and honor the needs and priorities of all participants. They offer useful techniques in building networks, such as: informing colleagues about the school's goals and plans; accepting questions non-defensively; utilizing discussions in future contacts; participating in social-professional activities. Maintaining and expanding contacts with professionals outside of nursing serves to give the dean important information and to expand authority and expertise. Sharing experiences and issues individually and collectively with other deans provides the forum for action plans. The second level of the network involves individuals and groups supraordinate to the dean, such as chief academic officers. Fagin and McGivern maintain that a dean must be certain that these individuals have information, knowledge, and understanding about the nursing profession, know and support their goals for the school, and are committed to assisting the dean to achieve the goals. At the same time deans need to demonstrate verbally and in other ways their support and understanding of the problems of chief academic officers. The third level of the support network incorporates individuals and groups subordinate to the dean. These include persons within the organization such as faculty, who fulfill goal oriented functions, but who also supply information and personal support to the dean and each other, as well as critically review action and reactions. Fagin and McGivern further discuss the mentor relationship a dean has, when democratic leadership is the mode of the dean, and the dean's role as a behavioral model.

The major components or skills a dean must use to develop and maintain networks are: the art of initiating, developing, and maintaining contacts; developing an appropriate mix of personal, social, and professional interests; the ability to project a successful, knowledgeable, and energetic image; and interpersonal competence, which is considered basic to the preceding skills. Four factors are indicated which impinge on network development and maintenance. These include the enormous amount of physical and emotional energy required, the diminished trust among deans and administrators due to intense competition for limited resources, ambivalent cultural socialization regarding the development and negotiation of power, which undermines efforts to be an influential leader, and socialization of women, which implies that women are not powerful, political, influential, analytical, or entrepreneurial.

Fagin and McGivern consider what happens when the dean's network of support fails. Areas for possible internal threat to a network are curriculum, faculty recruitment, governance, and the reward system used by the dean. Views of clinical and administrative preparation provided to students, competition for clinical resources or "turfs" in the hospital and university, and the *lack* of a highly developed collaborative relationship with the medical school by a nursing dean viewed as strong within his/her own school are all potential problem areas that may threaten a support network. Fagin and McGivern suggest some situations where behaviors may make the dean's position intolerable. A general review comprises strong differences of opinion concerning issues in nursing education, power struggles for control of the school either with external administrators, faculty members, or other candidates, and inability to resolve factional disputes in a school.

Fagin and McGivern maintain that resignation from a deanship position in and of itself does not suggest failure. They offer numerous conditions for resignation, such as a dean's incorrect original assessment of the situation, insufficient assessment of faculty candidates for positions, insufficient experience, education, or characteristics for the deanship of a particular school, and new executive officers being appointed who have set new goals and missions. Fagin and McGivern assert that no resignation should be offered without making a statement to the faculty, the university, and the nursing community at large. They recommend the "protest" type of resignation, which usually includes a set time for departure as well as a clear statement of cause. Fagin and McGivern conclude that the dean's personal needs and professional goals should receive great attention in timing the departure. The protest resignation is not the norm. They urge colleagues to consider a meaningful resignation as an alternative when a network of support is absent or has failed.

INTRODUCTION

Certainly one of the notable characteristics of the 1970s and 1980s will be the relationship between leaders and their constituents: a relationship marked by tension, high expectation, predictable disappointment, and disillusionment. Governments, corporations, and colleges and universities are experiencing the strain of exaggerated expectations for leadership and the difficulties encountered by top officials attempting to fulfill the personal and organizational expectations which have been defined overtly or inferentially. No doubt this is a by-product of the phenomenon of rapid change and unsettled goals and plans shared by organization leaders and members.

In accord with this view, we note that the rapid change and multiple goals apparent in our own profession are accompanied by great unrest in the academic scene. For example, recent events in nursing academic administration have been covered in various publications ranging from the most prestigious academic newspaper (The Chronicle of Higher Education) to student presses in several universities. Although nurses used to complain bitterly about lack of media notice, the print media, at the least, have focused increased attention on the profession in the past few years. A profession in motion brings visibility to formerly unnoted events, personalities, and actions. Opinions as to the future of the profession and the ways to shape the future may vary widely among practicing nurses, students, faculty, administrators, and members of professions interfacing with nursing.

Therefore, the facts about the status of nursing administrators are known to most of us and were well stated in the American Association of Colleges of Nursing (AACN) publication, "Academic Administration." This comments on the academic life expectancy of nursing deans and draws from data gathered in a 1979 AACN survey. Of the 170 respondents, 121 had held their positions for 5 years or less. That constituted 71 percent of the total population. Of this number, 85, or 50 percent, were in their positions 3 years or fewer. The AACN publication states that the mortality rate for deans (of nursing) is increasing and indicates further, as an example, that in the past year (according to public knowledge) five academic administrators have been relieved of their positions by their respective presidents. Four resigned in protest against administrative action. One of these had been in office fewer than 6 months. At least two were not reappointed on the basis of a faculty vote. The AACN publication asks whether this is a trend and adds

> To the best of our knowledge these administrators were not harridans who needed to be exorcised. They were colleagues who accepted the responsibility of academic administration

and met with a timely or untimely end depending upon your point of view. (1980:1)

In examining the present academic unrest, it is clear that whatever is one's point of view as to the smoothness of the dean's functioning or the timeliness of the dean's end, one or several important threads in the dean's support network were missing.

In this chapter we will examine the dean's leadership role; why a support network is crucial to success; what constitutes a network of support; what skills the dean must have to develop and participate in such a network; what the obstacles are to development of a network; and how the network of support or lack of it results in an alternative action, resignation.

LEADERSHIP

We are beginning with several basic assumptions: (1) to be an effective leader an individual must understand power; (2) a dean is a leader and as an effecitve leader must have the capacity to use power to influence goal attainment; and (3) a dean as a leader is viewed as a planner, energizer, and initiator who takes actions, accepts risks, and is accountable (Claus and Bailey, 1977:vii).

Discussion of the dean's leadership might be subtitled the trials and tribulations of deans. On the one hand one hears such comments as, "The dean is a weak leader and cannot pull the faculty together." On the other hand, one hears, "The dean wants to be too powerful and infringes on faculty rights."

The dean may be seen as an extremely strong leader within the school and show evidence of building a faculty and programs noted with respect by the nursing world. This same dean may be viewed in his or her own university as abrasive, uncooperative, isolationist, or having qualities described by many other negative adjectives.

Leadership is often "thought of as

> . . . a specific attribute of personality, a personality trait, that some persons possess and others

do not, or at least that some achieve in high degree and others scarcely at all... The truth would seem, however, to be quite different ... Leadership is not an attribute of the personality but a quality of one's role within a particular and specified social system." (Gibb, 1955:88)

Others have commented on the interaction of groups as the major factor in leadership. Kurt Lewin has stated "that the individual's characteristics and action change under the varying influence of 'the Social Field'" (Gibb, 1955:88). When viewed in this manner, leadership is not then an enduring role unless the organization is built in such a way that the individual is able to retain the role after the contextual purposes of the role are met. Looking at leadership from this perspective makes it possible to state the major functions of deans of schools of nursing and then to reflect upon the possible problem areas that would emerge based on the function. R. Lee Hornbake, in a paper presented to the AACN, stated six major functions as appropriate to dean of the professional school. These were:

1 The academic dean has the ultimate responsibility to define the major direction or the major thrust of a school or college, once reasonable alternatives have been identified.

2 The academic dean has the responsibility to verify that the instruction and research program of the school or college advances and fulfills the objectives decided upon.

3 The academic dean is responsible for maintaining an up-to-dateness with the profession, both the practicing component and the educational component.

4 The academic dean is responsible for maintaining a plan of internal governance which is based upon the principle of collegiality.

5 The academic dean is responsible for the up-to-dateness of the faculty, either through in-service learning opportunities or through a program of employment.

6 The academic dean is responsible for the overall quality control of the school or college which he or she administers as verified, in part, by professional accreditation (Hornbake, 1978:3).

It should be clear that the dean's leadership fit may be specific in relation to any one of these functions and may vary from one to the other. In other words, some deans' preparation in education and experience and considerable creativity with regard to the future of nursing help them to fulfill the first functions stated with a high degree of success. On the other hand, the same deans may have views of internal governance and the means to accomplish their goals which are out of keeping with those of the particular group holding the power in an institution or school. When defining the major direction or major thrust of the school or college requires programmatic changes, the means of accomplishing these changes must be seen within the context of the school, the subgroups most responsible for designing and implementing such changes, and whether or not general agreement exists among all the participants about the direction the dean has set. Specific examples of what may be perceived as weakness or domination could be offered for any one of the six functions that Hornbake has stated. We are sure that the readers (the audience) can develop their own sets or subsets of means to these functional ends, some of which may be congruent with each other and others of which will give evidence upon which to predict future controversies.

It is clear that whatever definition of leadership or description of decanal functions is subscribed to, it is essential for the dean to gain and utilize power to achieve all the personal, professional, faculty group, and institutional goals.

The demands of power, leadership, and management require that deans (1) make decisions based on knowledge gained through continual fact finding, (2) anticipate and rehearse a variety of scenarios with trusted and knowledgeable critics, (3) achieve goals through the motivation and guidance of a variety of work groups at several levels, and (4) renew physical and emotional energy, which is continually drained by the direction and support others expect from the leader.

We are also aware that leadership, decanal functions, and goals are increasingly difficult to negotiate. At this time individuals at top levels of management are required to gain a higher level of sophistication than in previous times as a result of the expanding science of management and increased competition for intra- and extrainstitutional resources. The pace of preparation and socialization for the role is not as rapid as the change in expectations, and the execution of functions and decision making frequently take place in an environment that is anxious, hostile, or without structure or precedent.

NETWORKS OF SUPPORT

In light of these factors it behooves the dean to marshal all the forces which will provide direct assistance in the work of "deaning." Development and maintenance of networks of support is a critical part of the assistance the dean is able to influence personally.

A *network of support* is a matrix or lattice of groups and individuals who provide the dean with information, critical review and feedback, completion of work which contributes to overall goals, and personal and professional support. These support network functions are important to the dean for reasons that are both personal and professional and contribute in the following ways:

1 Supportive structures assist the dean to enjoy the leadership position, develop personally and professionally, and achieve personal, institutional, and professional goals.

2 Networks of support for nursing deans are important to the profession since the attainment of personal, institutional, and educational goals is compatible with the growth of the nursing profession.

3 Insofar as networks of support contribute to the experience, growth, and longevity of individual administrators, they contribute to the nursing profession's collective understanding and use of leadership, power, and management.

4 The vast majority of deans in nursing are women, and networks of support are critical for development reasons as well. Men in all spheres have had vertical and horizontal supports and models. Men have been able to imitate and learn from the powerful and the decision makers around them. At a certain point, their contemporaries became their horizontal network. Most women have not learned the requisite skills from women above them on a hierarchy, and it is difficult if not impractical for women to attempt to imitate men. Therefore, the broadly horizontal networks of support developed by women in leadership positions are critical since in most instances they must compensate for the lack of earlier support groups and mentors.

THREE LEVELS OF A NETWORK

We have described networks of support as a latticework or matrix of individuals and groups. A matrix presupposes various levels of interaction. Three broad levels within the networks of support can be identified: (1) individuals and groups who are peers, (2) the supraordinate level, and (3) the subordinate level.

First, the dean must develop and maintain peer skills in order to establish and maintain an array of contacts with equals. Within this level three distinct categories emerge: (1) deans and administrators within one's institution and the formal councils of deans and administrators; (2) other professionals, including lawyers, corporation and foundation executives, business, social, and political figures, and all their respective organizations; and (3) deans of nursing, organizations of deans and administrators in nursing, and other colleagues in the nursing profession.

In building a network of support with colleagues and administrators in one's own institutional setting, certain ingredients are consistently found. These may be grouped under the category of *mutuality*: that is, "the return in kind or degree of what is given or demonstrated by the other" (Webster's New World 1968:970). The reciprocal nature of the support network cannot be underestimated. It must be recognized that to expect support, freely offered, for any length of time is naive and self-centered. All participants in the university atmosphere have their own needs and priorities, which need careful consideration by the dean of nursing. It is essential that the dean's ability to assess the scale of these needs and priorities for the various groups be carefully honored. The dean's recognition of the areas most crucial to the others will often spell the success or failure of her or his interpersonal endeavor. Deans who assess these crucial areas correctly are more able to argue on conflicting issues when these are higher on their own scale of values than on those of their colleagues. The importance of correct assessment and reciprocity of support must be stressed in all parts of the dean's network. Mutuality with administrators and other deans requires skills in communication, which include knowing what needs to be communicated as well as how and when to communicate. Clearly, the what varies considerably from group to group and within groups.

Expressing interest in the long-range goals of colleagues in other schools and sharing both successful and unsuccessful experiences relevant to their goals establishes the dean as an important person in his or her own networks. Having or making opportunities to inform colleagues about the goals of one's school and plans for meeting these goals, accepting questions and debate in a nondefensive manner, and utilizing discussions in subsequent contacts are all useful techniques in building a support network.

The social-professional activities in which the dean participates should also be included in the methodology for building support. In many institutions a range of professional-social functions occurs which may make the difference in relationships with both administrative officers and colleagues in other fields. The dean's participation in such events is crucial. Recognizing where nursing administrators and faculty may play an important role, the dean facilitates the addition of these persons to professional-social guest listings.

Maintaining and expanding the support network

with professional individuals and groups outside of nursing is extremely important. The information, criticial review, and expanded authority functions fulfilled by this category within the peer group level serve to give the dean important inside information and an expanded voice of authority and expertise. The dean's "in" with foundation heads, corporation presidents, and significant elected state and national officials at the least provides parity with other professionals and by virtue of mutuality may at times offer more substantive rewards.

The third category within the peer group level is the group of deans in nursing. Individually and collectively they share experiences, issues and threats, and the successful or less successful resolution of these should provide useful data. The collective impact of more than 350 deans and chairs of accredited programs should provide the forum for action plans helpful to a majority of causes.

Although deans and other colleagues in nursing are an important source of emotional and intellectual support to the dean of the school of nursing, we have not yet seen this group counted on to play an important role individually or collectively when a dean of a school of nursing is threatened. Thus, we have placed it last on our peer list because we are not able to develop an argument which would prove that this thread of the network can be as useful as the others. We have all had experiences of attempting to offer support to a dean whose immediate future in a particular institution was in our view, reprehensibly threatened. In certain situations the dean's role was so destructively impinged upon by outside persons that a resignation was the best alternative. The best statement the nursing community could make to such an institution would be to *ensure* that the dean's position remained open for some time until the structural problems were resolved. Unfortunately, we all know that often this does not occur and that even under the most difficult and widely publicized circumstances there is always someone who will walk into the position under the existing rules. Setting a direction for the profession requires a much larger group of committed colleagues in order for this part of our network to provide sufficient external support to compensate for some lacks in internal support. We believe, on the other hand, that it is possible to identify the ingredients of a strong network of support in the other threads.

The second level of the network of support involves individuals and groups supraordinate to the dean. Development and maintenance of this level draws on the dean's ability to understand and utilize channels of authority and communication to advantage. The dean develops alliances with individuals and groups inside and outside the institution who enhance the dean's authority, expertise, and position.

In professional relationships with the chief academic officers the dean first must be certain that these individuals have understanding about the nursing profession and its problems and potential, know and support her or his goals for the school, and be committed to helping the dean accomplish these. These individuals need to have information presented so that they buy into the programs the dean expects to establish. By the same token, the dean's helpful support toward these administrators, showing understanding of their problems and priorities, must be demonstrated verbally and by other appropriate means.

Similar concerns are basic to the dean's professional relationship to others within this level. It is important that the governor and state legislators understand nursing's characteristics and needs in the state. The dean's information and explanation about nursing are balanced by participation in the political process. Efforts on the part of political aspirants who support legislation and programs helpful to nursing must be acknowledged in an active participatory mode by the dean and his or her colleagues.

The third level in the dean's network of support incorporates individuals and groups subordinate to the dean. These tend to be people within the or-

ganization and require the dean's wide range of leadership skills. In general, individuals and groups within the organization are concerned about completion of activities designed to achieve organizational and professional goals.

While this level fulfills the goal-oriented work function of a support network, it also fulfills the other network functions by supplying information, critically reviewing actions and reactions, and supplying personal support to the dean and each other.

Building support among the faculty of one's own school has, in our view, all the ingredients already discussed and one additional characteristic not included in the concept of mutuality. This is the mentor relationship a dean has by design or by accident with faculty. We believe the essential characteristic of the administrator-leader is the building of leadership in others. This characteristic occurs only when democratic leadership rather than autocratic leadership is the mode of the dean. In a democratic group, leadership is shared as appropriate to the task and many members may influence goal setting and goal achievement. We believe this mode to be consonant with faculty rights and responsibilities, the provisions of support needed by faculty, and the building of leaders needed by the profession. While resulting in a support network to the dean, this is a by-product of rather than the purpose for the dean's efforts.

Building leaders and sharing leadership does not in any way diminish the leadership role of the dean. The dean's differentiated role as designated leader inside and outside the school of nursing is in part identified by structuring the democratic process and clearly identifying those roles and functions appropriate to the position. In addition, the dean is the behavioral model to faculty, whose organizational skills support individuals and groups; maintain group activities; promote cohesiveness; minimize destructive and divisive behaviors; and ultimately assist the group to goal attainment. Such groups will by their very nature seek to maintain themselves since multiple needs are being met. Hierarchical controversies and factionalism are deliberately kept to a minimum by the leadership method of the dean. The dean deals with such problems individually as well as in the group, in an open and constructive manner, focusing on the group goals to be met. Confronting negative behaviors on an individual basis from the standpoint of building the faculty member's professional potential is part of the dean's role as leader of leaders. Needless to say, we expect this kind of school to be characterized by a high degree of openness and trust.

NECESSARY SKILLS

We have described three levels within the dean's network of support. What are the common components or skills which the dean must utitize to develop and maintain these networks?

A major skill basic to this whole enterprise is the art of initiating, developing, and maintaining contacts. This requires the right blend of social and professional effort molded by a view of the function and purposes of these interactions. We have already discussed mutuality or the reciprocal flow of effort and support between the dean and the elements in her or his network of support.

Developing the appropriate mix of personal, social, and professional interest with each of the elements in the network is another critical skill. This component is, however, also one of the most individual aspects since each dean must be comfortable with the activities used, and the approach to the participants in one's network must "ring true" with the individual's personality and style.

According to all the clichés, success stimulates success, and a fourth skill requisite to the development and maintenance of networks is the dean's ability to project a successful, knowledgeable, and energetic image. These attributes make the dean desirable to work with and eligible for exchange of information, evaluation, and support.

Interpersonal competence is a skill that is basic to the preceding skill descriptions but one which must be examined independently as well. Interpersonal competence is a set of abilities which allows an individual to shape the responses he or she wishes or anticipates receiving or prompting in others. This includes the ability to extract and validate information and to disseminate it effectively and advantageously (Foote and Cottrell, 1955).

OBSTACLES TO DEVELOPMENT OF NETWORK

If the networks of support a dean needs to facilitate success are identifiable and the skills can be isolated and described, what prevents every dean, leader, or administrator from effectively employing networks of support? There appear to be several factors which impinge at different points in the network development and maintenance process.

The first by now must be very obvious; the planning, execution, and evaluation of all the activities with each of the components within the networks of support require a tremendous amount of physical and emotional energy. These demanding activities compete for one's energy and unless the dean gives network support top priority, the exhausting and conflicting demands of the dean's schedule will relegate network development to a low point on the list. Therefore, the dean must have high energy levels and a real commitment to network development.

A second obstacle to network development, particularly with the peer group level of support networks, is the diminished trust among deans and administrators due to the intense competition for limited resources within institutions or between institutions for government and/or private funding, for well-qualified faculty, and for students. Open sharing and cooperation is threatening if it means successful recruiting or monetary rewards for some administrators and thereby potentially less for the others.

A third obstacle to the development of networks of support for successful decanal work occurs as a result of our cultural socialization, which makes us ambivalent as to whether it is proper to want to develop a power base, negotiate power, take the initiative, or accept risk. Avoidance or at least ambivalence toward this aspect of our position or our aspirations potentially undermines efforts to be an influential leader.

The fourth obstacle stems from the third; our socialization implies that women and therefore nurses are not powerful, political, or influential. Women and thus most nurses do not control money, space, or other valued commodities. Women are also not viewed as analytical or entrepreneurial. These last two obstacles prevent female nurses from seeing themselves as influential leaders and bias others as nurses attempt to develop alliances.

There may be other obstacles, some general and some individual, but we should consider them just that; they are meant to be overcome because the network of support is so vital to success.

FAILURE OF THE NETWORK

The three levels of support previously discussed incorporate internal individuals and groups and those external to the dean's institution. Both the internal and external elements are essential to the dean's networks. We would like to consider what happens when the dean's network of support fails, particularly the support from the internal individuals and groups.

Possible problem areas within the school which may threaten faculty and subsequently bring threats to the dean's position may be in areas of curriculum, in faculty recruitment, in governance, and in the reward system the dean uses. Problem areas outside the school may also include the area of curriculum, particularly as it relates to the registered nurse program and the view of clinical and administrative preparation given to students. Other problem areas outside the school, and particularly with the medical school, are competition for clinical resources and competition for turfs both in the hospital and the university. Without a highly developed collaborative relationship with the medical school, a dean viewed as strong within his or

her own school in terms of curriculum development, strengthening faculty, and increasing powers to control nursing practice in clinical facilities may be viewed as a great threat to the power structure outside the school of nursing. It would be hard to find another professional school where the same example might be offered.

There are probably many administrators who are struggling with questions of their continuance in the role of dean of the school of nursing. Questions aroused by the numerous threats to the role and in some cases the powerlessness that has resulted from the threats make some deans decide to get out of a particular position. When the administrator to whom the dean reports wants the dean out, there are various behaviors and decisions which can be utilized to make the dean's life extremely uncomfortable. When a large and sufficiently powerful faculty wishes a dean replaced, faculty behaviors also may make the dean's position intolerable. As yet, no study has been done which might help us identify with certainty the common elements in the most extreme versions of this, but a review of those cited would suggest some factors: (1) a strong difference of opinion regarding the issues in nursing education such as entry level, registered nurse educational mobility, the external degree, etc.; (2) power struggles for control of the school with administrators external to the school; (3) power struggles for control of the school with faculty members representing controversial issues or other candidates; (4) inability to resolve factional disputes in a school. The latter problem, often identified as weakness on the part of the dean, will not be dealt with in this section. It has, however, been dealt with in the description of the characteristics of the dean's leadership in the previous section.

If all else fails, the dean in some instances is forced to consider the option of resigning from the position. Some have chosen this option with more or less success. Is it possible to use the word "success" in the context of resignation? Does not the resignation itself imply that the individual has failed?

We submit that the resignation in and of itself does not suggest failure. Rather, it stems from one or more of the following conditions: (1) The dean's original assessment of the situation was incorrect in that the assumption of internal supports was based on verbal promises and no data. (2) The dean's assessment of faculty candidates for positions did not utilize the covert as well as overt communication network in nursing and has not identified those persons whose own goals are not in keeping with group goals for the school and whose previous histories would have suggested subsequent problems in this area. (3) The position of the dean in this school requires more experience, education, or some other characteristic not part of the particular dean's repertoire. (4) New executive officers have since been appointed in the university who have set new goals and missions for the university. These goals are out of keeping with the goals of the school of nursing.

Knowing when and how to resign is an important aspect of success in a deanship, and in many instances the resignation cannot be construed as failure. Granted, resignation may not be a personal satisfaction; however professionally it can be used as a device to advance the school and its needs in situations where remaining in the position of dean[1] would only continue or even exacerbate the conflicts.

The remaining portion of a dean's support network could help to provide the dean with the necessary elements to make the resignation effective. Our view is that no resignation should be offered unless it makes a statement to faculty, to the university, and to the nursing community at large. This statement must be in keeping with the prevailing views of the profession and must indicate the factors which made the attainment of such goals impossible in this particular setting. Generally speaking, the dean should prefer to leave the institution at a point in time to be decided by the dean. However, even where the departure from the

[1] We are assuming that the dean of the school of nursing occupies a tenured position on the faculty.

deanship is immediate, the departure from professorial rank should be timed extremely carefully to provide the dean with the maximum latitude for meeting his or her own professional goals as well as permitting an effective statement at the school. At this time the dean's personal needs should receive considerable attention. As the AACN states "to the best of our knowledge, these administrators (who have left their positions) were not harridans who needed to be exorcised" (1980:1). Indeed for one or more of the reasons we have stated, the dean's life has probably been quite miserable for some period of time preceding the resignation.

A hasty escape from the situation may seem desirable at a particular moment but it will not serve the dean in his or her future professional goals nor will it serve the profession itself. Thus, we recommend the design sometimes termed a *protest resignation*. This type of resignation usually includes a set time for departure as well as a clear statement of cause. It can be more or less publicized depending upon the issues. It can also include the requirements for a sabbatical if this is desired or other period of paid leave. It should be recognized that the eventual resignation from the tenured position is seen as an economic advantage to the employer, and therefore negotiation for particular benefits is quite legitimate and timely. While we know of several who have utilized the protest resignation in recent years, it is still the exception rather than the norm. We strongly urge our colleagues, when a network of support is absent or has failed, to consider a meaningful resignation as an alternative.

CONCLUSION

In conclusion, we have discussed the leadership role of the dean and the importance of the networks of support to the success of the dean in attaining personal, institutional, and professional goals. The defined levels of networks include groups and individuals internal and external to the dean's institution.

We have identified why networks of support contribute to individual and collective professional development and specifically what functions these networks of support fulfill.

Some of the skills the dean must employ to establish support networks and what factors prevent network development have been described.

Last, we have discussed what occurs when the dean's networks of support fail in part and how resignation can be accomplished effectively, using the remainder of the dean's network of support.

EDITOR'S QUESTIONS FOR DISCUSSION

Describe the characteristics of the relationship between leaders and their constituents in academic and nursing care settings. How discrepant are expectations for leadership between leaders and their constituents? How can expectations for leaders and followers be more realistic? What changes have occurred within the profession of nursing that have impacted the academic scene? What is the quality of increased visibility on the nursing profession through the print and television media? What factors have influenced increased visibility?

What factors have influenced the increasing turnover rate for deans of nursing? How does the increasing rate for deans of nursing compare with the turnover rate for deans in other academic disciplines? If there are differences from deans in other disciplines, to what may the differences be attributed? What issues need to be addressed in preventing early or sudden resignations of nursing deans? What are the implications for preparation for the deanship role, academic nursing administration, and the profession in an increasingly short term of office for the dean?

What is the difference between leaders and managers? How do they differ in their orientations toward goals, work, human relations, and their selves? What strategies can be suggested for deans to successfully integrate the characteristics of leadership and management in their role? What strategies can be suggested for maintaining balances of power and converting "win-lose" into "win-win" situations? In face-to-face confrontations how can a dean and faculty member or members validate the distinction between preserving authority and debating issues? How can such validation demonstrate support for a dean, yet freedom to disagree without reprisal? What may be the significance of a sense of belonging and a sense of being separate for the kinds of investments managers and leaders make in their careers? What relationship is there between leaders who feel separate from their environment and those who search out opportunities for change in an organization or institution?

How can extremely divergent perspectives of a dean's leadership be reconciled? What significance is there for an organization, academic institution, and profession in the occurrence of extreme views regarding leadership at the highest level of administration? What remarks by Hegyvary (Chap. 49) and Editor's Questions for Discussion apply to Fagin and McGivern's discussion of leadership and appropriate match of a leader with an institution? According to Fagin and McGivern leadership is not an enduring role. How then can an individual retain a leadership role after the contextual purposes of the role are met? Discuss the advantages and disadvantages of deans retaining a position in a school or college once they have chosen to end their term of office. How can the talents, knowledge, and experience of a former dean be most effectively utilized? How might former deans effectively be mentors to aspiring deans of the future? How can former deans most effectively assist incumbent deans?

What factors influence the variation in degree to which a dean successfully fulfills the six major AACN functions appropriate to a dean? Designate the most appropriate means in your setting for a dean to fulfill the six functions. What criteria might be utilized in evaluation of a dean's role performance? Who should decide the criteria to be used? In developing an instrument for evaluation, what methodological considerations are essential? Who should participate in the development of such an instrument, how should it be administered, by whom should the data be interpreted, and to whom should the findings be disseminated? How different might criteria be for the performance evaluation of all academic administrative positions? To what extent should criteria be similar for general faculty as for faculty who hold administrative positions? Apply the same questions addressed to the construction of a performance evaluation tool for a dean to that developed for other academic administrative positions and faculty. What purpose should performance evaluations serve in academic settings? Design a performance evaluation instrument for a dean, academic nurse administrators, and faculty. Discuss the pros and cons and the methods for peer evaluation among faculty. Discuss the development of performance evaluation instruments for nurse administrators and professional staff in nursing and health care settings. What differences in purpose, methods, and criteria for measurement exist from those utilized in academic settings? Design performance evaluation instruments for nurse administrators and staff in nursing and health care settings.

Discuss the extent to which a dean realistically can achieve all personal, professional, faculty/group, and institutional goals. What are the most effective strategies for gaining and appropriately using power? What suggestions can be offered for a dean to sufficiently encourage and reward faculty without the deleterious effects of excessive competition and rivalry occurring between and among peers of faculty? What conditions are essential for the development of trust between a dean and faculty and among faculty? What suggestions can be offered to increase trust and interpersonal support between and among faculty?

What factors or variables which contribute to the criticalness of support networks are different for women than professional men who are deans in nursing? How does the lack of previous support groups and mentors for deans in nursing influence the means and methods utilized in developing a support network? How do professional men and women differ in developing support networks? Provide examples of the reciprocal nature essential to support networks. What suggestions can be offered to deans of nursing to assess accurately the needs and priorities of participants in a university in developing a support network? How can a dean accurately assess the climate and readiness of faculty for accepting proposed policies? Provide additional examples of techniques and avenues for building support. Why have deans and other colleagues in nursing not played a significant role individually or collectively when a dean of a school of nursing is threatened? What factors are most influential in whether collective support by colleagues in nursing is developed and demonstrated? What are the implications for the nursing profession when collective support does not exist?

What are the most effective means to develop alliances with individuals supraordinate to the dean? Provide examples of reciprocal understanding and demonstration of support. How can a dean accurately assess the balance that is needed and means to achieve mutuality in professional relationships with chief academic officers? What assessment is needed and suggestions may be offered when resistance is evident in building reciprocal support relationships? Under what conditions do faculties demonstrate resistance?

Provide examples of the dean as a behavioral model to faculty. How can discrepancies and difficulties be resolved between "espoused" theories of action and governance and the theory-in-use (observed behavior) phenomenon? What considerations are essential in developing a mentor relationship with faculty? What strategies can be suggested for minimizing destructive and divisive behaviors between and among faculty? What are the most effective methods for confronting negative behaviors? What is the role, function, and responsibility of the dean in conflict management?

What is the relationship between the skills discussed by Murphy (Chap. 55) and those outlined by Fagin and McGivern as essential to build and maintain support networks? What methods may be most effective for accurate self-assessment and developing interpersonal competence? What ethical implications are there in extracting, validating, and disseminating information by a dean?

How can obstacles to developing support networks be overcome? What other factors may impinge on the building of support networks? Provide specific examples of threats to a dean's position within a school in the areas of curriculum, faculty recruitment, governance, and reward system used. What additional areas within a school may be a source of threat? Provide suggestions as to how a dean may successfully resolve threats to their position.

How can nursing deans successfully negotiate for resolution of problem areas outside the school that may threaten their position? How can nursing deans successfully develop collaborative relationships with the medical school? Discuss the differences that exist when a school or college of nursing is located at and associated with a medical center campus versus a predominantly liberal arts campus or university. What strategies are essential in developing successful support networks by virtue of different settings in which the position of a nursing dean is located? Discuss the degree of autonomy a school or college of nursing, or nursing dean has in relation to the building of support networks. Are support networks more critical in settings where the nursing dean has less autonomy? What differences are there in building networks where there is less autonomy?

What are essential ethical considerations for relieving and replacing the position of a dean? How can limitations of a dean be strengthened? To what extent is there an obligation to support a dean's strengths and accept a dean's limitations? What are the obligations and responsibilities of faculty in supporting and strengthening the position of a dean? What other factors and conditions, in addition to those cited, may result in resignation? Address each of the conditions cited by Fagin and McGivern and provide suggestions for preventing the conditions or successfully dealing with the situations. How should the remainder of a dean's support network be used when resignation is to occur? What characterizes a "protest resignation"? What is meant by a "meaningful resignation"? How might a dean accurately assess when and how to resign? What are the characteristics of a "successful" resignation? How would you characterize a "successful" dean, indicating critical personal, institutional, organizational, and environmental variables?

How can this chapter be applied to the role of the chief nurse administrator who is ultimately accountable for the provision of professional nursing care in health care settings? Choose and respond to the editor's questions posed for discussion which are also relevant for the chief nurse administrator.

REFERENCES

American Association of Colleges of Nursing Executive Development Series
 1980 Academic Administration. Washington, D.C.: American Association of Colleges of Nursing.

Claus, Karen D. and June Bailey
 1977 Power and Influence in Health Care. St. Louis: The C.V. Mosby Co.

Foote, Nelson and Leonard Cottrell
 1955 Identity and Interpersonal Competence. Chicago: University of Chicago Press.

Gibb, Cecil A.
 1955 "The principle and traits of leadership." Pp. 87–95 in A. Paul Hare, Edgar F. Borgatta, Robert S. Bales (eds.), Small Groups. New York: Knopf.

Hornbake, R. Lee
 1978 "The academic dean as perceived by university administration." Pp. 3–10 in functions and Challenges to Deans of Nursing. Washington, D.C.: American Association of Colleges of Nursing, Publications Series 78, No. 3.

Webster's New World Dictionary
 1968 New York: The World Publishing Co.

Chapter 57

Future Social Planning for Nursing Education and Nursing Practice Organizations

Annettte Schram Ezell, R.N., Ed.D.
Associate Dean of Academic Affairs
College of Nursing
University of Utah
Salt Lake City, Utah

As evident in Fagin's and McGivern's chapter, strategic planning is critical to the construction of support networks for success and goal attainment in the role as a dean. Annette Schram Ezell proposes a method, developed by Donald Michael, that is applicable not only to the development of support networks, but also to numerous issues and concerns of the nursing profession. She applies the strategy as a means for planning, change, and generating greater congruence between nursing practice and nursing education, and the nursing profession and nursing organizations. Ezell's premise is that organizational goal conflicts and disparities in nursing may be clearer in using Michael's process. Long-range social planning (*lrsp*) is a strategy for organizational change and future-responsive societal learning (*frsl*). She raises five questions for discussion and application of *lrsp* and *frsl* in nursing. Long-range social planning (*lrsp*) and organizational future-responsive social learning (*frsl*) are examined. The interface of organization goals and learning, practice, and education are explored. Ezell emphasizes the importance of mutual goal setting for nursing organizations for movement toward *frsl*. She explicates six requirements and strategies for movement toward *frsl*: living with uncertainty, embracing error, accepting the ethical responsibilities of goal-setting, living with role ambiguity, boundary-spanning, and organizational restructuring. Evaluating the present in relation to the future, being open to change based upon evaluation of the present, and commitment to actions *now* to respond in the long range are also designated as requirements toward *frsl*.

Ezell cites some of the factors contributing to disparity in nursing. These include: the most highly qualified professional nurses pursuing the academic route; the federal financial support to prepare clinical specialists; the shortage of highly qualified nurse administrators to provide for the delivery of nursing care; resistance to information sharing; and preparing practitioners for the future rather than for current nursing practice settings. As a consequence, Ezell says, the gap between the purposes and goals of nursing education and practice organizations has widened. Resistance to collaboration and change has become an increasing problem. Ezell advocates (*lrsp*) as a remedy. For this process to occur, members of an organization need to become sufficiently uncomfortable with the present, encouragement for change must come from outside the organization, and deans of nursing and nurse administrators, who provide for the delivery of nursing care, need to allocate resources to plan for the future. Long-range social planning is a directed self-transformation, societal learning process. It is a means to achieve *frsl*.

Ezell provides examples of goal disparity between organizations of nursing practice and education. Goal disparity may occur due to different spatial relationships, variation in the amount of time required to achieve goals, and level of educational preparation for nurse administrators. Time lags in goal congruence between the two nursing organizational settings are predicted to continue. Organizational learning, which is critical to *frsl,* is contended to be intentionally rational. This is accomplished through communication structures, learning incentives, or belief structures. Distinctions are made between single-loop and double-loop learning. Both types detect and correct errors; however, double-loop learning further involves the changing of underlying values and policies. Ezell perceives that the nursing profession should be engaged in double-loop learning. She remarks that managerial technology has limited decision making to single-looped learning, such as routines. Ezell notes that few strategies have been taught to assist aspiring administrators of nursing organizations to transfer double-loop learning into constructive actions. This is related to the fact that double-loop learning surfaces contradictions, conflict, and undiscussable issues concerning values and policies.

Ezell discusses numerous issues involved with utilizing the six strategies to implement *frsl*. Although uncertainty is required for growth in organizational *lrsp,* there needs to be a balance of protection for the technical core in the organization. There should be a greater use of professionals in problem solving to reduce uncertainty. Acknowledging uncertainty, goal setting and provision of feedback are means for reducing uncertainty. Expecting and accepting errors increases the capacities for interpersonal support, revision of goals, and evaluation of programs. Value conflicts and ideological differences are expected, but require ethical responsibility in handling for goal setting. Anticipated stress, role conflict–ambiguity, and challenges to legitimacy are inherent in moving toward *lrsp*. The boundary spanner position (information carriers and generators between systems) is crucial to changing over to *lrsp.* Relationships between parts of and between the organization and its environment may need to change for *lrsp* to succeed.

In conclusion, Ezell views the movement toward *lrsp* and *frsl* being based on two organizational choices. Nursing organizations must continuously adapt to the environment at the expense of internal consistency or maintain internal consistency at the expense of environmental conflicts. She perceives the choice for nursing organizations to be revolution, not evolution, and opting for internal consistency. As a consequence self-transformation, different goals, and different directives can be envisioned for the nursing organizations of education and practice and the nursing profession in the 1980s.

The gap between nursing practice and nursing education has been extensively criticized, examined, researched, and bemoaned. The apparent conflict of goals reported to exist between nursing practice and nursing educational organizations and the functional realities of goal disparities have long been cited as major causes of communication problems. The conflicts that are experienced do not appear to arise from the lack of understanding of each other's intentions or goals but from a difference in perspective as to the purposes and procedures that are necessary to cope constructively with our changing society. I propose that the organizational conflicts and disparities seen and experienced in nursing may be more clearly viewed through a process currently utilized to determine social responsiveness and future organizational changes.

This chapter briefly examines the idea of long-range social planning (*lrsp*) as a purposeful strategy for organizational change and future-responsive societal learning (*frsl*).[1] Some issues which will be raised include:

- Are future-responsive goals needed for collaboration between nursing education and nursing practice organizations?
- What is organizational goal disparity and error?
- What might be the expected effects of long-range social planning on nursing organizations?
- How may future-responsive societal learning to reduce disparity and error occur?
- Why must those involved in the future of nursing contribute to a purposeful plan of directing nursing organizations toward future-responsive societal learning?

If nursing education and nursing practice organizations recognize that their goals are not appropriate to society and are not responsive to societal needs, should not their goals be modified? Are some less obvious needs being met by nursing organizations as they exist today? Information needs to be shared and goals redefined in order to achieve responsiveness by the nursing profession and nursing organizations. The application of

---

[1] The concepts of long-range social planning (*lrsp*) and future-responsive societal learning (*frsl*) have been described by Donald Michael in *On Learning to Plan—and Planning to Learn* (San Francisco: Jossey-Bass Publishers, 1976).

Michael's work to nursing is presented in this chapter as a strategy in future social planning and in generating greater congruence and unity between the nursing profession and nursing organizations (1976).

Before nursing education was transposed into organizations of higher education, the relationship between the worlds of nursing education and nursing practice was much closer. Now we are at a time when the best-prepared nurses in the United States are frequently those who are academicians. Some of these educators are extremely competent in a specialized area of nursing, and others are not. Most of these highly prepared professionals tend to pursue the academic route of research and teaching or to seek administrative posts in higher education.

Accompanying the movement of highly qualified nursing professionals into higher education has been a federal effort to support financially the development of clinical specialists. This has resulted in a decrease in the number of nurses being prepared for administration in health care delivery. Today we face a serious shortage of highly qualified nurses in the administration of nursing services throughout the country. Because of these changes, the gap between the purposes and goals of nursing education and nursing practice organizations has widened. Baker states that

> . . . loyalty to one or the other [education or practice] must be redirected and elevated to the profession as a whole. Separatism is no longer acceptable. Social and economic realities are forcing us to move toward more interdependence. Collaboration should enable both practice and education to benefit qualitatively by associating with each other and economically by allocating scarce resources to nursing's needs. (1981:35)

Yet, rigidity and resistance to collaboration and change have become an ever-increasing problem.

Much of the gap between nursing organizations appears to be related to dialogue disparity. Often there is resistance to information sharing. The

kinds of information sharing that *could* occur among various nursing organizations include the sharing of specific data, data sources, data collection methods, and data interpretation. Decisions about who has access to data and who is obligated to use what pieces of data and the decision rationale behind various organizational actions could also be shared, but such sharing is a scarce event.

Another source of disparity, somewhat related to the others, is that educators are preparing practitioners for the future, rather than for the current nursing practice settings. This concept of "future"—the faculty's interpretation of nursing roles and functions within a variety of settings—has been, at best, an estimate based on past experiences and the projection of current trends. This indirect method of professional goal setting emphasizes the future as an unavoidable arena for choice. Thus it has become the responsibility of the nurse-educator in the nursing education organization to become, in part, an astute futurist, sensitive and responsive to the implications of changes within the profession and nurse practice organizations. These changes have appeared in many forms: in technology, in the political and social climate, in long-range social planning, and in future-responsive societal learning.

LONG-RANGE SOCIAL PLANNING (*lrsp*)

As with all attempts to read the future, a professional group will often look to the past to predict the future, and some may even dare to think that the future is to be viewed very differently. However, for *lrsp* to become effective in any organization, the members must be sufficiently uncomfortable with the present [and the past] to begin to create radically different futures. During the planning process, great anxiety may surface, especially if the visionaries acknowledge that their organizations are weak and unable to deal with future societal change. Michael (1976:157–163) predicts that encouragement for organizational change will come predominantly from those *outside* the organization. If one is able to describe the future, the scenario will include dialectic and cybernetic thought. But these skills are not prevalent within nursing spheres.

Additionally, thinking into the future may produce information overload and a sense of uncertainty. These reasons alone demand that serious planning for the future be undertaken. Yet, few deans of nursing and few nursing service administrators have considered this task important enough to allocate some of their scarce financial resources for such faculty or staff efforts. The fear of uncertainty also contributes to resistance to giving serious attention to future planning and study.

Some experts advocate that future studies are merely methods for myth generation within the organizations (Michael, 1976:162; Kamens, 1977). Myth generation has been one method used to decrease organizational uncertainty. Through mythology, one becomes committed to a myth of the future, especially during periods of rapid social change, so that concerted group action increases the likelihood of realization. Therefore, for those organizations in nursing with chief executive officers who are willing to explore, a self-fulfilling prophecy of future-responsive societal learning might be attainable (Michael. 1976:163).

In identifying a framework for this chapter, I have searched through much literature and spent hours in thought. How can the nursing organizations effectively work together with the profession to create the best plan for the future evolution of nursing? Through the work of Michael (1976), March and Olsen (1976a; 1976b), Argyris (1980), and Bacharach and Lawlor (1980), strategies have been identified that may be effectively used in developing plans which will highlight the interrelationship of nursing organizations (education and practice) with the nursing profession.

Facing the future is a task filled with uncertainties—economic, political, and professional. How can one treat such a topic in new light without being caught up in old clichés? The issues posed in the beginning of this chapter provide a springboard for thought about the desired relationship between organizations of nursing and their environments, thought which should stimulate definition and interpretation.

ORGANIZATIONAL FUTURE-RESPONSIVE SOCIAL LEARNING (*frsl*)

One of the best comments on future responsivenes has been made by E. Dunn, who suggested that professionals must seek directed self-transformation.

> The principal problem of social organization that confronts advanced societies . . . can best be seen by contrasting the organizational consequences of normal problem solving and paradigm shifts. For normal problem solving, system reorganization is purposive, anticipatory, and controlled. In contrast, paradigm shifts have historically been primarily reactive, unanticipated, and uncontrolled. They tend to arise out of a reaction to exogenously and endogenously generated boundary crises. They are frequently unanticipated by the management elite of the system. The reorganization is often defensive in character—that is, it is directed toward preserving and extending the life of the system in the face of changes rather than taking the form of a directed self-transformation in pursuit of some higher order goal. (Dunn, 1971:214–215)

The means for purposeful or directed self-transformation that is addressed in this chapter is long-range social planning (*lrsp*) for the nursing profession and nursing organizations. Michael has warned us that the present turbulent and radical process of social change has made our routine problem-solving skills obsolete. Therefore, Michael (1976:17) views long-range social planning "as a societal learning process for learning how to do lrsp," where *lrsp* is a means of achieving future-responsive societal learning (*frsl*). In this sense Michael has used *lrsp* and *frsl* as interchangeable concepts in a dialectical process "to learn to change toward lrsp and to learn how to become sensitive in valuing frsl" (Michael, 1976:17–18).

Using Michael's model, let us examine the purposes and procedures for coping with a changing society, learn what can be anticipated and chosen, and learn to overcome the resistances inherent in all organizations which strive for *lrsp*.

ORGANIZATIONAL GOALS

Figure 57–1 has been schematically outlined to demonstrate the interface of nursing practice organizations (nursing clinics, hospices, birthing centers) with nursing organizations of higher education and the nursing profession. It is conceivable that the major nursing organizations of practice and education could be interested in similar goals, and yet these goals might be viewed in different spatial relationships according to a continuum of goal disparity and success (Sills, 1969:175–187). Goal continuums are valued as one function of legitimating organizational activities (e.g., doctoral education for administrators of nursing practice and education organizations). These decision processes, conscious or not, culminate in a choice among alternatives.

Another example of long-range goal disparity is shown in Fig. 57–2. The amount of time involved in the acquisition of organizational goals (considered on a continuum) is quite variable and often unknown. Complex organizations must inevitably come to terms with their environment—whether by rational or irrational processes. "Whether the process of adjustment is awkward or nimble becomes important in determining the organization's degree of prosperity" (Thompson and McEwen, 1961:190).

Figure 57–2 shows the use of "level of educational preparation for nursing administrators" as a variable affecting nursing organizations' priorities. Variables affecting time lag are often undocumented and unknown. Some variables contributing to time lag could include saliency, financial costs, available workers, and scope of professional practice expertise (Lum, 1979). These time lags in goal congruence may vary from several months to many years. Huckabay (1979) has completed one nationwide informal assessment of the time-lag

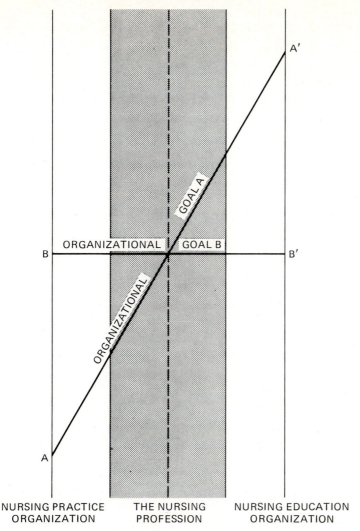

Figure 57-1 Organizational goals of nurse practice and nurse education organizations and overlap into the nursing profession.

phenomena. After interviewing 800 nursing administrators, Huckabay estimated that for some comparable areas of professional concern, nursing practice organizations were 15 to 20 years *behind* nursing education organizations.

These gaps of goal congruence and goal agreement will continue to be the central issues of *lrsp* throughout the 1980s. Administrators may find that the difference between effective and ineffec-

tive organizations of nursing may well depend upon the initiative they exercise in long-range planning.

ORGANIZATIONAL LEARNING

Another concept of importance in this matter is organizational learning. Learning is built upon a rational calculation of present and past experiences.

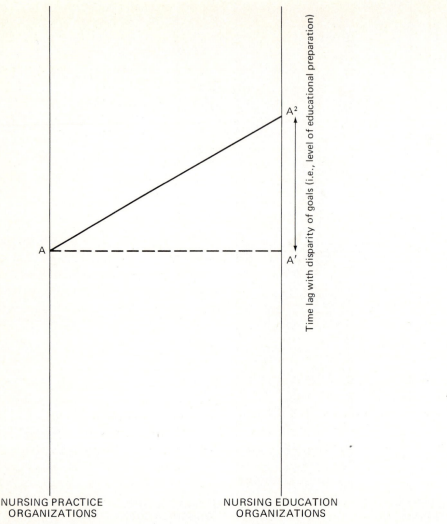

Figure 57-2 Time lag associated with disparity of nursing practice and education organizational goals (Example: Level of educational preparation for administrators).

In decision making, rational calculation includes choosing the best alternative and predicting consequences. Feedback from prior learning is the primary basis for making choices from among present alternatives. However March and Olsen (1976b:54-68) point out that, while organizations intend to be rational, they often act upon incomplete information and are not always aware of the alternatives. The authors state that "in learning from experience, organizations adapt their behavior

in terms of their experience and that the experience requires interpretation." March and Olsen also contend that organizational goals are usually ambiguous and unclear.

Kamen (1977) has referred to organizational learning as merely an example of organizational myth and illusion. But the concept of organizational learning has generally been viewed as one which produces wisdom and improved behavior. March and Olsen (1976b:659-60) have contended that organizational learning is intentionally rational. This notion includes several broad categories of ideas: organizational information and memory, learning incentive, and belief structures. More elaboratively, organizations are known to have communication structures through which information is transmitted and memory is stored. Certain incentives are known to be more desirable than others; therefore, organizations may select one interpretation for learning over another. This part of selection and interpretation is often dependent upon preexisting belief structures and related values. An example of such organizational learning occurred when the nursing profession stored in memory extensive information from the 1965 ANA proposal which depicted two levels of nursing practice. It was believed that this policy statement was the best alternative for the future. And the values and beliefs regarding professional nurse stratification codified in the 1915 proposal have been the foundation for many subsequent policy actions and concerns.

Argyris (1980:1-18) also has an interesting concept of organizational and individual learning—primarily as it occurs in professional schools. He defines learning as a circular process of discovery (of a problem), invention (of a solution), production (of a solution), and evaluation (of the production), a process which detects error or corrects it. He postulates that organizations learn through individuals (participants) acting as agents of the organization. Argyris categorizes two types of such learning. Single-loop learning is the detection and correction of error that does not alter underlying values or policies of the organization, while double-loop learning is the detection and correction of error that involves the changing of underlying values and policies. Single-loop learning focuses on routine acts, while double-loop learning is that from which routine acts are derived (Argyris, 1980:3).

The nursing profession should be currently engaged in the process of double-loop learning. The basic values and beliefs of nursing and of women in nursing need to be exposed and cited as significant issues for debate and analysis, issues in search of solutions. As noted by Argyris (1980:4), by limiting decision making to single-loop learning (routines), research on current managerial technology has acted to blind participants to the state of affairs which have resulted in the status quo. Although current professionals (e.g., those in nursing, medicine, and social work) are taught disciplined inquiry at the discovery or intervention level, few strategies have been taught which help aspiring administrators of nursing organizations to transfer double-loop learning into constructive action, primarily because contradictions and conflict would begin to surface. As in most professional organizations, intergroup conflict, contradictions, and problems exist and are handled through quasi resolution and a highly structured and limited search for solutions. Argyris predicts that these contradictions are, in fact, created to reinforce quasi resolution and limited search. This strategy usually results in a critical issue for valuing the undiscussable, and it is difficult to correct, let alone discuss, undiscussable issues (Cyert and March, 1963).

It is Argyris's belief that "neither the double-loop problems (values, policies) within or among organizations will be corrected unless the professionals are educated to detect and correct double-loop errors and create organizational learning systems that encourage such learning" (1980:17). Such is the task of nursing organizations today. They must get on with the process of initiating double-loop organizational learning environments. Nursing must initiate and articulate some of the undiscussable issues—i.e., new views of women in society, women as powerful entities, and women as a predominant force in the health care system in the United States—in order that the double-loop learning and changes in values can occur.

REQUIREMENTS FOR *lrsp*

Changing toward *frsl* in nursing requires that prominent nursing administrators and leaders of nursing organizations learn how to:

1 live with uncertainty;

2 embrace error;

3 accept the ethical responsibilities of goal-setting;

4 evaluate the present in relation to the future and commit actions now to respond long-range;

5 live with role ambiguity; and

6 be open to change based upon evaluation of ongoing activities and goals (Michael, 1976:18).

In acknowledging these six requirements for future-responsive social learning, nurses will also need to acquire new ways of viewing themselves, their environment (society), and the organizations that serve them. Approached from an *lrsp* strategy of learning rather than through social engineering, the task is accomplishable. Yet there are many obstructions to *lrsp*. These include limited funds, time constraints, contradictory and constricting laws, and physician control (Ginzberg, 1981). However, there is a strong core of nursing leaders who are choosing to direct their energies to *lrsp* and who are cautioning the rest of the profession not to resist some of the innovations and novel thinking, but to relax and "encourage organizational play by permitting (and insisting on) some temporary relief from control" (March, 1976:81).

GOAL SETTING FOR NURSING ORGANIZATIONS

Baker (1981) states that collaboration is absolutely necessary between the worlds of nursing education and nursing practice. There must be some agreed-upon and mutual basis for the selection of future direction, commitment of effort, and allocation of resources. The previous collaborative work of the American Nurses Association on credentialing and the development of a new organization, the Credentialing Center, was truly both novel and futuristic. But inherent in this meaningful and future-oriented activity is a force which threatens some individuals and some nursing groups. This threat has resulted in tremendous resistance to moving toward *frsl*. Yet, the profession of nursing cannot hope to evaluate whether it is approaching a desired future condition without having first collaboratively specified how that condition will be

recognized. Goals must be long-range and will require means and ends and reevaluation as movement is made toward the future. As previously stated, long-range goals may also be viewed as a future myth, a myth to which hopes and commitment can be attached (Michael, 1976:148). The goals contained and cited in the Credentialing Center concept provide a symbol for creating a different future and stand as an injunction to try. As a mode of societal learning, the concept provides an image of the future by providing guidance to the present.

MOVEMENT TOWARD *frsl*

Movement toward *frsl* has been derived from

> [a] philosophy of lrsp, with operational consequences, for going about learning how to act in the present, in light of continuously revised anticipations about the future. It is a philosophy of responsible, strategic decision-making in a complex and changing society; it is inherently open and tentative but strongly committed to acting in terms of chosen futures . . . [and] for thinking and acting in ways compatible with frsl. (Michael, 1976:57)

In order to accomplish the kind of organizational movement which is necessary for *lrsp*, *lrsp* must be treated as an *frsl* procedure with the following limitations:

1 Social technologies for these activities of learning are underdeveloped.

2 Requirements for *lrsp* must be introduced in ways that will not result in rejection.

3 New strategies will need to be developed to incorporate members of the environment into the process.

4 Which things in a turbulent world *can* be guided and regulated and which are *desirable* to regulate must be distinguished (Michael, 1976: 282–283).

Six strategies have been proposed for movement to facilitate *lrsp* toward *frsl;* these strategies are suitable for both nursing practice and nursing education organizations and their respective interface with the environment of professional nursing. (See Fig. 57-1).

Live with Uncertainty

There are several types or methods of organizational responses that can be viewed as "uncertainty reducers." The first response is that of organizational survival and of protection of the "technical core." In its conventional forms, this type of response is probably too protective because it sets organizational well-being ahead of environmental, or societal, well-being and is thus inadequate for societal learning through *lrsp*. The proper balance of protection and uncertainty is unclear; however, protection of the technical core (in this instance, the associate-degree nurse and the diploma nurse) will not suffice if the protection is at the expense of uncertainty and means denying the uncertainty that is required for growth in *lrsp*. Although the point of balance continues to remain an unknown factor, we should not shy away from the risk.

Secondly, there should be "greater use of professionals to discover, define, and to solve problems that otherwise would contribute to uncertainty" (Michael, 1976:122). Related to this, Argyris and Schon (1978) have completed research which demonstrates that professionals have "theories-of-action" in their heads about how to design and implement intended consequences; however, under observation they do not seem to behave according to the theories they describe. Their reported theories of action have been labeled "espoused theories." Their observed behavior has been referred to as "theory-in-use" phenomena. This performance discrepancy in professional practice has caused serious concern. Under these conditions, uncertainty and the discovery of novel solutions to problems will be greatly reduced and organizational double-loop learning will not likely occur. Because of these discrepancies or errors in the system it becomes the inevitable responsibility of nursing education organizations to reduce uncer-

tainty by the creative and realistic teaching of professionals to utilize double-loop learning.

The third constructive way of dealing with uncertainty relies simply on openly acknowledging and sharing the state of uncertainty. This acknowledgment reduces one's tendency to hide from oneself and challenges one to risk the threat of appearing incompetent during the learning process. Many nursing leaders still believe that competent administrators should always know what they are doing, so they go about *acting* as though they do.

Goal setting is also seen as a form of uncertainty reduction. When participants in nursing organizations and the profession can succeed in stating and agreeing on goals, the process of *frsl* becomes an open system of reduced ambiguity.

And lastly, feedback can be used to reduce uncertainty by clarifying organizational goals and specifying how the goals will be handled. Sometimes, however, feedback can produce anxiety and overload so that sorting and screening become necessary. Again, a balance of uncertainty is generally sought rather than eliminated.

Embrace Error

"Changing toward *lrsp* requires that instead of avoiding exposure to and acknowledgment of error, it is necessary to expect it, to seek out its manifestations, and to use information derived from failure (and success) as the basis for learning" (Michael, 1976:131). Therefore, nursing should experiment with alternatives in nursing practice in order to be able to establish clear and meaningful goals. With error embracing as a norm, it is possible to revise goals and evaluate programs without fear of being caught up in error. The concept of embracing error requires that nursing increase its capacities for trust and interpersonal support.

Accept the Ethical Responsibilities for Goal Setting

In addition to facing open conflict in others, participants in nursing organizations must be ready to handle value conflicts and ideological differences among themselves. Sabotage and resistance to serious goal setting may occur. Tactics which support such resistance will be seen in activities where goals are set in global or ambiguous terms; where there is myth generation with the top executive echelon only; where a scenario for the future is established which is very similar to the present scenario because too short a time frame has been allowed; where there is rejection of long-range future studies on the basis of little credibility; where there is avoidance of relevant feedback; where evaluations are based on a comparison of the present with the past; where feeling and values are excluded; and where there is support for disjointed incrementalism (Michael, 1976:152–156). Nursing organizations have scarcely begun to tap the surface of this organizational activity and to develop future goal-setting programs. Although a few studies have been reported (Lum, 1979), the literature is scant.

Live with Role Ambiguity

Those involved in *lrsp* will need to be prepared for anticipated stress, role conflict and ambiguity, and challenges to the legitimacy of who one is and what one is doing. This will be especially true in independent nursing practice and with new practitioner role definitions. One may also expect participant roles within the various nursing organizations to vary considerably. Value conflicts and philosophical differences will be observed in research and writing, nursing curricula, job specifications, definitions of role competence (within and without the nursing organizations), and designation of responsibility to multiple agencies through joint practice.

Boundary Spanning

Boundary spanning is that activity that occurs across boundaries within organizations and across boundaries between organizations. Boundary spanning is seen in joint nursing practice and collabora-

tion. Boundary spanners must be highly skilled because they tend to serve as information carriers and information-generating informants between systems. Therefore, spanners are vulnerable to error and subject to ambivalence. They function ambiguously and their communication may be distorted or rejected. "Boundary spanners perforate subsystem boundaries and threaten their autonomy, their secrets, their security, and their unexamined raison d'etre" (Michael, 1976:244). However, the boundary-spanner position is crucial to changing over to *lrsp*, and these individuals, in joint practice, serve as essential advocates who can influence peers and superiors throughout *lrsp* systems (Bacharach and Lawlor, 1980:90).

Organizational Restructuring

Changes in relationships between parts of the organization and between the organization and its environment may be required in order to succeed in *lrsp*. Some examples of these changes include the creation of task-oriented groups and of personal-need-fulfilling groups (support groups) and the integration of varous divisions and departments.

Nursing will also experience an increase in competition, collaboration, and redistribution of power (Baker, 1981). Nursing organizations will frequently undergo organizational and structural changes in order to respond to environmental needs—e.g., changes in management with primary care nursing, nursing pools, independent clinics, and joint practice. Other forms of organizational interaction with the environment will include various forms of cooperation, specifically, bargaining, co-optation, and coalition formation. Each of these strategies will influence the selection and choice of organizational goals (Thompson and McEwen, 1961).

SUMMARY

Through the skills of *lrsp* and *frsl*, Michael has proposed that new definitions of organizations (here, nursing) be developed for future successful existence. Linkages and resources will need to be acknowledged and maximized, so that *frsl* movement can be made

> . . . away from exploitation of self and others; away from compulsive needs to control and manipulate; away from the canons of logic and science as the only expressions of reason; away from valuing scientific rationality over feelings and intentions. . . . For individuals and organizations, the direction points toward openness, a much broader range of cognitive and affective experience and intercourse, and the shared development by responsible social evolution. (Michael, 1976:288)

Essentially, the movement toward *lrsp* and *frsl*

has been based upon two organizational choices. Nursing organizations can adapt continuously to the environment at the expense of internal consistency, or nursing can maintain internal consistency at the expense of environmental conflicts. In other words, the choice is between evolution and revolution. Most effective organizations of nursing will choose revolution. They will wisely opt for internal consistency and put up with brief periods of environmental disruption (Mintzberg, 1981:115). Through this self-transformation, different goals and directives can be envisioned for the nursing profession and nursing organizations of education and practice in the 1980s.

EDITOR'S QUESTIONS FOR DISCUSSION

What applications can be made from Ezell's discussion of *lrsp* and *frsl* to MacPhail's chapter (46) concerning collaboration/unification models? Discuss how can organizational conflicts and disparities in nursing through the process utilized to determine social responsiveness and future organizational changes as described by Ezell be resolved? Address each of the five questions raised by Ezell. What criteria might be suggested for deciding the goals to be modified? Which goals of nursing education and nursing practice should be modified? What suggestions can you offer for the process and acceptance of modifying goals of the profession?

Discuss the factors Ezell presents as contributors to disparity within the profession. What might be the perspectives of Williamson (Chap. 5), Sills (Chap. 42), Fralic (Chap. 48), and MacPhail (Chap. 46) regarding Ezell's discussion of the preparation of clinical specialists, shortage of prepared nurse administrators, and increasing gap between nursing practice and education organizations? How are nurse-educators preparing practitioners for the future rather than for current practice settings? What are the implications of Ezell's discussion concerning preparation for the future? Provide other examples of goal disparity and error in nursing.

What are the characteristics of the futurist? Provide examples of futurists in nursing. How have futurists in nursing utilized *lrsp* to move toward *frsl*? Define in your own terms *lrsp* and *frsl*. What are the essential characteristics of each? Provide examples in the administration of nursing education and provision for the delivery of nursing care where *lrsp* and *frsl* has been or could be utilized. What applications of these two processes may be made in the chapters by Conway (2), Peterson (7), Grace (12), O'Connor (13), Fawcett (14), Disbrow (18), Hardy (24), Newman (28), Roy (34), Bille (36), MacElveen-Hoehn (39), Corless (40), Klein (43), Cleland (44), Hegyvary (40), Malkemes (50), Stevens (52), Chaska (53), Froebe (54), Murphy (55), and Fagin and McGivern (56)?

What additional strategies can be suggested to reduce organizational uncertainty?

What strategies can be suggested to reduce time lags in goal congruence? Provide examples of organizational learning in nursing practice and education being intentionally rational. Suggest means for achieving double-loop learning in the profession of nursing. What are the implications of utilizing single-loop learning in the development of a scientific knowledge base for nursing? What are the relationships between double-loop learning and the construction of integrated conceptual models as discussed by Chaska (Chap. 53)? What implications does double-loop learning have for the development of such models?

Suggest strategies for negotiating and achieving mutual goals. How must the four limitations indicated by Ezell be accounted for in treating *lrsp* as a *frsl* procedure? In moving toward *frsl,* provide examples in nursing administration, nursing education, and nursing practice for each of the six strategies proposed by Ezell. Who are the "technical core" of an organization? How can a balance be achieved between protection of the technical core and uncertainty that is required for growth in *lrsp*? What are the consequences of discrepancies between espoused theories for behavior and observed behavior performance of professionals? What factors contribute to such discrepancies? How does Fagin's and McGivern's chapter (56) suggest a means for prevention and/or resolution of such difficulties for nurse administrators? What ethical implications are there for expecting, accepting error in nursing education and practice, and experimenting with alternative actions? What strategies can be suggested for effectively dealing with value conflicts and ideological differences in goal setting for nursing organizations of education and practice? Suggest additional strategies for facilitating *frsl* in an organization. Are there other organizational choices for adaptation than the two suggested by Ezell? Provide a rationale for the option you would choose.

REFERENCES

Argyris, C.
1980 "Educating administrators and professionals." Pp. 1–38 in C. Argyris and R. Cyert (eds.), Leadership in the 80's: Essays on Higher Education. Cambridge, Mass.: Institute for Educational Management, Harvard University.

Argyris, C. and D. Schon
1978 Organizational Learning. Reading, Mass.: Addision-Wesley.

Bacharach, S. and E. Lawlor
1980 Power and Politics in Organizations. San Francisco: Jossey-Bass.

Baker, C.
1981 "Moving toward interdependence: Strategies for collaboration." Journal of Nursing Administration 11:(4):34–39.

Cyert, R. and J. March
1963 A Behavioral Theory of the Firm. Englewood Cliffs, N.J.: Prentice-Hall.

Dunn, E.
1971 Economic and Social Development: A Process for Societal Learning. Baltimore: Johns Hopkins.

Ginzberg, E.
1981 "The economics of health care and the future of nursing." Nurse Educator 6(3): 29–32.

Huckabay, L.
1979 "Point of view: Nursing service and education: Is there a chasm?" Nursing Administration Quarterly 3,Spring:51–54.

Kamens, D.
1977 "Legitimating myths and educational organization: The relationship between organization ideology and formal structure." American Sociological Review 42, April:208–219.

Lum, J.
1979 "WICHE panel of expert consultants report: Implications for nursing leaders." Journal of Nursing Administration 9(7): 11–18.

March, J.
1976 "The technology of foolishness." Pp. 69–81 in J. March and J. Olsen (eds.), Ambi-

guity and Choice in Organizations. Bergen, Norway: University Press.

March J. and J. Olsen
1976a Ambiguity and Choice in Organizations. Bergen, Norway: University Press.
1976b "Organizational learning and the ambiguity of the past." Pp. 54–68 in J. March and J. Olsen (eds.), Ambiguity and Choice in Organizations. Bergen, Norway: University Press.

Michael, Donald
1976 On-Learning to Plan—and Planning to Learn. San Francisco: Jossey-Bass.

Mintzberg, H.
1981 "Organizational design: Fashion or fit." Harvard Business Review 59(1):103–116.

Sills, D.
1969 "The succession of goals." Pp. 175–187 in Amatai Etzioni (ed.), A Sociological Reader on Complex Organizations. New York: Holt.

Thompson, J. and W. McEwen
1961 "Organizational goals and the environment." Pp. 187–196 in Amatai Etzioni (ed.), A Sociological Reader on Complex Organizations. New York: Holt.

Chapter 58

Faculty Unionism:
Issues and Impact

Constance M. Baker, R.N., Ed. D.
Dean and Professor
College of Nursing
University of South Carolina
Columbia, South Carolina

As seen by Ezell, planning by nurse administrators is critical to the future of the nursing profession. There can be little doubt that the role of the nurse administrator in academia and in professional nursing care institutions has become increasingly complex. This section in the volume would not be complete without discussion of an issue that is gaining significant visibility—that is, collective bargaining. Although faculty unionism is a more recent phenomenon in academia than for nursing staff in health care facilities, there is every indication that it will increase in both settings. Professional nursing staff and faculty have similar major concerns that have led to collective bargaining. In addressing collective bargaining, Constance M. Baker focuses on faculty unionism in higher education. The term and process of collective bargaining is defined and described. She aptly and succinctly portrays the relevant issues, namely, governance, conditions of employment, and quality of education. Baker examines the impact of unionism on each of these major issues and proposes considerations for nurse educators in academia. Her chapter is based on two sources of data: personal experience in representing management on a bargaining team to negotiate the first union contract between administration and faculty in a four-year state college, and extensive review of the literature.

Collective bargaining is defined by the 1947 Labor Management Relations Act (Taft-Hartley Act). It involves negotiation between an employer and an organization representing a bargaining unit of employees concerning employment terms and conditions (an exclusive agent to represent employee interests), a written agreement, both conducted within a legal framework. In general, the process is subject to federal law, the National Labor Relations Act (NLRA), which is interpreted and administered by the National Labor Relations Board (NLRB), and federal courts. The NLRA covers *private* nonprofit institutions of higher education. Public colleges and universities are subject to state laws as interpreted and administered by state labor boards and courts. Baker identifies similarities and differences between the private and public sectors as to the bargaining process and legislation. She further delineates six assumptions in collective bargaining.

In higher education the first contract with a four-year institution was signed at City University of New York in 1969. Three national organizations have been the primary bargaining agents in higher education: American Association of University Professors (AAUP), American Federation of Teachers (AFT), and the National Education Association (NEA). The AAUP is the bargaining agent in over one-third of the four-year institutions.

According to the AAUP, academic decision making requires both the full-time efforts of administration and part-time efforts of faculty. Academic governance presumes a collegial model with shared authority demonstrated in the academic senate or council. Research findings indicate that most senates are ineffective in matters of substance. Findings of a study of 88 colleges of nursing offering baccalaureate and higher degrees indicate a low incidence of faculty and middle managers' expectations to participate in departmental decisions. A minimal understanding of the shared governance concept is also reflected. Baker asserts that faculty members are generally apathetic regarding governance. The Yeshiva decision rules that faculty and managerial employees are not entitled to bargain. This forces faculty to prove that even if they advise administration on educational and personnel policy, they do not have the power to implement their recommendations. Faculty collective bargaining would necessitate changes in an institution's governance system. Collective bargaining is essentially incompatible with the shared authority model of governance. A distinction would need to be made by unions and senates, between governance and economic issues, to coexist on a campus.

Personnel policies are reflected in diverse ways in higher education. Conditions of employment usually include criteria for appointment, promotion, tenure, nonreappointment, and termination. Personnel manuals often include statements on academic freedom, due process, faculty responsibilities, teaching load, and description of fringe benefits. Merit increases, peer review, and professional travel may also be mentioned. Job security is the major issue on unionized campuses, with higher salaries and fringe benefits of less importance. Unions have pressed for "due process" in decisions of nonreappointment and written, objective tenure procedures. Unions try to eliminate salary differentials within ranks, except those related to seniority. Given the declining economic state of academia, collective bargaining may be stimulated.

In discussing the issue of quality of education, Baker focuses on accountability and demands to evaluate faculty performance and productivity and to measure quality. Unions are opposed to peer review and student evaluation of faculty. Some academicians believe that this stance poses a threat to professionalism and quality education. Quality education requires that promotion and tenure be based on merit, incompetence be identified and handled, and students be involved in personnel decisions. Baker presents a report that indicates that unionization tends to be concentrated in institutions of lower quality. Union contracts that have clauses believed to be related to quality education include specific factors concerning teaching assignments of faculty, course preparations, contact hours, class size, professional development, continuing education, and travel. Baker believes higher education is confronted with two serious threats to survival: declining enrollments and the taxpayer revolt. Responses to these threats are related to how the three major collective bargaining issues are handled. Collective bargaining requires a great amount of time, money, and energy diverted from the primary purpose of academia. Governance patterns have serious implications for long-range survival.

Baker indicates similarities between all academicians regarding the three major issues and explores how nurses in academia differ from their colleagues. Nursing faculties have not been thoroughly socialized to higher education nor to the concept of shared governance. Nursing as an academic discipline lacks a tradition of shared authority, since it progressed through aggressive efforts of authoritarian nurse administrators who expected faculty to implement their policies and procedures. Most professional nurses have not had the opportunity to participate in decision making by consensus. Baker refers to Cleland's professional model of collective bargaining as being useful in socializing nurses for professional accountability. Shared governance is the mechanism for reconciling the inherent role conflict as a professional and institutional employee. Baker recommends that the American Nurses Association consider the economic needs of nurse-educators and suggests that nurse-educators might negotiate for representation through their state nurses' association.

Baker cites some advantages in collective bargaining for nurse faculty. Essentially, socialization of nurse faculty to higher education may be expedited; expectations of the academic community, including educational qualifications for appointment to each rank and requirements for promotion and tenure are specified in the contract. She indicates problem areas that are unique to nurse faculty that would require equitable resolution. These include the measurement of a faculty member's teaching load, issues related to distance and conditions of clinical agencies, and graduate preparation of nurse faculty. Baker contends that a nurse-educator is essential on the bargaining team in contact negotiations.

Faculty collective bargaining has achieved significant visibility in higher education during the past decade. Over 20 percent of all faculty in community colleges and senior colleges and universities are unionized. This has provoked the observation that collective bargaining is one of the significant areas of growth in higher education. There is every expectation that faculty unionization will continue to increase as student enrollments decline and the economic problems in higher education become more severe.

This chapter describes the collective bargaining process; considers its impact on governance, employment conditions, and quality of education; and posits some relevant ideas for nurse educators in academe. This paper is based on two sources of data. First, as head of the nursing department in a 4-year state college the author had the opportunity to represent management on the bargaining team and negotiate the first union contract between administration and faculty. This 11-month experience provided an extensive education about the collective bargaining process and the attitudes of administrators and faculty towards unionization. Despite efforts to be neutral this personal experience influences the objectivity of the paper. Second, extensive literature exists on collective bargaining in higher education. While there are limitations in the comprehensiveness of the literature, the amount is remarkable considering the recency of collective bargaining in higher education.

DEFINING COLLECTIVE BARGAINING

Collective bargaining is a decision-making process performed according to specific rules. In the 1947 Labor Management Relations Act (Taft-Hartley Act) collective bargaining is defined as:

> . . . the performance of the mutual obligation of the employers and representatives of employees to meet at reasonable times and confer in good faith with respect to wages, hours and other terms and conditions of employment . . . and the execution of a written contract incor-

porating any agreement reached . . . (Bureau of National Affairs 1953)

Thus collective bargaining involves negotiation between an employer and an organization representing a bargaining unit of employees regarding employment terms and conditions, followed by the development of a written agreement which usually includes an arrangement for settling disputes. The entire collective bargaining process is conducted within a legal framework.

At private colleges and universities the process is almost exclusively subject to federal law, the National Labor Relations Act (NLRA) as interpreted and administered by the National Labor Relations Board (NLRB), and the federal courts. The NLRA covers private nonprofit institutions of higher education having a gross annual revenue from all sources of not less than $1 million. Public institutions of higher education are not presently covered by the NLRA because they are excluded from the definition of *employer*. At public colleges and universities the process is subject to state laws as interpreted and administered by state labor boards and state courts. However, federal labor legislation does influence and guide state public employee bargaining legislation because there are many significant parallels and problems between the private and public sectors. Similarities include dealing with a request for recognition of a union, determining the bargaining unit, holding representation elections, defining the scope of bargaining, preparing for bargaining, negotiating the agreement, administering the agreement, and decertifying the union. Differences between the public and private sectors occur primarily because of differences in statutory framework and in decisions of the state public employment relations boards and the NLRB.

Collective bargaining is based on several assumptions (1) there are basic conflicts between the employer and the employees;(2) employees accept an organization as their exclusive representative; (3) sanctions (strikes) are used by employees to support their positions in disputes during the negotiations; (4) legal authorities beyond the institution enforce the agreements; (5) individual grievances are handled by prearranged procedures; and (6) the contract becomes a major force in managing the institution (Baldridge and Kemerer, 1977:269).

In Higher Education

Faculty unionism began in 1966 at Henry Ford Community College in Michigan, and in 1969 the first contract with a 4-year institution was signed at the City University of New York. Collective bargaining now occurs at 393 institutions on 650 campuses throughout the country, with nearly 170,000 faculty members unionized. Public institutions account for 80 percent of the signed contracts, one-fifth of which are at 4-year colleges and universities. Of the unionized private institutions, nearly 80 percent are 4-year colleges or universities (Garfin, 1980:iv).

Collective bargaining requires an exclusive agent to represent employee interests. Although some employees may become their own bargaining agent, usually they seek an experienced outside representative. In higher education three national organizations have been the primary bargaining agents: American Association of University Professors (AAUP), American Federation of Teachers (AFT), and the National Education Association (NEA). With its long history and prestige in higher education, it is not surprising that the AAUP is the bargaining agent in well over one-third of the 4-year institutions, while the NEA, with its very long history in public education, is the bargaining agent in nearly 60 percent of the 2-year institutions. The AFT represents nearly 30 percent of both 4- and 2-year institutions (Garfin, 1980).

While the doctrine of *exclusivity* fosters competition among the three national organizations, there is increasing evidence of collaboration. For example, agreements have been negotiated jointly by the local chapters of AAUP and the NEA at Kent State University, the University of Hawaii, and the University of Northern Iowa. Leaders of the three organizations have expressed some interest in a merger and currently are devising common litigation and legislative strategies (Bonham, 1977:32). Thus in 12 years faculty unionism has become a major force in higher education. In that short period three issues have recurred: governance, conditions of employment, and quality of education.

CONSIDERING THE ISSUES

Academic Governance

Traditionally operation of the academic enterprise has been based on the *shared authority* model. The 1966 AAUP "Statement on Government of Colleges and Universities" indicates that academic decision making in the university requires *both* the full-time efforts of the administration and the part-time efforts of the faculty. It is presumed that the variety and complexity of the tasks performed in academic institutions requires the professional expertise of both groups; thus an inescapable interdependence prevails. This collegial model is based on the beliefs that there is a consensus within academe regarding the purposes and goals of higher education and the role of faculty, that faculty has the necessary knowledge and therefore should be the key participant in governance; and that administrators and faculty have common interests which go beyond their role differences within the institution (Kemerer and Baldridge, 1975:14). Shared authority is demonstrated in the academic senate or council where faculty and administrators meet to decide on matters of mutual concern.

Despite the predominant commitment to shared authority and the academic senate, researchers of a national study of academic governance concluded that the importance of the senate has been overstressed because at most institutions senates do not deal effectively with matters of real substance. "The critical issues are generally handled by the faculty at the departmental level (curriculum, student relations, faculty hiring, firing, and promo-

tion) or by the administration at higher levels (budgets, overall staffing, physical plant, and long-range planning)" (Kemerer and Baldridge, 1977:139-40). While critical issues may be handled at the departmental level in some disciplines, one of the conclusions of a study of 88 large colleges of nursing offering baccalaureate and higher degrees was that the low incidence of faculty expectations to participate in departmental decisions, coupled with the low incidence of middle managers' expectations to involve them, reflect a minimal understanding of the concept of shared governance (Baker, 1981).

A crucial dilemma in relation to shared authority is created by the U.S. Supreme Court's 1980 decision in the case of *National Labor Relations Board v. Yeshiva University*. A divided court ruled that faculty are managerial employees and therefore not entitled to bargain under the federal labor law. Assuming that the faculty is the university, the court majority gave conclusive weight to the influence of the faculty upon personnel and educational policy and was not persuaded by the board's argument that faculty decisions are not managerial but independent professional judgments. Thus at this writing, in those private institutions where faculty members play a major role in governance they are not protected by the NLRA.

Challenges to the shared authority model of academic governance began in the political turmoil of the sixties and became more severe with the economic pressures of the seventies. The realities of decision making in academe are more accurately reflected when the shared authority model is coupled with other models of governance: the bureaucratic and the political (Baldridge, 1971). The bureaucratic model is characterized by a formal hierarchy, authority relationships, specific lines of communication, and policies and rules to guide such routine decision making as admissions, registration, course scheduling, and graduation procedures. The political model focuses on the process of policy formulation and the dynamics and conflicts of special interest groups. Policy decisions commit the institution to future goals which have varying degrees of implications for the participants, who, in turn, exert pressure to influence decisions in their favor. The interaction of the three governance models—collegial, bureaucratic, and political—creates a complex decision-making process.

Impact of Unionism Faculty collective bargaining will result in substantial changes in an institution's governance system. Collective bargaining is incompatible with the shared authority model of governance because the underlying assumptions of each are in conflict. Colleagues become adversaries and their relationships are determined by a legally binding contract developed by an outside agency. Research indicates that where faculty senates have been weak, and this seems to be the case on most unionized campuses, the union may protect and enhance faculty rights and collegial governance (Kemerer and Baldridge, 1975).

Whether or not unions and senates can distinguish between governance and economic issues and coexist on the campus remains to be seen. Since faculties are generally apathetic regarding governance and expansionism is characteristic of unions, it seems likely that future contracts will include more governance clauses, thus reinforcing the fears of some that campus life will be ruled by an outside agency (Mason, 1974:21-22). Yet, faculty at Boston University chose collective bargaining to reestablish traditional faculty rights of participation in academic governance which the administration was ignoring (Ringer, 1980). The Yeshiva decision forces the faculty to prove that even if they advise the administration on educational and personal policy, they do not have the power to implement their recommendations. Thus, the impact of collective bargaining on academic governance will be greatly influenced on a case-by-case basis as the Yeshiva decision is challenged, interpreted, and applied.

Employment Conditions

Personnel policies in higher education are reflective of the diversity among the colleges and universities. Institutions with long traditions of faculty participation in governance usually have comprehensive employment conditions, while younger institutions tend toward more limited policies. Conditions of employment usually include criteria for appointment, promotion, and tenure and for nonreappointment and termination. The personnel manual often includes a statement on academic freedom and due process, faculty responsibilities, including teaching load, and a description of fringe benefits. Manuals from some of the more mature institutions may also include reference to merit increases, peer review, professional travel, and research and clerical assistance.

During the rapid expansion of higher education in the 1960s, employment conditions also expanded, but only to be revised in the 1970s. The economic problems of the past decade are reflected in such changing employment conditions in higher education as terminating programs and faculty layoffs, salary freezes, and discontinuing such fringe benefits as tuition reimbursement for faculty children. One analysis of trends in faculty salaries during the 1970s led to the prediction that lower-ranking academicians could become part of the working poor in the 1980s and higher-ranking faculty would join them by 2000 (Abbott, 1980).

Impact of Unionism Two of the three issues dominating negotiations between administrators and unionized faculty are job security and economic compensation. Since 1975 job security has been the major issue on unionized campuses (Garfin, 1980). The unions' response to the financial problems in higher education has been to clarify procedures for layoffs and attempt to prevent layoffs that have already been ordered. Higher salaries and fringe benefits have been less important than faculty retaining their positions.

Tenure is the academic version of job security. Although tenure was developed to protect faculty from reprisal in their intellectual freedom in teaching and research, it does serve to protect faculty from dismissal for all but gross violations of law and ethics. Unions have provided considerable job security for nontenured faculty by pressing for "due process" in decisions of nonreappointment. Elaborate procedures for tenure have been written into contracts and include specification of evaluation procedures, open personnel files, stating reasons for denial, and providing for appeals. In institutions where faculty have had little influence on personnel policies the union has served a positive function by negotiating reasonable and objective tenure practices.

The impact of unions on the size of faculty salaries is difficult to assess with assurance because legislatures generally vote percentage increases in response to a variety of political pressures. In a study comparing matched sets of unionized and nonunionized institutions, it was concluded that the salary differences are narrowing and are due more to social, geographical, and political reasons than to collective bargaining (Birnbaum, 1974). There is consensus that salary parity can be attributed to collective bargaining because unions try to eliminate salary differentials within ranks except those related to seniority. Given the current declining economic state of academe, the belief that unions negotiate higher salaries may stimulate collective bargaining.

Faculty are confronted with a classic issue of organized labor in mandatory union dues. Many faculty have equated the concept of agency shop with infringement on academic freedom and have refused to cooperate. Legally, faculty are bound by the contract and the union is bound to represent them. However unions are spending considerable monies negotiating and processing grievances and arbitrations and will probably take a much stronger stand in the future on the agency shop clause. Examples of legal challenge by faculty to mandatory union dues can be found in Michigan, Hawaii, Minnesota, and New Jersey.

Quality of Education

Criticism of the quality of higher education intensified in the 1960s and gave rise to accountability demands from students, administrators, and governing boards. Faculty were accused of being unresponsive to students, abusing the privileges associated with academic freedom and tenure, and engaging in excessive outside employment. During budget hearings legislators began asking more questions about faculty workload and utilization of facilities. Educators responded to accountability demands by launching several projects to evaluate faculty performance, to measure "quality," and to assess faculty "productivity." Professional organizations representing specific disciplines, e.g., the American Sociological Association, developed mechanisms for the improvement of teaching its unique content. Colleges and universities began offering more opportunities for faculty development, and numerous curricula have been revised. Generally there have been substantial attempts to reform higher education during the 1970s.

Impact of Unionism It is extremely difficult to assess directly the impact of collective bargaining on the quality of education because there are few empirical data on the subject. The methodological problems of measuring quality are legion. Several authors have indirectly related the two variables by assuming certain relationships. For example, Begin "assumes there is a connection between the state of relationships among organizational members and the quality of education," examines the impact of adversarial relationships, and concludes that collective bargaining produces a mixed range of relationships, some of which may be beneficial to the education process (1979:91–92).

Egalitarianism is one of the guiding principles of collective bargaining. The Stanford research team expresses the fear that

> . . . unions will reduce the quality of the profession by substituting egalitarianism for meritocracy in personnel decision making . . . this possibility is the most serious negative aspect of faculty unionization . . . (because) . . . it stands in sharp contrast to many established and important academic traditions of quality. (Kemerer and Baldridge, 1975:12)

While faculty have obtained due process and job security in their union contracts, some academicians are lamenting the loss of peer review and the threat to academic professionalism. Evaluation by peers is not acceptable to the union because it is too subjective, yet peers are in the best position to judge quality academic work. Unions are also opposed to student evaluation of faculty, yet students are the recipients of the faculty's work. If job security can be obtained only by compromising evaluation procedures, then unions pose a serious threat to quality education. Quality education requires that promotion and tenure be based on merit, not seniority, that incompetence be identified and handled, and that consumers (students) be involved in personnel decisions.

In mid-1974 despite the small number of organized institutions and the difficulties in measurement, Garbarino attempted to analyze the relation between the quality of the institution and unionization. He reported that while "the pattern of unionization by quality category is not overwhelming, there appears to be a clear-cut tendency for unionization to be concentrated in the institutions that are in the lower tiers of the quality distribution" (1975:75).

Unions have negotiated several contract clauses believed to be related to quality education. Faculty must be assigned to teach in areas of their preparation. The number of different course preparations each year and the number of contact hours per week are specified in contracts. Class size continues to be a controversial item, although some states have made it a mandatory subject for bargaining. Professional development, continuing education, and travel are often included in negotiations. The relationship of these factors to the quality of education is yet to be established.

During the 1960s faculty unions in Great Britain introduced the idea of merit awards by tying salary increases to major improvements in teacher performance, either by accepting a more "exacting teaching load" or by raising the quality of teaching (Garbarino, 1975:226). It has been suggested that this experience may have relevance for faculty in the United States. The Stanford research team challenges administrators to demand higher standards of educational services in exchange for union demands of higher salaries, pointing out that in this way unionism can be tailored to improve the educational process and increase accountability (Kemerer and Baldridge, 1975:226).

Higher education is confronting two serious threats to survival: declining enrollments and the taxpayer revolt. Responses to these threats are intimately entwined with the manner in which the three collective bargaining issues are handled. Governance patterns have serious implications for long-range survival. Cooperation between administrators and faculty is imperative, especially in relation to dealing with the broader issues confronting higher education and setting priorities for the future. Collective bargaining has created such a proliferation of bureaucratic procedures that considerable amounts of time and money are diverted from the primary purposes of the institution. If collective bargaining is perceived by the public as totally self-serving, its acceptance will be difficult to achieve. The emphasis should be on improving the quality of higher education.

ORGANIZING NURSE EDUCATORS

Collective bargaining in nursing education has followed the pattern of the school of nursing's parent institution. It is estimated that faculty unionism exists at 10 percent of the baccalaureate and higher degree nursing programs and about 23 percent of the associate degree nursing programs (Garfin, 1980). Many of the issues confronting nurses in higher education are common to all academicians; defending academic quality, protecting academic freedom, and obtaining tenure. Despite these similarities nurses in academe differ from their colleagues in liberal arts and sciences and are confronted with unique issues in relation to governance, employment conditions, and quality of education.

Unlike other academic disciplines, nursing lacks a tradition of shared authority in governance.

Nursing's progress from an apprenticeship to academic discipline was made through the aggressive efforts of authoritarian nurse administrators. Nursing faculty were expected to implement the policies and procedures of the nurse administrator, and such expectations continue to prevail in many nursing schools today (Baker, 1981). Nursing faculty have not been thoroughly socialized to higher education and thus have a minimal understanding of the concept of shared governance in the collegium. Most nurses have not had the opportunity to participate in decision making by consensus and to constructively manage the conflict which often precedes that consensus (Baker, 1979). More often nurse faculty are threatened by conflicting opinions, are unable to take the institution's point of view, and respond in a maladaptive fashion (Barley and Redman, 1979). While collective bargaining is sometimes perceived in conflict with shared authority, Jacox says that if adequate safeguards are developed to protect these principles, "faculty in some schools of nursing may find their involvement in institutional decision making to be significantly increased, rather than decreased" (1973:703). In other words governance based on a written agreement reached through collective bargaining provides a context within which faculty and administrators are able to make decisions and to regularize policies and procedures that will henceforth govern their interaction.

A professional model of collective bargaining based on the principle of shared governance has been proposed for health care institutions (Cleland, 1978). Adopting the model from Baldridge's study of university governance, Cleland demonstrates its usefulness in educating and socializing nurses for professional accountability. Shared governance is the mechanism for reconciling the conflict between the role of the professional and the role of the institutional employee. Other professions, such as medicine and law, have tried to minimize these conflicts by selecting their professional association as their bargaining agent. The NLRB has recognized the dual professional status of selected faculty and has allowed faculty in professional schools to remain separate from other faculty members at their institutions, because their mission reflects a significantly different community of interest from the rest of academe. These professionals recognize that when they organize with others, they no longer speak as a united profession; in fact they are often in the minority and overruled.

Perhaps it is time for nurse-educators to negotiate for representation through the state nurses association. This notion takes on additional import when it is considered with the fact that the AFT and the NEA are using teacher dues to organize nurses in practice; thus inadvertently nurse-educators are contributing to undermining the ANA's economic security program. Before faculty unionism grows much larger, the ANA should consider the economic needs of nurse-educators, the threat to nursing's unity posed by teachers' unions, and a collective bargaining program to overcome professional fragmentation.

Comprehensive collective bargaining may expedite the socialization of nurse faculty to higher education because the expectations of the academic community are specified in the contract and all disciplines are treated equally. Contracts include educational qualifications for appointment to each rank and academic requirements for promotion and tenure. These standards should not be lowered for nursing faculty—rather efforts should be made to foster nurses' ability to meet them (Barley and Redman, 1979). Nurses must meet the educational qualifications for faculty appointment, work toward achieving all the institution's missions (teaching, research, and service), represent nursing on multidiscipline, collegewide committees, advise students on academic matters, and hold regular office hours.

Normally a faculty member's teaching load is measured by the number of student credit hours generated in a specified period of time, usually the academic year. Three factors compose the student credit hour formula: number of courses, number of credit hours, and number of students. Nursing faculties have low student credit hour production because in the clinical practice courses a low student-faculty ratio is prescribed by the accrediting agencies and in the classroom theory courses team teaching is frequently used. Thus this approach to measuring nursing faculty's teaching load lacks validity and requires interpretation in contract negotiations.

While defining *campuses* and *teaching site* may be routine for some disciplines, it is more complex for nursing and has relevance in negotiating conditions of employment. Consideration and equitable resolution must be found for such issues as distance of clinical agency from campus, travel time, mode of transportation, and requirements and conditions of the clinical agency. Interpretation of the uniqueness of nursing education requires that a nurse-educator participate on the bargaining team in contract negotiations.

During the past decade the quality of nursing education has been challenged by several forces. Kramer's research on "reality shock" revealed that students were not being appropriately socialized to the role of the nurse and the world of work (1974). In a time of fiscal austerity, nursing service administrators are confronted with very expensive orientation programs for inexperienced new graduates (Wagner, 1980). Similarly administrators in nursing education must attempt to overcome gaps in graduate preparation of nurse faculty. What is the relationship of these problems to the quality of nursing education? Whether or not collective bargaining has shown or will have an impact on the quality of nursing education are questions for study. With nearly one-fifth of all collegiate nursing programs unionized, questions related to quality could be examined.

SUMMARY

Collective bargaining is a new and controversial form of university governance which has occurred in response to changes in the external environment of higher education, to changes in the internal structure and functions of higher education, to changes in academic managerial styles, and to a failure of traditional forms of governance to solve current problems. Collective bargaining in nursing education is so recent that definitions, ground rules, and procedures are constantly developing. The heterogeneity of unionized institutions makes definitive conclusions very difficult. However, nurses in higher education need to be aware of what is transpiring so they can actively participate in future decision making in their own institutions. The advantages and disadvantages of unionism must be weighted against the goals and needs of the individual nurse-educator, the institution, and the profession of nursing.

EDITOR'S QUESTIONS FOR DISCUSSION

What factors have contributed to faculty collective bargaining in higher education? How different or similar are the collective bargaining issues between nurse faculty and professional nursing staff? Discuss the history of collective bargaining in nursing. What have been the major forces for and against unionization of nurses? What role conflicts have existed for nurses concerning collective bargaining? To what extent and how have these been resolved? What factors have contributed to a time lag in the organizing of professional nursing staff and faculty in higher education? What factors related to environment and geographic area have contributed to a time lag in the unionization of professional nursing staff and faculty? Discuss the advantages and disadvantages of collective bargaining for professional nurse-educators and nursing care staff. To what extent is quality of education and quality of nursing care the major issue in unionization by faculty and professional nursing staff versus economic security? What are the implications for professionalism of nursing in collective bargaining? How can the major issues related to collective bargaining be prevented in both professional education and practice settings? What alternative mechanisms have been developed in both settings in various geographic areas to deal effectively with the major issues? What is the role of the professional nurse administrator in prevention and/or participation in collective bargaining?

Provide examples of the six assumptions underlying collective bargaining in higher education and professional health care settings. What role have bargaining units played in the development of collective bargaining for nurses? Who initiates the request for recognition of a union? How is the bargaining unit and agent chosen to represent employees? Who are considered managerial employees, in professional nursing and health care institutions and in academia, and not entitled to bargain? What are the issues involved in the determination of managerial employees in both health care and academic settings? What issues are of concern for professional nurse administrators in being members of the American Nurses Association and collective bargaining? To what extent and how have these concerns or conflicts of interest been resolved? Provide suggestions as to resolution of the conflicts for nurse administrators in nursing and health care settings. Have similar conflicts presented themselves for nursing deans in academia? Should nurse-educators negotiate for representation through the state nurses association? How can conflict be resolved concerning the fact that the AFT and the NEA use teacher dues to organize nurses in practice?

Discuss the issues concerning academic governance. Provide examples of the three basic beliefs of the collegial model existing and not existing in academia. For the situations you indicate, examine how the collegial model could either be further promoted or initially developed. What factors contribute to ineffectiveness of institutional senates or councils? What suggestions can be recommended to prevent or counteract ineffectiveness of senates. What are the implications for the profession of nursing in the findings of Baker's study of 88 colleges of nursing? What challenges have been made to the shared authority model of academic governance? Discuss the impact of the Yeshiva decision in higher education. Discuss additional cases and results that have occurred since the Yeshiva decision. How has the Yeshiva decision been challenged, interpreted, and applied?

What factors are related to the amount of influence and power faculty have in the development and implementation of educational and personnel policy? Provide examples of faculty advising administration on policy but not having the power to implement recommendations. Given Baker's statement that faculty in general are apathetic regarding governance, how likely is that tendency to continue? How do faculties learn to recognize and effectively utilize their collective power in shared governance? What are the implications of the political model in shared governance? How are the underlying assumptions of shared authority and collective bargaining incompatible? To what extent do you agree or disagree with Jacox's statement regarding collective bargaining? Is there a relationship between academic freedom and shared governance. Suggest alternative models for shared governance. What additional mandates should faculty senates or councils fulfill in shared governance? What role should university faculty senates or councils have in the development of personnel policies for faculty? How has "due process" been carried out in academia and professional practice settings to this point in time? What changes have occurred in recent years? What factors or issues have contributed to those changes?

Suggest major performance areas for faculty appointment, promotion, and tenure (FAPT). For each performance area develop criteria progressively for each academic rank from the instructor level through to professor. Designate examples for each criterion as acceptable evidence for meeting the criteria. Should additional criteria be indicated for tenure? Should there be additional or different criteria utilized by FAPT committees for faculty members (nontenured or tenured) who hold an administrative position? How can the criteria for FAPT effectively be utilized for reappointment of nontenured faculty? What criteria should be indicated for nonreappointment of nontenured faculty or termination of tenured faculty? Refer to MacPhail's chapter (46) and recall the Editor's Questions for Discussion regarding tenure. Since reading Baker's chapter, address those questions again. How can the development of retrenchment policies and procedures, such as notification time required for lay-offs of nontenured and tenured faculty, be related to FAPT criteria?

Discuss the issue of academic freedom in relation to FAPT committee meetings. What are some of the current problems concerning FAPT meetings? Suggest means for preventing the difficulties concerning FAPT committee meetings and decisions. How might criteria for FAPT be related to areas and items included in the development of performance evaluation instruments for faculty? Should performance evaluation of professional staff and faculty be linked to merit increases in salary? Recall and address again the Editor's Questions for Discussion in Fagin's and McGivern's chapter (56) regarding performance evaluation.

Discuss the role and function of university faculty senates or councils in developing retrenchment policies and procedures, and grievance procedures. What is the process by which a university can judiciously and successfully complete those tasks? What process should be utilized in choosing representatives for faculty senates or councils. Suggest means for establishing equitable representation from schools or colleges in university or faculty senates or councils. What are the role, functions, and responsibilities of faculty councilor to the school they represent and to the senate or council on which they serve?

What should personnel manuals for faculty in academia include? How and by whom should they be developed? How are personnel policies monitored in a university? What should personnel manuals include in professional nursing care settings? Who should participate in the development of personnel manuals in nursing care settings? How can personnel policies effectively be monitored? In both settings—academia and professional nursing practice—whose responsibility is it for the development, implementation, monitoring, and updating of professional personnel manuals?

Suggest methodologies for addressing the issues in measuring quality of education. To what extent should students be involved in personnel decisions and evaluation of faculty performance? What factors may contribute to a relationship between unionization and the quality of an institution? How can unionism be tailored to improve the educational process and increase accountability? What alternative mechanisms can be suggested to accomplish the same goal without compromising academic professionalism?

Contrast professional nurses in academia with their colleagues from other academic disciplines. To what extent do you agree with Baker that nursing faculty have not been thoroughly socialized to higher education? Provide examples for your view. What factors may have inhibited the socialization process? Suggest strategies for expediting the socialization process of nursing faculty into higher education. To what extent are qualifications for faculty appointments, promotion, and tenure in schools and colleges of nursing higher, equal to, or lower than those of faculty from other disciplines? How different are nursing faculty in their concept of shared governance from their colleagues in other disciplines? What factors have contributed to minimal understanding of the concept in both nursing and other disciplines? How critical is the leadership style of nursing deans and executive nurse administrators in nursing care settings to the development and implementation; understanding of the concept; and participation in shared governance by faculty and professional nursing staff? Provide examples demonstrating a possible relationship between leadership style of the nurse administrator and shared governance. What applications of shared governance are evident or implied in the chapters by Williamson (5), Reeder (38), Cleland (44), Sills (48), Hegyvary (49), Malkemes (50), Mercadante (51), Murphy (55), and Fagin and McGivern (56)? What Editor's Questions for Discussion from Chaps. 55 and 56 pertaining to shared governance also can be applied to Baker's chapter? Provide examples demonstrating the usefulness of Cleland's model of collective bargaining based on the principle of shared governance in educating and socializing nurses for professional accountability.

Suggest valid means for measuring a faculty member's teaching load? How can the credit-hour formula approach be weighted with other factors as prescribed student-faculty ratio, team or collaborative project and thesis and/or dissertation advisement for an overall measurement of teaching load? With the additional professional mission of research and scholarly activity, how can these be included in measurement of faculty loads? How can service to the institution and professional community at large and professional development be considered in measuring overall responsibility and accountability of faculty? What factors and issues concerning the use of clinical agencies and location of campus sites should be considered in measuring accountability? How valid and reliable are current quarterly reports required by most universities for allocation of time and work loads of faculty? Suggest methods for improving the quality and utilization of such reports.

REFERENCES

Abbott, W. F.
1980 "Commentary: When will academicians enter the ranks of the working poor?" Academe 66:349–353.

Baker, C. M.
1979 "Role conflicts of middle managers in baccalaureate and higher degree nursing programs in the U.S." Pp. 147–159 in Power: Nursing's Challenge for Change. Kansas City: American Nurses' Association.
1981 "Departmental development and academic governance in colleges of nursing." Pp. 451–459 in J. C. McCloskey and H. K. Grace (eds.), Current Issues in Nursing. Boston: Blackwell Scientific.

Baldridge, J. V.
1971 "Power and Conflict in the University. New York: Wiley.

Baldridge, J. V., and F. R. Kemerer
1977 "Images of governance: Collective bargaining vs. traditional models." Pp. 252–271 in G. L. Riley and J. V. Baldridge (eds.), Governing Academic Organizations. Berkeley: McCutchan.

Barley, Z. A., and B. K. Redman
1979 "Faculty role development in university schools of nursing." Journal of Nursing Administration 9:43–47.

Begin, J.
1979 "Impact of faculty bargaining on the quality of education." Pp. 91–95 in J. A. Young (ed.), Proceedings of the National Conference on the Impact of Collective Bargaining on the Quality of Education Today. Amherst: University of Massachusetts Press.

Birnbaum, R.
1974 "Unionization and faculty compensation." Educational Record 55:29–34.

Bonham, G. W.
1977 "Three union leaders talk about the academic future." Change Magazine 9:30–36.

Bureau of National Affairs
  1953 Labor Policy and Practice. Washington: Bureau of National Affairs.
Cleland, V. S.
  1978 "Shared governance in a professional model of collective bargaining." Journal of Nursing Administration 8:39–43.
Garbarino, J. W.
  1975 Faculty Bargaining: Change and Conflict. New York: McGraw-Hill.
Garfin, M.
  1980 Directory of Faculty Contracts and Bargaining Agents in Institutions of Higher Education. New York: National Center for Study of Collective Bargaining in Higher Education.
Jacox, A.
  1973 "Collective bargaining in academe: Background and perspective." Nursing Outlook 21, 11:700–703.

Kemerer, F. R., and J. V. Baldridge
  1975 Unions on Campus. San Francisco: Jossey-Bass.
Kramer, M.
  1974 Reality Shock: Why Nurses Leave Nursing. St. Louis: Mosby.
Mason, H. L.
  1974 "Faculty unionism and university governance." Pp. 1–26 in J. H. Schuster (ed.), Encountering the Unionized University. San Francisco: Jossey-Bass.
Ringer, F.
  1980 "Academic governance and collective bargaining." Academe 66:41–44.
Wagner, D. L.
  1980 "Nursing administrators' assessment of nursing education." Nursing Outlook 28, 9:557–561.

Part Seven

The Future of
Nursing

A time for speaking

The future of nursing necessitates dialogue and planning. To be influential in affecting the future of nursing, the time is *now* to address the questions and reconcile the concerns that are relevant in and to the profession. Numerous suggestions have been made throughout the preceding chapters. Positive directions for the future of nursing are substantially evident. There are risks in speculating and making predictions regarding the future. However, nursing as a profession has demonstrated the ability to take risks in its endeavor to accomplish its mission sanctioned by society to provide a distinctive service in health care delivery. It is essential to anticipate the health and illness care needs of the future, in order for the profession to continue in growth and success in meeting obligations and efficiently plan for the future.

These sequential chapters propose considerable variation in perspective regarding the future of nursing. At the same time there are similar themes, such as the influence of technology and the economics of health care. Virtually every component of nursing is discussed. Thoughtfulness is clearly evident as projections for the future are made and risks are taken in proposing the future direction of nursing and health care delivery. Some persons may view the predictions with optimism or alarm. Others may perceive them as being pragmatic and foresighted. The diversity and dialogue shows that the profession indeed is alive, well, and prospering in contributing to the health care of society.

Chapter 59

Beyond the Horizon

Martha E. Rogers, Sc.D., F.A.A.N., R.N.
Professor, Division of Nursing
New York University
New York, New York

To speculate on a dream and believe in the impossible may well expedite as a reality the complete recognition of nursing as a science. It is heartening to have Martha E. Rogers set the tone and provide further incentive towards that goal and the future of nursing in this first chapter.

Martha E. Rogers shares her dream for nursing as she has watched it unfold. She assesses the escalation of change in science, technology, society, and nursing. Diverse obstacles, frictions, and turmoil towards achievement of that dream do not thwart Martha Rogers. She represents the epitome of optimism as she proposes a future for nursing. Rogers believes that to predict with any degree of certainty is to dare the impossible. However, vision promises the unexpected.

Rogers maintains that in spite of prophets of doom, jargon, and belief systems being threatened, the search for meaning goes on. Individuality marks the people of the new world. Synthesis and pattern seeing are the survival skills. Rogers asserts that transition requires new perspectives, thus for nursing a paradigm shift is explicit. To establish nursing as a science requires a phenomenon of concern unique to nursing. Rogers identifies the study of unitary man as unique to nursing. In essence, Rogers's theory contends that man is a unified whole having integrity and characteristics that are more than and different from the sum of his parts.

Rogers predicts that antieducationists will not survive. She identifies subterfuges that mislead the public to perceive a "nurse is a nurse is a nurse." These include grouping of all R.N.s, regardless of their initial preparation, as being qualified to practice at a baccalaureate level, certification procedures that ignore educational credentials, and nurse-practitioner courses which provide medical skills for nurses to function as physician assistants. Rogers believes the first undergraduate professional degree, regardless of the title, should prepare the student for beginning professional practice. Battle over entry levels to practice will disappear as substantive knowledge in nursing is recognized. Licensure exists to safeguard the public. Emphasis on certification may be confused with licensure and may result in overlooking the need for a knowledge base specific to nursing. Rogers insists nurses must cease using affectation in role terminology. She cites examples as: nurse practitioners are not practitioners of nursing; practitioners of nursing are not physicians' assistants; primary nursing is not primary medicine; the "expanded role" is a cover up for medicine's encroachment on nursing's practices established long ago; and the "unification model" is an euphemism for previous practices labeled as apprenticeship and joint appointments. Rogers states that the "practitioner-teacher" role is magnified and minimizes substantative knowledge in nursing. Nurses who have opted for medical skills as a way to save nursing and gain status will be interested in a report cited by Rogers.

The public is seeking alternatives in health services. A renewal of nursing leadership is essential. Rogers maintains that dependence on other fields denigrates professional autonomy. Although she believes referral systems will expand, she expects health measures derived from a science of unitary man to clash with practices directed toward treating parts of man or the sum of his parts. Rogers predicts nursing in the 21st century will have a new image; those who seek to perpetuate the past will not cross the horizon.

To peer into the future is to enlarge one's vision, to glimpse a becoming, to see with that "third eye." It is to speculate upon a dream and to watch that dream unfold. It is to create a new reality.

Man's advent into outer space made explicit this new world. Escalating science and technology help to underwrite new paradigms and to hasten the ending of the industrial age. Noise, confusion, and insecurities mount as the speed of change reaches a crescendo. Old values lie moribund among the detritus of famous last words. Man moves to transcend himself. A new scenario comes into view.

The information explosion looks embryonic as man's emerging capacities to communicate in hitherto undreamed-of ways come into focus. Seemingly instant transportation outdistances the speed of light. Illusory colors, shapes, sounds, smells, tastes diversify and proliferate in kaleidoscopic novelty. The impossible is possible.

Computers that can program themselves to produce a new race of "intelligent beings" superior to human life are serious subjects for workers in artificial intelligence. The United States Supreme Court has approved patent rights for new life forms. Civilian activities in outer space are not far off.

As the turmoil of change escalates, fanatic factions vie for supremacy. Violence is explosive. Prophets of doom clamor loudly. Iatrogenic and nosocomial ailments go hand in hand with hypochondriasis. Holistic jargon and multiplying medi-tative modalities give vague intimations of new vistas in the making. Ethical issues and human rights stir the bureaucratic ashes of mass mediocrity and portend a concern for the individual.

In this not so mythical mosaic nurses whisk through airless tunnels in very high speed transit tubecraft with Los Angeles only 21 minutes from New York City (Rosen, 1976). They travel to the moon in 13 seconds and to the nearest star in 43 years (Heppenheimer, 1977). They live and work and play in earth communities of multivariegated pattern and in space communities of incredible design. They are as diverse as the world they live in.

Individuality marks the people of the new world. Rhythmicities of extraordinary complexity weave pulsating patterns through threads of yesteryear and the "infinite now" expands. Alternatives in health care and health workers mushroom.

No utopia this. The search for meaning goes on. Beyond the horizon potentialities abound. J. B. S. Haldane's famous epigram comes to mind: "The universe is not queerer than we imagine, it is queerer than we can imagine."

Nursing changes coordinate with the larger world of man's perception. The confusion of nurses is the confusion of all people struggling to understand the contradictions, ambiguities, and uncertainties of a world caught up in a shifting panorama of infinite potentialities. Old securities have been shattered. Belief systems are threatened. Hierarchies are tumbling down. At the same time an optimistic view of man's future is beginning to permeate the current scene. Creative excitement is emerging out of the seeming chaos. New paradigms are taking hold.

To speculate upon the future can be an exciting game. To propose direction can be a dangerous one. To predict with any degree of certainty is to dare the impossible. The past presents no vistas of events to come. But people do have the capacity to participate in creation of this fabulous world of uncertainty. How little we know poses incredible hurdles. Errors in knowing magnify the problems. Nonetheless prediction gives direction to our gropings. Flexibility allows for fallibility. Vision promises the unexpected.

Let us peer beyond the horizon into a new world of nursing. A paradigm shift is explicit. People, long the center of nursing's purpose, appear as dynamic, irreducible wholes caught up in equally dynamic environmental wholes, together manifesting innovative patterns of growing complexity. And with Ferguson I would note that "synthesis and pattern-seeing are survival skills for the twenty-first century" (1980:300). An air of optimism is apparent.

The unfolding scene reveals a diversity of nursing personnel prepared for varying responsibilities of differing degrees of complexity in a multiplicity of settings on this planet and in outer space. All people fall within the scope of nursing. Principles and theories generated by nursing's new paradigm engage scholars and scientists in nursing as they seek to push back the frontiers of knowledge. Nursing educators incorporate the findings of nursing research into a rapidly growing body of substantive knowledge specific to nursing and transmit this knowledge to students seeking professional and technical careers in nursing. Practitioners of nursing translate this knowledge into novel and unexpected uses in their efforts to promote human health and welfare.

Nurses are not alone in this new world. A range of health workers participate in man's search for well-being. But the nature of health personnel and health services has changed dramatically. A new world view provides unity in diversity. Differences are held in high esteem. The public is oriented to health. People are active participants in the developmental process. Invasive therapies and drugs are rare. Health services issue from community centers as diverse as the life-styles of these variegated people. Facilities for sick services are notably diminished in number and are tangential to the primary purposes of a new design for health.

New perspectives reinterpret observable data. No longer is aging deemed a disease. Pregnancy is not a pathological event. Dying is a developmental process. Evolutionary emergence manifests individual differences that defy old norms. Innovation is viewed with enthusiasm. Problems are seen within a new context. Interventive modalities are directed toward promotion of health and well-being. Man and his world change together.

As nursing fulfills its social and professional responsibilities to people wherever they are, the dreams of tomorrow become today's reality. A clear, unambiguous commitment to nursing as a knowledgeable endeavor and a social necessity characterizes nursing personnel.

Education of nurses is firmly within the educational mainstream, but education itself manifests dramatic revisions. Man's past and future merge. Learning is broad, substantive, and exciting. Creativity is encouraged. Individual diversity and multiple career options abound. Theoretical knowledge specific to nursing provides a foundation on which to base practice. Career differences are valued and respected. A multiplicity of settings provides opportunity for testing theories. Imaginative concern for people is dominant.

Whatever the level of preparation or functional role or planetary or cosmic setting, a new sense of self and pride in nursing has taken hold. A new security embraces future uncertainties. The nature of nursing teems with innovations. Nursing is a major resource in its own right as people seek alternatives in health services.

These preliminary comments postulate a future for nursing as a basic science and public necessity. How realistic is this? Will there be nursing beyond the horizon? Multiple roads stretch into the future. Which ones lead to dead ends for nursing? What new alliances are in the making as fields encroach on one another's preserves in sometimes mighty territorial encounters? Will there be kaleidoscopic repatterning for new syntheses that can spell the disintegration of the traditional basic sciences and professional fields? What will people be like in this new world? These are heady questions.

In today's everyday world problems loom large, disagreements are common, and proposals for change are too often pedantic modifications of the past. Transition requires new perspectives. Practical realities demand imaginative resolution coordinate with accelerating change. Social responsibility is an indispensable adjunct in nursing's evolution. To realize nursing as an identifiable scientific field of endeavor dedicated to serving human kind requires creative action.

To establish nursing's identity as a science requires a phenomenon of concern unique to nursing, an organized conceptual system specific to the phenomenon, and unifying principles and hypothetical generalizations deriving from the system. The study of unitary man as an irreducible phenomenon is unique to nursing. It is not to be confused with the current ambiguities of holism, which is commonly associated with parts and sums of parts. A paradigm specific to nursing (and relevant to other fields concerned with man and environment) constitutes an organized abstract system. Principles and theories derive from the system. An aggregate of facts and theories drawn from various sciences do not provide a valid base for the practice of nursing. Neither do such aggregates contribute to knowledge of the unitary man. A firm belief in nursing as an organized body of abstract knowledge arrived at by scientific research and logical analysis is an essential prerequisite to nurses' ability to serve people knowledgeably.

Nursing as a science and an art rings the death knell for nursing's antieducationists. It is no longer tenable to proclaim "a nurse is a nurse is a nurse," whether this is done through misleading statistics that clump baccalaureate graduates indiscriminately with associate degree and hospital school graduates; or through the subterfuge that attends the New York State Nurses Association 1985 Resolution with its grandfather clause that would mislead the public into thinking that all R.N.s are qualified to practice at a baccalaureate level; or through certification procedures that ignore educational credentials; or through nurse-practitioner courses which provide medical skills for functioning as a physician's assistant to any R.N. in programs that range from 2 months to 2 years; or through other ways.

The uniqueness of nursing, like that of any other science, is found in the phenomenon of its concern. The practice of nursing derives from nursing's body of scientific knowledge specific to nursing. Justification for the education of nurses in institutions of higher learning, whether at the associate degree level or at the baccalaureate degree level, demands the transmission of substantive knowledge specific to nursing and appropriate to the student's level of study. Continued denial that education makes a difference leaves nursing vulnerable to proponents of trained subservience. Nor does the introduction of a professional doctorate in nursing change the issue or resolve the problem. The first undergraduate professional degree, whether it is labeled B.S. or M.N. or N.D., prepares for beginning professional practice. The confusion engendered by terminological differences only aggravates the situation. Antieducationists in nursing will not survive beyond the horizon.

Second, the battles over entry levels to practice will disappear as substantive knowledge in nursing is recognized. Nursing's educational system currently prepares persons for three different entry levels to practice. Licensure exists for the vocational (L.P.N.) and technical (R.N.) levels of preparation. Social responsibility demands that there be licensure for the professional (B.S.) level. Licensure exists to safeguard the public. It does not exist to serve the worker. Nor is certification to be confused with licensure. Moreover, as certification currently exists in nursing, there is little recognition of the need for a knowledge base specific to nursing or for the qualifications of those who certify (i.e., groups outside of nursing who claim to certify nurses to practice nursing). Proposals to place more control for certification with nurses continue to overlook a need for theoretical knowledge specific to nursing. Antieducationism in nursing denies safety to society and furthers the demise of nursing. "Beyond the horizon" demands a cohort of nurses firmly committed to "something to know in nursing" and ready and willing to assume the legal and personal responsibility it entails.

Next, nurses must get off the euphemistic merry-go-round. Nurse practitioners are not practitioners of nursing. Practitioners of nursing are not physicians' assistants. Primary nursing is not primary medicine. The "expanded role" might be better interpreted as a cover-up for medicine's encroachment on nursing's long established practices than as something new for nurses. Interestingly enough, many of those who have left nursing to become nurse-practitioner-physician Assistants are destined to wake up in a dead-end avenue as an already documented oversupply of medical doctors becomes increasingly explicit. Of further significance, it is reported that as the ratio of medical doctors and facilities to population increases, the death rate also increases, whereas as the ratio of nurses to population goes up, the death rate drops (Miller and Stokes, 1978). Such evidence suggests careful reexamination by those who have jumped on the bandwagon of medical skills as a way to save nursing and gain status.

The health care system is caught in a medical monopoly. Hospitals are big business (Goldsmith, 1980). Charges by hospitals and medical doctors have increased at a rate vastly in excess of the rest of the nation's economy. Too many hospital beds and frequent unnecessary hospitalizations are well documented. Hospitals are seeking to diversify their services and to advertise their wares, not unlike the products of the automobile, oil, and tobacco industries. A mammoth effort is ongoing to maintain a traditional power and profit structure replete with third-party payments. Meanwhile an awakening public is seeking alternatives in health services and personnel that they deem more effective as well as less costly.

Community-based health services developed under the aegis of nursing. A renewal of nursing leadership that will continue and enhance the broad scope of nursing's concerns and capabilities is essential. Nursing knowledge and nursing practice are the responsibility of nurses knowledgeable and competent to exercise such responsibility. Dependence on other fields denigrates professional autonomy, denies the identity of nursing, and leaves society without nursing services.

The *unification model* is a nurse-promulgated euphemism for earlier practices variously labeled as apprenticeships, joint appointments, and the like. The practitioner-teacher is magnified and substantive knowledge in nursing is minimized. Claims of economic and power pressures are used to excuse expediency. "A nurse is a nurse is a nurse" is avowed. Nurses are caught in a static web of their own shortsightedness. Some years ago Alfred North Whitehead stated that "when ideals sink to the level of practice, stagnation is the result" (McGlothlin, 1961). Those who seek to perpetuate the past, no matter how well-meaning they may be, are destined to fall by the wayside. They will not cross the horizon.

As nursing moves rapidly toward scientific identity and independent action, conflict with power and profit interests intensifies. Therapeutic modalities and health measures deriving from a science of unitary man can be expected to clash with practices directed toward treating part of man or the sum of his parts. Concomitantly the public is demanding freedom of choice, informed consent, and alternatives in health providers and health services. In the world of tomorrow autonomous nursing centers will augment independent professional practice in nursing. Referral systems within nursing and between nursing and other fields will expand. Emphasis on promotion of health will bring renewed optimism to a public too long deluged with threats of danger on every side.

The speed of change quickens. The horizon nears. Nursing in the twenty-first century has a new image. Problems of the twentieth century are no longer relevant. New concerns and new visions engage the nurses of tomorrow. Independence of thought and action, creative ideas, human compassion, and enthusiasm for the unknown abound. Diversity is a valued norm. Human health and welfare have new dimensions. Florence Nightingale said it rightly: "No system can endure that does not march."

EDITOR'S QUESTIONS FOR DISCUSSION

Speculate as to the future profession of nursing. Identify current trends in the profession. Trace the evolution of nursing toward these trends. What societal values and issues and technological, economic, and environmental factors influenced their development? What changes do you foresee for the enhancement of nursing as a profession, nursing education, nursing research, the establishment of a nursing theoretical knowledge base, nursing practice, and nursing administration? Provide specific examples in each area and indicate a rationale for your predictions.

Discuss the search for meaning and potential to be explored as encouraged by Rogers. What are some examples of contradictions, ambiguities, and uncertainties which contribute to that search? What options are available in the search for meaning? To what extent is it evident that persons are taking more personal responsibility for their lives than in previous decades? Discuss whether or not you agree with Rogers that an optimistic view of the future is beginning to permeate. What has been the impact on the profession of nursing of the search for meaning? What implications may exist in Ketefian's chapter (19) regarding the search for meaning? Do you agree with Rogers that the past presents no vistas of events to come? How can vision promise the unexpected?

Refer to Chap. 14 (Fawcett) and those in the section on nursing theory (Chap. 28–34). What does Rogers mean by a "paradigm shift"? How much agreement is there between Rogers and Hardy (Chap. 32) regarding the meaning of the term paradigm? How congruent is Rogers's proclaimed knowledge base for nursing as described by L. Walker (Chap. 30) with Rogers's statements in her chapter? Describe what is meant by "unitary man" as intended by Rogers. Do you agree with Rogers's statement that aggregates of factors and theories from various sciences do not contribute to knowledge of unitary man? How can "man be more than or different from the sum of his parts"? Provide specific examples in nursing to demonstrate this aspect of Rogers's theory. How can one treat "parts of man" without treating "the sum of his parts" if man is a unitary whole? Provide examples of health measures, derived from a science of unitary man, being expected to clash with practices directed toward treating parts of man or the sum of his parts as suggested by Rogers. Which questions for discussion by the editor in Newman's chapter (28) apply to Rogers's chapter? How congruent is Rogers's perspective on the development of a scientific knowledge base for nursing, with those scholars presenting in Chaps. 14, 28 to 24, and 52? To what extent is Rogers's theory a "grand" theory for nursing? What concepts of Rogers's theory are included in other nursing theories or conceptual models? What level of knowledge and method of reasoning is utilized in the construction of Rogers's theory? What are the assumptions underlying Rogers's theory? To what extent has unitary man been scientifically validated as a theory?

How much consensus is there between Rogers and Williamson (Chap. 5) regarding the first undergraduate professional degree? Provide examples of antieducationists in nursing? Provide additional examples of the use of euphemisms in nursing. Define the differences in the examples Rogers indicates, i.e., nurse practitioners versus practitioners of nursing. How much agreement would there be between Williams (Chap. 25), Brown (Chap. 26), and Rogers regarding the use of the terms nurse practitioners and primary care? What relationship is there between Fralic's discussion (Chap. 48) of an "expanded role" and Rogers's interpretation? How congruent is MacPhail's description (Chap. 46) of unification models with Rogers's reference to the term? Would Hegyvary (Chap. 49) agree with Rogers's view of the practitioner-teacher? What is the significance of the report concerning the ratio of doctors, nurses, and death rates? What further evidence and data are necessary before valid conclusions can be made?

To what extent do you agree with Whitehead's statement as cited by Rogers? What is the implication of the quote for nursing? Should not ideals and practice be reconciled? Is there a contradiction in advocating autonomy and independence in the professional practice of nursing and expansion of referral systems between nursing and other disciplines? To what degree do you affirm the speculations of Rogers?

REFERENCES

Ferguson, Marilyn
1980 The Aquarian Conspiracy. Los Angeles: J. P. Tarcher, Inc.
Goldsmith, Jeff C.
1980 "The health care market: Can hospitals survive?" Harvard Business Review September–October: 110–112.
Heppenheimer, T. A.
1977 Colonies in Space. New York: Warner Books, Inc.

McGlothlin, W. J.
1961 "The place of nursing in the professions." Nursing Outlook 4:216.
Miller, Michael K. and C. Shannon Stokes
1978 "Health status, health resources, and consolidated structural parameters: Implications for public health care policy." Journal of Health and Social Behavior September: 263–279.
Rosen, Stephen
1976 Future Facts. New York: Simon & Schuster.

Chapter 60

The Future of Nursing is Predicted by the State of Science and Technology

Luther P. Christman, R.N., Ph.D., F.A.A.N.
Dean, College of Nursing
Vice President of Nursing Affairs
Rush-Presbyterian–St. Luke's Medical Center
Chicago, Illinois

After Roger's eloquent introduction to the future of nursing, it is expedient to consider specific predictions. Similarity and diversity exist in nursing. Both are further emplified in views concerning the future. Luther Christman succinctly portrays a startling direction for the profession of nursing and the health care system. The basis for his predictions is related to rapid developments in science, technology, and the accretion and obsolescence of knowledge. The events Christman foresees are expansive.

There will be an increase in operational alliances between the disciplines and professions, with a decrease in territoriality. Doctoral preparation will be the entry level to practice for all the health professions, including nursing. All will have the same clinical base for their preparation, with emphasis on the application of science to practice. Whatever differences that may exist will evolve from the role expression of knowledge rather than from scientific content. Full democratization of the professions is foreseen, with equal sex ratios and appropriate representation of minority groups. As a result, personal competence and ability will be essential as each profession competes for the best talent. Nurses, like all clinicians, will limit their activities to clinical practice. Multidisciplinary efforts will necessitate 7-day, 24-hour coverage by all professions. Primary multidisciplinary teams will replace primary nursing.

Pluralism will be of more importance in the delivery of health care, with a system of hospitals without walls evolving to enable patients to remain at home. It is projected that this concept may level the costs of care to therapeutic services and home-making assistance. Out-of-hospital care systems would help two-career families and be a means to manage emotional illness and health care of the aged. Technological improvements, as in telemetry for monitoring care and miniaturing of computers, will facilitate this type of process in care.

Christman foresees health maintenance organizations flourishing to fulfill additional missions. Public policy mandates and means to shape personal life-styles are suggested to attain reduction of morbidity. Concern for patients' rights will increasingly grow. Thus, scientific precision and quality monitoring will be demanded in all designs and provisions of care. Norms of professional performance may become the means of maintaining licensure.

Christman does not indicate a time frame for the predictions to become a reality. However, he urges nurses to adequately plan for the future. Christman offers an insightful, extensive list of questions that require answers, which is critical to the emergence of nursing as a future-oriented profession.

The future direction of the health care system is tied inextricably to developments in science and technology. Thus the future of the health professions can be visualized as having a one-to-one correlation with the continuous accretion of knowledge. Experts assert that the amount of science and technology is doubling every 2 years. This concept is startling when the exponential nature of such growth is considered. For example, if this projection is correct, 8 years from now there should be 32 times the amount of science and technology available to the human race. The other side of the coin is equally astonishing. The obsolescence of knowledge is occurring at a rate fast enough to cause trepidation in all fields of scientific endeavor. In the mid 1960s the half-life of knowledge was about 5 years. Currently it is somewhere between 2 and 3 years. At this pace of erosion, conceivably a state of "instant obsolescence" will be attained before the turn of the century. New knowledge will be created faster than it can be learned and used. Uneasiness and ambiguity will become the steady state for all users of science.

One of the outcomes of this changing knowledge system will be the growth of operational alliances between the disciplines and professions. There will be a sharp decrease in territoriality and an equally sharp increase in cooperative enterprises. All the health professions, including nursing, will have doctoral preparation as the entry level to practice. All will take their preparation from the same clinical base. Dental science, nursing science, and medical science, for instance, will have more in common than they will have differences in their basic composition. All will emphasize the application of science to practice. Because they will all have highly similar educational requisites, communication difficulties will be reduced to the idiosyncracies between persons rather than dissimilarities between groups. The major differences, if they exist at all, will grow from the role expression of knowledge rather than from scientific content. As an example, nurses historically have had greater time and space binding with patients than have physicians. In all likelihood this structural phenomenon may persist.

The full democratization of the professions will be achieved. All the health professions will contain equal sex ratios, and minority groups will reach appropriate representation. The nursing profession will have to undergo one of the most radical changes of all the health professions because of its present undemocratic composition. The overwhelming white female makeup will have to yield to societal pressures. In addition, as many more opportunities for women to enter all the other scientific disciplines and professions arise, a brain drain from nursing may take place if the present pattern persists. Each profession will be competing avidly for the best talent. One of the desirable outcomes of this full democratization will be emphasis on growth of personal competence. All professionals will have to shape their development and careers on personal abilities rather than relying on more artificial claims in order to survive. Economic rewards will be tailored to individual competence rather than to professional membership.

The intense need to rely on scientific training will alter the organization of care into new patterns. Nurses, as all clinicians, will limit their activities to clinical practice. Because of the increasing need for rigorous training to transform science into socially useful outcomes, increased multidisciplinary efforts will necessitate that all the professions move toward 7-day, 24-hour coverage. A few of the health professionals, such as occupational therapists, may escape some of this pressure, but most will be caught in the intensity of the action. One may see primary multidisciplinary teams replacing primary nursing because this matrix form may be a basic requirement for effective management of patient care.

The delivery of health care will have a greater emphasis on pluralism. The increasing individualization of life-styles will stimulate the development of multiple forms of access to care and the operational delivery of care. The present in-hospital form will continue for some populations, especially those with tertiary care problems. Out-of-hospital care systems will develop as viable alternatives to current hospitalization patterns. However, out-of-hospital care will be based in hospitals to reduce overhead and to assure a fixed source of supplies, equipment, and health personnel. Out-of-hospital care will have many desirable characteristics as it will markedly reduce cross-infection and will cause the least violation of the life space of patients. A system of hospitals without walls will enable patients to remain at home in accustomed life-style patterns—familiar dietary intake and eating habits, pets, hobbies, family clusters—away from the bustle, rigid schedules, and life space–invading actions of hospital personnel. This concept also has the possibility of leveling the costs of care because the only cost will be for therapeutic care services and for homemaking assistance in two-career families. This type of care has the potential for producing the kind of ambience many persons desire when they are ill. Furthermore, the utilization of this modality for managing emotional and mental illness, which has been relatively unexplored, has such promise that it is certain to undergo intense development. All this inherent potential can be used to manage the health care of

the aged and to reduce further dependency on nursing home care. The whole field is an exciting setting for innovative nursing care.

The many improvements in technology may facilitate the growth of this type of care. The potential in telemetry alone for monitoring care and for precise assessment of physiological states will be a major support. The miniaturizing of technical equipment of all sorts, especially computers, to assist in care processes is another significant possibility. The two-way communiciation between team members temporarily separated by space or between a nurse-provider and the base hospital personnel will increasingly be made easier by new technology. Initiative for innovation will be hampered only by the predispositions to act and the imagination of specific nurses and other clinicians who are providing care.

Health maintenance organizations in their futuristic models should flourish if there are accompanying public policies to manage air pollution; industrial environments; addiction to tobacco; alcohol, and drugs; poor nutrition; inadequate highway safety; and similar major impediments to good health. One may envision a "sliding in and out" of different health-support organizations. Nurses' abilities will accommodate to the fluidity of the system and will predict the range of options available to their roles. Healthy young and middle-aged persons may utilize this form of care as long as they are in reasonably good health but will rely on other forms as they develop chronic illness unless this form also will supply a continuous 24-hour coverage. The reduction of illness morbidity may become a national goal, but its attainment seems more nearly bound to public policy mandates and personal life-styles than to differences in forms of care. One probable public policy undertaking is the integration of health fundamentals into the education of all children from kindergarten through twelfth year. This may be extended into the college years and beyond. Life-styles can be shaped much differently with underpinnings of this sort.

Patients' rights will continue to be a growing

concern. The impetus of attention will emanate from the general adversary climate of relationships in our nation, the attention of the media, the better education of all citizens, governmental regulations, the consumer movement, and the richer preparation of all providers. All designs of care will have to be put together with more scientific precision, and all providers will have to be very accountable for their actions. Nurses will no longer be able to hide behind physicians' orders, hospital policy, or routine procedures. Every act will have to be purposeful. Quality monitoring of care will be compulsory and surveillance will be intense. Computer-assisted practice will emerge in very sophisticated forms. By these means, the therapeutic actions and their appropriateness will be constantly and permanently tracked by every clinician around each patient. Norms of performance can be established nationally, and compliance with these norms may become the means of maintaining licensure. Nurses falling below accepted standards will likely be placed on probation or have their licenses suspended completely. Everyone will be involved in continuing education for a purpose instead of earning credits as a ritual.

From these easily foreseen events, can nurses plan adequately to become a vigorous component of the future? Can nurses overcome apathy and inertia? Can the educators from associate degree and hospital school programs forgo their own narrow self-interests and abandon their obstructionist behavior? Can the national organizations become effective instruments for keeping nursing in the mainstream of scientific evolution? Are nurses willing to democratize the profession? Are nurses willing to work openly for multidisciplinary cooperation? Can nurses replace confrontation with diplomacy in dealing with others? Are nurses willing to have a very high degree of accountability for their actions? Are nurses willing to develop nursing as an applied science? Will their research take this pathway or will it move toward areas of less productive research? Will nurses evolve a system of care that places the burden of direct delivery of care on the best educated nurses instead of the least prepared? Are nurses willing to shed their historical antiintellectualism to become prepared at the graduate level? Are nurses willing to give up their demonstrated rootlessness and develop careers instead of having a series of jobs? Will the dropout rate from the profession decrease to a manageable size? Will the studied aloofness from the other professions change to a community of interest? This list of questions is not exhaustive but poses a number of problems which require answers. Much of the positive response lies dormant in the bright young nurses now in graduate education. The way they shape their careers and provide leadership is critical to the emergence of nursing as a future-oriented profession. Furthermore, a large critical mass of nurses with graduate preparation must replace the present trickle, or the tempo of change will never reach the crescendo necessary for the profession to achieve its potential benefit to patients. The issues are straightforward; the solutions await responses.

EDITOR'S QUESTIONS FOR DISCUSSION

What are the similarities and differences between Rogers's (Chap. 59) and Christman's speculations and predictions? Compare the perspectives of the previous contributors with the outcomes of change predicted by Christman. How can autonomy as advocated by some authors be reconciled with an anticipated increase in cooperative enterprise and decrease in territoriality? How congruent is the mandate designated for nursing by Conway (Chap. 2) with Christman's discussion of the knowledge base for health professionals? What are the implications for the establishment of a scientific knowledge base for nursing given the predictions by Christman? Which of the contributors discussing research and nursing theory would agree with Christman regarding the emphasis on the application of science to practice? How can all health professionals be prepared from the same clinical base and simultaneously have the scientific content of their discipline be the knowledge base for their practice? What are the implications inherent in Christman's predictions for doctoral programs in nursing as discussed by Grace (Chap. 12)? How congruent is Christman's foreseeing of doctoral preparation as the entry level for professional practice with Williamson's view? Provide examples of the major difference among health professionals evolving from the role expression of knowledge. How much agreement would there be between MacPhail (Chap. 46), Fagin and McGivern (Chap. 56), and Christman regarding the development of operational alliances?

Suggest strategies for the democratization of the professions. What changes would need to occur for a democratic composition within nursing? What are the implications for the accountability of nurses and the profession with an increasing emphasis on personal competence? If nurses limit their activities to clinical practice, what are the implications for the organization and management of nursing care and professional education programs? What might be the composition of primary multidisciplinary teams to replace primary nursing?

Discuss the concept of a system of hospitals without walls. What application may exist from Ezell's chapter (57) in planning for such a system? What might be the impact on society, health care delivery systems, the health professions, and role preparation in implementation of out-of-hospital care systems? To what extent do such systems already exist? What are the implications for the humanization of patient care with the advances in technology? What are the ethical entailments for the professions concerning the use of technology? How might nurses be best prepared for flexible health care systems and a range of options to their roles? What is the process by which norms of professional performance can be established nationally to maintain licensure? Suggest public policy mandates for consideration in reducing morbidity. Given the difficulties in changing patterns of health and illness behavior, how can life-styles effectively be shaped through health education. Given Christman's assertion for scientific precision in future designs of care, who should participate in the planning, implementing, and evaluating of the designs?

Present arguments for and against the predictions indicated becoming a reality. Given Christman's foresight, what planning needs to occur within the profession of nursing and other health professions and disciplines to prepare for the future? Discuss and respond to each of the questions posed by Christman. Which queries pose a number of problems that need to be addressed? How might these issues be approached to prepare for the future? What additional questions might be suggested? What supplementary or alternative predictions can be proposed? Provide a rationale for those speculations.

Chapter 61

The Future Health Care Delivery System in the United States

Myrtle K. Aydelotte, R.N., Ph.D., F.A.A.N.[1]
Former Executive Director
American Nurses Association
Kansas City, Missouri

Given the provocative and exciting predictions of Christman, the challenge remains to explore further the health care delivery system which will be the base for the future. Myrtle K. Aydelotte explicates the exacting demands in the future delivery of health care. In so doing, she identifies future health care needs, examines the existing organization of health care services, poses questions to be resolved, indicates assumptions about health care delivery, describes the future structure of health care systems, and suggests the meaning of the demands for nursing and the preparation of nurses. Changes in population characteristics are cited as the bases for affecting both demands and satisfactory methods to meet the needs.

Aydelotte projects there will continue to be a decline in the birth rate with increasing life expectancy. The mix of diseases requiring treatment will change. However, chronic illnesses will increase, and cancer and heart disease will continue to be the major causes of death. The number of persons at high risk for mental illness will increase. More women and ethnic minorities in high level positions will be subject to greater job-related stress. Other needs and health problems that need to be resolved are provision of health-related services in child care for preschool- and school-age children, problem drinkers in early adolescence, epidemic proportion of sexually transmitted diseases among adolescents, increasing maternal death rates for adolescents, and increasing infant morbidity and mortality risks. Health needs of the aged are becoming more complex. With the increase of minority populations, a greater number of minority individuals who are sensitive to special problems of ethnic monorities need to assume health care roles. Drastic changes in family structure, roles, and functions have influenced health needs. The physical and socioeconomic environment have impacted on the health status of the public. There will be more emphasis on the responsibility for one's own health. Consequently there will be more demand for self-help programs, therapy-directed health services, as well as continued insistence on a higher degree of satisfaction and requests for more personal health services.

[1] This paper is not to be interpreted as a policy statement of the American Nurses' Association.

Aydelotte indicates eight factors as having influenced the organization of health care services in the past and contributed to changes, but serious problems still exist. Essentially, these are related to inadequate distribution of services and personnel resources, fragmentation of service, inflationary health care costs, and a focus on illness and crisis-oriented care. Recognizing the strengths and weaknesses of the current system, Aydelotte formulates six questions to be resolved. These pertain to constraints placed on growth of sectors of health care, area of emphasis (prevention or treatment), costs, value of technology, meeting gaps in the current system, and accommodations for illness versus disease care. Assumptions regarding trends that will influence the future structure include: little change in the value system of the affluent population for illness care and services provided by physicians; continued focus by physicians on curative rather than preventive aspects of care; greater emphasis for efficient utilization of existing personnel; decrease in government regulation and increase in competition between service units; more comprehensive services of higher quality; increase of HMOs and multiunit health organizations; diverse governance boards; and combining private and public/government funding for financing health care.

Aydelotte perceives health services continuing to be provided through primary, intermediary, and tertiary care centers. The purposes of each are described. She further discusses categories of multihospital arrangements: consortia for clinical service planning, contract management, lease, and corporate ownership. Characteristics of each type of multihospital arrangement are defined. Aydelotte foresees that the major portion of health care delivery will occur in ambulatory care; home and quasihome, occupational, child care centers; and school settings. Attention will be given to the proximity of clinics for convenient access. Primary care will focus on prevention and gerontology. In secondary care, the community hospital will provide more comprehensive services in multisettings, with an increase in technology and more corporate arrangements. Tertiary care will be more highly specialized and based on referral patterns. Physicians and nurses will practice through group arrangements or some type of corporate structure.

In foreseeing and preparing for the impact of these changes upon nursing, Aydelotte asserts there will be a greater need for nurses in primary and ambulatory care settings. There will be increased demands and expectations for nurses. For example, increased expertise in identifying behavioral changes, expanded communication skills, knowledge/acceptance of cultural diversity and change, and the utilization of technology in patient teaching will all be expected. Aydelotte predicts a great demand for well-prepared nurses in leadership positions of corporate structures. She specifies the knowledge base required for these nurses to address problems and issues, which affect the total organization, technology, structure, and management as they relate to health care organizations and the nursing profession. Aydelotte further insists there must be a basic, major difference in educational outcomes for each level of preparation in nursing. Education based on the *degree* of difference of the same dimension will no longer be tolerated. Aydelotte delineates the role for the associate and baccalaureate degree graduates as well as for those nurses who have advanced preparation. During the next 20 years, the growing complexity of health care delivery will require a different preparation from that currently offered in many colleges of nursing.

The need for and, in turn, the utilization of health care services depends upon the physical, emotional, social, and economic status as well as the cultural and environmental background of the consumer. During the next 20 years, changes in population characteristics will affect both demands upon the health care system and acceptable methods of meeting these demands. As a result of rising educational levels and greater affluence, the general public will demand better, more comprehensive health care services provided by more highly skilled personnel. Whether or not health care delivery systems can accommodate the exacting demands of a changing population is the issue at hand.

FUTURE HEALTH NEEDS

During the next 20 years, there will continue to be a decline in the birth rate coupled with advancing life expectancy. The emergence of a four-generation society will create new and different demands for health care and health-related services.

The mix of diseases requiring treatment will undergo change as the result of new medical technology and alterations in population characteristics. However, the number of persons with chronic illnesses who need surveillance will continue to increase, and cancer and arteriosclerotic heart disease will continue to be the leading causes of death.

There is new evidence to suggest that, at any one time, close to 15 percent of the population is in need of some form of mental health care. Community epidemiology studies show that a large number of persons suffer from mild to moderate depression, anxiety and psychophysiological discomforts, insomnia, loneliness, and other indicators of emotional disorders (President's Commission on Mental Health, 1978a:4). In the next 10 years, the number of people in the age groups at high risk for mental illness will increase substantially. In particular, youth and the aged will tend to suffer varying conditions related

to emotional disorder. Greater emphasis on a unisex approach to both work and domestic roles will increase psychological stresses for men and women. As more women and more ethnic minorities assume higher-level positions in the business world, they will be subject to greater job-related psychological stresses associated with higher rates of heart diseases and other related illnesses (Department of Health, Education and Welfare, Public Health Service and Health Resources Administration 1978:68). Social problems and changing mores will contribute to the increase in venereal diseases and the increase in self-damaging behavior such as alcoholism and drug abuse. Consequently, there will be a greater need for self-help programs and therapy-directed health services.

The special health needs of children and youth, the aged, and ethnic minorities are worth noting. In the future, these population subgroups must not be neglected.

Adults are increasingly unavailable to children. Since 1950, the proportion of mothers with school-age children working outside the home has doubled (from 26 to 51 percent) and the number of working mothers with preschool children has tripled (from 11 to 37 percent (President's Commission on Mental Health, 1978b:564.65). This has increased the need for provision of health-related services in child care and preschool settings as well as in elementary and secondary schools.

According to the President's Commission on Mental Health, mental health problems in childhood are clearly sufficiently common to constitute a major concern in the planning of health services and to make it impractical for them to be dealt with exclusively by child psychiatrists. (President's Commission on Mental Health, 1978a:7)

During the past 10 years, there has been an overall increase in drinking among youth. The trend has been toward the initiation of regular alcohol use in early adolescence (children as young as 10 to 11 years of age). In a 1974 nationwide survey of junior and senior high school students,

27.8 percent were found to be problem drinkers (President's Commission on Mental Health, 1978a: 6). This is a serious health problem, which must be dealt with and eliminated in the 1980s.

There is evidence to indicate that more and more young people are beginning sexual activity at earlier and earlier ages. It is estimated that there are 11 million sexually active adolescents in the age group 15 to 19. Sexually transmitted diseases have reached epidemic proportion among teenagers. During the period 1970-1977, the 300,000 cases of gonorrhea reported developed into 45,000 cases of pelvic inflammatory disease, leaving between 7000 and 18,000 victims sterile. Each year, 1.1 million American teenage girls aged 15 to 19 become pregnant. Maternal death rates are 60 percent higher for these young adolescents, and infant morbidity and mortality risks are twice as high (A Report on Hearings on the Unmet Health Needs of Children and Youth, 1979:3). New and innovative means must be found to teach sex education. Special screening and detection services and treatment clinics must be created to deal with these problems.

Like those of children and youth, the health needs of the aged are becoming more complex. By the year 2000, it is estimated that the average life expectancy will be 74 years of age and that one out of eight people in the United States will be 65 years of age and older. There will be as much as a 60 percent increase in the number of individuals over 75 years of age. This dramatic aging of the American population will greatly increase the demands for a more comprehensive, integrated system of gerontological services.

In the past few years, there has been a phenomenal increase in minority populations in this country because of increased birth and immigration rates. By 1995, it is projected that minority populations will reach over 50 million (Unpublished information compiled with ANA Graduate Fellowship Program in Nursing for Ethnic Minorities, 1980). These groups pose special problems for the health care system because of the limited number of health professionals who are sensitive to the special issues and problems faced by ethnic minorities. In the future, a greater number of minority individuals must be trained to assume health care roles. It will be extremely important that more minority individuals become alcohol and drug abuse counselors, psychologists, social workers, mental health nurses, and other trained mental health personnel.

There is evidence that family structure has a great bearing on health needs. Drastic alterations or abrupt major changes in the social dynamics of the family unit can create emotional stress severe enough to trigger serious illness (Department of Health and Human Services, 1979:2-3). The rising divorce rate, the increase in the number of single-parent families, the increase in the number of children born to unmarried parents, the decrease in the birth rate and in family size, and the changing roles of men and women in society are indicators of change in family functions, roles, and structures. In the future, it is likely that more persons will rely upon the health care system for support groups and substitutes for traditional geographical and extended family networks.

In the future, there will be increased concern about the impact of the physical environment on the health status of individuals. The American public will demand that more elaborate steps be taken to eliminate contamination of air, water, and food; workplace hazards; radiation exposure; excessive noise; dangerous consumer products; and unsafe highway designs. Greater emphasis also will be placed on upgrading the socioeconomic environment (income level, housing, and employment status) as a means for improving the health status of certain population subgroups.

There will continue to be demands for more personal health services and a greater degree of satisfaction with health services. A recent study indicates that factors contributing to the patient's overall satisfaction with services include doctor-patient interaction, cost of services, and convenience (location of health care facility and waiting time) (Aday et al., 1980:237-38).

Finally, in the future, there will be a greater

need to emphasize care of self and the assumption of responsibility for one's own health. There has been a significant decline in acute infectious diseases requiring special medications and highly specialized supportive therapy. Today's major health problems consist of chronic diseases which require constant self-monitoring. It is essential that patient education be included among the benefits of health care programs in the future.

EXISTING ORGANIZATION OF HEALTH CARE SERVICES

Over the past decade, a number of factors have influenced the organization of health care services. These factors include:

1 Increased government regulation and involvement through legislative action at all levels

2 Concern over costs of care and the costs of educating professionals in the health field

3 Efforts by professionals to protect selfish interests and to resist change

4 Increased sophistication of the public and its expectation for involvement in decisions regarding access to services and the quantity, quality, and cost of services

5 Increased concern of business regarding the productivity of workers and loss of production in the workplace

6 Increased concern on the part of workers and unions regarding provisions for more comprehensive "health" and insurance benefits

7 Increased concern on the part of insurance underwriters and the "blues" regarding the costs and utilization of premiums

8 Integration of the expanding body of scientific knowledge and technological innovations into the health care system

These and other factors have triggered changes within the health care system which include: proliferation of new types of health workers, greater specialization of existing health personnel, expansion of nursing roles, shifts in settings where health care is delivered, increasing use of automated procedures and devices based on technological advances, implementation of voluntary cost containment measures, closer governmental scrutiny of the accreditation of health personnel, introduction of regional health planning, and greater involvement of the public in health care planning.

Although efforts have been aimed at adapting to various factors affecting the delivery of care, serious problems do exist. The present health care system is characterized by an inadequate distribution of services and labor resources, fragmentation of services, and inflationary health care costs. Moreover, a focus on illness and crisis-oriented care has severely limited provision of primary care.

QUESTIONS TO BE ANSWERED IN THE NEXT DECADE

In light of predictions about future health needs and in recognition of the strengths and weaknesses of the current health care system, several questions must be resolved in the next decade:

1 Will there be constraints placed on the growth of major sectors of the health care system?

2 Will there be an increased emphasis on prevention of illness and health maintenance or will the emphasis continue to be on treatment and cure of illness and disease?

3 How will costs of prevention, care, and cure be met?

4 How will the value of technology be estimated?

5 By what means will gaps in the current health care system be met?

6 What accommodations(s) will be made for illness vs. disease care? How will illness requirements be met?

The formulation of answers to these questions will require careful study and analysis. However, several assumptions can be made regarding circumstances and trends which will influence the structure of health care systems during the next 20 years.

ASSUMPTIONS ABOUT HEALTH
CARE DELIVERY

The value system held by the affluent population will change very little. There will continue to be a great need for illness care and a high value will continue to be placed on physician services.

There will be little change in the orientation, services, and distribution of physicians. Physicians will continue to focus on the curative aspect of care rather than promotive, preventive, and rehabilitative care. They will continue to locate in prosperous medium-sized cities and in the wealthier districts of large metropolitan areas.

The supply of health personnel will not increase and there will be little change in overall distribution. Consequently, greater emphasis will be placed on more efficient utilization of existing personnel.

The emphasis placed by communities on self-contained organized services will not change markedly. Local interests, pride, and provincialism will continue to interfere with the efficient and effective planning and administration of health services.

Government regulation (as opposed to government stimulus) will decrease, and competition between service units, especially clinics, hospitals, and health maintenance organizations, will increase. As a result of increased competition, more comprehensive services of a higher quality will be made more readily accessible at more reasonable costs to the consumer. The number of Health Maintenance Organizations (HMO) across the country will continue to increase as more and more consumers are made aware of the benefits of this mode of delivering health care services. Studies have indicated that clients of health maintenance organizations have a markedly lower rate of hospital admissions and a shorter length of hospitalization than those covered by conventional health insurance plans. There also is evidence that subscribers receive an above average level of care at a below average cost (Department of Health, Education and Welfare, Public Health Service, 1976: 49-50).

With encouragement by forces from within the health industry, more health organizations (hospitals and HMOs) will become multiunit and national in scope. During the latter part of the seventies, multi-institutional arrangements received increased attention. In 1978, the American Hospital Association created the Center for Multihospital Systems and Shared Services Organizations to provide support in the development and improvement of these systems and organizations. To date, the majority of these arrangements have been confined to local or regional areas. In the next 10 to 20 years, more multiunit arrangements will become national in scope and will require different management and leadership skills. The governance boards of these units will be more diverse. They will be composed of representatives from across the country and this national representation will help to offset some of the problems created by efforts to protect local provincial interests.

The needs of the poor, ethnic groups, and the aged will not be met in the structured health care system unless marked intervention occurs. The private sector of the health care system will continue to focus its attention on the affluent. The special health needs of the poor, the aged, and ethnic groups will only be met through government-stimulated programs and services. The system for financing health care in the future will consist of a combination of private and public, i.e., government funding. Based on all these assumptions, certain observations can be made about the structure of health care systems in the future.

STRUCTURE OF HEALTH CARE SYSTEMS
IN THE FUTURE

Health services will continue to be provided through primary, intermediary, and tertiary care centers. The major purposes of primary care centers will be to provide: (1) entry into the system, (2) emergency care, (3) health maintenance, (4) long-term and chronic care, and (5) treatment of temporary malfunctioning that does not require hospitalization. Intermediary centers will exist to provide:

(1) the treatment of malfunctioning that is temporary but requires hospitalization of such a nature that highly skilled services and high-risk intervention are not required; (2) the evaluation of long-term and chronic illness to determine whether a change in intervention is required when the evaluation requires hospitalization; and (3) the provision of counseling and therapy that cannot be provided within the primary care center because of cost of services, equipment, or the infrequency with which it must be provided. Tertiary centers' major purposes will be: (1) the treatment of the esoteric illnesses of patients that occur infrequently and (2) the provision of personnel, new programs, new knowledge, and demonstrations of delivery for the total health delivery system. Very highly skilled personnel and equipment will be required in the tertiary center (Aydelotte, 1978: 352).

Initial entry into the system and basic emergency services for maintenance of life will be made available in all three centers. Thus, instead of the usual portrayal of a health delivery system as either a pyramid or satellite, it can be viewed as a series of concentric, overlapping circles encompassed within one field. The system may be thought of as a consortium of health institutions, agencies, and health care practitioners (Aydelotte, 1978:352).

There is evidence that the number and varieties of multi-institutional arrangements among health care facilities are on the increase. In the future, the scheme of health delivery will be arranged in larger multiunit and national networks. As a result, there will be marked improvement in the quality of care, comprehensiveness, and continuity between levels of care. Several types of multiunit arrangements may exist.

At least seven categories of multihospital arrangements have already been identified. These categories include: (1) consortia for clinical service planning, (2) contract management, (3) lease, and (4) corporate ownership but separate management. In the consortia for clinical service planning, groups of hospitals agree to meet separately from health systems agencies to plan which institution will provide which clinical service. In the contract management model, there is no change in the hospital's ownership, but there is a major change in top management and there is a systems influence on major policy decisions for the served institution. In the lease arrangement, policy making as well as full management are provided by a corporate board or agency that is separate from the ownership of the served institution. Under provision of most lease arrangements there is no change in ownership, but both board policy and management decisions are made in behalf of the benefiting institution by the serving agency. In corporate ownership but separate management, a corporation owns the system or several hospitals but it contracts for the administration of each of them with individual, independent managers. Under this arrangement owners do not interfere in the management of hospitals even though they have the legal authority to do so (De Vries, 1978:81–83).

In the future, the major portion of health care delivery will occur in newly developed ambulatory care settings, home and quasi-home settings, occupational settings, child care centers, and schools. Both the scope of services and the settings of primary care clinics will undergo change. Cultural diversity will be taken into account in the planning and delivery of primary care services. These services will be offered in a greater variety of settings, thus making access more convenient for all age groups and income levels. More attention will be given to the proximity of clinics to shopping centers, trade routes, and other well-trafficked areas. Services will be made available near apartment blocks, housing additions, and retirement settings. There will be a significant growth in arrangements for health services in industrial settings.

Government-stimulated programs and services will address the specific health needs of children, the aged, and ethnic minorities. There will be increased effort to establish well baby clinics and health services in child care settings, preschools, and elementary and secondary schools. There will be significant growth in the area of gerontological primary care. There will be multiple arrangements for the delivery of such care, including boarding homes and community day care centers. Greater emphasis will be placed on gerontological nursing. Prevention will continue to be a priority, and elaborate measures will be taken to collect and disseminate useful information on health and health services.

In the future, secondary care in hospitals will change significantly. The community hospital will evolve into a more comprehensive health care center delivering a wider spectrum of services in multisettings. The focus of ambulatory care will be enlarged. Gerontological care (skilled care) will become attached to secondary care in hospitals. Home care will be extended into the community as part of the hospital setting. More quasi-home settings will be created to provide protected environments in which more individuals can assume responsibility for health promotion, prevention of illness, disease protection, etc. There will be some increase in technology in secondary care centers. As a result of more corporate arrangements, specialization will be better planned.

Tertiary care will be more highly specialized and based on referral patterns from primary and secondary care sources. As a result of the very high level of specialization in intervention, patient requirements in tertiary care centers will be intense.

Finally, physicians and nurses will practice in group practice arrangements or through employment in some kind of corporate structure. Solo practice will be a thing of the past.

IMPACT UPON NURSING AND PREPARATION OF NURSES

In the next 10 to 20 years, there will be a much greater need for nurses to function in primary care and in ambulatory care settings. Moreover, there will be increased demands placed upon these nurses. They will be expected to acquire more skill in the identification of behavioral changes in patients and in assessment and evaluation. They will be expected to expand their communication skills (i.e., mastery of a second language, computerization of data, etc.). They will be expected to display an increased knowledge of cultural diversity and acceptance of cultures and change. They will be expected to utilize technology in the teaching of patients.

There will be increased demand for nurses skilled in gerontological and chronic disease care. Nurses will assume *major* responsibility for management of the chronically ill and for care of normal children and adults. Nurses employed in hospitals will be required to have a highly increased level of skill and scientific knowledge as well as the ability to assist the patient and family in adapting to a major change resulting from the application of intense medical intervention.

There will be a great demand for well-prepared nurses to function in leadership positions in corporate structures. These nurses will need to display clinical expertise as well as a command of knowledge of administrative concepts, organizational behavior, management processes, and legal matters as they pertain to health care organizations and to the nursing profession. They will need to be able to address problems and issues which affect the total organization, including goals and values, technology, structure, and management.

It is obvious that the growing complexity of health care delivery will increase the need for better prepared nursing personnel. Education for the preparation of nurses based on the *degree* of difference of the same dimension will no longer be tolerated. There must be a basic, major difference in educational outcomes for each level of preparation.

In addition to the general background, the associate degree program should provide an introduction to one clinical nursing specialty area where the associate degree graduate can learn to function comfortably with a large group of patients. The primary role of the associate degree graduate should be provision and evaluation of direct care to groups of patients (Aydelotte, 1978:356).

In future health care delivery systems, the baccalaureate graduate may best fit in as a beginning nurse-clinician in a specific clinical nursing field, where he or she will function in meeting special needs of patients, in planning programs for patients and nursing staff, and in evaluating effectiveness of care and the like. With increased maturity and experience and with continuing education, the baccalaureate graduate can move into leadership positions and become a professional in nursing practice. In order to function as a beginning nurse-clinician, the baccalaureate degree holder needs preparation vastly different from that currently being offered in many colleges of nursing. The baccalaureate graduate must possess pertinent, delineated knowledge, tested for its effectiveness, and must be able to synthesize knowledge and reduce it or translate it into action that is reality-oriented (Aydelotte, 1978:356–57).

Individuals with advanced preparation must assume the tasks of nursing leadership—the design of new nursing programs, their conduct and evaluation; the direction of personnel; the coordination of nursing with other disciplines; and the development of policy and direction. This is not to say that they are in administrative positions (although a number must be), but they are accountable for studying groups of patients to determine care requirements and for establishing the conditions that make it possible for nursing to contribute to the total programs of care (Aydelotte, 1978:356).

CONCLUSION

During the next 20 years, changes in population characteristics will affect both demands upon the health care system and acceptable methods of meeting these demands. The scheme of health care delivery will be arranged in larger multiunit and national networks. The major portion of health care delivery will occur in newly developed ambulatory care settings, home and quasi-home settings, occupational settings, child care centers, and schools. As a result of decreased government regulation and increased competition among service units, more comprehensive services of a higher quality will be made more readily accessible at more reasonable costs.

During the next 10 to 20 years, there will be a much greater need for nurses to function in primary care and in ambulatory care settings. It is obvious that the growing complexity of health care delivery will increase the need for better prepared nursing personnel. Education for the preparation of nurses based on the degree of difference of the same dimension will no longer be tolerated. There must be a basic, major difference in educational outcomes for each level of preparation.

EDITOR'S QUESTIONS FOR DISCUSSION

What factors have contributed to the increased number of persons in age groups at high risk for mental illness? Identify additional health needs for the future. Suggest alternatives for meeting the health needs of the future. How can Christman's concept (Chap. 60) of out-of-hospital care systems be developed and implemented to meet the needs identified by Aydelotte? Suggest means for evaluating self-help programs and therapy-directed health services. What strategies can be suggested for encouraging persons to assume responsibility for their own health? What societal, socioeconomic, technological, and family variables have influenced the trends toward alcohol abuse, earlier sexual activity and epidemic sexually transmitted diseases, and increasing maternal death rates among adolescents? Suggest means for dealing with these problems. What assessment and planning is needed to meet the health needs of the aged and ethnic minority groups? What relationship is there between physical and socioeconomic environment and health status? What alternatives can be suggested for the surveillance and/or treatment of persons with chronic illness? What application may be considered from Corless's chapter (40)?

How have the eight factors cited by Aydelotte influenced the organization of current health services? Provide examples of the result of these influences? Discuss the characteristics of the present system. What are the strengths and weaknesses of the current system? What suggestions can be made to resolve the six questions raised by Aydelotte? Discuss the assumptions indicated concerning trends that will influence the future structure of health care systems. To what extent do you agree with the assumptions? Suggest a rationale for the assumptions. What are the implications for the role of nurses if physicians continue to focus on curative aspects of care? Which contributors in previous chapters have defined the domain for nursing? What are the similarities and differences between Aydelotte's and Christman's view of the future? What might be the basis for decreased government regulation and increased competition between service units? What factors have contributed to the development of multiunit, national health organizations? What multiunit systems currently exist? Describe the governance boards of these units. How will health care be financed in the future? How can funding from private and public/government be effectively combined? What monitoring of health finances should or might occur? Who should do the monitoring? What policies may need to be established in combining two sources of funding?

Describe the differences between primary, intermediary, and tertiary care centers. What are the implications for nursing roles in these centers? What are the differences in the four categories of multihospital arrangements described by Aydelotte? Discuss the advantages and disadvantages of each type of system from the perspectives of the consumer and health professionals. How might each of these types impact on the quality of patient care and health services? What scope of services in settings of primary care would you suggest? What are advantages and disadvantages of increasing technology in health care services? What evidence is there that indicates solo practice will no longer exist? How would Sills's proposal (Chap. 42) for nurse-corporations relate to Aydelotte's prediction concerning group practice? Suggest additional alternatives for the structure of health care systems in the future.

Discuss the impact of future health care systems on the profession of nursing. What additional expectations of nurses and demands cited by Aydelotte can you suggest? To what extent do you agree with Aydelotte regarding the preparation of nurses for leadership positions in corporate structures? Delineate the basic major difference in educational outcomes for each level of preparation in nursing. How can this be distinguished from education based on the *degree* of difference of the same dimension? As presented by Aydelotte, what would be the difference in preparation and role of the associate and baccalaureate degree nurse? Is there a difference in performance between an associate degree student being introduced to one clinical nursing specialty area to provide direct care to groups of patients and a *beginning* baccalaureate nurse clinician in a specific clinical nursing field? Does Aydelotte imply that though the role expectations are different for the associate and baccalaureate degree nurse, their initial functioning is similar? How should baccalaureate preparation be different in colleges of nursing for a beginning nurse-clinician?

Does Aydelotte imply that the beginning nurse-clinician is not prepared for professional nursing practice? What content is suggested by Aydelotte for the advanced preparation of nurses to assume a nursing leadership role? How congruent is Williamson's

(Chap. 5) discussion of professional education with Aydelotte's prescriptions? What additional changes do you foresee that will affect both demands upon the health care system and the profession of nursing?

REFERENCES

Aday, LuAnn, Ronald Andersen, and Gretchen V. Fleming
  1980 Health Care in the U.S. Equitable for Whom? Beverly Hills: Sage Publications.

Aydelotte, Myrtle K.
  1978 "The future health delivery system and the utilization of nurses prepared in formal educational programs," Pp. 349–358 in N. L. Chaska (ed.), The Nursing Profession: Views Through The Mist. New York: McGraw-Hill.

DeVries, Robert A.
  1978 "Strength in numbers." Journal of the American Hospital Association 52:81–83, March 16.

Department of Health, Education and Welfare, U.S. Public Health Service
  1976 Healthy People. The Surgeon General's Report on Health Promotion and Disease Prevention. Washington, D.C.: U.S. Government Printing Office.
  1976 Forward Plan for Health, FY 1978–82. Washington, D.C.: U.S. Government Printing Office.

Department of Health, Education and Welfare, U.S. Public Health Service
  1978 Analysis and Planning for Improved Distribution of Nursing Personnel and Services: Final Report. Washington, D.C.: U.S. Government Printing Office.

President's Commission on Mental Health
  1978a Task Panel Reports. vol. II. Washington, D.C.: U.S. Government Printing Office.
  1978b Task Panel Reports, vol. III. Washington, D.C.: U.S. Government Printing Office.

A Report on the Hearings on the Unmet Health Needs of Children and Youth
  1979 Kansas City, Mo.: American Nurses Association.

Unpublished Information Compiled in Conjunction with the ANA Graduate Fellowship Program
  1980 Nursing for Ethnic Minorities.

Chapter 62

Public Health Nursing:
Now and as It Might Be

Dorothy M. Talbot, R.N., Ph.D., F.A.A.N.
Professor and Chairman
Department of Public Health Nursing
School of Public Health
University of North Carolina
Chapel Hill, North Carolina

Aydelotte's discussion of health care systems for the future has indicated the needs to be met. Alternative systems and changes in the delivery of health care are already on the horizon. Perhaps no one speciality or subdiscipline within nursing will be more affected by health care needs and changes in providing care than public health nursing. The premise of caring for defined populations, as families and community groups, is the unique feature of public health nursing. Dorothy M. Talbot presents a history of public health nursing practice, describes current practice, examines trends, and suggests alternative futures.

From the beginning of modern nursing, nurses have entered homes to assist with health care and cared for those in schools and industry. Public health nurses have historically focused predominantly on two populations at risk: mothers and children; sick and disabled. Their activities have included case-finding, referral, and mobilizing community resources. With the allocation of tax money, multiple new health services evolved, but so did regulations and categorical funding for selected social programs. Consequently, there is less home visiting for health promotion and prevention, and more clinics and home visiting for care of the sick. To assist in understanding the change in the public health nurse's role from a generalist to that of a specialist. Talbot reflects on Durkheim's theory regarding the division of labor in society. In essence, as society grows, organic solidarity comes into being. Labor becomes divided, and specialization increases; each part is autonomous but a vital part of the whole. Defined rules and regulations for relationships between groups occur. The more social ties are loosened, the easier it becomes for other components to enter. Talbot points out that as nursing has become more loosely tied to the health care collective, it has been easier for new elements, like nurse practitioners and nurse midwives, to be grafted onto public health nursing services. Specialization is causing public health nurses to diverge from caring for defined populations and total families to a program, that is, task orientation in caring of individuals. A major factor has been the growth of third-party payments and funding for separate programs in health departments, with clients seeing different nurses for different needs.

Thus, today the character of the work of public health nurses is more specialized. More nurses are practicing independently or in group practice settings. Primary care clinics are multiplying. Talbot expresses concern that no one professional is viewing nor caring for the family as the unit of service. There appears to be less commitment by many community nurses to meet the needs of families as a whole. She maintains that, although nurses are working in community settings, they are not practicing public health nursing as a specialty, which focuses on populations at risk with prevention and promotion of health as its primary aim.

Talbot cites trends which suggest probable futures. People are moving to smaller communities; values are changing; there is a growth in the spiritual dimension; self-help movements are multiplying. Economic instability is likely to continue. She foresees increased government and public control; machines replacing people; more low-status jobs and increased conflicts over territory; nursing associations serving increasingly as unions, with nursing becoming more political. Talbot arranges the trends that will affect public health nursing into five categories. *Political* forces include: legislators who determine what health programs are funded; social security regulations which decree who may receive home care; legislated cost containment; increasing numbers of persons who refuse to pay income tax; private physicians who thwart efforts of health departments to deliver primary care. *Economic* forces cited are: inflation; fewer dollars allocated to health programs; high interest rates; fixed incomes for many persons. *Demographic* information that pinpoints where services can be provided to reach the largest number of people indicates: half the population is 30 years old and over; the majority of the population live in suburbs, smaller cities, or rural areas. *Social-cultural* forces indicate that values are changing regarding sex, family structure, women, ethnic groups, and religion. Concern for ethics is increasing. Education is more emphasized as well as self-care. Computers are transforming all phases of life. Regarding *professional* forces which affect public health nursing, Talbot cites the move toward baccalaureate education and the provision of physical assessment skills for nurses to deliver primary care. She foresees leadership and management skills becoming the basis for promotion.

Talbot provides three scenarios of probable futures. The *surprise-free future* includes: proliferation of roles and responsibilities; lower standards of living; politically adept public health nurses; fragmented nursing care; satellite clinics; decreasing concern for populations as a whole. The *pessimistic future* includes: continued deterioration of the economy; below-poverty-level living standards; more nurses leaving nursing; public health nursing resembling the practice of the 1800s (illness oriented and no emphasis on prevention or caring for populations at risk). Health care generalists, with some education beyond high school, will do case finding and referrals to specialists. Specialists will provide the care, and develop the teaching and health care plans. The *optimistic future* includes: optimal decision making through the use of computers; increased efficiency due to technology; institutionalization of the hospice movement; public health nurses will be more educationally prepared as professionals—the gatekeepers to the health care system, managers of personal health services, and administrators of health care agencies. Health will be the focus of their work. Talbot concludes that the future will be the result of our choices today.

In Shinar, several thousand years ago, men were building a tower to heaven. Suddenly, through an act of God, they began speaking to each other in strange languages. Construction stopped on the tower of Babel because men became unable to communicate. There was much confusion. Today there is confusion among public health nurses and their publics over roles and responsibilities. It appears that specialization has created boundaries which has led to this phenomenon.

The purpose of this chapter is to describe present-day public health nursing practice and to suggest alternative futures based on signals heard today. An opening discussion of how confusion in role and responsibility evolved will lead to a discussion of present-day practice. Emile Durkheim's theory of the division of labor will be used to illustrate change (Durkheim, 1933). Trends portending probable futures will be presented, followed by scenarios describing how public health nursing might be practiced in the future.

Public health nursing is based on the premise of caring, the sine qua non of nursing, for populations, whether these be families or specified groups in a community, such as school children, workers in an industry, or teenage girls at risk for out-of-wedlock pregnancies. This premise of caring for defined populations is the unique feature of this type of nursing practice. The health needs of a defined population are assessed; plans for meeting them are made jointly by the client and nurse; there is implementation which is followed by evaluation. It is the process which all nurses use. Principles of practice include nursing the family as a unit, interdigitating one's practice with other community-based health and social service workers, and assisting clients to maximum self-management of their health. Prevention of disease and disability, together with promotion and maintenance of optimum health, is the goal. Public health nursing practice differs from other specialty nursing practices because it focuses on whole populations at risk rather than on single individuals. Providing the greatest help to the greatest number has been,

and continues to be, the benchmark of all public health practice, including nursing.

FACTORS LEADING TO PRESENT-DAY PRACTICE

Phoebe, who may be termed the founder of public health nursing, walked on the shores of Greece and cared for St. Paul and others who were sick and forlorn. Mothers, slaves, neighbors, the religious, and women like Dickens's Sairey Gamp, have cared for individuals outside of hospitals over the centuries.

From the beginning of modern nursing, nurses have entered homes to help persons manage their health care needs, concentrating on teaching principles of personal and environmental health and assisting families toward independence. The goal was, and is, development of an optimal plan of health care congruent with the client's life situation. So valued was this concept that, beginning in 1909, certain industries, for example, the Metropolitan Life Insurance Company, paid public health nurses to visit the homes of their ill or injured workers. For three-quarters of a century, public health nurses have also worked in schools and industries, caring for populations with defined health problems, for example, those with tuberculosis or some other form of communicable disease. There has been particular emphasis on two populations at risk—mothers and children and those who were sick and disabled in their homes. Public health nurses have been case finders, referral agents, teachers, counselors, providers of care, and mobilizers of community resources. They have been the constant and continuous link for clients in the health care delivery system, gatekeepers and pathfinders through an increasingly complex maze.

As social consciousness became aroused at the turn of the century, tax money was allocated to selected social programs, including those focusing on the health of mothers and children. Non-tax-supported voluntary agencies, stemming from the colonist's ethic of self-help, continued to care for the sick at home. Schools, developing in social responsibility, began providing for their sick and injured, as did more and more industries. Specialization had begun.

In the second quarter of this century, the impact of a social-minded government and World War II resulted in multiple new health services and new and different types of community health workers, such as health educators, nutritionists, and venereal disease investigators. With government money came regulations describing what services could be provided and for what clients. As programs developed, people began expecting the government to take care of them. "If the government wants my son immunized, then the government must provide."

Programs in which public health nursing is practiced have grown like Topsy. Medicare, Medicaid, family planning, mental health, chronic disease, home health, occupational health, school health, children and youth, adult health, and gerontology programs have proliferated, so that few regions of the United States are without them. For many of these programs there has been federal, state, and local tax money allocated, concomitant with regulations. These programs, each with different data and accountability requirements and regulations as to what clients may be served, are causing changes in public health nursing practice. There are fewer generalized nursing services provided by nurses practicing in defined geographical settings. Because categorical funding for programs has become the norm, nurses are more apt to be practicing in only one program. There is less home visiting for health promotion and prevention purposes. There is more home visiting for care of the sick, and there are many more clinics. New programs are frequently added; rarely is one deleted, at least not from the consciousness of the nurse.

These rapid changes have led to confusion over role and responsibility in the minds of public health nurses, their nurse colleagues, other profes-

sionals, and the public. It may help in understanding this state of affairs to reflect on Emile Durkheim's ideas regarding the division of labor in society.

DIVISION OF LABOR: THEORETICAL CONSIDERATIONS

Although Adam Smith was the first to attempt a theory explaining division of labor, Emile Durkheim, a French social thinker, wrote the first definitive work on the topic in 1893 (Durkheim, 1933). Durkheim saw work in a society organized in one of two ways; he differentiated these work modes according to what he termed mechanical or organic solidarity. Individuals of primitive societies were dependent upon the collective. All of the members had the same customs, did the same things. There was little division of labor, little or no specialization. This is how public health nursing was organized in the earlier parts of the present century. Public health nurses were generalists; they cared for families and other populations at risk in defined geographical districts. All practiced in more or less the same manner. There was mechanical solidarity.

As a society grows, however, organic solidarity comes into being. Labor becomes divided and specialization increases; each part is autonomous, yet a vital part of the whole. Durkheim likened this phenomenon to that system which is observed in the anatomical structure of higher animals; each organ has its own shape and autonomy, yet it is vital to the life of the whole organism. The whole has freedom of movement, as does each of its elements. Durkheim saw more creativity in this type of society than in the one characterized by mechanical solidarity, for the yoke of social control is less heavy. Durkheim believed, however, that each type, mechanical and organic, has unity in purpose and direction.

Health care is big business today; it has organic solidarity, and within it, public health nursing has shape and function. But the chasm which used to separate occupations is being filled in. At the same time, within each occupation, differences are growing. To illustrate, nurse practitioners, nurse midwives, and nurse anesthetists have blurred the line between medicine and nursing, while at the same time they demonstrate differences within nursing.

Although labor may become more divided, the different parts of the aggregate, because they fill different functions, cannot be easily separated from the whole. Nor can new elements be grafted on without upsetting the equilibrium and altering relationships. Accordingly, society resists intrusions that produce disturbance. However, the more the social ties to the central society are loosened, the easier it becomes for foreign elements to become part of that society.

Nursing, as it strides toward autonomy as an occupation, is becoming more loosely tied to the health care collective. New elements are entering in and are being grafted on the public health nursing services. Nurse practitioners and nurse midwives, as new elements, are practicing in large numbers in public health settings. New types of workers, such as pharmacists and mental health workers, are becoming a regular part of public health nursing services. The equilibrium is upset, and one should expect resistance within the health care collective as roles and responsibilities get sorted.

Durkheim explained that society attempts to define and govern relationships between groups through rules and regulations. When a society no longer imposes upon all members certain uniform practices, more rules and regulations emerge. The increase in principles of conduct resulting from new workers in the field of public health nursing has led to breakdowns in communication, which in turn have created confusion over roles and responsibilities. Although humans like change, despite its difficulties, a change of existence, whether sudden or expected, brings crisis. It is hard to pull up roots of habit.

Durkheim believed that work becomes more divided as societies become more voluminous and

dense. Different occupations are able to coexist as long as they have different aims. The closer, however, functions come to one another, the more there is apt to be conflict, as observed, for example, in the debate at state levels over the licensing of nurse midwives and nurse practitioners. Durkheim also believed, however, that functions, when sufficiently in contact with one another, tend to stabilize and regulate themselves, and this mode of adaptation becomes the norm when consecrated by authority. Conflict causes growth; specialization occurs only if society has a need for it. The enormous growth in numbers of nurse practitioners and other nurse specialists attest to society's need. As nurses, however, take on more of the functions formerly in the domain of physicians, there will be conflict. Economics will come into play with the predicted surfeit of physicians in America; more clients will turn to nurses for affordable health care and fewer turn to physicians for expensive medical care.

Durkheim believed it was one's duty to specialize. He saw activity becoming richer and more intense as it became more specialized. Public health nurses, although some yearn for the days of the generalist role, are becoming specialized. What is happening? Specialization is causing public health nurses to diverge from their emphasis on caring for defined populations with health needs. As an ever-increasing tide of people present themselves for care at clinics, as inflation takes its toll, and as health workers become fewer, public health nurses are overwhelmed with work. A major factor has been the growth of third-party payments, which provide more people with the means to seek care. Categorical funding has created separate programs in health departments, each with its own staff. In most health departments, clients see different nurses for different needs. A mother visiting a family planning clinic brings her baby with her. The baby needs immunizations but cannot be given them there. These are only given in the pediatric clinic, often on another day. It makes one think of the lady who telephoned the grocery store manager and asked to speak to the man in charge of the peaches. The manager, willing to help, asked, "Which one, dried or fresh?" There are exceptions. In rural areas and smaller health departments nurses work very hard to maintain the generalist approach, but in the larger agencies it is becoming very difficult to do.

Durkheim believed the reason labor became progressively divided was the human desire for happiness, happiness which was thought to come through productive work. He recognized though, that pleasure lies between the two extremes of insufficient and excessive activity. For this reason, the happiness of individuals does not increase indefinitely: it fades when demands become too heavy. Today public health nurses are faced with heavy demands and multiple new relationships, two reasons which help explain their frustration.

PRESENT-DAY PUBLIC HEALTH NURSING PRACTICE

Nursing is practiced in many community settings— homes, schools, industries, prisons, migrant camps, rest homes, outpatient departments of hospitals, and neighborhood clinics—as well as in tax-supported public health departments. An increasing number of nurses are practicing independently, often working in group practice settings. The process is the same, that is, health needs of clients are assessed and plans for meeting the needs are made, implemented, and evaluated. The character of the work has changed, however, in that public health nurses are more specialized. Home visits are made to care for the sick; few visits are made for prevention of disease or disability or for health promotion, even to new mothers with babies. Many different nurses, as well as home health aides and chore workers, are entering the patient's home. Just recently, a 76-year-old lady met the home health nurse at the door as she came to administer care to the lady's 100-year-old mother. "Nurse, my mother is very agitated because you are new. Why can't the same nurse visit her each day?" Just when hospital nursing is turning toward primary care nursing, with one nurse responsible for the 24-hour

care of his or her patients, community nursing seems to be going the task-oriented route. How does one develop a nurse-patient relationship when contacts are so brief and the care so fragmented?

Primary care clinics are multiplying. In these clinics there is decreased concern with the family as the unit of service and an increased number of specialists. Nutritionists provide diet counseling; laboratory workers collect specimens; pharmacists dispense medications and counsel clients on their use; health educators do client education and mobilize communities for self-help measures. Physicians' assistants and nurse practitioners examine, diagnose, and treat the multiple conditions seen.

Because of this fragmentation and program orientation, no one worker is taking a look at the total family. Emphasis is on the individual. There appears to be less commitment on the part of many community nurses to look at the health needs of a family as a whole. Although home health nurses generally take excellent physical care of their home-bound clients, they frequently fail to do health teaching or to see other health needs in the immediate environment. Clinic nurses, too, for the most part give quality care to individuals. Both categories are nurses working in community settings. They are not practicing public health nursing, which is a specialty that focuses on populations at risk with prevention and promotion of health as its primary aim.

There are many programs, many settings, many technological developments. Specialization is the only way nurses can hope to know enough to care well for the clients they serve. People are living longer and new health problems, together with new treatments, emerge. Individuals are getting better care. People, though, are receiving less continuity of care and are faced with adjusting to multiple health workers. As Durkheim explained, specialization leads to more specialization.

What then is the future of nursing in the community as it becomes increasingly specialized and its emphasis on the care of individuals, not populations, increases? Is a new specialist in public health nursing emerging, one who is primarily concerned with populations at risk?

One cannot predict the future, but one can suggest probable futures based on trends which today are whispers in society. The future is formed by decisions made by people today—and tomorrow and the day following.

TRENDS IN SOCIETY THAT IMPACT ON PUBLIC HEALTH NURSING

Humans have always been fascinated with the future. Oracles, fortune-tellers, and astrologers were consulted in attempts to peer into the future. The images thus created guided human behavior. Today, however, probability takes precedence over prophecy as we try to create, rather than merely to endure, our future. There are trends in today's society that affect nursing practice in community settings. The future is based on their interaction and on the decisions made by those in power.

Plato's *Republic* (1973:234–263) is probably the best known example of the human attempt to envision an ideal future. And Jules Verne (1870, 1888) and H. G. Wells (1906, 1913, 1923, 1939) made uncannily accurate forecasts. The Rand Corporation's "think tank" concept, however, marks the beginning of modern forecasting. Today it is accepted management practice to plan and forecast. The future can be imagined and then created from choices made. The future is fluid, not fixed nor frozen. To know where one is going, it is helpful to know where one has been. Forecasters are helped by people who are familiar with the past and who will be practicing in the future.

Social change in our lifetime has been tremendous. A world community has evolved through rapid air travel and television satellites. In the remote parts of the world, natives have transistor radios. Computers enable humans to transcend earlier intellectual accomplishments. Family planning advances are releasing women from devoting themselves completely to reproductivity. Women everywhere are denouncing the myth that ours is a patriarchal society.

Today we see no increase in human kindness; we are multiplying too fast in most of the world; the number of suicides is increasing. Bureaucratic structures are having breakdowns as they become larger and less able to plan centrally for unmet needs of the periphery.

People are moving to smaller communities where they are able to be more self-sufficient by growing their own food and producing other necessities. Values are changing, with simplicity becoming the preferred life-style. Mutual aid is a growing phenomenon, and there is a growth in the spiritual dimension. Self-help movements are multiplying.

Localism is developing. This boundary setting can become dangerous as it brings less effective communication. With computers, however, there will be few secrets, and the ability to communicate health information will reside with all who can use computers.

It is likely that economic instability will continue to make long-range plans impossible. Probably there will be increased government control in our lives and constant crises in leadership. Unemployment will grow as inflation continues and machines replace humans. There will be more low-status jobs and more problems of turfdom. There will be a "blue jeans doctor," who just may be the neighborhood nurse practitioner. Our nursing associations will serve increasingly as unions, and nursing will become more political.

The entire health community is watching nursing as we continue to look to ourselves and our own vested interests and look less to our collective future. There are whispers in society that will affect the future of public health nursing. These whispers have political, economic, demographic, social-cultural, and professional overtones.

Political

Political forces are those stemming from government. In America there are frequent changes in legislators, and all are influenced by partisan and economic interests. Legislators determine what health programs are funded; thus they determine, to a large extent, the types of public health nursing programs offered. Social security regulations decree in a large measure those who may receive home care; presently they are the ill. Less than 1 percent of the health care dollar is spent on prevention. One effect of legislated cost containment is fewer health care personnel. As nurses retire or move, the likelihood increases that their positions will be frozen. There is growing distrust of government; the number of people refusing to pay income tax is increasing. Private physicians often thwart efforts of health departments to deliver primary care. Paradoxically, public health nurses, with a commitment to quality, family-centered care based on the promotion and prevention of health, work within the constraints of government-funded programs that provide care only to those who have health conditions that fit the regulations.

Economic

Economic forces are those that pertain to the production, distribution, and consumption of wealth. Inflation is eroding personal wealth. Gasoline and fuel have skyrocketed in price. Fewer dollars are allocated to health programs, and supplies and services are being altered. With the high interest rates, fewer people can afford homes and cars. People on fixed incomes, and this is the majority of those over 65, are able to purchase less each year. People are losing their jobs, thus compounding the stress prevalent in society. Skills are becoming obsolete, and continuing education is needed; such education is expensive. Mandatory retirement is disappearing, and a generation of workers from the "baby boom" are finding fewer opportunities for work.

Demographic

The population of the United States is moving to less-populated towns in the Sun Belt. As the 1980 census is tabulated one learns that half of the population is 30 years old and over. Only one-quarter of the population lives in central cities. The vast

majority live in suburbs or smaller cities and rural areas. The numbers of single parents and of those over age 65 have increased dramatically. This information is useful in pinpointing where services can be provided to reach the largest number of people in need.

Social-Cultural

Social-cultural forces are those that affect the mind and behavior of a community. Values are changing regarding sex, family structure, women, ethnic groups, and religion. Social factors that affect public health nursing practice include the increased incidence of unmarried teenage mothers, many of whom want and keep their babies; a greater incidence of venereal disease from increased promiscuity; more singles living together in permanent relationships; open deviant sexual practices; and more working mothers.

Ethics are of increasing concern. The unfortunate dilemma of the "Death Angel" only punctuates fears and uncertainties as public health nurses deal with the hopelessly ill.

The move toward increased education, both formal and continuing, for nurses has an impact on practice. Education makes expensive demands in both time and money.

There is more emphasis on self-care. People appear to be eating more wisely, smoking less, drinking alcohol less, exercising more, and treating their minor ills and injuries themselves. Individuals are being trained to care for themselves. The neighborhood drug store has self-help supplies available. People are using ways of caring for their health other than the traditional medical methods. They are using touch, meditation, herbs, prayer, and biofeedback to help themselves.

Computers are transforming all phases of life. Desk-top computers aid health workers with diagnoses by determining drug dosages and synergistic effects. Machines are becoming available for use at home in monitoring such things as one's blood pressure. Video cassettes are often the present-day health educators.

Professional

Nursing is awakening. Although still primarily a female occupation, the profession is shedding the yoke of male authority. Nurses now carry out many activities once the province of physicians. The movement toward providing more nurses with physical assessment skills, thus making them more skilled in delivering primary care, is seen in the trend to include development of these skills in nursing education programs, both basic and graduate. With the move toward baccalaureate education, fierce competition is expected to emerge among nurses for leadership positions. Leadership and management skills will become the basis for promotion, rather than seniority.

SCENARIOS

Based on these trends and prevailing forces, three probable futures can be forecast. By considering several alternatives, one can keep an open mind and be ready for whatever occurs, a stance that permits contingency planning and allows futures to be created.

The Surprise-Free Future

Our present-day practice, with proliferation of roles and responsibilities, will continue. The population is slowing its growth, so increases in personnel and programs will not be needed. Living standards, despite inflation, will remain the same and the proportion of "haves" and "have-nots" will not change markedly. Everyone, except the very wealthy, will have a lower standard of living. Although electronic communication devices will continue to develop, their development will be slowed because of restricted availability of petroleum and metal ores. Public health nurses will become more politically adept. More of them will become specialized. Nursing care will continue to be fragmented, with less emphasis on continuity. Home visits will be a thing of the past except in the care of the sick. There will be more satellite clinics, more work in rest homes, and more primary care delivered in clinics. Essentially, services will remain the same and they will be available for individuals. There will be less and less concern for populations as a whole.

The Pessimistic Future

The economy of the United States will continue to deteriorate, with inflation soaring. Oil will become more expensive. Living standards of large numbers will fall below the poverty level, particularly in the rapidly growing population over 65 years of age. Political unrest will continue unabated. There will be massive unemployment, and the recession will result in a depression greater than that of the 1930s. A nuclear holocaust, possibly World War III, will threaten. Nurses' salaries will not keep pace with inflation. Motivation for self-development will decrease, and nurses will leave the field for other types of work. Other types of health care workers will increasingly take over the role of nurses now working in community settings. Pharmacists and their aides will administer drugs, counsel concerning their effects, and question clients for side effects. Nutritionists and their aides will take over diet counseling for all clients. Health educators will teach people at home through video cassettes. Social workers will do psychological and social counseling. Health care needs of larger numbers of people will place more demands on a system which cannot be enlarged because of economic factors. Public health nursing will become more illness-oriented and focus primarily on individuals. It will begin to resemble that which was practiced in the 1800s, a one-to-one practice. The emphasis on prevention, promotion of health, and caring for populations at risk will be forgotten. Burnout will increase as stresses increase and resources decrease. By the year 2000, there will be personnel in the health care services known as health care workers, generalists, young men and women with some education beyond high school, who will do the case finding, referrals, and follow-up for clients who have been guided to specialists. Specialists, some of whom will be former public health nurses who have become highly specialized in health care, will provide the care and develop the teaching and health care plans. Data concerning client needs and services will be coordinated and computerized, so details will not be forgotten. Nostalgia will exist in the minds of those clients who once had "their" nurse coordinating their care and providing aid to the family as a whole.

The Optimistic Future

New technological devices will emerge to increase the efficiency with which energy is used. Homes will be warm; cars will be driven. Optimal decision making will be made through the use of computers. Homes, schools, and industries will have communication computers so that health education and counseling are easily obtained. Breakthroughs in the prevention and treatment of cancer will occur. Heart disease will go the way of polio, once proper nutrition, more exercise, and less stress become the norm for people. More attention will be paid to people's emotional needs, and the hospice movement will become institutionalized. The over-65 population will be active participants in society; many will be working. Public health nurses will be better educated, more able to command higher salaries, and thus have more self-esteem. The general population and other health care professionals will view them as trusted and capable health care providers. They will be gatekeepers to the health care system, managers of personal health services, and administrators of health care agencies. Health will be the focus of their work, leaving diagnosis and cure of disease to medicine. Population-based nursing, based on needs of de-

fined groups at risk, will be practiced, led by capable nurses with an epidemiological point of view. Many will become specialized in the various branches of health care management, where they will be policy makers and decision makers. Research will be a respected and sought-after role. There will still be public health nurses in the year 2000. Their goal will still be health for everyone, a goal which is no more unobtainable than our American dream of equality for all.

CONCLUSION

By considering trends in society and alternative pathways to the future, one can view the future as a realm built upon present-day choices. Public health nursing values that must be thoughtfully considered before being irrevocably lost are consideration of the family, and other defined populations at risk, as the units of service; continuity of care, with a single nurse coordinating services; and emphasis on prevention of disease and promotion of optimum health. Whatever the future, one fact is clear. That future will be the result of our choices today.

During the Ice Age, glaciers came down from the north. Living things had to adjust to a colder climate and other environmental alterations. The human survived; many species did not. Perhaps the most important qualifications for adaptation are brains and heart. It takes intelligence and courage to spring from a familiar place to a strange one.

"Where there is no vision, the people perish." (Proverbs 29:18).

EDITOR'S QUESTIONS FOR DISCUSSION

Compare the historical role of the public health nurse with the present and with the predicted future as presented by Talbot. What additional factors may have contributed to present-day practice? How has categorical federal funding for programs been established? Who provides the professional input for categories to be established? What data base is utilized for establishing national, regional, state, and local needs for specific programs? How can public health nursing utilize its power base to influence the development of programs that should be funded in health care delivery? How should caring for an individual be interrelated with caring for families as a unit or caring for groups in a future health care delivery system? What suggestions can be offered for linking the health care of groups to a total population?

Apply Durkheim's theory explaining the division of labor to the nursing profession, other health professions, and the health care delivery system. What is the difference between mechanical and organic solidarity? Are there examples for each being present today in health care? To what extent were all health professionals generalists in the early history of their discipline? How did a health care system evolve? Which type of society has less social control: mechanical or organic solidarity? How is that demonstrated today?

As Talbot suggests, nursing in striving toward autonomy is becoming less tied to the health care collective. What examples and/or evidence can you provide of this occurrence? What are the possible or evident outcomes? Suggest avenues for resolution of possible conflict between being autonomous and being part of a health care system. How does Durkheim's explanation of increasing rules and regulations in a society apply to the health care system? Provide examples of conflict stimulating growth versus disintegration or destruction. Under what conditions and for whom would nurses assuming more functions formerly in the domain of physicians cause conflict? Are there other factors which contribute to specialization other than a need of society? Who determines the health care needs of society? How is the need for specialization established?

What are the critical issues in public health nursing? In practice and education? How is the generalist versus specialist view expressed in professional education programs? Review Williams's (Chap. 25) and Brown's (Chap. 26) Editor's Questions for Discussion. What issues are addressed in those chapters that apply to Talbot's discussion of present day and future practice in public health nursing? Having read *all* the previous chapters, what additional issues may need to be addressed that may impact public health nursing? How much consensus is apparent among the contributors regarding the role of nurse practitioners and primary care? Do nurses in primary care utilize physical assessment skills differently from physicians? What is the difference between health and physical assessment? How can the debate as to whether primary care provided by nurse practitioners is medical or nusing practice be resolved? Would you include nurse midwives under the umbrella of public health nursing or maternal-child health? What criteria can be suggested for delineating the areas, roles and boundaries included as public health nursing? Should health educators, occupational, school, home health, and family health nurses and nurse practitioners (specialized in psychiatry, maternity, child and/or adult care) all be under the aegis of public or community health? How would you define a family health practitioner? How would you define psychosocial nursing? Should professionals from both public health and psychiatric nursing be represented and content integrated from both subdisciplines in developing professional education programs? If public health nursing continues to be fragmented, what common, core knowledge base is essential to educationally prepare public health nurses for professional practice? What additional knowledge base would be essential in preparation for the various roles in public health nursing? Refer to Bullough's chapter (45) and consider the legal issues involved in preparing professional nurses. Discuss the advantages and disadvantages of all the possible options in developing professional programs for public health nursing.

Discuss additional, political, economical, demographic, social-cultural and professional forces which impact on public health nursing and the future health care delivery system. What similarity exists between the predictions by Rogers (Chap. 59), Christman (Chap. 60), and Aydelotte (Chap. 61)? To what extent would you agree that public health nurses in the future will be the gatekeepers to the health care system, managers of personal health services, and administrators of health care agencies? If you perceive that is the future role for public health nurses, what is essential to plan, prepare, and implement that role? Identify the restraining and driving forces in developing that role. Suggest strategies for reducing the restraining forces. Which of the three possible futures appears the most likely to occur? Provide a rationale for your choice. What additional characteristics would you suggest for each of the three? Given that the future is the result of choices today, what choices can you make to prepare for and contribute to the future you would like to foresee?

REFERENCES

Bible, The Holy
  1937 Authorized King James Version. New York: Collins Clear Type Press.
Durkheim, E.
  1933 The Division of Labor in Society. Tr. G. Simpson. New York: Macmillan.
Plato
  1973 The Republic and Other Works. Book VIII. Tr. B. Jowett. New York: Anchor Press, Doubleday.
Verne, Jules
  1870 From the Earth to the Moon and Round the Moon. New York: Burt.
  1888 20,000 Leagues Under the Sea. New York: Pollard and Moss.
Wells, Herbert George
  1906 The Future in America: A Search After Realities. New York: Harper.
  1913 Discovery of the Future. New York: Huebsch.
  1923 The First Man on the Moon. London: Collins.
  1939 The Fate of Man. New York: Alliance.

Chapter 63

Professional Nursing: The Drive for Governance

Myrtle K. Aydelotte, R.N., Ph.D., F.A.A.N.
Former Executive Director
American Nurses Association
Kansas City, Missouri

The future for health professionals and the health care delivery system, Talbot has affirmed, will be the result of choices made today. Inherent in an effective health care delivery system is the professionalism of the providers for care. Myrtle K. Aydelotte examines the status of nursing as a profession, identifies obstacles in nursing's drive for governance, and discusses movements and arrangements to enhance nursing's role in governance.

Aydelotte reviews the characteristics of a profession as indicated by Shephard, Bixler, and Hall. According to Aydelotte, one predominant theme prevails: In order to achieve full professional status, an occupational group must exercise autonomy within its defined area of practice. She contends that without governance, there is no autonomy, thus full professional status is unattainable. Governance refers to the establishment and maintenance of social, political, and economic arrangements by which practitioners maintain control over their practice, self-discipline, working conditions, and professional affairs.

According to Aydelotte, the establishment of the American Nurses Association in 1896 was the first real indication of nursing's desire to be accorded professional status. Since then, nursing has achieved other professional characteristics: nurse practice acts in every state; a pool of licensing examinations for state boards of nursing; a code of ethics; and standards for organized nursing services, practice, and education. Although progress has been slow, there have been signs of movement toward clarification of the scope of nursing practice. More emphasis has been placed on defining a well-organized body of scientific knowledge. The ANA's Commission on Nursing Research has developed priorities for research in nursing to improve practice and advance the knowledge base of the profession. The ANA's *Nursing: A Social Policy Statement* examines the social context of nursing, the nature and scope of practice, and specialization in nursing practice. There has been a need to achieve consensus on a national system of

---

*The views expressed in this chapter represent the personal observations of the author and do not necessarily reflect the positions of the American Nurses Association.

nursing education for standardization of expected competencies and educational preparation. Innovation in the educational system has been advocated through numerous studies: the 1923 Goldmark Report, Esther Lucille Brown's 1948 report, and a 1970 study of the National Commission for the Study of Nursing and Nursing Education. As a result there has been a definite trend toward implementation of baccalaureate preparation in nursing as entry into professional practice. Nineteen seventy-two was the first year that more nurses graduated from collegiate schools of nursing than hospital programs. In 1980, the ANA House of Delegates adopted guidelines for educational mobility of individuals seeking academic nursing degrees. In addition, the house adopted a mechanism for deriving a comprehensive statement of the roles, functions, and competencies of two categories of nursing practice.

Aydelotte views credentialing mechanisms as essential for public accountability through establishing standards which qualified practitioners must meet. She indicates that deficiencies in the system have been related to a fragmented approach. She reviews the recommendations and report of *The Study of Credentialing in Nursing: A New Approach.* The study's recommendations include a proposal for a national credentialing center to study, develop, coordinate, provide services for, and conduct credentialing in nursing. Finally, she justifies the need for nursing to achieve greater autonomy for full professional status.

Aydelotte devotes considerable discussion to examining nursing's drive to achieve governance as the means toward autonomy. Three major obstacles have been the bureaucratic organization of hospitals which prevents autonomous roles for nurses, the insufficient number of well-prepared leaders in nursing, and the drive of labor unions to secure the right to represent and bargain for nurses. It is contended that nurses always have had equity but not parity—equality in the execution of power and influence in decision making regarding the care process. She cites Wandelt's study that indicates that inability of nurses to exercise control over clinical practice produced feelings of career stagnation, caused nurses to leave nursing, and brought about the end result: a nurse shortage. Aydelotte maintains that the lack of appropriate arrangements for governance not only has contributed to the nurse shortage but fostered the growth of supplemental nursing services with additional associated problems in the delivery of nursing services.

Aydelotte asserts that the divisiveness that exists within the profession and slow resolution of issues is indicative of the inadequate preparation of leaders for nursing. The confrontation-negotiation style of leadership is considered necessary. Two requisites for the leadership role and these broad sets of knowledge by the nurse leaders are indicated. Regarding the drive toward unionization, Aydelotte argues that it is the professional association, rather than trade unions, that is best equipped to represent the professional interests and concerns of nurses.

Finally, Aydelotte examines the movement toward implementing arrangements for nursing governance. There are efforts aimed at decentralizing the nursing organizational structure. In considering potential arrangements for nursing organization, Aydelotte delineates seven characteristics, from a series of 20, deemed desirable for a professional nursing department by the ANA's Commission on Nursing Services. Examples of the trend toward governance are the creation of a nursing staff organization, adoption of nursing staff bylaws, formation of joint practice councils/committees, and application of the primary nursing concept. Additional evidence of enhancing nursing's role in governance in other settings are cited. This includes changes in nurse practice acts, formation of nursing private practice groups, nurse practitioners collaborating with physicians in primary care, and collective action through the professional association. Aydelotte provides five major reasons for trends toward governance to continue and increase. She concludes that in the future nursing needs to continue to define and test models of governance, but also that nurses must acquire the knowledge and preparation essential to assuming the responsibilities implied in the concept of governance.

What is a profession? What are the basic characteristics of a profession? What are the criteria for professionalization? These and similar questions have been explored and debated for many years as individuals and occupational groups attempt to determine the magic formula for achieving professional status. Many books have been written on professionalization, yet it is difficult to find a succinct definition of the word "profession." A study of various professions does reveal that the aim of a profession is altruistic rather than materialistic. Members of a given profession are motivated more by a commitment to the provision of service of a high quality than by considerations of economic gain.

A profession is best explained as a composite of characteristics. According to Shephard, a profession, among other things, must (1) satisfy an indispensable social need and be based upon well established and socially accepted scientific principles; (2) develop a scientific technique which is the result of tested experience; and (3) require the exercise of discretion and judgment as to time and manner of performance of duty (in contrast to the kind of work which is subject to immediate direction and supervision) (1948:146). Bixler and Bixler contend that a profession (1) utilizes a well-defined and well-organized body of specialized knowledge in its practice, (2) enlarges the body of knowledge it uses and improves its techniques of education and service, (3) entrusts the education of its practitioners to institutions of higher education, and (4) strives to compensate its practitioners by providing freedom of action, opportunity for continuous professional growth, and economic security (1959:1142-1146). Hall reports that, to be considered a profession, a group must (1) educate its own practitioners, (2) set its own standards, (3) adapt its services to meet changing needs, (4) accept responsibility for safeguarding the public it serves, (5) promote the welfare and well-being of its practitioners and safeguard their interests, (6) adhere to a code of conduct based on ethical principles, and (7) unite for strength in achieving its larger purposes (1973: 89-92).

Careful examination of these and other characteristics assigned to a profession reveals one overriding theme: *In order to achieve full professional status, an occupational group must exercise autonomy within its defined area of practice.* To be accorded true professional status, a group must function autonomously in the formulation of policy and in the control of its activity. Merton once observed that an occupation does not become a full-fledged profession unless the members of that occupation are "the ones who make the final decisions in the field of activity in which they are engaged" (1958:298). As long as one occupational group is basically subordinate to some other occupational group, it will not likely be accorded unequivocal status as a profession.

To be an autonomous body implies that an occupational group has been granted the *authority* to define its scope of practice, delineate its specific functions and roles, and determine its goals and responsibilities in delivery of its services. It also implies that the group has acquired the *power* to have a positive influence on the environment in which its services should and must be delivered. It is the author's contention that the degree of professional autonomy accorded an occupational group depends on the effectiveness of the group's efforts at governance. Without governance, there is no autonomy. Without autonomy, full professional status is unattainable.

Governance refers to the establishment and maintenance of social, political, and economic arrangements by which practitioners maintain control over their practice, their self-discipline, their working conditions, and their professional affairs. Knowledge is absolutely essential in the domain of governance. For seeking a greater role in policy making and decision making in a designated area, knowledge can open the door to power and authority. Above and beyond mastery of the body of specialized knowledge in the designated practice area, there is a need for practitioners who are knowledgeable in the cultural, political, social, and economic considerations which must be dealt with in policy program development. Politically and economically astute leaders and well-informed, skillful practitioners are an essential ingredient to ensure effective governance and, in turn, to guarantee professional autonomy.

The purposes of this chapter are (1) to examine the status of nursing as a profession; (2) to identify some of the obstacles in nursing's drive for governance; and (3) to discuss several arrangements under which nurses may organize in order to achieve greater self-determination of parameters of practice and of accountability, better conditions of employment, and greater influence in shaping the policies and positions under which institutions operate.

Describing nursing before the turn of this century, Robb observed:

Among the nurses there was no professional feeling, not even among graduates of the same school; there was simply nothing organized or professional about us. Collectively, we could neither qualify as a profession, a calling, or a trade. For to be a member of a profession implied more responsibility, more serious duties, a higher skill, and work demanding a more thorough education than was required in many other vocations in life. But two things more were needed—organization and legislation. . . . We were, therefore, a most indefinite quantity. (1976:326–327)

In the span of 100 years, nursing has grown from "a m... group of h... health wo... gredient i... to compre... formation... of nurses... of other... public. W... Nurses A... a vehicle,... which to... factors impacting upon... services. This was, in effect, the first real indication of nursing's desire to be accorded professional status. The establishment of a strong effective association is viewed as one step in a series of events aimed at professionalization (Carr-Saunders, 1966:6).

As a result of the efforts of the American Nurses Association, nursing has achieved several basic characteristics attributed to professional status: nurse practice acts in every state; a pool of licensing examinations for state boards of nursing; a code of ethics for professional practice; standards for organized nursing services, nursing practice, and nursing education; and such legislation as the Nurse Training Act. There are, however, certain interrelated areas in which nursing's progress has been slow: clarification of the scope of nursing practice; standardization of nursing education; development of a coherent, effective system of credentialing nurses; and implementation of arrangements to enhance nursing's role in governance.

Over the years, one of nursing's greatest shortcomings has been its failure to clearly define and specifically delineate its functions and unique contributions to the delivery of health care. The fact that nursing has not produced a well-defined, well-organized body of specialized knowledge has contributed to this problem. Much of the existing knowledge in nursing has been arrived at intuitively and experientially rather than through systematic inquiry and observation. Considering the knowledge explosion which has occurred in other fields, this fact has serious implications for nursing's

834

...f nurses are to be accorded ...s, they must be able to iden-...sly add to the theoretical body ...on which nursing is based.

...e past few years, there have been ...movement toward clarification of the ...f nursing practice. Greater emphasis has ...placed on increasing the scientific knowledge ...hich forms the basis for practice. More nurses have been encouraged to research and study nursing at the master's and doctoral degree levels. ANA's Commission on Nursing Research has developed priorities for research in nursing to focus attention on the development of information that is essential to the improvement of nursing practice and the advancement of nursing as a profession. In addition, ANA, speaking on behalf of the profession, has issued definitive statements regarding standards of practice and definitions and descriptions of specific nursing roles. Most recently, ANA's Congress for Nursing Practice published *Nursing: A Social Policy Statement*. This statement examines the social context of nursing, the nature and scope of nursing practice, and specialization in nursing practice. These and other documents can be utilized not only by the nursing profession, but by other health professions, health consumers, and legislators to clarify nursing's role in the health care system.

Since the turn of this century, there has been a need to achieve consensus on a national system of nursing education in order to upgrade and standardize the expected competencies and the educational preparation for each category of nursing practice. Nursing's slow transition into higher education has diminished its standing among other professions. It is the only major health occupation which does not require a minimum of a baccalaureate for entry into practice. Moreover, the tension among nurses over the entry-into-practice issue has, in large measure, weakened nursing's influence in the health care arena.

Numerous studies have pointed to the need for innovation in the educational system. As early as 1923, a study of nursing and nursing education (Goldmark Report) revealed the need to develop and strengthen collegiate schools of nursing in order to keep pace with other professions. In 1948, Brown, in her report to the National Nursing Council, concluded that the term "professional" should only be applied to nursing education provided by schools that were able to furnish professional education as the term had come to be understood by educators. According to Brown, professional schools in most other fields were established within degree-conferring institutions (1948:42–43). As recently as 1970, the National Commission for the Study of Nursing and Nursing Education recommended that (1) hospital schools endowed with a qualified faculty and suitable educational facilities should be encouraged to seek and obtain regional accreditation and degree-granting power, and (2) all other hospital schools of nursing should move systematically to effect arrangements with collegiate institutions.

Fortunately, there have been signs of movement toward implementation of baccalaureate preparation in nursing as entry into professional practice. As a result of greater emphasis on preparation in institutions of higher learning, there has been a gradual increase in the number of baccalaureate programs in nursing and a corresponding growth in the number of graduates of these programs. In 1972 more nurses graduated from collegiate schools of nursing than from hospital programs for the first time in the history of nursing education. In keeping with its 1965 position statement on educational preparation, the ANA House of Delegates, in 1980, adopted guidelines for educational mobility to promote increased accessibility to nursing education programs for individuals seeking academic degrees in nursing. The House also adopted a mechanism for deriving a comprehensive statement of the roles, functions, and competencies of the two categories of nursing practice.

Resolution of the entry-into-practice issue is essential if improvements are to be made in nursing's credentialing system. Credentialing mechanisms provide for public accountability. Their ultimate purpose is to protect the public by establishing standards which qualified practitioners must meet. The effectiveness of any credentialing system rests upon the conceptualization of a basic level of competence in a given occupation and the delineation of various levels of competence as they relate to occupational roles. If this information cannot be measured, the system cannot protect the public from incompetent practitioners. The existence of multiple kinds of basic nursing education programs leading to licensure has created tremendous confusion regarding minimal educational requirements necessary to assure the safe and effective practice of nursing.

The shortcomings of nursing's credentialing system have been compounded by the fact that too many governmental and nongovernmental bodies have been credentialing nurses, nursing education programs, and nursing services without respect to cost, duplication of effort, or apparent gaps in the system. Rather then establishing an effective system for defining and documenting the proficiency of nurses, mechanisms have been developed in isolation from one another, thus creating a complex, fragmented approach to credentialing. As a result, questions and doubts have been raised about nursing's accountability for the public's welfare. Unfortunately, accountability is an essential consideration in evaluation of professional status.

Recently, there have been signs of movement toward delineation of a more coherent, comprehensive system of credentialing. A 22-month study was undertaken in 1977 and 1978 to examine all aspects of credentialing, including accreditation of basic, graduate, and continuing education; accreditation of organized nursing services; certification; and laws that regulate nursing practice. The recommendations and reports from this study were published in a two-volume work, *The Study of Credentialing in Nursing: A New Approach* (1979). Among the study's recommendations is a proposal for a national credentialing center to study, develop, coordinate, provide services for,

and conduct credentialing in nursing [1979 (I): 75-81]. This study and its recommendations are receiving careful scrutiny from the nursing community. A special task force has been established (1) to convene cooperating groups to study and gain acceptance of the study's recommended principles and positions, (2) to educate nurses and the public about the study, and (3) to sponsor a cost-analysis study of credentialing as a basis for developing the fiscal operation of a national credentialing center.

Finally, it must be acknowledged that there has been a need for nursing to achieve greater autonomy. The growing number of nurses and the increased demands for nursing services have not produced a corresponding rise in the profession's power and authority within the health care arena. This is due to the fact that, until recently, nursing has been unable to implement effective arrangements for governance, unable to organize nurses in an effort to achieve greater self-determination and greater influence in decision making and policy making in the planning and delivery of nursing and health care services. As stated earlier, power and authority are a reflection of professional autonomy. The degree of professional autonomy accorded an occupational group depends on the effectiveness of the group's efforts at governance. Without governance, there is no autonomy. Without autonomy, full professional status is unattainable. In light of the significant relationship of governance to professionalization, the remainder of this chapter is devoted to an examination of nursing's drive to achieve governance.

The foremost obstacle in nursing's drive for governance has been the bureaucratic organization of hospitals which prevents nurses from assuming autonomous roles in the delivery of nursing services. Today, approximately 66 percent of all registered nurses are employed by hospitals (McCarty, 1980:6). Hospitals have been the primary employers of nurses since the mid-1930s. It is interesting to note that, prior to the 1930s, the nursing labor force exercised a high degree of autonomy as self-employed private duty nurses. However, during the mid-1930s, the autonomy of private practice gave way to institutional nursing, which was characterized by regimentation, rigid division of labor, and intense supervision. Upon investigating nursing between 1932 and 1946, Wagner reported that "nursing history has been characterized not by a rise in professional autonomy, responsibility, and prestige . . . but by a diminution of independence, increasing stratification and division of labor, and growing revolt against assembly-line conditions (1980:272).

Several authors contend that nurses always have had equity (a stake) in the health care system, but they have not enjoyed parity, that is, equality of power and influence in decision making regarding the care process. Under the traditional hospital hierarchy, the medical staff is recognized as a self-governing body, responsible and accountable to the hospital board of trustees for its professional practice, while the nursing staff bears its primary relationship to the hospital administration. Physicians and administrators alike have shown reluctance to allow any shift in this power structure.

Studies indicate that nursing is a high-stress profession because nurses are delegated significant responsibilities without being accorded the opportunity to influence the many factors which determine the quality of nursing. Wandelt et al. (1981) report that conditions in the structure of hospital organization actually inhibit professional nursing. As a result, conflict arises as "nurses perceive themselves as professionals engaging in nursing practice while administration views them as employees carrying out the jobs of nursing" (Wandelt et al., 1981:76). According to Wandelt, the inability to exercise control over clinical practice produced feelings of career stagnation. This and related factors have caused nurses to leave nursing and remain outside the work force. The end result has been a nurse shortage. The absence of appropriate arrangements for governance has not only contributed to the nurse shortage, it has fostered the growth of supplemental nursing services. A number of problems have been associated with the use of temporary nursing personnel; these problems include the inability to enforce standards and to ensure sustained care of a high quality. If appropriate arrangements for governance were in place, it is likely that the delivery of nursing services could be planned and organized in such a way as to avoid reliance upon nursing personnel from outside sources. Many of the problems associated with the shortage of nurses in the hospital setting (e.g., unrealistic workloads, lack of job satisfaction, and involvement in nonnursing tasks) could be resolved if nurses were in control of nursing.

A second major obstacle in nursing's drive for governance has been the insufficient number of well-prepared leaders in nursing. The divisiveness that exists within the profession and the slow movement on resolution of issues is an indication of this shortcoming. According to Leininger, the nursing profession needs "politically and economically astute leaders who are good risk-takers, fairly aggressive, and adept in using a variety of management and interpersonal strategies" (1974: 29). Leininger contends that mid- and top-level nursing leaders have not been prepared to undertake the confrontation-negotiation style of leadership necessitated by the times (1974:28).

Two requisites of the leadership role in nursing are an understanding of the social, political, and economic influences affecting programs of health care and competence in dealing with problems in the relationships of professional practitioners and those within the complex social system in which nursing operates. Three broad sets of knowledge are needed by the nurse leader: (1) knowledge of nursing and nursing practice, (2) knowledge of the realities inside and outside the organization that affect the accomplishment of purpose, and (3) knowledge of research method and study which can be used to obtain or review data needed to make decisions and to influence others (Aydelotte, 1976:16–17). The effective implementation of mechanisms to facilitate governance depends on skillful management by nursing's leadership.

A third major obstacle in nursing's drive for governance has been the recent push by labor unions, such as the American Federation of Teachers, to add nurses (the largest body of health care workers) to their membership ranks. These groups have launched expensive campaigns to secure the right to represent and bargain for nursing and nurses on all issues. The efforts of these groups have created tension and discord within nursing and, in some instances, hindered the effectiveness of nursing organizations. It is the professional association that is best equipped to represent the professional interests and concerns of nurses. Should more and more nurses grant trade unions the right to speak for them, nursing would ultimately relinquish control of its own affairs.

To be accorded true professional status, nurses at all employment levels and in all patient care settings must participate in determining the terms and conditions of their employment and must share in decision making which affects the quality of nursing care they provide, whether as employees or as self-employed individuals. It is obvious that, in the past, the limitations of nursing's leadership and the absence of appropriate arrangements for governance have prevented such involvement. More recently, nursing's problems have been compounded by the drive of labor unions to secure the right to represent and bargain for nurses. However, in keeping with the movement toward clarification of the scope of practice, standardization of nursing education, and development of a coherent credentialing system, there also have been signs of movement *toward* implementation of arrangements to enhance nursing's role in governance.

Many hospitals across the country are experimenting with various arrangements to strengthen nursing's position on the health care team. Current efforts are aimed at decentralizing the nursing organizational structure in order to increase nurses' control over nursing practice. Ironically, these "innovative" measures are in keeping with basic principles set forth by Florence Nightingale as early as 1860. Nightingale viewed the establishment and operation of a school of nursing and the organization and delivery of nursing services in the hospital as the sole responsiblity of nursing. In the Nightingale system, the matron had final authority for the entire nursing education program as well as the utilization of the hospital's nursing staff. Unfortunately, the authority given the matron in the Nightingale system was never accepted or exercised in the United States. In America's modified Nightingale pattern, this position was regarded as subordinate to a hospital superintendent or some other individual or committee (Notter and Spalding, 1976:14–16).

At the outset of an examination of new and potential arrangements for nursing organization within the hospital setting, it would be wise to delineate some of the desired characteristics of a professional nursing department. Recently, ANA's Commission on Nursing Services set forth a series of 20 such characteristics (1981). Seven of these characteristics are listed below:

- Sufficient autonomy and budgetary control to be able to assume responsibility and accountability for the quality of nursing practice and the outcomes of nursing care
- A system of direct communication with the board of trustees, mechanisms for shared governance, including (1) either contracted agreements bylaws approved by the board of trustees or (2) rules and regulations to provide for clinical privileges and accountability to the governing body and to the patient
- Institutional policies which assure shared responsibility between the institution and the individual nurse for development and maintenance of competence of the practitioners
- A joint practice committee to promote collegial relationships between physicians and nurses
- Full participation of nursing administration, by title and actions, in top-level administrative decision making and with the governing body
- A nursing management information system and other resources to develop and manage plan-

निष्

ning, budgeting, and monitoring quality of nursing care

- A plan (in operation) to maintain and enhance the competence of nurses through promotion strategies, scholarship resources, and continuing education programming (ANA, 1981:4-8)

Recently, greater interest has been shown in the creation of a nursing staff organization which would be comparable in structure and function to the medical staff organization. It is proposed that all registered nurses who practice in the institution, regardless of the means of reimbursement, would be members. The purpose of the nursing staff organization would be to provide advice and recommendations directly to the board of trustees as well as to the hospital administration in matters involving the care of patients. According to Kimbro and Gifford, membership in the nursing staff organization would document "the hospital's recognition of the reality that nurses' legal responsibility for their own practice exists as a separate entity and cannot be assumed by physicians or agents of hospital administration" (1980: 613-614).

In several hospitals across the country, nursing staff bylaws have been adopted. These bylaws set forth rules by which to regulate internal affairs and dealings with other personnel and to govern the nursing staff. They provide the vehicle for nurses to be self-directed and self-governed within a department and within an institution. Establishment of nursing staff bylaws helps to reinforce the idea that the nursing service of a hospital is an organization and the nursing staff is its membership (Carson and Ames, 1980).

At the urging of the National Joint Practice Commission, a number of hospitals also have created joint practice councils to provide a forum for nurse-physician dialogue. Composed of equal representation from nursing and medicine, the purposes of these joint bodies are (1) to review and assist in the resolution of professional practice issues that create conflict between nurses and physicians and (2) to clarify the roles and rela-

tionships between nurses and physicians in providing health care of a high quality. Several sources have reported that the focus of some joint practice councils is evolving from that of conflict resolution to that of a medium for planning and implementing changes (Brunner and Singer, 1979).

Moreover, the application of the concept of primary nursing in some hospitals has reinforced nursing's autonomy, authority, and accountability in these settings. According to Anderson and Choi, in primary nursing emphasis is on "one nurse having professional/organizational autonomy in assuming responsibility and retaining accountability for planning and, when possible, personally administering total care to designated patients throughout their hospitalization" (1980:29). Primary nursing is characterized by decentralized decision making. In effect, each nursing unit becomes autonomous, and each nurse in that unit has a voice in determining what constitutes quality care and what administrative procedures will be developed. Preliminary studies indicate that, where primary nursing is practiced, there is no nurse shortage and the overall quality of care is higher.

All of the measures examined above reflect a significant departure from the traditional nursing organization characterized by centralized authority and a closed communication system. These and similar types of rearrangements are essential if nurses are to experience freedom of practice; if nurses are to collaborate with physicians; if nurses are to control (reasonably) their practice environment. It must be stressed that changes leading to structural rearrangements in the hospital setting must occur at more than one level; such changes must be evident in unit, middle management, and executive levels if they are to have a lasting effect.

There also have been signs of implementation of arrangements to enhance nursing's role in governance in other settings. In the last 10 years, changes have been made in many nurse practice acts in order to place greater emphasis upon the independent practice aspects of nursing. Since 1971, some 15,000 registered nurses have hung out shingles as independent nurse practitioners. Others have formed nursing private practice groups to provide low-cost, prevention-oriented health care services. There also has been a growing acceptance of the concept of nurse practitioners working in concert with physicians. While there is no universally accepted definition of the term "nurse practitioner," it is being used increasingly to refer to an expanded nursing role, e.g., pediatric nurse practitioner. The concept of the expanded role of the nurse implies assumption of more responsibility for delivery of primary health and nursing care and the coordination of preventive services. Moreover, during the 1970s, the National Joint Practice Commission launched a campaign to encourage joint practice in primary care. The commission issued numerous statements expressing the belief that "the provision of primary care to the public is best accomplished by the joint efforts of specially educated nurses and physicians, and that the relationship should be that of colleagues in professional practice, regardless of individual employment status" (National Joint Practice Commission, 1977:2).

Finally, there have been concrete indications that collective action through the professional association has enabled nurses to effect desirable changes within a given employment setting. When handled properly, collective bargaining provides an organized, democratic framework within which nurses, working together in their respective employment situations can develop and agree upon collective goals. Through written agreement, nurses, working together in their respective employment situations, can develop and agree upon conditions of employment. Reports appear routinely in the *American Journal of Nursing* acknowledging the success of nurses in bargaining for the implementation of practice standards and for improvements in general working conditions, as well as for the establishment of equitable compensation systems.

There are several reasons to assume that these trends will continue to gain momentum in the future:

- During the past 20 years, alternations in population characteristics, scientific and technological advancements, changing disease patterns, and diverse life-styles have had a profound impact on the organization of health care services and the scope of practice of health professions. In an attempt to meet the existing and projected demands for health care, a number of study groups have recommended that nurses assume greater responsibility for delivering primary health and nursing care, coordinating services, and promoting continuity of care.
- Since 1965 there have been some dramatic changes in the nursing education system. As more nurses are prepared at the baccalaureate and higher degree levels, they will be better equipped to be held accountable for nursing practice.
- There are indications that nursing's leadership is becoming more sophisticated and more willing to take risks and assume greater responsibility to ensure nursing's professional autonomy.
- In light of the nurse shortage, recruitment and retention of nurses, especially in the hospital setting, are receiving close scrutiny. Numerous studies have indicated that changes are needed in the organization and management structures to alleviate conditions which cause nurses to leave nursing and remain outside the field. Lack of control over nursing practice has been identified as a key factor.
- Currently, the American Nurses Association represents more registered nurses for collective bargaining purposes than all other labor organizations combined. The association is making every effort to ensure that the nursing profession will remain united within the professional association and that the professional association will continue to speak for nursing and nurses.

In conclusion, professionalization is a dynamic process. At the heart of this concept is autonomy within a defined area of practice. It is the author's contention that the degree of professional autonomy accorded an occupational group depends on the effectiveness of the group's efforts at governance. Governance refers to the establishment and maintenance of social, political, and economic arrangements by which practitioners maintain control over their self-discipline, their working conditions, and their professional affairs. These arrangements may take a variety of forms, but regardless of form, they enable a practitioner to have a strong and rightful place in policy making and decision making in the practice setting.

Until recently, nursing has been unable to implement effective arrangements for governance. Fortunately, there has been some experimentation recently with the establishment of such mechanisms as nursing staff bylaws and joint practice councils. In the future, nursing needs to continue to define and test models of governance. It also needs to ensure that nurses will be equipped and prepared to assume the responsibilities implied in the concept of governance. Knowledge is absolutely essential in the domain of governance. There is need for increased knowledge in clinical nursing practice and its delivery. This knowledge must be based on research and clinical investigation and the testing of the application of knowledge to nursing practice and its consequences. Nurses also must acquire knowledge which enables them to analyze power structures and to identify means of access to power centers. They must develop the skills which enable them to discern when certain types of interaction, such as compromise and confrontation, are in order.

EDITOR'S QUESTIONS FOR DISCUSSION

Discuss the characteristics of a profession. Provide examples of the degree to which nursing possesses the characteristics outlined by Shephard, Bixler, and Hall. What has handicapped the development of one or more of those characteristics in nursing? What are other commonly cited characteristics of a profession? Which characteristics are considered essential for a profession? To what extent are the essential characteristics possessed by nursing? Should any one occupational/professional group be subordinate to another? How can parity be developed within and between occupational/professional groups and maintain an autonomous body? To what extent have nurses had equity (a right) in the health care system without parity? How is governance essential to autonomy? Provide examples of governance in other occupational/professional groups. How has the lack of knowledge of the social, political, and economic influences affecting programs of health care contributed to the lack of governance in nursing? What factors have influenced recognizing sufficiently the need for such knowledge in nursing? What factors have contributed to insufficient interest and/or participation in political and legislative activities concerning health care and program and policy development by nurses? Suggest means for promoting the consciousness of that need in nursing.

Trace the history of nursing's desire and attempts to be accorded professional status. What early efforts were initiated and thwarted? What has been the impact and implications for the profession with the ANA being established in 1896 as a means to influence factors impacting upon the delivery of nursing services? Is there any relationship between the earliest efforts of nursing focusing on the delivery of nursing care and the lag in developing a scientific knowledge base for practice? What evidence exists in the previous chapters by contributors that a scientific knowledge base for the profession is being identified and implemented into practice? Discuss the major contributions of the ANA toward achieving professional status. What has been the role of the ANA in clarifying the scope of nursing practice, setting standards of nursing practice and nursing education, and developing policy? What changes have occurred concerning the role and function of the ANA to the present day? What factors influence the degree to which nurses are members of and participate in and contribute to their professional association? What suggestions can be offered to resolve issues concerning nonmembership or nonparticipation? What effect(s) has the continuation of the present trilevel membership structure had on the ANA and the profession? What was the mechanism adopted by the 1980 ANA House of Delegates for deriving roles, functions, and competencies of two categories of nursing practice? What new resolutions would you propose to be addressed at the 1983 ANA convention? Provide a rationale for those resolutions and strategies for acceptance. What outcomes would you predict for the 1983 meeting? How do you foresee the entry into practice issue being resolved?

What relationship exists between Christman's views (Chap. 60) concerning establishing national norms of professional performance to maintain licensure and credentialing? How congruent is credentialing with Rogers's view (Chap. 59) of certification? What is the difference between licensure, certification, and credentialing? How can professional competency validly and reliably be measured? What has been the progress of the task force established as a result of *The Study of Credentialing in Nursing?* What are the significant issues regarding the development of a national credentialing center? Present arguments and rationale for and against the establishment of such a center.

Discuss the obstacles in nursing's drive for governance. Suggest strategies for departments of nursing to achieve parity—equality in the execution of power and influence in decision making. What relationships and comparisons can be made between Aydelotte's discussion of governance and those views expressed by Cleland (Chap. 44), Sills (Chap. 48), Malkemes (Chap. 50), Mercadante (Chap. 51), Murphy (Chap. 55), Fagin and McGivern (Chap. 56), and Baker (Chap. 58)? What are the implications for nursing practice, nursing administration, and the profession concerning Wandelt's findings as to the discrepant perceptions about professional nurses? Provide examples of professional nurses' inability to exercise control over clinical practice resulting in a nurse shortage. Suggest alternatives to correcting these problems. How has divisiveness within the profession prevented the resolution of issues? What factors or conditions contribute to divisiveness? Propose solutions to promote unity. How would divisiveness inhibit the development of appropriate arrangements for governance?

Would you agree that the lack of well-prepared leaders in nursing has been an obstacle for governance? How necessary is a confrontation-negotiation style of leadership today? Compare the requisites and knowledge base, indicated by Aydelotte, for leadership with those suggested by Murphy (Chap. 55) and Fagin and McGivern (Chap. 56). What issues addressed and Editor's Questions for Discussion in those chapters apply to leadership and governance? Compare Aydelotte's view of collective action through the professional association with Baker's (Chap. 58). What issues raised and questions posed for discussion by the editor in Baker's chapter apply to collective bargaining through the professional association? With the ANA representing more registered nurses for collective bargaining than all other labor organizations, how is the ANA making every effort to ensure that the profession will remain united within the association and that the ANA will continue to be the spokesperson for nursing and nurses? What are the predominant issues concerning collective bargaining that may be more effectively dealt with by a professional association bargaining unit than other labor organizations? What are the major purposes of collective bargaining through the professional nursing association? To what extent do nurses perceive collective bargaining through their professional association being related to quality-of-care issues more than governance, "due process," conditions of employment, and/or economic security? Suggest avenues by which misconceptions most effectively may be clarified or conflicts resolved concerning nurses being represented by their professional association for collective bargaining purposes. What other obstacles than those cited by Aydelotte inhibit the development of governance in nursing?

Discuss arrangements to enhance nursing's role in governance. What strategies can a nursing organization employ to implement the 20 desired characteristics of a professional nursing department set forth by the ANA's Commission on Nursing Services? Evaluate your professional nursing department as to the degree seven of the characteristics exist, as listed by Aydelotte. What criteria should be used in prioritizing the implementation of the characteristics? What process has been utilized to establish nursing staff organizations, nursing staff bylaws and joint practice councils/comcittee in hospitals? Discuss the restraining and driving forces in the planning implementation of these mechanisms to enhance nursing's role in governance. What are the most effective strategies for reducing the restraining forces and obtaining the acceptance of these arrangements? How has the concept of primary nursing contributed to nursing governance? What alternative arrangements have been employed and can you suggest to enhance nursing's role in governance in hospitals and other settings?

REFERENCES

American Nurses Association
  1979 The Study of Credentialing in Nursing: A New Approach. Vols. I and II. The report of the committee. Kansas City, Mo.: ANA
  1981 "Organizing structure and management to recruit and retain nurses." Testimony presented to the National Commission on Nursing, February.
Anderson, Marcia and Thomas Choi
  1980 "Primary nursing in an organizational context." Journal of Nursing Administration 10 (March):26–31.
Aydelotte, Myrtle K.
  1976 "The emergence of nursing leadership in the United States." A paper prepared for the King's Fund Seminar of Nurses, July.
Bixler, Genevieve K. and Roy W. Bixler
  1959 "The professional status of nursing." American Journal of Nursing 59 (August): 1142–1146.
Brown, Esther Lucille
  1948 Nursing for the Future. Report prepared for the National Nursing Council. New York: Russell Sage Foundation.
Brunner, Nancy A. and Lillian E. Singer
  1979 "A joint practice council in action."

Journal of Nursing Administration 9 (February):16–20.
Carr-Saunders, A. M.
  1966 "Professionalization in historical perspective." Pp. 3–9 in Howard Vollmer and Donald Mills (eds.), Professionalization. Englewood Cliffs, N.J.: Prentice-Hall.
Carson, Frances E. and Adrienne Ames
  1980 "Nursing staff bylaws." American Journal of Nursing 80 (June):1130–1134.
Goldmark, Josephine
  1923 Nursing and Nursing Education in the United States. New York: Macmillan.
Hall, Catherine M.
  1973 "Who controls the nursing profession? The role of the professional association." Nursing Times 69 (June 7):89–92.
Kinbro, Clara D. and Alice J. Gifford
  1980 "The nursing staff organization: A needed development." Nursing Outlook 28(October: 610–616.
Leininger, Madeleine
  1974 "The leadership crisis in nursing: A critical problem and challenge." Journal of Nursing Administration 4 (March–April): 28–34.
McCarty, Patricia
  1980 "Survey shows a million RNs employed." The American Nurse 12 (October):6.

Merton, Robert K.
  1958 "Issues in the growth of a profession."
       P. 298 in Summary Proceedings of the
       1958 Convention of the American Nurses
       Association. New York: ANA.
National Joint Practice Commission
  1977 "Joint practice in primary care: Defini-
       tion and guidelines." June. Chicago:
       NJPC.
Notter, Lucille E. and Eugenia Kennedy Spalding
  1976 Professional Nursing: Foundations, Per-
       spectives, and Relationships. Philadel-
       phia: Lippincott.
Robb, Isabel Hampton
  1976 "A general review of nursing forces." Pp.
       326–327 in Lyndia Flanagan (comp.),
       One Strong Voice: The Story of the

American Nurses Association. Kansas
City, Mo.: ANA.
Shephard, William
  1948 "The professionalization of public
       health." The American Journal of Public
       Health and The Nation's Health 38
       (January):146.
Wagner, David
  1980 "The proletarianization of nursing in the
       United States, 1932–1946." International
       Journal of Health Services 10 (February):
       271–290.
Wandelt, Mabel A., Patricia M. Pierce, and Robert
  R. Widdowson
  1981 "Why nurses leave nursing and what can
       be done about it." American Journal of
       Nursing 81 (January):72–77.

Chapter 64

Nursing and the Politics of Health

Sister Rosemary Donley, R.N., Ph.D., F.A.A.N.
Dean and Associate Professor
School of Nursing
The Catholic University of America
Washington, D.C.

It is evident from Aydelotte's discourse on governance that access to power centers is a prime requisite to the enhancement of social, political, and economic arrangements by which practitioners maintain control over their practice and professional concerns. So too, nurses are realizing that access is the key in using the political process to influence health legislation and policy development. Sister Rosemary Donley foresees that nurses will strive for more active roles in health legislation, education and reimbursement of nurses, and formulation of policy about planning, delivery, and evaluation of care. She examines the relationships between policy and politics in the health field, traces the impact that nursing has made on the direction of federal policy, and suggests strategies for effective working relationships with policy makers.

The most common evaluative statement regarding the history of nursing activism in political areas is that nurses do not sit at policy tables. Being excluded from the inner circle of decision making, their knowledge is secondhand. Nurses are said to react rather than to initiate. Reasons cited for the status of nurses in the policy area are historical, sociological, religious, and biological. Title VIII of the Public Health Service Act, the Nursing Training Act, is the only federal law which speaks specifically to nursing. Validation of nurses' perceptions of their power and politics in the political arena of legislation and policy may be seen in comparing their influence with other health providers.

Donley uses Parsons's definition of power: the ability to amass resources and direct them toward goal accomplishment. Politics is defined as the sharing of limited resources. Federal health priorities identify three scarce resources: money, personnel, and health services. The espoused goal of health policy is to design a system whereby health personnel and services are equitably distributed and appropriate care is given to the right people at reasonable costs. Donley believes the actual objective is to save federal dollars, decrease federal expenditures for health, and contain health care costs. To demonstrate the tension between policy and politics, Donley portrays the revolution in health care caused by the passage of Medicare and Medicaid Acts as public laws in 1965. A large group of Americans who had lost access to the health care system became eligible and entitled to a wide range of services; physicians were entitled to a fee for service; hospitals were reimbursed for reasonable costs; consumers over 65 developed a new set of expectations. During the same period of time, federal money was appropriated for training of traditional health providers and allied health workers. With the mushrooming of health and social programs since the enactment of Medicare, policy makers in the eighties are faced with inflation in services, costs, workers, technology, and insurance coverage. In addition health and illness care has become more complex with increased expectations and demands for care, particularly for the aged. Donley compares the Johnson and Carter administrations concerning health policy. Policy decisions during Johnson's administration focused on spending money to improve health, i.e., Medicare and Medicaid, with increased funding for research and training of health personnel, whereas the thrust during Carter's administration was to reduce expenditures for the health entitlement legislation, support for research, and develop health professionals to reconcile policy decisions of the two. Democratic policy makers now espouse access to services rather than provision, improving distribution of health personnel instead of increasing personnel, and designing new systems of payment rather than enhancing reimbursement. Given the obligation government has by law to pay for care provided to persons who qualify for the benefit package, Donley maintains it is essential to ask how the dollars for health can be reallocated to preserve the integrity of the public health service programs. She cites four options.

Donley focuses on the cost containment proposals to reduce expenditures for medical and hospital care, and reduction of fraud and abuse. She portrays the tug of war between voluntary hospitals and the administration. The intertwining of power and politics and strategies for working with policy makers is evident. Hospitals entered voluntarily into programs to curtail costs; federal policy strategists lost control of the cost containment agenda. A key factor was the well established connections to members of Congress through representatives from hospitals.

Donley explores the appropriation process in nursing, specifically raising questions concerning the Nurse Training Act and the role of government. Currently, questions about future relationships of the federal government to programs of nursing education are under study by the Institute of Medicine. The nursing shortage has become a major concern of nursing and hospital associations, although Secretary Patricia Harris has insisted that a shortage does not exist. Due to the continued assault on the Nurse Training Act, the nursing lobby has been limited in issues it has addressed. Donley asserts that there is an effect from the fact that nurses are not concerned about health legislation or policy but only about continuing support for nursing education.

She delineates the position of nursing and nurses within the federal hierarchy. Access to the executive level of government is a different experience for nursing. Few nurses have been well placed in policy, social circles or residential complexes with presidents of corporations and leaders in industry and government. Recognizing this phenomenon, remedial action is ongoing. The ANA recommends nurses to federal advisory panels and study sections; congressional fellowships have been sponsored by the ANA and the NLN (National League for Nursing); mentorship has become one way to develop nurses for participation in health policy. However, Donley maintains the absence of an organized system of nursing as more of a constraint to overcome than any other. As a collective, nurses lack a shared identification or socialization process. Nurses do not agree on the essence of a professional education and practice in a schizophrenic pattern of relationships. The internal confusion continues to surface each time the nursing lobby tries to organize a constituency, e.g., the debate concerning the position of the Nurse Training Act.

Donley perceives the key to a position of influence in society is linked to the advancement of women in nursing, religious, economic, and social spheres. Entrance of nurses into the policy arena is a significant part of a social movement. She urges nurses, who aspire to participate in health policy decisions, to analyze their personal and corporate assets, and examines the credentials of those with whom they will work and compete. Career patterning and development is essential for success. Donley likens policy development to the nursing process: policy is to legislation as planning and evaluation are to assessment and implementation. For the nursing community to engage in legislative activity, policy analysis is a prerequisite to long-term success.

In recent years there has been a growing awareness among nurses of the effects of government intervention in health care. Interest in health policy has been cultivated in the nursing community. As a result nurses strive for more active roles in health legislation and policy development. No longer are they satisfied to "write to Congress" about a particular bill or regulation. Some, who have undertaken serious study of the policy implications of federal health laws of the past decade, want to develop legislative initiatives. This chapter is dedicated to those nurses who are interested in health policy as a field of study or research. In the future more nurses will use the political process to influence federal support for the education and reimbursement of nurses. They will also formulate policy about planning, delivery, and evaluation of care. Consequently it is important to examine systematically the relationships between policy and politics in the health field; to trace the impact which nursing has made on the direction of federal policy; and to suggest strategies for working effectively with policy makers.

The words *power* and *politics* are familiar to anyone who reads contemporary nursing literature. These terms are used in discussions about the place and role of nursing in hospitals and academic institutions as well as in discussions of local elections or legislative activity. Usually nurses are presented in the literature as disenfranchised and angry (Ashley, 1980). The history of nursing's covert activity in health policy areas gives the same

impression (Davis and Maraldo, 1980). The evaluative statement in most analyses of nurse activism in the political areas is that nurses do not sit at policy tables. They are excluded from the inner circles of decision making. Consequently their knowledge base is always secondhand and inferential. Nurses are said to react rather than initiate. They "wait and see" rather than advance their programs. They respond to ideas rather than set the agenda. The reasons given for the status of nurses in the policy area are historical, as in, "Who signed the Declaration of Independence?"; sociological, as in, "Woman's place is in the home"; religious, as in the story of Adam and Eve; biological, as in the traditional idea that most nurses are women, ergo, they feel rather than think.

If one moves beyond the commentaries and examines, for example, the compendium of laws in the Public Health Service Act, it is difficult to identify in public law the word "nurse" or that professional activity called "nursing service," "nursing practice," or "nursing care" (Government Document, 1977c). In fact Title VIII of the Public Health Service Act, the Nursing Training Act, is the only federal law which speaks specifically to nursing (Wehr, 1980). Given the direction of the Ninety-sixth Congress, it seems that this title will soon disappear from the listing of health titles even in the Public Health Service Acts. For if support for nursing education survives the authorization, appropriations, rules, and recession processes of the Ninety-sixth Congress, it will be just one section of a comprehensive occupational training bill for doctors of medicine, osteopathy, podiatry, veterinary medicine, optometry, and dentistry (the MOD-VOP legislation) (Government Document, 1976a).

Another way of charting or validating nurses' perceptions of their power and politics in the health field is to trace nursing's influence on legislation and policy in comparison with that of other well-known providers such as physicians and hospitals. This academic exercise reveals a pessimistic view of the importance of nursing on the health agenda. Another, and perhaps less frustrating exercise is to look at the prevailing directions in health policy formulation and to suggest political strategies for the future.

What are the national priorities for health? A cursory reading of the federal priorities for health suggests a familiar refrain of improving access to health services, decreasing costs, and improving the distribution of health personnel (Rushmer, 1980). These goals are familiar to any student of health policy. They are worthy of examination, however, in this framework because they speak to the important theme of politics and power in the health care area. *Power*, according to Parsons (1960:181), is the ability to amass resources and direct them toward goal accomplishment. *Politics* is the sharing of limited resources (Donley, 1979). Federal health priorities identify three scarce resources: money, personnel, and health services.

It becomes important to examine the relationship between politics and policy within the federal government. The stated (or espoused) goal of health policy is to design a system whereby health personnel and services are equitably distributed and appropriate care is given to the right people at reasonable costs. This lofty goal, which requires power and political acumen, seems to be beyond the reach of the public and private sector. What, then, is the practical goal, or as Argyris (1976:21) would say, the theory of practice? The real objective of health policy, I believe, is to save federal dollars, to decrease federal expenditures for health, and to contain health care costs. The purported

difference between what is stated as the espoused policy and what seems to be the actual policy (policy in use) deserves attention in any discussion about the tension between policy and politics. As the federal government struggles to achieve a balance among trained personnel, people in need, health services, technological advances, and costs, it encounters an inheritance of policy and political decisions. The legacy worthy of greatest attention was the passage of Medicare and Medicaid acts which became public laws in 1965. Medicare and Medicaid, Titles XVIII and XIX of the Social Security Act, caused a revolution in health care. People over 65 and those who qualified for medical assistance became entitled by law to a health care package. Under the Medicare program, people who had lost the protection of health insurance benefits when they retired became eligible again for a variety of hospital-based services. The Medicare provision which stated the reimbursement for care would be given if the person over 65 were treated in a semiprivate room had an immediate effect on hospital construction. Medicare, with its unattainable promise of 100 days posthospital care, gave great impetus to the nursing home industry and encouraged the development of a variety of home nursing programs (Somers, 1967; Government Document, 1977a).

In short, a group of Americans who had lost access to the health care system were eligible and entitled to a wide range of services. Physicians who gave care to the Medicare beneficiary were entitled to a fee for service, and hospitals came to be reimbursed after a retrospective review for reasonable costs. In this instance a new group of consumers (those over 65) entered existing facilities with a new set of expectations. In this same period the federal government also spent billions of dollars in the training of health personnel. Money went to the traditional providers (doctors, dentists, and nurses). However, the initiation of care also offered a provision for the reimbursement of physicians in training. New federal money was invested in the education of medical professionals. During these years new money was appropriated to prepare a host of allied health workers (Government Document, 1977d). In this period of the Great Society a large number of health and social programs were set in place.

In the years since the enactment of Medicare the incremental changes in this program have been additive. Consequently in the eighties policy makers face existing programs which have become more elaborate and expensive as a result of inflation, the increase in the number and preparation of health workers, new technology, improved services, and the high level of insurance coverage (Government Document 1977d). Accompanying this has been a growing sophistication in the care of the aging and the application of complex surgical and medical interventions to their disease states. This has had the impact of increasing public expectations about the treatment of the aging and intensifying the demand for care. Upon examination, the development in health care expenditures in the first 10 years of Medicare resemble a growth curve. In 1965, for example, total health care expenditures were $38.9 million. These expenditures accounted for 5.9 percent of the gross national product (GNP), and $2.8 million of the total amount was spent by the federal government. In 1975, the total bill for health was $118.5 billion. The federal contribution was $28.6 billion and 8.3 percent of the GNP was expended for health (Government Document, 1976b:2). Examined from another perspective, in the period from 1965 to 1978 expenditures for hospital care increased from $13.9 to $76 billion. During the same years expenditures for health care rose at a rate 1.5 times higher in the public sector than in the private sector in the same period (Freedland et al., 1980:12).

In reviewing the direction of programs started in the Johnson administration, it seems that the thrust of policy decisions was to spend federal money to improve health. This was accomplished through dramatic increases in spending for research and in increased expenditures for the training of health personnel. The most significant change, however, was the inauguration of a wide spectrum of health and socially oriented programs. The most notable of these was Medicare. The present-day outcomes of these decisions challenge the contemporary policy maker. It is generally conceded that it is almost impossible to eradicate a federal program. How then, in a more conservative age, can the Congress or the administration curtail and contain the burgeoning health care system and simultaneously achieve some rapprochement between the provision of service and people in need of care?

Modern health policy, viewed from the perspective of health financing, does not seem that dissimilar from the motivation of the Johnson administration. There is, of course, a dramatic difference in outcome. Where Johnson advocated expenditure of federal dollars for health, Carter era democrats wished to reduce the dollars to be expended to purchase health care services, to reduce support for biomedical and nursing research, and to decrease spending to develop health professionals. Whereas policy in the Johnson administration was a set of decisions to spend money for health, policy under Carter was a set of decisions to withhold or limit federal dollars for health. What are the political consequences of this policy direction? Phrased another way, how does one reconcile a policy decision to withhold support with political expectations of traditional Democratic voters such as the aged, the minorities, and the poor? One uses the language of the sixties with a different emphasis. For example, policy makers now espouse access to services rather than provision of services, improving the distribution of health personnel rather than increasing their supply, and designing new systems of payment rather than enhancing the reimbursement of services. The end that is achieved is that the policy issues and goals remain the same while the means actualizing the goals are altered radically. It is a case of being idealistic about the ends but pragmatic about the means.

If the Johnson era could be described as the seven fat years, the present period can be symbolized as the seven lean ones. Given this vision, it is not surprising that one major thrust of the

Carter administration was to reduce expenditures for the health entitlement legislation. Given the nature of the entitlement which supports Medicare and Medicaid, the government is obligated by law to pay for care that has been rendered to persons who qualify for the benefit package. Consequently, as the costs of medical and hospital care have escalated, the federal government has found that increasing shares of the health budget are being engulfed by Medicare and Medicaid. When Theodore Cooper was the Secretary of Health, Education, and Welfare, he noted, before a Senate committee, that Medicare and Medicaid were growing at annual rates in excess of 15 percent. He estimated in 1976 that the costs of the programs would soon equal the entire Public Health Service budget—a budget which supports research, personnel training, resource development, direct services, and formula and grant programs (Freedland et al., 1980:12). Cooper was prophetic. If dollars for health are limited and Medicare and Medicaid consume more health dollars each year, it is essential to ask how the dollars for health can be reallocated so that public health service programs are not sacrificed to the consuming capacity of Medicare and Medicaid. How can the integrity of the public health service programs be preserved?

It seems the options are restricted: repeal Medicare and Medicaid laws; change the financing of the programs by disassociating these programs from the Social Security System; control and contain expenditures for medical and hospital care; reduce fraud and abuse. The Carter administration opted for the third and fourth alternatives. In fact, the major health initiative of the Carter administration was the struggle to advance cost containment legislation (Inglehart, 1977). The rise and fall of cost containment proposals captivated the Ninety-sixth Congress during its first session. The program, which was proposed to reduce the federal burden of Medicare and Medicaid payments, was focused on the voluntary hospitals. In retrospect, this is not remarkable. The hospital is the most visible structure in the health service setting. It is the amphitheater for the gathering of a vast array of health technology, the temple of computerized axial tomography. Hospitals receive a sizable slice from the Medicare-Medicaid budget and the "hospital day" is generally acknowledged to be a well-defined expensive category in the reimbursement formula (Government Document, 1976b:3). When reasoning from a policy framework, hospital cost containment made sense.

The concern with fraud and abuse in Medicare and Medicaid programs had its roots in the political environment of a post-Watergate Congress. Coupled with the public interest in identifying those who misused public funds was the desire to manage federal programs more efficiently. The existence of the information which had been developed for the management of Medicare-Medicaid gave federal investigators the technical access to audit records at will. Investigative activity creates an energy and life of its own. Certain abusers are identified, embarrassed, and punished. Some are frightened into more careful practices. Others are discouraged from ever manipulating the system. The bottom line of these efforts is that some money is saved. The significant savings, however, occur during the investigation because new programs are not initiated. The Congress is doing something in the public interest. Oversight and evaluation are substituted for authorization and appropriations. In the case of legislative and executive initiatives against fraud and abuse, the policy direction was clear and coherent (Government Document, 1977b). As was noted earlier, the political climate was supportive of investigative activity. The anti-fraud and abuse legislation also supported efforts to reduce federal spending through efficient management. Pursuit of this option by the Carter administration illustrates good policy and good politics.

What happened when hospital cost containment legislation came to town, however, provides a view of the "flip side" and gives increased credibility to the underlying theme of the interrelationship between politics and policy in the field of health legislation. The controversy evoked by the "hospital cap legislation," as the bill came to be known, was a tug of war between the voluntary hospitals and the administration. Although everyone agreed that the reduction of health care costs was a desirable goal, hospital officials vehemently opposed the decision to apply arbitrarily the cap to hospitals. They argued too that hospitals could accomplish voluntarily what the government wished to mandate—cost containment. As the debates continued labor unions joined with the hospitals in protesting the proposed cap. They contended that the cap would result in a wage freeze for the ancillary hospital workers who were already at the bottom of the economic ladder. Eventually the powerful lobby of the hospital association defeated and discredited the cap motion as fiscally simplistic, unnecessary, and detrimental to care (Report, 1980). As the drama developed in the media and before the committees of Congress, the operative principles of access to policy makers and organization of efforts and ideas became manifest. Jones (1977:32-34) speaks to these factors as essential for bringing and keeping an idea before the Congress or administration. With cost containment, they became successful strategies for removing an idea from the legislative agenda.

Access is the key to bringing a message to the policy makers. It means in practice that those who are informed on the issue have the opportunity to tell their story in the right setting. Hospital executives and fiscal managers possess high levels of technical knowledge about the management of hospitals. They are often the single source of information about the hospital industry. Hospitals are important to the development of a community. As a result of the Hill-Burton legislation few congressional districts are without a hospital. In rural areas, hospitals are major sources of employment as well as the sole source of institutional health care. For all these reasons, representatives from hospitals have well established networks to members of Congress. In this case the organized hospital lobbies were able to use their presence in local communities and their contact "on the hill" to bring their message before the Congress. From the beginning of the debate, the hospital association

was certain that the cost containment proposal was not in the best interests of the hospitals or the public. They had strong internal consensus on this issue. Documentation and defense of this position developed later. Other groups, such as the labor unions, were helped to see that the passage of a cost containment law would jeopardize the interests of their constituencies. The issue was further expanded as the hospital industry reached out to others with an interest in the financial operation of hospitals: suppliers, designers of hospital technologies, pharmaceutical manufacturers, organized medicine, and nursing. In the attack on the hospital cost containment bill, ideas and constituencies were well organized.

The hospital lobby also executed a political coup as hospitals around the country entered voluntarily into programs to curtail costs. The federal policy strategists found that they had lost control of the cost containment agenda. Voluntary cost containment programs supplanted the major health initiative of the administration.

It is not surprising to learn that policy and politics are intertwined in other efforts to reduce federal spending for health. As has been noted earlier in this chapter, the federal dollar for health is unequally divided between the entitlement programs and other health programs. When the Carter administration failed to control or reduce spending for the "uncontrollable" components in the health budget, the entitlement programs, they turned serious attention to the research and personnel budgets. These programs are more accessible to the Congress and the administration. Authorized for specified periods and reviewed yearly in the budgetary and appropriation processes, both medical and nursing research and personnel programs have come under intense scrutiny in the past several years. In the case of nursing, funding for the nursing educational programs has been provided through the Nurse Training Act. In recent years, support for the program has been threatened. Funds have been impounded by Nixon, vetoed by Ford, and subjected to pocket veto and a chain of recommendations to delete and rescind budgetary outlays by Carter. The funds for nursing research have been treated similarly. The major policy issue which has been raised in discussions about the Nurse Training Act is the question of the role of government. Is government intervention essential in the support of nursing education? Has the Nurse Training Act achieved its goal? Are the questions of nurse supply and distribution best addressed by support for nursing education? The question raised about nursing research is more basic: What is it? How is it different from medical research? Currently, under congressional mandate questions about future relationships of the federal government to programs of nursing education are under study by the Institute of Medicine.

The political implications of the attack on the nurse training program are difficult to tease into perspective. It seems that the nursing lobby has found a more sensitive hearing with the legislative branch of government. It also appears that repressive efforts by several administrations have been directed toward nursing more than medicine. The political image which has been synthesized and sustained in the history of the nurse personnel debates is the concept of shortage. This issue was raised provocatively by the former Secretary of Health, Education, and Welfare, Joseph Califano (1978). He suggested that there were too many nurses. Citing teachers as a profession in which there was an evident oversupply, Califano quipped that if the federal government continued to support the training of nurses, nurses would soon be on the bread lines. These words were a battle cry for the nursing community. The Nurse Training Act developed around a different statement of a chief officer for health. The act developed from the surgeon general's study which indicated that the number of nurses graduating from programs was significantly too few to meet the nation's need for nursing care. Since 1964 federal money has been made available to students and to schools of nursing (Thompson, 1972). Evaluation studies have demonstrated a steady growth in the numbers of students who graduated

from schools of nursing over the years (Government Document, 1978). Secretary Califano's data did not match the perceptions or the real-world experiences of hospital administrators, nursing service directors, and nurses in practice (Special AJN Report, 1979).

In the time since Califano's controversial statements, the nursing shortage has become a major concern of nursing and hospital associations. In the summer of 1980 the Health and Longterm Care Subcommittee of the House Select Committee on Aging held hearings on the effect of the nursing shortage on the elderly. However, as the hospital and nursing collective has struggled with unfilled positions and turnover of nurses, the administration has remained firm in its unwillingness to continue support for nursing education. Rather, it has addressed itself to encouraging such programs as medication courses for unlicensed personnel and supporting nurse-practitioner programs. Patricia Harris, who succeeded Joseph Califano as the Secretary of Health, Education, and Welfare, now the Department of Health and Human Services, insisted that a shortage does not exist (1980). She agreed that the inability of hospitals to find nurses is secondary to nurses' leaving active practice for more desirable or lucrative employment. Whether one uses the oversupply explanation of Califano or dropout analogy of Harris, the administration remained firm in its position to withdraw support from nurse training. Interest in nursing research has also been tenuous.

Through its various struggles with the administration over the value of the Nurse Training Act, the nursing lobby found a friend in Congress. The American Nurses Association successfully defeated vetoes, recessions, and impoundment. However, these victories have a price. Repeated federal efforts to alter the funding for nurse training and research have evoked a repetitive response from the American Nurses Association. As a consequence of responding to the continued assault on the Nurse Training Act, the nursing lobby has been limited in the issues it has addressed. Energy, budget, and personnel have been diverted to one policy issue. The lobby realizes that it becomes increasingly difficult to arouse passion about an issue that is constantly on the agenda.

Another unfortunate but understandable spin-off of nursing's preoccupation with the personnel legislation is facing the accusation of self-interest (Isaacs, 1980). In this critique nurses are presented as "Johnny one-notes"—persons interested in one issue. There is some truth in this accusation; nurses are interested in the Nurse Training Act. However all special interest groups have, by definition, special interests. A survey of the existing legislation reveals that nursing has only one law which it seeks to protect. The intensity with which this law and the concept of federal support for nursing education have been debated has effectively aroused more than ordinary protective behavior. However the criticism carries with it the implication that nurses are not concerned about health legislation or policy but only about their single interest—continuing support for nursing education.

Perhaps the most critical dilemma facing nursing can be understood within the context of access and organization. It is generally accepted that nurses as individuals and nursing as an organization have access to the Congress. Compared with hospital and medical groups the lobby is under-developed and minimally financed. It remains effective, despite these limitations, because of the number of nurses and the *credat emptor* attitude which prevails on the Hill.

Access to the administration, however, is a very different experience. As is evident in this discussion, the viewpoints of nursing and the attitude of the executive branch diverge on the issue of continuing the role of the federal government in nursing education. If the concept of access is linked to voice and vote—that is, a visible verbal presence at the right time and place, it is important to pause and reexamine the position of nursing and nurses within the federal hierarchy. Few nurses are well placed in policy circles. Nurses sit as experts in the Division of Nursing, in the Alcohol, Drug Abuse and Mental Health Agency (ADAMHA), and in the Public Health Service. However nurses

are not members of the domestic policy staff, the upper echelon of the Health Care Financing Administration (HCFA), or the policy staff of the Secretary of Health and Human Services. Physicians operate in these areas.

Moreover the financial social status of physicians places them in social and residential complexes with presidents of corporations and leaders in industry and government. Since Washington is a town where business is conducted at social gatherings as well as in caucus rooms, the presence of physicians at private clubs and elite receptions places them in advantageous positions to raise their viewpoints. The Women's Movement has certainly enhanced the mobility of women. However inflation has had a dampening effect on social change. The unstable economy has made those who sit in positions of influence less willing to expand the circle or abdicate their places. It is a period when those who have power struggle to retain it. Then, too, nurses are seen as dependent semiprofessionals. Employed in institutions, limited by state law in their scope of practice, uncommitted to a career, salaried and undereducated, the average nurse is not a peer of the physician, industrialist, or administrator. All these factors mediate against access to the executive level of government. This phenomenon is recognized within the nursing community.

Remedial action is ongoing. An "old girls network" is developing within nursing. The American Nurses Association has assumed a proactive role in recommending nurses to federal advisory panels and to study sections. Congressional fellowships have been sponsored by the American Nurses Association and the National League for Nursing. Mentorship has become a fashionable activity among nursing's elite (Vance, 1979). A group of Washington- and New York-based nurses has organized a Washington Round Table. Its mission is to develop nurses for participation in health policy.

More difficult to overcome than the demographic and sexual constraints highlighted under the heading of access to policy makers is the absence of an organized system of nursing. Nurses face tragic sequelae from their struggle to professionalize. As a collective, nurses lack a shared experience of socialization or identification. They are yet to achieve the autonomy which flows from professional definition.

Physicians, on the other hand, graduate from college and medical school. They complete an internship and many pursue a residency in a specialized field of study. Although there may be academic disputes about credit distribution in premedical and medical education, no one argues that physicians can be trained on the job or that hospitals should define the curriculum in medical schools. Physicians agree that the doctor-patient relationship is sacred. They believe in the autonomy of the physician. They support, with vigor, the right of the physician to practice medicine and protect the fee-for-service model of reimbursement. Certainly the medical community has agnostics and heretics. However there is an amazing degree of faith in the creed of the American Medical Association on the issues of physician authority, autonomy, and compensation.

As is evident in the confusion occasioned by the 1985 proposal of the American Nurses Association, nurses do not agree on the essence of a professional education (Zarett, 1980). Most nurses who practice in institutional settings engage in a schizophrenic pattern of relationships with physicians, hospital administrators, nursing administrators, and patients. Lines of responsibility and accountability are blurred. It is practically impossible for a group of nurses to establish a nursing practice. Medical and nurse practice acts, the cost of malpractice insurance, and third-party reimbursement schemata confine this model of practice to risk takers. The public sees nurses within the framework of the acute care hospital. The internal confusion within nursing usually surfaces when the nursing lobby tries to organize a constituency. The debate about the future governmental support for nursing education has provoked new evidence that nursing is still a house divided against itself. This is unfortunate because it did seem that nurses

had achieved consensus around the Nurse Training Act.

In the late days of President Carter's administration, this agreement began to disintegrate. The shortage debate polarized nurses, physicians, and hospital administrators. In some rhetoric it appeared that the nursing shortage was a direct outcome of federal support for nursing education. Illustrative of this view is a study commissioned by the Division of Health Manpower, Department of Health and Human Services. This study will examine the effects which the Nurse Training Act has achieved upon the "mix and match": Do nurses who are educated in Schools of Nursing have the ability and skill to work in hospitals, ambulatory care settings, and long term care units?

In some areas, baccalaureate education is held accountable for the closure of the hospital-based school and by extension the nursing shortage. Senator (now Health and Human Services Secretary) Schweiker, in a bill introduced in the Senate in late 1979 proposed that those schools of nursing which gave evidence of hospital-based clinical training for students should qualify for federal support (Government Document 1979). In fact, the position of the Nurse Training Act toward 2-, 3-, and 4-year students has been neutral. Schools within each category have qualified for support. Increasingly, in newsletters of local hospital associations there is a bias toward reopening diploma schools. The American Nurses Association, on the other hand, insists that the baccalaureate degree in nursing is the criterion for entrance into practice. This example of disorganization within nursing and its community of interest around the solitary nursing issue on the federal agenda places, in bold relief, the problem that nurses face in authoring their destiny.

How can nurses better manage their own agenda and place it on the policy table? The analysis in this chapter seems to suggest that the key to access to position of influence in society is irrevocably linked to the advancement of women, not just in nursing, but in religious, economic, and social spheres. This is not to argue that nurses should wait until other women succeed. It is a statement that the entrance of nurses into the policy arena is not an isolated happening but rather a significant part of a social movement. If nurses wish to participate in decisions about the allocation of resources, an analysis of personal and corporate assets is imperative. In the area of health policy it is important to examine the credentials of those with whom nurses will cooperate and compete.

Career patterning and development are orientations by professionals. Vance (1977) in her study of nursing influentials, found that successful nurses were career-oriented, academically certified, and assisted by others as they developed in their profession. However these qualities were attributed to a relatively small number of nurses. What is atypical behavior must become normative if nurses are to win the right to participate in policy deliberations. In its education, and to some degree its practice, nursing is moving from a crisis orientation. It is generally recognized that preventive activity, although somewhat difficult to document, is more effective than treatment or rehabilitation.

Work at the level of policy is a form of prevention. In addition to nurse activism in the world of legislation and regulation, the epidemiology of health policy requires that some nurses take a view from backstage. Less stimulating and less frenetic than the world of the House and the Senate, the work of policy development is analytic and evaluative. Phrased within the framework of the nursing process as defined by Yura and Walsh (1973), policy is to legislation as planning and evaluation are to assessment and implementation. As the nursing community mobilizes to engage in legislative activity, it is imperative to underline the significance of policy analysis as an essential prerequisite to long-term success.

EDITOR'S QUESTIONS FOR DISCUSSION

What factors have influenced nurses striving for more active roles in health legislation and policy development? How does Sills (Chap. 42) view the political activism of nurses? Is there a trend developing by nurses to advance their programs rather than to "wait and see"? Provide examples for your response. In light of Christman's predictions of fewer differences between the education of health professionals and evolvement of multidisciplinary teams in primary nursing, how likely is it that reimbursement of nurses for practice will continue to be an issue for federal support? What type of policies might nurses be influential in formulating regarding planning, delivery, and evaluation of care? Compare nursing's influence on health legislation and policy with such other health providers as physicians and hospitals; what have been nursing's contributions? What constraints have been evident for nurses? How have nurses and the profession responded to the constraints? What alternative responses can be suggested and/or encouraged? How are federal health priorities established? What influence should nurses and nursing have on the identification of priorities and allocation of resources?

Discuss the impact of Medicare and Medicaid on society, the consumer, and the professions. What have been the advantages and disadvantages of these acts which became public laws? What has been the impact on the quality of care provided to the elderly? What set of expectations evolved by consumers? What effect has Medicare had on nursing homes, the hospice movement, and home health programs? How can the integrity of public health service programs be preserved, while maintaining the government's obligation by law to support Medicare and Medicaid? How effective has been the option of voluntary cost containment by hospitals?

What are the implications for society, the consumer, and the health professions regarding differences between espoused policies and actual policy? What obligations and/or responsibilities do health professionals have to the consumer and the professions regarding discrepancies between the ideal and practical goal in providing care? What differences are there in health policy statements, formulation, and expenditure between the administrations of Johnson, Carter, and Reagan? As Donley has examined previous administrations, do you foresee differences between espoused and actual health policy in the Reagan administration? Indicate the rationale for your response. To what extent do you foresee the health policy issues and goals remaining the same but the means to achieving these goals being greatly altered? What health policies do you predict will be developed in the future? What are the ethical considerations essential in development of health policy? What role do you foresee for nurses and nursing in the development of those policies? What outcomes do you predict for health policies developed within the next 10 years? What are the critical variables related to outcomes of health policy?

What applications can be made to nursing as a profession concerning the organization of constituencies to attack the hospital cost attainment bill? Provide examples in nursing as a profession where policy and politics are intertwined? What have been the strategies utilized? How successful were the strategies in achieving a desired goal? To what extent was there difficulty in organizing as a collective? What factors, in addition to those cited by Donley, inhibit unification of nursing concerning a major issue? What are the issues of concern in the debate within nursing, pertaining to future governmental support for nursing education? How can the bias, indicated by Donley, of local hospital associations toward reopening diploma schools most effectively be addressed? Respond to Donley's queries regarding the role of government and the Nurse Training Act. What representation exists from the nursing profession on the research team for the study being conducted by the Institute of Medicine concerning the federal government and programs of nursing education? What are the political and professional implications for nursing as a profession concerning the qualifications of the research investigators, methodology utilized, and interpretation of data? How willing is the present administration to continue support for nursing education? What response might be offered to those who insist a shortage of professional nurses does not exist? What evidence is available to support your response? Refer to the chapters by Braito and Caston (27) and Aydelotte (61) for factors related to a nursing shortage. How true is the inference that nurses are not concerned about health legislation or policy but only about continuing support for nursing education? Provide examples of the successful lobbying by nurses and the ANA?

What additional factors mediate against access of nurses to the executive level of government? What alternative strategies can be suggested for entry into the field of health policy? In addition to factors cited by Donley, what variables contribute to differences between medicine and nursing when trying to organize a constituency to lobby? What factors mitigate against the development of a collective identification by nurses? Provide examples, as suggested by Donley, that nursing is still a house divided against itself. What underlies the basis for the division and/or divisiveness within nursing? Suggest strategies for decreasing the division and capitalizing on the collective strength of the profession. Provide examples of issues where nursing as a profession was or is united. How is the entrance of nurses into the policy arena a significant social movement? What are the implications for the profession, other professions, and society in this movement? How might career patterning and development prepare professional nurses for success in policy analysis? What personal and educational qualifications and preparation may be most enabling in the field of health policy? Should health policy and analysis be a subspecialty or specialty in professional nursing education programs? At what level in professional education might this field of study be incorporated in a curriculum?

REFERENCES

Argyris, Chris and Donald Shon
1976 Theory in Practice: Increasing Professional Effectiveness. Washington, D.C.: Jossey-Bass.

Ashley, JoAnn
1980 "Power in structured misogyny: Implications for the politics of care." Advances in Nursing Science 2 (April):3–22.

Califano, Joseph
1978 Informal Statement. February 4.

Davis, Carolyne and Pamela Maraldo
1980 "Who determines health manpower policy." Nursing and Health Care 1 (July–August):27–33.

Donley, Sr. Rosemary
1979 "A nurse's experience in Washington." Journal of the Association of Operating Room Nurses 29 (July): 1270–1283.

Freedland, Mark, George Calat and Carol Ellen Schendler
1980 "Projections of national health expenditures, 1980, 1985, 1990." Health Care Financing Review 1 (Winter):1–117.

Government Documents
1976a Health Professions Educational Assistance Act of 1976 (PL 94-484). Washington: U.S. Government Documents Office.
1976b "Inflation of Health Care Costs, 1976." Hearings before the Subcommittee on Labor and Public Welfare, United States Senate, Ninety-fourth Congress. Washington: U.S. Government Printing Office.
1977a "Medicare-Medicaid." Washington: Library of Congress Congressional Research Service.
1977b Medicare-Medicaid Anti Fraud and Abuse Amendments (PL 95-142). Washington, D.C.: Government Documents Office.
1977c "Public Laws Under the Jurisdiction of the House of Representatives Committee on Interstate and Foreign Commerce." Washington, D.C.: U.S. Government Printing Office.
1977d Special Analysis K: Federal Health Progress. Washington, D.C.: U.S. Office of Management and Budget.
1978 First Report to the Congress, Feburary, 1977, Nurse Training Act of 1975. Washington, D.C.: U.S. Department of Health Education and Welfare, publication #78-38.
1979 The Health Professions Educational Assistance and Nurse Training Act (S2144). United States Senate, 96th Congress. Washington, D.C.: U.S. Government Printing Office.

Harris, Patricia
1980 Informal Statement. March 6.

Inglehart, John
1977 "And now it's Carter's turn to try to control costs." National Journal 9 (April 9): 551–556.

Isaacs, Marion
1980 "Nurse political action: Interview with Marge Colloff." Advances in Nursing Science 2 (April):89–95.

Jones, Charles
1977 An Introduction to the Study of Public Policy. Massachusetts: Duxbury Press.

Parsons, Talcott
1960 Structure and Process in Modern Societies. Glencoe, Ill.: The Free Press of Glencoe.

Report
1980 "Nelson drops fight to pass hospital cost control bill." Hospital Week 16:1–4.

Rushmer, Robert
1980 National Priorities for Health: Past, Present and Projected. New York: Wiley.

Special AJN Report
1979 "Nursing shortage? Yes!" American Jour-

nal of Nursing 79 (March):469–480.

Somers, Herman and Anne Somers
  1967 Medicare and the Hospitals: Issues and
         Prospects. Washington, D.C.: The Brook-
         ings Institute.

Thompson, Julia
  1972 The ANA in Washington. Kansas City:
         The American Nurses Association.

Vance, Connie
  1977 "A Group Profile of Contemporary In-
         fluentials in American Nursing." Unpub-
         lished doctoral dissertation. New York:
         Teachers College, Columbia University.

  1979 "Women leaders: Modern day heroines or
         societal deviants?" Image 11 (June):
         37–41.

Wehr, Elizabeth
  1980 "Committees retool health professions
         aid." Congressional Quarterly 38 (July 5):
         1882–1884.

Yura, Helen and Mary Walsh
  1973 The Nursing Process. Englewood Cliffs,
         N.J.: Prentice-Hall.

Zarett, Anita
  1980 "Is the BSN better?" RN 41 (March):
         28–33, 78.

Chapter 65

Changing Perspectives on Health Care

Rosalee C. Yeaworth, R.N., Ph.D., F.A.A.N.
Dean and Professor
College of Nursing
University of Nebraska Medical Center
Omaha, Nebraska

The significance of health policy, policy analysis, and political influence, as delineated by Donley, grows as one reflects on the past and plans for the role of the nursing profession within the future health care delivery system. Rosalee C. Yeaworth captures the essence of the past to project and offer a promising and refreshing perspective for nursing and the future of health care. She reviews the changes in health care through the years, assesses the results, analyzes the climate and concerns of the 1980's, discusses the influence changing perspectives will have on nursing and offers a challenging role in the future of nursing. She emphasizes that changes in perspectives, plans, and institutions will increase the importance of political influence.

Yeaworth cites the rapid advances in knowledge and technology, and major changes in attitudes, values, and beliefs concerning health and care. A reverence for physicians, hospitals, and miracle drugs occurred prior to the 1970s with rising expectations in care. During the 1970s, life expectancy increased, infant mortality was reduced, and intensive care units and trauma centers were introduced. There were also significant problems, such as skyrocketing health care expenditures, reports of higher death rates in areas concentrated with physicians, and longer hospital stays in areas with an oversupply of beds. Advances in technology required high utilization for cost-effectiveness. Increasing concerns evolved related to chemical technology. It became apparent that there were serious health threats outside the scope of traditional medical care. Yeaworth reports a study which indicates that life-style accounts for 48 percent of the contributing factors of mortality.

In the early 1980s, concerns about health care and preparing adequate numbers of health professionals gave way to anxiousness about energy, national defense, and inflation. Capitation grants were eliminated and funds greatly reduced for health professions students. Yeaworth cites the major change that has occurred is that people are being expected to assume overall responsibility for their own health, not just seek treatment and cure for disease. The 1980 Surgeon General's report lists 15 priority activities for health in the areas of disease prevention, health protection, and health promotion. Yeaworth indicates key preventive services needed in each area. She em-

858

phasizes that a new perspective is emerging in relation to priorities, therefore in relation to dollars. Yeaworth provides examples of the health dollar being focused for the 15 priority activities. Plans of local health system agencies, the Center for Disease Control, and the W. K. Kellogg Foundation are presented. In addition, Congress has appropriated financial support to test the ability of community long-term care projects to correct the fragmentation of care and unnecessary institutionalization of the elderly.

Yeaworth predominantly addresses the influence these changing perspectives will have on nursing and nursing education. Nursing has previously stressed disease prevention and promotion of optimal general health. Home and community health care became the domain of nursing with the advent of modern medicine. Nursing was conceived of as consisting of dependent functions related to medical regimen and independent functions related to disease prevention, health promotion, and maintenance. Yeaworth maintains that the changing emphases should be the impetus which nursing needs to gain recognition of its contribution to health care, justify billing for third-party payment for nursing service, and assure appropriate funding for nursing research and demonstration projects. She identifies and explores two areas which can present major obstacles to nursing's role in health promotion: the efforts of other disciplines to lay claim to disease prevention, health promotion, and counseling as part of their mission, and the reluctance of much of nursing to embrace this aspect as part of nursing. Some of the numerous obstacles are: colleges of education are developing programs for health educators and counseling, colleges of pharmacy are promoting the pharmacist as health educator, and physicians' assistants are laying claim to the health teaching–counseling role.

There are additional obstacles within nursing. In nursing education, the emphasis on wellness and community health has occurred primarily at the baccalaureate level; more than 80 percent of present nurses were prepared in educational programs that focused on illness with a major portion of clinical experience provided in illness settings. The sanctions for fostering the health promotion image for nursing are not too positive. Yeaworth provides examples: the schism within the profession and misinterpretation from hospital associations and physicians concerning the level of entry into professional practice; assertions that baccalaureate graduates in nursing are not prepared to function effectively in hospital settings; support for a resurgence of diploma education with some hospitals attempting to become degree granting institutions.

Yeaworth further discusses problems and cites examples in obtaining support for the professionalization of nursing in academic health centers. Competition for scarce resources exists for which some disciplines have an advantage, e.g., generation of fees for services provided by dental students. Nursing faculty cannot bill for services to supplement nursing educational funds. Hospital nurses may not have the academic credentials for faculty appointments to teach to reduce the cost. Academic health center hospitals may cost account expenses for nursing education back to the schools of nursing. However, schools of nursing may need to contract with 50 different agencies to gain clinical experience for nursing students, thus may not have the same investments as other disciplines to ensure that the hospital receives a fair share of the health center budget. Yeaworth quotes Morris to illustrate how other disciplines may not always view nursing as a good ally.

Yeaworth maintains that nursing needs to realize it cannot hold a special claim on health promotion; however, the generalist preparation of nurses enables a role for health promotion. She urges nurses and nurse-educators not to abandon hospitals, hospitals not to stress preparing nurses primarily for illness care, and a return to diploma education as an answer to the hospital nursing shortage. Health promotion provides hospitals with new directions for growth and revenue. This can be accomplished with more collaboration among the health care disciplines and expansion of more independent roles for professional nurses in hospitals. Safe self-care presupposes also knowledge in order to decide when professional help is needed. Although health promotion should be less costly, Yeaworth believes it should not be used to justify cuts and underfunding of health care. Yeaworth concludes it is essential for nursing to exert political influence to define its role and share in the health promotion movement. However, nursing needs to restore the breaks and unify the profession if nurses' increasing adeptness in political influence is to be effective.

A new decade, new leadership, or major individual and institutional changes are cause for looking back as well as planning ahead. Long-range planning is a required task of all organizations, even if rapid change quickly obliterates many of the assumptions on which plans are based. The literature and most institutional budgets tell us that the 1980s will emphasize changes in perspectives, plans, and institutions. These changes come framed in discussions of "retrenchments" and "survival," increasing competition for scarce resources, and increasing importance of political influence.

EMPHASES PRIOR TO AND INTO THE 1970s

If we look back over the 1970s and into the years preceding, it becomes obvious that there have not only been rapid advances in medical knowledge, treatment techniques, equipment and technology, but there have also been major changes in attitudes, values, and beliefs in regard to health and health care. As medical breakthroughs eased many of our agonies, corrected severe injuries and deformities, and prolonged our life expectancies, we developed a certain reverence for physicians, hospitals, miracle drugs, and medical research. We also developed rapidly rising expectations as to what could be accomplished.

The thinking in regard to our personal obligations for our own health centered closely around having medical and hospitalization insurance,

going to a physician at the first sign of illness or pregnancy, following this medical advice unquestioningly, and taking medications as prescribed. There was public support for Congress to make large amounts of tax dollars available for medical research, for the building and equipping of hospitals, for subsidizing education of increased numbers of physicians, nurses, dentists, pharmacists and allied health personnel, and for Medicare and Medicaid to make health care available to all.

RESULTS OF PREVIOUS APPROACHES

These approaches brought certain successes. Between 1968 and 1977, life expectancy increased, the infant mortality rate decreased by slightly over 35 percent, and death rates from all causes decreased by just over 9 percent (Kellogg Foundation, 1980). In areas where such measures as specially trained paramedics and emergency medical personnel, mobile intensive care units, and trauma centers were introduced, deaths from accidents were reduced almost eightfold.

But with progress, there were also problems. With skyrocketing inflation, ethical, political, and economic questions began to arise. Health care expenditures reached $200 billion, or about 9 percent of the gross national product, and represented one of the most rapidly rising costs in the economy. While studies can be misleading, there began to be reports indicating that there were higher death rates in areas with concentrations of physicians, more surgery in areas where surgeons were concentrated, and more hospitalizations with longer stays in areas with an oversupply of hospital beds.

As most larger cities developed an oversupply of hospital beds, hospitals competed to obtain CAT scanners, megavolt radiation therapy units, cardiovascular units, trauma units, renal dialysis units, kidney transplant capabilities, and other technology which might increase hospital utilization. They purchased helicopters and small aircraft to transport emergency cases. But this technology also required high utilization for cost-effectiveness. As it became obvious that expenditures and resources for health care were not unlimited, troubling questions regarding the amounts spent on critical and chronic care for limited numbers versus the amounts spent on public health measures began to arise.

Our chemical technology was not without its problems as increasing incidences of drug reactions, drug interactions, drug dependency, and drug abuse received attention. Food additives and processing came under scrutiny. Insecticides, pesticides, and fertilizers became concerns not only in regard to direct handling, but also in the food chain and in runoff into the water supply. Hazards in the work place, pollution, and nuclear accidents presented additional threats.

Not only were these health threats outside the usual disease treatment realm, but they made it apparent that much of what kills people falls outside the scope of traditional medical care. Heart and vascular disease, cancer, stroke, accidents, cirrhosis of the liver, and suicide are among the leading killers, and alcohol and drug abuse are often factors in the accidents, cirrhosis, and suicide. In fact, alcohol is a factor in more than 10 percent of all deaths (U.S. Surgeon General's Report, 1979). The Center for Disease Control has done a proportional allocation of contributing factors of mortality from the ten leading causes of death in the United States, and problems arising from life-style account for 48 percent of the national death rate (Kellogg Foundation, 1980). Better medical treatment is obviously not the answer to lowering this mortality rate.

CLIMATE AT ENTRY TO THE 1980s

Whether it was disillusionment, complacency, a bit of both, or unrelated factors, with the advent of the 1980s, concerns about health care and about preparing adequate numbers of health professionals lost ground to concerns about energy, national defense, and inflation. President Carter's fiscal 1981 budget counted on $1.3 billion in savings from hospital cost containment. It called for elimination of the capitation grants program for health professionals and attempted to rescind $88 million in capitation funds and $16.5 million for student loans in the health professions from the already approved 1980 budget. Carter's budget also sought a $77 million decrease in nurse training monies at a time when shortages of nurses were being experienced throughout most of the country. Medical research through the National Institutes of Health was to be limited to a 4 percent increase which, with inflated dollars, translated to a decrease.

It has been gradual, but a major change has occurred in thinking and planning in regard to health and medical care. People are now expected to assume overall responsibility for their own health, not just seek treatment and cure for their diseases. Community health planning is being mandated to prevent duplication of costly services. In attempts to offset the rising costs of health insurance and decreased productivity due to illness, major companies are providing their employees with gymnasiums and other facilities for exercise, diet clinics, stress-management workshops, and special incentives and assistance in stopping smoking or overcoming alcohol abuse. Both federal and private foundation funding is beginning to be directed toward disease prevention, health promotion, and keeping people out of institutions. Clearly, prevention is less costly in dollars, and, more importantly, it enhances human productivity and life quality.

The Surgeon General's Report on Health Promotion and Disease Prevention (1979) lists 15 priority activities for health and breaks them down into disease prevention, health protection, and health promotion. Key preventive services need to be provided in the areas of: family planning, pregnancy, and infant care; immunizations; sexually transmissible diseases; and high blood pressure control. For health protection, attention must be focused on toxic agent control, occupational safety and health, accidental injury control, flouridation of community water supplies, and infectious agent control. Health promotion activities include promoting cessation of smoking, which is the largest single preventable cause of illness and premature death in the U.S.; reducing misuse of alcohol and drugs; and encouraging improved nutrition, exercise and fitness, and stress control.

Increasing numbers of people are becoming more knowledgeable about health and more concerned about exercise and fitness. Many adults are succeeding in ceasing smoking, conquering problems with alcohol consumption, and losing weight. Community agencies are providing education and support to assist such efforts. The health promotion and disease prevention activities listed in the Surgeon General's Report are not that revolutionary. Family planning, pregnancy and infant care, immunizations, services for sexually transmissible diseases, and high blood pressure control have been pretty much standard practice in health department and community clinics for a number of years. It is not that something new has been discovered, but that a new perspective is emerging in relation to priorities and hence in relation to dollars.

"Currently only four percent of the Federal health dollar is specifically identified for prevention related activities" (Surgeon General's Report, 1979:9). There now is evidence however that federal and private dollars will follow the priorities set by the surgeon general. Local health systems agencies are developing plans that relate closely to the activities listed by the surgeon general. The Center for Disease Control has announced that as

much as $2 million will be available in fiscal 1980 to support as many as 15 new grants for venereal disease research, demonstration, and public information and education projects. The W. K. Kellogg Foundation's January, 1980, report on its health programming activities states: "The current emphasis [for Foundation funding] is on identifying strategies which have the potential for yielding a balanced program to demonstrate the most effective approach to promoting health" (1980:21). The Health Resources Administration opened the 1980s by announcing the availability of $1.7 million in grants to develop curricula in environmental and humanistic health.

In January, 1976, the Report of the Subcommittee on Health and Long-Term Care of the Select Committee on Aging of the House of Representatives, Ninety-Fourth Congress stated, as one of two priorities, the need to correct the emphasis which was put on institutionalization by federal statutes and by the Department of Health, Education, and Welfare (Select Committee, 1976). The report set forth the need to establish a comprehensive system of home health and supportive services designed to permit the elderly person, often inappropriately institutionalized, to remain in the dignity of his or her own home and community. Four years later, in January, 1980, DHHS's Health Care Financing Administration and the Administration on Aging announced the intent to initiate the "National Long-Term Care Channeling Demonstration Program." Congress appropriated approximately $20 million to support coordinated demonstrations to test the ability of community long-term care projects to correct the fragmentation of care and unnecessary institutionalization of the elderly. Such projects require a coordinated case management system for home and community care.

INFLUENCE ON NURSING AND NURSING EDUCATION

How much influence will these changing perspectives have on nursing? Nursing, in its attempts to escape the image and expectations associated with the role of "handmaiden of the physician" and to attain recognition as a profession, has stressed that nursing focuses on disease prevention and promotion of optimal general health, while medicine focuses on disease detection and cure. With the advent of modern medicine, much of home and community health care, especially in more rural areas, became the domain of nursing. The physician's time was too valuable to be spent in health teaching, so more and more nurses took on health teaching and counseling roles. Nursing was conceptualized as consisting of dependent functions related to carrying out treatments which were part of the medical regimen and of independent functions related to disease prevention, health promotion, and health maintenance. Thus, the current emphases of the surgeon general and of federal and private foundation funding should be just the impetus nursing needs to gain recognition of its contribution to health care, to justify billing for third-party payment for nursing service, and to assure appropriate funding for nursing research and demonstration projects.

Nursing's gain from the health promotion emphasis cannot be taken as a given, however. Major obstacles lie in two areas: (1) the efforts of other disciplines to lay claim to disease prevention, health promotion, and health counseling as part of their mission, and, thus, to vie for the monies associated with these roles; and (2) the reluctance of much of nursing to really embrace this aspect as part of nursing. These two obstacles should be considered in more detail.

Educators, researchers, and health practitioners tend to adjust to do what they are funded to do. In times of inflation and tightening budgets for medical care, research, and education, acquiring grants and demonstration projects can represent answers for funding positions that might otherwise be cut. With the depressed job market for teachers, schools and colleges of education are developing programs for health education, special education, and specialized counseling. Colleges of pharmacy, in an attempt to develop new and expanded roles

and, hence, more positions for pharmacists, are promoting the pharmacist as the one who should administer medications, teach about drug actions, interactions, and reactions, and serve as health educator. As physicians' assistants become better organized, they, too, are laying claim to the health teaching and counseling role. Jobs have tended to be plentiful in business administration, but schools and colleges of business are developing programs in health services administration to prepare nurses and nonnurses to administer health clinics and long-term care institutions. Colleges of medicine have had to meet stipulations in regard to preparing physicians for family medicine and for rural, occupational, and family health.

In nursing education, the emphasis in wellness and community health has occurred primarily at the baccalaureate level of preparation and has been reinforced by the availibility of positions in community and public health or health maintenance agencies. The 1977 National Sample Survey of Registered Nurses (Moses and Roth, 1979) indicated that three-fourths of the registered nurse population initially graduated from a diploma program and 11 percent from an associate degree program. Only 12.3 percent were initially graduates from a baccalaureate program. Slightly over 61 percent of working R.N.s are employed by hospitals, and an additional 8.1 percent are employed by nursing homes. Only 7.9 percent of working nurses are employed in public health and only 2.5 percent in occupational health. This means that more than 80 percent of nurses employed at the time of the survey were prepared in educational programs that focused on illness and provided the major portion of clinical experience in illness settings. The majority of nurses are employed in settings where the values and the role expectations communicated by others in their role set relate to illness care. The public image of the nurse portrayed by the media reinforces these expectations.

Aside from the minority of nurses who work in community, public, and occupational health settings, the sanctions for fostering the health-promotion image of nursing have not been particularly positive. The effort to make the baccalaureate degree the level of entry into professional practice has created schisms within the profession and has been subject to major misinterpretations by hospital associations and physicians. Nursing educators are being told by nursing service administrators that they are not preparing graduates to function in hospital nursing service. Hospital associations in many areas are mustering forces to gain economic and political support for a resurgence of diploma education, and some hospitals are trying to become degree-granting institutions. They are justifying their efforts by saying that they would supply the need for in-depth clinical education, which generally translates into care in acute illness situations.

In academic health centers, where the most advanced creativity in health education, service, and research should be fostered, nursing should be supported in its efforts toward professionalization, but there are problems. Nursing schools are in competition for scarce resources with the other health center units, including the hospitals. Some disciplines have certain advantages in that competition. With inflation and decreasing federal support, it is predicted that there will be a higher reliance on fees for services. Unlike dental students, who may generate an income of several thousand dollars a year from the patients they care for in dental clinics, nursing students do not earn fees for their services. In fact, many academic health center hospitals help justify their budgets by cost-accounting expenses for nursing education back to the nursing schools, making nursing education look even more expensive.

Unlike faculty in medical schools who can bill for professional services performed while teaching medical students who are seeing patients, most nursing faculty cannot supplement nursing educational funds by billing for their services. Some even donate time in clinical agencies to keep their skills current and promote good working relationships in the agencies. Since most hospital nurses do not have the academic credentials for faculty appointments, nursing cannot even follow the model used by many schools of pharmacy, where the hospital pharmacist does much of the clinical teaching, thereby reducing educational costs. All of these things tend to make the other units of the academic health center believe that the school of nursing is not pulling its weight. Since the nursing school may be contracting with 30, 40, or 50 different agencies in order to gain clinical experience for nursing students, it does not have the same investments as the other disciplines of the health center in seeing that the hospital gets its fair share of the health center budget.

Although academic health centers do not necessarily provide a climate that fosters nursing's professional development as a discipline with a unique claim on health promotion, they might at least allow for alliances to balance the power in the competition for resources. But other disciplines do not always view nursing as a good ally. Morris (1980) likens nursing in academic health centers to the Third World. He states that academic nurses believe as do the developing nations that "the rest of the world owes them a better future since they lack the resources to solve their own problems independently." He goes on to say that "academic nurses are so absorbed with their own challenges that they display very little interest in the problems of others. They tend to view every issue in terms of whether it is good or bad for nursing" (Morris, 1980:158).

If nursing is to reap particular gains from the changing perspectives in regard to health and the changing funding priorities, it must realize that it cannot hold a special claim on health promotion activities. It may be better able to compete, but it must realize that the competition will be rigorous. Some of nursing's disadvantages are also its advantages. There are probably no nursing functions, taken individually, which cannot be performed by a nonnurse, if one disregards the risk of being charged with practicing without a license. Some specific functions which are performed by nurses can be performed as well or better by pharmacists, dentists, physicians, and allied health workers who have had specialized preparation for the function. These specialists cannot, however, perform the broad spectrum of functions encompassed in the nursing role. Indeed, it is difficult to speak of "the nursing role"if one thinks of all of the various levels of preparation of nurses and the settings in which they function.

It is the broad generalist preparation which makes it possible for nurses to be the most numerous of all the health discipline practitioners—1.4 million nurses are licensed to practice—and for there still to be a critical shortage of nurses. This general preparation does mean that work settings will have to provide orientation for specifics and that graduates may indicate that the curriculum did not adequately prepare them for their jobs. It is also a factor in turnover. It is still probably less costly for society for nurses to be prepared as generalists rather than as specialists. The generalist preparation can be good preparation for health promotion functions.

Despite the multifaceted problems in hospitals and in the many other agencies in which nurses work and with which schools of nursing must affiliate, nurses and nurse educators cannot afford to abandon hospitals, for it is here that others are least able to adequately replace the nurse. The acutely ill and the severely injured need nurses with skill and expert knowledge. Hospital risk-management programs cannot afford underprepared staff. Hospital administrators and physicians must realize that a return to diploma education, with its educational mobility difficulties and its reduced career options, is not an answer to the hospital nursing shortage. Hospitals cannot afford to stress preparing nurses primarily for illness care, since hospitals are also attempting to shed the acute- and chronic-care-only functions in order to move with the emphasis on health promotion and disease prevention. Because of utilization reviews, excess hospital beds in most urban areas, inflating costs, and attempts to reduce federal and state budgets, hospitals are caught in a tightening financial squeeze. Government-operated hospitals are especially threatened. Philadelphia General Hospital has closed. Homer G. Phillips Hospital in St. Louis has closed except for outpatient services (Freidman, 1980).

Health promotion is viewed as providing hospitals with new directions for growth and revenue.

The Chicago Hospital Council, representing 104 member-hospitals, has begun marketing health promotion programs to businesses. The Wellborn Baptist Hospital in Evansville, Indiana, holds a spring fitness festival to emphasize its preventive health program (Idea Forum, 1980). Just as much of the general public believes we already have a health care system which is called medicine, they also believe that we already have health centers called hospitals. The various health care disciplines may gain more by collaborating to provide solid foundations for the latter belief than by pointing out the fallacies and attempting to establish something different. If hospitals are to be successful as health promotion agencies, there will certainly have to be more expanded, independent roles for nurses, roles which could help hospital nursing gain better rewards and more control over how nursing is practiced in the hospital setting.

Nursing will have to be able to exert political influence at all levels—federal, state, and local—if it is to gain its share of the health promotion move. But little influence can be successfully effected in the larger arena if nursing cannot heal the rifts within its own ranks. Nurses have become more skilled at being assertive and more willing to confront and make demands, but as a group, they are still not inclined toward careful fact gathering and toward formally co-opting prestigious intermediaries in their efforts to negotiate and persuade. Nursing is becoming more adept at utilizing political influence, but leaders must learn not to spend that influence on every issue of value, since influence, like money, is not unlimited. Careful calculations must be made in utilizing it for the greatest overall benefit for the profession.

PLANNED PROGRESS OR REACTIVE PLOY

The utilization of scarce resources automatically involves ethical and value judgments as well as economic and political ones. It is doubtful that it could really be determined how much the increasing relevance of health promotion has been influenced by the beliefs and values associated with utilizing our health care resources to provide the best health for the greatest numbers, and how much it has been influenced by the crunch of spiraling health care costs at a time when our national resources are being hard pressed by other needs. Perhaps only a cynic would even consider the question. As one who spent a number of years planning and implementing graduate nursing curricula in gerontology and gerontological mental health to prepare nurses to meet the specialized health care needs of this at-risk population, I feel a twinge of cynicism when I see an official NIH publication entitled "A Guide to Medical Self-Care and Self-Help Groups for the Elderly" (National Institutes of Health, 1979). While, in the final analysis, people must assume responsibility for their own health, I hope the changing emphasis does not herald the tendency for heath care professionals to abdicate responsibility or for government to avoid health funding. Safe self-care presupposes a great deal of knowledge in order to decide when professional help is needed. Health promotion should ultimately be less costly, but this new emphasis should not be used merely to justify underfunding of health care.

EDITOR'S QUESTIONS FOR DISCUSSION

Discuss the changes in health care perspectives from the 1960s to the present time. What have been the most influential factors contributing to change? What have been the most significant problems related to change? Could the problems have been foreseen for intervention or prevented? Suggest mechanisms for controlling costs of health care. What variables are essential to consider in controlling costs to provide quality care? What factors have contributed to persons assuming overall responsibility for their health? How congruent is that expectation with the previous social consciousness concerning health care needs? Suggest services for disease prevention, health protection, and health promotion additional to those indicated by Yeaworth. What evaluation and planning should occur before implementing those services? Project into the future and cite health care needs and services to be provided. Given the current federal investment in long-term care programs for the elderly, what direction can you foresee in health care policy?

Discuss the impact of changing perspectives on nursing. How do the history and issues concerning public health nursing as portrayed by Talbot (Chap. 62) relate to Yeaworth's perspective of home and community health care? What evidence is there to suggest nursing's reluctance to embrace health promotion as part of nursing? Provide examples of educators, researchers, and health practitioners adjusting their role to what they are funded to do. Provide other examples of disciplines claiming disease prevention, health promotion, and health counseling as their mission. How can territorial claims or domains be negotiated or legitimately be defined? In the past, on what basis has professional domain or boundaries been established?

To what extent has wellness and community health actually been emphasized at the baccalaureate level? What are the implications for the role of nursing in health promotion and the nursing profession given the data presented by Yeaworth concerning the registered nurse population? Given that 80 percent of present nurses were initially prepared in educational programs that focused on illness, what effects may be evident in present faculty and curricula? What differences are there in faculty perspectives in teaching that may be related to their initial nursing education program and experiences? Should these differences in perspectives be reconciled among faculty? If you perceive differences should be reconciled, suggest avenues for attaining that goal. How are divergent perspectives in teaching related to academic freedom? How can qualifications for teaching in an academic program be distinguished from perspectives regarding the content being taught and the mode of teaching? What relationship may there be between quality of teaching and a nursing faculty's undergraduate preparation, and professional graduate education? What means are utilized for faculty development in most schools of nursing?

Given that the socialization of nurses into the profession usually occurs during their professional education, may the divisiveness that is said to exist within nursing be related to their education experience? Suggest alternative avenues to explore related to dissension within the profession. Refer to Dalme's chapter (11) for possible clues.

How can the divergent expectations for graduates employed in hospital settings be resolved? How can the profession most effectively counter the forces supporting a resurgence of diploma education and/or hospitals trying to become degree-granting institutions? Rather than react, as Donley says (Chap. 64), how can the profession set the agenda to advance professional education programs? What applications may be drawn from Donley's chapter for effectively meeting the issues concerning the education of professional nurses?

Discuss the advantages and disadvantages of schools of nursing in academic health centers. What applications can be made from Fagin and McGivern's chapter (56) regarding the development of alliances between nursing and constituents? What alternative approaches can you suggest for schools of nursing in competing for scarce resources with other health center units? How much responsibility and accountability does nursing have for the situations and/or conditions, as portrayed by Yeaworth, existing for schools of nursing in academic health centers? Suggest means to prevent or alleviate such situations. To what extent do you agree with the quote by Morris as cited by Yeaworth? If that view is accurate, what are the implications for nursing deans, nursing education, and the image of the nursing profession?

Discuss the generalist approach to the professional education of nurses. What are the advantages and disadvantages of a generalist preparation? Refer to the chapters by Williamson (5), Peterson (7), Santora (8), Sargis (9), Clayton (10) and Dalme (11) before responding. What are the implications for meeting patients' and clients' needs if illness care is the predominant focus of professional education programs in nursing rather than health care, *or* if health care is the major emphasis instead of illness care? How can the two approaches be effectively combined to sufficiently prepare a nursing student for professional practice? How might a generalist preparation contribute to a shortage of nurses? What are the implications for the number of role options nurses may have or attempt to fulfill? What relationship may there be between a generalist preparation and the "burn-out" phenomenon? With the increasing emphasis on specialization, should a generalist preparation be supplemented? Provide arguments for your response. How can a generalist preparation best prepare nurses for a role in health promotion?

Present arguments for and against nursing claiming disease prevention, health promotion, and health maintenance as the domain of nursing. How congruent would this be with the domain of nursing as discussed in previous chapters by Palmer (1), Fawcett (14), Newman (28), Chinn (29), L. Walker (30), Roy (34), Bille (36), La Monica (37), and Bullough (45)? Should a single or multiple domains be defined as nursing? What role can nurses specifically develop in hospital settings concerning health promotion? How should illness care and health care be combined in hospitals? Suggest mechanisms for collaboration with other health disciplines in planning and implementing health centers. What strategies and political influence is needed to organize health centers. Suggest methodologies to evaluate health centers. What critical variables should be included in evaluation of health promotion?

Review the chapters contributing to this section of the text concerning the future of nursing. What are the common themes evident between and among Rogers (50), Christman (60), Aydelotte (61 and 63), Talbot (62), Donley (64), and Yeaworth (65)? What divergent perspectives exist? Review all the previous chapters in this volume. What relationship exists between the predictions of the authors in this section and the contributions of authors in previous sections? Which of those authors in other sections suggest further evidence for the speculations or predictions offered in this section? What other predictions of the future are suggested by authors in previous chapters? How do you perceive the future of nursing? Provide a rationale for your arguments.

REFERENCES

Freidman, Emily
  1980 "Public hospitals: Is 'relevance' in the eye of the beholder?" Hospitals 54(9):83–93.
Idea Forum
  1980 "Community and industry ready for health promotion." Hospitals 54(9):35–38.
Morris, Alvin L.
  1980 "Inter-school relationships in academic health centers." Pp. 155–165 in The Organization and Governance of Academic Health Centers. Position Papers. Vol. 3. Washington, D.C.: Association of Academic Health Centers.
Moses, Evelyn and Roth, Aleda
  1979 "Nursepower: What do statistics reveal about the nation's nurses?" American Journal of Nursing 79(10):1745–1756.

National Institutes of Health
  1979 A Guide to Medical Self-Care and Self-Help Groups for the Elderly. Washington, D.C.: U.S. Government Printing Office.
Select Committee on Aging of the House of Representatives, 94th Congress
  1976 Report of the Subcommittee on Health and Long-Term Care. Washington, D.C.: U.S. Government Printing Office.
United States Surgeon General
  1979 Healthy People. The Surgeon General's Report on Health Promotion and Disease Prevention. Washington, D.C.: U.S. Government Printing Office.
W. K. Kellogg Foundation
  1980 Viewpoint: Toward a Healthier America. Battle Creek, Mich.: Kellogg Foundation.

Part Eight

Summary and Conclusions

A time for healing; . . .
a time for embracing, . . .
a time for loving, . . .
a time for peace

Nursing as a profession has shown the tenacity to endure and thrive in this society of discontent. However, there have been and are splinters visible within the profession, and distress evident among and between its members and other health professionals in nursing's endeavor to progress as a profession. It is the time for healing the wounds of individual members and groups within the profession and a time of embracing for the entire profession. Splinters, pain, and wounds are inevitable in growth and development towards maturity. The unfinished business of resolving the past needs to be completed before the profession can effectively move forward to confront and meet the multiple demands which are bound to be presented in the future. It is the time for loving to be demonstrated through a network of professional support in accomplishing the present and future tasks of the profession. It is a time for peace to exist and be nurtured within and between members of the profession and with all other health professions and disciplines. In essence, all health professions have a common goal—to provide for and contribute to the health care of the consumer and society. That goal

869

cannot be achieved without the united efforts of all health professions. It cannot effectively be attained without unity and peace within each health profession—more appropriately, the nursing profession, for which this volume was written.

In this final chapter, the editor reflects in general on some issues cited or alluded to in each of the sections in this volume: professionalization, nursing education, nursing research, nursing theory, nursing practice, nursing administration and the future of nursing. Possible answers or avenues to pursue in resolving perplexing situations for nursing are suggested. Observations are offered from the perspective of the sociology of professions. Particular attention is given to the professionalization of nursing and concerns about the professionalism of women. Support networks are strongly advocated. The comments, observations, suggestions, and speculations should stimulate others to raise additional questions and potential answers. The editor proposes the analogy of a tapestry for the strength and continued perseverance of nursing as a profession.

Chapter 66

Winter of Discontent and Invincible Springs

In the depth of winter, I finally learned that within me there lay an invincible summer.[1]

Albert Camus

Norma L. Chaska, R.N., Ph.D., F.A.A.N.
Associate Professor
Chairperson, Nursing Administration
Coordinator, Nursing Research
School of Nursing
Medical College of Georgia
Augusta, Georgia

The excerpt from Camus's essay offers an application and meaning for the profession of nursing. From the earliest history of nursing through to the present day, nursing, as it continues to mature as a profession, has experienced numerous "winters" complete with blizzards and frigid temperatures with seemingly no relief or assistance and warmth in sight. Nursing is learning that *within* the profession is the key, not only for endurance, but for the tranquility essential for remaining steadfast in purpose and mission through the storms and darkness that are inevitable for growth and progress. Nursing is realizing that the strength of the profession lies within the collective strength and unity of its members. In unity *within* the profession nursing will know it has an

invincible summer to withstand the external forces of "winter" confronting it from every direction. As suggested by a quotation cited by Yeaworth in Chap. 65 (Morris, 1980:158), the time is past for expectations for assistance in resolving the problems of the profession by other disciplines and professions. Nursing must realize it is responsible for its own difficulties and divisiveness within the profession. Neither as individuals nor as collective members of a profession can nurses truly give of themselves in providing service and care to others unless internal conflicts have been reconciled. Resolution of dissonant issues lies in emphasizing the positive strengths and talents of the individual members of the profession. The numerous concerns and discontents, as well as hopes and ideals, of the profession are evident throughout the chapters of this volume. In Irene Palmer's chapter, Nightingale's belief in the wisdom of small beginnings is indicated. The profession may well recon-

[1] Camus, Albert. "Return to Tipasa." Pp. 169–171 in Lyrical and Critical Essays, edited by Philip Thody; translated by Ellen Conroy Kennedy. Used by permission of Alfred Knopf, Inc., N.Y. Copyright 1968.

sider the wisdom of small beginnings as it looks within itself and realizes it has an invincible summer.

To condense the major points of the contributors in a summary chapter may be an injustice to the authors and misleading to the reader, as well as a formidable task. Specifically to address the Editor's Questions for Discussion requires a volume in its own right. Thus, the editor chooses to reflect briefly and in general about some of the issues and concerns the authors have discussed and to present some additional thoughts on the current state of the profession. Finally, by speaking of a winter of discontent moving toward a spring of hope the editor offers an analogy for the profession in actualizing an invincible summer.

PROFESSIONALIZATION

The process by which and extent to which nursing has assumed the attributes of a profession are referred to throughout this volume. This issue is particularly addressed in the sections on professionalization, nursing education, nursing research, nursing theory, the future of nursing, and chapters in the sections on nursing practice and administration. For the purpose of review, attributes commonly cited as indicative of professionalization are those designated by Greenwood (1957): the presence of systematic theory, formal and informal community sanction, a code of ethics, and a professional culture. Furthermore, Myrtle K. Aydelotte (Chap. 63) has presented a composite of characteristics from several authors, which should refresh one's memory in considering the professionalization of nursing. A number of recurring themes are evident in the contributor's chapters. Some of the predominant topics are necessity for the development of a scientific knowledge base for nursing, delineation of nursing's domain, exercise of professional autonomy, enhancement of a professional culture, and adherence to academic and professional standards in education and practice. Some of these themes are more appropriately mentioned in other portions of this chapter, i.e., the section on nursing education.

In the quest of a scientific knowledge base for nursing, it may be more fruitful to promote further collaborative efforts between nurse practitioners and researchers. As separation of nursing education from practice has resulted in a dichotomy within the profession, so too the seclusion of nurse researchers from the practice arena may have inhibited the evolution of a scientific knowledge base. Obvious efforts are being made to unify nursing research and practice similar to the endeavors of nurse-educators and nurse practitioners. Arguments persist regarding the value and identification of a knowledge base that is unique to nursing. It would appear that the extent to which the search for knowledge occurs in isolation from the practice setting may indeed be knowledge that is not nursing.

Furthermore, it remains debatable whether nursing should draw from other disciplines in the development of its knowledge base. It is generally agreed that nursing has a unique service to offer for the patient (client). Whether nursing should utilize knowledge from other disciplines in assisting the definition of that service based on a scientific knowledge base appears to be a moot question. *How* the knowledge is integrated may be what is unique to nursing in definition and practice. It also should be the prerogative of the professional practitioner uniquely to apply that knowledge in order to most effectively practice professional nursing.

The lack of consensus as to the domain of nursing has been a source of discontent within nursing and frustration to the public as well as to other health professionals. There is increasing awareness of an evolving role for nurses in disease prevention, health care, and health maintenance. There appears to be less focus on the curative aspects of care and more emphasis on the caring-teaching role for nurses. That is not to say that, particularly in areas where physicians are in short supply, nurses will not have included in their role the treatment of disease and illness. However, state nurse practice acts, defining the scope of nursing practice, and state medical practice acts have profound implications for nurses, who do not adhere to what is defined and interpreted as nursing practice. It would appear that professional education programs to prepare nurses for practice in areas where other health professionals are scarce may become more demanding in quality, standards, and performance expectations. With increased litigation over provision of health care, nurses may well become more cautious in choosing the type of educational preparation and arena for practice.

Nurses appear to be less interested in providing medical care and concerned more with nursing care. The differentiation between a nursing and medical diagnosis perhaps has raised the consciousness of nurses as to their role and the domain of nursing. The evolution of primary nursing in settings that have appropriately been conducive for effective implementation also has further nurtured the role of nurses in providing professional nursing care. Nurses should not abandon the care of the ill and swing to the extreme opposite of caring for the well. A balance is needed in defining the territory, domain, and role of nursing. It is evident that nurses and nursing, in returning to the "roots" of their heritage, through the writings of Nightingale and the evolution of the knowledge base in nursing, are clarifying their role.

Perhaps the most predominant attribute of professionalization, which is of the utmost concern to the profession and nurses today, is that of autonomy for professional practice. There are various points of view regarding the issue. Control over one's professional practice is without a doubt essential for professionalization. At the same time there is potential danger in focusing on one particular attribute of a profession more than others. No single health professional, with the complexities in providing health and illness care today, can afford to claim absolute autonomy. Perhaps at no other time in our society has collaboration and negotiation been more essential between and among professionals—whether it be in education, research, or practice. No one health professional or health profession can begin effectively to meet all of the needs of patients/clients in providing care. The knowledge explosion and rapid obsolescence, technology, economics, and costs of health care

have had a tremendous impact on the provision of health care. It is demanded that every health professional be more accountable than in the past in every aspect of his or her professional status. No single health profession can afford to stand alone or predominate.

To a point, the consensus of some nurses, and in some respects the profession, on autonomy as essential for practice may be a reflection of a professional and cultural lag. Nurses may now have had their "consciousness" significantly raised about the historical dominance of the medical profession in providing care that the "reaction "timing" of that reaction may not be as effective or appropriate in this current era of health care crisis as it might have been had the drive for autonomy displayed itself sooner. Due to the external forces that are compelling cooperation and collaboration, pushing for complete autonomy may alienate rather than integrate the efforts of all health professionals in providing for health care. The increased emphasis on autonomy may be related to the discontent and distress within the profession. It is usually easier to look for an outside agent or agents as the source of problems which may be essentially internal to a profession. Calling attention to external sources related to the distress can restrain a profession from effectively resolving discordent issues that exist within the core of a profession. This is not to imply that either nurses or the profession should not strive for increased professional autonomy, such as through governance structures, nursing bylaws, and reimbursement for nursing services. The plea is for balance and realism in the degree to and manner by which autonomy is contended for. Collaboration, cooperation, and negotiation are in order.

A phenomenon is coming to light in the evolution of professionalization—the lack of support, compassion, and empathy for one another as professionals. It shows itself in intense competitiveness and dissension within the profession. This has been alluded to by some of the authors in this text; for example, Ezell (Chap. 6), Fagin and McGivern (Chap. 56), and Yeaworth (Chap. 65). Williamson (Chap. 5) discusses the phenomenon and uses the term "professional bonding." The lack of professional bonding may be the most significant source for the conflicts and problems within the profession.

A basic premise suggested by Harragan is that women as young girls are never socialized to be part of a team or team players (1977:73). Women essentially are socialized to care about and for men not women. Many women have not had the opportunity to progress through the developmental stages to cooperative teamwork. This can severely handicap a profession, such as nursing, whose membership is mostly women. Inadequate development of ability to cooperate shows itself in sharklike behavior among and between professionals.

Sharklike behavior is best described by Johns (1975). Johns portrays an analogy between sharklike behavior and group behavior in the academic world. Johns reviews a brief satire entitled, "How to Swim with Sharks: A Primer," originally attributed to Cousteau (1973), as a basis for his later essay. Johns presents the rules of the primer as a prelude to his dinner address entitled: "How to Swim with Sharks: The Advanced Course." Briefly, the rules are: Assume that unidentified fish are sharks; do not bleed; counter any aggression promptly; get out if someone is bleeding; use anticipatory retaliation; and disorganize an organized attack (1975:45–48). The advanced course is addressed to those who have control over, influence upon, or some responsibility for the pervading atmosphere in an environment (Johns, 1975:52). His essential message is to discourage swimmer-type, sharklike behavior. In so doing, Johns's final sentence is a plea to strive to change the environment so that this behavior is unnecessary (1975:54).

Johns's message is most applicable for the profession of nursing. In striving for professionalism, some professionals may have found themselves swimming with sharks and desperately trying to survive the experience. Others may realize they have tried to prevent the development of a sharklike environment—or contributed to it. In pursuing

professionalism, some nurses may make specific choices that affect not only their personal lives but also the profession and environment in which they practice.

The challenges nursing offers, perhaps even the competitiveness, may so intrigue some nurses that a professional career is placed ahead of a marriage, family, or personal life. Although there are numerous variables involved, it appears that more professional nurses than in the past, who are women, are making the choice for a career rather than sustain the commitment of a marriage. Many are finding it difficult to maintain effectively a stable balance between the two major roles. Some nurses discover—all too late—that the choice of abandoning a marriage for a career was too great a price to pay. This awareness may occur as the lack of true support systems within nursing becomes evident; the rewards are fewer, less enjoyable, and less satisfying. For some, the choice to invest more of their lives in a profession was the most viable for them, albeit an altruistic one. For others, there may have been little or no choice in the paths of their lives. The identity crisis of nurses has been noted (La Monica, Chap. 37). Part of that crisis may be related to the multiple roles professional women are attempting to fulfill. It may be that the identity crisis for professional nurses may exist more for those who are women than for those who are men.

Regardless of these questions, it is becoming more difficult to preserve the privacy and resources available through one's personal life, to sustain a separation between one's personal and professional life. This author perceives it is essential not only to the health and holism of the person as a professional, but also for the profession, to keep the areas of one's life in balance and as distinct as possible. Each area, personal and professional, should complement the other. Fulfillment in each area will enrich the totality of the person and enable people to give more of themselves. Most often the greatest source of strength and support lies within the treasure of one's personal life. If one jeopardizes the quality of that life,

not only may professionals lose a primary resource in exclusive sharing and sustaining themselves, but also the profession stands to lose the
contributions of a productive member.

For self-actualization, reasonableness is essential as one weighs and balances the importance and
efforts in being a professional with one's personal
values, needs, and life. The professional is first a
person and secondarily a professional. To compromise needs as a person for the status of a professional can be disastrous. The search for meaning
is primarily within oneself. It is essential for effective professionals to know *who* they are as persons, their predominant personal strengths and
needs, and their professional strengths and limitations. Peace and fulfillment within, then, enables
one really to contribute as a professional; the
profession benefits, and the individuals have something more to give and offer in their personal lives.

Professional women and men need to take
heed. Each is responsible for her or his own behavior. As a professional role model, each nurse
has an impact on the profession and environment.
It may be that the "workaholic" professional is
more a detriment to the professionalization of
nursing than an asset. For some, there is a goal to
be attained that *will* be achieved no matter what
the cost to themselves or to others. Unfortunately,
some professionals never realize that some goals
are not attainable, and that other goals once
achieved will never bring true satisfaction—more is
always wanted. This author perceives that the
more balanced a professional's life is, the less dissonance exists within the environment. "Worka-
holics" may find that their professional lives leave
them empty, depleted of both internal and external resources, unable to give or to receive from
others.

Professional nurses who have not developed,
nurtured, and maintained strong support systems
may also be the ones who have exceedingly unrealistic expectations for nursing staff and faculty,
as well as for themselves. Needs, which have not
been fulfilled or effectively sublimated, may then
manifest themselves in adverse or distorted profes-

sional relationships with nursing staff, faculty, and
other health professionals and disciplines. Each
professional has a responsibility for preventing the
sharklike environment as well as changing it if it
appears. The choice and means is the responsibility
of each member of the profession. As a professional, each member is accountable to the profession and society to provide the most conducive
atmosphere possible to the enhancement of self-
actualization, professionalism, and the professionalization of nursing. Integrity, respect for others,
compassion, and caring are essential for nurses to
become "professionally bonded" in establishing a
community culture for professionalization.

NURSING EDUCATION

Controversy continues to abound internally and
externally regarding nursing education. The entry
level for professional practice in nursing remains
the central issue. One of the reasons this is a
constant source of division within nursing is
related to the lack of sufficient empirical evidence documenting the differences in nursing
practice of graduates from the three entry levels
—diploma, associate degree, and baccalaureate
degree programs. Although there is consensus
that the baccalaureate degree should be the entry
into professional practice, criticism still exists of
the competence of these graduates in performing
nursing skills and professional practice.

Part of the controversy is connected to the present nature of the baccalaureate degree programs
themselves. It is perceived by some educators, i.e.,
Williamson (Chap. 5) that nursing has developed
technical baccalaureate programs for technical
practice, not professional programs. If this perception is accurate, it appears that there is a contradiction between the perceptions of those who
employ new baccalaureate graduates and nurse
educators. It also suggests that baccalaureate
curricula may not be sufficiently integrated to
prepare professional practitioners. With the increased emphasis on and need for holism in providing nursing care, it would appear more likely

that a totally integrated curriculum may prepare the professional practitioner.

The criticism of integrated curricula—that the beginning practitioner is not sufficiently prepared for professional practice—may be related more to inappropriate organization of critical content (including insufficient or inadequate content), teaching strategies, and clinical experience utilized. Integrated curricula require significant coordination and a holistic approach in nursing care. They demand nursing faculties who do not work conceptually from a holistic framework but are extremely adept in transmitting the depth of essential principles of nursing care for application in the care of a broad range of patients. It prescribes faculties themselves to have deeply integrated a general knowledge base in all areas of nursing practice. Faculties would need to have specialized nursing and clinical knowledge and skill to be able to enforce the concepts and principles of an integrated curriculum.

It should be accepted as a given fact that the integrated curriculum should evolve from conceptual nursing models or theories. The more eclectic the conceptual approach utilized and strands employed throughout an integrated curriculum, the more the professional nursing student should be prepared for general professional practice in a broad range of settings. The key may be the extent and degree to which the various conceptual nursing bases are evident throughout the core of the baccalaureate curriculum and the consistency with which they are realized. To utilize only one nursing model as the base for an integrated curriculum may severely limit the future professional practitioner. On the other hand, to incorporate multiple concepts, theories, or models may thoroughly confuse the student, prevent sufficient internalization of a nursing orientation to health and illness care, and ill prepare the student to meet the variety of patients' needs in numerous settings. Reasonableness is essential in choosing the degree of exposure to one or more theories or models. Time, length of programs, abilities of the student population, and faculty are critical variables.

The criticism of integrated curricula may more

accurately reflect the *lack* of academically prepared faculties who are nursing conceptually oriented and who possess in-depth clinical knowledge and competence in nursing skills. This liability can severely handicap the effective implementation and employment of integrated curricula. To implement an integrated curriculum requires a sophisticated ability among and between staff to coordinate in order to transmit sufficient depth of nursing clinical knowledge and skill to professional nursing students. Another criticism of integrated curricula may be that insufficient *time* is given for successful development, implementation, and employment of integrated curricula. Obviously, the orientation and approach in many faculties' baccalaureate and graduate preparation and the integrated approach to curriculum are disparate. Thus, time is essential for adequate preparation of faculty to use an integrated approach as well as for valid evaluation of the outcomes expected in performance of baccalaureate graduates. It would appear that, given the present-day needs of society and the focus on wellness and health maintenance as well as on care of the acutely ill, an integrated approach in baccalaureate curricula is in order. The need is evident for holism to provide effectively for health and illness needs in this highly fragmented and technological society.

Perhaps an anology might be found in the work of committees. Committees require a tremendous amount of time, effort, and coordination to achieve a goal. The more complex the problem, the more sophisticated and expert the members of the committee need to be, and the more likely the complex problem can be most effectively resolved through the pooled knowledge base of the committee structure. Perhaps there is nothing more complex than the human person, ill or well. Thus, the integrated approach in baccalaureate nursing curricula with the pooled knowledge base of expert faculty members, may more effectively prepare the professional practitioner to meet the complex health and illness needs of patients/clients for humanistic holism in care.

The baccalaureate degree should be the entry into professional practice, but inclusive of content recommended by Williamson (Chap. 5). Assessment of the needs of the public it serves should be the basis for the content taught from a nursing conceptual framework. It does not appear that it will ever be economically feasible or realistic to expect a postbaccalaureate degree, however it is titled, to be the entry requirement. The whole dilemma of how to qualify nurses for professional practice who have graduated from diploma programs or associate degree programs or obtained a baccalaureate degree in another discipline needs to be resolved. This author suggests that two levels of licensure be developed: the associate degree graduate and the professional baccalaureate degree graduate. The content of associate degree programs should be sufficiently general to enable them to care for a large group of patients/clients who do not have complex health/illness problems in a variety of settings. Intensive care settings are an inappropriate place for the associate degree graduate nurse. Suggestions that such settings are predominantly technological, and therefore that the focus of care is essentially technological, implies a lack of awareness of the total complexities of needs in holistic intensive care.

The justifiable frustrations and paradoxical situation of the diploma graduate who wants to obtain the nursing credential of a baccalaureate degree are well known. Indirectly, the diploma nurses have been told since 1965 that they are not appropriately prepared for professional practice (See Sargis, Chap. 9). The inadequacies of R.N. (registered nurse) completion programs or incorporation of diploma nurses with generic baccalaureate nursing students are also well understood. So too are known the frustrations of R.N.s who obtain a nonnursing baccalaureate degree and those nonnurses who have a baccalaureate degree from another discipline. The R.N. who has a non-nursing baccalaureate degree is unable to gain entry into an NLN (National League for Nursing) accredited graduate program in nursing. The only viable option for the latter is to enter a postbaccalaureate professional nursing doctorate program, such as offered at Case Western Reserve University. Perhaps the real solution to these problems,

including that of the nursing shortage, is the offering of nontraditional nursing education programs, such as external baccalaureate degree programs. The New York Regents External Degree Bachelor of Science in Nursing Program is the first B.S.N. program, based entirely on assessment of learning acquired outside the institution awarding the degree, to achieve accreditation by the profession on September 1, 1981 (U.S.N.Y., 1981).[2] External degree programs, not only at the baccalaureate level but at the master's and doctoral level, may well become the most viable and legitimate option for professional education acquired outside the institution awarding the degree. With the decreased funding of nursing programs at all levels in academic institutions, increased demands for professional preparation at all levels, limited access to superior academic institutions, family limitations in mobility, difficulties in adapting nurses' needs to meet formal institution schedules, it would seem that further efforts will evolve to provide high-quality external degree programs with superior academic credibility.

Given that the entry level for professional nursing practice will be a baccalaureate degree in nursing, the present need of the public for holistic health care, and the development of integrated baccalaureate curricula to prepare practitioners for holistic health care, some comment is necessary concerning master's and doctoral education. Specialists are needed, prepared at the master's and doctoral level for education, practice, and research. If the undergraduate curriculum is integrated and the practitioner sufficiently prepared as a generalist, faculty and practitioners need to be specialized at the master's level. Master's programs should prepare nurses for advanced knowledge as clinical specialists, nurse administrators, and nurse-educators. This author does not view these specialty areas as "functional" roles, but rather as ad-

---

[2] For information about the program write:

Regents External Degree (NG 501)
Cultural Education Center
Albany, New York 12230

vanced specialties that should build upon an integrated baccalaureate curriculum.

Nursing seemingly was in error when master's programs in administration and education began to be deleted over a decade ago, and the entire focus in master's education was directed toward preparation of clinical specialists. Consequently, in this decade the profession has found itself without sufficiently qualified executive administrators, managers, and leaders in health care and academic settings. It is suggested that master's programs for clinical specialists focus on providing the concentrated, coordinated content in an integrated baccalaureate curriculum and the advanced clinical knowledge for role models in clinical practice.

Master's programs in nursing administration need to concentrate on preparing both the nurse executive and middle manager of nursing for professional practice. Ideally, programs in nursing administration should be developed from an undergraduate curriculum which has significant management and leadership concepts integrated throughout the curriculum. However, few undergraduate curricula include such preparation. Therefore master's programs in nursing administration need to include sufficient depth in order to prepare students to practice at either the middle or executive level of management.

The argument has been made that such programs should be offered in schools of health care management. Until two-track systems (for nurses and nonnurses) are available in schools outside of nursing, there is potential danger that the essential linkage of nursing with administration and management concepts, principles, and content will be lost. The integration of both nursing and management for application in the clinical practice of nursing administration at this time can most effectively be offered in master's programs in schools or colleges of nursing. Ideally, a master's program in nursing administration should include one core course that offers advanced clinical core concepts from each of the other four traditional clinical areas. In turn, master's programs in nursing administration should offer two courses which

include the content of administrative theory and organizational behavior, and management of human resources plus a role practicum for the mid-level nurse manager.

Given the expressed need for numerous practitioners of nursing administration at the executive level, the master's curriculum developed by this author at the School of Nursing, Medical College of Georgia in Augusta, is comprehensive. In addition to three required courses, for all master's students (Nursing Theory, Methods of Nursing Research, and Advanced Methods in Nursing Research), seven major courses for nursing administration are required: Theory of Administration, Organizational Behavior, Management of Human Resources in Health Agencies, Accounting and Financial Analysis for Nurse Administrators, Health Information Systems, Role Practicum: Programming for Quality Assurance, and Role Practicum: Nursing Administration.[3] All the courses are taught by doctorally prepared nurse-faculty members, with the exception of the two courses offered prior to the role practicum. Those doctorally prepared faculty members have a substantial knowledge base of nursing for administrative practice. Three electives are also available in the program. The curriculum was formulated in accordance with the guidelines suggested by the Council of Graduate Education for the Administration of Nursing (CGEAN, 1980). CGEAN is not officially connected with a national nursing organization, but meets annually prior to either the ANA or NLN national conventions.

It would appear that master's preparation for nursing education is more appropriately offered either as an elective in schools/colleges of nursing or schools of education. Perhaps those persons who would pursue an academic administration of nursing program should have available to them an academic administration track in a master's program in nursing administration.

In the future, it may be ideal to have a totally

---

[3] The author acknowledges Muriel A. Paulin, Ed.D., F.A.A.N., Professor and Chairperson, Nursing Administration, Boston University, for information exchange toward program development.

integrated master's curriculum with the three specialty areas of clinical nurse specialist, nursing administration for the first-line and mid-level manager of nursing service and for the mid-level academic administrator, and nurse educator. The master's clinical nurse specialist curriculum in an integrated program might include advanced clinical concepts and knowledge from each of the traditional clinical areas of medical–surgical, maternal–child health, psychiatric–mental health, and community nursing.

At the doctoral level, in the future, again, concepts could be built from an integrated master's curriculum and developed from a nursing conceptual structure. In addition, two-track systems should be available (see Grace, Chap. 12). The doctoral level should prepare the nurse for advanced clinical practice in various settings in one specialty area, executive administration and management in service and academic settings, or research for clinical practice, administration, and nursing education. At the doctoral level it has been more appropriate to pursue programs in higher education offered by schools of education. Although in the future that option may still be chosen, significant electives may be taken in nursing doctoral programs for nursing administration in service and academic settings. There are few doctoral programs in nursing administration for either service or academic settings. Even more scarce are doctoral programs for nursing administration, where both tracks—service and academic—are options. Leadership for service or for academic settings should be emphasized in administrative doctoral programs.

Given the current state of the economy, it does not seem realistic or wise to develop future doctoral programs without assurance of adequate resources. This includes the existence of sufficient doctorally prepared faculty members who are conducting research and a clinical practice as well as teaching. The proportionate amount of time allotted for each needs to be reasonable. It is an unrealistic expectation for faculties to perform equally as well or to be simultaneously productive in the three areas of research, teaching, and prac-

tice, yet produce scholarly publications as the result of their professional work. Negotiation and trade-offs among and between teachers concerning workloads are essential. However, compromise on the matter of academic credentials and qualifications for faculty jeopardizes the legitimacy of graduate programs and the profession. The path of the future in doctoral education for nurses appears to be through the development of cooperative or collaborative arrangements between colleges of a university system or universities. This requires careful assessment of the need, resources, and resolution of potentially difficult issues through considerable negotiation before a commitment is made to plan and implement a cooperative or collaborative arrangement. Though the need for doctoral programs in nursing exists, the profession is accountable to society for the projected role graduates of doctoral programs are to fulfill and the quality of the educational program offered to prepare the doctoral student for that anticipated role.

NURSING RESEARCH

Nursing research is the basis for defining the scientific knowledge base of nursing as a profession and the construction of theories to be tested and applied for nursing practice. There has been considerable discussion regarding the development of prescriptive theory and applied research. Prescriptive (situation-producing) theory identifies goals and specifies actions needed to achieve goals (see Fawcett, Chap. 14). Applied research is viewed as the application of knowledge to achieve a particular goal. Distinctions have been made between the two on the assumption that prescriptive theory is generated by goal-oriented research, whereas applied research uses knowledge generated by nongoal-oriented research and does not generate new knowledge.

This author perceives that in reality there is little difference between the two, and it may not be relevant as to *how* the knowledge is obtained. The critical point is that both prescriptive theory and applied research apply knowledge for practice. It is of more value to know whether or not the knowledge was effective in application to practice. Applied research does try to achieve a particular goal in practice. Furthermore, as a result of evaluating the effectiveness of that knowledge in practice, new knowledge may be obtained. For example, the professional practitioner may define a goal of evaluating the effectiveness of a prescribed nursing action for a patient. The practitioner may have taught patients a method of organizing their daily life to make the best use of time the patients have to communicate with their families. In prescribing the nursing action—the method of organizing time—the professional nurse may have used knowledge derived from the testing of prescriptive theory. The professional may have previously conducted or used the findings of specific goal-oriented research to determine actions that maximize the quality of time in family communication. The variable that appears to be most relevant is the organization and management of time. The practitioner may have further found that some methods are more effective than others in organizing time. Thus one specific method that appears most appropriate was recommended to the patient. Though, greatly oversimplified, this example is indicative of using knowledge through the development of prescriptive theory to identify an activity to achieve a specific goal.

The professional nurse may have recommended the same method based on knowledge obtained from counseling numerous dual-career families in communication and time management, and from reviewing professional literature. The professional nurse is trying to achieve a specific goal (applied research), though the professional nurse may not have initially derived the knowledge for application from utilizing a systematic research process. However, evaluating the results of the recommended method for time management may gain new knowledge regarding methods of time management as well as communication within a family. The new knowledge attained concerning the recommended method for time management

may lend itself to empirical testing and further development of prescriptive theory. The professional nurse should evaluate the effectiveness in goal achievement and outcomes of any recommended nursing action.

It would seem that prescriptive theory development and applied research should be combined. If there is indeed any difference between the two, it would be the degree to which a scientific method is utilized in obtaining the initial knowledge for application. For those who adhere to the Dickoff and James schema (1968) for the development of nursing knowledge, applied research might be an additional fifth and highest level in the development of nursing theory. In that event, applied research would have included all the previous steps of the hierarchy in the development of knowledge: factor-isolating, factor-relating, situation-relating, and situation-producing (prescriptive). The mode of testing theory at each of these levels varies, beginning with descriptive through quasi-experimental research. Although applied research may not be the same as prescriptive testing research, experimental designs could be utilized to test applied research as, or for, prescriptions.

Prescriptive theory testing through research may not contribute to the identification of nursing knowledge in itself, but studies should indicate how it relates to the building and testing of a given nursing theory. Nursing research should have a theoretical or conceptual base that pertains to the identified phenomena relevant for study: person, environment, health, and nursing. Otherwise the further development of nursing knowledge is inhibited.

With the tremendous decrease in federal funding for research, it is likely that applied research will be of more interest. Broad subject areas of nursing which warrant substantial study are: evaluation of the quality of nursing care utilizing nursing conceptual frameworks and theories; measures of structure, process, and outcome; modes of providing nursing care; roles and methods of professional nurses in health teaching and maintenance; nursing interventions utilized in care; risk-taking behaviors of nurses in providing care; holistic nursing care; ethical issues in nursing; performance expectations and outcomes of nursing students at all levels of preparation; and nontraditional modes of providing for nursing education. Finally, it is to the benefit of the profession to promote collaborative and interdisciplinary research to achieve the goals of research.

Students and professional practitioners can learn from research that is well designed as well as that conducted with poor design or under adverse conditions. This author has frequently cautioned students that perfection neither exists nor is possible in research. There are always limitations. Published research reports frequently present condensed information from a study. Most often this is due to necessary limitations in space and the need to present only the essence of a study. This can create confusion for learners in evaluating a research report. To enable the evaluation of a research report, the author developed guidelines for critique (Table 66-1) as a tool for graduate students studying nursing research methods. In summary and conclusion, it is offered for consideration in reviewing published research articles and reported studies.

NURSING THEORY

It is evident throughout this volume that there is an intricate relationship between nursing research, theory, and practice. A scientific knowledge base is essential to substantiate nursing interventions; a shared understanding of nursing practice is critical for the development of nursing knowledge; and research is the basis for establishing both the knowledge and practice of nursing. Perhaps the greatest impediment for appreciating the value of nursing theory is the tremendous lack of clarity in the use of theoretical terminology. In some respects, nurse-scholars rarely use the same or similar definitions for terms. Although differences in the use of terms are to be expected, it is most helpful for the learner and scholar when the terms are defined.

This permits a shared understanding of the proposed theory, evaluation for relevance in nursing practice, and understanding the current status of nursing knowledge. The differences in manner by which the term "theory" can be defined can be seen in reviewing Meleis's (Chap. 33) and Roy's (Chap. 34) clarifications. To prevent possible confusion in presenting some thoughts about theory in or for nursing, the author will attempt to refrain from using theoretical language.

There are various perspectives, methods, and stages in the formulation of nursing theory. In nursing there does not appear to be a consensus on one perspective for theory development. At best, there is considerable agreement to focus on the phenomena of person, health, environment, and nursing. This may be due to the influence of Nightingale, who emphasized the situation that the nurse and patient are in and their purpose for being together—namely the health of the patient (see Palmer, Chap. 1). It is doubtful that there will be one unified perspective in nursing knowledge other than consensus on the purpose of nursing itself. A distinction is being made that one of the differences between the disciplines of medicine and nursing is the frame of reference for problem definition and resolution (see Williams, Chap. 25). Medicine may tend to focus more on surgical and pharmacological interventions, whereas nursing tends to center on interpersonal interactions and interventions. Consequently, some commonalities are found to exist among nurse-scholars regarding the nature of nursing practice. For example, the nature of the interaction between the nurse and patient has received considerable attention. (For one example, see La Monica, Chap. 37.) The patient's ability to adapt to the environment is another predominant theme. The emphasis given to any one of the four phenomena in the formulation of theory varies.

It would appear that a variety of perspectives and methods for the development of nursing knowledge is beneficial. The diversity of academic and experiential backgrounds of nurses with doctorates, who are contributing to nursing knowl-

Table 66-1   Guidelines for the Critique of a Research Report

I Author's (or Authors') Credentials
To what extent are these appropriate for the expertise needed for the type of research conducted?

II Title of the Report
To what extent does it clearly indicate the nature of the study?

III Statement of the Problem
  a Identify the research question.
  b Comment to what extent it is clearly stated.
  c To what extent is it a significant problem for nursing research?
  d Has the investigator clearly stated the limitations and delimitations of the research? What are they?

IV Assumptions
  a What assumptions are stated? Are they documented?
  b Are some assumptions implied but not stated? What are they?
  c Evaluate those assumptions.

V Review of Relevant Literature
  a Comment on the thoroughness of the literature review.
  b Are original sources of previous research indicated?
  c To what extent is the present status of knowledge in the area of investigation indicated?
  d What linkage is there between the present status of knowledge and the research question?
  e Are findings of *relevant* studies included?
  f Is the review presented in a logical manner?

VI Conceptual or Theoretical Framework
  a Identify the conceptual or theoretical framework.
  b Is it a nursing conceptual or theoretical framework?
  c To what extent is it clearly stated?
  d To what degree are concepts clearly defined?
  e Are definitions generally accepted by those knowledgeable in the discipline (intersubjectivity)?

VII Hypotheses
  a Identify the hypotheses.
  b To what extent are the hypotheses clearly stated?
  c To what extent do the hypotheses appear to be derived from the conceptual or theoretical framework? Are they logical? Are they testable?
  d Identify the independent and dependent variables.
  e If there are no hypotheses stated, to what degree or how is that justified?

VIII Linkages
  a What linkage(s) are there between the literature review, conceptual framework, and the construction of the hypotheses?
  b How adequate, clear, and logical are the linkages?

IX Design and Method
  a Assess the appropriateness of the design and method in terms of the research problem. To what extent is it adequately explained?
  b What type of sampling was used? Was it justifiable?
  c What were the criteria for the sample?
  d How representative of the population under investigation was the sample?
  e Identify any threat(s) to internal validity.

X Operational Measures
  a Comment on the validity and reliability of any instruments utilized.
  b To what extent were validity and reliability obtained through pretesting?
  c Comment on the extent to which the validity and reliability of instruments have been previously documented.

Table 66-1   Continued

XI   Method of Data Collection
  a   How appropriate was the method?
  b   Were there other ways data could have been obtained that would have been more appropriate?
  c   Comment on the quality versus quantity of the data.
  d   To what extent did the investigator protect the rights of human subjects?

XII   Data Analysis
  a   How appropriate were the methods used for the type of data obtained *and* the research question?
  b   How clearly did the investigator present the analysis?
  c   If statistical testing was utilized, to what degree were statistically significant findings presented as well as nonsignificant findings?
  d   If qualitative analysis was utilized, to what extent was the coding logical and clearly presented?

XIII   Findings and Conclusions
  a   To what degree are hypotheses supported?
  b   To what degree are inferences made which are not supported by the data?
  c   How well do data support the conclusions drawn?
  d   To what extent is there statistically significant support for the conclusions?
  e   Could the findings be due to other variables?
  f   Were other variables accounted for in the discussion of the findings?
  g   Identify any bias introduced in the interpretation of the findings.
  h   Comment on the clarity of the discussion.
  i   Does the investigator state the degree to which findings can be generalized? Is the statement justifiable?
  j   How well do the conclusions serve to answer the research question originally proposed?

XIV   Implications and Recommendations
  a   To what degree does the investigator clearly state the nursing practice relevance of the findings?
  b   To what degree does the investigator clearly state the *theoretical* relevance for nursing practice of the findings?
  c   What are the implications for future nursing research?
  d   What recommendations were made for future research?
  e   Were the recommendations relevant for future nursing research?

edge, may enable further insight into the development and application of nursing knowledge in a variety of situations. In addition multiple theories may more likely evolve through numerous approaches. Perhaps Rogers's theory of unitary man (person) may include specific formulations by other theorists, for example, Roy's adaptation model. The comprehensive involvement of practitioners in nursing is essential for providing critical information as nursing theory is formulated, tested, and evaluated. From the experiential base of these practitioners, concepts that are most relevant for nursing practice can be identified and verified. The classification of nursing diagnoses is one step in eliciting the contributions of practitioners (see Gordon, Chap. 41, and Roy, Chap. 34). However, future linkage needs to be established between nursing diagnoses and formulations of nursing theory for nursing practice. The ultimate desirable consequence of all of the combined, collaborative efforts is that the consumer will be the receiver of the highest quality in nursing care. The profession of nurse scholars and practitioners will have uniquely defined nursing knowledge as a scientific discipline.

NURSING PRACTICE

In this decade there has been increasing unification of nursing practice with education as well as recognition to include nursing research within a triad. The changing course of events in nursing has resulted from realizing the results of distinct separation of those three aspects of the nursing profession. In essence, the patient/consumer has been the victim of the division. The profession has also suffered in the lack of an integrated professional community. Wholeness (holism) in health and illness care, education, and the profession was virtually lost.

Fortunately, the profession is endeavoring to correct the errors of the past by focusing on the consumer (patients/clients, professional nursing students) and practitioners. Efforts are being redirected to provide holistic (humanistic) nursing care and education, increase control over and improve the practice of nursing, and enhance a unified profession of nursing.

First, it is obvious the emphasis on consumer needs and the most effective means of servicing the consumer is a central focus of the profession. That is as it should be since it reflects the profession's concern to fulfill its primary mission and purpose. Humanism in care is the key significant variable evident in this decade. The emphasis on involving consumers (patient/client and professional students) in their own care and education is obvious. It appears in the increased quality of patient education/teaching programs, redefining the role of a nurse as a "helper," and professional curricula being developed to prepare students better for professional, holistic practice.

Consequently, the role of professional nurses is changing to focus more on illness prevention, health maintenance, and education, but at the same time acute-illness care is not being neglected. The clinical specialist role is being more fully developed to be not only experts of clinical care, but also first-line and middle managers in providing nursing care. Their roles differ in settings where primary nursing has been implemented as

well as in settings where they are being employed to provide primary care as nurse practitioners. In settings where primary nursing has been implemented, clinical specialists are assuming increased responsibility and accountability for care. In settings for primary care, clinical specialists who have received additional professional preparation as nurse practitioners need to take heed regarding the scope of their role. It does not appear viable—either as a professional nurse or legally—that nurse practitioners will be the predominant care provider for primary care. In general, legal definitions and interpretations of the scope of nursing practice may more clearly define how a nursing diagnosis and therapeutic plan is different from a medical diagnosis and treatment by a physician. The outcome for the role of nurse practitioners related to their professional education and settings for practice remains to be seen and evaluated.

Without a doubt new modes of providing nursing care are increasing. Primary nursing has previously been discussed in relation to professionalization. It should be noted that it is essential to consider the setting, the resources available, and the professional level of nurses to provide primary nursing before it is implemented. Increased use of cooperative dyads and triads in providing nursing care should significantly increase the quality of humanistic patient/client care. The increased involvement of the patient, significant family member, and the nurse in planning nursing care needs to be tested and evaluated in all types of settings. The patient, nurse, and physician are another example of triad cooperative care, whereas dyads of care would exist between all participants. The central point is that the professional nurse would be the focal coordinator in the collaboration for nursing care. Increased adherence of patients to plans of care and the quality of care provided should be improved. Finally, holistic and humanistic health and illness care should be the outcome.

Governance systems in nursing and reimbursement for nursing practice are strongly being advocated within the profession. Sills's (Chap. 42) suggestion for the development of nurse corporations is unique. It may not only enable direct reimbursement for nursing practice and increase the autonomy of professional nurses, but even more, ensure that patients/clients receive the quality of professional nursing care suitable to their level of need. Furthermore, it may be a possible solution to the nursing shortage and superior to the quality and continuity of care and control of nursing practice that currently is being offered through utilizing temporary nurses from outside sources. To project the impacts on the profession and consumer in implementing professional nurse corporations are issues themselves. Nurse corporations would require great planning, coordination, collaboration, and evaluation.

Job satisfaction in nursing is increasing in importance. It is related to high turnover rates and the shortage of nurses in service and academic settings. However, data indicate (see Braito and Caston, Chap. 27) that the intrinsic, self-fulfilling rewards of nursing are more significant variables than extrinsic factors, such as salary and fringe benefits. It would appear that autonomy and more control of one's practice through nursing governance mechanisms would be related to the intrinsic rewards of nursing. The development of clinical ladders, based on professional performance, competency levels, and professional education, for upward mobility in clinical practice is also increasing the intrinsic as well as extrinsic rewards for nurses. However, job satisfaction is a complex issue, with numerous variables to be considered, which requires further extensive nursing research. The environment within which a professional practices is without a doubt a significant variable. Professional career counseling offered within hospital, ambulatory, and other settings where health and illness care are provided, as well as in academic institutions for professional faculty may greatly increase job satisfaction as well as prevent dissatisfaction.

New models for providing nursing care are being advocated. The hospice movement has been an initial step in that direction. Hospice care for long-term and chronic illness needs to be seriously considered with the increased longevity of today. The problems and issues indicated by Corless (Chap. 40) require resolution before further means of providing hospice care and other patient populations are included as being eligible for hospice care. Home care for health and illness needs to be anticipated in planning professional education programs for practice. It would be expected that with the increase in the costs of care every effort will be made to receive optimal care in the home.

Finally, the practice of nursing has become increasingly professionalized. Roles are being redefined, the domain and territory of nursing is becoming more distinct, and nursing is returning to where it originated as a profession—directly providing humanistic nursing care with and for the patient, a purpose it uniquely serves.

ADMINISTRATION: NURSING SERVICE AND EDUCATION

Effective nursing administration, management, and leadership to provide for the delivery of nursing care and nursing education are central to the cooperation and collaboration in health care and education. The development of leadership skills for the executive nurse administrator and mid-level manager in service and academia is essential for successful orchestration of all the functions in providing nursing care and education. There is a difference between administration management and leadership. It is ideal, and perhaps rare, for one person to have the essential innate qualities to fulfill these roles equally well. However, the integrated conceptual base of nursing and management should enable increased success in performing those combined roles. Preparation for these roles of ultimate accountability for nursing, to the consumer and public, has previously been mentioned in reflecting upon nursing education. Additional comment is in order, regarding specific issues related to administration, management, and leadership in service and academic settings.

Every effort needs to be made to further increase the collegial relationships between service and academic settings. Persons who possess the qualifications for academic clinical appointments should be provided with criteria for them to enable achievement of promotion and tenure within an academic system. Furthermore, two-track systems for promotion and tenure should be considered in academia. Two-track systems would affect not only professionals in practice settings who serve a reasonable amount of time fulfilling academic roles in clinical nursing, but also teachers who are expert professional clinicians. Some teachers, for various realistic and legitimate reasons, are not able to pursue doctoral study. In most major universities, a doctoral degree is a requirement for tenure. Yet to lose the expertise of professionally competent clinicians of nursing practice and nursing management in service and academic settings due to the lack of one formalized credential is an injustice to the professional, deprives the professional student of valuable learning experiences and possible mentor relationships for practice, and could inhibit the further professionalization of nursing.

This is not to imply that academic credentials and qualifications for a faculty rank and tenure should be decreased. The contrary is proposed. First of all, most professionals who might qualify for a clinical academic track for promotion and tenure would have demonstrated continued expertise as teachers and clinicians as well as have evidence of ongoing continued education through other mechanisms. Secondly, it is suggested that the criteria for promotion and tenure that are developed for clinicians be equally demanding as those for faculty members with earned doctorates. However, the emphasis in the criteria may be different. Most doctorally prepared faculty members are expected to demonstrate continued evidence of research as principal or coinvestigators or in interdisciplinary collaboration in scholarly publications, besides expertise in teaching and competence in clinical practice. Clinicians may be expected to provide stronger and more evidence of their clinical nursing knowledge and expertise in practice and teaching in academia,

service settings or continuing education programs. Furthermore, for clinicians, some evidence should exist of significant involvement in nursing research, most appropriately with persons who are doctorally prepared and in some scholarly publications. There are numerous issues to be addressed in the consideration, planning, and implementing of a two-track system. Two potential pitfalls must be avoided. A two-track system should not be an avenue for devaluing the importance of doctoral education and the contributions of doctorally prepared nurses in the nursing care of patients, in the education of professional students, in nursing research, and to the profession. Secondly, it should not be a means for discouraging the number of persons who enter and complete doctoral programs for nursing or for those who choose doctoral programs in another discipline to return to nursing faculties. Thus, criteria for those who might *qualify* for or choose a clinical track, as well as equitable criteria for those who are on an academic, research track, require the utmost consideration.

It is essential for administrators and managers to assess accurately the *climate* of an organization before any change is planned. Accurate assessment requires time, verification of data obtained, and anticipation of and preparing for obstacles in planning and implementing change. Critical pacing of the amount and degree of change and evaluation is vital throughout the process for change to be accepted and effective. Participative management, particularly in processes of change, is salient today. However, this varies in the role and degree utilized as well as according to the institutional environment and structure, leadership style of the executive, and the situation itself that requires change and constant planning. Shared authority and governance systems are being demanded and utilized today in both service and academic settings. It is critical, not just for planning and accountability for numerous variables affecting health care and education, but for participative decision making by nursing staff in professional practice and academic faculty.

A brief comment is offered regarding the role of ethics in administration. There is no doubt that people differ in the normative ethical system which they have internalized. A major issue is the resolution of conflict when ethical stances differ in a situation. Ethical differences may arise, whether it is in the direct care of patients, the teaching of professional students, or the marketing for nursing staff, faculty, and nursing administrators for service and academic settings. There are no simple answers to the question of resolving differences. However, professional persons do have a number of choices. Some include compromising one's own basic normative ethical stance, leaving the situation entirely, or attempting to understand and respect the differences and negotiate for a mutually satisfactory resolution. There is little doubt that ethics will become of increasing concern in administration and management. Particularly as executive and mid-level manager role models, nursing staff and faculty will have high expectations in ethical decision making by the nurse administrator and managers of nursing care and education at all levels.

THE FUTURE OF NURSING

The future of nursing will continue to present complexities and challenges, but at the same time springs of hope for an invincible summer are present within the profession. Nursing continues to evolve in its status towards full professionalization as members review and renew their commitments to each other and negotiate with other health professionals for true collegial, collaborative relationships. Efforts to achieve autonomy are being realized through effective governance mechanisms. Emphasis is increasing toward growth of personal professional competence. As a result, professionals may be called upon to produce evidence in order to maintain licensure for practice. The impact of a national nursing credentialling center has the potential to support professionalization further, if it is established and maintained primarily by professional nurses, comprising a coalition of professional nursing organizations, particularly the American Nurses Association. The National Council of State Boards of Nursing may further ensure uniform expectations in knowledge and competency for professional practice.

Recognition of the diversity in perspectives and approaches in the development of nursing knowledge may result in concerted efforts to integrate the efforts of scholars and practitioners. Consequently, a shared understanding and definition of nursing may be the outcome. The domain of nursing has been more clearly defined, with distinctions between the practice of medicine and nursing clearer.

Economics and technology will have tremendous impact on the profession in nursing education, research, and practice. Cost-effective mechanisms for all three missions in nursing are certain to be advocated. Nontraditional modes of professional nursing education may greatly increase with increased cooperation and collaboration between schools and colleges of nursing. The profession will need to be concerned with the socialization process and role identification of nursing students as new modes are proposed. Mentor systems may not only evolve in nursing education, but also increase in nursing research and nursing administration. Integrated curricula for baccalaureate and graduate degrees should further evolve.

Nursing research may become focused on the effectiveness of the application of knowledge and integrated with efforts to define the unique knowledge base of nursing. Communication and collaboration in the two purposes of obtaining knowledge—for defining the base for nursing and application for nursing practice—could further unite the profession. Nursing research may also be directed toward the cost-effectiveness of all modes and roles in providing nursing care, as primary nursing and nurse practitioners. The role of nurses in primary care for quality care and cost-effectiveness is being examined. The effects of specialization in nursing care may be further explored from the perspective of holistic health care, economics, and technology.

In nursing practice a balance is likely to occur between the nursing clinical and management expertise of practitioners. In the future the former head nurse role may be redefined or replaced by clinical nurse specialists with management expertise. This may more likely occur if primary nursing proves to be not only cost-effective in providing high quality nursing care, but if means to provide sufficient professional resources for nursing care are developed. Patient classification systems developed from the classification of nursing diagnoses may further enable the appropriate use of professional nursing personnel in nursing practice. Present nursing roles may be expanded to coordinate the movement toward preventive care and health maintenance. The likelihood of reimbursement for nursing practice on a fee-for-service basis appears somewhat slim, due to the government becoming increasingly concerned with reimbursing institutions and health professionals. However, the prospect is still viable and an overdue legitimate goal. The great increase in computer technology in care is bound to place new demands on all nursing roles and the profession, as well as to provide great assistance.

Multiple settings for providing nursing care in wellness and illness are on the scene. In addition new organizational structures are evolving via multihospital systems and corporate structures. Leadership centers to prepare nurse executives for corporate roles in service and academic settings are needed. Increased familiarity and involvement with legislation and health policy analysis are essential for the nurse administrator of the future.

There is an analogy that can be made between the artistry by which a tapestry is created and the evolvement of nursing into a full profession.[4] The real makings of a tapestry can actually be seen only by viewing its "back side." While the tapestry is being created, we only see and work with its back side. There are threads, strands, and many knots all going in different directions. When the tapestry is complete, we view the front part of that tapestry and the picture that was made. It strikes this author that that back side of a tapestry is similar to all that we see as we work together in developing the profession. The tapestry back side of a profession is made up of all kinds of different threads and colors. This represents the tremendous diversity and talent within the profession. Some threads and colors are thicker, brighter, and longer than others—all according to the significance they have for contributing and developing the profession. At the end of a particular thread—again, some are longer and are more significant—there is a knot. To this author, that is the end of a trend, a certain confusion, a change, or the achievement of a professional goal. However, there is always a new thread that is started from that knot *until* the "picture" of a profession is complete on the other side. The difficulty is that we do not usually *know* when a trend, confusion, or change is to end or a goal is to be achieved, and/or when it has indeed ended or started, because that is the most difficult to accept or believe. But as that new thread begins, it is easier to accept that one trend, confusion, or change has been completed, or one goal achieved and another started.

The key factor in all of this is to believe and trust in someone or something beyond our individual selves for "professional bonding" to occur; this serves as an artist in shaping the picture of our profession. Mingled with all of those threads, there is one clear golden strand of the professional bond. It is woven in our united efforts of mission (theme) and purpose, all through the varying strands of different brilliance, thickness, and length—as well as through all of the knots. This is the only explanation, if you will, for being able to accept and deal with all the events and uncertainties, and/or some adversities or tragedies that do occur in the evolution of a profession. In effect, we can *never* know the answer to the "whys"

---

[4] Modifications were made from an address titled "The Tapestry," which was originally presented by this author at the Annual Eisenhower Prayer Breakfast, February 6, 1981, Dwight David Eisenhower Army Medical Center, Fort Gordon, Georgia.

until the picture of a profession is complete. It calls for complete trust and belief in a professional bond to guide us as to the unique service and actualization as a profession, through all the threads and knots.

We do have choices as to what directions we may take with those strands, and at times try out and test varying directions, sometimes simultaneously. Perhaps, some "mistakes" have been made, as they too show up in the strands and knots on the back side of the tapestry. Perhaps, "mistakes" can be viewed as events or occurrences that were positive for strengthening the professional bond and individual members.

The point is that the professional bond is there between us in and through *all* the events that we have no control of as well as those we do. The end product is what we are accountable for in the expectations of the public we serve and the profession we represent. To the extent we realize or actualize our own potential as total persons— through the guidance and direction of the professional bond, a belief system beyond ourselves, and choices made individually and collectively— the picture of the profession will be complete and to the liking of the public we serve and to the profession. Each of us *is* unique—in terms of what and who we are, what we are given in abilities, and choices we make. All the diversity is needed for an unique profession.

The point also is that we all have to "hang in there" at times; otherwise the picture we are creating will really be "fouled up." There may be times that we fear we will run out of thread, or that the thread will break before a knot is tied, and/or a trend, confusion, change is ended or a goal achieved. But that clear golden strand of the professional bond and belief system beyond ourselves sustains the weak points of the thread to carry it through to the knot. Some professions more than others have all kinds of knots, colors, and strands on the back side of the tapestry, but the challenge is to keep going so that the picture does get made. We may never live to see the total picture on the other side. But each of us can be

assured that our contributions are there. Most tapestries have numerous crooked lines and strands that make no sense to us. The name of the game is to trust and support each other, and believe we are creating a beautiful tapestry of a unique profession with a unique contribution until the picture is complete. This author offers the analogy of the tapestry as a key for the success and invincibility of the nursing profession.

REFERENCES

CGEAN Council of Graduate Education for the Administration of Nursing
  1980 Unpublished document.
Cousteau, Voltaire
  1973 "How to swim with sharks: A primer." Perspectives in Biology and Medicine 16:(Summer)525-528.
Dickoff, James and Patricia James
  1968 "A theory of theories: A position paper." Nursing Research 17:197-203.
Greenwood, Ernest
  1957 "Attributes of a profession." Social Work 2(3):45-55.
Harragan, Betty Lehan
  1977 Games Mother Never Taught You. New York: Warner Books, Inc.
Johns, Richard J.
  1975 Dinner Address. How to Swim with Sharks: The Advanced Course. Pp. 44-54 in Transactions of the Association of American Physicians. Eighty-Eighth Session. Atlantic City, New Jersey: May 5-6.
Morris, Alvin L.
  1980 "Inter-school relationships in academic health centers." Pp. 155-165 in The Organization and Governance of Academic Health Centers. Position Papers. Vol. 3. Washington, D.C.: Association of Academic Health Centers.
U.S.N.Y. (The University of the State of New York)
  1981 Press release: NLN Accredits First External Baccalaureate Degree Nursing Program. Regents External Degree Program, Cultural Education Center, Albany, New York 12230.

Name and Title Index

Subject Index